PRINCIPLES & PRACTICE OF

VETERINARY ANESTHESIA

PRINCIPLES & PRACTICE OF

VETERINARY ANESTHESIA

edited by

Charles E. Short

D.V.M., M.S., D.A.C.V.A.

Professor and Chief, Anesthesiology, Department of Clinical Sciences
The New York State College of Veterinary Medicine, Cornell University, Ithaca, New York

Professor, Anesthesiology, Department of Anesthesiology, College of Medicine
Cornell University, New York, New York

Adjunct Professor, Anesthesiology, Department of Anesthesiology
Upstate Medical Center, Syracuse, New York

WILLIAMS & WILKINS
Baltimore • London • Los Angeles • Sydney

Editor: Jonathan W. Pine, Jr.
Associate Editor: Victoria M. Vaughn
Copy Editor: S. Lohmeyer
Design: JoAnne Janowiak
Illustration Planning: Asterisk Group
Production: Raymond E. Reter

Accurate indications, adverse reactions, and dosage schedules for drugs are provided in this book, but it is possible that they may change. The reader is urged to review the package information data of the manufacturers of the medications mentioned.

Printed in the United States of America

Library of Congress Cataloging-in-Publication Data

Principles and practice of veterinary anesthesia.

Bibliography: p.
Includes index.
1. Veterinary anesthesia. I. Short, Charles E. SF914.P74 1987
636.089'796 86-15649
ISBN 0-683-07702-3

Composed and printed at the
Waverly Press, Inc.

87 88 89 90 91
10 9 8 7 6 5 4 3 2 1

Dedication

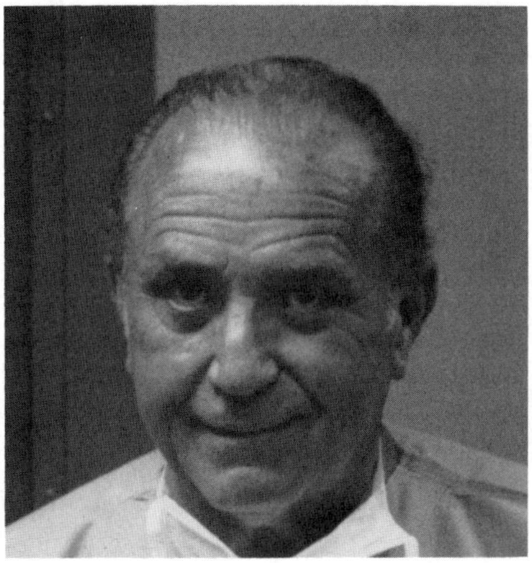

In 1948, Arthur Stanley Keats, M.D., became a Clinical and Research Fellow in Anesthesia at Massachusetts General Hospital in Boston, Massachusetts, under the very capable direction of Dr. H.K. Beecher, one of the major contributors to the advancement of anesthesia in human patients. At the beginning of Dr. Keats' training program in anesthesia, it was highly unlikely he was aware that later, his activities might influence the development of veterinary anesthesia as well. In 1954, Arthur Keats completed his examination to become a Diplomate of the American Board of Anesthesiology.

After the completion of 2 years of service as an anesthesiologist at Mary Imogene Bassett Hospital in Cooperstown, New York, and after serving as an associate in anesthesia at Columbia University College of Physicians and Surgeons in New York City, Dr. Keats became Professor and Chairman of the Department of Anesthesiology at Baylor College of Medicine in Houston, Texas, a position he held from 1955 to 1974. From 1974 until the present time, he has been Chief of the Division of Cardiovascular Anesthesia, Texas Heart Institute, Texas Medical Center, Houston, Texas, and serves as Clinical Professor of Anesthesiology at the University of Texas Health Science Center in Houston, Texas.

Included among the many accomplishments of Dr. Keats are a term from 1963 to 1969 as Editor of the journal *Anesthesiology* and a term from 1970 to 1973 as Editor-in-Chief of *Anesthesiology*. In 1967, he became a director of the American Board of Anesthesiology and served as its president from 1975 to 1977. It is of interest that Dr. Keats was President of the American Board of Anesthesiology during the same time that the American College of Veterinary Anesthesiologists was approved by the American Veterinary Medical Association for its initial official recognition.

Dr. Keats has made many presentations, including a number of Distinguished Lectureships, among which was the prestigious Rovenstine Lecture for the American Society of Anesthesiologists in 1983. In 1984, he was selected to receive the Distinguished Service Award by the American Society of Anesthesiologists.

Dr. Keats has been active throughout his career in the pursuit of new information and in the development of anesthetic procedures, and an understanding of analgesics and anesthetics. In the early 1950s, his work with Dr. Beecher concentrated on the relief of pain through the use of various medications, including a variety of opiate and nonopiate analgesics. He was concerned not only about the effectiveness of these medications, but also about their mechanisms of action. In the late 1950s, Dr. Keats became involved in the development of anesthetic techniques to be used in conjunction with cardiac catheterization and for cardiopulmonary bypass and open-heart surgical procedures. Among his responsibilities was the anesthetic management of patients undergoing open-heart surgeries, while he worked with a number of outstanding cardiovascular surgeons, including Drs. Denton A. Cooley and Michael E. DeBakey. After the initial development of many of these techniques, the interest of Dr. Keats continued into mechanisms of action of medications used in open-heart surgery and the effect of these medications and techniques on patient responses. As a result, he has authored or co-authored over 100 publications.

Dr. Keats is a long-time member of the American Society of Anesthesiologists, American Society of Pharmacology and Experimental Therapeutics, Association of University Anesthetists, American Society of Clinical Pharmacology and Therapeutics, the Society of Academic Anesthesiology Chairmen and, in addition, an honorary diplomate of the American College of Veterinary Anesthesiologists.

I was fortunate to become acquainted with Dr. Keats in 1965. With his encouragement and support, I was able to complete a training program which resulted ultimately in a Master's Degree from Baylor University College of Medicine with a major emphasis on developing anesthetic techniques and experimental cardiovascular surgery. I found in Arthur Keats a physician anesthesiologist who was extremely dedicated to providing excellent clinical anesthesia for his patients, teaching for his students, leadership, encouragement for learning new information, and enthusiasm for life. His efforts not only made it possible for me to complete a program on which I was to build my career in veterinary anesthesiology, but also provided stimulation and encouragement to my contribution toward the development of the specialty of veterinary anesthesiology and the encouragement for the development of the American College of Veterinary Anesthesiologists.

His high standards of anesthetic care helped establish the goals that we hope to achieve during the administration of quality anesthesia to our animal patients. Because of his encouragement and contributions, it is a pleasure for me to dedicate this text to my teacher and friend, Arthur Stanley Keats, M.D.

Preface

In the unique world of veterinary medicine, relief or prevention of suffering in the animal kingdom is one of our primary objectives. Our activities must be accomplished without the benefit of verbal communication with the patient. As a result, perhaps we are already mentally conditioned to monitoring patients under the influence of anesthetics and analgesics, during which we must relate to the signs of physiological responses.

What is anesthesia? The appropriate selection of anesthetic and related agents renders the patient unaware and unresponsive to painful stimuli, including existing trauma and surgery. Anesthesia is the pharmacological manipulation of physiological functions. It allows the accomplishment of diagnostic and surgical procedures that otherwise would be impossible or inhumane.

Anesthesiology is conceived by some to be a narrow specialty consisting of the mere administration of a few medications to make the patient unconscious, after which the patient arouses from the effects. In real terms, the practice of anesthesia is one of the most complex of the sciences. In addition, the safe practice of anesthesia demands that the veterinarian has an understanding of internal medicine, including cardiology and neurology, along with pharmacology, physiology, physics, mathematics, and mechanics. There are no totally safe anesthetics. Safe anesthesia is administered by those who understand anesthesiology, administer anesthetics carefully and selectively, and diligently monitor the patient. There is both a science and an art to the safe practice of anesthesia.

The owners of the animals receiving anesthetics are frequently very apprehensive about the procedure. They may have had bad experiences in the past because of complications in an animal or a family member. Others are quite unaware of the risks involved. Appropriate client relations should be established prior to the administration of agents. The establishment of such a relationship not only results in less emotional situations, but may gain valuable information for the care of the patient.

The practice of anesthesia has been described as periods of boredom spiced with other periods of sheer panic. I would like to believe the progress made in anesthesiology has greatly reduced both of these situations. Appropriate monitoring of the patient reduces both boredom and panic because it provides fine adjustment in the anesthetic regimen and allows one to anticipate complications and correct them before they become disastrous.

I appreciate the efforts of the many people who have contributed to anesthesiology. My own efforts in the specialty have been gratifying, and I feel fortunate to have been involved at a time when so much advancement has been made. The opportunity to know and work with other anesthesiologists and benefit from their efforts has made the challenges more interesting and rewarding. Many have shared their knowledge in this text.

The first meeting of American veterinarians to discuss organized efforts to improve veterinary anesthesia was held in conjunction with the American Veterinary Medical Association in July 1970 in Las Vegas, Nevada. Over 40 people from academia and private practice attended the meeting, which resulted in the formation of the American Society of Veterinary Anesthesiology. This was the forerunner to the American College of Veterinary Anesthesiologists, which was approved by the American Veterinary Medical Association in 1975. This organization, the goals of which include improvements in veterinary anesthesia by obtaining new information through research, the teaching of anesthesiology in veterinary colleges, and the presentation of information on anesthesia to our profession through presentations, journals, and texts, has now grown to over 50 Diplomates.

The efforts of these Diplomates to provide information on anesthesiology is appreciated, and a number have contributed to this text. It is important to recognize that a number of veterinary practitioners have contributed by obtaining information relative to anesthesia, and the quality of practice of anesthesia in private hospitals has dramatically improved during the past 25 years.

The medical profession has played an important role in animal anesthesia as well. Countless research projects have been completed in medical centers throughout the country. The data from animal research in these laboratories have been instrumental in many of the improvements that have been made in clinical veterinary anesthesia. Data from these studies have been included in a number of the chapters of this text. In addition to the many contributing scientists in the medical community to date, the encouragement of veterinary anesthesiologists by many physician-anesthesiologists has been significant. Drs. Robert Dripps, G.W.N. Edgars, Jr., Arthur Stanley Keats, and Edmond I. Eger II have been recognized as Honorary Diplomates of the American College of Veterinary Anesthesiologists for their contribution to the science and organization of veterinary anesthesiology.

Industrial efforts in the development of anesthetic equipment, anesthetic agents, and adjunct medications and cooperation and support of veterinary medicine are greatly appreciated. The development of new drugs and equipment has been highly instrumental in the amount of progress we have been able to achieve.

This text has been prepared both for the student in the professional curriculum and for the graduate using it for continuing education. I would like to consider that we are all still learning. Without this philosophy, how can we continue to make progress and obtain new knowledge? Many more senior members of the profession effectively maintained patients with barbiturates or ether, but we still welcomed new anesthetics with excitement. Many learned to monitor anesthesia by reflexes and heart/lung sounds, where we now also use monitoring for the electrocardiogram, blood pressure, and other parameters. Progress in anesthesiology has been evident.

This book provides the details of the progress made in the principles and practice of veterinary anesthesia. *Veterinary Anesthesia*, an earlier text by my friend Dr. Lawrence R. Soma of the University of Pennsylvania, was an excellent addition to the veterinary literature. He chose not to revise *Veterinary Anesthesia* for its second edition. I was honored to be asked by Williams & Wilkins to edit this edition. It has been quite interesting to review the extensive information relating to anesthesia and analgesia, and I am very pleased to share these efforts with the profession.

The opportunities I have enjoyed in the specialty of anesthesiology would not have been possible without the support of my family. To Kathie Anne, Chuck, Janie, and Steve, to my parents, and to my wife Kathie, thanks for your support.

Charles E. Short, D.V.M., M.S., D.A.C.V.A.

Acknowledgments

The editor of a new text always recognizes the contributing authors of each chapter. In this text, 30 authors have contributed from their work to the subject material on veterinary anesthesia. I'm pleased to acknowledge two other important contributors.

An effort of this magnitude required not only my professional input, but also extensive assistance in preparing manuscripts and related efforts. Without the dedicated efforts of Mrs. Linda Ritzler to provide that support, this text would not have been completed. Many thanks to her for an effort well done and most appreciated.

The cover is by Inger Jorgensen, Designer. She has chosen to represent the various animals in veterinary anesthesia with the horse, since it is used for work, sport, or companionship. All forms of anesthesia are represented by the anesthesia unit. Her design is appreciated and appropriate.

Contributors

M. Sawkat Anwer, Ph.D.
School of Veterinary Medicine, Tufts University, North Grafton, Massachusetts

G. John Benson, D.V.M., M.S., D.A.C.V.A.
Anesthesiology Section, Department of Veterinary Clinical Medicine, College of Veterinary Medicine, University of Illinois, Urbana, Illinois

Julia T. Blue, D.V.M., Ph.D., D.A.C.V.P.
Assistant Professor of Clinical Pathology, Department of Pathology, The New York State College of Veterinary Medicine, Cornell University, Ithaca, New York

William J. Boever, D.V.M.
Senior Staff Veterinarian and Director of Research, St. Louis Zoological Park, St. Louis, Missouri, and Adjunct Assistant Professor, College of Veterinary Medicine, University of Missouri, Columbia, Missouri

Charles X. Connick, Esq.
Rosano, Mosé, Garden City, New York

Joseph N. Cunningham, Jr., M.D., A.B.S., A.B.T.S.
Head, Cardiovascular Surgery Section, Department of Surgery, Maimonides Medical Center, Brooklyn, New York

Nicholas H. Dodman, B.V.M.S., M.R.C.V.S., D.A.C.V.A.
Associate Professor, School of Veterinary Medicine, Tufts University, North Grafton, Massachusetts

Larry R. Engelking, Ph.D.
School of Veterinary Medicine, Tufts University, North Grafton, Massachusetts

Robin D. Gleed, B.V.Sc., M.R.C.V.S., D.V.A., D.A.C.V.A.
Assistant Professor of Anesthesiology, Department of Clinical Sciences, The New York State College of Veterinary Medicine, Cornell University, Ithaca, New York

Stephen A. Greene, D.V.M., M.S.
Assistant Professor, Department of Veterinary Small Animal Medicine & Surgery, College of Veterinary Medicine, Texas A&M University, College Station, Texas

Sandee M. Hartsfield, D.V.M., M.S., D.A.C.V.A.
Professor, Department of Veterinary Small Animal Medicine & Surgery, College of Veterinary Medicine, Texas A&M University, College Station, Texas

Ralph C. Harvey, M.S., D.V.M.
Assistant Professor of Anesthesiology, Department of Urban Practice, College of Veterinary Medicine, University of Tennessee, Knoxville, Tennessee

Steve C. Haskins, D.V.M., M.S., D.A.C.V.A.
Associate Professor, Department of Surgery, School of Veterinary Medicine, University of California at Davis, Davis, California

S.V. Hildebrand, D.V.M., D.A.C.V.A.
Associate Professor, Department of Surgery, School of Veterinary Medicine, University of California at Davis, Davis, California

Thomas J. Kern, D.V.M., D.A.C.V.O.
Assistant Professor of Medicine, Department of Clinical Sciences, The New York State College of Veterinary Medicine, Cornell University, Ithaca, New York

Lin V. Klein, V.M.D., D.A.C.V.A.
Associate Professor of Anesthesiology, School of Veterinary Medicine, New Bolton Center, University of Pennsylvania, Kennett Square, Pennsylvania

Kathleen A. Linn, D.V.M.
Sinclairville, New York

Charles J. McGrath, D.V.M., D.A.C.V.A.
Professor of Anesthesiology, Virginia-Maryland Regional College of Veterinary Medicine, Virginia Polytechnic Institute and State University, Blacksburg, Virginia

Robert E. Meyer, D.V.M., D.A.C.V.A.
Assistant Professor of Anesthesia, School of Veterinary Medicine, North Carolina State University, Raleigh, North Carolina

N. Sydney Moise, D.V.M., M.S., D.A.C.V.I.M.
Assistant Professor of Medicine, Department of Clinical Sciences, The New York State College of Veterinary Medicine, Cornell University, Ithaca, New York

Robert R. Paddleford, D.V.M., D.A.C.V.A.
Associate Professor and Director of Anesthesia Services, Department of Urban Practice, College of Veterinary Medicine, University of Tennessee, Knoxville, Tennessee

Peter J. Pascoe, B.V.Sc., M.R.C.V.S., D.V.A., D.A.C.V.A.
Associate Professor, Department of Clinical Studies, Ontario Veterinary College, University of Guelph, Guelph, Ontario, Canada

Mark E. Peterson, D.V.M., D.A.C.V.I.M.
Animal Medical Center and The Center for Research Animal Resources, Department of Medicine, Cornell University Medical College, New York, New York

Marc R. Raffe, D.V.M., M.S., D.A.C.V.A.
Associate Professor of Veterinary Medicine, Department of Small Animal Clinical Sciences, College of Veterinary Medicine, University of Minnesota, St. Paul, Minnesota

D.H. Riedesel, D.V.M., Ph.D., D.A.C.V.A.
Professor of Veterinary Clinical Sciences, Department of Veterinary Clinical Sciences, College of Veterinary Medicine, Iowa State University, Ames, Iowa

Urs Schatzmann, Prof. Dr. med. vet.
Professor of Anesthesiology, Faculty of Veterinary Medicine, University of Berne, Berne, Switzerland

Richard V. Shawley, D.V.M., M.S., D.A.C.V.A.
Associate Professor, Boren Veterinary Medical Teaching Hospital, College of Veterinary Medicine, Oklahoma State University, Stillwater, Oklahoma

Charles E. Short, D.V.M., M.S., D.A.C.V.A.
Professor and Chief of Anesthesiology, Department of Clinical Sciences, The New York State College of Veterinary Medicine, Cornell University, Ithaca, New York; Professor, Anesthesiology, Department of Anesthesiology, College of Medicine, Cornell University, New York, New York; and Adjunct Professor, Anesthesiology, Department of Anesthesiology, Upstate Medical Center, Syracuse, New York

Roman T. Skarda, Dr. med. vet., PH.D., D.A.C.V.A.
Associate Professor, Department of Veterinary Clinical Sciences, College of Veterinary Medicine, Ohio State University, Columbus, Ohio

J.C. Thurmon, D.V.M., M.S., D.A.C.V.A.
Professor and Head, Anesthesiology Section, Department of Veterinary Clinical Medicine, College of Veterinary Medicine, University of Illinois, Urbana, Illinois

William J. Tranquilli, D.V.M., M.S., D.A.C.V.A.

Cynthia M. Trim, M.R.C.V.S., D.V.A., D.A.C.V.A.
Professor of Anesthesiology, College of Veterinary Medicine, University of Georgia, Athens, Georgia

Alan Van Poznak, M.D., F.A.C.A., D.A.B.A.
Professor of Anesthesiology, Professor of Pharmacology, Department of Anesthesia, The New York Hospital-Cornell Medical Center, New York, New York, and Adjunct Professor of Veterinary Anesthesiology, The New York State College of Veterinary Medicine, Cornell University, Ithaca, New York

James Walberg, D.V.M.
Experimental Pathology Service, Mattenz (Basel), Switzerland

A.I. Webb, B.V.Sc., Ph.D., M.R.C.V.S., D.V.A., D.A.C.V.A.
Associate Professor of Anesthesiology, College of Veterinary Medicine, Department of Medical Sciences, University of Florida, Gainesville, Florida

Contents

SECTION 2. Special Clinical Considerations

SECTION 3. Related Clinical Topics

Introduction

Some of the most exciting advances in veterinary medicine during the past 25 years are in anesthetic management. The practice of anesthesia prior to that time consisted primarily of the administration of barbiturates or diethyl ether, usually by face mask, to induce or maintain anesthesia in small animals. Either ultrashort or short-acting barbiturates were chosen depending on the duration of the procedure. Chloroform was occasionally used in the horse, but more frequently chloral hydrate-magnesium sulfate combinations were used. Little attention was given to monitoring of anesthesia by means other than determining responsiveness to painful stimuli and whether the animal was breathing. Frequently, the awareness of adverse reactions during anesthesia was an observation of cyanosis by the veterinary surgeon during the operative procedure. Deaths were often explained as "surgical shock."

Inductions with the barbiturates were usually rapid. Maintenance of anesthesia did not assure adequate oxygenation or control of true anesthetic responses, and recoveries were frequently associated with a degree of excitement. This excitement during recovery, especially following injectable anesthesia in horses, contributed to standing procedures in horses with local blocks or use of the casting harness to avoid total anesthesia in the horse.

Predominantly, control of pain was accomplished by the administration of morphine sulfate. Some surgical procedures were completed using morphine sulfate alone or in combination with a nerve block in small animals.

Eventually, the availability of methoxyflurane and halothane began to play a significant role in the improvement of anesthetic management in animal patients. By the late 1960s, utilization of methoxyflurane in relatively simple anesthetic units was gaining popularity in small animal practices. The approach appeared to be safe, not too expensive, and easy to use. In contrast, halothane was utilized for anesthesia in large animals, especially the horse. The conversion of ether-type vaporizers to some of the early home-made anesthetic machines for large animals resulted in high sudden major variation in concentration of halothane delivered by the coarse adjustment vaporizers. Higher than desired concentrations of halothane resulted in fast depression of the responses of the horse and, in some instances, cardiac arrest. It became obvious that precision vaporizers were needed. By the middle 1970s, methoxyflurane was an anesthetic of choice in small animals and halothane was the inhalant agent of choice in the horse. It was not until after this time that excellent quality anesthetic units for small animals and large animals were commercially available. The most difficult equipment problems to resolve were the large animal anesthetic units. The production of these units was relatively expensive, especially because the number of units that could be sold was limited.

With the extensive improvements in technique and the unbelievable volume of information published in the literature, it was only appropriate that a new text on the principles and practice of veterinary anesthesia should be considered. This text has a perhaps impossible set of objectives. First was the need to provide a text for the veterinary student learning the pharmacology of anesthetic agents and related medications and the clinical significance of those medications in use. We also wanted to consider the veterinary practitioner as a user of this information. As a result, it was appropriate to consider the various animal species, the clinical environments, and the types of complications that the practitioner might encounter. It was further important to consider that a number of people, especially in academia, would use the text as a reference for a better understanding of veterinary anesthesia and as a part of training programs. Finally, we anticipated that some readers would be administering anesthetics to animals in research projects in veterinary medicine or at medical centers. As a result, an attempt was made to organize this text to provide an opportunity for each of these four segments of the medical profession to use the material as it applies to their needs.

The authors selected to contribute to this text included not only veterinary anesthesiologists, but also a clinical pathologist, an ophthalmologist, a cardiologist, an endocrinologist, a physician, and an attorney. Anesthesia is not just the administration of medications to produce unconsciousness. Knowledge of pharmacology, physiology, internal medicine, and pathophysiology is desirable for the practice of anesthesiology. The contributors represent concepts of anesthesia from America, Canada, England, and Europe, resulting in an international composite of information.

The first part of the text is concerned with the basic concepts in anesthesia and pharmacokinetics. The second part considers clinical anesthesia relative to body systems and the special considerations for different species. The third part of the text relates to clinical topics such as critical situations that may occur in conjunction with anesthesia.

Preanesthetic evaluation and clinical pathology values are included in the text. These values will serve as guidelines because we are accustomed to the good practice of analysis of the parameters that may influence the selection of anesthetic agents that can be given by clinical pathology values. Chapters 2 through 7 address the issues of anticholinergics, tranquilizers and sedatives, medications for pain, barbiturates, and inhalant anesthesia. Pharmacology and clinical usage are described. Not only is local anesthesia discussed, but also the author has illustrated the anatomical structure involved in making local and regional blocks. Concept and practice in the use of muscle relaxants have changed tremendously during the past 25 years. Although the concept is not yet widely utilized by practitioners, its popularity in veterinary anesthesiology is growing with better understanding of its usage.

As we have attempted to provide quality anesthesia, more drug combinations have been used. This results in concern about drug interactions. The section on the concepts of anesthetics and pharmacokinetics would not be complete without dissociative anesthesia. Dissociative anesthetics are discussed in a separate chapter because they represent a form of anesthesia that is symptomatically different from the injectable barbiturates or the inhalant anesthetics.

The considerations and complications that represent special clinical situations merit concern. Due to the complexities of ophthalmic surgery and the sensitivity of the eye, special attention should be given to anesthesia for these patients. There is a considerable contrast in the needs of anesthesia for central nervous system conditions in animals and humans. In animal patients, we are seldom asked to provide anesthesia for surgery of the brain, although this is more common for canine spinal surgery. Seldom is anesthetic consideration given to the central nervous system problems discussed in veterinary texts. It was our good fortune that Dr. Van Poznak agreed to provide us with comparative information on anesthesia of the central nervous system of animals and man.

The management of cardiac arrhythmias and dysfunctions related to anesthetics has been provided jointly as a cardiology-anesthesiology concept. This was considered critical because the anesthetics and related medications may have such dramatic effect on cardiovascular function. The same is true for the pulmonary system. Under most circumstances, when adequate control and maintenance of the function of cardiopulmonary systems are provided, there is assurance that other organ systems will be protected by perfusion and ventilation.

In response to the editor's request, this text provides extensive information on the hepatic system, information that is frequently unavailable. The majority of anesthetics and anesthetic-related medications undergo some degree of biotransformation in the liver. In the detoxification and elimination process, hepatic function is one of the most critical of all organ systems to the anesthesiologist. As a result, the authors have provided a thorough understanding of the hepatic system. In addition to biotransformation by the hepatic system, renal elimination of medications is quite critical. It was considered very appropriate that detailed information of anesthetic relationships to the renal system should be understood by the veterinarian administering anesthetics.

The endocrine system can greatly influence the animal's function during anesthesia. Perhaps it is not as likely to influence the immediate response during the induction phase, but it can certainly affect the responses during anesthesia and in recovery. Most veterinary texts do not fully cover this subject.

Until recent years, anesthesia for surgical correction of problems in the gastrointestinal system were not considered as critical as procedures of the thoracic cavity. This was before the emphasis on such dynamic syndromes as equine colic or gastric torsion and dilatation in the dog. These procedures require critical anesthesia for surgical correction to be ultimately successful.

There are many differences in anesthetic management of various species and breeds of animals. Attention has been given to the horse, the ruminants, dogs and cats, swine, and wildlife. We must give attention not only to the various breeds, but also to young and old, the pregnant and the well-conditioned animal. The traditional laboratory animal has many functional differences. We must understand its responses when it is anesthetized for research purposes; additionally, often "laboratory animals" are presented as pets for surgical procedures requiring anesthesia.

The related clinical topics obviously include anesthetic equipment. The advances in anesthetic equipment are well illustrated, and it is anticipated that the reader will have a better understanding of the utilization of this equipment. Information is provided on controlled ventilation and how it influences pulmonary function because this is so much influenced by available equipment.

A simplistic approach to cardiovascular medications used during veterinary anesthesia would be to give a brief overview of those medications and to list them with the dosages for various species. It was thought that a better understanding of the autonomic system and how the anesthetics and the cardiovascular medications relate to the control of function by the autonomic nervous system was needed, so an excellent review of the autonomic system and its responses to anesthetics has been provided. Anesthetic management includes the utilization of fluids and electrolytes and maintenance of acid-base balance and blood replacement. Often the primary care of fluid and electrolyte balance occurs during anesthesia in animal patients.

Unfortunately, not all patients react to medications with a normal physiological response. Some patients have inherited characteristics that may result in highly detrimental responses. A class of patients in this category are those susceptible to malignant hyperthermia. These patients will be seen rarely; however, should the problem occur, immediate knowledge of and response to this complication are essential if the patient is to survive.

Special diagnostic and surgical procedures often require modifications in technique or choice of medications. Appropriate postoperative care is a crucial part of total anesthetic management. Anesthetic management includes the period from the first premedication until the animal has returned to its preanesthetic condition.

Emergency care medicine could be discussed as patients presented to the veterinarian in shock, trauma, or other complications. They may need analgesia, anesthetic management, or supportive therapy. Unfortunately, the crisis may occur intraoperatively or in the postoperative period. As a result, our discussion includes patients' responses to shock and trauma and the factors leading up to potential cardiopulmonary arrest. This understanding should provide the reader with more knowledge of the total management of the critical patient, including cardiopulmonary resuscitation.

Immune responses and allergic reactions do not occur often. When they do, the crisis develops rapidly. Without an understanding of the problem, loss of life can result.

We would not consider this text complete if we provided only information on the medications to use and an understanding of the responses to them by the animal patient. Information to protect the veterinarian and other medical personnel involved in providing anesthetic care from the effects of anesthetic waste gases is essential, and we have made recommendations on ways to reduce anesthetic exposure of personnel.

A thorough understanding of anesthesia and its various components is very helpful in providing excellent anesthetic care of each animal. Unfortunately, the owner is not always convinced that the best of anesthetic care has been provided. As a result, in our final chapter, guidelines for avoiding medical/legal problems or defending against actions are provided.

On behalf of the contributors, it is my hope that this text will provide better understanding of the principles and practice of anesthesia and the relationship of anesthetics to many patient conditions. This can result in further improvements in the management of veterinary anesthesia.

Charles E. Short, D.V.M., M.S., D.A.C.V.A.
Editor

Section

1

Basic Concepts in Anesthetics and Pharmacokinetics

CHAPTER 1

Preanesthetic Evaluation and Clinical Pathology

JULIA T. BLUE, D.V.M., Ph.D., D.A.C.V.P., AND
CHARLES E. SHORT, D.V.M., M.S., D.A.C.V.A.

Introduction

One of the responsibilities of the veterinarian prior to the administration of an anesthetic is the assessment of the patient to optimize development of an anesthetic management plan, coordinate of anesthesia and surgery, and assure high quality patient care. The purpose of this chapter is to present an approach to preanesthetic considerations. No attempt will be made to cover the myriad of possible congenital or acquired anomalies that occur. It should be apparent that a cursory examination of the animal is not as adequate as a thorough evaluation to provide useful information.

If disease or abnormal function is detected during the preoperative assessment, further evaluation is needed to determine the extent of the problem and a safe approach to anesthesia. If irregular cardiac sounds or abnormal pulse pressures are detected, further evaluation with electrocardiographic recordings may well be indicated. The detection of respiratory difficulties in the horse, for example, may lead to endoscopic evaluation of the upper airway. Specific consideration of patients with existing disease is discussed in Section 2.

The following outline can be used as a suggested preanesthetic evaluation except in those situations where complete preanesthetic evaluation is not possible.

Preoperative Assessment

PATIENT HISTORY

Age is important, because the usual response can be anticipated with knowledge of normal growth and development. The chief complaint and planned procedure are evaluated. Past medical history of operations, allergies, medications, and systems review will be helpful. Previous response to anesthesia is often more useful than general guidelines, such as drug doses, tube sizes, type of surgery, or recovery complications. Concerning allergies, a previous exposure to an agent is not necessary for an adverse reaction. Medications are a good screen for general medical problems (i.e., iron for anemia, phenobarbital for seizures, steroids for allergy, phenylbutasone for pain and inflammation, or antibiotics for infection. Review of systems can be a minimal screening; it should be more extensive for specific problems. The following should be considered: general health, development compared with similar age for the species and breed; respiratory, pneumonia, bronchiolitis, nasal discharge, and rales; cardiac, history of murmur or exercise intolerance; hepatic, jaundice or hepatitis; hemodynamic, bleeding postsurgery, dental work, or trauma and previous transfusions; gastrointestinal, last meal, regurgitation, vomiting, and feeding problems; and neurological, seizures, motor or sensory abnormality, and behavioral problems. Finally, background information should be collected. The history of related animals may suggest problems. Previous anesthetic problems, neuromuscular diseases, malignant hyperthermia susceptibility, bleeding disorders, allergies, prolonged recoveries, or drug interactions should be queried.

PHYSICAL EXAMINATION

Vital signs include weight, for drug dosages and assessment of nutritional state; temperature, normal temperature for species and breed at rest; heart rate, blood pressure, respiratory rates, and respiratory pattern; general health, well or sick, assessment of attitude and level of activity; extremities, edema or bruising, identification of sites for intravenous access, peripheral pulses for blood pressure monitoring, and temperature; and head and face, including asymmetry of pupils, amount and quality of nasal discharge, and mobility, tongue size, dentition, cynosis, and capillary refill time of the month. The neck should be examined for mobility and length. The asymmetry, pectus, respiratory effort, and lung fields of the chest and cardiac pulses, color, and murmurs should be assessed. The abdomen should be examined if indicated for hepatomegaly, splenomegaly, mass, and distension. Observation is all that is usually necessary for neurological evaluation.

LABORATORY DATA

The inclusion of laboratory data in the preanesthetic evaluation of the animal will provide a more complete understanding of the condition of the animal and aid in a more accurate selection of medications, and anesthetic techniques that may improve the safety of the entire anesthetic-surgical procedure.

The reference ranges shown in Tables 1.1 through 1.4 should be considered as general guidelines that may not be applicable in all situations. Whenever possible, test results should be interpreted by comparing the patient's result to a reference range for the species established by the laboratory performing the test. Most commercial laboratories that test many samples from veterinary practices will have established their own references ranges for the four major species. However, many veterinarians who use office clinical chemistry instruments or who use laboratories that infrequently test animal blood do not have species-specific reference ranges for their instrument or laboratory. These veterinarians must rely on published reference ranges to guide them in interpreting results. With consideration of certain cautions expressed in the following paragraphs, Tables 1.1 through 1.4 should be helpful guides to the interpretation of routine laboratory tests during preanesthetic evaluations.

The reference ranges in the tables are presented both in conventional units presently used in the United States and in units of the International System of Units (SI), which is now in use in Canada and European countries and may become standard in the United States in the future. For those tests in which the units are the same in both systems or in which the number value is the same but the units are different, the number values are given once and both units are indicated. For other tests in which the number values as well as the units are different, the reference range in conventional units is listed above the range in SI units.

Table 1.1
Hematology Test Reference Ranges[a]

Test	Units	Dog	Cat	Horse	Cow
PCV	%	37–55	24–45	32–52	24–46
	L/L	0.37–0.55	0.24–0.45	0.32–0.52	0.24–0.46
Hemoglobin	g/dL	12–18	8–15	11–19	8–15
	g/L	120–180	80–150	110–190	80–150
RBC	$10^6/\mu L$ or $10^{12}/L$	5.5–8.5	5–10	6.5–12.5	5–10
MCV	fl	60–77	39–55	34–58	40–60
MCHC	g/dL	32–36	30–36	31–37	30–36
	g/L	320–360	300–360	310–370	300–360
MCH	pg/red cell	19.5–24.5	13–17	13–19	11–17
Reticulocytes	%	0–1.5	0–1	0	0
WBC	$10^3/\mu L$ or $10^9/L$	6–17	5.5–19.5	5.5–12.5	4–12
Segmented Neutrophils	$10^3/\mu L$ or 10^9L	3–11.5	2.5–12.5	2.7–6.7	0.6–4.0
Band Neutrophils	$10^3/\mu L$ or $10^9/L$	0–.3	0–.3	0–.1	0–.1
Lymphocytes	$10^3/\mu L$ or $10^9/L$	1.0–4.8	1.5–7.0	1.5–5.5	2.5–7.5
Monocytes	$10^3/\mu L$ or $10^9/L$	0.1–1.4	0–0.8	0–0.8	0–0.8
Eosinophils	$10^3/\mu L$ or $10^9/L$	0.1–1.2	0–1.5	0–0.9	0–2.4
Platelets	$10^3/\mu L$ or $10^9/L$	200–500	300–800	100–350	100–800
Plasma Protein (by refractometry)	g/dL	6.0–8.0	6.0–8.0	5.8–8.5	7.0–8.5
	g/L	60–80	60–80	58–85	70–85

[a] Source of ranges: Schalm OW, Jain NC, Carroll EJ: *Veterinary Hematology*, ed 3. Philadelphia: Lea and Febiger, 1975.

Table 1.2
Serum Biochemistry Test Reference Ranges[a]

Test	Units	Dog	Cat	Horse	Cow
Glucose	mg/dL	62–108	61–124	62–114	42–75
	mmol/L	3.4–6.0	3.4–6.9	3.5–6.3	2.3–4.1
Urea nitrogen	mg/dL	9–26	15–31	10–25	8–25
Urea	mmol/L	3.1–9.2	5.5–11.1	3.7–8.8	2.8–8.8
Creatinine	mg/dL	0.5–1.6	0.5–1.9	0.9–2.0	0.6–1.8
	mmol/L	44–138	49–165	77–175	56–162
ALT (GPT)	U/L	8–57	8–53	3–21	7–35
AST (GOT)	U/L	9–49	9–40	116–287	45–110
Total protein	g/dL	5.5–7.5	5.7–8.0	5.7–7.9	6.2–8.2
	g/L	55–75	57–80	57–79	62–82
Albumin	g/dL	2.6–4.0	2.4–3.7	2.5–3.8	2.8–3.9
	g/L	26–40	24–37	25–38	28–39
Globulin	g/dL	2.1–3.7	2.4–4.7	2.4–4.6	2.9–4.9
	g/L	21–37	24–47	24–46	29–49
Albumin/globulin		0.7–1.9	0.6–1.2	0.5–1.5	0.6–1.3
Alkaline phosphatose	U/L	11–100	12–65	70–227	18–153
Gamma glutamyl transferase (GGT)	U/L	1–10	2–12	3–22	5–26
Total bilirubin	mg/dL	0.1–0.6	0.1–0.5	0.3–3.0	0.0–0.8
	μmol/L	1–11	1–8	5–51	1–14
Sodium	mEq/L or mmol/L	140–154	146–159	133–147	135–148
Potassium	mEq/L or mmol/L	3.8–5.6	3.8–5.3	2.8–4.7	4.0–5.8
Chloride	mEq/L or mmol/L	102–117	108–130	97–110	96–109
Total CO_2 (bicarbonate)	mEq/L or mmol/L	18–25	16–22	22–29	21–29
Calcium	mg/dL	8.7–11.8	7.9–10.9	10.4–13.4	8.4–11.0
	mmol/L	2.2–3.0	2.0–2.7	2.6–3.3	2.1–2.8
Phosphorus	mg/dL	2.9–6.2	4.0–7.3	2.3–5.4	4.3–7.8
	mmol/L	1.0–2.0	1.3–2.4	0.7–1.7	1.4–2.5
Creatine kinase (CK, CPK)	U/L	14–120	17–150	34–166	14–107
Amylase	U/L	270–1462	371–1193	47–188	41–98
Lipase (lipase-turbidometric method, Boehringer Mannheim Diagnostics, Houston, Texas)	U/L	16–200[b]	0–50[b]		
Lipase (Sigma Serum Lipase, Sigma Chemical Co., St. Louis, Mo.)	Sigma Teitz U/dL	0–1.0[b]			

[a] Source of ranges except as noted otherwise: Boyd JW: The interpretation of serum biochemistry–Test results in domestic animals. *Vet Clin Path* 13(2):7–14, 1984.
[b] Range determined at New York State College of Veterinary Medicine, Cornell University.

The reference ranges for hematology data in Table 1.1 are widely used ranges that can be applied to results from many laboratories. However, veterinarians should be aware that the reference ranges for packed cell volume (PCV) in this table are for PCV measured by spinning blood in a microhematocrit centrifuge, and the ranges for mean corpuscular volume (MCV) are based on MCV calculated from a spun PCV and red cell count (RBC) using the formula

$$MCV = PCV \times 10/RBC.$$

Newer electronic cell counters, which are used in many large laboratories, measure PCV and MCV electronically. Reference ranges for electronically measured PCV (or hematocrit) and MCV may not coincide exactly with the reference ranges from spun PCV and calculated MCV as shown in Table 1.1.

The ranges shown in Table 1.2 were derived by calculating the means of the upper and lower limits of the reference ranges of many veterinary diagnostic laboratories; they therefore represent a composite list of reference ranges. For many of the tests, particularly those that measure the concentration of a serum constituent, the ranges of this table are similar to the ranges for individual laboratories and other published ranges. For enzyme activities, however, there may be marked differences between the ranges in Table 1.2 and the reference range for a particular laboratory or instrument. Therefore, special caution should be exercised when using this table to interpret enzyme activities.

The reference ranges for prothrombin time (PT), activated partial thromboplastin time (APTT), and fibrinogen are based on results for normal animals measured at one laboratory. Results produced by other methods may be somewhat different. It is recom-

Table 1.3
Acid/Base Test Reference Ranges[a]

Test	Units	Dog	Cat	Horse	Cow
pH		7.31–7.42	7.24–7.40	7.32–7.44	7.35–7.50
Partial pressure oxygen (pO_2)-arterial	mmHg KPa	80–100 10.64–13.30	80–100 10.64–13.30	80–100 10.64–13.30	80–100 10.64–13.30
Partial pressure carbon dioxide (pCO_2)	mmHg KPa	29–42 3.86–5.59	29–42 3.86–5.59	38–46 5.05–6.12	35–44 4.66–5.85
Bicarbonate (HCO_3)	mEq/L or mmol/L	17–24	17–24	24–30	20–30
Total CO_2	mEq/L or mmol/L	18–25	18–25	25–31	21–31
Sodium	mEq/L or mmol/L	141–157	147–156	134–140	131–144
Potassium	mEq/L or mmol/L	4.0–5.3	4.3–5.6	2.2–4.5	3.5–5.3
Chloride	mEq/L or mmol/L	105–115	117–123	99–109	97–111
Anion Gap (AG)[a]		15–25	5–30	6–15	14–21

[a] Source of ranges, New York State College of Veterinary Medicine, Cornell University.
[b] Anion Gap calculated as ([Na] + [K]) − ([Cl] + [HCO_3].

Table 1.4
Coagulation Test Reference Ranges

Test	Units	Dog	Cat	Horse	Cow
Prothrombin time (PT)[a] (Fibrosystem, Becton Dickinson & Co., Rutherford, N.J., and Simplastin, General Diagnostics, Morris Plains, N.J.)	sec	5–8	6–10	7–11	10–15
Activated partial thromboplastin time (APTT)[a] (Fibrosystem, Becton Dickinson & Co., Rutherford, N.J., and Automated APTT, General Diagnostics, Morris Plains, N.J.)	sec	12–19	12–19	28–64	24–49
Fibrinogen[a] (Fibrosystem, Becton Dickinson and Co., Rutherford, N.J., and Data Fi Dade Diagnostics, Aquada, P.R.)	mg/dL g/L	100–500 1.0–5.0	60–300 0.6–3.0	110–450 1.1–4.5	130–500 1.3–5
Activated Whole Blood (Clotting Time (ACT) 37° C incubation (Vacutainer 6522, Becton Dickinson and Co., Rutherford, N.J.)	sec	60–100[b]	<65[c]	120–190[b]	120–180[d]
Fibrin (ogen) Degradation Products (FDP)[a] (Thrombo-Wellcotest, Wellcome Diagnostics, Dartford, England)	μg/mL	<10	<10	<10	<10

[a] Ranges determined at New York State College of Veterinary Medicine, Cornell University.
[b] Values from Duncan JR and Prasse KW: *Veterinary Laboratory Medicine*, ed 2. Ames, The Iowa State University Press, 1986.
[c] Greene CE and Meriwether E: Activated partial thromboplastin time and activated coagulation time in monitoring heparinized cats. *Am J Vet Res* 43:1473–1477, 1982.
[d] Riley JH and Lassen ED: Activated coagulation times of normal cows. *Vet Clin Path* 8:31–33, 1979.

mended that a control sample from a clinically healthy animal of the same species as the patient be collected, handled, and tested with the patient sample. If the coagulation test results for the control animal are well within the reference ranges given in Table 1.4, then these ranges may be used to interpret the patient's results.

Since an unanticipated failure of normal clotting can turn the most routine surgical procedure into a complicated problem, veterinarians should be aware of the methods available to screen patients for such defects. Ideally, a minimum coagulation profile consisting of platelet count, PT, and APTT is performed on each patient before surgery. However, for several reasons, such a set of tests is not practical for routine screening. These tests are not readily available to many veterinarians, and the cost is too high to justify performing these tests in apparently healthy animals. Fortunately, there are other methods that are inexpensive, readily available to the practitioner, and likely to detect many of the patients at risk to bleed during or after surgery. These tests are the estimate of platelet count and the whole blood activated clotting time (ACT).

The platelet count can be estimated with reasonable accuracy from a well-made blood smear by determining the average number of platelets per field using an oil immersion objective magnifying 100 times. The smear should be scanned first at low magnification to detect clumps of platelets, which if present make the estimate nonvalid. The area of the smear to use for the platelet estimate should be one in which leukocytes are evenly distributed and red cells are touching but not overlapping to any great extent. The average number of platelets per oil immersion field is multiplied by 15,000 to give the estimated number of platelets per microliter of blood. For example, if the average number of platelets per oil immersion field is 15, then the estimated platelet count is 225,000/μl. Platelet counts of 100,000/μl are sufficient for normal clotting unless there is a concurrent defect in platelet function.

ACT is a test to detect defects in the intrinsic and/or common coagulation pathways. Clinically significant deficiencies in Factors XI, IX, VIII:C, X, or II or fibrinogen, whether congenital or acquired, should result in prolongation of the ACT. Factor XII deficiency, which is not a cause of clinical bleeding, also can prolong the ACT. Because the test requires some platelets, severe thrombocytopenia (platelet count $<$10,000/μl) may prolong the ACT slightly. The ACT is not prolonged with Factor VII deficiency and may be normal in patients with vonWillebrands disease. An ACT tube (No. 6522 Vacutainer, Becton Dickinson and Co., Rutherford, New York), a 37°C heating block or water bath, and a timer are needed to perform the ACT. The ACT tube is warmed to 37°C, exactly 2 ml of blood from a large vein is drawn cleanly into the tube, and the tube is inverted five times and placed in the 37°C heating block or water bath. Time 0 is the time at which blood first enters the tube. At 60 seconds for dog blood, 45 seconds for cat blood, or 120 seconds for horse and cow blood, the tube is picked up, tilted and examined for the first sign of clot formation. If there is no clot at the first examination, the tube is replaced in the heating unit and the procedure is repeated every 5 seconds until a clot begins to form. The endpoint is the beginning of clot formation, not a solid clot. The ACT results for normal animals are shown in Table 1.4.

Application of the platelet estimate and ACT to all surgical patients would increase the likelihood of detecting asymptomatic thrombocytopenic patients, patients in disseminated intravascular coagulation (DIC), and patients with unsuspected congenital deficiencies of clotting factors. For patients with abnormal results on screening tests, surgery should be postponed, if possible, and additional testing should be done to define the problem. If surgery cannot be postponed, then appropriate preparations can be made to manage anticipated bleeding.

EXCEPTIONAL CIRCUMSTANCES

Not all animals will cooperate in preanesthetic examinations; this group most obviously includes wild and exotic animals. There is an increase in anesthetic risk in this group of animals because complete assessment of preanesthetic information cannot be accomplished. Neither can complete assessment of range animals or untamed domestic species be expected before medication to at least calm the unruly.

It is obvious that the guidelines for preanesthetic evaluation will be different for patients for elective surgery and those with trauma, severe shock, an acute abdomen, or other life-threatening conditions requiring rapid action. The acute patient requires not only rapid evaluation, but also rapid correction of a critical malfunction. One should proceed in the following sequence: assess airway and gas exchange; assess hemodynamics and blood volume; and perform a gross physical examination of chest, abdomen, head and neck, neurology, long bones, spine, and pelvis. Then initiate therapy: intubate, administer oxygen; place intravenous lines; treat persistent severe hypotension; and initiate corrective measures for head and airway injuries. If there is cardiac arrest, initiate cardiopulmonary resuscitation (CPR). One must control hemorrhage and start fluid infusion when indicated. The critical patient may need to be moved to the operating room if CPR is successful. After the patient is stable, more complete evaluation and administration of preanesthetic or anesthetics may be considered.

CHAPTER 2

Anticholinergics

CHARLES E. SHORT, D.V.M., M.S., D.A.C.V.A.

Introduction

Anticholinergic agents may be indicated prior to the administration of a variety of anesthetic and related agents, including sedatives, narcotics, barbiturates, and inhalant anesthetic agents. Naturally occurring anticholinergic drugs are alkaloids of the plant *Atrpa belladonna*. The plant has potent poisonous characteristics, but in spite of these toxic effects, low dosage administration of the *belladonna* alkaloids has beneficial medicinal effects (1). Efforts have continued to find and develop new anticholinergic agents that can duplicate the desired peripheral antimuscarinic effects and at the same time avoid potential toxicity. Atropine sulfate, scopolamine, and glycopyrrolate are the three principle anticholinergics that merit attention. In animal usage of anticholinergics, comparisons are normally made between atropine and glycopyrrolate as preanesthetics and for their effects on cardiovascular and other organ functions. Scopolamine has not become a popular anticholinergic agent in animal anesthesia.

Chemistry and Pharmacology

The *belladonna* drugs are widely distributed in various plants such as *Atrpa belladonna* and the deadly night shade plant, which yields the alkaloid atropine. The same alkaloid can be found in Jimsonweed. The scopolamine alkaloid is found predominantly in *Hyoscyamus niger*, the henbane scrub. Glycopyrrolate is a synthetic substitute for the belladonna alkaloid. The chemical structure for these three predominant anticholinergic agents are shown in Figure 2.1.

Antimuscarinic Medications

These medications have little effect on acetylcholine (ACh) at the nicotinic receptor sites. Related quaternary ammonium analogues, in contrast, can exhibit various degrees of nicotinic blocking activity. The quaternary ammonium compounds also have more difficulty penetrating blood-brain barriers; as a result, they do not show extensive central effects. These drugs do have varying degrees of sensitivity at the neuroeffector junction of the parasympathetic nervous system affecting different organs. The administration of these products can depress salivary and bronchial secretions; they frequently dilate the pupil of the eye and in the process may interfere with vision. They also may affect the heart rate due to the blockade of vagal tone. Larger doses inhibit the parasympathetic responses for control of the urinary bladder and the gastrointestinal tract. The predominant effect on the gastrointestinal tract is reduced gastric secretion at low dosages. However, at higher doses, parastyolic movement may be reduced in varying degrees and for various periods of time. As a result, a lower dose of anticholinergic agents will affect heart rate by reducing vagal activity, whereas higher doses will be required for changes in gastrointestinal motility. These are the general responses of animals to this class of medication. For a better understanding of the anticipated responses to specific anticholinergics, a deeper understanding of the response to atropine sulfate and glycopyrrolate is indicated.

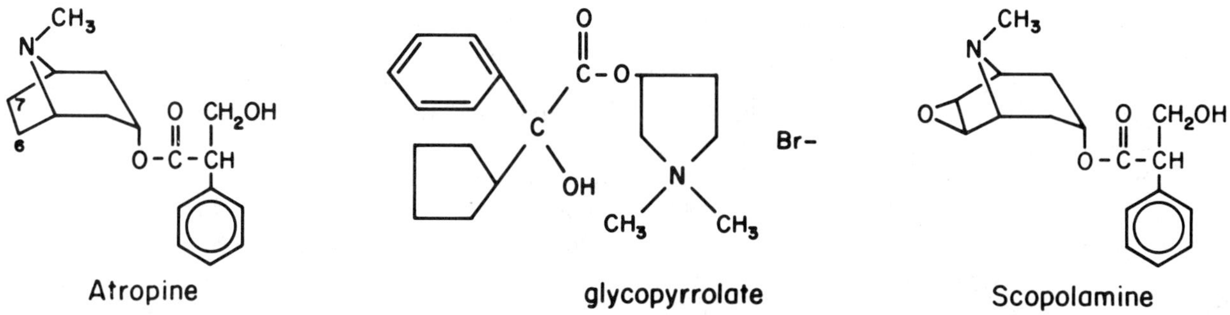

Figure 2.1. Chemical structure of atropine, scopolamine, and glycopyrrolate

Responses to Atropine Sulfate Administration

During the era of diethyl ether anesthetic technique, excessive salivation was considered an undesirable side effect of anesthesia. Atropine was considered as an important anticholinergic agent to control salivation. Atropine is very effective for this purpose, having been demonstrated even to control nicotine-induced salivation in cats. Its control of salivation is via central receptors that have muscarinic properties (2).

In addition to the control of salivation during certain anesthetic procedures, it was discovered that atropine was beneficial in preventing severe bradycardia. this was especially important during the administration of potent narcotics, heart rate-depressing general anesthetics, and agents such as xylazine with known characteristics of reducing heart rate. Atropine sulfate at adequate dosages can prevent or correct xylazine-induced bradycardia in dogs and other species. In the dog, for example, atropine sulfate 0.045 mg/kg i.m. increased both arterial blood pressure and heart rate but did not always prevent xylazine-induced bradycardia. Higher dosage rates of atropine sulfate (an additional 0.01 mg/kg i.v.) corrected xylazine-induced bradycardia previously uncorrected by intramuscular use of atropine (3). Although atropine corrects xylazine-induced bradycardia, in studies of the effects of atropine on dogs receiving xylazine and pentobarbital anesthesia, a marked tachycardia and an increase in the $PaCO_2$ was observed. That atropine may contribute to respiratory depression should be considered (4). Atropine has been used effectively during halothane anesthesia in many species to prevent excessive slowing of the heart during clinical anesthesia. It has also been shown to be effective in preventing bradycardia during the effect of narcotics or neuroleptanalgesia, especially in the presence of Innovar. Because atropine is normally administered prior to the administration of potent narcotics, sedatives, or anesthetics, an understanding of the response of conscious animals to atropine is of importance.

A slowing of the heart rate in atrioventricular conduction may be observed after the administration of lower doses of atropine (6.26 mcg/kg i.v. in dogs). Higher doses will result in an acceleration of heart rate and atrioventricular conduction time (5). Heart rates in conscious dogs are higher after the administration of atropine than after bilateral vagotomy. Atropine sulfate at 0.1 mg/kg i.v. can result in excess tachycardia (6). Atropine has also been shown to produce tachycardia in conscious cats. A cat receiving a beta-blocking agent in conjunction with atropine does not demonstrate as severe a degree of tachycardia. It is suggested that there is a linkage to changes in sympathetic-vagal balance to activation of sympathetic centers and to the muscarinic antagonistic effects of atropine in sympathetic nerves (7). This is further explained by vagal stimulation prolonging the frequency-dependent sinus nodal cycle length and atrioventricular nodal conduction. Atropine eliminates the effects of vagal stimulation (8). The bradycardic response to arginine-vasopressin in conscious dogs has been blunted by atropine (9). Even in fetal bradycardia, atropine has been demonstrated to substantially correct bradycardia caused by vagal activity during hypoxia to the fetus. The use of atropine to block this activity can cause marked tachycardia, but no increase in fetal oxygen uptake (10). This evidence supports the hypothesis that the tachycardia associated with the administration of atropine sulfate is due both to blockade of vagal inhibition of heart rate and greater influence on heart rate by the sympathetic system. It may also further explain the instances of observed improvement in blood flow or blood pressure after the administration of the anticholinergic.

Atropine has been shown to prevent increased cerebral blood flow during hypertension in newborn pigs. Atropine does effectively cross the blood-brain barrier (11).

Atropine characteristically causes dilitation of the pupil. This dilitation may last for up to 24 hours after systemic injection. One is cautioned in the utilization of atropine to avoid exposing the animal patient to excessive light. Chronic mydriasis in kittens and adult cats has shown that pupil size can be altered permanently by chronic usage of atropine (12), and there are organic changes in the retinal blood vessel pattern during chronic administration of atropine in cats (13). In addition to the dilitation of the pupil in animals after atropine sulfate, tear production is decreased, usually within 10 minutes after subcutaneous administration. This has been demonstrated in cats during ketamine hydrochloride and acetylpromazine anesthesia (14). The combination of reduced tear formation and dilitation of the pupil indicates the need for maintaining moisture in the eye and avoidance of undesirable light and heat during the anesthesia-surgical procedure to avoid potential complications to eyesight.

Bronchial-tracheal responses are influenced by administration of anticholinergic agents. The influence of atropine to counter the effects of 4-aminopyridine on the electrical activity and cable properties of canine tracheal smooth muscle reflects chiefly on an activation of muscarinic receptors in contrast to interference with potassium conductance (15). Using strong cholinergic and beta-adrenergic antagonists, the afferent arms of two reflex arcs that relax tracheal smooth muscle in dogs showed that relaxation of the muscle was due to withdrawal of a tonic cholinergic input. Beta-adrenergic pathways played little role in causing these reflex responses (16). In contrast, atropine completely blocked the response of canine trachealis muscle strip's contractual responses induced by histamine or electrical stimulation of cholinergic nerves. The effect of atropine on the smooth muscle of the canine trachealis muscle is probably completely due to cholinergic nerve stimulation with no histaminic effect (17). In further studies, atropine derivatives produced antiasthmatic effects by their persistent anticholinergic activity in sensitized dogs, in addition to anticholinergic activity. It was postulated that antihistamine action in the broncheous and broncheos was also present (18). Atropine also appears to block antigen-induced contractions in canine bronchial rings by its antimuscarinic effect on reflex cholinergic activity (19). These studies indicate atropine can reduce the extent of bronchial construction, hypermuscular activity in the trachea, and other responses to the upper airway.

Unfortunately, in addition to these beneficial effects, there may also be some undesirable characteristics. Perhaps the one of most concern is the prolongation of the presence of viable bacteria in the trachea in rare circumstances. Atropine may impair mucociliary clearance or cause other alterations in the mucosal function, thus predisposing the airway to a higher incidence of tracheitis. This would be of greater concern in those animals with prolonged anesthesia or potential drying of the trauma to the airway by the placement of or prolonged contact with the endotracheal tube.

Gastric smooth muscle is sensitive to the administration of atropine. Normal smooth muscle contractions can be blocked by atropine. These mucosal sites of stimulation may be related to intramural excitatory cholinergic neurons blocked by the anticholinergic atropine (21). Also, in further studies in the cat, anticholinergics have been shown to inhibit centrally mediated gastric acid and pepsin secretion by depressing muscarinic receptors (22). Atropine has been effective in countering the stimulating effect of codeine on circular muscular contractions of the gastrointestinal tract causing both a dose-dependent reduction in amplitude and frequency of burst-phase contractions (23). It has also been demonstrated in the dog that intestinal absorption is in part mediated through cardiovascular influence by cholinergic control. In contrast, the tonic parasympathetic activity primarily has direct effect on gut absorption, as demonstrated in the dog (24). At higher levels of atropine administration, the alteration in circulation and absorption from the gut will give further support to gastrointestinal problems, including intestinal stasis, which may occur in equine subjects inadvertently given atropine after eating. The incidence of ileus or colic is remarkably lessened in animals given atropine without food in the gastrointestinal tract. Acetylpromazine has been shown to greatly reduce the electrical activity of the equine small intestine, as has meperidine and methadone. It is understandable horses receiving both acepromazine and atropine or acepromazine, narcotic and atropine would experience changes in intestinal motility patterns (25).

Atropine increases latency by secretions of hydrochloric acid and pancreatic fluid (26). At the same time, atropine significantly increases heart rate. This effect on the pancreas further influences the digestive process when food is present (27).

The alpha-adrenergic receptor blockade by atropine via the muscarinic chlonoreceptor depresses contractions of the urethra (28). Small doses of atropine can abolish voiding of urine from the bladder from some species, such as humans and monkeys, but not in most other species (29). This contributes to the urinary response of animals during anesthesia.

Response to the Anticholinergic Glycopyrrolate

PHARMACODYNAMIC EVALUATION OF GLYCOPYRROLATE IN ANIMALS

In anesthetized dogs, intravenous doses of 5 to 10 mcg/kg of glycopyrrolate markedly reduced intestinal tone and markedly inhibited amplitude of intestinal contractions. There was no determined effect on respiration or carotid arterial blood pressure. The intestinal activity was depressed, and response of the urinary bladder to the parasympathetic stimulating agents was inhibited. The 5 to 10 mcg/kg doses of glycopyrrolate reduced bradycardia, hypotension, and intestinal hyperactivity resulting from peripheral vagal stimulation. Studies in vitro showed that glycopyrrolate in low concentrations antagonized the spasmogenic effect of acetylcholine. The potency of this response was comparable to atropine sulfate. Glycopyrrolate, like atropine, is a weak antagonist of histamine-induced spasm. In unanesthetized dogs, glycopyrrolate lowered intestinal tone and decreased the amplitude of intestinal contractions. Glycopyrrolate produced an inhibition of intestinal activity at dosages lower than required to cause mydriasis or dryness of oral mucous membrane. Tachycardia can occur with high levels of glycopyrrolate administration, but it is probably due to some level of excitement in unanesthetized animals, because during anesthesia in dogs, higher doses of glycopyrrolate are not as likely to produce tachycardia. Intestinal hyperactivity and salivation were reduced with dosages as low as 10 mcg/kg glycopyrrolate i.v. Glycopyrrolate significantly decreased gastric hypertenicity secretions induced by histamine. This reduction was in both volume and acidity of secretions. Glycopyrrolate does not readily penetrate the central nervous system. This has been demonstrated in several species including the cat. This lack of penetration of the central nervous system is related to the difficulty of glycopyrrolate in crossing blood-brain barrier.

Glycopyrrolate is an antagonist of various parasympathetically mediated responses. Its effect is derived predominantly from motor and secretory activity of the gastrointestinal tract because these functions are the easiest to inhibit. Glycopyrrolate has no central nervous system stimulating effect. This is not an unexpected finding; it is a quaternary ammonium compound. These products do not normally cause central nervous system stimulation (30).

After the determination of the chemical and pharmacodynamic characteristics of glycopyrrolate, studies determined the dosage level of this product in small animals. A dosage level of 0.011 mg/kg as a preanesthetic in dogs was determined as appropriate after studies at 0.0055, 0.011, and 0.022 mg/kg levels, respectively. The determination of effective dosage of glycopyrrolate in cats was studied using 0.005, 0.011, and 0.22 mg/kg. As in the dog, 0.011 mg/kg was determined to be the effective dose level (31, 32).

Glycopyrrolate has been shown to reduce the incidence of respiratory complications in man after aspiration of gastric secretions, frequently referred to as Mendelson's syndrome. The incidence of silent regurgitation in dogs was determined as 13.3% of animals with barbiturate anesthesia for routine surgical procedures compared to 13.5% of animals with an abdominal manipulation (32). Of the patients receiving atropine, 82.4% had gastric pH of less than 2.5 versus 34.1% of those receiving glycopyrrolate. Aspiration of gastric secretions with a pH below 2.5 can produce extensive acute inflammation and pulmonary changes within seconds after the aspiration. Glycopyrrolate has been used to control the hypertenicity, reduce parastolysis, and increase gastric pH. It was shown in dogs that gastric secretions averaged above 2.5 pH when glycopyrrolate is used, whereas gastric secretions were 3.5 from dogs after atropine. After mechanical administration of these gastric secretions to the airway, patients continued to breath, but there was a change in minute respiratory volume in all groups. Initially, arterial blood pressure drops with an increase in $PaCO_2$. However, PaO_2 values were relatively stable. There was an increase in respiratory rate after aspiration of gastric secretion; this was more pronounced in the atropine group with the lower pH. Glycopyrrolate had a longer lasting effect and provided more smooth muscle relaxation and less adverse cardiovascular effect when compared to atropine (33).

Glycopyrrolate is compatable with many other medications. Tests have been run, as shown in Table 2.1, to determine the compatibility of glycopyrrolate in the same syringe with other agents commonly used in anesthesia. It is incompatable in the same syringe with the barbiturates, pentazocine, diazepam, and dramamine.

Atropine Sulfate and Glycopyrrolate Compared

Atropine sulfate is a less expensive product than glycopyrrolate; however, atropine has been associated with a variety of cardiac arrhythmias including sinus tachycardia and premature ventricular contractions. More frequently than glycopyrrolate, it has been accused of contributing to intestinal stasis or equine colic. In the dog, the respiratory pattern is similar for atropine or glycopyrrolate; blood pressure is similar for controls, dogs given atropine and ultrashort barbiturates, and dogs given glycopyrrolate and ultrashort barbiturates. When sodium thiamylal was given alone or with atropine, heart rates decreased markedly during the first 5 minutes after induction and then increased progressively in the atropine-treated dogs. The heart rate remained stable during early maintenance of anesthesia. Glycopyrrolate was not as completely effective in preventing sialorrhea and intestinal parastolysis at dosage levels of 0.005, 0.011, or 0.022 mg/kg i.m. Levels of 0.011 and 0.022 mg/kg did suppress sialorrhea and intestinal parastolysis. Dogs showed no salivation or bronchial secretions during anesthesia and recovery. None demonstrated cardiac arrhythmias or respiratory

Table 2.1
Compatibility of Glycopyrrolate and Other Drugs (0.2 mg/ml) When Mixed in a Syringe[a]

Drug Product	Concentration	Compatibility[b]
	per ml	
Acepromazine maleate	[c]	C
Chlorpromazine (Thorazine)	25 mg	C*
Codeine Phosphate, U.S.P.	30 mg	C
Diazepam (Valium)	5 mg	I
Dimenhydrinate (Dramamine)	50 mg	I
Diphenhydramine (Benadryl)	10 mg	C
	50 mg	C
Droperidol and fentanyl (Innovar)	2.5 and .05 mg	C
Hydromorphone (Dilaudid)	2 mg	C
Ketamine HCl (Ketaset)	[c]	C
Lidocaine HCl, U.S.P.	10 mg	C
	20 mg	C
Meperidine HCl (Demerol)	40 mg	C
Methohexital Na (Brevital)	10 mg	I
Morphine sulfate, U.S.P.	15 mg	C
Neostigmine (Prostigmin)	0.5 mg	C
Oxymorphone (Numorphan)	1.0 mg	C
	1.5 mg	C
Pentazocine (Talwin)	30 mg	I
Pentobarbital Na (Nembutal)	50 mg	I
Procaine HCl, U.S.P.	10 mg	C
	20 mg	C
Prochlorperazine (Compazine)	5 mg	C*
Promazine (Sparine)	50 mg	C
Promethazine (Phenergan)	25 mg	C
Pyridostigmine (Mestinon)	5 mg	C
Secobarbital Na (Seconal)	50 mg	I
Sodium bicarbonate, U.S.P.	75 mg	I
Sodium Thiamylal (Bio-tal)	[c]	I
Thiopental Na (Pentothal)	25 mg	I
Xylazine (Rompun)	[c]	C

[a] Evaluation performed by the A. H. Robins Pharmacy Research and Analytical Services Department.
[b] C, physically compatible; I, incompatible, unsuitable for administration; C*, physically compatible, but mixing these drug products with other agents in a syringe is not recommended. Note that physical compatibility does not assure absence of chemical degradation.
[c] Mixtures of glycopyrrolate injection with this drug product were prepared to contain the highest and lowest dosage levels of the drug based upon the average animal body weights that would normally be encountered in practice.

dysfunction. Blood pressures remained normal. Atropine was administered at 0.04 mg/kg (31).

In a study to compare glycopyrrolate and atropine as a preanesthetic in cats undergoing a variety of surgical and anesthetic procedures, glycopyrrolate was effective in control of bradycardia and sialorrhea in over 95% of cats, whereas atropine was successful in controlling sialorrhea in 92% and bradycardia in 88% of animals studied. Glycopyrrolate was shown to be an effective preanesthetic agent as a result. The concentration of glycopyrrolate administered was 0.011 mg/kg compared to 0.067 mg/kg of atropine sulfate (34). Glycopyrrolate and atropine have been administered as preanesthetics before anesthesia for Caesarean section in dogs and other species (35). Because glycopyrrolate and atropine have similar indications but glycopyrrolate is not as likely to cross the placental barrier or cause an excessive increase in heart rate, it is probably preferred over atropine during Caesarean section. Especially in Caesarean section in brachycephalic breeds of dogs, the increase in gastric pH created by glycopyrrolate versus atropine is of advantage to prevent aspiration of acidic gastric secretions and resulting respiratory difficulties.

The penetration of the blood-brain barrier by glycopyrrolate and atropine has been compared (36). Glycopyrrolate, a quaternary ammonia anticholinergic agent, appears in cerebral spinal fluid and serum after a single intravenous dose, as does atropine. Glycopyrrolate was administered at 0.1 mg/kg to dogs during barbiturate anesthesia; dogs treated with similar doses of atropine were compared. The cerebral spinal fluid levels of atropine averaged 10.3 ng/ml of spinal fluid, whereas glycopyrrolate levels were restricted to 0.9 ng/ml. There was a further comparison of the crossing of the placental barrier by atropine and glycopyrrolate (36). Atropine crosses the placental barrier, representing 30% of the corresponding maternal serum concentration. The fetal serum level was 13 ng/ml within 10 minutes after a single intravenous dose. The peak glycopyrrolate level obtained was 0.63 ng/ml of fetal serum as late as 4 hours after administration, with the peak reached in 4 hours. Anticholinergic effects of atropine and glycopyrrolate compared in placental and blood-brain barrier crossage indicate that glycopyrrolate is a selective peripheral anticholinergic agent and that it is more resistant than atropine to penetration across these barriers.

Clinical Usage of Anticholinergics

A wide range of dosage recommendations have been made for the use of atropine sulfate; the most frequent range from 0.02 to 0.1 mg/kg body weight. In the comparative studies completed by this author, an average dose of 0.044 mg/kg of atropine i.v. has been used as the standard for comparing glycopyrrolate at varying dosages. The glycopyrrolate equivalent dose determination made by the author is 0.011 mg/kg i.m. Intravenous doses studied in dogs, cats, and horses have been 50% of the i.m. dosage used. In contrast to years past, anticholinergics are not now routinely administered to each animal to receive anesthetics. Rather, a clinical preanesthetic evaluation is completed on the animal, and anticholinergics are administered selectively, according to the determined needs of the individual patient, the anticipated response to the anesthetic medication, and the tendency to develop bradycardia or excessive salivation. Atropine or glycopyrrolate are frequently used to avoid bradycardia with xylazine, heavy dosages of narcotics, or potent inhalant anesthetics, which have a tendency to reduce heart rate. They are used with ketamine anesthesia to reduce salivation. There is greater tendency to sinus tachycardia and ventricular arrhythmias with atropine than with glycopyrrolate; as a result, the popularity of glycopyrrolate has increased. Anticholinergics are still used fairly often in dogs and cats. Anticholinergics are seldom used and are not as effective in ruminants because of the very short duration of the atropine-like products in the ruminant.

The use of anticholinergics in horses is controversial at best. Although glycopyrrolate has been used in horses with chronic obstructive pulmonary disease as a long-lasting bronchodilator (37), controversy over the use of anticholinergics still exists (38). There is concern that the incidence of postoperative ileus and increased myocardial oxygen consumption are not justified by the intraoperative response to anticholinergic agents. Anticholinergics in the horse are beneficial if atrial ventricular conduction disturbances, bradycardia, or interference dissociation with heart rates less than 25 beats per minute are observed. This is especially true if concurrent hypotension is present. In horses which have received xylazine and ketamine inductions followed by halothane maintenance without the addition of anticholinergics, sudden severe bradycardia or cardiac arrest has been observed at 15 to 18 minutes after induction. The influence of ketamine on heart rate is no longer present. Resuscitative or other corrective efforts have been difficult or unsuccessful with the appearance of a heart block-like phenomenon. After xylazine and ketamine induction and halothane maintenance, the ocular cardiac reflex activity during ocular surgery has a greater tendency to produce severe bradycardia or cardiac arrest than with other anesthetic techniques or when anticholinergics have been administered as premedications.

Efforts to demonstrate the detrimental effects of atropine in producing postoperative ileus or colic have frequently involved dosages that exceed those normally used as preanesthetics. In addition, postoperative ileus or colic has been observed in anesthetized horses during and after surgery when there has been inadequate time for gastrointestinal emptying after food consumption without the presence of anticholinergics. Nevertheless, the utilization of anticholinergics in the horse should be selectively evaluated and given by indication, in contrast to routine administration. Because it is more likely that the horse will not receive anticholinergics to protect against bradycardia, control of anesthetic concentration and selection of drugs with potential to depress the heart must be considered more critically in the horse than in other species. This is especially true if small incremental doses of xylazine during halothane anesthesia are used to reduce excitement during anesthesia recovery or to provide partial analgesia during the surgical procedure.

Anticholinergic Contraindications

Use of anticholinergics as premedication or in conjunction with anesthesia is contraindicated in situations in which tachycardia exists prior to administration. One must proceed with caution in any situation where ventricular arrhythmias such as premature ventricular contractions or other high sensitivity ventricular arrhythmias exist. These precautions are justified because further reduction in vagal tone or heart rate and sensitivity by the anticholinergic agent may allow the heart rate to increase and thereby produce further reduction in diastolic time. Major ventricular arrhythmias may then occur. Such products as propranolol, isoproterenol, and atropine significantly reduce the percentage of time in diastole (39, 40). These factors can play a role in the development of myocardial ischemia. Myocardial ischemia may be diagnosed as cardiac dysrrthymia and may be enhanced by anticholinergic therapy, especially with atropine (41). Great caution should be exercised in the utilization of atropine in patients in which myocardial ischemia is known to exist. If an anticholinergic is needed in patients with myocardial excitability, glycopyrrolate is the drug of choice because it is not as likely to produce major increases in heart rate and has a more gradual onset. Our experiences agree with those recorded on the incidence of cardiac arrhythmias caused by atropine (42).

Postoperative Utilization of Anticholinergics

Anticholinergics may be necessary in the postoperative period to avoid excessive salivation or in instances, in which narcotics are used for postoperative control of pain, especially if those narcotics are administered before complete recovery from potent inhalant anesthetics. At the end of the surgical procedure, those receiving balanced anesthesia or inhalant anesthetics with concurrent utilization of paralytic agents such as pancuronium, gallamine, or other reversible muscle blockades for which neostigmine is being considered should receive an anticholinergic prior to the administration of the reversal agent. The administration of neostigmine without atropine or glycopyrrolate will frequently result in severe bradycardia. The administration of the anticholinergic of choice prevents this problem. The selective utilization of anticholinergics in dogs and cats will be common, and selective use of anticholinergics in the horse can add to the safety of the anesthetic procedures, but the ruminant is not likely to respond effectively to anticholinergic therapy.

References

1. Weiner N: Atropine, scopolamine, and related antimuscarinic drugs. In Gilman AG, Goodman LS, and Gilman A (ed): *The Pharmacological Basis of Therapeutics.* New York, Macmillan Publishing Co., 1980, ed 6, pp 120–137.
2. Beleslin DB, Krsti'c SK, Tomi'c-Beleslin N: Nicotine-induced salivation in cats: effects of various drugs. *Brain Res Bull* 12(5):585–587, 1984.
3. Hsu WH, Lu ZX, Hembrough FB: Effect of xylazine on heart rate and arterial blood pressure in conscious dogs, as influenced by atropine, 4-aminopyridine, doxapram and yohimbine. *JAVMA* 186(2):153–156, 1985.
4. Hsu WH: Effects of atropine or xylazine-pentobarbitol anesthesia in dogs: preliminary study. *Am J Vet Res* 46(4):856–858, 1985.
5. Kantilip JP, Alatienne M, Gueroguieu G, Duchene-Marullaz P: Chronotropic and dromotropic effects of atropine and hyoscine methobromide in unanesthesized dogs. *Br J Anaesth* 57(2):214–219, 1985.
6. Rigel DF, Lipson D, Katona PG: Excess tachycardia: Heart rate after antimuscarinic agents in conscious dogs. *Am J Physiol* 246(2):H168–173, 1984.
7. Samonina GE, Hakumäki MO: The role of the sympathetic nervous system in atropine-induced tachycardia in conscious cats. *Scand J Clin Lab Invest* 43(5):389–392, 1983.
8. Takabashi N, Zipes DP: Vagal modulation of adrenergic effects on canine sinus and atrioventricular nodes. *Am J Physiol* 244(6):H775–781, 1983.
9. Liard JF: Atropine potentiates the pressor effect of arginine-vasopressin in conscious dogs. *J Cardiovasc Pharmacol* 6(5):867–871, 1984.
10. Parer JT: The effect of atropine on heart rate and oxygen consumption of the hypoxic fetus. *Am J Obstet Gynecol* 148(8):1118–1122, 1984.
11. Brubakk AM, Bratlid D, Oh W, Yao AC, Stonestreet BS: Atropine prevents increases in brain-blood flow during hypertension in newborn piglets. *Pediatr Res* 18(11):1121–1126, 1984.
12. Smith EL 3rd, Redburn DA, Harwerth RS, Maquire GW: Permanent alterations in muscarinic receptors and pupil size produced by chronic atropinization in kittens. *Invest Ophthalmol Vis Sci* 25(2):239–243, 1984.
13. Crewther DP, Crewther SG, Cleland BG: Is the retina sensitive to the effects of prolonged blur? *Exp Brain Res* 58(3):427–434, 1985.
14. Arnett BD, Brightman AH 2nd, Musselmen EE: Effect of atropine sulfate on tear production in the cat when used with ketamine hydrochloride and acetylpromazine maleate. *JAVMA* 185(2):214–215, 1984.
15. Kannan MS, Jager LP, Daniel EE, Garfield RE: Effects of 4-aminopyridine and tetraethylammonium chloride on the electrical activity and cable properties of canine tracheal smooth muscle. *J Pharmacol Exp Ther* 227(3):706–715, 1983.
16. Rybicki KJ, Kaufman MP: Atropine prevents the reflex tracheal relaxation arising from the stimulation of intestinal and skeletal muscle afferents in dogs. *Brain Res* 270(1):159–161, 1983.
17. Skoogh BE, Nadel JA, Fabbie lM, Sheppard D, Hotzman MJ: Antihistaminic versus anticholinergic effects of atropine on canine trachealis muscle. *Am Rev Respir Dis* 128(4):603–606, 1983.
18. Yanaura S, Mizuno H, Goto K, Kanoi J, Kosokawa T, Ohtani K, Misawa M: Effects of 8-(2-fluorethyl)-3 alpha-hydroxyl-1 alpha H, 5 alpha H-tropanium bromide benzilate (Ba598Br) on allergy and drug induced asthmas. *Jpn J Pharmacol* 33(5):971–982, 1983.
19. Simonsson BG, Laitenen LA: Does atropine block antigen-induced contraction in canine bronchial rings? A preliminary report. *Eur J Respir Dis* 64(8):588–590, 1983.
20. Whiteside ME, Lairredo I, Chapman GA, Ratzan KR, Abraham WM, Wanner A: Effect of atropine on tracheal mucociliary clearance and bacterial counts. *Bull Eur Physiopathol Respir* 20(4):347–351, 1984.
21. Delbio D, Lisander B, Andersson SA: Atropine-sensitive gastric smooth muscle excitation by mucosal nociceptive stimulation—the involvement of an axon reflex? *Acta Physiol Scand* 122(4):621–627, 1984.
22. Browning JG, Heathcote BV: A comparison of pirenzepine and cimatidine inhibition of centrally-mediated gastric acid and pepsin secretion in the gastric fistula cat. *Arch Int Pharmacodyn Ther* 263(2):288–296, 1983.
23. Fox DA, Bauer R, Bass P: Use of gut cyclic motor activity to evaluate a stimulant (narcotic) and inhibitor (anticholinergic) of gastrointestinal-tract activity in the unanesthetized dog. *J Pharmacol Methods* 13(2):147–155, 1985.
24. Mailman D: Effects of atropine and guanethidine on canine intestinal absorption and blood flow. *Life Sci* 34(14):1309–1315, 1984.
25. Davies JV, Gerring EL: Effect of spasmolytic analgesia drugs on the motility patterns of the equine small intestine. *Res Vet Sci* 34(3):334–339, 1983.
26. Singer MV: Latency of pancreatic fluid secretory response to intestinal stimulants in the dog. *J Physiol (Lond)* 339:75–85, 1983.
27. Singer MV, Niebel W, Uhde KH, Hoffmeister D, Goebell H: Dose-response effects of atropine on pancreatic response to secretion before and after truncal vaogtomy. *Am J Physiol* 248:G532–538, 1985.
28. Larsson B, Anderson KE, Mattiasson A: Influence of antimuscarinics on alpha-adrenoceptors in the female rabbit urethra. *Acta Physiol Scand* 120(4):537–542, 1984.
29. Craggs MD, Stephenson JD: Bladder electromyograms and function in monkeys after atropine. *Br J Urol* 57(3):341–345, 1985.
30. Franko BV, Alphin RS, Ward JW, Lunsford CD: Pharmacodynamic evaluation of glycopyrrolate in animals. *Ann NY Acad Sciences* 99(1):131–149, 1962.
31. Short CE, Miller RL: Comparative evaluation of the anticholinergic agent glycopyrrolate as a preanesthetic agent. *Vet Med/Sm An Clin* 1269–1272, 1978.
32. Short CE, Martin R, Tracy CH: Effective dosage levels of glycopyrrolate injectable in cats. *Vet Med/Sm An Clin* 1377–1380, 1983.
33. Short CE, Paddleford RR, Cloyd GD: Glycopyrrolate for prevention of pulmonary complications during anesthesia. *Mod Vet Practice* 3:194–196, 1974.
34. Short CE, Martin R, Henry CW Jr: Clinical comparison of glyco-

pyrrolate and atropine as preanesthetic agents in cats. *Vet Med/ Sm An Clin* 10:1447;–1560, 1983.

35. McIntyre TAJ: Anesthetic management of the canine cesarean section. *The Animal Health Technician* 3(1):15–23, 1982.
36. Proakis AG, Harris GB: Comparative penetration of glycopyrrolate and atropine across the blood-brain and placental barriers in anesthetized dogs. *Anesthesiology* 48(5):339–344, 1978.
37. Goetz TE: Successful management of equine chronic obstructive pulmonary disease. *Vet Med* 8:1073–1077, 1984.
38. Hubbell JAE, Robertson JT, Muir WW, Gobel AA: Perianesthetic considerations in the horse. *Comp Cont Educ Pract Vet* 6(7):401–413, 1984.
39. Conrad KA: Effects of atropine on diastolic time. *Circulation* 63(2):371–377, 1981.
40. Hirshman CA, Donnes H: A possible undesirable interaction of propranolol and atropine. *Anesthesiology* 53:521, 1980.
41. Mirakhur RK: Reversal of neuromuscular blockade: dose determination studies with atropine and glycopyrrolate given before or in a mixture with neostigmine. *Anesth Analg* 60(8):557–562, 1981.
42. Muir WW III: Effects of atropine on cardiac rates and rhythms in the dog. *JAVMA* 172:917–921, 1978.

CHAPTER 3

Tranquilizers and Sedatives

ROBIN D. GLEED, B.V.Sc., M.R.C.V.S., D.V.A., D.A.C.V.A.

Tranquilizers and sedatives are widely used in veterinary practice. The appropriate use of these drugs, either alone or in conjunction with others, has helped improve veterinary practice and the life of the practicing veterinarian.

These drugs are principally used to depress the central nervous system (CNS) for chemical restraint or preanesthetic medication. Many animals show signs of fear and anxiety when they are handled in an unfamiliar way or have their environment changed by transportation or hospitalization. This fear and anxiety cannot always be relieved by physical and vocal efforts by veterinarians or their assistants. The use of tranquilizers and sedatives enables the veterinarian to minimize the stress of such necessary interference. From a humane point of view, and especially in the light of the increasing concern of society for animal rights, it is beneficial for the veterinary profession to be concerned about minimizing such stress.

Reduction of stress is also useful for more pragmatic reasons. Fear causes increased levels of circulating catecholamines, which may be counterproductive; for example, catecholamine-induced dysrhythmias may occur as a result of drug interactions with some anesthetics (1). The calming effect of these drugs also makes fractious animals more tractable, thus making handling less hazardous. With the exception of the thiazine derivatives (xylazine and detomidine), these compounds have no significant analgesic activity, so painful interference must be avoided unless a narcotic analgesic or local anesthetic is used in addition. Increased stimulation (for example, loud noises) will usually reverse the calming effect of these drugs at clinical dose levels; care should be taken to provide a quiet environment after administration in order to see the maximum effect of any of these drugs. If using the tranquilizers and sedatives as preanesthetic agents, sufficient time should pass for maximum effect to be produced before anesthesia is induced.

Intravenous administration generally produces peak effects in the shortest time and with the smallest dose. The tranquilizers and sedatives also have additive or synergistic effects with many other compounds acting on the CNS. These permit reduction in the required dose of barbiturate induction agents, general anesthetics, and narcotic analgesics, for example. This is beneficial in that the possibility of adverse side effects from large doses is reduced. It is also possible that the total cost of a procedure may be reduced by decreasing the amount of more expensive compounds used (2).

Recovery from general anesthesia can be made quieter by the use of tranquilizers and sedatives. Usually, they are given as part of a preanesthetic regimen, but they may also be selectively administered after anesthesia. All of the tranquilizers and sedatives have the general characteristics mentioned above; however, each drug and group of drugs has its own diverse pharmacological properties and contraindications. Knowledge of these characteristics aids the rational choice of an agent for specific circumstances. Phenothiazines, for example, have antidysrhythmic properties (3) and thus might be indicated when ectopic myocardial activity is anticipated; however, they may also cause hypotension (4, 5) and thus should be avoided in hypovolemic patients.

The distinction between tranquilizers and sedatives is a question of semantics and is of little value except that increased doses of tranquilizers may tend to produce side effects but not loss of consciousness, whereas increased doses of sedatives produces more profound CNS depression that resembles anesthesia.

The tranquilizers used in veterinary practice include the phenothiazine derivatives, the butyrophenones, and the rauwolfia alkaloids. Other words used synonomously with tranquilizer and "neuroleptic" and "ataractic." An ataractic is a compound that produces a state of stoical indifference. This is a good description of the signs produced by these drugs under ideal circumstances. The sedatives used include the barbiturates, benzodiazapines, chloral derivatives, and thiazine derivatives. Because an increase in dosage of sedatives produces a state similar to sleep, these drugs are also called "hypnotics." As of March 1986, the number of animal tranquilizers and sedatives approved by the United States Food and Drug Administration (FDA) is fairly limited. Table 3.1 gives a list of these approved drugs. From this list, it is evident that use of unapproved drugs is extensive in veterinary practice in the United States of America.

Phenothiazines

NERVOUS SYSTEM ACTIONS

The phenothiazines are among the most widely used veterinary drugs. They are utilized extensively to make animals more tractable, as preanesthetics, and also as antiemetics. Acepromazine is probably the most familiar drug in this group of compounds.

Table 3.2 give a list of some commonly used tranquilizers and doses that have been shown to be satisfactory. It should be noted that doses of acepromazine currently given in manufacturer's data sheets are often considered excessive for preanesthetic medication.

Phenothiazines act on the CNS by depressing the brain stem and connections to the cerebral cortex (6). Most reports describe the actions of acepromazine maleate, chlorpromazine hydrochloride, or promazine hydrochloride. All of the phenothiazines in clinical use, however, seem to act qualitatively in a very similar manner, i.e., they produce general calming and reduction in motor activity.

The stereoscopic structure of phenothiazines is similar to that of the catecholamine neurotransmitter dopamine. It is likely that at least some of the activity of phenothiazines is associated with antagonism of dopamine excitatory receptors (6). The emetic action of narcotic analgesics in some species (e.g., dogs) may be due to stimulation of these dopamine excitatory receptors, and antagonism of this emetic action is one reason why phenothiazines have been included with narcotic analgesics in neuroleptanalgesic combinations. The piperazine derivatives of phenothiazine (e.g., prochlorperazine and perphenazine) are especially potent antiemetics.

Phenothiazines, especially in high doses, may cause extrapyramidal signs, such as rigidity, tremor, and catalepsy. The antiemetic piperazine phenothia-

Table 3.1
Tranquilizers and Sedatives Approved by the United States Food and Drug Administration for Use in Animals (March 1986), with Approved Routes of Administration and Subject Species

Generic Name of Drug by Parent Compound	Species	Route of Administration
Phenothiazines		
Acepromazine (acetylpromazine)	Dog, cat, and horse	i.v., i.m., s.c., p.o.
Chlorpromazine	Dog and cat	i.v.
Ethylisobutrazine	Dog	i.v., i.m., p.o.
Piperacetazine	Dog and cat	i.v., i.m., s.c., p.o.
Prochlorperazine[a]	Dog and cat	s.c., p.o.
Promazine	Dog, cat, and horse	i.v., i.m., p.o.
Propiopromazine	Dog and cat	i.v., i.m., p.o.
Triflupromazine maleate	Dog	p.o.
Triflupromazine HCl	Dog, cat, and horse	i.v., p.o.
Butyrophenones		
Azaperone	Pig	i.m.
Droperidol (with fentanyl)[b]	Dog	i.v., i.m.
Lenperone	Dog and cat	i.v., i.m., p.o.[c]
Benzodiazepines		
Zolazepam (with tiletamine)	Dog and cat	i.m.
Thiazines		
Xylazine	Dog, cat, and horse	i.v., i.m., s.c.
Others		
Chloral hydrate[d]	Horse and cattle	i.v.
Pentobarbital sodium[e]	Dog, cat, and horse	i.v., i.p.

[a] In combination with isopropamide.
[b] Innovar Vet.
[c] Dogs only.
[d] In combination with magnesium sulfate and pentobarbital (Chloropent, Fort Doge Laboratories).
[e] Used as general anesthetic or sedative (Somnopentyl Injection, Pitman-Moore, and Pentobarbital Injection, Carter-Glogau).

Table 3.2
Dosage and Route of Administration for Tranquilizers

Drug	Animal	Dosage (mg/kg)		
		i.v.	i.m.	p.o.
Acepromazine	Dogs	0.03–0.05	0.03–0.05	1.0–3.0
	Cats	0.03–0.05	0.03–0.1	1.0–3.0
	Horses	0.02–0.05	0.04–0.09	
	Pigs		0.03–0.4	
	Cattle		0.1	
Chlorpromazine	Dogs	0.55–4.4	1.1–6.6	0.55–8.8
	Cats	0.55–4.4	2.2–6.6	2.2–8.8
	Horses		1.1–2.2	
	Pigs		1–2	
	Cattle	0.2–1.1	0.2–2.2	
	Goats/Sheep	0.55–4.4	2.2–6.6	
Promazine	Horses	0.44–1.1	0.44–1.1	1–2
	Pigs	0.44–2.0	0.44–4.0	
	Cattle	0.44–1.1	0.44–1.1	
	Goats/Sheep	0.44–1.1	0.44–1.1	
Azaprone	Pigs		0.4–8.0	
Droperidol	Dogs	0.7–1.7	2.2–2.9	
	Pigs		0.1–0.4	
Lenperone	Dogs	0.22–0.88	0.44–1.8	0.55–2.2
	Cats	0.22–0.88	0.22–0.88	
	Pigs		0.22–0.88	

zines seem more prone to this side effect (6). Increasing dosage of phenothiazines does not produce a proportional increase in tranquilization but may produce extrapyramidal signs. Horses have become excited after chlorpromazine administration; this may be extrapyramidal in origin, but it could also be a response to hypotension or inadvertent carotid injection, among other things (4).

Chlorpromazine augments epileptiform activity on the electroencephalogram (7, 8). For this reason, Holliday says that phenothiazines should not be used in animals that have had seizures or that may convulse for any reason (9). Phenothiazine premedication should thus be avoided in animals undergoing myelography because intrathecal injection of radiographic contrast agents is often associated with seizures (10).

Any analgesic activity that the phenothiazines may have is very mild and cannot be relied upon except as an adjunct to specific analgesic therapy. However, one member of this group, Methotrimeprazine, may have some analgesic action in its own right (11).

Thermoregulation is depressed by these drugs, probably due to depletion of catecholamines in the region of the hypothalamic thermoregulatory center (6). Premedication with phenothiazines may thus render animals under anesthesia more susceptible to changes in environmental temperature, and this may help account for the hypothermia reported in small animals (12).

CARDIOVASCULAR EFFECTS

The most important and obvious effect of phenothiazines on the cardiovascular system is hypotension (4, 5). This effect is dose dependent and can be seen with clinically useful doses. Relative and absolute overdosage of these chemicals is associated with hypotension. This hypotension is usually ascribed to alpha-adrenergic blockade causing vasodilation and decreased systemic vascular resistance. Phenothiazines may also cause hypotension by depressing those areas of the hypothalamus responsible for vascular tone and by direct action on vascular smooth muscle (13).

Hypotension from phenothiazines may be severe enough to cause collapse of the animal. Muir has observed this adverse response in fearful or hypovolemic patients (14). A reflex tachycardia with weak pulse pressure is usually noted in such animals. The hypotension may be ascribed to phenothiazine alpha blockade preventing the vasopressor effect of endogenous catecholamines. The beta-2 stimulating properties of these endogenous catecholamines is simultaneously unmasked, causing vasodilation in vessels supplying skeletal muscles and a further decrease in systemic vascular resistance and blood pressure. This leads to orthostatic hypotension. Therapy for animals that collapse after phenothiazine administration should include fluid administration for blood volume replacement and specific alpha sympathomimetics (e.g., methoaxamine and phenylephrine). Epinephrine is obviously contraindicated because it has both alpha- and beta-agonistic activity, and the latter may led to further hypotension.

Cardiac output and heart rate are usually not changed significantly by clinically useful doses of promazine or acepromazine in the horse. This is probably the case with other phenothiazines in other species. The hypotension observed is probably thus associated with decreased systemic vascular resistance and redistribution of perfusion. Peripheral vasodilation caused by phenothiazines may permit increased heat loss through the skin and potentiate the hypothermia mediated through central thermoregulatory depression.

Tranquilization of animals with phenothiazines before epidural or spinal anesthesia is contraindicated (6). The normal physiological response to segmental anesthesia is compensatory vasoconstriction in unanesthetized segments and increased cardiac output. This response is obtunded by phenothiazine tranquilizers, and their use may thus lead to severe hypotension.

The use of phenothiazines to premedicate an animal with known or even suspected hypovolemia is potentially hazardous because the animal's ability to respond to this challenge is reduced. The use of intravenous fluids in cases undergoing general anesthesia is widely advocated, and this is helpful in those receiving a phenothiazine (14).

Acepromazine reduces the sensitivity of canine myocardium to circulating catecholamines, and chloropromazine also has antiarrhythmic activity (3, 6). This antidysrhythmic action of phenothiazines has been attributed to sympathetic blockade, local anesthetic-like action, and quinidine-like action (14). The use of preanesthetic phenothiazines is rational when drugs known to sensitize the myocardium (e.g., halothane) or cause dysrhythmias (e.g., epinephrine) are to be used.

RESPIRATORY EFFECTS

The respiratory effects of phenothiazines are minimal at clinically used doses. A decrease in respiratory rate is seen, but this is often compensated for by an increase in tidal volume (15). Blood gas tensions rarely change much, and there is little evidence of resetting of the carbon dioxide threshold for respiratory stimulation.

OTHER EFFECTS

One of the most dramatic and unpleasant adverse reactions to phenothiazines is penile prolapse in the horse. The addition of the potent narcotic agonist etorphine (M99) to a phenothiazine may increase the possibility of this condition being permanent (16). The mechanism behind permanent penile prolapse after phenothiazines is poorly understood, but it may involve a central sympatholytic action causing paralysis of the retractor penis muscle. Permanent penile prolapse may render a horse impotent; consequently phenothiazines should be avoided in breeding stallions.

Hyperglycemia has been observed after these drugs. It is attributed both to release of epinephrine from the adrenal medulla causing utilization of glycogen (6) and direct inhibition of insulin (17). Horses given promazine and acepromazine show a decrease in packed cell volume (PCV) and total protein (18). These effects are thought to be related to increased storage of red cells in the spleen and decreased hydrostatic pressure in the arterioles (hypotension), the latter allowing increased access of interstitial fluid to the circulation and thus producing hemodilution. Phenothiazines have been shown to cause thrombocytopenia and platelet dysfunction (19); until the significance of this in a veterinary clinical situation is clarified, phenothiazines should be avoided in animals known to have a platelet disorder.

Urine production increases after low doses of phenothiazines have been given to healthy animals (20). This may be secondary to a decrease in antidiuretic hormone (ADH) or a result of redistribution of perfusion to the kidney cortex. Animals which have severe pre-existing or drug-induced hypotension will, however, have lower urine production due to decreased glomerular filtration.

Phenothiazines have variable H_1 antihistaminic activity. Promethazine hydrochloride is one of the more potent antihistaminic phenothiazines (21). Phenothiazines must be avoided in animals undergoing intradermal testing for allergy because the response may be masked. Their antihistaminic property may be useful, however, in patients undergoing mast cell tumor removal, where manipulation of the tumor may cause degranulation of mast cells and consequent histamine release.

As with most drugs effecting the CNS, the phenothiazine tranquilizers cross the placenta to the fetus. Their significance to the fetus is now known; however, it should be anticipated that they will contribute to neonatal depression if they are used to premedicate the mother before Caesarean section.

Decreased stomach and intestinal motility has been observed in dogs after phenothiazine administration (22). This may be explained by the slight anticholinergic activity that these drugs possess as well as direct action on smooth muscle. Premedication of ruminants with phenothiazines may be inadvisable because cardiac sphincter relaxation could lead to increased regurgitation of rumen contents after recumbency (23).

At high doses, prophylactic acepromazine prevented the occurrence of halothane-induced malignant hyperthermia in susceptible pigs. The percentage of pigs so protected was dose-related at 1.1 mg/kg and 1.65 mg/kg of acepromazine such that 40% and 73% of the pigs, respectively, did not develop hyperthermia (24). Phenothiazine premedication may thus be beneficial if a patient is thought to be susceptible to malignant hyperthermia.

An obvious sign of the onset of sedation in dogs is protrusion of the nictitating membrane. The phenothiazines are mostly metabolized in the liver; consequently, their action may be prolonged in patients with functional liver disease.

Butyrophenones

The butyrophenones have many properties in common with the phenothiazines. Most importantly, both groups have general sympatholytic activity that can account for many of their effects. The butyrophenones of major clinical importance are azaperone, droperidol, fluanisone, and lenperone. The butyrophenones are considered safe drugs with higher therapeutic ratios than the phenothiazines. The therapeutic ratio of the phenothiazine chlorpromazine is 850, whereas that of droperidol is 68,000. However, the butyrophenones do seem to be more likely to produce extrapyramidal signs of rigidity, tremor, and catalepsy in clinical usage; for this reason, they are less popular than the phenothiazines. These signs may not appear until several hours after the drug has been administered (25).

Azaperone is licensed in the United States for use in swine. It is used to reduce fighting when mixing batches of feeder and weanling pigs. It is also popular as a premedication before general or local anesthesia in this species.

Droperidol is not licensed for sole use in animals, but is combined with fentanyl in the proprietary neuroleptanalgesic combination Innovar-Vet (20 mg/ml of droperidol and 0.4 mg/ml of fentanyl) which is used in dogs. Fluanisone has been used in combination with fentanyl (10 mg/ml and 0.345 mg/ml, respectively) in the proprietary neuroleptanalgesic Hypnorm. Lenperone is licensed in the United State for use in dogs and cats and has been used in swine (26).

ACTIONS ON THE NERVOUS SYSTEM

Like the phenothiazines, the butyrophenones produce tranquilization in the form of indifference to their surroundings and decreased motor activity. Increasing dosage of the butyrophenones produces rigidity, tremor, and catalepsy, the so-called extrapyramidal signs. This adverse reaction may occur even at recommended doses. In humans, the butyrophenones may cause unpleasant reactions including hallucinations, dysphorea, frustration, and aggression that only become apparent after recovery from the drug. Because of this, Hall and Clarke question whether these drugs should be used alone in animals (27). Certainly, occasional animals will become unexpectedly excited or even aggressive after butyrophenone administration either alone or in combination. These personality changes fortunately are usually temporary and disappear over several days. Sometimes these temperament changes are accompanied by signs of tremor, nystagmus, and rigidity. However, low doses of droperidol (butyrophenone) and fentanyl citrate combination (0.005 ml/kg i.v.) given once daily to dogs produced adequate tranquilization for electroencephalography (EEG) (28). The EEG showed a consistent response to this drug combination that did not change over a 5-day period, nor was there any evidence of behavioral change in these dogs. The pathogenesis and incidence of personality changes after butyrophenone administration is not known in animals.

The probable mechanism of action of these drugs is via blockade of catacholamine neurotransmitters in the CNS (6). Butyrophenones are very potent inhibitors of the emesis produced by narcotic analgesic stimulation of the chemoreceptor trigger zone (CTZ). They have consequently been used in neuroleptanalgesic combinations consisting of butyrophenone and a narcotic analgesic, where the former antagonizes the emetic action of the latter.

The butyrophenones decrease the dosage of agents necessary for induction of anesthesia and potentiate the action of anesthetics and narcotic analgesics. Like phenothiazines, they probably have negligible analgesic activity of their own. Because they apparently stimulate extrapyramidal pathways at least as much as the phenothiazines/derivatives, it is prudent to avoid their use in patients with a history of seizures or who may have seizure activity as a result of interferences being performed, such as (myelography).

CARDIOVASCULAR EFFECTS

Butyrophenones cause hypotension. The degree of hypotension is probably comparable to that caused by the phenothiazines. However, the genesis of this hypotension may be slightly different in the two groups of drugs. In one study in anesthetized dogs, 0.4 mg/kg of either acepromazine or lenperone was required to produce a similar significant drop in blood pressure (29). This was easily reversed with phenylephrine, an alpha-sympathetic agonist in those dogs receiving lenperone. However, in the dogs receiving acepromazine, a much higher dose of phenylephrine was required to reverse the hypotension. This led Muir and Hubble to conclude that hypotension caused by lenperone is mediated less through alpha blockade than hypotension caused by acepromazine, and phenylephrine more likely reverses such hypotension when it occurs subsequent to butyrophenone administration (29). This may also indicate that lenperone and possibly the other butyrophenones are preferable to phenothiazines in stressed patients (see the section on cardiovascular effects of phenothiazines). Decreases in cardiac output and heart rate have been reported in pigs given large doses (2.5 mg/kg i.m.) of azaperone (30). In general, butyrophenones and phenothiazines depress cardiac output to a comparably small extent. The butyrophenones also provide some protection against epinephrine-induced ventricular arrhythmias.

RESPIRATORY EFFECTS

Clinically useful doses of azaperone (1.1 to 3.5 mg/kg i.m.) may cause slightly increased respiratory rates and decreased $PaCO_2$ in pigs (31), whereas large doses of droperidol (4 mg/kg i.v.) caused slowing of respiration (6). Small changes in respiratory parameters may be anticipated with currently recommended doses of butyrophenones on their own. Droperidol is said to antagonize the respiratory depressant effects of narcotic analgesic compounds (27). This is, at best, incomplete in the case of the proprietary droperidol and fentanyl combination (Innovar-Vet), which causes decreased minute volume leading to respiratory acidosis in dogs (32).

Other Effects

Azaperone given to ponies did not produce changes in plasma protein concentration, but lowered packed cell volume and hemoglobin concentration for 4 hours after administration (6). Azaperone does produce ataraxis in horses, but there may be excitement, especially after intravenous injection (33). This may be related to panic from muscle weakness, hypotension, or central stimulation. Azaperone may also produce sweating in horses, making it unsuitable for sedation for clipping horses (34). Excitement in horses is always dangerous, and the risk associated with azaperone is so great that alternative agents are invariably more suitable. Droperidol (0.2 mg/kg i.m.) given prophylactically has been shown to delay the onset of halothane-induced malignant hyperthermia in susceptible pigs (24). Azaperone (2.5 mg/kg i.m.) has been used in Europe extensively to premedicate pigs before metomidate (Hypnodil), an imidazole hypnotic induction agent (2.5 mg/kg i.v.) (35). This has proved satisfactory for surgical procedures such as Caesarean section when combined with regional anesthesia.

Rauwolfia Alkaloids

Reserpine and metoserpate hydrochloride are the two rauwolfia alkaloids of importance in veterinary medicine. Neither is commonly used. Metoserpate is sometimes used in young chickens as a water additive (150 ppm) to facilitate flock replacement (6). The use of reserpine has all but disappeared; it has been replaced by other tranquilizers, sedatives, and neuroleptanalgesic combinations. However, in some horse circles reserpine is still used to quiet excitable horses, and occasional instances of overdosage are seen in practice. Reserpine administration, especially if undetected, may cause dangerous drug interactions (for example, with other sedatives, tranquilizers, and anesthetic agents). The difference between a safe and toxic dosage of reserpine is rather small. For these reasons, it is prudent to be cognizant of the properties of reserpine.

GENERAL EFFECTS OF RESERPINE

Reserpine causes tranquilization by depleting levels of 5-OH tryptamine, dopamine, and other catecholamines in certain parts of the brain (36). After a single dose of reserpine in a rabbit, serotonin levels were substantially depressed for nearly 7 days (37). The action of reserpine is prolonged both upon the CNS and the rest of the body. reserpine causes prolonged hypotension that may be associated with vasodilation and bradycardia. General anesthesia administered to horses under the influence of reserpine might be hazardous because of this cardiovascular impairment. Signs of toxicity and overdosage in horses include hypotension and violent colic.

Benzodiazepines

Diazepam is the most commonly used benzodiazepine in veterinary practice, but it is not approved by the FDA for animal usage. It is used primarily to treat seizures or is given prophylactically to prevent the anticipated seizure activity of other drugs such as ketamine hydrochloride. Other benzodiazepines include zolazepam and midazolam. Zolazepam is licensed by the FDA for use with tiletamine (a dissociative anesthetic agent) in the proprietary combination Telazol. Midazolam has been compared favorably with other agents for induction of anesthesia (38), and its further evaluation in clinical situations is warranted.

ACTIONS ON THE NERVOUS SYSTEM

Nearly all of the actions attributable to the benzodiazepines can be traced to their CNS-depressing properties. Benzodiazepine receptor sites have been found within the CNS. As yet, no definitive endogenous agonists of these receptors have been isolated, although some compounds, such as purines, have slight activity at these sites. It is hypothesized that benzodiazepine protagonism of these receptors potentiates the action of GABA (gamma aminobutyric acid), which is generally an inhibitory neurotransmitter. The safety of these drugs in relatively large doses may thus be explained because the extent of depression they cause is ultimately dependent upon the release of an endogenous neural inhibitor, GABA (39). The benzodiazepines and especially diazepam have found little clinical support as sole agents for sedation or chemical restraint. Administration to normal dogs and cats is often associated with a dramatic increase in excitability, which is an unpleasant surprise if the animal has been given the drug for premedication or restraint. This unusual response to a sedative is explained by the benzodiazepines' known ability to reveal behavior patterns that have previously been suppressed by punishment in animals. Other sedatives and tranquilizers either do not release such unsuppressed behavior or do so only at doses that may produce ataxia.

The use of diazepam (5 to 40 mg i.v. total dose) to treat dogs in status epilepticus is described (40, 41). Tolerance to the long-term use of diazepam for treatment of epilepsy has also been described. Failure of diazepam to control epileptic seizure activity may occur after myelography; in such cases, it should be supplemented with a barbiturate, such as pentobarbital or phenobarbital. Diazepam is an effective appetite stimulant. It has been used intramuscularly and orally at doses ranging from 0.05 mg/kg to 0.4 mg/kg to treat anorexic cats (42).

The benzodiazepines are important as adjuncts to other agents used in anesthetic practice. There is mutual potentiation of the effects of barbiturates, the anticipated induction doses of which may be reduced after diazepam premedication. This effect is also likely even if increased excitement occurs after the benzodiazepine alone. The CNS actions of narcotic analgesics may also be potentiated. The dissociative anesthetic agents, such as ketamine and tiletamine, produce very poor muscle relaxation when used alone. If they are either preceded or accompanied by a suitable dose of benzodiazepine, then much more satisfactory muscle relaxation may be produced. Telazol is approved for use in the dog or cat and is a proprietary combination of tiletamine and zolazepam. Diazepam (0.36 mg/kg) and ketamine (3.6 mg/kg) given together intravenously after a parasympatholytic premedication produces chemical restraint for short procedures in dogs. It should be remembered, however, that neither agent is approved by the FDA for use in dogs and that the extent of analgesia produced by this combination alone is debatable. A slightly different mixture (0.27 mg/kg diazepam and 5.5 mg/kg ketamine i.v. together) may be used in cats, but with similar constraints; ketamine is not FDA approved for use in cats by the intravenous route.

Muscle relaxation produced by benzodiazepines is probably mostly central in origin. although some of this action is also attributable to direct activity at the postsynaptic neuromuscular junction. Doses of more than 0.2 mg/kg in horses produce ataxia and muscle weakness; however, doses need to exceed 0.4 mg/kg in normal horses before significant cardiopulmonary changes occur (43). High doses of benzodiazepines may cause hypnosis with minimal cardiopulmonary depression. Midazolam has been administered to dogs and people to induce hypnosis for induction of general anesthesia. It is apparently rapidly active, but it is not as quick as thiopental and produces less cardiopulmonary depression (38). It is metabolized rapidly (44). The further evaluation of this drug in clinical situations is warranted on the grounds of this and other evidence.

CARDIOVASCULAR EFFECTS

The cardiovascular depressant effects of the benzodiazepines are not usually important at low doses. In horses, Muir et al. reported that more than 0.4 mg/kg i.v. was necessary to produce significant changes in cardiopulmonary dynamics, whereas only one-half of this dose was sufficient to produce recumbency (43). Diazepam decreases catecholamine release, and this accounts for some antidysrhythmic properties that have proven useful in treating certain kinds of myocardial hyperexcitability. Most injectable preparations of diazepam contain propylene glycol, a substance that unfortunately causes dysrhythmias and cardiovascular depression (45). New preparations of diazepam or other benzodiazepines that do not contain propylene glycol may be superior antidysrhythmic drugs. Coronary blood flow also increases after benzodiazepine administration. This may prove beneficial if diazepam, for instance, is used as an anesthetic adjunct for cases with myocardial ischemia (e.g., dogs with gastric distention volvulus). Although the cardiovascular depressant effects of diazepam have generally been considered to be less than many other tranquilizers or sedatives, evidence now suggests that when administered with a narcotic analgesic (fentanyl) the combination may have a supra-additive or synergistic effect, decreasing cardiac output, peripheral resistance, and arterial blood pressure (46–48).

OTHER EFFECTS

The respiratory effects of these drugs are very small. However, in large doses or when given during anesthesia, they may cause decreased alveolar ventilation, PaO_2, and increased $PaCO_2$.

Thiazine Derivatives

Two compounds are used in this group for sedating animals, xylazine and detomidine. Detomidine is currently under investigation in the United State for use as an equine analgesic. Experience suggests that its properties are qualitatively similar to those of xylazine. Further information regarding detomidine may be found in the section on analgesics in this book. This chapter will restrict its discussion to properties of the thiazine derivative xylazine.

Xylazine is very widely used in veterinary medicine in many species. It is approved in the United States for use in dogs, cats, horses, deer, and elk. In Europe, it is also approved for use in cattle. It is used as a sole agent and also in combination with other drugs to premedicate before anesthesia and for chemical restraint. Its use has become so routine that its profound physiological effects are often forgotten. The safe use of xylazine requires knowledge of its properties and potential side effects.

There is a wide variation in susceptibility to xylazine (Table 3.3). In general, ruminants are 5 to 10 times more susceptible than horses. There may also be unexpected differences in susceptibility associated with breed and sex.

EFFECTS ON THE NERVOUS SYSTEM

Xylazine produces a more or less dose-related depression of the CNS. Decreased motor activity and ataxia are evident. In some animals, especially ruminants, recumbency is produced easily at clinically acceptable doses. Xylazine most likely acts by activation of central presynaptic alpha-2 receptors (49). Activation of these central alpha-2 receptors seems to regulate central dopamine and norepinephrine storage or release. Xylazine is a potent analgesic for certain types of pain. However, the analgesia produced by a dose of xylazine is shorter-lived than either the sedation or cardiovascular effects it produces. At least for the relief of the signs of equine colic, xylazine compares very favorably with narcotic analgesics and other non-narcotic analgesics (50). In this situation, however, it may mask clinical signs used for patient monitoring. In horses, xylazine is usually very reliable as a sedative, rarely causing recumbency or unmanageable excitement. However, some horses will become sensitized, especially around their hind quarters, and well-sedated horses will occasionally kick with unexpected venom. Excitement and seizures are the sequelae to inadvertent intracarotid injection of xylazine in the horse. The occasional reports of adverse reactions to jugular injection of xylazine may be subsequent to inadvertent arterial injection. If such a dangerous reaction occurs, the treatment of choice is anesthesia, intubation, and oxygenation. Recovery from this anesthetic should take place in a padded recovery stall.

Table 3.3
Dosage and Route of Administration for Sedatives

Drug	Animal	Dosage (mg/kg) i.v.	Dosage (mg/kg) i.m.
Diazepam	Dogs	0.1–0.5	0.3–0.5
	Cats	0.1–0.5	0.3–1.0
	Horses	0.05–0.2	
	Pigs		0.5–10
	Cattle		0.5–1.1
	Goats/Sheep		0.5–1.1
	Chicken		5.5–11.0
Xylazine	Dogs	0.5–1.0	1–2
	Cats	0.5–1.0	1–2
	Horses	0.3–1.1	1–3
	Pigs		2–3
	Cattle	0.03–1.0	0.05–2.0
	Sheep	0.05–0.1	0.1–0.3
	Goats	0.01–0.5	0.05–0.5
	Birds		5–10

Emesis is common in cats and occurs occasionally in dogs after xylazine administration (51). This effect is apparently due to central stimulation of the emetic center (52). Muscle relaxation produced by xylazine may be related to decrease in intraneural and synaptic transmission in the CNS (51, 53). This property of xylazine is made use of when the drug is given as an adjunct to ketamine, which produces extremely poor muscle relaxation in many species when used alone.

The dose of anesthetic agents may be substantially reduced after xylazine premedication. Administration of otherwise conventional amounts of barbiturates or inhalational agents after xylazine may result in serious overdosage.

CARDIOVASCULAR EFFECTS

Xylazine has a profound effect on the cardiovascular system. It causes bradycardia, decreased cardiac output, and increased central venous pressure. After intravenous administration, there is an initial transient increase in arterial blood pressure and myocardial contractility followed by subsequent hypotension and decreased myocardial contractility (54, 55). The initial hypertension is most likely due to the alpha protagonistic effects of the drug. Sinus bradycardia and first, second, and third degree heart block have been observed in horses and dogs. Substantial decreases in cardiac output observed after xylazine are probably mostly attributable to the decreased frequency of ventricular contraction. These bradyarrhythmias are usually reversible with parasympatholytics such as atropine. Atropine at 0.045 mg/kg i.m. was, however, insufficient to reliably prevent bradycardia in dogs given 1 mg/kg of xylazine (56). Additional intravenous doses of atropine (0.01 mg/kg) were necessary to achieve this end. Therefore, unexpectedly large doses of parasympatholytic agents may be necessary to treat xylazine-induced dysrhythmias. Xylazine also increases the susceptibility of the myocardium to circulating catecholamines during halothane anesthesia (3); therefore, its use in conjunction with halothane in animals known to have certain types of dysrhythmias (e.g., dogs with traumatic myocarditis) is inadvisable. Xylazine is successfully used in conjunction with a variety of agents to produce anesthesia or chemical restraint. In order to avoid potential adverse drug interactions, the properties and doses of these other drugs should be carefully considered when using them with xylazine in any particular case.

RESPIRATORY EFFECTS

In clinically useful doses, xylazine does not cause great changes in respiratory parameters. Respiratory rate and PaO_2 are decreased and $PaCO_2$ is increased, but the changes are usually small. The larynx is relaxed and facilitates laryngeal examination by fiberoptic endoscope. Xylazine aids diagnosis of left laryngeal paresis in the horse because excitement produced by examining the unsedated animal may override the effects of partial paralysis (Cook, W.R., personal communication). Occasionally, increased upper airway noises may be observed after xylazine administration.

OTHER EFFECTS

Xylazine depresses gastrointestinal and ruminal motility. This depression may be prolonged (57). In ruminants, this side effect is a potential hazard because ruminal tympany may follow the use of xylazine. It is important to ensure that a ruminant is able to eructate safely before leaving it unobserved after sedation with xylazine. Decreased motility may help xylazine treat the signs of equine colic. This is, however, a two-edged sword in that important diagnostic signs may also be masked or changed (51).

Xylazine causes hypoinsulinemia with subsequent hyperglycemia (58). It is not known if the hypoinsulinemia is related to decreased synthesis or inhibited release of insulin. Glycosuria has also been reported. Urine volume is increased after xylazine administration. This effect lasts for 5 hours subsequent to administration in cattle.

Xylazine causes increased intrauterine pressure in cows (59), and this response is greater during pregnancy (60). These effects are very similar to those caused by oxytocin. Dose-related contractions have also been observed in vitro in bovine uterine strips exposed to xylazine (16). Xylazine has not been fully evaluated in pregnant animals; however, some authors suggest it may be contraindicated in pregnancy. However, many pregnant cows have received xylazine at the New York State College of Veterinary Medicine without subsequent abortion.

Thermoregulation in cats is depressed by xylazine (62). This effect lasts for several hours after sedation is no longer evident. This being the case, animals should not be exposed to extremes of temperature, as are often encountered in parked cars or open fields, after treatment with this drug.

Barbiturates

The barbiturates, particularly short-acting ones such as pentobarbital, have been used in veterinary medicine for many years. Pentobarbital is usually used in high doses for anesthesia (e.g., 28 mg/kg i.v. in dogs). It may, however, be used as a sedative and premedicant; it is given orally, intramuscularly, or intravenously. In horses, an i.v. dose of 0.5 to 1.1 mg/kg will produce sedation and facilitate some procedures under local anesthesia (14). Pentobarbital has also been used in mixtures with chloral hydrate or chloral hydrate and magnesium sulfate. An example of the latter is Equithesin, which may be used for sedation or general anesthesia in horses. Low doses of pentobarbital have also been used to sedate dogs and cats. The use of preanesthetic pentobarbital greatly reduces the requirement of other anesthetic drugs. There is a wide variability in individual response to pentobarbital; this makes it an unreliable sedative. In general, the duration of sedation will be shorter in horses, sheep, and goats than in pigs, dogs, and cats (27). This is probably related to differences in rate of metabolism. The use of barbiturates for sedation has largely disappeared; they have been replaced by other sedatives and tranquilizers.

Chloral Derivatives

Chloral hydrate is an effective, reliable sedative hypnotic in animals. Low doses are rarely reported to cause excitement. In the blood, chloral hydrate is metabolized to 2,2,2-trichloroethanol (27). Its CNS depressant effects are mostly attributed to this metabolite. It has poor analgesic properties even at anesthetic doses, but it may be used in combination with local anesthetics for standing procedures in horses. Three grams given i.v. to a 500-kg horse will usually produce fairly profound standing sedation (14). Additional doses may be given to prolong this sedation. Exceedingly high doses, however, may be associated with ataxia. Chloral hydrate has also been used as a chemical restraint in horses when mixed with either pentobarbital or pentobarbital and magnesium sulfate. The toxic dose of chloral hydrate is very close to the anesthetic dose, and an inadvertent overdose is a real possibility. For this reason, coupled with its poor analgesic properties, chloral hydrate is now rarely used for general anesthesia. It is still a useful agent, however, for standing sedation in horses, at which dosage level adverse side effects are much less likely.

Chloral hydrate is an irritant when injected perivascularly but may be given i.v. and by mouth. Similarly, mucous membranes are sensitive to this drug, and for this reason it is best administered orally by a stomach tube or in gelatin capsules. Chloral hydrate has largely been replaced for sedation by other drugs in most species other than the horse and cattle. In cows, it is often used to treat the excitement of nervous ketosis (30 to 60 g p.o.) (63).

Reversal of Tranquilizers and Sedatives

A compound that completely reversed the effects of a tranquilizer or a sedative would hold many attractions. It would allow elective cessation of depressant effects and effectively bypass the time constraints imposed by normal distribution and elimination of the tranquilizer or sedative. Such an agent would also have a place in treatment of inadvertent overdosage. Needless to say, the perfect reversal agent has not yet been found; however, some drugs may be used for counteracting the effect of tranquilizers and sedatives mentioned in this chapter.

Atropine is used to reverse some of the cardiodepressant effects of xylazine, particularly when it is used as a preanesthetic. Doxapram hydrochloride is used to stimulate respiration by its direct action upon the peripheral chemoreceptors. It has also been used to decrease the duration of xylazine sedation in dogs (64), although the underlying mechanism is poorly understood. Although not observed by the author, doxapram has been reported to cause muscle tremors, spasms, and periodic outbursts of aggressive behavior when used to reverse xylazine sedation in dogs (65). Doxapram (5.0 mg/kg i.v.) has also been used to reduce the duration of acepromazine-thiopental anesthesia in dogs (66).

Yohimbine is an alpha-2 adrenergic blocking agent that easily penetrates the blood-brain barrier (67). As such, it can enhance the central neural release of norepinephrine without blocking peripheral postsynaptic alpha receptors and producing vasodilation. Currently, it is undergoing extensive trial as a potential reversing agent for xylazine. Because detomidine is so closely related to xylazine, it is likely that yohimbine will be useful as an antagonist for this compound as well. Yohimbine is being used either or alone or in conjunction with other dogs (e.g., doxapram and 4-aminopyridine) to reverse xylazine effects in several species, including cats (0.1 mg/kg i.v.) (68), dogs (0.1 mg/kg i.v.) (69), cattle (70), and white-tailed deer (71). This drug also abbreviates the anesthesia or chemical restraint produced by xylazine in combination with other agents (e.g., pentobarbital and ketamine) (72–74). Yohimbine is also used to reverse the gastrointestinal stasis produced by xylazine (75), an especially serious side effect in ruminants, which are prone to tympany. Because of wide variation in susceptibility to xylazine and the widely different concentrations in which the drug is prepared (20 mg/ml and 100 mg/ml in the United States), accidental overdosage with xylazine is not uncommon. The availability of yohimbine has made this event slightly less serious. It should be noted that yohimbine is not approved for use in animals in the United States.

The drug 4-aminopyridine crosses the blood-brain barrier and causes CNS-stimulating effects. It has been used alone and in combination with other drugs (e.g., yohimbine, doxapram, and naloxone) to reverse various anesthetic agents, tranquilizers, and sedatives. For instance, 4-aminopyridine (0.5 mg/kg i.v.) with naloxone (0.04 mg/kg i.v.) reverses the neuroleptanalgesic combination of Innovar-Vet (76). A mixture of doxapam (1.0 mg/kg i.v.) and 4-aminopyridine (0.3 mg/kg i.v.) was found effective in reversing xylazine sedation in steers (70), and a combination of 0.4 mg/kg of yohimbine and 0.5 mg/kg of 4-aminopyridine smoothly reversed meperidine-acepromazine-pentobarbital anesthesia, xylazine-pentobarbital anesthesia, or acepromazine-pentobarbital anesthesia in cats (77, 78). Some benzodiazepine competitive compounds appear to act by competitive inhibition at the benzodiazepine site. The clinical significance of such competitive compounds in veterinary medicine has not been evaluated, but the potential for benzodiazepine-reversing drugs exits.

References

1. Price HL, Ohnishi ST: Effects of anesthetics on the heart. *Fed Proc* 39:1575–1579, 1980.
2. Bednarski RM, Bednarski LS, Muir WW III: Cost comparison of anesthetic regimens in the dog and cat. *J Am Vet Med Assoc* 185:869–872, 1984.
3. Muir WW III, Werner LL, Hamlin RL: Effects of xylazine and acetylpromazine upon induced ventricular fibrillation in dogs

anesthetized with thiamylal and halothane. *Am J Vet Res* 36:1299–1303, 1975.
4. Hall LW: The effect of chlorpromazine on the cardiovascular system of the conscious horse. *Vet Rec* 72:85–87, 1960.
5. Muir WW, Skarda RT, Sheehen WC: Hemodynamic and respiratory effects of xylazine-acetylpromazine drug combination in horses. *Am J Vet Res* 40:1518–1523, 1979.
6. Booth NH: Psychotropic agents. In Booth NH, McDonald LH (eds): *Veterinary Pharmacology and Therapeutics*. Ames, The Iowa State University Press, 1982, pp 321–345.
7. Redman HC, Wilson GL, Hogan JE: Effect of chlorpromazine combined with intermittent light stimulation in the electroencephalogram and clinical response of the beagle dog. *Am J Vet Res* 34:929–936, 1973.
8. Holliday TA, Cunningham JG, Gutnick MJ: Comparative clinical and electroencephalographic studies of canine epilepsy. *Epilepsia* 11:281–293, 1970.
9. Holliday TA: Therapeutics of convulsive states. In Phillipson AT, Hall LW, Prtichard WR (eds): *Scientific Foundations of Veterinary Medicine*. London, William Heinmann Medical Books, 1980, pp 201–213.
10. Wright JA, Clayton-Jones DG: Metrizamide myelography in sixty-eight dogs. *J Small Anim Pract* 22:415–435, 1981.
11. Hall LW, Clark KW: *Veterinary Anaesthesia*, ed 8. London, Bailliere Tindall, 1983, p 55.
12. Waterman A: Accidental hypothermia during anaesthesia in dogs and cats. *Vet Rec* 96:308–313, 1975.
13. Klein L, Sherman J: Effects of preanesthetic medication, anesthesia and position of recumbency on central venous pressure in horses. *J Am Vet Med Assoc* 170:216–219, 1977.
14. Muir WW: Drugs used to produce standing chemical restraint in horses. *Vet Clin N Am* 3:17–44, 1981.
15. Muir WW, Hamlin RL: Effects of acetylpromazine on ventilatory variables in the horse. *Am J Vet Res* 36(10):1439–1442, 1975.
16. Pearson H, Weaver BMQ: Priapism after sedation, neuroleptanalgesia and anaesthesia in the horse. *Equine Vet J* 10:85–90, 1978.
17. Proakis AG, Borowitz JL: Blockade of insulin release by certain phenothiazines. *Biochem Pharmacol* 23:1693–1700, 1974.
18. Persson SGB: Blood volume and work performance. *Proceed 1st Symposium Equine Hematology*, 1975, pp 321–326.
19. Davenport DJ, Breitschwerdt EB, Carakostas MC: Platelet disorders in the dog and cat. Part I. Physiology and pathogenesis. *Comp Cont Educ* 4:762–776, 1982.
20. Baldessarini RJ: Drugs and the treatment of psychiatric disorders. In Gilman AG, Goodman LS, Gilman A (eds): *The Pharmacological Basis of Therapeutics*, ed 6. New York, Macmillan Publishing, 1980, p 403.
21. Adams HR: Histamine and antihistamines; Serotonin and antiserotonins. In Booth NH, McDonald LH (eds): *Veterinary Pharmacology and Therapeutics*. Ames, The Iowa State University Press, 1982, pp 388–389.
22. Zontine WJ: Effect of chemical restraint drugs on the passage of barium sulfate through the stomach and duodenum of dogs. *J Am Vet Med Assoc* 162:878–884, 1973.
23. Hall LW, Clarke KW: *Veterinary Anaesthesia*, ed 8. London, Bailliere Tindall, 1983, p 54.
24. McGrath CJ, Rempel WE, Addis PB, Crimi AJ: Acepromazine and droperidol inhibition of halothane-induced malignant hyperthermia (porcine stress syndrome) in swine. *Am J Vet Res* 42:195–198, 1981.
25. Wood-Smith FG, Vickers MD, Stewart HC: *Drugs in Anaesthetic Practice*, ed 4. Boston, Butterworths, 1973, p 70.
26. Cloyd GD, Gilbert DL: Dose calibration studies of lenperone, a new tranquilizer for dogs, cats, and swine. *Vet Med/Small Anim Clin* 68:344–348, 1973.
27. Hall LW, Clarke KW: *Veterinary Anaesthesia*, ed 8. London, Bailliere Tindall, 1983.
28. Katherman AE, Knecht CD, Redding RW: Effects of fentanyl citrate and droperidol on electroencephalographic findings in dogs. *Am J Vet Res* 46:974–976, 1985.
29. Muir WW, Hubbell JAE: Blood pressure response to acetylpromazine and lenperone in halothane anesthetized dogs. *J Am Anim Hosp Assoc* 21:285–289, 1985.
30. Porter DB, Slusser CA: Azaperone: A review of a new neuroleptic agent for swine. *Vet Med/Small Anim Clin* 80:88–92, 1985.
31. Clarke KW: Effect of azaperone on the blood pressure and pulmonary ventilation in pigs. *Vet Rec* 85:649–651, 1969.
32. Krahwinkel DJ, Sawyer DC, Eyster GE, Bender G: Cardiopulmonary effects of fentanyl-droperidol, nitrous oxide and atropine sulfate in dogs. *Am J Vet Res* 36:1211–1219, 1975.
33. Dodman NH, Waterman AE: Paradoxical excitement following the intravenous administration of azaperone in the horse. *Equine Vet J* 11(1):33–35, 1979.
34. Serrano L, Lees P: The applied pharmacology of azaperone in ponies. *Res Vet Sci* 20:315–323, 1976.
35. Jones RS: A review of tranquilization and sedation in large animals. *Vet Rec* 90:613–617, 1972.
36. Booth NH: Psychotropic agents. In Booth NH, McDonald LE (eds): *Veterinary Pharmacology and Therapeutics*. Ames, The Iowa State University Press, 1977, p 395.
37. Pletscher A, Shore PA, Brodie BB: Serotonin as a mediator of reserpine action in the brain. *J Pharmacol Exp Ther* 116:84–89, 1956.
38. Crawford ME, Carl P, Andersen RS, Mikkelsen BO: Comparison between midazolam and thiopentone-based balanced anaesthesia for day-case surgery. *Br J Anaesth* 56:165–169, 1984.
39. Harvey SC: Hypnotics and sedatives. In Gilman AG, Goodman LS, RAll TW, Murad F (eds): *The Pharmacological Basis of Therapeutics*. New York, MacMillan, 1985, pp 339–371.
40. Turner T: Treatment of convulsions in dogs. *Vet Rec* 81:386–387, 1967.
41. Averill DR: Treatment of status epilepticus in dogs with diazepam sodium. *J Am Vet Med Assoc* 156:432–434, 1970.
42. Macy DW, Gasper PW: Diazepam-induced eating in anorexic cats. *J Am Anim Hosp Associ* 21:17–20, 1985.
43. Muir WW, Sams RA, Huffman RH, Noonan JS: Pharmacodynamic and pharmacokinetic properties of diazepam in horses. *Am J Vet Res* 43(10):1756–1761, 1982.
44. Amrein R, Cano JP, Eckert M, Coassalo P: Pharmacokinetics of midazolam after IV administration. *Arzneim-Forsch/Drug Res* 31:2202, 1981.
45. Gross DR, Kitzman JV, Adams HR: Cardiovascular effects of intravenous administration of propylene glycol and of oxytetracycline in propylene glycol in calves. *Am J Vet Res* 40:783–791, 1979.
46. Stanley TH, Webster LR: Anesthetic requirements and cardiovascular effects of fentanyl-oxygen and fentanyl-diazepam-oxygen anesthesia in man. *Anesth Analg* 57:411–416, 1978.
47. Flacke JW, Davis LJ, Flacke WE, Bloor BC, Van Etten AP: Effects of fentanyl and diazepam in dogs deprived of autonomic tone. *Anesth Analg* 64:1053–1059, 1985.
48. Reves JG, Kissin I, Fournier SE, Smith LR: Additive negative inotropic effect of a combination of diazepam and fentanyl. *Anesth Analg* 63:97–100, 1984.
49. Hedler L, Stamm G, Weitzall R, Starke K: Functional characterization of central alpha-adrenoceptors by yohimbine diastereomers. *Eur J Pharmacol* 70:43–52, 1981.
50. Pippi NL, Lumb WV: Objective tests of analgesic drugs in ponies. *Am J Vet Res* 40:1082–1086, 1979.
51. Knight AP: Xylazine. *J Am Vet Med Assoc* 176:454–455, 1980.
52. Colby ED, McCarthy LE, Borison HL: Emetic action of xylazine on the chemoreceptor trigger zone for vomiting cats. *J Vet Pharmacol Ther* 4:93–96, 1981.
53. Booth NH: Nonnarcotic analgesics. In Booth NH, McDonald LH

(eds): *Veterinary Pharmacology and Therapeutics*. Ames, The Iowa State University Press, 1982, pp 297–320.

54. Muir WW, Piper FS: Effect of xylazine on indices of myocardial contractility in the dog. *Am J Vet Res* 38:931–934, 1977.
55. McCashin FB, Gabel AA: Evaluation of xylazine as a sedative and preanesthetic agent in horses. *Am J Vet Res* 36:1421–1429, 1975.
56. Hsu WH, Zheng-Xing L, Hembrough FB: Effect of xylazine on heart rate and arterial blood pressure in conscious dogs as influenced by atropine, 4-aminopyridine, doxapram, and yohimbine. *J Am Vet Med Assoc* 186:153–156, 1985.
57. Seifelnasr E, Saleh M, Soliman FA: *In Vivo* investigation on the effect of Rompun on the rumen motility in sheep. *Vet Med Rev* 2:158–165, 1974.
58. Benson GJ, Thurmon JC, Neff-Davis CA, Corbin JE, Davis LE, Wilkinson B, Tranquilli WJ: Effect of xylazine hydrochloride upon plasma glucose and serum insulin concentrations in adult pointer dogs. *J Am Anim Hosp Assoc* 20:791–794, 1984.
59. LeBlanc MM, Hubbell JAE, Smith HC: The effects of xylazine hydrochloride on intrauterine pressure in the cow. *Theriogenology* 21:681–690, 1984.
60. LeBlanc MM, Hubbell JAE, Smith H: The effect of xylazine hydrochloride on intrauterine pressure in the cow. *Proceed Am Coll Vet Anesthesiol* 1982.
61. Minoia P, Mitolo-Chieppa D: Pharmacological and clinical properties of xylazine (in cows and rats). *Vet Bull Abstr* 47:559, 1977.
62. Ponder SW, Clark WG: Prolonged depression of thermoregulation after xylazine administration in cats. *J Vet Pharmacol Ther* 3:203–207, 1980.
63. Hall LW: *Veterinary Anaesthesia and Analgesia*, ed. 7. London, Bailliere Tindall, 1971, p 179.
64. Short CE, Gleed RD, Bristol D, Meyer RE, Harvey RH: Antagonistic effects of Dopram-V on xylazine and acepromazine in dogs. *Vet Med/Small Anim Clin* 77:1761–1764, 1982.
65. Hatch RC: Effects of doxapram in dogs given atropine and xylazine. *J Am Vet Med Assoc* 183:948–950, 1983.
66. Hatch RC, Wilson RC, Jernigan AD, Clark JD, Brown J: Reversal of thiopental-induced anesthesia by 4-aminopyridine, yohimbine, and doxapram in dogs pretreated with xylazine or acepromazine. *Am J Vet Res* 46:1473–1478, 1985.
67. Weiner N: Drugs that inhibit adrenergic nerves and block adrenergic receptors. In Gilman AG, Goodman LS, Rall TW, Murad F (eds): *The Pharmaceutical Basis of Therapeutics*, ed 7. New York, Macmillan, 1985, p 190.
68. Jensen WA: Yohimbine for treatment of xylazine overdosing in a cat. *J Am Vet Med Assoc* 186:627–628, 1985.
69. Hatch RC, Kitzman JV, Zahnar JM, Clark JD: Antagonism of xylazine sedation with yohimbine, 4-aminopyridine, and doxapram in dogs. *Am J Vet Res* 46:371–375, 1985.
70. Zahner JM, Hatch RC, Wilson RC, Booth NH, Kitzman JV, Brown J: Antagonism of xylazine sedation in steers by doxapram and 4-aminopyridine. *Am J Vet Res* 45:2546–2551, 1984.
71. Hsu WH, Schulaw WP: Effect of yohimbine on xylazine-induced immobilization in white-tailed deer. *J Am Vet Med Assoc* 185:1301–1303, 1984.
72. McGruder JP, Hsu WH: Aantagonism of xylazine-pentobarbital anesthesia by yohimbine in ponies. *Am J Vet Res* 46:1276–1281, 1985.
73. Hsu WH: Xylazine-pentobarbital anesthesia in dogs and its antagonism by yohimbine. *Am J Vet Res* 46:852–858, 1985.
74. Kitzman JV, Wilson RC, Hatch RC, Booth NH: Antagonism of xylazine and ketamine anesthesia by 4-aminopyridine and yohimbine in geldings. *Am J Vet Res* 45:875–879, 1984.
75. Hsu WH, McNeel SV: Effect of yohimbine on xylazine-induced prolongation of gastrointestinal transit in dogs. *J Am Vet Med Assoc* 183:297–300, 1983.
76. Booth NH, Hatch RC, Crawford LM: Reversal of the neuroleptanalgesic effect of droperidol-fentanyl in the dog by 4-aminopyridine and naloxone. *Am J Vet Res* 43:1227–1231, 1982.
77. Hatch RC, Zahner JM, Booth NH: Meperidine-acepromazine-pentobarbital anesthesia in cats: Reversal by 4-aminopyridine and yohimbine. *Am J vet Res* 45:2658–2662, 1984.
78. Hatch RC, Kitzman JV, Clark JD, Zahner JM, Booth NH: Reversal of pentobarbital anesthesia with 4-aminopyridine and yohimbine in cats pretreated with acepromazine and xylazine. *Am J Vet Res* 45:2586–2590, 1984.

CHAPTER

4

Pain, Analgesics, and Related Medications

CHARLES E. SHORT, D.V.M., M.S., D.A.C.V.A.

Pain in Animals

In mammalian animals, pain is considered universal, protective in nature, and part of the flight and fright mechanism. The clinical assessment and evaluation of the intensity of pain is based on signs exhibited by the animal that we interpret as pain. Our judgment of the intensity of pain is based on observation of animals and our perception, due to personal experience and observation after various procedures (1).

The type of surgical procedure or manipulation performed is important in determining the type of sedation or analgesics that can be helpful during the immediate postoperative or postmanipulative period. Surgical procedures that include the eye or surrounding structures are distressing to most animals; care must be taken to protect the area from rubbing and pawing. Operative procedures in and around the ears are similar to orbital and eye surgery. Head tilt, shaking of the head, pawing at the ears, or rubbing on an object are commonly exhibited signs of eye and ear pain. Vocalization and motor activity may also be noted when recovering from general anesthesia.

Invasion of the femur and humerus are obviously painful to animals; pain may be due more to the trauma to large muscle masses than to direct manipulation of bone. This is also seen when high limb amputations are performed as a result of trauma or malignant tumors. Whether the distress noted by the animal is due only to muscle trauma or if there is a loss or a phantom limb component as seen in humans is not clear (1). Attempting to escape, guarding the area, trying to bite the handler, or crying upon manipulation of a painful site can be an expression of acute pain.

Emergence delirium after general anesthesia may be due to postoperative pain or excessive noise or may be related to the behavioral characteristics of the animal. Highly nervous, generally timid, and easily frightened animals are more likely to have a stormy recovery. If extensive surgery has been done and pain is suspected, narcotics should be administered. The personality of the animal may require that tranquilizers or sedatives be combined with narcotics to ease recovery. Emergence delirium includes vocalization, paddling, lunging against the walls of the recovery cage or stall, and attempting to rise prematurely (1).

Another behavioral response to acute pain is reluctance to move in an animal that is normally active or moves when the handler approaches. Abdominal pain can be manifested by looking or kicking at the abdomen, lying down and getting up, and general restlessness, especially in the larger animals. Sweating, pacing, and restlessness are all signs of acute pain in the horse; these and attempts to lie down or throw itself to the ground are signs of acute abdominal pain in this species. The "tucking up" of the abdomen is a common sign of abdominal pain in many species (1).

Nociceptors

The work of Perl (2) in the 1960s revealed the presence of large numbers of cutaneous receptors in anesthetized animals that responded selectively to noxious (i.e., tissue-threatening or damaging) mechanical or thermal skin stimuli. These and subsequent studies indicated that subcategories of nociceptors exist. These include the polymodal type with a slowly conducting unmyelinated or C-fiber afferent that responds to noxious mechanical (squeeze or pricking), thermal (>43°C), and chemical (e.g., acidic) stimulation of skin in the small spot-like receptive field and the mechanical nociceptor with thinly myelinated (A delta) afferent fiber that responds to intense mechanical deformation of several discrete spots of skin (2).

Although efferent control of sensory transmission is a well-established concept, a specific network for nociceptive modulation has only recently been discovered. This network includes interconnected components at midbrain, medullary, and spinal levels. At the midbrain level, electrical stimulation of the periaqueductal grey (PAG) inhibits spinal neurons that respond to noxious stimuli as well as nociceptor-induced reflexes and escape behavior in a variety of species. Midbrain stimulation also produces analgesia in patients with clinically significant pain. The rostral ventral medulla (RVM) has similar behavioral and physiological effects and mediates midbrain antinociceptive actions at the level of the spinal cord. Endorphins are present at all levels of this nociceptive modulating network. Opiate microinjections at PAG, RVM, or spinal levels produce analgesia, presumably by mimicking the actions of the endorphins. The nociceptive modulatory system is diffusely organized and highly interconnected and appears to act as a unit whether activated by opiates or electrical stimulation. There are two classes of RVM neurons the activity of which are correlated with the occurrence of reflexes induced by noxious stimulation. One class (the on-cell) accelerates, the other class (the off-cell) pauses just before tail flick. Both classes project to the spinal cord and are excited by electrical stimulation of the midbrain. However, when morphine is injected either systemically or into the PAG, the off-cell is excited and the on-cell stops firing. The off-cell is probably the RVM output cell that inhibits nociceptive transmission at the level of the spinal cord. The function of the on-cell is not clear. The nociceptive modulatory system can be activated by a variety of stressful environmental factors, which are often, but not necessarily, noxious. The idea that the system acts as a simple negative feedback circuit is not consistent with its known properties (2).

The primary afferent fibers of nociceptors, like other somatic receptors, consist of a peripheral branch innervating the end organ, a cell body in the dorsal root ganglion, and a central branch entering the spinal cord through the dorsal root (3). It is conceivable that both "nocicpetive specific" and "multireceptive" spinal neuronal types transmit nociceptive information.

The morphology, background activity, and responses to stimulation of primary afferent inputs of small neurons in the superficial dorsal horn that could only be excited from the skin by noxious stimulations were investigated by intracellular recording and ionophoresis of horseradish peroxidase (HRP). Neurons that gave similar responses to afferent stimulation were morphologically heterogeneous with respect to dendritic tree geometry and axonal projection, but were located around the Lamina I/II border. Cutaneous excitatory receptive fields responding to noxious stimulation were generally small; most neurons had more extensive inhibitory fields responding to innocuous mechanical stimulation, in many cases overlapping the excitatory fields. Generally, stimulation of the inhibitory field resulted in hyperpolarization. Electrical stimulation of peripheral nerves revealed the existence of converging excitatory inputs carried by different fiber groups, and all neurons received an inhibitory input activated at low threshold. Excitatory responses were short-lived and occurred consistently in response to repeated stimulation. Central delay measurements gave evidence of a number of A delta monosynaptic inputs but only one A beta monosynaptic input; inhibitory inputs along A beta fibers were polysynaptic. The constant latency and regularity of the C response suggested monosynaptic connections. Low intensity stimulation of inhibitory inputs elicited a short-lived inhibitory postsynaptic potential (IPSP) that increased in amplitude with increasing stimulus strength until it disappeared into a more prolonged hyperpolarization. This was associated with inhibition of background action potentials and increased in duration with increasing stimulus strength up to C levels, indicating an A delta and C component. It is suggested that the level of excitability of these neurons depends on the relative amounts of concurrent noxious and innocuous stimulation and that the resultant output, which is conveyed mainly to other neurons within the spinal cord, could modulate reflex action at the spinal level as well as affecting components of ascending sensory pathways (4). Although some mechanoreceptors or thermoreceptors can respond to stimuli in the noxious range, an important distinguishing characteristic of nociceptors is their ability to encode increasing intensities of noxious stimuli with increased firing rate (2).

Information about tissue-damaging subjectively painful stimuli is transmitted to the central nervous system by specific receptors. Histologically, they are supposed to be free nerve endings connected to the spinal cord by thin myelinated (A delta or Group III) and nonmyelinated (C or Group IV) fibers. Nociceptive information is transferred to secondary cells mainly in the surface layers (Lamina I and II) and the neck (Lamina V) of the dorsal horn; it then ascends the anterolateral funiculus contralaterally in axons of the spinothalamic tract. One portion of this tract ends in the ventroposterior and posterior thalamus. It is assumed that it mediates the discriminative component of a pain sensation. The emotional-affective component of a pain sensation is supposed to be produced by that portion of the spinothalamic tract that terminates in the intralaminar nuclei and by the spinoreticular tract. The existence of a cortical pain center has not yet been proved, nor is it clear where in the cerebrum pain is consciously felt. The descending pain-inhibiting systems, originating in the brain stem, may block the transfer of nociceptive information at a spinal level, probably using enkaphalin as a transmitter. It is probable that they mediate morphine-induced analgesia. Lesions of tissue release endogenous substances, such as serotonin and certain prostaglandins, which sensitize receptors. The analgesic effect of nonsteroidal anti-inflammatory drugs, such as aspirin, can be explained by the inhibition of prostaglandin synthesis and the desensitization of nociceptors (5).

It has long been assumed, but not yet demonstrated unequivocally, that transduction by nociceptors involves noxious stimulus-evoked intradermal release of some chemical intermediate, such as histamine, substance P, or bradykinin, leading to nociceptor excitation. Sensitization may likewise involve chemical intermediates, because it is reduced by antagonists of bradykinin, histamine, and serotonin (2).

The existence of nociceptors lends support to specifity theories of pain, which hold that pain is a sensation, like vision or hearing, mediated by specialized receptors linked to a discrete pathway whose activation results only in the sensation of pain (2).

Some cutaneous multireceptive dorsal horn neurons additionally receive afferent input from muscle, joint, and/or visceral receptors. Viscerosomatic convergence onto spinal neurons has been suggested as the basis for referred pain (pain in a somatic structure resulting from injury or disease of a visceral organ), whereby normally infrequent visceral input excites spinal neurons, whose activity is interpreted by association as originating from the more frequently stimulated cutaneous receptive field (2).

In the cat, there is no convincing evidence that a particular compound mediates a supraspinal control of spinal transmission of nociceptive information. There is good evidence that opioid peptides are released segmentally in response to nociceptive input to the spinal cord and that this acts to inhibit motor neurons and to reduce transmission of nociceptive information to supraspinal areas. In the cat, there is no evidence that stimulation at supraspinal sites producing analgesia results in a spinal release of opioid peptides. In the rat, evidence for the latter has been obtained, but there are no data from other species. Tonically present supraspinal inhibition of spinal transmission of nociceptive information in the cat does not involve opioid peptides. Indirect evidence favors a role for 5-hydroxytryptamine (5-HT) and noradrenaline in supraspinal control of spinal processing of nociceptive transmission. Peripheral antagonists of 5-HT have reduced spinal inhibition from stimulation of supraspinal sites, but the site of action is unknown. Progress with noradrenaline involvement has been hindered by lack of a suitable antagonist. Although the amino acids, glycine, and gamma-aminobutyric acid (GABA) are involved in segmental inhibition of transmission of nociceptive information, no convincing evidence has indicated their involvement in supraspinal controls (6).

The major ascending pathway for pain and temperature sensibility in primates is the spinothalamic tract, which originates primarily from spinal neurons in Laminae I and IV–VI and the medial ventral horn (2).

A role for thalamic structures in the processing of signals of nociception and pain has been suggested on the basis of clinical data since the turn of the century. Searches for a "pain center" by lesion or stimulation were often disappointing, and electrophysiological data were rare and usually contradictory. However, recent electrophysiological anatomical and neuropharmacological studies made in various species (mainly rat and monkey) appear to give some clues to the understanding of the pain process at the thalamic level. These studies have been mainly concerned with the areas receiving projections from ascending spinal pathways conveying noxious inputs, either directly by the spinothalamic tract or indirectly by the spinoreticulothalamic pathway (7).

Another ascending pathway probably involved in nociception is the spinoreticular tract, which originates from more ventrally situated spinal neurons and projects in the ventral white matter bilaterally to the brain stem reticular formation. Some spinoreticular neurons also have an axonal branch terminating in the thalamus and are functionally similar to spinothalamic neurons (2).

In a recent study, 11 Macaque monkeys underwent a variety of lesions in the trigeminal afferent system; these were tractotomy, rhizotomy, and radiofrequency destruction of various components of the bulbospinal trigeminal nuclear complex. Behavioral responses were evaluated before and after the lesions using a quantitative paradigm that measured lever pressing in response to electrical stimulation of the dental pulp or facial skin and by assessing adhesive responses to facial cutaneous and intraoral pin-scratch. Thresholds for lever pressing in response to cutaneous facial stimulation were elevated by tractotomy; elevated further by a combination of tractotomy and rhizotomy of the 7th, 9th, and 10th cranial nerves and cervical dorsal roots C1–3; and maximally elevated by complete radiofrequency destruction of the trigeminal nucleus caudalis. These lesions also abolished adversive responses to cutaneous facial pin-scratch. None of these lesion combinations, however, altered lever pressing responses to dental pulp stimulation. Radiofrequency destruction of the trigeminal nuclei principalis, oralis, and interpolaris caused elevations of lever pressing thresholds in response to dental pulp stimulation and also smaller but statistically significant elevations on cutaneous electrical stimulation. Mild reductions in adversive responses to cutaneous pin-scratch were also produced by these rostral nuclear lesions, suggesting analgesia. The experiments suggest that primary afferent fibers for dental pain perception travel only in the trigeminal nerve and that these fibers relay via the trigeminal brain stem nuclei principalis, oralis, and interpolaris. Primary afferent fibers for cutaneous facial pain perception travel in the trigeminal, facial, glossopharyngeal, and vagus nerves and the upper cervical dorsal and ventral roots, and these afferents relay mainly in the trigeminal nucleus caudalis (8).

Other ascending pathways that have been proposed to play a role in nociception, but for which there is little evidence in humans, include the spinocervical tract (especially in carnivores), the postsynaptic dorsal column pathway, and short polysynaptic propriospinal connections (2).

Opioid peptides derived from proenkephalin and prodynorphin are differentially distributed in the spinal cord. Proenkephalin peptides are preferentially located in the sacral portion of the cord, whereas prodynorphin peptides are concentrated in the cervical spinal cord. Mu opioid receptors are highly concentrated in superficial layers of the dorsal horn in all the spinal cord. Delta opioid receptors are more diffusely distributed in the gray matter of the spinal cord. These sites are principally located in cervical and thoracic portions of the spinal cord. Kappa opioid receptors are highly concentrated in the superficial layers of the lumbosacral spinal cord. Its density decreases in the upper levels of the spinal cord. It appears that mu opioid receptors are indifferentially activated by thermal, pressure, and visceral nociceptive inputs. Delta receptors are more likely to be involved in thermal nociception, whereas kappa opioid binding sites are associated with visceral pain nociceptive inputs (9).

Spinopetal pathways may be activated by a variety of brain stem manipulations, including microinjections of morphine, which are known to modulate spinal nociceptive processing. Based on the ability of these manipulations to release spinal noradrenalin, the ability to reverse the antinociceptive effects by intrathecal adrenergic antagonists, and the fact that intrathecal injections of noradrenaline mimic the antinociceptive effect, it appears that the descending modulation may be mediated by descending noradrenergic systems. Examination of the spinal receptor systems with intrathecally administered agents indicates that spinal alpha, but not beta adrenergic, receptor agonists produce a powerful analgesia as measured on a variety of reflex and operant measures in mouse, rat, cat, primate, and human. On the basis of agonist and antagonist structure-activity relationships, it appears that a significant effect can be produced in the absence of any detectable effect on motor function by the occupation by spinal alpha 2 receptors. Distinguishable alpha 1 receptors also appear "analgetically-coupled," but their effects are uniformly contaminated by signs of cutaneous hyperreflexia at doses required to produce analgesia. The ordering of potency with which intrathecal adrenergic antagonists reverse the effects of intrathecal noradrenalin is indistinguishable from that of the reversal by these intrathecal agents of the antinociceptive effects evoked by brain stem morphine. This suggests that the population of spinal receptors acted upon by exogenously administered adrenergic agonists and endogenously released noradrenaline has indistinguishable characteristics (10).

Another important impetus for analgesia research was the discovery in the early 1970s of the opiate receptor and its natural ligands, the endorphins and enkephalins (11). Endorphinergic neurons certainly play a role in the brain's processing of painful stimuli. Endorphins act to alter pain appreciation at many levels within the central nervous system, including spinal cord, midbrain, thalamus, and cortex. The activity of this pain-suppressing system may play a role in individual differences in the experience of pain. Endorpinergic mechanisms play a major role in analgesia associated with stress and acupuncture and perhaps mediate placebo-induced analgesia. Chronic pain influences endorphinergic function, perhaps depleting endorphinergic neurons of their neurotransmitters. Endorphin function and pain sensibility are prominently affected in affective illness and schizophrenia. It may be that endorphinergic neurons play a fundamental role in selective attention, a kind of sensory filtering of information flow, in somatosensory and other sensory modalities (12). Endogenous analgesia systems might function continually to regulate nociceptive and/or other sensory inputs (2).

A review of pharmacological, neuroanatomical, electrophysiological, and behavioral data indicates that systems controlling cardiovascular function are closely coupled to systems modulating the perception of pain. This view is directly supported by experiments showing that activation of either the cardiopulmonary baroreceptor reflex arc or the sinoaortic baroreceptor reflex arc induces antinociception. The outcomes of studies using pharmacological treatments, peripheral nerve stimulation, peripheral nerve resection, and central nervous system (CNS) lesions are also presented as a preliminary means of characterizing cardiovascular input to pain regulatory systems. The network formed by these systems is proposed to participate in the elaboration of adaptive responses to physical and psychological stressors at various levels of the neuroaxis and possibly to participate in "diseases of adaptation." In particular, the present analysis suggests that the inhibition of pain brought about by elevations in either arterial or venous blood pressure may provide a form of psychophysiological relief under situations of stress and contribute to the development of essential hypertension in humans (13).

Effects of gallbladder distention on blood pressure, heart rate, and T-2–T-4 dorsal horn cell activity were determined in 18 cats anesthetized with alpha-chloralose. Distention of the gallbladder (10 to 100 mm Hg) increased blood pressure in 17 of 18 cats, but heart rate was altered in only 2. The gallbladder pressure-blood pressure relation was derived for 11 cats. Pressor responses were greater with greater distending pressures over the gallbladder pressure range of 20 to 80 mm Hg. The maximum increase in blood pressure was 21 ± 6 mm Hg at a gallbladder pressure of 80 mm Hg. Effects of gallbladder distention were tested on 64 T-2–T-4 dorsal horn neurons that had a somatic receptive field and were excited or inhibited by electrical stimulation of the left greater splanchnic nerve. In addition, all 64 neurons responded to stimulation of cardiopulmonary sympathetic afferent fibers. Gallbladder distention excited 17 cells and inhibited 9 cells. Responses usually consisted of phasic and tonic components. Significant increases or decreases in cell activity were elicited at a gallbladder pressure of 40 mm Hg. Pressor responses as well as changes in cell activity were abolished or greatly attenuated when both greater splanchnic nerves were sectioned. Vagotomy had no effect. Gallbladder pressure thresholds for a change in blood pressure (27 ± 3 mm Hg) and cell activity (29 ± 4 mmHg) were not significantly different. Cells responding to gallbladder distention were located in Laminae IV to VII of the T-2–T-4 segments. We conclude that gallbladder distention alters cell activity in the upper thoracic spinal cord and increases blood pressure. These findings may explain the phenomenon of chest pain that results from disease of the gallbladder (14).

In the last two decades, there have been substantial advances in our knowledge of the scientific basis of the mechanisms of pain. Nociceptors or pain receptors are widespread in the skin and tissues of animals; chemical mediation of nociceptor excitation may provide a key for understanding the peripheral phenomena related to pain. The expression of pain in animals involves multiple ascending and descending branches, as well as specialized pain-signaling mechanisms in the spinal cord. The importance of these different pathways varies with species and circumstances. Endogenous neural systems in the brain stem and forebrain, including both opioid and nonopioid mechanisms, may modulate the central transmission of nociceptive signs in animals. Noxious stimuli mediate a variety of different functions; each animal has a consistent response to noxious stimuli or a consistent pattern of escape from pain. As we better understand the mechanisms of pain, the humane treatment and alleviation of pain in experimental animals can be placed on a much firmer scientific basis (15). Unfortunately, new analgesics and the understanding of pain cannot progress without use of animals in pain studies. Tests have been designed to study pain and its control.

Experiments using three analgesic tests, the tail-punch, hot-plate, and tail-flick methods, were done to evaluate the roles of the spinal noradrenergic and serotonergic systems in the production of morphine analgesia in rats. To deplete noradrenaline or serotonin in teh spinal cord, 6-hydroxydopamine or 5,6-dihydroxytryptamine was given intrathecally. 6-Hydroxydopamine suppressed the antinociceptive effects of morphine injected systemically or intracerebrally into the nuclei reticularis gigantocellularis and paragigantocellularis or into the periaqueductal gray matter in the tail-pinch test, but not significantly in the hot-plate and tail-flick tests. Conversely, 5,6-dihydroxytryptamine suppressed the antinociceptive effects of systemically given morphine in the hot-plate test, but not significantly in the tail-pinch and tail-flick tests. The results not only provide further evidence for the involvement of the descending inhibitory systems in morphine antinociception, but also show that the extent of participation of the spinal noradrenergic and serotonergic systems in the effects of morphine has to be carefully assessed because different analgesic tests (tail pinch, tail flick, and hot plate) yield different results (16).

The cortical projection of tooth pulp afferents has been investigated by extracellular recordings in lightly chloralose-anesthetized cats. The results indicate two different projection systems from the tooth pulp afferents terminating on the cortical cells. One system appears to be specific with topographical distribution; it activates cells mainly in Lamina IV in a restricted region of the coronal gyrus. The cells in this area also receive excitation from restricted cutaneous fields. At stimulation of the tooth pulp with single electrical pulses, cells are activated with high discharge probability and with a stable latency. The other system projects mainly to cells in the superficial cortical laminae in a much larger area. These cells receive input from large bilateal cutaneous fields, but show less discharge probability and often require temporal summation to discharge at tooth pulp stimulation (17).

Analgesics are not only used to control pain without the use of anesthetics, but as part of the anesthetic management, as a preanesthetic, and for the relief of postoperative pain. Efforts over hundreds of years have developed medications for the control of pain. The most common are opioid analgesics, a group of medications with morphine-like responses. Opioids interact with related receptors and have some of the same properties as enkephalins and endorphins (18).

Opium, derived from the juice of the poppy, *Papaver sommiferum*, has been known since the 3rd century B.C. Although it was not then known as an analgesic or anesthetic, its use in the control of dysenteries and relief of suffering was fairly well understood. Opium contains more than 20 distinct alkaloids, of which morphine became a standard for comparison of analgesics. Morphine was widely used for control of pain among the wounded Civil War soldiers during the middle 1800s (18).

The adverse responses of respiratory depression and addiction stimulated interest in the development of analgesics free of these problems. In 1915, Pohl observed that *N*-allylnorcodeine reversed morphine-induced respiratory depression. Several years later, the morphine-antagonizing properties of nalorphine were described, but they were not clinically explored until 1951 (18).

The search for useful compounds led to the discovery of new drugs, including the relatively pure antagonist naloxone and compounds with mixed actions such as pentazocine, butorphanol, and buprenorphine. Such agents not only have enlarged the range of available therapeutic entities, but also, in conjunction with the subsequent discovery of receptors for opioids and endogenous peptides that bind to these receptors, have helped to change our views about the actions of the opioids (18).

The term "opiate" was once used to designate drugs derived from opium, such as morphine, codeine, and the many semisynthetic congeners of morphine. There is, at present, no entirely satisfactory classification of the opioids and the antagonists that have been studied.

The term "narcotic" was obsolete long before the discovery of endogenous opioid-like ligands and receptors for these substances. Derived from the Greek word for stupor and at one time applied to any drug that induced sleep, it was for a number of years used to refer to morphine-like strong analgesics. With the development of mixed agonist-antagonists, some of which do not suppress morphine-like physical dependence, and with the increasing use of the term in a legal context to refer to any substance that can cause dependence, the term "narcotic" is no longer useful in a pharmacological context to describe the analgesics used in animal anesthesia (18).

The potency of analgesics is compared to morphine as a means of understanding pain-relieving qualities. Table 4.1 illustrates a number of established opioid analgesics and their relative potency, assigning morphine a value of 1. Oxymorphone is then 10 times as potent as morphine (18). Newer agents are many times more potent. As an example, etorphine has 1000 times the potency of morphine.

Table 4.1
Comparison of Opioid Analgesics

Nonproprietary Name	Trade Name	Dosage Index	Duration of Action
			hr
Morphine		1	4–5
Oxymorphone (dihydrohydroxymorphinone)	Numorphan	7.5–10	4–5
Codeine		0.08	4–6
Hydrocodone (dihydrocodeinone)	Hycodan	1–2	4–8
Dihydrocodeine	Paracodin	0.16	4–5
Levorphanol	Levo-Dromordan	3–5	4–5
Methadone	Dolophine	0.75–1	3.5
Meperidine	Demerol	0.08–0.1	2–4

Structure-Activity Relationship of the Opioids

In addition to morphine, codeine, and the semisynthetic derivatives of the natural opium alkaloids, there are a number of other structurally distinct chemical classes of drugs with pharmacological actions similar to those of morphine. These diverse groups share the capacity to produce analgesia, respiratory depression, gastrointestinal spasm, and morphine-like physical dependence. Toxic doses produce convulsions, and the analgesic, gastrointestinal, depressant, and convulsant effects can be antagonized by naloxone and related antagonists (18).

The pupillary effects of morphine vary with the species. Cats (excited by morphine) and monkeys (sedated by morphine) show mydriasis. Therapeutic doses of morphine increase accommodative power and lower intraocular tension in both normal and glaucomatous eyes.

EXCITATORY EFFECTS

Extremely high doses of morphine and its surrogates produce convulsions. The mechanism is unclear, and different opioids may produce different patterns of seizures. Supraspinal structures are more sensitive to the convulsant effect than is the spinal cord because convulsant doses produce seizures above the level of a cord transection but not below it. With most opioids, convulsant effects are seen only at dose levels far in excess of those required to produce profound analgesia. The convulsant effect of opioids can be reversed by naloxone, but the dose required varies considerably among the agents. The seizures may not involve the same receptors that are responsible for opioid-induced analgesia.

In some species, relatively low doses of morphine produce gross excitation and hyperthermia. After high doses of opioids, mice show increased locomotor activity. Animals stimulated rather than sedated by morphine include pigs, cows, sheep, goats, lions, tigers, bears, horses, and cats. Reduction in dosage or combining with other medications such as xylazine or diazepam diminishes the incidence of excitement or seizures.

Cerebrospinal fluid (CSF) opioid activity was measured in dogs before and after morphine administration in order to investigate whether morphine results in an increase in CSF endogenous opioid levels. CSF was fractionated on a gel filtration column, and these fractions were assayed using a radioreceptor assay. Several peaks of opioid activity were seen in dog CSF both before and after morphine treatment. The predominant change in opioid peak patterns was the appearance after morphine treatment of a large peak in the elution position of morphine itself. Radiotracer studies verified that micromolar concentrations of morphine were present in CSF, which is enough morphine for potent binding activity. In addition to the increased activity in the elution position of morphine, several peaks of endogenous opioid activity showed increases that were statistically significant after morphine treatment (19).

The electrophysiological effects of morphine, naloxone, and capsaicin were studied on C fiber reflex and heat-evoked discharge in adult spinal cats. C fiber reflex was recorded from the L-7 ventral root at the time of superficial peroneal nerve electric stimulation. Heat evoked discharge was recorded from the L-7 ventral root at the time of hind paw heating. The drugs were injected slowly into the right cephalic vein. Results can be summarized as follows: morphine depressed the excitatory neuronal activity of capsaicin; morphine followed by capsaicin was antagonized by 0.4 mg/kg of naloxone; at the C fiber reflex, 2 mg/kg of morphine depressed the neuronal activity; and at heat evoked discharge, 4 mg/kg of morphine depressed the neuronal activity. These findings suggest that morphine depressed the effect of capsaicin and this effect was antagonized by naloxone. At the C fiber reflex, morphine was more sensitive than at heat-evoked discharge (20).

The effects of acute opiate receptor stimulation on regional cerebral oxygen consumption and blood flow were examined in nine regions of the artificially respired, alpha-chloralose-anesthetized cat. Regional cerebral arterial and venous oxygen saturation was examined microspectrophotometrically, and regional cerebral blood flow was monitored using radioactively tagged microspheres (15 ± 3 μm in diameter). Oxygen consumption was calculated as the product of flow and oxygen extraction in eight cats, control cerebral blood flow was obtained. The same measurement was obtained 40 minutes after the administration of 1.5 mg/kg morphine sulfate. Systolic and diastolic blood pressure were significantly decreased by treatment. The heterogeneity of venous oxygen saturation was significantly reduced by morphine. Average cerebral blood flow and oxygen extraction and consumption were not altered significantly by morphine. Regional cerebral blood flow in the hypothalamus, thalamic oxygen extraction, and hypothalamic and thalamic oxygen consumption were significantly decreased by treatment. This low dose of morphine may produce changes in cerebral neuronal and/or synthetic activity that lowers oxygen consumption in some regions rich in opiate receptors while not affecting overall brain oxygen supply or consumption (21).

Intraocular pressure is expected to increase after morphine injection, especially during emesis. In contrast, it has been shown that acute intraocular injection of morphine or D-ala-met-enkephalinamide (D-ala-E) in rabbits caused a sustained decrease in intraocular pressure. Conjunctival instillation of naloxone solution prevented the lowering effect of morphine or D-ala-E on intraocular pressure. Aqueous outflow facility appeared to be significantly higher in patients addicted to morphine or heroin than in healthy volunteers. Intraocular pressure was significantly lower in addicted patients than in control subjects. Conjunctival instillation of naloxone solution decreased aqueous outflow facility and increased intraocular pressure in addicted patients. Patients with chronic open angle glaucoma showed a significant decrease in intraocular pressure after conjunctival instillation of morphine solution. It is concluded that intraocular opiate receptors are involved in the regulation of intraocular pressure in animals and humans (22).

Epidural morphine has found increasing popularity in clinical trials for the relief of chronic and postoperative pain relief. A study was conducted to determine if there was any adverse tissue reaction when morphine was applied to the epidural space of dogs. Sixteen dogs were given 0.07 mg/kg of morphine in a volume of 2 ml of normal saline in the epidural space. Gross and microscopic studies of the epidural space, dura mater, and spinal cord did not show any adverse tissue reaction (23).

RESPIRATORY RESPONSES

Morphine is a primary and continuous depressant of respiration, at least in part by virtue of a direct effect on the brain stem respiratory centers. The respiratory depression is discernible even with doses too small to disturb consciousness and increases progressively as the dose is increased. The diminished respiratory volume is due primarily to a slower rate of breathing. Morphine and related opioids may also produce irregular and periodic breathing; in man, this is often seen even after therapeutic doses.

Maximal respiratory depression occurs within approximately 7 minutes after intravenous administration of morphine, but may not be seen for as long as 30 minutes after intramuscular administration or as long as 90 minutes after subcutaneous administration. The sensitivity of the respiratory center begins to return to normal within 2 to 3 hours; however, respiratory minute volume is still considerably below normal for as long as 4 to 5 hours after therapeutic doses (18).

The mechanism of respiratory depression by morphine involves a reduction in the responsiveness of the brain stem respiratory centers to increase in carbon dioxide tension (pCO_2). Opioids also depress the pontine and medullary centers involved in regulating respiratory rhythmicity and the responsiveness of medullary respiratory centers to electrical stimulation (18).

The influence of various afferent stimuli on the respiratory center is not affected to the same degree. Hypoxic stimulation of the chemoreceptors may still be effective when the respiratory center shows decreased responsiveness to CO_2. When the main stimulus to respiration is hypoxia, the inhalation of high tensions of O_2 may produce apnea. In addition to a marked depression of the automatic regulation of respiration, voluntary control of respiration may also be altered.

Within minutes after an intravenous therapeutic dose of morphine, there is a decrease in minute volume, followed by an increase in CO_2 in the blood and alveolar gas. As CO_2 accumulates, it again drives the respiratory center to a degree dictated by the opioid. Thus, respiratory rate and sometimes even minute volume can be unreliable indicators of the degree of respiratory depression.

The patient with severe pain may tolerate larger doses of morphine (three to four therapeutic doses over a period of a few hours). However, such a patient may exhibit subjective and respiratory depression should the pain suddenly subside (18).

Patients with reduced blood volume are considerably more suceptible to the hypotensive effects of morphine and related drugs, and these agents must be used cautiously in patients with any type of hemorrhage. The respiratory depressant effects of morphine and the related capacity to elevate intracranial pressure may be markedly exaggerated in the presence of head injury or an already elevated CSF pressure produced by trauma (18).

Morphine and related opioids must be used with great caution in any situation in which there is decreasd respiratory reserve, such as emphysema or other forms of chronic or acute lung disease. Opioids can precipitate attacks of asthma in anesthetized patients, but the risk does not seem to be high. (See Chapter 23.)

CARDIOVASCULAR SYSTEM

In the supine patient, therapeutic doses of morphine or synthetic opioids have no major effect on blood pressure or cardiac rate and rhythm. Despite obvious respiratory depression from doses that cause toxicity, the blood pressure is usually maintained until relatively late in the course of intoxication and falls largely as a result of hypoxia. Thus, artificial respiration or administration of oxygen may cause the blood pressure to rise despite the persisting medullary depression. Morphine and related opioid agonists dilate resistance and capacitance vessels and thereby decrease the capacity of the cardiovascular system to respond to gravitational shifts. The peripheral arteriolar and venous dilatation produced by morphine involves several mechanisms. Morphine and most opioids provoke the release of histamine, which sometimes play a large role in the hypotension; vasodilatation is usually only partially blocked by histamine-receptor (H_1) blocking agents. Morphine also induces arteriolar dilatation by a central suppression of adrenergic tone and blunts the reflex vasoconstriction caused by increased pCO_2.

Effects on the myocardium are not significant; the cardiac rate is either unaffected or slightly increased, and there is no consistent effect on cardiac output (18).

In coronary artery-ligated conscious dogs, intravenous injection of both morphine (8.0 mg/kg) and pethidine (12.0 and 24.0 mg/kg) inhibited the cardiac arrhythmia, whereas naloxone (1.0 mg/kg) facilitated it. Intravenous pretreatment with naloxone completely blocked the morphine-induced inhibition of the arrhythmia. Pethidine, however, elicited significant inhibition of the arrhythmia in the naloxone-pretreated animals, but its duration of action was markedly reduced. The temporal effect of i.v. injection of xylocaine (24.0 mg/kg) was parallel to that of pethidine (24.0 mg/kg) injected i.v. in the naloxone-pretreated animals. In cervical spinal cord-transected and bilaterally vagotomized dogs, i.v. injection of only 50.0 μg/kg of morphine elicited significant inhibition of the arrhythmia that was completely blocked by intrathecal pretreatment with a small dose (1.0 μg/kg) of naloxone. The same dose of naloxone, when given intravenously, failed to block the effect of morphine. The antiarrhythmic activity of morphine against the cardiac arrhythmia induced by coronary artery ligation appears to be due to activation of spinal opioid receptors. The local anesthetic activity of pethidine contributes its early phase of antiarrhythmic activity (24).

Morphine and related agents should be used with caution in patients who have a decreased blood volume because they are prone to develop hypotension. The concurrent use of certain phenothiazines may increase the risk of morphine-induced hypotension.

Cerebral circulation is not directly affected by therapeutic doses of morphine. However, respiratory depression and CO_2 retention result in cerebral vasodilatation and an increase in CSF; the pressure increase does not occur when pCO_2 is maintained at normal levels by artificial ventilation (18).

Fetal hemodynamics may be effected by morphine or other opiates. Meperidine hydrochloride (MHCl) is one of the most widely used analgesics today. Its effect upon maternal and fetal sheep hemodynamics and acid base were investigated in 13 experiments after maternal i.v. administration of 100 mg (approximately 2 mg/kg) of the drug. Blood samples were taken at base line and at 7.4, 15, 30, 45, 60, 75, 90, and 120 minutes postinfusion. Significant changes were an increase in maternal pH at 45 minutes, $P < 0.01$, at 120 minutes, $P < 0.01$, accompanied by a decrease in pCO_2 at 45 minutes, $P < 0.01$. No changes in maternal pO_2, O_2 saturation ($O_2\%$), base excess (BE), hemoglobin (Hb), heart rate (HR), blood pressure (BP), and uterine blood flow (ut, BF) were noted. Fetal pH, pO_2, pCO_2, $0_2\%$, bicarbonate, BE, Hb, HR, and BP remained unchanged. It is suggested that MHCl causes transient maternal respiratory alkalosis without any significant changes in uterine blood flow. With the dose used in this study, no adverse effect was observed in the fetus. Therefore, based upon this study, MHCl seems to be tolerated well by both ewe and fetus (25).

NAUSEANT AND EMETIC EFFECTS

Nausea and vomiting produced by morphine and its derivatives are unpleasant side effects caused by direct stimulation of the chemoreceptor trigger zone (CTZ) for emesis in the area postrema of the medulla. Apomorphine, a dopaminergic agonist, also causes vomiting by stimulation of the CTZ. The emetic effect of morphine is counteracted by some phenothiazine derivatives, particularly those with a potent dopamine-blocking action (18).

GASTROINTESTINAL TRACT

The use of opium for relief of diarrhea and dysentery preceded by many centuries its use for analgesia. The observed effects of morphine and related drugs on the bowel may vary widely, depending on the species, the dose, and the experimental techniques.

Stomach

Morphine and related drugs cause some decrease in the secretion of hydrochloric acid. A more pronounced effect is the decrease in motility of the stomach and the first part of the duodenum (18).

The effects of intravenous and intracerebroventricular (i.c.v.) administration of the opiate-like drugs morphine and cyclazocine on gastrointestinal motility were investigated in conscious fasted dogs chronically fitted with strain gauge transducers on the antrum, the jejunum, and the colon. Intravenous administration of morphine (100 mcg/kg) induced a disorganization of the cyclic motility of the antrum, a premature phase of regular activity on the jejunum, and a stimulation of colonic motility. Intracerebroventricular administration of morphine at a 10 times lower dose induced a short (10 to 15 minutes) stimulation of gastric motility followed by a prolonged (2 to 3 hours) inhibition associated with a disorganization of the jejunal motility and a stimulation of colonic motility. Cyclazocine at the same doses (10 mcg/kg) induced identical effects after administration by i.v. and i.c.v. routes; these effects consisted of an inhibition of gastric and jejunal motility and a stimulation of colonic motility. These results show peculiar motor responses at each level of the digestive tract to central and peripheral administration of an opiate-like drug (26).

The effects of opioids and naloxone on cyclical forestomach motility were determined in anesthetized and conscious sheep. To assess central or peripheral opioid actions, differential routes of administration were used. Possible dynamic effects along the innervating vagovagal reflex arc were investigated electrophysiologically at the cervical level of the vagus nerve. Further, direct influences on the smooth muscle were evaluated in vitro on isolated longitudinal reticular strips. Additionally, the effects of some spasmogenic agents were studied for comparative purposes. In anesthetized sheep, opioids depressed in an identical manner both the amplitude of spontaneous cyclical contractions and contractions evoked by electrical stimulation of the distal end of the cut cervical vagus. In conscious sheep, low doses of normorphine and loperamide inhibited frequency and amplitude centrally (20 μg/kg and 4 μg/kg via carotid artery, respectively), whereas locally higher dose levels (200 μg/kg and 10 μg/kg via coeliac artery, respectively) affected only the amplitude of cyclical contractions. Furthermore, the opioid peptides leu-, met-enkephalin, and (D-ala2-met4)-enkephalinamide preferentially depressed the amplitude of cyclical motility most efficiently if administered via the coeliac artery. These results indicate the presence both of a central opioid action depressing frequency and amplitude and of a local opioid action depressing only the amplitude of cyclical reticuloruminal motility. Opioids did not alter the resting discharge of afferent tension units and similarly failed to modulate the tone of reticular strips in vitro, suggesting that the opioids act locally on the intramural neuronal plexus, possibly by diminishing the output of excitatory transmitter. The central opioid mechanism is probably not situated within the gastric centers; it is likely elsewhere in the brain. Naloxone (greater than or equal to 100 μg/kg, jugular vein) stimulated the frequency of cyclical ruminal motility only in well-defined experimental conditions, probably via a central mechanism (27).

Gastroesophageal sphincter (GES) pressure was 47.9 ± 1.2 mm Hg in nontreated dogs. Treatment with atropine, acepromazine, and xylazine reduced GES pressure to 13.2 ± 1.19 mm Hg. Treatment with meperidine resulted in phasic contractions with minimum and maximum pressures of 27.9 ± 4.55 and 98.9 ± 9.16 mm Hg, respectively. Drugs used in anesthetic procedures can reduce GES pressure in dogs (28).

The effects of intravenous infusions of morphine, met-enkephalin, and leu-enkephalin on gastric acid secretion, gastrin release, and gastric emptying were investigated in four dogs with gastric cannulas stimulated by a liquid peptone meal. The actions of a potent opiate antagonist, naloxone, used alone or combined with opiates, were also studied. Morphine, met-, and, leu-enkephalin decreased the fractional gastric emptying rate. Acid secretion was decreased by enkephalins and increased by high doses of morphine. Enkephalins and to a lesser degree morphine inhibited gastric release during the first hour after the administration of the meal. Only leu-enkephalin decreases significantly the integrated gastrin response. Naloxone at the doses used antagonized partly or totally the effects of opiates on gastric emptying, but not those on gastric secretion or gastrin release. Naloxone infused alone had no significant effect on the gastric functions tested. These studies indicate that in dogs stimulated by a liquid test meal, enkephalins inhibit gastric emptying, acid secretion, and gastrin release. Morphine inhibits gastric emptying and gastrin release and enhances acid secretion (29).

Intestinal Na and H_2O fluxes and blood flow were determined in extrinsically denervated or innervated ileum of fed dogs during intra-arterial (0.2, 2, or 20 mcg/min) or intraluminal (4, 40, or 400 mcg/ml) morphine sulfate infusion. ^3H_2O and ^{22}Na were used to determine unidirectional fluxes, and ^3H_2O clearances were used to determine total segmental and absorptive site blood flow. Net Na and H_2O absorption decreased with time in innervated gut segments, but were unchanged in denervated segments. Intra-arterial morphine prevented the decrease in net segments. Intra-arterial morphine prevented the decrease in net Na and H_2O absorption in innervated segments due to increases in unidirectional absorptive fluxes. Intra-arterial morphine did not affect absorption in denervated segments. Intraluminal morphine increased net Na and H_2O absorption from both innervated and denervated ileal segments due to increases in the unidirectional absorptive fluxes. Absorptive site blood flow was linearly related to unidirectional absorptive Na fluxes in each group although not with the same slopes. The increment in absorptive site blood flow vs. absorptive Na flux was greatest with luminal morphine, intermediate with intra-arterial morphine and in denervated segments without morphine, and least in innervated segments. It was concluded that intra-arterial morphine inhibits an antiabsorptive effect of extrinsic nerves and that intraluminal morphine promotes an absorptive effect that could be direct or mediated through intrinsic nerves (30).

The infuence of fentanyl and morphine on the intestinal circulation was evaluated in an isolated loop preparation in 37 dogs anesthetized with pentobarbital intravenously. Selected intestinal segments were pumped with aortic blood at a constant pressure of 100 mm Hg. A mixture of ^{86}Rb and 9-μm spheres labeled with ^{141}Ce was injected into the arterial cannula supplying the intestinal loop while mesenteric venous blood was collected for activity counting. A strong correlation was found between the clearances of rubidium and microspheres ($r = 0.97$, $P < 0.0001$), suggesting that the shunting of 9-μm spheres through the intestines reflects the shunting of blood through nonnutritive vessels. Intravenous fentanyl decreased oxygen uptake (O_2), and vascular resistance (VR), and increased blood flow (BF), ribidium and microsphere clearances (Cl-Rb and Cl-Sph, respectively), and permeability-surface area produce (PS) in a dose-related fashion. Intravenous morphine in a dose of 1 mg/kg increased Cl-Rb (nutritive BF) without changes in total (nutritive and nonnutritive) BF. This increase in nutritive BF is probably related to morphine-induced histamine release. Morphine in a dose of 5 mg/kg was accompanied by vasoconstriction that was completely abolished by alpha-adrenoceptor blockade. Morphine-induced intestinal vasoconstriction is mediated via a release of epinephrine, apparently from the adrenal medulla. It was concluded that changes in the intestinal circulation during anesthesia with narcotics might play a certain role in the cardiovascular homeostasis during anesthesia and surgery. An increase in oxygen content in portal venous blood, resulting from a decrease in intestinal oxygen uptake, should facilitate hepatic oxygenation (31).

Other studies show a potent opiate with morphine-like effects can lower glucose in dogs by enhancing peripheral glucose utilization independently of hormonal changes (32).

INTERACTIONS WITH OTHER DRUGS

The depressant effects of some opioids may be exaggerated and prolonged by phenothiazines, monoamine oxidase inhibitors, and tricyclic antidepressants; the mechanisms of these supra-additive effects are not fully understood, but may involve alterations in the rate of metabolic transformation of the opioid or alterations in neurotransmitters involved in the actions of opioids. Some, but not all, phenothiazines reduce the amount of narcotic required to produce a given level of analgesia. However, the respiratory depressant effects seem also to be enhanced, the degree of sedation is increased, and the hypotensive effects of phenothiazines become an additional complication. Some phenothiazine derivatives enhance the sedative effects, but at the same time seem to be antianalgesic and increase the amount of opioid required to produce satisfactory relief from pain (18).

ABSORPTION, DISTRIBUTION, FATE, AND EXCRETION

Absorption

The opioids are readily absorbed from the gastrointestinal tract; they are also absorbed from the nasal mucosa and the lung and after subcutaneous or intramuscular injection. With most opioids, including morphine, the effect of a given dose is less after oral than after parenteral administration, due to significant first-pass metabolism in the liver.

When morphine and most of its congeners are given intravenously, they act promptly. However, the more lipid-soluble compounds have a somewhat more rapid onset of action after subcutaneous administration due to differences in the rate of absorption.

Distribution and Fate

When therapeutic concentrations of morphine are present in plasma, about one-third of the drug is protein-bound. Free morphine rapidly leaves the blood and accumulates in parenchymatous tissues, such as the kidney, lung, liver, and spleen. Skeletal muscle has a somewhat lower level of morphine, but because of its mass it accounts for the major fraction of the drug in the body. Morphine does not persist in tissues; 24 hours after the last dose, tissue concentrations are quite low.

The major pathway for the detoxication of morphine is conjugation with glucuronic acid. After the intravenous administration of morphine, the concentrations of free morphine in tissues decline progressively, whereas those in conjugated morphine (morphine-3-monoglucuronide) increase and then decline more slowly.

Excretion

Small amounts of free morphine and larger amounts of conjugated morphine are found in the urine, and these account for most of the administered drug. Use with N_2O, inhalant anesthetics, or injectable anesthetics results in combined responses to produce analgesia and anesthesia. It should be evident that combined drug action can result in extensive depression of vital physiological function in many species.

Meperidine

Meperidine is a synthetic, analgesic drug introduced by Eisleb and Schaumann in 1939 (Fig. 4.1). Originally studied as an atropine-like agent, it was soon discovered to have considerable analgesic activity. Meperidine, like other opioids, binds to opioid receptors and exerts its chief pharmacological actions on the CNS and the neural elements in the bowel.

The analgesic effects of meperidine are detectable about 15 minutes after oral administration, reach a peak in about 2 hours, and subside gradually over several hours. The onset of analgesic effect is faster (within 10 minutes) after subcutaneous or intramuscular administration and reaches a peak in about 1 hour. In clinical use, the duration of action is shorter than that of morphine, being approximately 2 to 4 hours.

In equianalgesic doses, meperidine depresses respiration to the same degree as does morphine. Peak respiratory depression is observed within 1 hour after administration. In therapeutic doses, meperidine has no significant untoward effects on the cardiovascular system, particularly when patients are recumbent; myocardial contractility is not depressed, and the electrocardiogram (ECG) is unaltered. After the intravenous administration of meperidine, there is an increase in peripheral blood flow and a decrease in peripheral arterial and venous resistance; these effects are not blocked by prior oral administration of antihistamines. Meperidine crosses the placental barrier.

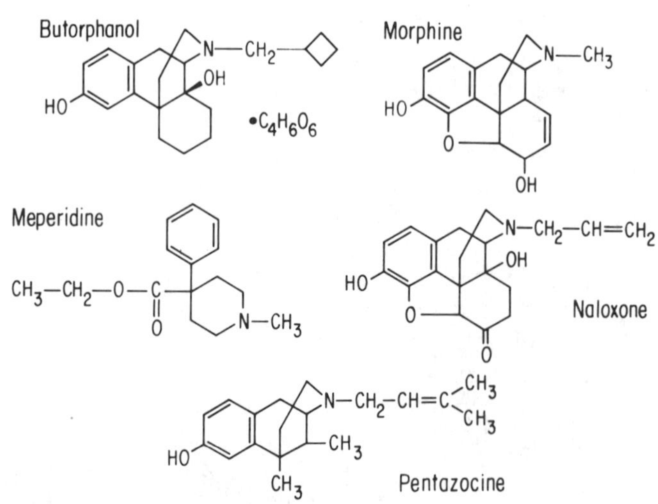

Figure 4.1. Structural formulas of butorphanol, morphine, meperidine, pentazocine, and naloxone

Meperidine is absorbed by all routes of administration. Although peak concentrations in plasma are usually observed between the first and second hour after oral administration, only about 50% of the drug escapes first-pass metabolism to enter the circulation.

Meperidine is metabolized chiefly in the liver. After intravenous administration, the rapid decline of the concentration in plasma due to distribution is followed by a slower phase with a half-life of about 3 hours (18).

Methadone

Methadone was synthesized by German chemists and came into clinical use at the end of World War II. The pharmacological properties of methadone are qualitatively similar to those of morphine.

PHARMACOLOGICAL ACTIONS

The pharmacological actions of single doses of methadone are qualitatively identical to those of morphine. The outstanding property of methadone is its effective analgesic activity. Methadone produces respiratory depression, miosis, antitussive effects, and effects on the secretion of pituitary hormones that are qualitatively similar to those of morpine.

SMOOTH MUSCLE

Methadone, like morphine, increases intestinal tone, diminishes the amplitude of contractions, and produces a marked decrease in propulsive activity; it is constipating and causes biliary tract spasm. After therapeutic doses, the ureters become quiescent, perhaps because of the antidiuretic effect. The uterus at term is not significantly affected.

ABSORPTION, FATE, AND EXCRETION

Appreciable concentrations of methadone can be found in the plasma within 10 minutes after its subcutaneous injection. After therapeutic doses, about 85% of methadone is bound to plasma proteins; only a fraction enters the brain. Peak concentrations occur in the brain within 1 or 2 hours after subcutaneous or intramuscular administration.

Methadone undergoes extensive biotransformation in the liver. The major metabolites, the results of N-demethylation and cyclization to form pyrrolidines and pyrroline, are excreted in the urine and the bile along with small amounts of unchanged drug.

Pentazocine

Pentazocine is one of the many compounds synthesized as part of a deliberate effort to develop an effective analgesic with little or no abuse potential (Fig. 4.1). A benzomorphan derivative, pentazocine has both agonistic actions and weak opioid antagonistic activity.

PHARMACOLOGICAL ACTIONS

Pentazocine exerts its major effects on the CNS and smooth muscle. The pattern of CNS effects is generally similar to that of the opioids, including analgesia, sedation, and respiratory depression. A dose of approximately 20 mg, administered parenterally, produces the same degree of respiratory depression as does a 10-mg dose of morphine.

The effects of low doses of pentazocine on the gastrointestinal tract are qualitatively similar to those of the opioids. The cardiovascular responses to pentazocine differ from those seen with the morphine-like opioids in that high doses cause an increase in blood pressure and heart rate.

ABSORPTION, FATE, AND EXCRETION

Pentazocine is well absorbed from the gastrointestinal tract and from subcutaneous and intramuscular sites. Concentrations in plasma coincide closely with the onset, duration, and intensity of analgesia; peak values occur 15 minutes to 1 hour after intramuscular administration. First-pass metabolism in the liver is extensive, and somewhat less than 20% of pentazocine enters the systemic circulation (18).

Newer Analgesics

Butorphanol tartrate is a parenteral synthetic opioid agonist-antagonist analgesic of the nalorphane-cyclazocine class. Its chemical structure is similar to morphine (Fig. 4.1). It acts on opioid receptor sites. As previously indicated, there are three types of opioid receptors: mu, kappa, and sigma. Morphine, meperidine, and fentanyl interact with mu receptors. Mu receptors are associated with respiratory depression, supraspinal analgesia, euphoria, and physical dependence. The drugs effecting Mu receptors are opioid agonists. Kappa receptors cause spinal analgesia, miosis and sedation. Sigma receptors cause dysphoria, hallucinations, and respiratory and vasomotor stimulation.

The competitive antagonists such as naloxone compete with the agonists for binding to mu, kappa, and sigma receptors. The agonist-antagonists have competitive antagonist activity at the mu receptor but also agonist activity at the kappa and sigma receptors. Butorphanol, pentazocine, and nalbuphine are agonist-antagonist agents (33).

Butorphanol has 17 times the potency of morphine in rats and 50 times that of pentazocine. It has 0.1 to 0.025 the potency of naloxone for reversal of opioid agonists. Butorphanol is metabolized by the liver and excreted predominantly via the kidney (33).

Butorphanol, like other opioids, is a dose-related respiratory depressant. At 1.25 mg/kg, butorphanol does not depress respiration. Subcutaneous doses of 2.5 to 10 mg/kg produce slight increases in $PaCO_2$ and decreases in arterial pH in dogs. In similar procedures in dogs, morphine 5 to 20 mg/kg caused significant decreases in arterial pH. The same trend is observed with intravenous administration, but the change is more significant (33).

In conscious dogs, intravenous doses of butorphanol (0.03 to 1.0 mg/kg) produced small decreases in systemic pressure (22). Morphine (1.0 mg/kg) produced its well-known cardiovascular effects of hypotension due to direct and central effects and histamine-mediated vasodilation. These initial effects sometimes elicited reflex hypertension and tachycardia. Morphine is known to stimulate the central vagal nuclei; over time, heart rates were significantly reduced in these animals. Butorphanol also produced decreases in heart rate, but they were of lesser magnitude.

Subcutaneous 5-, 10-, 20-, and 40-mg/kg doses of butorphanol produced a dose-related depression of spontaneous motor activity in mice, although the effect was minimal at 5 mg/kg. At 10, 20, and 40 mg/kg, the depression was two- to four-fold. In the rat, depression occurred only at the 40-mg/kg dose. These doses were 100 to 1000 times those required to produce analgesia in rodents, as shown by the phenylquinone writhing test. In squirrel monkeys, subcutaneous butorphanol doses of 1 to 5 mg/kg produced only mild to moderate behavioral depression that did not appear to be dose related.

In the cumulative dose range of 0.1 to 3 mg/kg i.v., butorphanol minimally affected cortical voltage output in the curarized cat. In the conscious and unrestrained cat, behavioral changes were observed after administration of 3 mg/kg butorphanol i.v. The animals initially showed marked ataxia, salivation, and piloerection, but less than 10 minutes later appeared alert and responsive to sound stimulation (33).

In dogs, 1 minute after rapid i.v. administration of 0.5 mg/kg butorphanol, whole blood histamine levels were essentially unchanged from control values, whereas in the animals receiving an equinalgesic dose of morphine (2 mg/kg), the levels were 77% above control (33).

Butorphanol-produced pain relief is good to excellent with parenteral administration in 90% of patients with moderate to severe pain. Surgical anesthetic indications involve preoperative and preinduction supplementation, balanced anesthesia, and postoperative pain. Side effects are sedation, nausea, elevated pulmonary vascular pressures, and, rarely, CNS excitation. Limited respiratory depression exists. Butorphanol is a potent analgesic agent with a favorable side effect profile (34).

USE AS PREANESTHETIC

The analgesic and behavioral effects of butorphanol (0.22 mg/kg), flunixin (2.2 mg/kg), levorphanol (0.033 mg/kg), morphine (0.66 mg/kg), and xylazine (2.2 mg/kg) given i.m. were observed in eight ponies. These ponies were equipped with instrumention to measure response to painful superficial and visceral stimuli objectively. Effects on the cardiopulmonary system and rectal temperature also were evaluated in six of these ponies. Observations were conducted before drug injection (base line values) and after injection at 30, 60, 120, 180, and 240 minutes. Xylazine provided the highest pain threshold for the first 60 minutes and a sedative effect for 105 minutes. The effects for superficial pain and visceral pain persisted 3 and 4 hours, respectively. Morphine produced good analgesia for superficial pain (30 minutes), whereas butorphanol provided good effect for visceral pain (4 hours). A slight degree of analgesia for visceral pain was obtained after morphine (1 hour) and levorphanol (4 hours); flunixin did not induce analgesia. Butorphanol, levorphanol, and morphine stimulated motor activity. Behavioral effects did not occur after flunixin was given. Xylazine decreased systolic, diastolic, and mean blood pressures. Marked increases in these pressures, heart rate, and respiratory rate were observed after morphine was given. Changes of central venous pressure, rectal temperature, and blood gas values remained within base line limits after both drugs were given. Butorphanol increased heart rates for 1 hour; flunixin and levorphanol did not alter any of the above values (35).

In a recent study in our laboratories, it was concluded that butorphanol at 0.05, 0.1, and 0.2 mg/lb could be safely administered to dogs. There can be a dramatic reduction in the dosage of sodium thiamylal required, indicating that butorphanol and its analgesic effect does indeed reduce the dosage requirements of other anesthetic agents. It can be further concluded that the 0.1 mg/lb dosage level is a more ideal dosage rate because of the relationship of heart rates, reduction in dosage of other anesthetics, and response of the animal. At the 0.5 mg/lb level, there is less reduction in dosage of other medications required, and at the 0.2 mg/lb level, there was a greater tendency toward depression. It is concluded that butorphanol can be an adequate compound for postoperative pain.

Naloxone and Similar Medications

CHEMISTRY AND STRUCTURE-ACTIVITY RELATIONSHIP

Relatively minor changes in the structure of an opioid can convert a drug that is primarily an agonist into one with antagonistic actions at one or more of the receptor subsites (Fig. 4.1). The most common such substitution is that of a larger moiety (e.g., an allyl or methylcyclopropyl group) for the *N*-methyl group on an opioid such as codeine, morphine, or levorphanol. Such substitutions sometimes produce congeners that are relatively pure antagonists, such as naloxone, but more often produce drugs that are agonist-antagonists.

ANTAGONISTIC ACTIONS

Small doses (0.4 to 0.8 mg) of naloxone given i.m. or i.v. prevent or promptly reverse the effects of morphine-like opioid agonists. In patients with respiratory depression, there is an increase in respiratory rate within 1 or 2 minutes. Sedative effects are reversed, and blood pressure if depressed returns to normal. Antagonistic effects last from 1 to 4 hours, depending on the dose of naloxone. It can also reverse the psychotomimetic and dysphoric effect of agonist-antagonists such as pentazocine, but higher doses (10 to 15 mg) are required.

Although the antagonistic effects of opioid antagonists are seen most dramatically in the presence of opioid agonists and agonist-antagonists, antagonism of the analgesic and respiratory depressant effects of nonopioids in both animals and man has been reported. In rats, naloxone antagonizes the analgesia produced by nitrous oxide. Nalorphine also prevents or abolishes opioid-induced CNS and gastrointestinal effects, with certain minor exceptions. The antagonism of severe opioid-induced respiratory depression is seen within 1 or 2 minutes after the intravenous injection of 4 to 10 mg of nalorphine and lasts 1 to 4 hours.

The degree of opioid antagonism observed depends not only on the dose of the antagonist but also on which opioid has been given and the degree to which physical dependence has developed. Thus, 10 mg of nalorphine does not antagonize the relatively mild respiratory depression produced by 10 mg of morphine, perhaps because its antagonistic effects at the mu receptor are counterbalanced by its own weak respiratory depressant activity. However, smaller doses of nalorphine antagonize the severe depression produced by 70 mg of morphine. In patients who are physically dependent, very small doses (2 to 5 mg) of nalorphine or small doses of naloxone may be sufficient not only to antagonize respiratory depression but also to precipitate withdrawal phenomena. In such individuals, large doses of opioid antagonists can produce severe withdrawal symptoms (18).

Fentanyl

Fentanyl is a synthetic opioid related to the phenylpiperidines. As an analgesic, it is estimated to be 80 times as potent as morphine. Its respiratory depressant effect is of shorter duration than that of meperidine; its analgesic and euphoric effects are antagonized by opioid antagonists, but are not significantly prolonged or intensified by droperidol, a neuroleptic agent with which it is usually combined for use (18).

Relationships between plasma concentrations of fentanyl and its analgesic, respiratory, and cardiovascular effects were determined in unanesthetized dogs. To avoid drug interactions, trained unanesthetized spontaneously breathing dogs were used. After a control period in the awake state, fentanyl was injected in increasing amounts (2.5, 5, 20, 40, and 100 micrograms/kg) at 5-minute intervals to a cumulative dose of 167.5 micrograms/kg administered over 20 minutes; its effects were studied on pain responses (heart and blood pressure changes and somatic responses to tail clamping), respiration (respiratory rate, oxygen consumption, and blood gas tensions), and circulation (heart rate and blood pressure). Plasma concentration/effect curves were derived by relating the changes in variables from the awake state to the corresponding plasma concentration (range, 2 to 453 ng/ml). Maximum effects occurred at plasma concentrations at and around 30 ng/ml. Oxygen consumption decreased only slightly and remained well above the basal metabolic rate. Cardiac output, heart rate, respiratory rate, and arterial oxygen tension were almost halved during the full action of fentanyl. In dogs, fentanyl's analgesic action cannot be separated from its respiratory and cardiovascular effects. All receptor-mediated effects are maximal at the same plasma concentration, a phenomenon suggesting saturation of the opiate receptors (36).

Pain perception and its alteration by analgesic drugs is difficult to measure in the horse. The latency to onset of flexion of a limb in response to a noxious thermal stimulus has been used as a nociceptive end point for analgesic studies in many species. Although this method has been used in the horse, it may be confounded by the spontaneous locomotor activity observed after administration of narcotic analgesics. Consequently, an alternative method of assaying narcotic analgesia that did not involve the equine locomotor apparatus was developed. Heat-evoked skin-twitch reflex as a reproducible measure of pain threshold and its alteration by the narcotic analgesic fentanyl was studied. This method is compared with the heat-evoked hoof-withdrawal reflex. Fentanyl, administered at intravenous doses of 0.010, 0.005, and 0.0025 mg/kg, produced a dose-related prolongation of the skin-twitch reflex but failed to alter the latency to hoof withdrawal after noxious thermal stimulation. The skin-twitch reflex is therefore a more sensitive assay of narcotic analgesia in the horse than is the hoof-withdrawal reflex (37).

The effects of fentanyl and sufentanil with and without N_2O on left ventricular myocardium supplied by a critically narrowed and normal coronary artery were studied in 16 dogs. Regional ventricular function was measured by recording ventricular segment length with the use of ultrasonic length detectors in the left anterior descending (LAD) and the left circumflex (LC) coronary artery territories before and during critical stenosis of the LAD. Critical stenosis was documented by the absence of a hyperemic response after a 10-second total occlusion of the LAD. Hemodynamic variables (aortic flow and pressure, left ventricular pressure, heart rate, and coronary blood flow) were measured, and the first derivative of left ventricular pressure (LVdP/dt) and coronary perfusion pressure was derived. Eight dogs received fentanyl (100 μ/kg) followed by an infusion of 1 μg/kg/min while ventilated with O_2:N_2 (1:2), and 8 dogs received sufentanil (30 μg/kg) with an infusion of 0.3 μg/kg/min. Replacement of N_2 with N_2O produced evidence of mild systolic myocardial depression but no dysfunction in either group. After application of the critical constriction, the addition of N_2O rapidly produced evidence of dysfunction with significant postsystolic shortening only in the LAD area. This was not accompanied by hypotension or a decrease in coronary flow from either opioid. Fentanyl, 2 and 4 μg/kg/min, and sufentanil, 0.6 and 1.2 μg/kg/min in the absence of N_2O did not produce dysfunction but had no protective effect when N_2O was added (38).

The colonic motility index was measured in dogs using strain-gauge transducers before and after administration of opiate agonists. Fentanyl, a mu-compound, ethylketazocine (EKC), a kappa-compound, and (D-Ala2,Leu5) enkephalin (DADLE), a delta-agonist, were administered by intravenous (i.v.) or intrathecal (i.t.) routes. Fentanyl (2 to 10 nmol × kg i.v.) induced a dose-related period of hyperactivity characterized by an increase in both tone and frequency of contractions in the distal portion of the colon, whereas a period of hypomotility following a short-lived period of increased activity was elicited on the proximal colon. Fentanyl (0.1 or 0.2 nmol × kg i.t.) had inhibitory effects on both proximal and distal colon. Small doses of EKC (2 to 4 nmol × kg) administered i.t. or larger doses (20 to 40 nmol × kg i.v.) inhibited colonic motility for a dose-related duration, the effects of EKC being more marked on the distal colon than on the proximal colon. The administration of DADLE, 1 to 2 nmol × kg i.t. and 20 to 40 nmol × kg i.v., inhibited and stimulated the colonic contractions, respectively, in both proximal and distal colon. The results demonstrated that the colonic opiate-mediated responses may vary according to the route of administration, the portion of the colon studied, and the opioid agonist used. Opiate agonists when administered centrally show a tendency to modulate colonic activity in a similar way whatever the type of agonist (39).

The effect of prior administration of reserpine on fentanyl dose-response curves for loss of the righting reflex and prevention of purposeful movement response to noxious stimulation was studied in rats. It was found that reserpine (4 mg/kg, 3 hours before the tests) antagonized the effect of fentanyl on purposeful movement response to the tail clamp and, at the same time, strengthened its effect on the righting reflex. As a result, reserpine pretreatment reversed the order of fentanyl potency regarding these two effects. Reserpine changed fentanyl ED_{50} values for the purposeful movement response from 8.2 to 20.3 μg/kg ($P < 0.0001$) and for the righting reflex from 20.5 to 13.7 μg/kg ($P < 0.0001$). The results suggest that reserpine dissociates the analgesic action of fentanyl from its anesthetic action, defined as a loss of the righting reflex. This may be regarded as an indication that the analgesic action of narcotics may not adequately reflect their anesthetic potency (40).

The effects of fentanyl, nitrous oxide, and their combination on myocardial contractility were investigated in the papillary muscle preparation perfused by a donor dog. With a conscious donor, fentanyl infused directly into the arterial blood perfusing the papillary muscle produced a dose-related depression of developed tension. However, blood concentrations of fentanyl required to obtain the depression were in the range of 30 to 120 μg/ml. Fentanyl produces a direct negative inotropic effect only in concentrations that are two to three orders of magnitude higher than its blood concentrations in fentanyl-induced anesthesia. When fentanyl and nitrous oxide are used together, their interaction is not significantly different from additive effects (41).

Since the demonstration of opiate receptors in the spinal cord in the middle 1970s, investigators have been looking for the most effective epidural narcotic. With the use of the chronically catheterized maternal sheep model, we injected two different doses of preservative-free fentanyl (40 and 100 μg) into the epidural space. No statistically significant changes were observed, either in maternal or fetal arterial pressure and acid-base status or in maternal central venous pressure, systemic and pulmonary vascular resistance, cardiac output, and intrauterine pressure ($P > 0.05$). With a dose of 50 μg of fentanyl, maternal levels of fentanyl peaked at 60 minutes (50 pg/ml) and the fetal levels of fentanyl peaked at 45 minutes (20 pg/ml). With a 100-μg dose of fentanyl, maternal levels of fentanyl peaked at 45 minutes (230 pg/ml) and the fetal levels peaked at 15 minutes (110 pg/ml). We conclude that the injection of 50 and 100 μg of fentanyl into the maternal epidural space has no adverse effects on mother or fetus in the sheep model (42).

Most fentanyl used in animal anesthesia is combined with a tranquilizer or may be used as part of balanced anesthesia or preanesthesia prior to inhalant anesthesia.

Sufentanyl, Alfentanil, and Carfentanil

Newly developed analgesics (opioids) similar to fentanyl include sufentanyl citrate, carfentanil, and alfentanil. This group of analgesics are very potent and must be used with this understanding (Table 4.2).

Dr. Paul Janssen has been instrumental in the development of fentanyl, and a group of clinically related compounds. Fentanyl is an opiate agonist of the 4-anilinopipridine series (42). The fentanyls are all more potent than morphine. Structural formulas are shown in Figure 4.2. Much of the difference in potency can be explained in terms of access to central opiate receptors (42). In contrast to the majority of other opiates, the fentanyls are most frequently given intravenously, and absorption studies of other routes of administration are understandably limited.

In a study of pharmacodynamics after intramuscular injection of fentanyl, peak analgesic effects generally occurred at 1 hour and lasted for a shorter period than morphine. Under these conditions, the analgesic potency ratio of fentanyl:morphine was estimated at 25:1. Although pharmacokinetic data were not studied, the time at which peak analgesic effects occurred

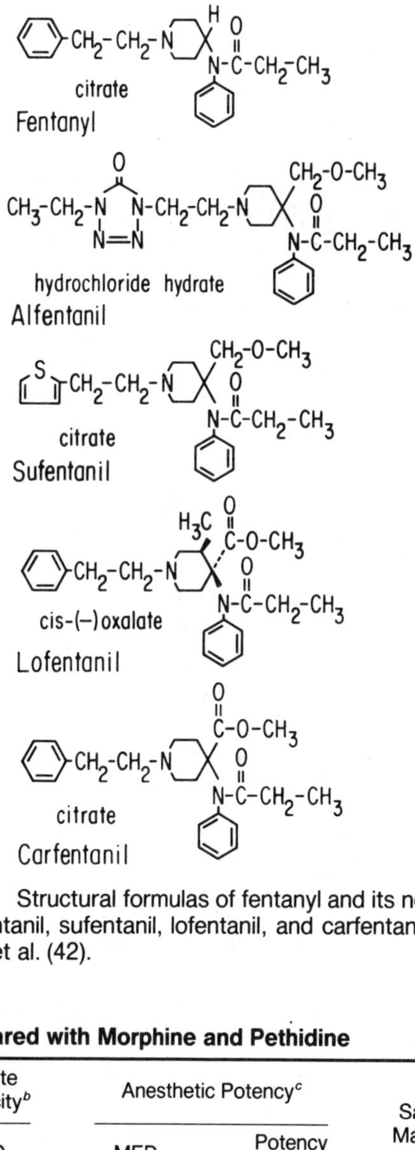

Figure 4.2. Structural formulas of fentanyl and its newer derivatives: alfentanil, sufentanil, lofentanil, and carfentanil. Adapted from Craft et al. (42).

Table 4.2
Animal Pharmacological Data for Fentanyl and Its Newer Derivatives Compared with Morphine and Pethidine

Opiate	Analgetic Potency[a]			Acute Toxicity[b]	Anesthetic Potency[c]		Safety Margin[d]
	MED_{50} (mg/kg)[e]	$TMED_{50}$	Potency Ratio	MLD_{50}	MED_{50}	Potency Ratio	
	mg/kg	*hr*		*mg/kg*	*mg/kg*		
Fentanyl	0.011	0.093	292	3.5	0.0012	125	160
Alfentanil	0.044	0.03	73	47.5	0.005	30	50
Sufentanil	0.00071	0.14	4521	17.9	0.00025	625	800
Lofentanil	0.00070	0.55	4586	0.20	0.000025	6250	10000
Carfentanil	0.00032	0.29	10031	3.39	na	na	na
Pethidine hydrochloride	6.04	0.11	0.53	29	0.45	0.3	0
Morphine sufphate	3.21	0.31	1	223	0.15	1	33

[a] Rat, tail withdrawal from 55°C water.
[b] Rat, intravenous bolus.
[c] Dog, awake intubation with no increase in blood pressure.
[d] Dog, ratio of single intravenous dose for surgical anesthesia (20 × MED_{50}) to dose producing severe cardiovascular side effects (alternating hyperactivity and depression) together with acidosis and hypermetabolism, convulsions, and EEG exhaustion.
[e] Abbreviations: MED_{50}, minimum ED_{50}, intravenous administration; $TMED_{50}$, time to maximum effect after single intravenous (5-second) bolus; MLD_{50}, mean value of LD_{50}; na, not available. Adapted from Mather (43).

would suggest that the rate of absorption was similar to pethidine (43).

PHYSIOLOGICAL DISTRIBUTION

The physiological distribution of fentanyl was reported in a series of animal studies during the late 1960s and early 1970s. Animal studies provide the key to understanding the use of these agents.

In keeping with other drugs with high lipid solubility at physiological pH, fentanyl is widely distributed to organs and tissues of the mammalian body. After intravenous injection, high concentrations occur quickly in well-perfused tissues, notably the lung, kidney, spleen, heart, and brain. Maximum concentrations in the intestine wall, liver, and muscle lag slightly behind the well-perfused tissues, and the maximum concentrations in fat occur in approximately 30 minutes after injection. This reflects the high affinity and low perfusion of the adipose tissue compared with the other tissues named. Not unexpectedly, after intramuscular injections lower concentration gradients are presented to these well-perfused tissues (especially the lung, which receives all of the dose) than after intravenous injection. This results in a several-fold lower concentration 5 minutes after injection than after the same dose given intravenously (42).

Both N-O-dealkylation of alfentanil and sufentanil are the dominating biotransformations in the dog and rat (42).

Development of the newer derivatives of fentanyl would seem to be an important step. The range of duration of actions has been extended from ultrashort (alfentanil) and short (fentanyl and sufentanil) to intermediate/long (lofentanil). Carfentanil is yet to find a use in humans; at present it is proving an interesting agent in veterinary medicine trials as a "capture" agent for wild animals. Early animal experiments have suggested it may have a possible role in clinical anesthetic induction via topical application to the nasal mucosa (42).

The hemodynamic changes, plasma norepinephrine levels, pupil size, and rapidity of postoperative mental recovery were measured and compared in 72 patients randomly assigned in a double-blind manner to receive either morphine, meperidine, fentanyl, or sufentanil as supplements to nitrous oxide anesthesia. Meperidine, unlike the other opioids, which did not change heart rate, consistently increased it. Hemodynamic responses to laryngoscopy and intubation were suppressed by fentanyl and sufentanil, but not by morphine or meperidine. The sufentanil group was the only group in which median norepinephrine levels remained consistently below preinduction values. The frequency with which opioids had to be administered (doses per hour) was significantly less with sufentanil than with morphine and meperidine. Meperidine produced less constriction of the pupils than the other opioids, and the duration of nuosis was shorter. Fentanyl and sufentanil were associated with a more rapid return of mental function than morphine and meperidine. Meperidine caused deleterious effects on objective tests of psychomotor and cognitive skills that were not reflected by subjective evaluation of rate of recovery from anesthesia. It was concluded that moderate doses of fentanyl and sufentanil are better supplements to nitrous oxide anesthesia than morphine or meperidine and that fentanyl and sufentanil are equally satisfactory. Subjective effects of the opioids correlated well with changes in pupil diameter (44).

The cardiovascular and some respiratory effects of alfentanil, a potent short-acting morphinomimetic, were studied in conscious and anesthetized, artificially ventilated dogs. The compound was injected intravenously in increasing doses of 12.5, 12.5, 25, 50, 100, 200, 400, and 800 μg/kg in the conscious dogs and 0.16, 0.32, 0.64, 1.25, 2.5, and 5 mg/kg in the anesthetized animals. In the conscious dogs, the heart rate decreased significantly, reaching a maximum decrease after the injection of 400 μg/kg × pCO_2; arterial and venous lactate concentration increased, although pO_2, pH and base excess decreased significantly. At higher dose levels (100 to 400 μg/kg), short periods of convulsions were seen. The most pronounced change in the anesthetized dogs was a significant fall in LVdP/dt max and LVdP/dt max/P, associated with a rise in left ventricular end-diastolic pressure after the injection of 5 mg/kg, suggesting negative inotropic properties at this high dose level. Most of the animals showed atrial-ventricular (A-V) dissociations that disappeared at higher doses. All animals survived. These findings indicate that alfentanil is a safe analgesic as far as the effects on the cardiovascular system are concerned. High doses are tolerated well, especially when the animals are artifically ventilated. The short periods of convulsions, seen only in the awake dogs, may have been facilitated by the low pO_2 levels reached (median value, 9 kPa) (45).

The hemodynamic effects of alfentanil were investigated in six dogs receiving verapamil, 0.5 mg/kg, and six dogs receiving saline in equal volume. Basic measurements were done after 30 minutes, and the dogs were then given alfentanil, 160 μg/kg, with measurements at 5, 15, and 30 minutes. Significant increases in central venous pressure (CVP), mean pulmonary arterial pressure, and pulmonary wedge pressure (PWP) were found 30 minutes after verapamil. After verapamil-alfentanil, increases were seen in CVP and PWP at 5 and 15 minutes and in PWP at 30 minutes. Mean arterial pressure and cardiac index were unchanged; decrease in heart rate was fully compensated by an increase in stroke volume. Indices of contractility

Table 4.3
Dosage of Analgesia in Animals

	Dog	Cat	Horse
Morphine	10–50 mg/kg s.c.	0.1 mg/kg s.c.	0.75 mg/kg i.m.
Oxymorphone	0.2 mg/kg i.v.	0.2 mg/kg i.v.	0.02–0.03 mg/kg i.m. or i.v.
Levorphanol			0.03 mg/kg i.m.
Methadone	1.0 mg/kg s.c. or i.v.		0.5 mg/kg i.v.
Meperidine	10 mg/kg s.c. or i.m.	3 mg/kg s.c. or i.m.	1 mg/kg s.c.
Pentazocine	2–3 mg/kg i.m.		0.5–3.0 mg/kg i.v. or i.m.
Butorphanol	0.22 mg/kg i.m.		0.22 mg/kg i.v.
Naloxone	0.04 mg/kg i.v., i.m., or s.c.	0.04 mg/kg i.v., i.m., or s.c.	
Fentanyl	0.04 mg/kg i.v.		0.055 mg/kg i.v.

were unchanged. All values were within the limits of normal hemodynamic function. High-dose alfentanil has no adverse effects on hemodynamic parameters during calcium blockade (46).

Sufentanil in 10 to 30 mcg/kg doses in severe coronary artery disease patients maintained on their preoperative medications does not adversely affect the coronary circulation. In some patients, however, regional myocardial metabolic imbalances may occur independent of sufentanil dose in association with a decrease in perfusion pressure (47).

Stable hemodynamics were maintained after a sufentanil bolus induction followed by an infusion flow anesthetic maintenance technique in patients with valvular heart disease. Isolated incidences of hypertension and bradycardia occurred particularly in those patients with aortic valve disease. Of note is the attenuation of the previously described stress response during CPB in CABG patients. Perhaps this is related to the underlying physiology as well as stable sufentanil levels by infusion (48).

The effects of intravenously administered fentanyl (25 and 50 μg/kg) and alfentanil (12.5 and 25 μg/kg) on the noxiously evoked, single-unit activity of cells in the nucleus reticularis gigantocellularis (NRGC) were studied in decerebrate cats. Only cells of the NRGC excited exclusively by supramaximal electrical stimulation of A delta fibers (noxious stimulation) of the superficial radial nerve were studied. The noxiously evoked activity of all cells in the NRGC was suppressed by the administration of opioids (by 58 and 88% for fentanyl, 25 and 50 μg/kg, respectively; by 35 and 78% for alfentanil, 12.5 and 25 μg/kg, respectively). Fentanyl and alfentanil effects were antagonized by the intravenous administration of naloxone. These results indicate that opioid suppression of noxiously evoked activity is seen in neurons located in the brain stem, and thus suppression of brain stem neurons may be important in the production of fentanyl and alfentanil analgesia (49).

No single anesthetic agent has been shown to encompass rapid onset, short duration of action, amnesia, analgesia, cardiovascular stability, and freedom from side effects. Narcotics can be given as an adjunct to a thiopental anesthetic induction to take advantage of each agent's useful properties. The analgesic properties of the narcotics can be combined with the rapid hypnotic effect of the barbiturates. Low-dose sufentanil, 0.5 and 1.0 μg/kg, reduced the thiopental requirements by 50 to 68% and improved hemodynamic stability during laryngoscopy and intubation in healthy patients (50).

The use of opioids as preanesthetics prior to inducing general anesthesia may dramatically effect dosage requirements as well. As an index to usage of opioid and other analgesics in animals, the dosage guide shown in Table 4.3 may be used.

Dosage adjustments should be made when there is evidence of disease or conditions influencing the response to these agents. Of special concern are those conditions which result in depressed respiratory function.

References

1. Soma LR: Behavioral changes and the assessment of pain in animals. *Proc 2nd Intl Cong Vet Anes* 38–41, 1985.
2. Carstens E: Neurophysiological mechanisms of nociception. *Prof 2nd Intl Cong Vet Anes* 48–52, 1985.
3. Fields HL, Heinricher MM: Anatomy and physiology of a nociceptive modulatory system. *Philos Trans R Soc Lond (Biol)* 308(1136):361–374, 1985.
4. Steedman WM, Molony V, Iggo A: Nociceptive neurones in the superficial dorsal horn of cat lumbar spinal cord and their primary afferent inputs. *Exp Brain Res* 58(1):171–182, 1985.
5. Mense S: Basic neurobiologic mechanisms of pain and analgesia. *Am J Med* 14;75(5A):4–14, 1983.
6. Duggan AW: Pharmacology of descending control systems. *Philos Trans R Soc Lond (Biol)* 308(1136):375–391, 1985.
7. Guilbaud G: Thalamic nociceptive systems. *Philos Trans R Soc Lond (Biol)* 308(1136):339–345, 1985.
8. Young RF, Perryman KM: Pathways for orofacial pain sensation in the trigeminal brain-stem nuclear complex of the Macaque monkey. *J Neurosurg* 61(3):563–568, 1984.
9. Quirion R: Pain, nociception and spinal opioid receptors. *Prog Neuropsychopharmacol Biol Psychiatry* 8(4–6):571–579, 1984.
10. Yaksh TL: Pharmacology of spinal adrenergic systems which modulate spinal nociceptive processing. *Pharmacol Biochem Behav* 22(5):845–858, 1985.
11. Bloom FE: The endorphins. *Ann Rev Pharmacol Toxicol* 23:151–

170, 1983.

12. Davis GC: Endorphins and pain. *Psychiatr Clin North Am* 6(3):473–487, 1983.
13. Randich A, Maixner W: Interactions between cardiovascular and pain regulatory systems. *Neurosci Biobehav Rev* 8(3):343–367, 1984.
14. Ammons WS, Foreman RD: Cardiovascular and T2-T4 dorsal horn cell responses to gallbladder distention in the cat. *Brain Res* 321(2):267–277, 1984.
15. Erickson HH, Kitchell RL: Pain perception and alleviation in animals. *Fed Proc* 43(5):1307–1312, 1984.
16. Kuraishi Y, Harada Y, Aratani S, Satoh M, Takagi H: Separate involvement of the spinal noradrenergic and serotonergic systems in morphine analgesia: the differences in mechanical and thermal algesic tests. *Brain Res* 273(2):245–252, 1983.
17. Roos A, Rydenhag B, Andersson S: Activity in cortical cells after stimulation of tooth pulp afferents in the cat. Extracellular analysis. *Pain* 16(1):61–72, 1983.
18. Jaffe JH, Martin WR: Opioid analgesics and antagonists. *The Pharmacological Basis of Therapeutics*. New York, Goodman and Gilman, 6th ed., 494–534.
19. Noel MA, Byrne WL: The effect of morphine upon CSF opioids in dogs. *Neuropeptides* 5(4–6):429–432, 1985.
20. Matsumiya T, Sawa A, Ishizuka Y, Oka T: The effects of morphine, naloxone and capsaicin on C-fiber reflex and heat evoked discharge in acute spinal cats. *Tokai J Exp Clin Med* 9(1):13–20, 1984.
21. Buchweitz E, Grandison L, Weiss HR: Effect of morphine on regional cerebral oxygen consumption and supply. *Brain Res* 291(2):301–308, 1984.
22. Drago F, Panissidi G, Bellomio F, Dal Bello A, Aguglia E, Gorgone G: Effects of opiates and opioids on intraocular pressure of rabbits and humans. *Clin Exp Pharmacol Physiol* 12(2):107–113, 1985.
23. King FG, Baxter AD, Mathieson G: Tissue reaction of morphine applied to the epidural space of dogs. *Can Anaesth Soc J* 31(3 Pt 1):268–271, 1984.
24. Pant KK, Gurtu S, Sinha JN, Tangri KK, Bhargava KP: Spinal site of antiarrhythmic action of morphine and pethidine in normal and spinal cord transected dogs. *J Auton Pharmacol* 4(1):11–15, 1984.
25. Ayromlooi J: Hemodynamic and acid-base effects of meperidine on unanesthetized pregnant sheep and fetus. *Pediatr Pharmacol (New York)* 5(1):49–55, 1985.
26. Fioramonti J, Fargeas MJ, Bu'eno L: Comparative effects of morphine and cyclazocine on gastrointestinal motility in conscious dogs. *Arch Int Pharmacodyn Ther* 270(1):141–150, 1984.
27. Maas CL, Leek BF: Central and local actions of opioids upon reticulo-ruminal motility in sheep. *Vet Res Commun* 9(2):89–113, 1985.
28. Strombeck DR, Harrold D: Effects of atropine, acepromazine, meperidine, and xylazine on gastroesophageal sphincter pressure in the dog. *Am J Vet Res* 46(4):963–965, 1985.
29. Kostritsky-Pereira A, Woussen-Colle MC, De Graef J: Effects of morphine, enkephalins and naloxone on postprandial gastric acid secretion, gastric emptying and gastrin release in dogs. *Arch Int Physiol Biochim* 92(1):19–26, 1984.
30. Mailman D: Morphine-neural interactions on canine intestinal absorption and blood flow. *Br J Pharmacol* 81(2):263–270, 1984.
31. Tverskoy M, Gelman S, Fowler KC, Bradley EL: Influence of fentanyl and morphine on intestinal circulation. *Anesth Analg* 64(6):577–584, 1985.
32. Werther GA, Joffe S, Artal R, Sperling MA: Opiate modulation of glucose turnover in dogs. *Metabolism* 34(2):136–140, 1985.
33. Pircio AW, Gylys JA, Cavanagh RL: The pharmacology of butorphanol, a 3,14-dihydroxymorphinan narcotic antagonist analgesic. *Arch Int Pharmacodyn Ther* 220:231–256, 1976.
34. Pachter IJ, Evens RP: Butorphanol. *Drug Alcohol Depend* 14(3–4):324–338, 1985.
35. Kalpravidh M, Lumb WV, Wright M, Heath RB: Effects of butorphanol, flunixin levorphanol, morphine, and xylazine in ponies. *Am J Vet Res* 45(2):217, 223, 1984.
36. Arndt JO, Mikat M, Parasher C: Fentanyl's analgesic, respiratory, and cardiovascular actions in relation to dose and plasma concentration in unanesthetized dogs. *Anesthesiology* 61(4):355–361, 1984.
37. Kamerling SG, Weckman TJ, DeQuick DJ, Tobin T: A method for studying cutaneous pain perception and analgesia in horses. *J Pharmacol Methods* 13(3):267–274, 1985.
38. Philbin DM, Föex P, Drummond G, Lowenstein E, Ryder WS, Jones LA: Postsystolic shortening of canine left ventricle supplied by a stenotic coronary artery when nitrous oxide is added in the presence of narcotics. *Anesthesiology* 62(2):166–174, 1985.
39. Bardon T, Ruckebusch Y: Comparative effects of opiate agonists on proximal and distal colonic motility in dogs. *Eur J Pharmacol* 110(3):329–334, 1985.
40. Kissin I, Brown PT: Reserpine-induced changes in anesthetic action of fentanyl. *Anesthesiology* 62(5):597–600, 1985.
41. Motomura S, Kissin I, Aultman DF, Reves JG: Effects of fentanyl and nitrous oxide on contractility of blood-perfused papillary muscle of the dog. *Anesth Analg* 63(1):47–50, 1984.
42. Craft JB Jr, Robichaux AG, Kim HS, Thorpe DH, Mazel P, Woolf WA, Stolte A: The maternal and fetal cardiovascular effects of epidural fentanyl in the sheep model. *Am J Obstet Gynecol* 148(8):1098–1104, 1984.
43. Mather LE: Clinical pharmacokinetics of fentanyl and its newer derivatives. *Clinical Pharmacokinetics* 8:422–446, 1983.
44. Ghoneim MM, Dhanaraj J, Choi WW: Comparison of four opioid analgesics as supplements to nitrous oxide anesthesia. *Anesth Analg* 63:405–412, 1984.
45. D'Aubioul J, Van Gerven W, Van de Water A, Xhonneux R, Reneman RS: Cardiovascular and some respiratory effects of high doses of alfentanil in dogs. *Eur J Pharmacol* 100(1):79–84, 1984.
46. Lehd Pedersen J, Strom J, Berthelsen P, Eriksen J, Rasmussen JP: Hemodynamic effects of alfentanil in verapamil-treated dogs. *Acta Anaesthesiol Scand* 29(3):354–357, 1985.
47. Lappas DG, Palacios I, Athanasiadis C, Mastrocostopoulos G, Hilgenberg A, O'Young J, Elia S, Skonitis C: Sufentanil dosage and myocardial blood flow in metabolism in patients with coronary artery disease. *Anesthesiology* 63(3A):A58, 1985.
48. Samuelson PN, Reves JG, Kirklin JK, George J, Bradley EL, Wilson KD, Barker S, Oparil S, Adams ML: Sufentanil infusion anesthesia in patients undergoing valvular heart disease. *Anesthesiology* 63(3A):A74, 1985.
49. Yuge O, Kitahata LM, Collins JG, Matsumoto M, Tabatabai M, Suzukawa M, Tanaka A: Fentanyl and alfentanil suppress brainstem pain transmission. *Anesth Analg* 64(6):595–600, 1985.
50. Brizgys RV, Morales R, Owens B: Low-dose sufentanil: Effects on thiopental requirements and hemodynamic response during induction and intubation. *Anesthesiology* 63(3A):A377, 1985.

CHAPTER

5

Neuroleptanalgesia and Alpha-Adrenergic Receptor Analgesia

CHARLES E. SHORT, D.V.M., M.S., D.A.C.V.A.

Neuroleptanalgesia is often considered as the altered state of consciousness and inhibited responses resulting from a combination of tranquilizer and analgesic medication. Although neuroleptanalgesia will be influenced by the medications used and their dosages, it should accomplish two basic objectives: the patient should be free from pain and in a state of euphoria. In neuroleptanalgesia, the tranquilizer is used to reduce fright and calm the animal while the analgesic controls pain.

Neuroleptanalgesia is used for those procedures that require less than total anesthesia but more central nervous system (CNS) control than can be accomplished by a tranquilizer or analgesic alone. The most widely used commercially prepared neuroleptanalgesia is Innovar Vet, a combination of fentanyl and droperidol. This combination is more often used in dogs than in other species. The usual dosage in dogs is 1 ml/7 to 9 kg i.m. or 1 ml/10 to 25 kg i.v. Maximum effects are normally observed within 5 to 10 minutes of intravenous and 20 to 30 minutes of intramuscular administration. The dogs have adequate analgesia for minor procedures. They tend to sleep, but they are responsive to noise or sudden movement (1). The most pronounced effect lasts 30 to 60 minutes depending on route of administration.

Unless an anticholinergic has been administered, heart rates slow with Innovar Vet. The electrocardiographic (ECG) pattern is usually that of sinus bradycardia with Innovar Vet; however, one may observe heart block in an occasional dog. Blood pressure does not significantly increase. During profound bradycardia, tissue perfusion may suffer. This is further complicated by depression of ventilation. The respiratory rate may increase, but tidal volume decreases. With Innovar Vet, a decrease in arterial pH and PaO_2 with increases in $PaCO_2$ may occur.

ECGs recorded in dogs receiving Innovar Vet demonstrated adequate narcosis for up to 60 minutes. Tail wagging can begin within 30 to 40 minutes after i.v. administration of the drug (2).

Because electroencephalographic studies did not show adverse responses, added emphasis must be placed on the role of cardiopulmonary function as contributing to post-Innovar personality changes in dogs. Some dogs show alteration in behavioral patterns (which some fail to recognize) during the 24-hour to 1-week period after Innovar Vet. Most changes do not last more than 1 week. These behavioral changes have occurred more often in dogs receiving no anticholinergic or those receiving higher dosages of Innovar Vet without reversal with an antagonist. Dogs presented for Caesarean section receiving Innovar Vet, placed in dorsal recumbancy, and receiving no supplemental oxygen are prime candidates for related hypoxia and postdrug behavioral changes. Narcotic antagonists only affect the fentanyl component of the combination. Innovar Vet provides longer tranquilization than analgesia. This becomes significant when repeat dosages are given, because these dogs may undergo prolonged periods of tranquilization.

Innovar Vet may also be used in swine, especially pigs, at the same dosage as in dogs. It has been used in laboratory animals, particularly the rabbit. Use in cats or horses has not produced acceptable results. Analgesia is produced in the horse, but unpredictable CNS responses were observed. The fixed ratio of Innovar Vet and the somewhat casual attitude toward its use in humans has led to complications due to inadequate maintenance of cardiopulmonary and CNS function. Use of the components as separate injections has resulted; in animal neuroleptanalgesia, separate administration of fentanyl and droperidol did not follow as a popular use.

Other drug combinations became popular. The combination of oxymorphone and acetylpromazine became widely used in dogs and cats. Acetylpromazine is administered at 0.05 to 0.10 mg/kg i.m. or i.v. followed by 0.2 mg/kg of oxymorphone i.v. Total dosages of over 6 mg of oxymorphone are seldom used. Bolus injections are usual, but slow i.v. infusions provide a means of control of dosage. The onset by bolus technique is within 5 minutes, with a duration of up to 3 hours. Tranquilization may last up to 24 hours. This same combination can be used in horses; however, other combinations are more frequently employed.

In the horse, acetylpromazine, 0.06 mg/kg, and methadone, 0.04 mg/kg, i.v. was the first popular neuroleptanalgesia combination. Acetylpromazine and meperidine, acetylpromazine and pentazocine, xylazine and butorphanol, xylazine and morphine, and xylazine and methadone have been used (3).

The responses observed are reasonably predictable if the characteristics of each drug in the combination are evaluated. In neuroleptanalgesia, using xylazine as a component will result in greater analgesia than if acetylpromazine is used, but there is a greater chance of reduced heart rate. Meperidine use in the horse was associated with a higher incidence of CNS excitement than methadone. Butorphanol did not produce as much depression as morphine. Morphine and xylazine were shown to produce a very effective level of analgesia in the horse, but there were three areas of concern. The heart rate slows as a result of the influence of xylazine, and respiration is depressed due to the influence of morphine. If inadequate levels of xylazine are used, CNS excitement from morphine could occur in the horse. Corrective anticholinergic administration to prevent or control bradycardia and oxygen to correct hypoxia were effective.

Combinations to produce neuroleptanalgesia in ruminants have been used on rare occasions, but extensive development has not progressed, probably due to the effectiveness of xylazine as a single agent in this group of animals. One study has been completed in sheep. The immobilizing action of Immobyl (fentanyl and azaperone, 5:1) in six sheep has been analyzed on the basis of the changes in dopamine, noradrenaline, adrenalin, homovanillic acid, and 5-hydroxytryptamine (5-HT) concentrations in the corpus striatum, frontal motor cortex, pons, cerebellum, and lumbosacral spinal cord as compared to control animals given saline. Forty minutes after i.m. injection of an immobilizing dose of 0.19 mg/kg body weight, Immobyl caused a significant decrease in dopamine, noradrenaline, and 5-hydroxytryptamine concentrations and a similarly large decrease in homovanillic acid concentration (47%) in the corpus striatum, with a simultaneous but insignificant increase in the concentrations of these substances in the frontal motor cortex region. With Immobyl neuroleptanalgesia, sheep showed a significant increase in dopamine concentration with an equally significant decrease in homovanillic acid concentrations in the lumbosacral part of the spinal cord. It is suggested that fentanyl stimulates the presynaptic dopamine receptors in the corpus striatum in sheep, significantly decreasing synthesis and release of dopamine and noradrenalin and intensifying an inhibitory effect of the corpus striatum on locomotor activity and thus causing the immobilization of the animal (4).

Neuroleptanesthesia

Neuroleptanalgesia is not always adequate for planned procedures. Should more drug be given, or should other agents be administered? Efforts to provide appropriate anesthesia after the use of neuroleptanalgesia have resulted in a state of neuroleptanesthesia. This state of anesthesia may also be referred to as balanced anesthesia. Neuroleptanesthesia often provides a means to reduce the undesirable responses of the animal to potent anesthetics that may depress cardiac function. It should be evident that the usage of concurrent medications increases the need for patient monitoring and an understanding of the interactions of each of the medications involved.

Neuroleptanesthesia usually includes tranquilizer, analgesic, nitrous oxide, and oxygen. In many cases, muscle relaxants are used to provide convenience for the surgical procedure. An example of neuroleptanesthesia in the dog is glycopyrrolate and acetylpromazine as preanesthetics, oxymorphone or fentanyl for anesthesia, nitrous oxide for additional analgesia, and pancuronium, a paralytic muscle relaxant, to provide complete muscle relaxation. This procedure will require controlled ventilation. Because nitrous oxide is relatively inpotent in animals, supplemental administration of the opioid analgesics is still necessary (5).

In animals deeply anesthetized with fentanyl and nitrous oxide, the arterial blood pressure and heart rate were increased using dopamine, atropine, electrical pacing, and phenylephrine in order to study the accompanying change in whole body oxygen consumption. Seven dogs (16 to 24 kg) were anesthetized with fentanyl, 1 μg/kg/min. After completing instrumentation, a dopamine infusion was started at a rate of 39 μg/kg/min. After the mean blood pressure reached 18.6 kPa, the infusion was reduced to 10 μg/kg/min and maintained for 10 minutes. After waiting 45 minutes, an infusion of atropine 20 μg/kg/min was started. When the heart rate reached 120 b.p.m., the infusion was slowed to 1.25 μg/kg/min and maintained for 10 minutes; 25 minutes later, the heart rate was increased to 140 b.p.m. and maintained at that level for 10 minutes using electrical pacing. The pacing was removed, and an infusion of phenylephrine, 5 μg/kg/min, was started. When the blood pressure reached 21.3 kPa, the infusion was reduced to 2.5 μg/kg/min and maintained for 10 minutes. The results show increases in oxygen consumption of 14% with dopamine, 19% with atropine, and 16% with phenylephrine. All changes were significantly different from the control values (6).

The responses of the horse to xylazine-morphine or Immobin show effective analgesia, physical control, and reversability. Reversal of the opioid as the procedure is completed will contribute to improvement in cardiopulmonary function.

Fifteen to 20 years ago, neuroleptanalgesia was considered preferable to barbiturate anesthesia in dogs at high risk because of greater cardiovascular stability and a more controllable duration of action. However, in some situations when used alone or for major surgery in the dog, cardiovascular instability and prolonged depression was found to occur due to the depressant effects of the tranquilizer. As a result, the trend has been to use neuroleptanalgesia only for minor procedures (7).

The inclusion of an opioid as a component of balanced anesthesia offers many advantages, with the major effect being less fluctuation in cardiovascular dynamics. The decreased requirements for potent inhalation agents and provisions for postoperative analgesia are also advantageous (7).

For major surgery in high risk patients, sedatives and hypnotics may be used with a narcotic, a muscle relaxant, nitrous oxide, and/or a potent inhalation anesthetic to produce desired levels of anesthesia with concurrent stability of cardiopulmonary function. This approach to anesthesia for major surgery can be safe and effective. It does, however, require close attention to the details of anesthesia and patient monitoring. The addition of muscle relaxants requires controlled ventilation, and monitoring of vital functions with equipment is justified. In humans these requirements are met; however, in veterinary anesthesia, equipment and personnel availability may limit the use of neuroleptanalgesia to shorter procedures.

Alpha-adrenoceptor Analgesia

One of the problems associated with large animal anesthesia is the selection of medications for anesthesia for standing procedures or for prolonged surgical procedures requiring injectable medications rather than inhalant anesthetic approaches. Various combinations that suffice for this purpose include tranquilizers and narcotics to produce neuroleptanalgesia, as discussed earlier. Included in this group of agents have been combinations of acepromazine and methadone, acepromazine and meperidine, xylazine and morphine (8, 9, 10, 12), and a host of others (8, 11, 13). Such combinations should provide adequate analgesia for minor surgical procedures and at the same time produce a horse that is calm and easily handled. When standing procedures are not considered appropriate, combinations of preanesthetic agents followed by agents such as ketamine or combinations of muscle relaxants and barbiturates including sodium thiamylal and guaifenesin have been used for induction of general anesthesia. Supplemental dosages, either intermittently or by continuous intravenous drip, have been used to prolong such anesthesia for surgical procedures lasting more than 5 to 10 minutes. The need for profound analgesic agents that will facilitate safe standing surgical procedures and analgetic combinations that can precede the administration of safe and effective field anesthesia continues. The alpha-adrenoceptor analgesics have been represented by xylazine.

Observations of the responses in laboratory animals (14) and in horses (15, 16) to a new analgetic/sedative injectable, detomidine hydrochloride, showed profound relaxation and analgesia, but with subjective changes of cardiovascular function. The responses were related to those observed with xylazine (7, 12, 17), but with more profound sedation, due to activation of alpha-2 adrenoceptors (16, 18, 19, 20, 21).

Detomidine was discovered during the development of alpha-adrenoceptor agonists. It is appropriate to consider xylazine as a tranquilizer and sedative because it is so frequently used for those purposes. It is discussed in Chapter 3. Xylazine is also our first major alpha-adrenoceptor agonist. An awareness of the characteristics of these medications is necessary. What is an alpha-adrenoceptor?

INTRODUCTION TO ADRENOCEPTOR PHARMACOLOGY

The sympathetic "fight or flight" response of an animal is evoked by hormonal and neuronal impulses coordinated by the CNS. These peripheral impulse pathways mainly use different transmitters and reach different targets through different distribution (innervation or vascular bed) and receptors (alpha or beta adrenoceptors) (22).

The pharmacological compounds reach their targets from the vascular bed depending on their physiochemical characteristics. Thus, for instance, small lipophilic compounds reach the CNS effectively and therefore have a targeting of the response.

Another factor in targeting the pharmacological effect is the specific binding of the compound to adrenoceptors. Alpha-adrenoceptors for noradrenaline can be divided to definite subtypes alpha-1 and alpha-2 using specific agonists and antagonists. This specificity cannot be reached with compounds having an indirect effect on adrenergic transmission, such as reserpine, amphetamine, or monoamine oxidase (MAO) inhibitors.

It is obvious that the adrenoceptor subtypes have different mechanisms on the cell membrane. Alpha-2 adrenoceptor activation seems to inhibit the release of Na and other neurotransmitters by inhibiting CA^{++} influx in the membrane. However, they have similar effects on some other secretory cells, such as platelets, gastric mucosa, and endocrine pancreas. A further classification of alpha-2 adrenoceptors on different cells is anticipated in the future.

The adrenoceptor agonists and antagonists are thought to transmit or block sympathetic responses. However, the discovery of presynaptic regulation of transmitter release opened a new level of specific effects: modulation of reactivity in different neurotransmitter systems. Modulation of neuronal activity became even more interesting after the finding of cotransmitters in neurones (22).

SUBTYPES AND FUNCTIONS OF ALPHA-ADRENOCEPTORS

The alpha-adrenoceptors may be subdivided based on a pharmacological characterization in which selective agonists and antagonists are used or on their anatomical distribution within the synapse. The $alpha_1$-adrenoceptor is stimulated preferentially by methoxamine, cirazoline, and phenylephrine and blocked selectively by prazosin and corynanthine. The $alpha_2$-adrenoceptor is stimulated preferentially by agonists such as clonidine, and the responses mediated by these agonists are selectively blocked by the $alpha_2$-adrenoceptor antagonists yohimbine, rauwolscine, and idaxozan (23).

In blood vessels, both the $alpha_1$ and $alpha_2$-adrenoceptor subtypes are present postsynaptically, where they mediate vasoconstriction, although the $alpha_1$-adrenoceptor is the predominant receptor in vascular smooth muscle. Presynaptically, on noradrenergic nerve terminals, the stimulation of inhibitory $alpha_2$-adrenoceptors reduces the depolarization-evoked release of the transmitter. The alpha-adrenoceptors in the central nervous system that mediate the central hypotensive and sedative effects of clonidine and related drugs are probably of the $alpha_2$-subtype. These central $alpha_2$-adrenoceptors are probably similar to $alpha_2$-adrenoceptors in the periphery (23).

Although there are several unresolved issues, $alpha_1$- and $alpha_2$-receptor activation at a cellular level may possess different mechanisms for signal transduction. Thus, postjunctional $alpha_2$-receptors that mediate the contraction of some vascular preparations appear to be more dependent upon the entry of extracellular calcium. The activation of $alpha_1$-adrenoceptors may initiate a train of events in which the breakdown of inositol phospholipids somehow brings about a mobilization of calcium within the stimulated cells.

ALPHA-ADRENOCEPTOR ROLE IN VIGILANCE AND PAIN REGULATION

Alertness correlates with increased activity in cortical neurons and release of noradrenaline (NA) from cortical terminals is one contributing factor. Activation of $beta_1$-receptors increases cAMP and cellular metabolism, but $alpha_1$-agonists are at least as effectively arousing. $Alpha_2$-agonists such as xylazine, clonidine, detomidine, and medetomidine are sedative and may be counteracted with $alpha_2$-antagonist drugs (24).

Noradrenergic neurons in the locus coeruleus project diffusely to the forebrain, probably modulating cortical and limbic activity in conjunction with other ascending transmitter systems from the brain stem. The locus coeruleus neurons are inhibited by systemic $alpha_2$-agonists; in addition, however, their terminals are inhibited by $alpha_2$-receptor activation. Sedation is conceivably the result of diminished activity in the ascending NA projection. However, as neonatal destruction of this projection does not normally disturb regulation of vigilance in the adult, it is apparent that there are other regulating systems that may counteract $alpha_2$-agonist sedatives during prolonged medication (24).

The noradrenergic involvement in the modulation of pain is more complex. Like 5-HT, noradrenaline inhibits spinal nociceptive neurons, but the anatomical origin of the descending NA projection is unclear. Whereas 5-HT and NA thus may act synergistically on pain modulating in the spinal cord, some NA neurons in the brain stem inhibit those 5-HT neurons in the raphe nuclei that are pain-modulating. While the alpha-antagonist phentolamine reduces pain when injected into the raphe, its effect is blocked by 5-HT antagonists, showing that it acts through 5-HT. Systemic administration of $alpha_2$-agonists has an analgetic effect. The action may be spinal, but it may also result from direct depression of such NA neurons in the brain stem as inhibit the pain-modulating 5-HT system (24). In addition, there is interaction between opiate and NA mechanisms.

PHARMACOLOGY OF DETOMIDINE AND OTHER ALPHA$_2$-ADRENOCEPTOR AGONISTS IN THE CNS

Detomidine (Fig. 5.1) is a very potent agonist at pre- and postsynaptic alpha$_2$-adrenoceptors. In receptor binding experiments with rat brain membranes, detomidine shows strong affinity to alpha$_2$-receptors. There is some binding affinity toward alpha$_1$-receptors also, but only negligible or no affinity toward dopamine, opiate, and adenosine receptors. In electrically stimulated mouse vas deferens preparation, detomidine causes a concentration-dependent inhibition of the twitch response, which effect can be antagonized by alpha$_2$-blocking agents. In rat anococcygeal muscle and rabbit aorta preparations, detomidine was shown to have partial alpha$_1$-stimulating effects at high concentrations (25).

Detomidine causes a dose-dependent inhibition of NA (but not dopamine or 5-HT) turnover and release in rat CNS. This effect can be antagonized by administration of alpha$_2$-adrenoceptor blocking agents. Inhibition of sympathetic tone in the CNS by alpha$_2$-agonists leads to a characteristic pattern of pharmacological responses. Cardiovascular effects such as bradycardia and initial hypertension of detomidine are partly of central origin. Detomidine has no hypnotic properties even after high doses. An in vivo receptor binding study in the rat showed that a detomidine-induced decrease in spontaneous activity was significantly correlated with ^{3}H-clodine but not with ^{3}H-prazosin displacement in brain membranes. Accordingly, it has been shown that the sedative effects of detomidine can be inhibited by antagonists of alpha$_2$ but not alpha$_1$-adrenoceptors (25).

CARDIOVASCULAR EFFECTS OF DETOMIDINE IN LABORATORY ANIMALS

Detomidine is a potent sedative and analgesic drug that has proved to be clinically efficient, especially in horses and cattle. Its mechanism of action has been related to an alpha$_2$-adrenoceptor-stimulating property in the CNS. Because the underlying mechanism of the sedative and analgesic action of detomidine seems to involve stimulation of the same subpopulation of alpha-adrenoceptors as that of clonidine and related drugs that are well-known antihypertensive agents, it was reasonable to expect detomidine to have cardiovascular effects. Can detomidine be used to separate "sedative" alpha$_2$-adrenoceptors from "antihypertensive" alpha$_2$-adrenoceptors (26)? Xylazine, which is a sedative and antinociceptive drug already widely used in veterinary practice, has a similar mechanism of action.

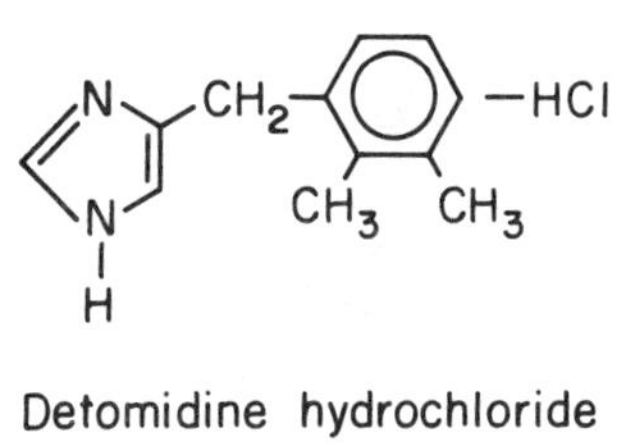

Figure 5.1. Detomidine hydrochloride

After i.v. administration of detomidine (1 to 3 μg/kg) and xylazine (10 to 1000 μg/kg) to anesthetized normotensive Wistar rats, a hypotensive and bradycardic effect in a dose-dependent manner was observed. On the other hand, when detomidine (30 to 1000 μg/kg) was given s.c. to conscious spontaneously hypertensive Okamoto-Aoki rats, relatively high doses had to be used to obtain a significant decrease in blood pressure, although heart rate was reduced with much lower doses. Xylazine (1 to 10 mg/kg s.c.) had both antihypertensive and bradycardia effects. In pithed rats, both detomidine (0.3 to 30 μg/kg i.v.) and xylazine (3 to 1000 μg/kg i.v.) induced alpha$_2$-adrenoceptor-mediated postsynaptic responses and presynaptic sympathoinhibitory actions. The alpha$_2$-adrenoceptor-mediated hypotensive and bradycardic effect was shown directly in anesthetized cats by infusing a low dose of detomidine into the vertebral artery. The effect was greater than after systemic application; it could be antagonized by idazoxan, an alpha$_2$-adrenoceptor-blocking drug (26).

The results indicate that detomidine is an agonist of central and peripheral alpha$_2$-adrenoceptors that exerts hypotensive and bradycardic effects via activation of the central alpha$_2$-adrenoceptors. In conscious rats, detomidine did not decrease blood pressure as readily as xylazine, but the basic mechanism for the observed difference was not demonstratable in these experiments.

PHARMACOKINETICS OF DETOMIDINE

The pharmacokinetics of detomidine after the administration of a single dose was studied in laboratory animals and cattle with tritium-labeled molecules and in horses using radioimmunoassay (RIA). The results showed a rapid distribution into rat tissues, including the brain, after a subcutaneous dose. In the plasma/serum curves of each species, a first distribution phase with a half-life of a few minutes and a redistribution with a half-life of 0.5 to 2.5 hours were found. These distribution phases seem to be important factors controlling the fast onset and evidently dose-dependent termination of the clinical effects. The apparent volumes of distribution ranged from 6.8 to 37.7 liter/kg, and plasma clearances ranged from 44.4 to 34.6 ml/min/kg. Elimination half-lives were between 9.7 and 22.1 hours depending on the species and method of analysis (27). Elimination from tissues of the rat followed approximately the time course of elimination from plasma. Excretion into urine seemed to be a major elimination route, although a small fraction was also excreted into feces. The total excretion ranged from 60 to 81% of the dose in 3 days. Residues observed in calf tissue 24 hours postdose were at the p.p.b. level. Peak concentration was reached in 15 minutes after i.m. doses to calf, indicating rapid absorption. No differences in elimination were found between i.v. and i.m. doses; neither was there any dose dependence in the kinetic parameters within the 50 to 300 mcg/kg range used in cattle (27).

PHARMACOLOGICAL PROFILE OF DETOMIDINE IN HORSES AND CATTLE

The hemodynamic effect of detomidine is hypertensive at the dose levels above approximately 20 μg/kg and hypotensive at the lower doses. Bradycardia is found at all clinical dose levels. Conductivity disturbances (second degree atrioventricular (AV) blocks and sinoatrial (SA) blocks) have been observed in horses. Atropine, 0.01 mg/kg, does not abolish them, but the duration of their existence shortens (28).

Respiratory effects of detomidine are variable. The frequency of respiration varies. On average, a slight respiratory stimulation in horses and a depression in cattle has been observed. However, changes in the blood gas (pO_2 and pCO_2) values have not been observed.

In addition to the sedative, analgesic, cardiovascular, and respiratory effects, detomidine has still other effects that are attributed to the alpha$_2$-adrenoceptor agonism mechanism of action. These effects are common to all drugs acting via the same mechanism. Piloerection and sweating has been observed in horses, as has salivation and tympany in cattle. Preliminary work *in vitro* and *in vivo* give clues to the fact that detomidine does not contract the uterus muscle. Furthermore, detomidine has no proved teratogenic or mutagenic properties (28). Detomidine has been successfully combined with other sedatives (xylazine and phenothiazine derivatives), local anesthetics (lidocaine), and general anesthetics (ketamine, barbiturates, guaifenesin, and halothane).

ANALGESIC AND SEDATIVE EFFECTS OF DETOMIDINE

Using a balloon-induced colic model in a double-blind study on 10 ponies, 4 dose levels and placebo were compared in 50 i.v. and 50 i.m. trials. Ten i.v. and 10 i.m. trials using the same ponies were also conducted to compare recommended levels of xylazine to detomidine. Excellent analgesia/sedation was obtained and appeared dose-related at 20, 80, and 160 μg/kg. Mean duration of effect for i.v. routes was 45, 105, and 239 minutes and for i.m. routes, 25, 90, and 225 minutes. Five μg/kg was ineffective by either route. Xylazine was effective by either route, but of short duration compared to detomidine (29).

Single blind studies were completed to objectively determine the strength and duration of analgetic and/or sedative effects of detomidine over a range of doses (0, 5, 20, 80, and 160 μg/kg BW) and in comparison with xylazine. Six animals were used in a Latin-Square design. For analgesia, a method to measure changes in pain threshold to electrical pain stimulation was adapted from rodents. Pain was inflicted on the left coronary band of the front and hind legs and to the perineal area (30).

At a dose level of 20 μg/kg or higher given i.v., all animals responded with deep sedation. Although the strength of sedation did not increase much with higher doses, duration did. Depending on the parameters used, duration increased from 0 to almost 4 hours. After giving detomidine i.m., strength and duration of sedation was similar, but of shorter duration. Xylazine provided a short-lived sedation of 15 to 30 minutes when given i.v. and an unsatisfactory sedation when given i.m. (30).

Analgesia with detomidine was dose-dependent in strength and duration. Duration was longest at the front legs and shortest at the perineal area; 20 μg/kg i.b. provided analgesia to the front legs only; 80 μg/kg i.v. reduced pain at all locations from 0.70 to 0.80 hours; 160 μg/kg i.v. reduced pain from 1.5 to 3.00 hours ($r = 0.95$). After i.m. injection, 20 μg was ineffective; the analgesic effects of 80 and 160 μg were shorter (0.25 and 0.75 hours) and changes in pain thresholds were smaller ($r = 0.89$). Peak levels of sedation occurred later after i.m. administration. Xylazine provides analgesia that was significantly less pronounced than that with 20 μg/kg of detomidine when given i.v. Xylazine administered i.m. had no measurable analgetic effects (30).

The effect of the potent alpha$_2$-adrenoceptor agonist detomidine on brain potentials and pain reactions evoked by electrical stimulation of the chorium of the hoof has been compared to xylazine. Evoked potentials (EPs) were recorded from scalp electrodes in three horses with implanted electrodes for electrical stimulation of the chorium of the hoof. A recording with previously implanted electrodes for corticography was made in one horse for comparison. EPs to single pulses of 2 and 5 ms duration at 10-second intervals were tape-recorded and selectively averaged. Reaction thresholds (RTs) were visually observed. Recording was made before drugs and at half-hour intervals after 10, 20, and 60 μg/kg of detomidine i.v. In one horse, xylazine was tested at 300, 600, and 900 mg/kg; in another horse, it was tested at 600 mg/kg i.v. Doses were given in random order at several-day intervals (31).

Detomidine induced sedation within 5 minutes; 10 μg/kg increased the RT 2- or 3-fold for 30 to 60 minutes; 20 μg/kg increased the RT more, and the effect lasted about 90 minutes. After 60 μg/kg, the RT remained high for 3 hours. With respect to the effect on RTs, 300 μg/kg xylazine was comparable to 10 μg/kg detomidine and 900 μg/kg xylazine to 20 μg/kg detomidine.

Reproducible EP waveforms, not obscured by reflex artifacts, had latencies around 90 to 130 ms. Mean amplitudes were consistently dependent on stimulus strength. EPs could sometimes be seen to stimuli that were slightly subthreshold by observation. Detomidine at 10 μg/kg depressed the EEG and EPs profoundly, with a maximum effect between 10 and 30 minutes. After 20 μg/kg, EPs could not at first be elicited even with strong stimuli. After 1 hour, stimuli 5 to 10 times the predrug threshold could evoke similar EPs, and they gradually returned during the second hour after injection. After 60 μg/kg, there was total absence of EPs for 90 minutes, and total recovery took 4 hours. In comparison, restitution of EP amplitudes took place in 30 minutes after 300 mg/kg xylazine, 90 minutes after 600 mg/kg, and 90 minutes after 900 mg/kg. Detomidine was thus effectively analgetic at much lower doses than xylazine, and its effect could be considered to be prolonged by increasing the dose (31).

Specific data for parameters that would be influenced by the drug as an analgetic/sedative, as a preanesthetic prior to barbiturate muscle relaxant induction and maintenance, and as a preanesthetic for a similar induction followed by halothane maintenance have been developed. Mature female horses were used in the study. The treatment groups considered were 20 mcg/kg, 80 mcg/kg, and 160 mcg/kg detomidine hydrochloride i.v. without anesthetic induction and dosage levels of 20 and 60 mcg/kg as a preanesthetic followed by two types of general anesthesia.

Before the studies, each horse had undergone a surgical procedure to exteriorize a carotid artery for collection of arterial samples. Arterial blood gases were determined from samples collected from the carotid artery and analyzed on a Radiometer blood gas analysis system. Other clinical pathological values were made using standardized laboratory instrumentation. Blood pressures were determined using a noninvasive system with a cuff placed on the tail-head for measurements over the coccygeal artery.

During treatments with detomidine alone, the horses were studied for up to 4 hours or until the animal would not tolerate attachments to leads to recording equipment after the calming effect of the drug had disappeared. The parameters evaluated included: ECG, blood pressure (systolic, mean, and diastolic), heart rate, rate pressure product (heart rate × systolic blood pressure as an index to myocardial O_2 demand), and respiratory rates. These parameters were evaluated at 5-minute intervals during the first hour and then at 30-minute intervals until the completion of each experiment. Clinical pathological data included blood, serum, and urine analysis. Each horse had a pretrial evaluation of packed-cell volume, hemoglobin, blood urea nitrogen (BUN), blood glucose, blood gases, pH, liver enzymes, and electrolyte values. At 15 and 30 minutes after the administration of the drug, blood glucose, blood gases, and pH values were determined. One hour after the start of the procedure, BUN, blood glucose, blood gases, pH, and urinalysis were completed; at 4 hours, BUN, blood glucose, blood gases, pH, urinalysis, liver enzymes, and electrolytes were evaluated.

Each horse had a pretrial evaluation of packed cell volume, hemoglobin, BUN, blood glucose, blood gases and pH, liver enzymes, and electrolyte values in Treatments 4 and 5. At 15 and 30 minutes after administration of the drug, blood glucose, blood gases, and pH values were determined. At the time, anesthetic induction with an ultrashort acting barbiturate and muscle relaxant, guaifenesin (glyceral guaicolate), was made. In one-half of the horses, anesthesia was prolonged by maintenance with halothane for 1 hour after induction while monitoring continued. Anesthetic recovery patterns were reviewed. BUN, blood glucose, liver enzymes, and electrolytes were repeated at 4 hours.

Arterial blood gases were determined on samples collected from the carotid artery. Halothane anesthesia was maintained using a large animal anesthetic unit with precision vaporizer. An oxygen flow of 1 liter/100 kg minimum in a semiclosed system with spontaneous breathing was used.

RESULTS

Use as Primary Agent

Each of the eight horses receiving the three dosage levels of detomidine hydrochloride as a sole agent demonstrated the clinical signs of sedation and major analgesia within 2 to 4 minutes after the administration of the drug. Lack of response to external stimuli (i.e., response to pinch, placement of forceps, or other pain stimulus), drooping of the head, a relaxed lower lip, and reduction in coordination was noted. The ability to maintain a standing position in each of the eight horses at each dosage level, especially at 20 mcg and 80 μg/kg, was evident. The horses at 160 μg/kg had more difficulty with coordination. The animals were in restraining stocks. This was an advantage in recording information because the animals did not change position as frequently. In all eight horses at three dosage levels, the inclination to kick, paw, or become excitable was not evident. The duration of analgesia and sedation was 60 minutes at 20 $\mu g/kg$, 180 minutes at 80 $\mu g/kg$, and 210 minutes at 160 $\mu g/kg$. Each animal at each dosage level demonstrated increased urine production, with voluminous urination occurring usually about 60 minutes after the administration of the drug.

Respiratory responses included an initial slowing of respiration within a few seconds to 1 to 2 minutes after the administration of the drug. At the 160 $\mu g/kg$ dosage level, slow respiration lasted up to 5 minutes after the administration of the drug. After this, respiratory rates increased to control values or higher. There was an initial decrease followed by an increase in tidal volume. The respiratory pattern frequently could be described as pauses of up to 30 seconds between breaths, which might be followed by three to eight breaths in a close pattern. Mucous membrane color as an index to tissue level oxygenation deteriorated primarily at the 160 $\mu g/kg$ dosage level. This was confirmed by reduced arterial blood oxygen levels. At the deepest level of analgesia and sedation, usually 14 minutes postinjection, arterial blood gas analysis indicated the lowest level of oxygen available. The arterial pH stayed normal or slightly elevated; in some horses there was evidence of increased ventilation reflected by lower CO_2 values than in controls. Acidosis was not evident in these studies. Fortunately, the myocardial oxygen demands dropped at the same time.

There was an initial drop in blood pressure at the 20 $\mu g/kg$ dosage level, as well as a drop in heart rate. Heart rates also dropped with the 80 and 160 $\mu g/kg$ administrations. At the 80 $\mu g/kg$ level, systolic blood pressures increased within 5 minutes of administration of the drug. The heart rates dropped within 30 to 60 seconds after the administration of detomidine hydrochloride; in some instances, rates dropped as low as 10 to 15 beats/minute. Heart block occurred in several instances. Compensation for drop in heart rates was exemplified in these horses by an increase in systemic blood pressure. In some horses, the heart block or bradycardia that was present was very transient, and in others the bradycardia lasted for up to 60 minutes.

The blood glucose levels increase in the detomidine-treated horses at each dosage has been demonstrated as with xylazine-treated horses. All horses made uneventful recoveries. The most obvious clinical difference in dosage levels was duration of response.

Use as Preanesthetic

Detomidine was used as an effective preanesthetic for either injectable anesthesia or for injectable anesthetic induction followed by halothane maintenance. Studies at 20 mcg/kg as a preanesthetic showed reduction in dosage requirements for induction. Heart rates were slowed with evidence of bradycardia or heart block, as was shown in earlier results of this study. There was reduction in available oxygen but oxygen demand by the myocardium was also decreased during the same period of time.

Blood pressure increased during detomidine use, but dropped during induction of anesthesia. Spontaneous respiration was maintained. Arterial O_2 dropped, but because the horses were exhaling into the atmosphere, arterial CO_2 did not elevate sufficiently for concern. This resulted in an arterial pH that was acceptable.

When halothane was added, low concentrations were required to maintain anesthesia, but heart rates were not further reduced. Respiration slowed, but oxygen levels increased because the horses were breathing an oxygen-enriched mixture.

Blood pressures became stable during halothane maintenance. There was a tendency toward hypotension; myocardial oxygen demand was stable. Arterial CO_2 increased because respiration was depressed with the combination of medications for general anesthesia. With the accumulation of CO_2, arterial pH dropped, although not to the extent of respiratory acidosis.

Similar responses were observed when 60 $\mu g/kg$ of detomidine was used. The main differences were slower recovery and that halothane requirements were lower during the first 40 minutes. There was a lower myocardial oxygen demand due to slower heart rates within 60 $\mu g/kg$. Oxygen levels were not as high with 60 $\mu g/kg$; because neither was $PaCO_2$, acceptable pH levels were maintained. The blood glucose levels increased during the response to detomidine, as was the case when detomidine was used alone.

The characteristics of induction were exemplified by a gradual relaxation and a slow calm drop to recumbency. Heart rates characteristically increased during induction at 30 minutes. During early pretrials to determine types of expected responses, induction of anesthesia at 5 minutes postdetomidine resulted in slow, shallow respiration and weaker blood pressure. This was not demonstrated when induction was delayed 30 minutes after administration of detomidine.

Detomidine can be an effective preanesthetic. Induction of anesthesia 30 minutes after detomidine was characterized by profound relaxation, reduced dosage of other medications, reduced myocardial O_2 demands, reduced respiration, and a trend toward CO_2 accumulation and acidosis. This has been characteristic of other forms of general anesthesia in the horse. One can conclude that detomidine hydrochloride is an effective analgetic with potential for use in a variety of surgical procedures in the standing horse and that its duration is dose-dependent. Detomidine can be used as a safe and effective preanesthetic. It can produce a smooth induction and recovery. Induction should be delayed up to 30 minutes after detomidine for safety. Detomidine dramatically reduces the dosages of other anesthetics that may be used. Increased safety can probably be obtained by administering anticholinergics to control bradycardia or heart block. Careful attention to dosage should be maintained.

If complications do occur, they are most likely relative to overdose of drug combinations with the following potential complications: excessive depression of respiration with associated hypoxia, slow heart rates or heart block, changes in blood pressure, elevation of blood glucose, excessive urination (diuretic) if the horse is dehydrated, or prolonged recovery due to pain relief and sedation. These complications can occur with other anesthetic combinations; although detomidine was shown to be a safe and effective preanesthetic with both injectable and inhalant anesthesia, it does not eliminate the need for monitoring of the patient and professional judgement to provide safe and high quality anesthesia in the horse.

Detomidine has been used as a premedicant prior to ketamine anesthesia in the horse. Horses and ponies were given detomidine (20 mcg/kg i.v.) followed at least 5 minutes later by ketamine (2.2 mg/kg i.v.) compared to xylazine (1.1 mg/kg i.v.) followed by ketamine. The type and quality of induction and anesthesia was similar with both regimes. Xylazine-ketamine recoveries were sudden and complete, while detomidine-ketamine took significantly longer. The animal tended to remain in lateral or sternal recumbancy for several minutes after apparently regaining awareness after detomidine-ketamine. If this extra period of recumbancy did not occur, recovery was quiet, but the animal was sometimes very ataxic.

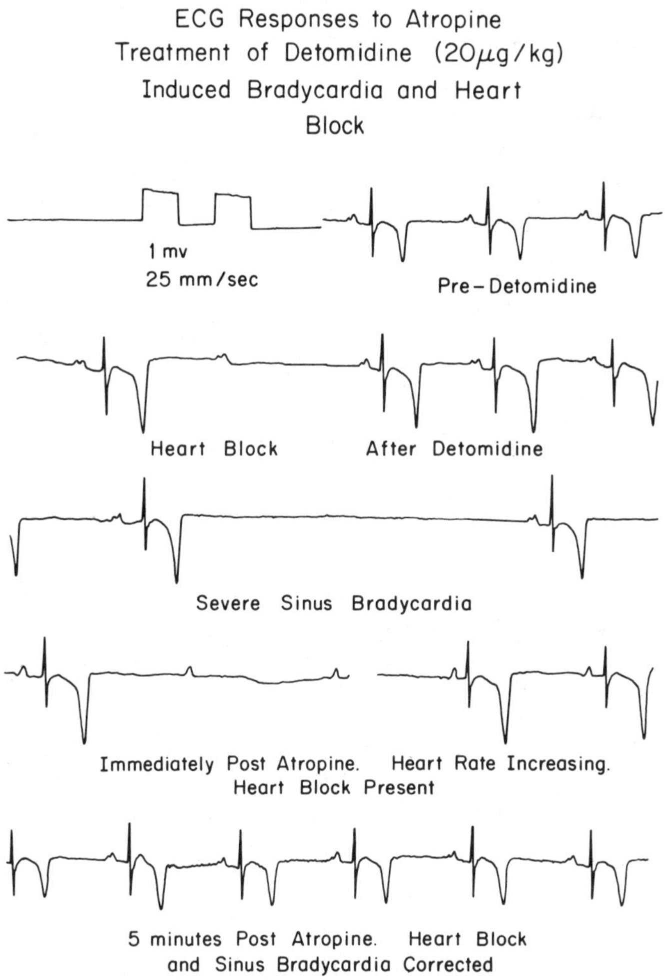

Figure 5.2. ECG responses to atropine treatment of detomidine-induced (20 μg/kg) bradycardia and heart block

Cardiovascular and respiratory measurements were made in horses and ponies receiving detomidine and ketamine. Although the hypertension and bradycardia induced by detomidine was reduced after the administration of ketamine, arterial blood pressure still remained significantly above that before sedation. Respiratory rates were very variable, but arterial blood oxygen tensions were always reduced after ketamine administration and recumbancy (32).

Detomidine has been given as a preanesthetic at the dosage level of 10 mcg/kg body weight i.v. before a 5% solution of guaifenesin was infused under pressure via an intravenous catheter after 20 to 30 minutes. The infusion was interrupted when the horse began to sway after administration of 17.5 to 30 mg/kg guaifenesin, and an intravenous bolus of thiopentone sodium at the dosage level of 3 to 4 mg/kg body weight was administered. After induction, the anesthesia was maintained with halothane (33). Satisfactory results were observed, however, because detomidine can dramatically reduce anesthetic requirements of halothane. Careful monitoring is encouraged.

In cattle, the sedative and analgetic effect was equal to xylazine. The dose varied in the first clinical trials from 10 to 250 μg/kg, with a dose range of 20 to 80 μg/kg producing desired effects (34).

An antagonist to detomidine, MPV-1248, has been used to correct cardiorespiratory parameters as well as behavior. MPV-1248 at dose levels ranging from 0.06 to 0.36 mg/kg was administered 20 minutes after an initial dose of 0.03 mg/kg of detomidine, and the horses were observed for the following 30 minutes.

Immediately postantagonist blood pressures decreased and heart rates increased toward rest values; they reached these values at a dose of 0.24 mg/kg and above. These effects were, however, of a very short duration, and values 30 minutes postantagonist did not differ from those observed using detomidine alone. Respiratory rate did decrease further postantagonist, and this tendency persisted throughout the testing period (35).

Behavior changed immediately postantagonist; the horse raised its head, looked around, and reacted to the environment. A tendency to fall back to a stage of

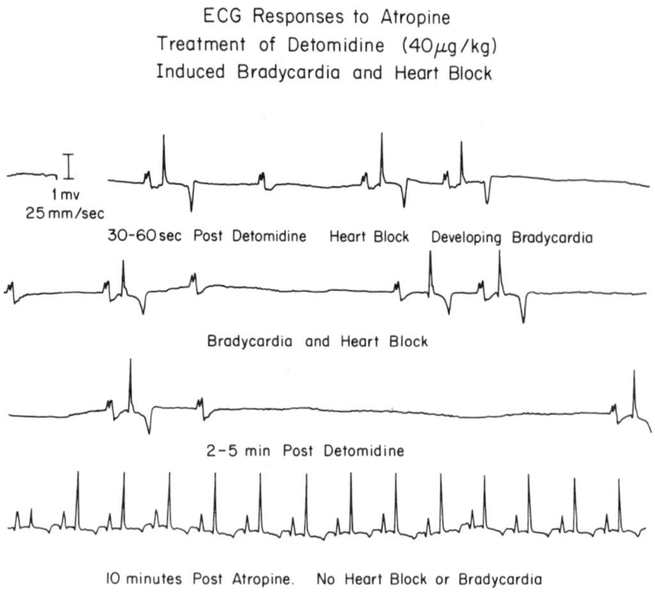

Figure 5.3. ECG responses to atropine treatment of detomidine-induced (40 μg/kg) bradycardia and heart block

light sedation was noted at the dose levels of antagonist below 0.24 mg/kg. At all dose levels, two horses were able to walk steady and relaxed at the dose levels of 0.24 mg/kg and above (35).

Early investigations of the use of detomidine in the horse revealed the development of bradycardia with or without an associated heart block. The occurrence of the slowing of the heart was within seconds to 5 minutes after the intravenous administration of the detomidine and might occur at a wide range of dosages from 20 to 160 μg/kg of intravenous detomidine. The duration of bradycardia appeared to be somewhat dose-related. However, this was not always the case. The observance of bradycardia after detomidine administration in the horse was not unexpected because a similar phenomenon had been observed after the administration of xylazine.

Since this response was observed, it was appropriate to determine if the administration of an anticholinergic agent such as atropine sulfate could be used for control of the bradycardia with or without heart block or if it could be used to prevent the occurrence of this phenomenon. Atropine was selected for use in this study as a representative of the anticholinergic group due to its approved usage in a large number of countries and due to the lack of specific approval for use of glycopyrrolate in the horse. It was anticipated that similar responses for the use of anticholinergics to correct or prevent bradycardia during detomidine use in horses would be expected from either anticholinergic agent.

Bradycardia occurred within 30 seconds to 2 minutes in each of the horses administered detomidine without premedication with atropine. The characteristic ECG pattern is shown in Figure 5.2 for 20 μg/kg detomidine and in Figure 5.3 for 40 μg/kg detomidine. The most severe drop in heart rate occurred within 2 minutes, but slow heart rates were still in existence at 5 minutes. Atropine was effective in correcting the reduced heart rate at both 20 and 4 μg/kg detomidine in horses.

Neither bradycardia nor heart block occurred in horses receiving atropine as a premedication before administration of detomidine. Heart rates were accelerated, but abnormal electrocardiographic wave patterns were not observed in either horse.

Respiratory rates were stable in either of the experimental groups. Arterial blood pH was within normal limits in all groups, as was $PaCO_2$. PaO_2 levels were acceptable for awake horses without oxygen supplementation. Systolic blood pressures were stable or elevated, with the exception of the 40 μg/kg group, which had a brief period of reduced systolic blood pressure. Systolic blood pressure increased in all horses. Atropine 0.02 mg/kg i.v. as a representative to the anticholinergic group was effective as both a preventative of bradycardia and heart block during 20 and 40 μg/kg dosage levels of detomidine in the horse and for the correction of bradycardia and heart block when they occurred and anticholinergics had not been used as the preanesthetic prior to the administration of the detomidine.

The usage of neuroleptanalgesia, neuroleptanesthesia, or alpha-adrenergic agonist analgesia offers an opportunity for versatile approaches to anesthesia.

References

1. Soma LR, Shields DR: Neuroleptanalgesia produced by fentanyl and droperidol. *J Am Vet Med Assoc* 145:897–901, 1964.
2. Katherman AE, Knecht CD, Redding RW: Effects of fentanyl citrate and droperidol on electroencephalographic findings in dogs. *Am J Vet Res* 46(4):974–976, 1985.
3. Nolan AM, Hall LW: Combined use of sedatives and opiates in horses. *Vet Rec* 114(3):63–67, 1984.
4. Kania BF: Presynaptic stimulation of dopaminergic CNS structures in sheep as a mechanism of immobilising action of Immobyl (fentanyl + azaperone). *Res Vet Sci* 38(2):179–183, 1985.
5. Hunter JM, Jones RS, Utting JE: Effects of anaesthesia with nitrous oxide in oxygen and fentanyl on renal function in the artificially ventilated dog. *Br J Anaesth* 52(3):343–348, 1980.
6. Westenskow DR, Huffaker JK, Stanley TH: The effect of dopamine, atropine, phenylephrine and cardiac pacing on oxygen consumption during fentanyl-nitrous oxide anaesthesia in the dog. *Can Anaesth Soc J* 28(2):121–214, 1981.
7. Sawyer DC: Neuroleptanalgesia and anesthesia. *Proc 2nd Intl Cong Vet Anesth* 1–4, 1985.
8. Kalpravidh M, Lumb WV, Wright M, Heath RB: Effects of butorphanol, flunixin, levorphanol, morphine and xylazine in ponies. *Am J Vet Res* 45:217–223, 1984.
9. Klein LV, Baetjer C: Preliminary report: Xylazine and morphine sedation in horses. *Vet Anesth* 2:2-C, 1974.
10. Muir WW, Skarda RT, Sheehan WC: Hemodynamic and respiratory effects of xylazine-morphine sulfate in horses. *Am J Vet Res* 40:211–216, 1979.

11. Kalpravidh M, Lumb WV, Wright M, Health RB: Analgesic effects of butorphanol in horses: Dose-response studies. *Am J Vet Res* 45:211–216, 1984.
12. Kerr DD, Jones EW, Huggins K, Edwards WC: Sedative and other effects of xylazine given intravenously in horses. *Am J Vet Res* 33:525–532, 1972.
13. Robertson JT, Muir WW, Sams R: Cardiopulmonary effects of butorphanol tartrate in horses. *Am J Vet Res* 42:41–44, 1981.
14. Virtanen R, Ruskoaho H, Nyman L: Pharmacological evidence for the involvement of alpha-2 adrenoceptors in the sedative effect of detomidine, a novel sedative-analgesic. *J Vet Pharmacol Therap* 8:30–37, 1985.
15. Clark KE, Hall LW: Xylazine—a new sedative for horses and cattle. *Vet Record* 85:512–517, 1969.
16. Vainio O: Detomidine hydrochloride. A novel imidazole-type sedative analgesic. In Ruckebusch T, Toutain PL, Horitz GD (eds): *Veterinary Pharmacology and Toxicology*. Lancaster, MTP Press Ltd., 1983, pp 798–799.
17. Hsu WS: Xylazine-induced depression and its antagonism by alpha adrenergic blocking agents. *J Pharm Exp Therap* 218:188–192, 1981.
18. Clough DP, Hatton R: Hypotensive and sedative effect of alpha-adrenoceptor agonists: relationship to alpha-1 and alpha-2 adrenoceptor potency. *Brit J Pharmacol* 73:595–604, 1981.
19. Delbarre B, Schmitt H: Sedative effects of sympathomimetic drugs and their antagonism by adrenergic and cholinergic blocking drugs. *European J Pharmacol* 13:356–363, 1971.
20. Delini-Stula A, Baumann P, Buch O: Depression of exploratory activity by clonidine in rats as a model for the detection of relative pre- and postsynaptic central noradrenergic receptor selectivity of alpha-adrenolytic drugs. *Nauuyn-Schmiedeberg's Arch Pharmacol* 307:115–122, 1979.
21. van Zweiten PA, Thoolen MJMC, Timmermans PBMWM: The pharmacology of centrally acting antihypertensive drugs. *Br J Clin Pharmacol* 15:455S–462S, 1983.
22. Lammintousta R: Introduction to adrenoceptor pharmacology. *Proceedings Domosedan Symposium*, Turku, Finland, 1985, 1.
23. Ruskoaho H: Subtypes and functions of alpha-adrenoceptors. *Proceedings Domosedan Symposium*, Turku, Finland, 1985, 2.
24. Stenberg D: The role of alpha-adrenoceptors in the regulation of vigilance and pain. *Proceedings Domosedan Symposium*, Turku, Finland, 1985, 3.
25. Virtanen R, MacDonald E, Nyman L: Pharmacology of detomidine and other alpha adrenoceptor agonists in the central nervous system. *Proceedings Domosedan Symposium*, Turku, Finland, 1985, 4.
26. Savola J-M: Cardiovascular effects of detomidine in laboratory animals. *Proceedings Domosedan Symposium*, Turku, Finland, 1985, 5.
27. Salonen JS: Pharmacokinetics of detomidine. *Proceedings Domosedan Symposium*, Turku, Finland, 1985, 6.
28. Vainio O: Pharmacological profile of detomidine in horses and cattle. *Proceedings Domosedan Symposium*, Turku, Finland, 1985, 7.
29. Lowe JE: Analgesic and sedative effects of detomidine compared to xylazine in a colic model using IV and IM routes of administration. *Proceedings Domosedan Symposium*, Turku, Finland, 1985, 9.
30. Hamm D, Jochle W: Analgesia and sedation in horses: Dose response studies with domosedan. *Proceedings Domosedan Symposium*, Turku, Finland, 1985, 8.
31. Stenberg D: Sedative and analgetic action of detomidine in horses as evaluated from evoked potentials. *Proceedings Domosedan Symposium*, Turku, Finland, 1985, 10.
32. Clarke KW, Taylor PM, Watkins SB: Detomidine-ketamine anaesthesia in the horse. *Proceedings Domosedan Symposium*, Turku, Finland, 1985, 15.
33. Saarinen H: Preanesthetic use of detomidine in horses—some clinical observations. *Proceedings Domosedan Symposium*, Turku, Finland, 1985, 14.
34. Alitalo I: Clinical experience with domosedan in horses and cattle. *Proceedings Domosedan Symposium*, Turku, Finland, 1985, 17.
35. Nilsfors L, Kvart C: Cardiorespiratory effects of detomidine: preliminary study. *Proceedings Domosedan Symposium*, Turku, Finland, 1985, 12.

CHAPTER 6

Barbiturate Anesthesia

CHARLES E. SHORT, D.V.M., M.S., D.A.C.V.A.

PHARMACOLOGY AND USE OF THE ULTRASHORT-ACTING BARBITURATES

Because of their versatility, the barbiturates have enjoyed a long period of popularity in veterinary medicine. They are classified as hypnotic sedatives. Their dose-dependent actions can range from simple sedation to hypnosis to general anesthesia. In recent years the use of the ultrashort-acting barbiturates has increased for the induction of general anesthesia that is to be followed by maintenance with an inhalant anesthetic and for short surgical and diagnostic procedures requiring a light plane of barbiturate anesthesia.

The ultrashort-acting barbiturates are derivatives of barbituric acid, which is a combination of malonic acid and urea (Fig. 6.1). This parent compound was derived in 1867 by von Bayer. It lacks central nervous system (CNS) depressant activity unless additional groups are present at Position 5 on the barbituric acid ring. If these clinical groups have carbon chains greater than 2 but no more than 5 carbons long, the onset and duration of action of the drug is shortened.

The commonly used ultrashort-acting agents are created by replacing the oxygen molecule with sulfur at Carbon 2 on the barbituric acid ring. This substitution markedly increases the lipid solubility of these drugs and their subsequent transfer across biological membranes, resulting in rapid onset and short duration of action. Although only compounds having a barbituric acid ring with an oxygen molecule at Carbon 2 are properly called barbiturates, the common practice is to call both types of compounds barbiturates and to differentiate them as thiobarbiturates and oxybarbiturates.

The most commonly used thiobarbiturates are thiamylal sodium (Bio-Tal, Bio-Ceutic, and Surital, Parke-Davis) and thiopental sodium (Pentothal, Abbott). These popular thiobarbiturates are used for short procedures as an ultrashort-acting anesthetic. The principle chemical difference between thiamylal and thiopental is that thiamylal has an allyl group attached at Carbon 5 and thiopental has an ethyl group attached at that position (Fig. 6.2).

Methohexital sodium (Brevane, Squibb) is an oxybarbiturate that is also classified as an ultrashort-acting agent. It has an allyl group and a long chained methyl-pentyl group at Carbon 5 and a methyl group at Nitrogen 3, which markedly increase its lipid solubility and shorten its duration of action (Fig. 6.2). Methohexital is commonly referred to as a methylated oxybarbiturate.

The sodium salts of these barbituric acid derivatives dissolve easily in water, resulting in a relatively unstable, pharmacologically inactive solution that has a strong alkaline pH of 11 or 12. The alkalinity is caused by the addition of sodium carbonate. After it is injected into the body, the sodium carbonate is neutralized by buffers in the blood. Thiamylal sodium and thiopental sodium when given intravenously are converted to nonionized, acidic forms. They do not precipitate readily in blood but bind to plasma proteins, particularly albumin.

Solutions of thiamylal sodium or thiopental sodium are pale yellow. Solutions of methohexital sodium are clear. Most ultrashort-acting barbiturates are supplied in 1- or 5-g containers. Sterile diluents should be used to reconstitute these products. The diluent should not contain pyrogens, dextrose, or acid chemical substances that may precipitate the sodium salts of the anesthetic agent. The amount of diluent added is used to determine the concentration of the agent, which ranges from 1 to 5% for small animals and up to

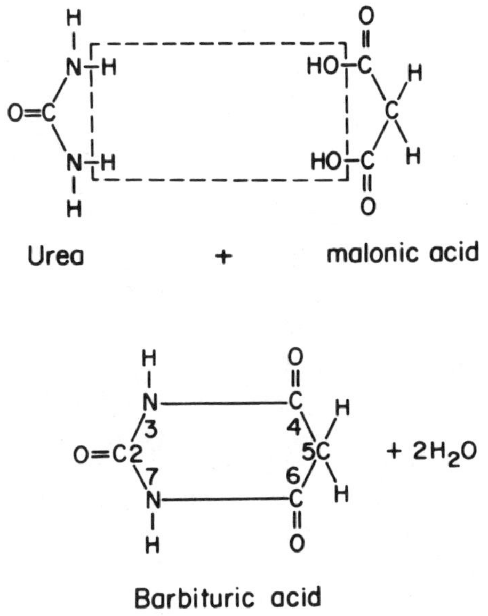

Figure 6.1. Urea and malonic acid are combined to form barbituric acid, the parent compound of the barbiturate anesthetics.

10% for large animals. To avoid mistakes in dosage, containers should be labeled with the date of reconstitution and the concentration.

ADMINISTRATION

Although barbiturates have been administered orally or rectally to human infants, in veterinary practice the most commonly used and appropriate route for anesthesia and for management of convulsive emergencies is by intravenous injection. Injection into muscle or other tissue should be avoided because the extreme alkalinity of the barbitures causes inflammation, pain, and potential necrosis at the injection site. Likewise, intra-arterial injection causes immediate endothelial damage and can lead to gangrene in an extremity.

Ultrashort-acting barbiturates can be used successfully as sole agents for anesthesia without using other medications that may alter the amount of barbiturate required to produce unconsciousness. Induction of anesthesia is normally rapid; it is accomplished by quickly administering one-third to two-thirds of a calculated dose to reduce excitement during the early phases of anesthesia. The amount of drug necessary to produce the desired state of anesthesia can vary from 10 to 18 mg/kg in small animals to 6 to 10 mg/kg in large animals.

Lower doses administered rapidly can result in a brief period of unconsciousness followed by rapid recovery, whereas slower adminstration of the drug may produce the need for more anesthetic, resulting in a longer duration of activity. Unconsciousness usually begins between 30 and 90 seconds after administration in the dog and cat. This depends on the speed with which the injection is given. The duration of action can vary from 5 to 15 minutes for the same reason. Rapid injection in large animals will produce unconsciousness in about 30 seconds.

Giving other drugs concurrently or administering barbiturates to animals that have been premedicated with tranquilizers, narcotics, or other types of medication results in variations in response and dosage requirements. The presence of disease or toxic conditions may dramatically reduce the amount of anesthetic required to produce unconsciousness. Because barbiturates are poor analgesics, signs of sympathetic response, such as increased blood pressure in response to surgical stimulation, should be closely monitored.

Protein Binding

There are several methods to determine the degree of binding of the ultrashort-acting barbiturates to plasma proteins (1–5). The binding of the ultrashort-acting barbiturates in plasma influences the uptake and distribution of the anesthetic, the duration of anesthesia, and the recovery pattern. Other medications, techniques, and conditions can influence protein-binding potential in plasma and thus the concentration of the anesthetic available to the brain. The protein bind-

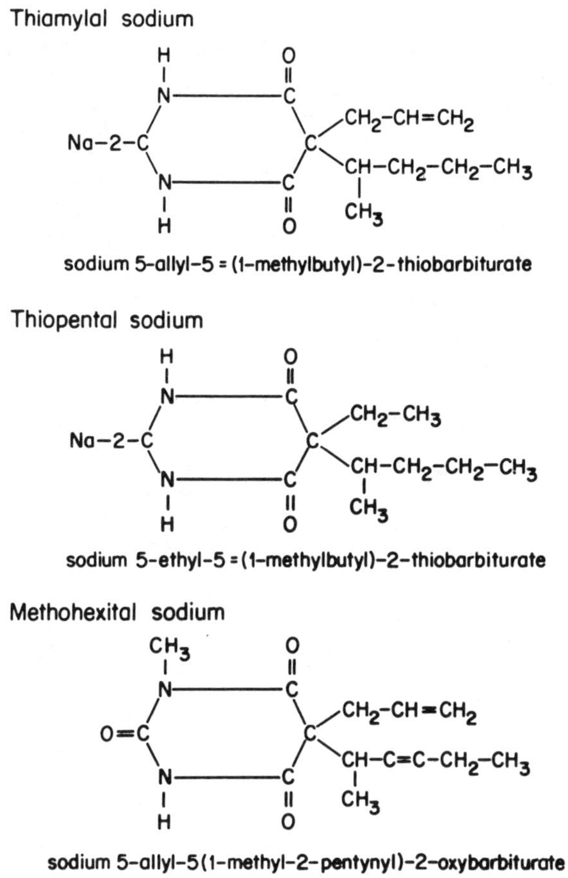

Figure 6.2. The chemical structures of three ultrashort-acting barbiturates.

ing of ultrashort-acting barbiturates is concentration-dependent (6), and there is a strong correlation between the concentration of barbiturate in the plasma and the speed of recovery relative to the induction dose (7).

In rabbits, recovery is slower after a bolus induction dose is given rather than when slower repeated doses are used (8). It has been theorized that peak concentration of the drug in the blood of the rabbit after injection of a bolus is higher than after slow injection and that this results in an increased concentration of the ultrashort-acting anesthetic in the brain, which extends the duration of anesthesia. The author has not observed prolonged sleep in dogs and cats after injection of a bolus, but has seen the opposite—longer sleep after slower inductions. In fact, in one study it was determined that recovery from ultrashort-acting barbiturate anesthesia was quicker when the concentration of plasma proteins was increased (9).

The protein-bound, ultrashort-acting barbiturates can be displaced by various other drugs, resulting in prolongation of anesthetic sleep. Sodium methiodal, a product used for canine myelography (10), and the analgesic phenylbutazone have been clinically observed to cause this phenomenon at the New York State College of Veterinary Medicine. In rare instances, phenylbutazone was administered at a sufficiently high dose after recovery from anesthesia to cause a return of anesthesia. The antibiotic sulfadimethoxine does not affect the tissue binding of the ultrashort-acting agents, but it does influence the distribution and the total clearance of these drugs, resulting in a slower elimination time (11). Mice given thiamylal sodium and chloramphenicol slept 10 times longer than mice given thiamylal sodium alone (12). Such an extensive prolongation of anesthetic time has not been observed in the dog or cat. Products that complete with ultra-short-acting agents for protein binding can lengthen the time of anesthesia by increasing the amount of unbound drug.

Recovery

Recovery from barbiturate anesthesia begins with redistribution of the anesthetic to various parts of the body. On initial injection, a major portion of the agent is rapidly delivered to such highly perfused tissues of the body as brain and heart. This produces the initial unconsciousness. The drug is then redistributed from the vessel-rich organs to tissues that receive a smaller proportion of the animal's blood supply, the moderately perfused tissues such as muscle. Ultimately, the drug is redistributed to vessel-poor areas such as fat and skin. Once the redistribution takes place and the concentration of anesthetic in the brain has dropped below the level necessary for unconsciousness, recovery begins.

The initial recovery phase for the thiobarbiturates is primarily the result of redistribution of the drug within the body and is not a consequence of active metabolism and elimination. For total recovery to occur, the agent must be biotransformed by the liver, and the metabolites and by-products must be eliminated from the body via the renal system. Interference with any of these processes lengthens the anesthetic recovery period. The short action of methohexital, an ultrashort-acting methylated oxybarbiturate, is due to rapid metabolism and not to redistribution.

For dogs and cats, recovery time is frequently defined as the time required before the animal can maintain itself in a sternal position. This is a predictable index, and it would be difficult to use a more definitive test to determine when the animal has fully recovered. Even human volunteers anesthetized with methohexital or thiopenthal sodium were unstable for 1 to 7 hours after anesthesia, depending on the medication administered (13). It was difficult to determine when total recovery had been made and the patient could resume normal activity.

For horses and other large animals, recovery time is determined by when they can stand. Recovery from thiobarbiturates alone is stormy; therefore, use of tranquilizers in horses is especially recommended.

Cardiac Response

Changes in cardiovascular function may be observed after the administration of ultrashort-acting barbiturates. Heart rate and total peripheral resistance usually increase, unless a large overdose causes cardiac arrest. Mean arterial pressure initially falls and then usually rises to preanesthetic levels or above in 30 to 60 minutes. It is believed that the increase in heart rate frequently seen after the administration of the ultrashort-acting agents is a reflex action secondary to stimulation of the baroreceptors and chemoreceptors; they have been shown to be affected by these agents (14).

Cardiac arrhythmias may occur when ultrashort-acting barbiturates are administered, especially during the first few minutes of induction. Bigeminy is the most characteristic of these arrhythmias (Fig. 6.3). In more severe cases, premature ventricular contractions occur. These arrhythmias are not caused by sensitization of the myocardium to catecholamines, as with inhalant anesthetics. They are frequently associated with corresponding decreases in ventilation, and more than 90% of affected animals will respond to the administration of oxygen. In fact, most animals recover from these arrhythmias before the condition is discovered by the anesthetist and before corrective measures can be instituted. The rate of administration of drug, concentration, and total dosage given will be factors in

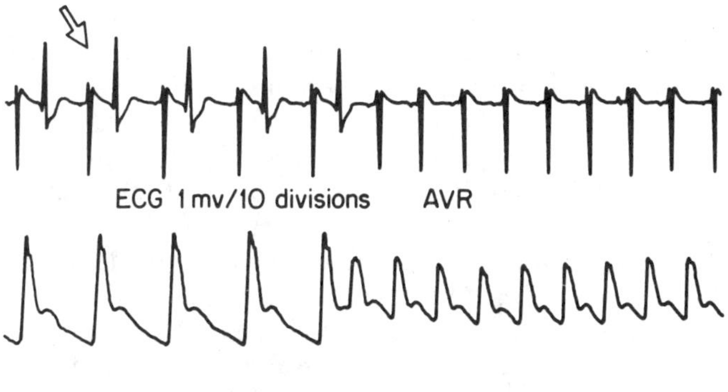

Figure 6.3. Bigeminy during induction with correction after oxygenation.

the incidence of arrhythmias. Obviously, when using higher concentrations, rapid injection can produce a higher probability of respiratory depression and cardiac arrhythmias.

The administration of lidocaine is appropriate when supplemental oxygen does not stop the arrhythmias. Lidocaine, in addition to controlling ventricular arrhythmias associated with ultrashort-acting barbiturates, is a local anesthetic and can serve as an adjunct to the barbiturate anesthetic (15). When lidocaine is used, slightly less general anesthetic may be needed to achieve the required degree of relaxation.

The effect of the method of induction (e.g., bolus or incremental administration) on the cardiovascular system should be considered. In studies done to compare the cardiovascular effects of these two methods of administration for ultrashort-acting agents, only slight differences between arterial pressures, heart rates, systolic time intervals, and measurements of end tidal carbon dioxide (CO_2) levels were found (16). Efforts were made in the study to produce the same depth of CNS depression in all of the healthy subjects. The effects of miscalculations of drug dosages or the effects of accurately calculated dosages on unhealthy subjects were not taken into account.

Body temperature may also affect the cardiovascular depression that occurs in an animal under the influence of ultrashort-acting barbiturates or combinations of an ultrashort-acting barbiturate and a gas anesthetic. This has been evaluated in a number of clinical situations, including a study of harbor seals that showed that cardiovascular responses were depressed during hypothermia (17).

In a nonclinical situation, the mitochondria of the heart were studied in animals under the effects of thiopental anesthesia (18). Evidence indicated that the ultrashort-acting barbiturates could be administered safely in a variety of circumstances without undue effect on the heart. In other studies, however, it was determined that thiopental does have a negative inotropic effect on the heart secondary to reduced availability of calcium to the myofibrils (19). Another team of investigators found that thiobarbiturates could indeed cause a moderate drop in serum calcium (20). However, in another study it was found that the effect of thiobarbiturates on cardiac performance, coronary hemodynamics, and myocardial oxygen consumption in patients with ischemic heart disease was not detrimental. Despite the calcium exchange problems, myocardial oxygen demand could be matched with supply, and the degree of cardiac depression was clinically insignificant (21).

Respiratory Response

Levels of barbiturates sufficient to produce anesthesia cause some respiratory depression. If the dosage is controlled, anesthesia can be maintained using continued spontaneous ventilation and a tidal volume adequate to support the oxygen demands of the patient. Rapid and excessive administration of the drug can result in respiratory depression and a corresponding reduction in respiratory volume. When tidal volume is reduced, the respiratory rate may compensate by increasing to provide an adequate minute volume and level of oxygenation. Compensation is not always adequate or present, however, and the administration of increasing dosages of drug may result in apnea. A high incidence of dose-related apnea occurs after induction of anesthesia with a thiobarbiturate (22).

The ideal therapy for depressed or arrested respiration is the administration of supplemental oxygen and the application of mechanical ventilation. Artificial respiration performed by compressing the chest may be adequate for minor respiratory depression, but is not as effective as the administration of oxygen.

When respiratory effects of anesthetics given to rabbits were studied, it was found that the anesthetic caused a decrease in minute and tidal volume and an increase in the tension of carbon dioxide (PCO_2) (23). Another study showed that cardiovascular and respiratory responses to induction of anesthesia with a barbiturate were related and that a significant tachycardia was frequently observed secondary to respiratory depression (24). Recommendations were made to supplement the patient with oxygen during induction and to monitor respiratory effort closely to make overall anesthetic management safer.

In veterinary medicine, when anesthesia is induced with an ultrashort-acting barbiturate, the animal frequently is not provided with supplemental oxygen before administration of the anesthetic. As a result, when enough drug is administered to cause anesthesia and depression of the CNS, there is a corresponding depression of cardiopulmonary function that can lead to hypoxia, hypercarbia, and irritation of the heart. In this situation, oxygen should be administered and cardiopulmonary responses should be monitored during the induction and maintenance of anesthesia. When there is an oxygen deficit, accumulation of CO_2, and the potential for a major increase in metabolic demand, the administration of epinephrine or other stimulants that primarily affect the cardiovascular system or the administration of medications that affect the CNS are usually not indicated. They frequently may be contraindicated.

CNS Response

Ultrashort-acting barbiturates can be used for the production of anesthesia or for the control of CNS hyperactivity, such as a convulsion. The dose of a thiobarbiturate needed to treat status epilepticus and other milder convulsions is frequently larger than the amount needed to induce anesthesia.

Barbiturates have also been used to protect the brain against excessive cerebral edema after periods of ischemia (25). In studies designed to determine how long cerebral ischemia can exist before irreversible brain injury and death occur, barbiturates were found to afford some protection against irreversible brain injury, but adequate blood pressure and ventilation still had to be maintained (26). In most instances, 2 minutes or less of cerebral ischemia can result in some damage to the nervous system. Irreversible damage occurs after 5 to 7 minutes.

Another drug that may help protect the brain during prolonged cerebral ischemia after cardiac arrest is lidocaine. In studies of cardiac arrest that occurred during induction of anesthesia, it was found that there is an increase in extracellular potassium within the brain and that administration of thiopental had no effect on the influx of this potassium during an ischemic crisis in the dog (27). Lidocaine, however, did help to protect the brain, but its use for this purpose is controversial, and lidocaine is not recommended for preventing cerebral ischemia during cardiac arrest in clinical patients. The effectiveness of lidocaine given intravenously for the rapid control of acute intracranial hypertension had also been studied. The administration of lidocaine did not lower intracranial pressure as much as the administration of thiopental, but it did have a less adverse effect on mean arterial pressure (28).

Studies were done to evaluate alterations in cerebral blood flow, oxygen metabolism, and electrical activity produced by giving high doses of ultrashort-acting barbiturates (29). Initially, systemic arterial pressure and cardiac output decreased. Cerebral metabolic depression and vasoconstriction reached a plateau when sufficient barbiturate was administered to suppress burst activity on the electroencephalogram (EEG) for 30 and 60 seconds. At this point no further cardiovascular depression was noted, and cerebral rate of oxygen metabolism and the cerebral blood flow stabilized.

Cerebral circulatory responses to changes in blood CO_2 levels during the administration of ultrashort-acting barbiturates in the dog were investigated (30). Vasoconstriction of the cerebral circulation tends to occur during the administration of anesthetic sufficient to produce unconsciousness and cause burst suppression on the EEG. Hyperventilation from mechanically assisted respiration can increase intracranial pressure, but this increase can be offset somewhat by the effects of the barbiturates (31). A balance of these two effects can be anticipated if barbiturate anesthesia and assisted respiration are used concurrently.

During anesthesia, brain function is dependent on continuation of appropriate glycolysis and the stabilization of the glucose levels needed to support brain tissues. Key enzymes of glycolysis in the brain were found not to be significantly changed when a barbiturate was administered (32).

Other investigators were concerned about the effect of catecholamines on the CNS. Catecholamines are frequently released by animals during anesthetic induction secondary to the excitement associated with restraint. Although catecholamines are known to affect cardiac function, they do not appear to influence the acute effects of barbiturates (33).

Hypothermia has been shown to prolong EEG suppression caused by ultrashort-acting barbiturates (34). This partially explains the prolonged anesthesia that sometimes occurs in smaller breeds of dogs and cats, which are most prone to hypothermia during anesthesia. The same can occur in young colts, lambs, calves, and pigs, but is not as likely to occur in adults. Care should be taken when large animals are undergoing prolonged anesthesia in conditions of extreme ambient temperatures.

The ultrashort-acting barbiturates can be effective for rapid, short-duration control of seizure activity in the brains of dogs and cats. They have been used in horses to effectively control seizures caused by inadvertent intracarotid artery injections of tranquilizers. They can be used to control intracranial pressure, and they have a beneficial effect on cerebral blood flow and metabolism. There is convincing evidence that ultrashort-acting barbiturates can be safely used to produce unconsciousness, as demonstrated by the classic clinical signs of anesthesia and EEG recordings of animals experiencing seizures. The brain's uptake of ultrashort-acting barbiturates is rapid, as indicated by the quick onset of anesthesia and loss of reflexes. The principal concerns in using the ultrashort-acting barbiturates for production of unconsciousness and anesthesia are the problems that can occur from preexisting

CNS depression caused by toxins, other medications, or pathological lesions.

Muscle Relaxation

The degree of relaxation of the musculature achieved with ultrashort-acting barbiturates is usually adequate for minor or short surgical procedures. If relaxation sufficient for delicate surgery is achieved by using ultrashort-acting barbiturates alone, cardiopulmonary function will often be compromised and recovery will be prolonged. The administration of muscle relaxants during a surgical procedure when ultrashort-acting barbiturates are used may produce additional detrimental effects on total cardiopulmonary function. The animal's ability to ventilate adequately without manual or mechanical support may be hampered. The use of centrally acting muscle relaxants in conjunction with thiobarbiturates in large animals is a common practice in veterinary medicine. The use of paralytic agents without capability to support ventilation should be avoided.

The ultrashort-acting barbiturates cannot effectively control the neuromuscular junction, as shown by a study in which succinylcholine-induced fasciculations were reduced, but not entirely eliminated, by using ultrashort-acting barbiturates (35). Furthermore, the action of barbiturates on acetylcholinesterase activity suggests that they can change the interactions between lipids and proteins in the cell membranes (36). During recovery from ultrashort-acting barbiturate anesthesia, extensive movement of the extremities may occur without tranquilizers or other medications to reduce muscle activity. Also, coordination may not have returned completely when the animal attempts to stand.

Liver and Kidney

The use of barbiturates causes induction of the microsomal enzymes system of the liver (37). It has been reported that barbiturates combine with cytochrome p-450 to competitively interfere with the biotransformation of many substrates of this enzyme. The biotransformation process can also be affected by the presence of other medications or hepatic dysfunction. Although most of their biotransformation takes place in the liver, thiobarbiturates can also be biotransformed, to a small extent, in the kidney, brain, and perhaps other tissues. Barbiturates are transformed by oxidation of the radical groups at Carbon 5. These may appear in the urine as alcohols, ketones, phenols, or carboxylic acids. Renal and hepatic function are important in the fate of the barbiturate because malfunction of the liver can influence biotransformation and renal malfunction can influence elimination of the drugs.

Placental Transfer

Barbiturates are transferred across the placenta and can cause respiratory depression in the newborn. When the pharmacokinetics and plasma binding of thiopental given to pregnant animals were studied, it was found that for any given dose, a higher plasma concentration of the drug was present in pregnant than in nonpregnant individuals. Apparently, pregnancy is a greater determinant of differences in drug concentrations than the amount of drug administered (38).

Another study showed that when ultrashort-acting barbiturates were used as the anesthetic during Caesarean section, concentrations in the venous blood of the newborn were only slightly less than in the mother, ranging from 1.7 to 6.0 μg/ml in mothers and from 1.3 to 5.5 μg/ml in blood from the fetal cord (39). The half-life of the barbiturate in maternal blood ranged from 21 minutes to 9.9 hours, whereas in the newborn it ranged from 10.3 to 42.7 hours. Although the concentration of drug in the blood of the newborn is not as high as in maternal blood, the length of time required for elimination of the agent is considerably longer. Thus, the effects of a barbiturate will be prolonged in the neonate.

When the placental transfer of anesthetic agents that could be used in performing Caesarean sections was evaluated, it was found that the concentrations of thiopental in maternal blood rose during the 5- to 10-minute period after injection of the barbiturate (40). The amount of ultrashort-acting barbiturate transferred, however, was not large enough to be detrimental to the newborn at birth. When thiopental and methohexital were evaluated using equally potent doses, as induction agents for a Caesarean section, it was noted that there was no clinical or biochemical difference in the neonates relative to the agent used (41). Because there is free transfer of a barbiturate across the placenta, the amount of the drug used should be limited to the amount needed for a procedure. The stress caused by obstetric procedures will not be improved by the administration of an agent such as an ultrashort-acting barbiturate.

Gastrointestinal Response

The effects of anesthetic agents on the gastrointestinal motility of greyhounds was studied. Electrical and mechanical activities of the stomach, duodenum, jejunum, and ileum were monitored with strain gauge transducers and implanted bipolar electrodes (42). The activity of the duodenum and jejunum increased when anesthetic was administered, but the activity of the stomach and the ileum remained the same. The duodenal and jejunal activity could be prevented by premedication and atropine. Clinically, it has been observed that ultrashort-acting barbiturates do not cause prolonged decreases in gastrointestinal tract activity.

Immune Response

Adminstration of an anesthetic may affect immune response, as shown by the effects of ultrashort-acting barbiturates and inhalant agents on tumor growth (43). Thiopental impaired the afferent immune response, and halothane impaired the efferent immune response to such growth.

Morbidity and Mortality

The evaluation of clinical case material involving ultrashort-acting anesthetics revealed two important considerations. First, pre-existing pathological conditions frequently contributed to morbidity or mortality. Second, healthy subjects that succumbed to a relative overdose of ultrashort-acting barbiturates usually did not show any major pathological lesions of diagnostic value (44).

Unusual Adverse Reactions

Allergic reactions to the ultrashort-acting barbiturates may occur during induction of anesthesia. During the past 27 years, the author has observed three of these reactions. Frothy secretions occurred immediately in the bronchial and tracheal areas. These signs subsided quickly when the animal was given supplemental oxygen via an endotracheal tube. Anaphylactic reactions caused by thiopental sodium have also been observed (45). Administration of barbiturates will rarely produce cutaneous reactions or severe acute reactions, such as cardiovascular emergency, at the time of induction of general anesthesia.

Venous complications can occur after injection of ultrashort-acting barbiturates (46). The most usual problems is extravascular tissue reactions after inadvertent injection outside the vein. Complications have arisen from improper care or poor initial placement and contamination of intravenous catheters. Phlebitis is more common in patients that have catheters inserted than in patients that receive the anesthetic agent via a needle and syringe.

Because of their high alkalinity, pain has frequently been reported after injection of ultrashort-acting barbiturates. Administration of a local anesthetic before injection of the barbiturate will reduce the pain (47). However, this process is involved and does not seem to warrant serious consideration in animals.

Barbiturates have been accidentally injected intra-arterially, this can cause major difficulties, including arterial spasm, emboli, loss of vessel, gangrene, and loss of limb (48). Also, if the injection is made into the carotid artery, as is sometimes done in large animals, excessive CNS activity can occur rapidly. This can cause major convulsions, cerebral edema, ischemia, or death. If a carotid artery is injected inadvertently, ultrashort-acting barbiturates should be given intravenously at the dosage necessary to control the seizure activity. This should be followed by treatment with intravenous anti-inflammatory medications and diuretics.

Conclusion

Intravenous administration of 10 to 18 mg/kg of ultrashort-acting barbiturates such as sodium thiamylal or thiopental sodium or 5 to 9 mg/kg of methohexital sodium can produce anesthesia in 30 to 90 seconds. The anesthesia should last 5 to 15 minutes in dogs and cats. Intravenous administration of 6.6 mg/kg of ultrashort-acting barbiturates such as sodium thiamylal or thiopental sodium in tranquilized horses can produce anesthesia in 30 seconds and usually lasts 5 to 10 minutes. Adjustments in dosage must be made for sick, injured, debilitated, or premedicated animals.

CONCURRENT USE OF OTHER AGENTS WITH ULTRASHORT-ACTING BARBITURATES

Combining different drugs to produce anesthesia is referred to as balanced anesthesia. Veterinarians using these combinations generally want to reduce the amount of each required, complement the predominant anesthetic with products that make the anesthetic regimen safer, and produce certain desirable responses. The use of these combinations is summarized in Table 6.1.

Anticholinergics

Anticholinergics are often given before the administration of ultrashort-acting barbiturates. An anticholinergic such as atropine sulfate or glycopyrrolate is used to protect the animal against bradycardia and hypersalivation. It is more important that an animal be given an anticholinergic if it is receiving the ultrashort-acting barbiturate in conjunction with other medications such as xylazine or the narcotics, which tend to slow the heart rate. Several diseases and conditions, including bradycardia and cardia arrhythmias such as heart block, may or may not respond to administration of anticholinergics. A transient bradycardia caused by a vagal reflex response may be affected, whereas congenital or acquired heart block caused by cardiovascular damage may not.

The use of anticholinergics in the horse and rum-

Table 6.1
Medications Used Concurrently with Ultrashort-Acting Barbiturates[a]

Drug	Purpose	Dosage		Effect on Barbiturate Response
		Dog	Cat	
Atropine[b]	Reduce salivation, prevent bradycardia	0.044 mg/kg s.c., i.m. 0.022 mg/kg i.v.	Same as dog Same as dog	Less tendency for bradycardia. May increase incidence of arrhythmias.
Glycopyrrolate[b]	Reduce salivation, prevent bradycardia	0.011 mg/kg i.m.	Same as dog	Less tendency for bradycardia. Not likely to increase incidence of arrhythmias.
Morphine	Analgesia, reduce anesthetic dose	0.11–6.6 mg/kg s.c.	Not recommended	Major reduction in anesthetic dose required. Reduced heart rate unless anticholinergic used. Vomiting may occur.
Methadone	Analgesia, reduce anesthetic dose	0.11–0.55 mg/kg i.m., i.v.	Not recommended	Reduced respiratory response. Reduced anesthetic dose required.
Meperidine	Analgesia, reduce anesthetic dose	2.2–6.6 mg/kg i.m., s.c.	4.4–8.8 mg/kg i.m., s.c.	Reduced heart rate.
Oxymorphone	Analgesia, reduce anesthetic dose	0.22 mg/kg i.m., i.v., s.c.	0.88–3.3 mg total dose s.c., i.m., i.v.	Reduced heart rate.
Pentazocaine	Analgesia, reduce anesthetic dose	2.2–3.3 mg/kg i.m., s.c.	Same as dog	Reduced anesthetic dose required. Less cardiopulmonary depression than narcotics.
Innovar-Vet	Neuroleptanalgesia	1 ml/7–9 kg i.m.	Not recommended	Major reduction of dose required. Use ultrashort-acting agents with extreme caution and at low doses (10% of calculated dose or less).
Chlorpromazine	Tranquilization	1.1–2.2 mg/kg i.m., i.v.	Same as dog	Calm animal during induction and recovery. Reduced dose of anesthetic required.
Promazine	Tranquilization	2.2–4.4 mg/kg i.m., i.v.		Calm animal during induction and recovery. Reduced dose of anesthetic required.
Acetylpromazine	Tranquilization	0.11 mg/kg i.v. 0.22 mg/kg i.m.	0.06 mg/kg i.v.	Calm animal during recovery. May also produce hypotension. Reduced dose of anesthetic required.
Xylazine	Tranquilization, sedation, analgesia	0.22–1.1 mg/kg i.v. 0.55–2.2 mg/kg i.m.	0.5–1.1 mg/kg i.v.	Calm animal, may cause vomiting, can cause bradycardia and heart block. Reduced dose of anesthetic required.

[a] All these medications except the anticholinergics will reduce the dosage of ultrashort-acting barbiturate needed for induction or maintenance. Individual animals may require from 25 to 90% reduction in dosage of barbiturate when compared to animals not receiving medications.
[b] An anticholinergic administered with narcotics, neuroleptanalgesics, or xylazine will greatly reduce the possibility of severe bradycardia or cardiac arrest during ultrashort-acting barbiturate induction.

inants prior to barbiturates is controversial. The concern with the horse is that the anticholinergics will cause a reduction in gastrointestinal activity, leading to the development of colic. These problems, however, are frequently due to the presence of ingesta in the gastrointestinal tract and not to the administration of an anticholinergic and an ultrashort-acting barbiturate. If ingesta is absent, the incidence of gastrointestinal problems is tremendously diminished. It is the author's observation that induction of anesthesia unaccompanied by concurrent administration of anticholinergic agents can still result in colic if the horse has been fed recently. This problem is not as pronounced in the dog and cat, but it is advisable to keep these animals off feed for 6 to 8 hours before they are anesthetized.

Tranquilizers

Tranquilizers are also used as premedicants. They are used to calm animals so that they are safer and easier to handle. Normally, less anesthetic is required when an animal has been premedicated with a tranquilizer. Also, when ultrashort-acting barbiturates are used alone to provide anesthesia, tranquilizers usually ensure a quieter, more pleasant recovery period. Acetylpromazine, promazine, diazepam, and xylazine are the most commonly used tranquilizers in veterinary medicine.

A concern in human anesthesiology is the reduction of a patient's anxiety before induction of anesthesia. In veterinary anesthesiology, tranquilizers are used not only to reduce the anxiety of the patient, but also to reduce the anxiety of the person administering the anesthetic. Because potent tranquilizers are used in veterinary medicine, some of the possible adverse effects of these products must be considered. The dosage of ultrashort-acting barbiturates must be reduced in proportion to the effect of the preanesthetic tranquilizer.

The phenothiazine-derivative tranquilizers, such as acepromazine and promazine, not only produce tranquilization, but may also cause hypotension by alpha blockade. This fall in blood pressure may result from high doses of these drugs, and it may be enhanced by the use of ultrashort-acting barbiturates. The dose of acetylpromazine given before administration of an ultrashort-acting barbiturate is usually reduced to 0.1 to 0.2 mg/kg in dogs and cats and to 0.06 mg/kg in horses and cattle. This is far less than the dose recommended by the manufacturer for use in dogs and cats but will still greatly reduce the dose of barbiturate needed for induction. The label recommendation of 0.25 to 0.5 mg/lb (0.6 to 1.1 mg/kg) can result in profound tranquilization that may last for as much as 48 hours without the addition of other anesthetic agents.

Xylazine

A combination of xylazine and an ultrashort-acting barbiturate has been used for short-term anesthesia in the horse, dog, and cat. Xylazine is a very potent tranquilizer, sedative, and analgesic that produces tranquilization for several hours and dose-related pain relief lasting 10 to 15 minutes. It can also tremendously depress heart rate, even to the point of causing heart block, unless anticholinergic agents are used concurrently. The author has found that the slowing of heart rate caused by giving xylazine can last as long as 6 hours in some dogs, but it is not unusual for this effect to last only 15 to 30 minutes. The practitioner should remember that xylazine can have detrimental effects on the heart; consequently, the concurrent administration of an ultrashort-acting barbiturate may be unsafe.

After studying numerous referrals concerning complications that have occurred during or after preanesthetic treatment with xylazine and induction with ultrashort-acting barbiturates, the author found that the two most common causes of complications were failure to adequately reduce the dosage of the induction agent after preanesthetic tranquilization and the lack of anticholinergic therapy to prevent heart block. Xylazine can reduce the amount of anesthetic (thiamylal or thiopental) required by 25 to 50% of the original dosage, depending on the amount of xylazine administered, the species, and the speed with which the anesthetic is given. Ruminants are more sensitive to xylazine than are horses, dogs, and cats. This must be considered if ultrashort-acting barbiturates are also planned.

Diazepam

Diazepam is a popular tranquilizer in human medicine, and its popularity as a preanesthetic in veterinary medicine is growing. Diazepam depresses the CNS but has a less severe effect on the cardiopulmonary system than some of the more potent tranquilizers and sedatives currently in use. However, there is some hesitancy to use this drug in veterinary medicine because dosage regimens are not as clearly established for animals as they are for humans. Diazepam is effective in controlling seizure activity at an intravenous dose of 0.04 mg/kg, so this dose or less is probably appropriate for preanesthetic tranquilization before use of an ultrashort-acting barbiturate. The combination of diazepam, which depresses the CNS, and an ultrashort-acting barbiturate, which produces unconsciousness, may have synergistic effects and produce profound relaxation and anesthesia.

Narcotics

Current data indicate that narcotics produce analgesia when used in animals. Another advantage of using a narcotic for premedication is reduction in the amount of anesthetic required.

A detrimental effect of narcotics is depression of the cardiopulmonary system, especially when they are given at high levels. Some narcotics such as morphine cause vomiting. Although vomiting in some instances is desirable, usually it is not.

The use of narcotics dramatically reduces the amount of ultrashort-acting barbiturate needed to produce unconsciousness. The dose of ultrashort-acting barbiturates depends on the condition of the animal, the narcotic used, and the dose of the narcotic.

Neuroleptanalgesics

Neuroleptanalgesia is produced by administering a combination of a tranquilizer and a narcotic. Even though it may seem that combining tranquilizers and narcotics is safe, extreme bradycardia and hypotension can occur when they are used concurrently. Anticholinergics are frequently given along with these combinations to protect against extreme slowing of the heart, and oxygen is administered to correct tissue hypoxia.

Only in rare circumstances should neuroleptanalgesics be used as premedications before induction with ultrashort-acting barbiturates. They should be used together with extreme caution because cardiac arrest has occurred when 10% or less of the calculated barbiturate dose is given. It is usually much safer to use inhalant anesthetics to induce anesthesia in animals premedicated with neuroleptanalgesics.

Muscle Relaxants

In large animals, the use of an ultrashort-acting barbiturate such as thiamylal or thiopental in combination with a centrally acting muscle relaxant such as guaifenesin allows for an easier induction of anesthesia. The guaifenesin is usually given in a 5% solution with 2 to 3 g of ultrashort-acting barbiturate added. Anesthesia can be induced by giving a tranquilized horse approximately 1 to 2 ml/kg i.v. of this mixture. In tranquilized cattle, the dosage can be reduced even further. The effects of anesthesia are easily prolonged by additional administration of the mixture by slow intravenous flow. The animal usually awakes from anesthesia 30 to 40 minutes after administration is discontinued. This combination is not used in the dog or cat.

Paralytic agents such as succinylcholine, pancuronium, gallamine, and other curare products have been used in small animals. If succinylcholine is administered in conjunction with ultrashort-acting barbiturates for induction, and appropriate oxygen is administered by intermittent positive pressure, cardiac arrhythmias usually do not occur. However, if oxygen is not administered manually or mechanically by a positive-pressure method, tissue hypoxia of the myocardium can cause extreme tachycardia, ventricular arrhythmias, and possibly ventricular fibrillation or cardiac arrest. In some animals in which these problems resulted in death, myocardial hemorrhage was evident.

When administering paralytic agents in conjunction with ultrashort-acting barbiturates, the animal must be intubated to provide a patent airway for oxygen. Manual and/or mechanical ventilation must be provided during the anesthetic and paralytic period to ensure the maintenance of adequate ventilation.

Ketamine

Ketamine is a dissociative anesthetic that typically produces an incoherent, cataleptic state in cats, subhuman primates, and humans. Used alone, the agent produces incomplete visceral and muscle relaxation, excellent somatic analgesia, and partial visceral analgesia. Cardiac rate is usually increased with ketamine. In many species an increase in CNS activity, even to the extent of seizure, can occur. Ketamine can slightly depress the respiratory response for approximately 40 minutes. This can be observed as an apneustic pattern. Associated with it are an increase in tension of arterial carbon dioxide ($PaCO_2$), a reduction in tension of arterial oxygen (PaO_2), and a corresponding drop in pH.

If ultrashort-acting barbiturates are administered to produce greater relaxation in conjunction with ketamine anesthesia, the veterinarian should take into consideration that a very small dose of barbiturate is required and that the safety of this combination is questionable.

Ultrashort-acting or longer-acting barbiturates can be used to reduce the seizure activity or major convulsions that can occur if ketamine is inadvertently administered to the wrong species or if the response of animals such as cats or subhuman primates is abnormal. The dosage required is unpredictable, but the amount of ultrashort-acting barbiturate required to anesthetize a subject and reduce CNS effects caused by ketamine is usually quite small. Supportive therapy should include supplemental oxygen and the administration of fluids to allow elimination of the ketamine by the renal system. Body temperature should be maintained under these circumstances to avoid prolonged recoveries.

Conclusion

Ultrashort-acting barbiturates can be used in combination with a variety of products, many of which reduce the amount of barbiturate needed to depress the CNS to the level required for surgical anesthesia. The duration of the effects of these other products varies. Many of them enhance ultrashort-acting barbiturate anesthesia by altering the heart rate, influencing the degree of relaxation and analgesia, and altering the characteristics of induction and recovery. Their corresponding detrimental effects must be taken into account. It is the responsibility of the veterinarian who selects these combinations to determine the effect of each of the products separately and in combination.

The dosage of each drug and the ultimate responses that the veterinarian wishes to achieve with each animal are critical. With these considerations in mind, ultrashort-acting barbiturates can be used safely as a major component of balanced anesthesia. If these considerations are not taken into account, detrimental results can occur, and it becomes difficult to ascertain which product is contributing to the adverse effects.

ULTRASHORT-ACTING BARBITURATE INDUCTION FOLLOWED BY MAINTENANCE WITH INHALANT ANESTHETICS

To use ultrashort-acting barbiturate induction followed by maintenance of anesthesia with an inhalant agent, an understanding of the ultrashort-acting agents is needed to ensure that safe anesthetic induction and support of the patient is accomplished. The veterinarian must know how to maintain the physiological function of the animal while appropriately using equipment for intubation, support of respiration, and control of anesthetic concentrations. Also, an understanding of the individual inhalant agents and how they interact with the barbiturates is necessary.

Induction and Maintenance

Before using ultrashort-acting barbiturates such as thiamylal or thipoental to induce anesthesia, appropriate equipment and supplies should be available to administer the inhalant anesthetic. The amount of barbiturate needed to induce anesthesia under these circumstances is frequently less than that required when using the ultrashort-acting barbiturate alone. The reduction may vary from 10 to 50%, depending on the rapidity with which the ultrashort-acting barbiturate is administered. In healthy dogs and cats, rapid administration of 50% of the calculated dose of ultrashort-acting barbiturate is usually enough to produce unconsciousness that is adequate for intubation and the maintenance of anesthesia until the concentration of inhalant agent is sufficient to prevent arousal. If the dog or cat is premedicated with a tranquilizer, narcotic, or other sedative, even less barbiturate is necessary for induction. The importance of using an anticholinergic as a preanesthetic depends on the type of inhalant anesthesia used.

The anesthetic unit, complete with a filled vaporizer, supply of oxygen, and either a rebreathing or a nonbreathing system, should be properly prepared before the induction of anesthesia. Endotracheal tubes and any devices such as a laryngoscope needed to facilitate intubation should be available. The patient should be completely evaluated, and any therapy needed during anesthesia should be initiated.

After induction, the animal should be intubated immediately and connected to the anesthetic unit if inhalants are to be used. If the patient will be maintained on injectable medication, consideration of the anesthetic administered and the uptake and redistribution characteristics is necessary.

Acknowledgments

Portions of this chapter were reproduced with permission from Short CE: Practical Use of the Ultrashort-Acting Barbiturates and from Bioceutics Laboratories, St. Joseph, MO, and from Veterinary Learning Systems Co., Inc., Princeton, NJ.

References

1. Christensen JH, Andreasen F, Jansen FB: The binding of thiopental to serum proteins determined by ultrafiltration and equilibrium dialysis. *Acta Pharmacol Toxicol* 47(1):24–32, 1980.
2. Helliwell M, Flanagan RJ: Thiopentone infusions. *Anaesthesia* 35(1):78–79, 1980.
3. Jung D, Mayersohn M, Perrier D: Gas-chromatographic assay for thiopental in plasma, with use of a nitrogen-specific detector. *Clin Chem* 27(1):113–115, 1981.
4. Jung D, Mayersohn M, Perrier D: The "ultra-free" ultrafiltration technique compared with equilibrium dialysis for determination of unbound thiopental concentrations in serum. *Clin Chem* 27(1):166–168, 1981.
5. Salvadori C, Farinnoti R, Duvaldestin P, Dauphin A: Liquid chromatography determination of thiopentone in human plasma. *Ther Drug Monit* 3(2):171–176, 1981.
6. Morgan DJ, Blackman GL, Paull JD, Wolf LJ: Pharmacokinetics and plasma binding of thiopental. I: Studies in surgical patients. *Anesthesiology* 54(6):468–473, 1981.
7. Tarnow J, Hess W, Klein W: Etomidate, alfathesin and thiopentone as induction agents for coronary artery surgery. *Can Anaesth Soc J* 27(4):333–344, 1980.
8. Kurz H, Fichtl B: Interrelation between plasma protein binding, rate of injection and the anesthetic effect of thiopental. *Biopharm Drug Dispos* 2(2):191–196, 1981.
9. Torri G, Stella L, Pradella G, Maestrone E, Martani C: Plasma protein concentration and recovery from anesthesia in man. *Br J Anaesth* 53(12):1281–1284, 1981.
10. Bonhaus DW, Sawyer DC, et al: Displacement of protein-bound thiopental by sodium methiodal may contribute to anesthetic complications during canine myelography. *Am J Vet Res* 42(9):1612–1614, 1981.
11. Yu H, Sawada Y, Sugiyana Y, Iga T, Hanano M: Effect of sulfadimethoxine or thiopental distribution and elimination in rats. *J Pharm Sci* 70(3):323–326, 1981.
12. Azadegan A, Johnston DW, Stowe CM: Influence of time interval between administration of chloramphenicol and thiamylal on the sleeping time of mice. *Am J Vet Res* 4(6):976–977, 1980.
13. Korttila K, Ghonemin MM, Jacobs L, Lakes RS: Evaluation of instrumented force platform as a test to measure residual effects of anesthetics. *Anesthesiology* 55(6):625–630, 1981.
14. Blake DW, Korner PI: Role of baroreceptor reflexes in the hemodynamic and heart rate responses to althesin, ketamine and thiopentone anesthesia. *J Auton Nerv Syst* 3(1):55–70, 1981.
15. Sorrell JF: Intravenous lidocaine: An adjunct for nitrous oxide thiopental anesthesia. *AANAJ* 48(5)477–481, 1980.
16. Seltzer JL, Gerson JI, Allen FB: Comparison of the cardiovascular effects of bolus v. incremental administration of thiopentone. *Br J Anaesth* 52(5):527–530, 1980.
17. Sinnett EE, Wahrenbrock EA, et al: Cardiovascular depression and thermoregulatory disruption caused by pentothal/halothane anesthesia in the harbor seal, Phoca Vitulina. *J Wildl Dis* 17(1):121–130, 1981.
18. Dutkiewicz T, Chelstowski K: Comparative studies on the influence of decapitation, ketamine and thiopental anesthesia on rate heart mitochondria. *Basic Res Cardiol* 76(2):136–143, 1981.
19. Frankl WS, Poole-Wilson PA: Effects of thiopental on tension development, action potential, and exchange of calcium and potassium in rabbit ventricular myocardium. *J Cardiovasc Pharmacol* 3(3):554–565, 1981.
20. Heitz C, Dulac H, Cuisinier-Gleizes P, Stoclet JC: Parathyroid hormone effects on calcium metabolism in the rat are impaired by 5-ethyl-5′-(1-methylpropyl)-2-thiobarbiturate(inaktin). *Eur J*

Pharmacol 75(2–3):161–166, 1981.

21. Reiz S, Alfors E, Friedman A, Aggmark S, Peter T: Effects of thiopentone on cardiac performance, coronary hemodynamics and myocardial oxygen consumption in chronic ischemic heart disease. *Acta Anaesthesiol Scan* 25(2):103–110, 1981.
22. Bowe EA, Wolf S: Prevention of intracranial hypertension during the insertion of a pulmonary artery catheter. *Neurosurgery* 9(5):562–565, 1981.
23. Bellman MH, Pleuvry BJ: Comparison of the respiratory effects of ICI 35 868 and thiopentone in the rabbit. *Br J Anaesth* 53(4):425–429, 1981.
24. Dionne RA, Driscoll EJ, Gelfman SS, Sweet JB, Butler DP, Wirdzek PR: Cardiovascular and respiratory response to intravenous diazepam, fentanyl, and methohexital in dental patients. *J Oral Surg* 39(5):343–349, 1981.
25. Belopavlovic M, Buchthal A: Barbiturate therapy in the management of cerebral iscaemia. *Anaesthesia* 35(3):271–278, 1980.
26. Rose DM, Bassell GM, Eugene J: Complete neurological recovery after 13 minutes of hypovolemic hypotension. *Crit Care Med* 9(2):101–103, 1981.
27. Astrup J, Skovsted P, Gjerris F, Sgrensen HR: Increase in extracellular potassium in the brain during circulatory arrest: Effects of hypothermia, lidocaine, and thiopental. *Anesthesiology* 99(3):256–262, 1981.
28. Bedford RF, Persing JA, Poberskin L, Butler A: Lidocaine or thiopental for rapid control of intracranial hypertension? *Anesth Analg* 59(6):435–437, 1980.
29. Kassell NF, Hitchon PW, Gerk MK, Sokoll MD, Hill TR: Alterations in cerebral blood flow, oxygen metabolism, and electrical activity produced by high dose sodium thiopental. *Neurosurgery* 7(6):598–603, 1980.
30. Kassell NF, Hitchon PW, Gerk MK, Sokoll MD, Hill TR: Influence of changes in arterial pCO_2 on cerebral blood flow and metabolism during high-dose barbiturate therapy in dogs. *J Neurosurg* 54(5):615–619, 1981.
31. Moss E, Gibson JS, McDowall DG: The use of anesthetic drugs to reduce ICP changes in head-injured patients. *Acta Anaesthesiol Belg* (Suppl) 31:43–48, 1981.
32. Bielicki L, Krieglstein J, Wever K: Key enzymes of glycolysis in brain as influenced by thiopental. *Arzneim Forsch* 30(4):594–597, 1980.
33. Bourn WM, Reigel CE: Lack of influence of brain catecholamines on acute effects of barbiturates. *Pharmacol Biochem Behav* 13(5):733–735, 1980.
34. Quasha AL, Tinker JH: Hypothermia plus thiopental: Prolonged electroencephalographic suppression. *Anesthesiology* 55(6):636–640, 1981.
35. Manani G, Valenti S, Sharbrough FW: The influence of thiopentone and alfatahesin on succinylcholine-induced fasciculations and myalgias. *Can Anaesth Soc J* 28(3):253–258, 1981.
36. Pastuszko A: Action of barbiturates on activity of acetylcholinesterase from synaptosomal membranes. *Neurochem Res* 5(7):769–776, 1980.
37. Harvey SC: *Hypnotics and Sedatives*, ed 6. In Goodman AG, Gilman A (eds): New York, Macmillan Publishers, 1980, pp 339–375.
38. Morgan DJ, Blackman GL, Paull JD, Wolf LJ: Pharmacokinetics and plasma binding of thiopental, II. Studies at caesarean section. *Anesthesiology* 54(6):474–480, 1981.
39. Christensen JH, Andreasen F, Jansen JA: Pharmacokinetics of thiopental in caesarean section. *Acta Anaesthesiol Scand* 25(2):174–179, 1981.
40. Bakke OM, Haram K, Lygre T, Wallem G: Comparison of the placental transfer of thiopental and diazepam in caesarean section. *Eur J Clin Pharmacol* 21(3):221–227, 1981.
41. Morgan M, Holdcroft A, et al: Comparison of thiopentone and methohexitone as induction agents for caeserean section. *Anaesth Intensive Care* 8(4):431–435, 1980.
42. Healy TE, Foster GE, Evans DF, Syed A: Effect of some IV anesthetic agents on canine gastrointestinal motility. *Br J Anaesth* 53(3):229–233, 1981.
43. Lovett EJ III, Alderman J, Munster E, Lundy J: Suppressive effects of thiopental and halothane on specific arms of the immune response. *J Surg Oncol* 15(4):327–334, 1980.
44. Campbell RL, Satterfield SD, Dionne RA, Kelley DE: Post anesthetic morbidity following fentanyl, diazepam and methohexital sedation. *Anes Prog* 27(2):45–48,1980.
45. Dolovich J, Evans S, Rosenbloom D, Goodacre R, Rafajac FD: Anaphylaxis due to thiopental sodium anesthesia. *Can Med Assoc J* 123(4):292–294, 1980.
46. Korttila K, Aromaa U: Venous complications after intravenous injection of diazepam, flunitrazepam, thiopentone and etomidate. *Acta Anaesthesiol Scand* 24(3):227–230, 1980.
47. Millar JM, Barr AM: The prevention of pain on injection. A study of the effect of intravenous lidocaine before methohexitone. *Anaesthesia* 36(9):878–890, 1981.
48. Mazumder JK, Metcalf IR, Holland AJ: Inadvertant intra-arterial injection of thiopentone. *Can Anaesth Soc J* 27(4):395–398, 1980.
49. Butera ST, Garner HE, Moore NJ, Amend JF: Xylazine/sodium thiopental combination for short-term anesthesia in the horse. *VM/SAC* 75(5):765–770, 1980.
50. Tammisto T, Aromaa U, Korttila K: The role of thiopental and fentanyl in the production of balanced anaesthesia. *Acta Anaesthesiol Scand* 24(1):31–35, 1980.

CHAPTER 7

Inhalant Anesthetics

CHARLES E. SHORT, D.V.M., M.S., D.A.C.V.A.

Introduction

Almost 20 different inhaled anesthetics have been used in man since the first development of nitrous oxide and ethyl ether. In 1844, Horace Wells saw a nitrous oxide demonstration, noted its analgetic properties, and then used it clinically for dental work. He gave a public demonstration of its use for dental extraction at the Massachusetts General Hospital in 1845 (1).

W. E. Clark used diethyl ether for extraction of a tooth in 1842. Several months later, Crawford W. Long used it for clinical anesthesia in Athens, Georgia. The first public use of ether anesthesia was William T. G. Morton's removal of a tumor in Boston in 1846 (1).

Anesthetic properties of chloroform were discovered in animals in 1847 (1). Both ether and chloroform were administered by the open drop method and were to influence anesthetic management in veterinary medicine. Nitrous oxide was to play a minor role during the early years of veterinary inhalant anesthesia because its lack of potency in animals required a minimum concentration of 100% for anesthesia; thus it was considered toxic in animals.

Diethyl ether and chloroform were potent anesthetic agents. Diethyl ether had disagreeable properties, at high concentrations could cause profound depression or cardiac arrest, and was flammable and explosive. Chloroform at higher concentrations was highly toxic, producing respiratory depression and cardiac arrhythmias. These characteristics limited interest in chlorinated anesthetics. The available equipment did not improve control of anesthetic concentrations or assist with needed ventilation. This resulted in a fear of the use of inhaled anesthetics in veterinary medicine. Most surgical procedures prior to the development of halothane and methoxyflurane were completed using injectable anesthetics or combinations of injectable medications including narcotics (2).

Cyclopropane, first used clinically in humans by Ralph Waters at the University of Wisconsin in 1933, was beneficial in the development of anesthesia (1). However, it did not significantly change the course of modern veterinary anesthesia because the gas was highly flammable and its blood solubility was almost identical to that of nitrous oxide (1).

Fluroxene (2,2,2,trifluroroethyl ether) was prepared by Shukyse in 1951 (1). It was an anesthetic that produced anesthesia rapidly but also produced cardiopulmonary depression. There was a danger of arrhythmias, and it could induce vomiting. Fluroxene was more toxic in animals than in humans, especially after repeat anesthetic administration; in such a case, death was not uncommon. It also was highly flammable.

It was only after the discovery of halothane (2-bromo-2 chloro-1,1,1-trifluoroethane) by Sweking (1951) (3) that the modern era of inhalant anesthesia in veterinary medicine began. Halothane was a nonexplosive anesthetic and was a more stable, colorless, pleasant liquid. It possessed many of the qualities of a desirable anesthetic, including rapid induction and recovery. It was less toxic than previous agents. Unfortunately, it was a potent cardiopulmonary depressant and was suspected of causing hepatic dysfunction.

Methoxyflurane (2,2-dichloro-1,1-difluoroethyl methyl ether) had been synthesized in 1940 (1), but not until Dow Chemical Company produced the anesthetic in 1958 was there a major interest in the development of this agent. It was first used clinically by Joseph Artusio (4) and Alan Van Poznak (5) of Cornell University College of Medicine, in New York City in

1960. Methoxyflurane was a potent, nonflammable anesthetic with remarkable analgesic properties. It was potent at low concentrations and provided excellent muscle relaxation, especially in small animals. Its high blood and tissue solubility showed induction and recovery and made it difficult to maintain anesthesia in large animals. It had properties that indicated potential renal and hepatic toxicity.

The use of halothane and methoxyflurane in veterinary medicine began to increase significantly during the 1960s, although there was a need for anesthetic equipment to safely administer the anesthetics. Methoxyflurane was safely administered to small animal patients utilizing ether-type vaporizers; however, halothane administered by similar equipment was too often associated with difficult anesthetic management. The early efforts of William V. Lumb, E. Wynn Jones, Lawrence R. Soma, John C. Thurman, and others to use inhalant anesthesia in veterinary medicine in the United States included adaptations of equipment as well as development of an understanding of comparative anesthetic responses in various species. This was to influence teaching programs in veterinary colleges.

In part due to equipment availability and drug solubility, methoxyflurane became a popular anesthetic for use in dogs and cats and halothane gained acceptance for use in the horse. Although halothane in many species and methoxyflurane for small species have provided quality anesthesia, there is a continuing interest in the development of new inhalants.

Ross Terrell synthesized over 700 halogenated compounds. Presently, the two most notable discoveries in the methyl ethyl series are enflurane (2-chloro-1,1,2-trifluoroethyl-difluoromethyl ether) and isoflurane (1-chloro-2,2,2-trifluorethyl difluoromethyl ether) (1, 6–8). These two compounds produce rapid induction and recovery. They are potent agents but appear to have much less toxic effects on the renal and hepatic systems because there is minimal biotransformation. These agents show promise in veterinary medicine for high risk and selected cases.

Anesthetic Uptake and Distribution

The work of Eger (9) has contributed greatly to the understanding of anesthetic action. The uptake and distribution of inhalant anesthetics is dependent on many factors. These include partial coefficients, minimum alveolar concentrations, physical-chemical properties, absorption, and delivered concentrations of the anesthetics. Corresponding to minute volume exchange, alveolar partial pressure, pulmonary blood flow, cardiac output, perfusion, and lipid content of tissues are anatomical and physiological mechanisms that influence spread of uptake, tissue distribution, and final elimination.

The anesthetic vaporizer settings will directly effect the rise in alveolar concentration of anesthetic gases. Higher inspired concentrations will result in more rapid rise in alveolar concentration due to concentration, especially compared to lower inspired concentrations. This is apparent because the absolute alveolar rise in concentration has a direct relationship to the concentration inspired. Lower inspired concentrations will reflect closer correlation to the solubility coefficients of the individual anesthetic gases. Alveolar ventilation is a contributing factor to the alveolar rise in anesthetic concentration. The effect of alveolar ventilation will be influenced by the functional residual capacity of the individual patient. When there is a high oxygen flow and high anesthetic inspired vapor concentration relative to FRC, rapid rise in alveolar concentration will occur. Thus, this rise in alveolar concentration may be influenced by increasing the vaporizer setting or utilization of assisted or controlled ventilation to artificially increase ventilation (10). Even with increased ventilation, there will be maximum rates at which uptake of inspired anesthetic concentrations can influence alveolar concentration. The ultimate alveolar concentration will be a reflection of the difference between the inspired concentration and the concentrations in the gases in the alveoli being exchanged with new gases and a time constant. Eger (9) has indicated that the time constant is the time required for the flow through the lungs to equal the capacity of the lung. It is also the time required for 63% washin or washout of new gas from the lungs. Ventilation adds anesthetic to the alveoli, whereas uptake by the pulmonary circulation removes anesthetic (10).

The solubility of inhalant anesthetic influences the induction time and speed of arousal from anesthesia. A relatively low solubility allows a rapid increase in alveolar concentration of anesthetics during induction and a rapid decrease during recovery. Isoflurane has low levels of solubility, whereas methoxyflurane represents an agent with high levels of solubility. Solubility is defined as a concentration distribution ratio between alveolar concentrations and the concentration in other tissues (Table 7.1).

Thus, in order to achieve sufficient anesthetic concentration in the brain to produce unconsciousness, it is necessary for sufficient anesthetic tension to occur between the inspired anesthetic gas and the alveoli. The blood gas coefficients indicate how easily the agents pass from the alveoli to blood and then to other tissues. Not only does nitrous oxide pass quickly across the alveolar membrane, its solubility is so low that rapid establishment of concentration in tissues will occur. In dramatic contrast is methoxyflurane, with high blood gas coefficients for slow uptake; the high

Table 7.1
Solvent/Gas Partition Coefficients at 37°C

Solvent	Cyclopropane	Nitrous Oxide	Isoflurane	Enflurane	Halothane	Diethyl Ether	Methoxyflurane
Blood	0.4–0.6[a]	0.47	1.4	1.9	2.4	12.1	12.0–13.0
Tissue							
Brain	0.76	0.50	2.6	2.9	6.7	1.12	24.2
Liver	1.16	0.38	3.5	3.7	6.0	1.01	22.8
Kidney	0.62	0.40	1.8	1.9	3.7	1.06	11.2
Muscle	1.16	0.54	5.2	4.6	8.0	0.98	16.1
Fat	12.9	1.08	60	63	138	3.7	635
Oil	11.8	1.4	91	96	224	65	970

[a] Adapted from Eger (2, 11).

blood tissue coefficient will reflect high levels of absorption into body tissues. This results in slow induction and recovery patterns (9, 10).

Cardiac output will influence the uptake of anesthetics. As cardiac output increases, there will be a tendency to distribute the anesthetic from the alveoli to body tissues. At least initially, the gradient of anesthetic will be directed to vessel-rich organs (brain, liver, kidney, heart, and endocrine glands), which receive the major portion of cardiac output. The concentration in these organs will move more rapidly to reach equilibrium with arterial anesthetic tension than other tissue groups. Seventy to eighty percent of the cardiac output is directed to these tissues, which comprise less than 10% of body mass (9, 10).

The skin and muscle comprise the next group of tissues to reach equilibrium with blood anesthetic tension. This represents more of the body mass, but receives proportionately less of the cardiac output. The body fat is slower to saturate than more highly perfused tissues. The body fat is a critical consideration in uptake distribution and elimination because some agents are highly fat-soluble (diethyl ether and methoxyflurane); prolonged anesthesia not only results in higher tissue concentration, but highly delayed recoveries (9, 10). The vessel-poor tissues (bones, cartilage, tendons, and ligaments) do not significantly influence anesthetic uptake and distribution.

Concerning the alveolar to mixed venous anesthetic partial pressure difference, during induction with inhalant anesthetics, the alveolar concentrations will initially be much higher than the mixed venous anesthetic partial pressures. Venous concentrations do not appreciably rise until there is uptake from the lung by arterial blood during the induction or early maintenance of anesthesia; body tissues remove most of the anesthetic agent supplied to them by the blood. The venous anesthetic partial pressure during that time will be far below the partial pressure in the arterial blood. This results in a large initial partial pressure difference. As the venous partial pressure of the anesthetic agent increases with time, one observes the development of a smaller difference between arterial and venous concentrations. This results in less uptake of anesthetic from the alveoli and a reduction in the amount of anesthetic that needs to be delivered by the vaporizer. More dramatic changes in these factors will be noticeable either during induction or during maintenance in short-term anesthetic procedures than during prolonged anesthetic procedures.

Tissue uptake of anesthetic will influence the amount of anesthetic removed from the lung. If for various reasons, including shunts (especially in the horse), hypovolemic shock, and poor profusion of body tissues does not result in removal of anesthetic agent from the blood to tissues. There is a return by venous blood of higher concentrations than when tissue uptake is high. Tissue uptake will increase during physiologically normal cardiopulmonary function; two major factors influencing tissue uptake will be tissue perfusion (blood flow) and tissue solubility of the anesthetic agent used. Tissues with high fat content can be expected to absorb higher concentrations of anesthetic agents, especially those with high levels of fat solubility such as methoxyflurane. As the tissues become saturated with anesthetic agent, the arterial-to-tissue partial pressure difference will lessen. Likewise, by the time tissue concentrations have increased to equilibrate with the supply of anesthetic agent in arterial blood, there will be an increase in partial pressure of anesthetic agent in venous blood leaving the tissues. Theoretically, an ultimate equilibrium of anesthetic partial pressure in blood and tissues could eventually be established. This, however, does not occur during normal surgical anesthetic procedures and could only occur during chronic exposure of steady state inspired concentrations over hours (10).

The administration of high concentration and large volumes of nitrous oxide may increase the total volume of anesthetic gases inspired by patients. Nitrous oxide easily crosses the alveolar membrane. Utilization of nitrous oxide and potent anesthetic agents during induction will therefore result in an increase in inspiratory volume of the concurrently administered anesthetic gases. This can hasten the increase in alveolar concentration of the second gas. This second gas effect during the use of nitrous oxide and such other agents as halothane or methoxyflurane can result in rapid inductions. The second gas effect is significant only during induction and when a second gas is used in conjunction with either nitrous oxide or diethyl ether.

The rate of anesthetic induction can be influenced by factors controlling cerebral blood flow. Even though the brain is a highly perfused organ, conditions relative to anesthetic management, such as hyperventilation versus hypoventilation, can influence cerebral blood flow. When cerebral blood flow is reduced, the production of unconsciousness and surgical anesthesia may be delayed because of reduced availability of anesthetic to cerebral tissues. Factors such as hyperexcitement in animal patients without tranquilization or careful restraint may cause rapid uptake of anesthetic in brain tissue due to increased blood flow to the brain. This may result in crash inductions and the potential for undesirable adverse responses (10).

Anesthetic uptake will be influenced by ventilation perfusion abnormalities. These include the presence of arterial venous shunts across the lung. Difficulties of anesthetic uptake in horses with ventilation perfusion mismatch have been observed on numerous occasions. Difficulties with anesthetic uptake during these ventilation perfusion mismatches can be confirmed by evidence of poor ventilation with elevated $PaCO_2$ and reduced PaO_2 values in spite of efforts to improve ventilation.

After adequate uptake of anesthetic agent to body tissues to produce general anesthesia, maintenance of anesthesia is provided by supplying an inspired concentration that will maintain the desired level in the compartments of the body influenced by anesthetics, especially the brain and other compartments. Elimination of anesthetics at the completion of the anesthetic period will be inversely related to the uptake of the anesthetic during induction and early maintenance. As the inspired anesthetic concentration is reduced or eliminated, the available alveolar concentration will diminish and the uptake of anesthetic to the arterial blood to be supplied to the perfused tissues will diminish. Venous return of blood will carry anesthetics from the tissues to be either eliminated unchanged by the lung or undergo biotransformation by the hepatic system (10). Solubility in body tissues, anesthetic concentrations, duration of anesthesia, and saturation of body tissues will be factors influencing the amount of any anesthetic agent that undergoes biotransformation. An increase in ventilation usually accelerates arousal from anesthesia, especially if the anesthetic agents used do not have high levels of solubility (9).

During recovery from anesthetic regimes that include nitrous oxide, an awareness of the rapidity which nitrous oxide diffuses to the lung will aid in avoiding diffusion hypoxia. Nitrous oxide is four times more soluble than nitrogen. There is often depression of cardiopulmonary responses at the completion of the anesthetic regime; converting from oxygen/nitrous oxide and anesthetic mixtures to breathing atmospheric air with 80% nitrogen can result in less than 20% oxygen availability in the lung. A period of 5 to 10 minutes of respiration without nitrous oxide is recommended to avoid diffusion hypoxia.

Minimum Alveolar Concentration

The use of minimum alveolar concentration (MAC), which is the concentration of anesthetic at one atmosphere that produces a lack of response in 50% of subjects to a standard stimulus, has become an index of anesthetic potency (11). The most obvious sign of no response to a standard stimulus is lack of movement. As a result, the concurrent use of paralytic agents during studies to determine minimum alveolar concentration values is invalid. The utilization of minimal MAC has been very helpful in providing some assessment of the appropriate concentrations to use in veterinary anesthesia. We do not have the benefit of discussing the recall of unpleasant experiences after anesthesia with animal patients as with humans. Knowledge of relative values and potencies of various anesthetic agents thereby provides the veterinarian with a greater opportunity to assure that sufficient concentrations of anesthetic agents are being administered to produce both immobility and lack of pain during surgery. MAC is equally adaptable to all inhaled anesthetics and can be used in all species. It is substituted for the classic Guedel signs and our efforts to standardize responses of animals to various anesthetic agents. MAC relates to the partial pressure of anesthetic available at the site of action. It does not account for situations in which the alveolar concentration of anesthetic is not transmitted across the alveolar membrane to arterial blood, nor can it compensate if inadequate time has been allowed for equilibrium to be established between alveolar concentrations and tissue levels to provide surgical-plane anesthesia. The adjustment of the anesthetic vaporizer to deliver inspired concentrations of anesthetic vapors does not guarantee that certain MACs of anesthetic agents always exist at the time of surgery. The concentration of anesthetic agent in the alveoli does not necessarily coincide with the concentration in other body tissues, including the brain.

MAC has been determined for many species. Animals are anesthetized with the agent to be evaluated, the alveolar concentration is measured after 15 minutes, and the animal is stimulated and observed for movement. The most common means of stimulation are the application of a hemostat to the tail or the use of a standardized electrical current. MAC is then established as the concentration somewhere between the concentration that allows movement and the concentration that prevents all movement. As a result, there can be slight variation in the MAC values reported for various animal species by different investigators. Table 7.2 shows MAC values for volatile anesthetics for various species.

Nitrous Oxide

Nitrous oxide is the oldest anesthetic gas or vapor available for use in anesthesia. At standard pressure and temperature, it is a colorless inert gas (11). Although it is nonflammable, it can support combustion. Nitrous oxide can exist as a liquid under pressure at room temperature, which explains its cylinder pressure as it is usually stored. The cylinders when filled normally are stable at 750 cm of water pressure and should be handled accordingly.

Nitrous oxide has analgesic properties. The potency of this analgesia is much greater in humans than in animals. There is evidence to suggest that nitrous oxide and narcotics interact selectively with the opiate receptor endorphin system to produce analgesia; the mechanisms may be related to central nervous system depression as part of the result produced by nitrous oxide in analgesia in animal and human subjects (11). Nitrous oxide has been used as the principle agent for dental procedures in humans; often levels of 80% nitrous oxide and 20% oxygen are required. Although the anesthetic potency of nitrous oxide has been demonstrated in humans, potency in animal subjects is probably less than one-half that shown in man (12). The MAC for nitrous oxide is more than 100% in animals; monkeys, cats, dogs, calves, and horses require more than 100% nitrous oxide to achieve 1 MAC (12). Because nitrous oxide is not anesthetic at less than 1 atmosphere, its use as a principle agent in veterinary anesthesia is extremely limited. It has been used effectively in selected cases of severe CNS depression as the sole agent for painful procedures. In animals without extensive CNS depression, nitrous oxide must be combined with potent injectable analgetics, injectable anesthetics, or potent inhalant anesthetics to provide effective surgical anesthesia (13). Its predominant use in veterinary medicine has been as a part of balanced anesthesia or as a carrier gas to provide additional uptake of anesthetic by second-gas effect, allowing reduction in concentration of potent anesthetics that may give greater depression of cardiopulmonary function when used alone. A minimum of 50% nitrous oxide and oxygen is necessary to contribute significantly to the analgesia and anesthetic mixtures. The selection of concentration of nitrous oxide and oxygen requires the simultaneous delivery of inadequate oxygen supply. The supply of oxygen needed in human patients, especially for dental procedures, may be adequate when 20 to 30% oxygen is supplied. The addition of potent opioids or anesthetics to supplement the analgetic effect of nitrous oxide is not as necessary in humans as in animal subjects. The additional respiratory-depressing effects of potent agents administered to animals in conjunction with nitrous oxide may interfere with adequate uptake of oxygen unless the simultaneous delivery of oxygen to the animal subject is at high flow rates. If high levels of nitrous oxide are to be delivered to animal subjects, oxygen analyzers should be incorporated into the delivery system to assure a safe concentration of oxygen. Assisted or controlled respiration may be needed if the combination of N_2O and other agents result in reduced tidal volume.

Table 7.2
MAC Values in Various Species

Agent	Dog (2)	Cat	Pig	Horse	Rat (2)
Halothane	0.87%	0.75 (2)	1.25 (24)	0.9	0.95
Methoxyflurane	0.23%	0.16 (2)		0.3	0.22
Enflurane	2.2%	1.2 (2)	1.66 (104)	2.1	
Isoflurane	1.5%	1.61 (126)	1.47 (139)	1.3	

There is a rapid uptake of nitrous oxide to body systems. It has a low partition coefficient and is relatively insoluble in body tissues (12); thus its elimination is also very rapid. Nitrous oxide may affect the concentration of concurrently administered potent anesthetic agents because some of the nitrous oxide will be absorbed into the liquid anesthetic as it passes through the vaporizer. Nitrous oxide appears to have a concentrating effect on the anesthetic vapor in the pulmonary system. Little nitrous oxide is metabolized in the system (11). Nitrous oxide moves very readily through the tissues; this can affect function because nitrous oxide diffuses through tissues faster than nitrogen and thus may increase intracellular osmolarity. It is apparent that nitrous oxide diffuses into closed gas spaces. This is particularly significant in instances of pneumothorax, gas-filled pockets of strangulated intestine, or other gas-filled spaces. Nitrous oxide diffuses into these spaces faster than carbon dioxide or nitrogen is removed. This increases the potential for distention secondary to the administration of nitrous oxide in intestinal obstruction. The volume of gas in closed spaces can double within 10 minutes and triple within 30 minutes during the concurrent use of nitrous oxide (11). This impact on ventilation and circulation can contraindicate the use of nitrous oxide as part of anesthetic management.

Nitrous oxide is a respiratory depressant. It limits the level of arterial oxygenation, partially by its depressing effect and partially by the reduced inspired oxygen concentration. In instances of expansion of gas-filled spaces, either from gastrointestinal gas or from pneumothorax, diaphragmatic activity is impaired, further reducing the animal's ability to maintain adequate arterial oxygenation (13).

Ventilation perfusion difficulties are known to occur relatively frequently in large animal subjects. Expansion of rumen gases by nitrous oxide or ventilation-perfusion mismatch in equine subjects limits the usefulness of nitrous oxide as a part of the anesthetic regime. Postoperative arterial oxygen appears to be lower when nitrous oxide has been used. There may also be diffusion hypoxia during the early recovery period from nitrous oxide anesthetic combinations because nitrous oxide diffuses into the lung more rapidly and interferes with the uptake of inspired oxygen.

The cardiovascular system is not significantly depressed by nitrous oxide. Nitrous oxide has the ability to depress myocardial function directly, especially in human subjects. However, the indirect action of nitrous oxide in animal subjects may cause an increase in cardiac output and arterial blood pressure. Animals receiving nitrous oxide as part of their anesthetic regime are not as likely to have depression of the sympathetic activity influencing cardiac function (13). The degree of depression of nitrous oxide anesthetic mixtures versus oxygen anesthetic mixtures may be expected to be somewhat proportional to the percentages of the total anesthetic levels attributed to either the nitrous oxide or the potent anesthetic agent. For example, more cardiovascular depression is expected with halothane and oxygen than with a reduced halothane concentration in conjunction with nitrous oxide and oxygen. In animal subjects, when nitrous oxide is used as a part of balanced anesthesia including paralytic agents, higher levels of cardiac output and arterial blood pressure can be considered as associated with inadequate total anesthesia rather than lack of depressant effect of nitrous oxide (13).

The financial involvement in veterinary practice is important. The limited potency of nitrous oxide does not justify the increased cost of administering nitrous oxide in most situations. If nitrous oxide is to be used in large animals with high flow rates, greater justification of the cost of nitrous oxide usage can be made in small animals.

The principal advantage of using nitrous oxide in veterinary medicine is to reduce the amount of potent inhalant anesthetics, which are more depressing to the cardiovascular system when used at lower concentrations with nitrous oxide than when used alone with oxygen (13). Due to its extremely low potency in animals and the compromise of oxygenation, it is difficult to justify the physiological benefits of nitrous oxide in veterinary practice, especially in large animals where the disadvantages appear to outweigh the advantages.

Because nitrous oxide is a colorless, odorless gas and occupational exposure to nitrous oxide may impose significant health hazards, it is necessary to insure that concentrations less than 25 ppm in the operating room do not occur. Efforts should be made to minimize the veterinarian's exposure to nitrous oxide as well as other anesthetic gases.

Although nitrous oxide is widely used in human anesthesia and possesses some unique qualities that may be beneficial in veterinary medicine, its lack of potency, potential toxicity, potential contributions to hypoxia, and the problems associated with gas-filled spaces in veterinary subjects make it much less useful in animal anesthesia. Its use therefore appears to be limited to those patients in which the characteristics of nitrous oxide can justify its use as part of anesthetic management and appropriate measures are taken to assure adequate oxygenation has been accomplished.

Diethyl Ether

Diethyl ether is a colorless, high volatile liquid with a pungent odor; it yields an irritating vapor (1). Its high flammability means it must be handled with care. It has an ignition temperature of 304°C in air. One pound of ether mixed with air can give 277 cubic feet of flammable mixture. The MAC for ether is 1.92%. Induction of anesthesia may be somewhat prolonged. Its irritation to mucous membranes results in extensive salivation unless anticholinergics are used. It produces cortical depression of the electroencephalogram (EEG) with decreased early vagal activity. However, vagal depression and tachycardia may be replaced with increased concentrations; these may be associated with varied arrhythmias. There is progressive depression of the respiratory center due to its irritating affect. Respiratory movements may increase in amplitude during the early induction phases. The heart rate may also increase due to autonomic nervous system stimulation. Catecholamines are increased in the blood. This increased release of epinephrine and norepinephrine aids in preventing myocardial depression.

Hepatic and renal function are decreased during surgical plane anesthesia, body temperature decreases due to depression of metabolic rate, and there is heat loss through the skin due to vasal dilatation. Postanesthetic nausea and vomiting are common in man. This is not as pronounced in animal subjects.

The utilization of diethyl ether as an inhalant anesthetic dramatically diminished after the development of nonexplosive, nonflammable agents with greater ease of control of physiological function, such as methoxyflurane, halothane, enflurane, and isoflurane.

Extreme care must be taken to avoid occupational dangers to personnel. Prolonged periods of chronic exposure to inhaled ether may adversely effect human health. Diethyl ether use in areas where conductive floors, appropriate equipment, exhaust systems, and other facilities are not maintained for the appropriate handling of highly inflammable explosive products is extremely dangerous.

Methoxyflurane

Methoxyflurane is a potent inhalation anesthetic agent. It is chemically 2,2-dichloro-1,1-difluoroethyl methyl ether (2). It has a molecular weight of 165.9 and a specific gravity at 25°C of 1.41. The boiling point of methoxyflurane is 104.7°C with a vapor pressure of 20°C of 22.8 mm Hg. The chemical formula for methoxyflurane is:

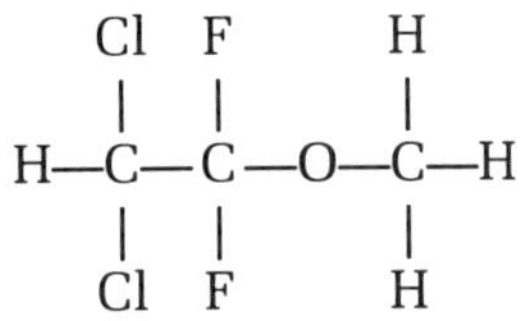

Methoxyflurane has a fruity odor, reacts with metal, and decomposes in ultraviolet light. It has a flash point in air of 62.8°C and in oxygen of 32.8°C. Methoxyflurane contains an antioxidant butylated hydroxytoluene to insure stability. This, however, will oxidize to a yellowish-brown and may accumulate on the wick of the vaporizer. This material can cause malfunction of vaporizers and may be cleaned by rinsing the wick with diethyl ether. Methoxyflurane is very soluble in rubber and soda lime, and its uptake and release by these substances can prolong recovery time (2).

The vapor concentration of methoxyflurane is limited by its vapor pressure at room temperature to a maximum of approximately 3.5% regardless of vaporizers used. Even this concentration is difficult to obtain during use in anesthetic units. Fortunately, the MAC value of methoxyflurane is quite low, having been established at 0.23. Methoxyflurane is approximately 4.7 times as potent as halothane (2).

The CNS depression of methoxyflurane is dose-related. There is smooth and gradual depression as the uptake of anesthetic is accomplished. Mask induction can be used in small animals; however, induction with injectable anesthesia followed by methoxyflurane maintenance is considerably more convenient. Maintenance is usually accomplished in small animals at 1 to 2 MAC. At light surgical planes of anesthesia or more, profound analgesia is present.

CARDIOVASCULAR RESPONSES

The heart rate and rhythm during methoxyflurane anesthesia is not adversely affected except at high concentrations, where there is some decrease in blood pressure with or without bradycardia. Hypotension is usually associated with reduced cardiac contractual force and a drop in cardiac output. Profound cardiovascular depression is not usually observed unless assisted breathing with encircled vaporizers has been utilized, forcing higher inspired concentrations of anesthetic into the alveoli. The myocardium is sensitized by methoxyflurane to epinephrine, but not as extensively as with halothane anesthesia. Concurrent use of epinephrine in patients under methoxyflurane anesthesia can result in cardiac arrhythmias and ventricular standstill. Patients are not as prone to superventricular arrhythmias, ventricular tachycardia, or ventricular fibrillation as with halothane (1).

RESPIRATORY RESPONSES

Ventilation should be carefully assessed during methoxyflurane anesthesia. Methoxyflurane can produce sufficient reduction in respiratory minute volume to result in respiratory acidosis during prolonged deep surgical anesthesia. Carbon dioxide may accumulate (14). There is usually sufficient ventilation to maintain arterial oxygen levels at or above awake arterial oxygenation values. Stimulation of bronchial or salivary secretion is not noticeable (15). Methoxyflurane does not have a tendency to produce laryngeal spasms. In most patients, even with deep anesthesia, respiratory efforts continue even though minute volume may be depressed (16).

There is significant uptake of methoxyflurane by body tissues. It is the most fat-soluble inhalant anesthetic agent available. Concentrations of methoxyflurane uptake in the obese patient during prolonged anesthesia can be very high. The recovery patterns are slow after prolonged methoxyflurane anesthesia. This also results in a greater volume of methoxyflurane to undergo biotransformation by the liver. If prolonged anesthesia has been maintained with methoxyflurane, especially in debilitated or obese patients or patients suffering from hepatic and renal dysfunction, they may demonstrate adverse metabolism effects. The biotransformation of methoxyflurane by the liver results in a release of the fluoride ion (17). Concentrations of fluoride ion may be toxic to the kidney (18). This toxicity increases if there is concurrent medication with antibiotics, such as tetracycline. This has resulted in nonreversible renal toxicity with high volume water output in human patients and a limited number of animal subjects (19–23). Due to the extent of biotransformation by the liver and the renal toxicity of the fluoride ion of methoxyflurane, there was a rapid decrease in popularity of methoxyflurane for use in human patients (19–23).

Methoxyflurane's use in veterinary medicine had been predominantly for small animal subjects (16). Use in horses has been limited to those areas where the atmospheric temperature is usually high. Under ideal situations, it is virtually impossible to obtain over 3.5% delivered concentration of methoxyflurane. Attempts to maintain anesthesia in horses and ponies where atmospheric temperatures are 20°C or less resulted in difficulty in maintaining surgical plane anesthesia. Anesthetic procedures requiring less than 2 MAC hours of anesthesia in dogs and cats are usually not associated with hepatorenal toxicity. Some of the cases of postanesthetic complications after methoxyflurane anesthesia in small animal patients have been related to low flow delivery of oxygen. Low oxygen flow anesthetic regimes can be used with methoxyflurane, but it is important to assure adequate oxygenation of the individual patient. This is especially true in small subjects with low tidal volume where adequate exchange of oxygen does not necessarily occur with the equipment used.

Methoxyflurane is a potent inhalant anesthetic agent that provides excellent analgesia and muscle relaxation even at low concentrations. Its role in veterinary medicine has been predominantly in small animal subjects. Its undesirable effects on the hepatic and renal systems can be reduced when it is selectively used in shorter surgical procedures. It does not affect the cardiovascular system as adversely as many other anesthetic agents.

Halothane

Halothane is a potent inhalant anesthetic (1). It possesses many qualities of an ideal anesthetic, including nonflammability and the capacity to provide excellent muscle relaxation with a rapid, pleasant induction and recovery. Its chemical formula is:

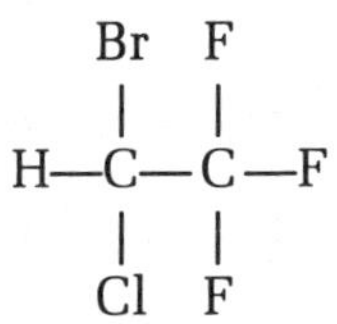

It does not cause extensive irritation to mucous and secretory membranes. It has a molecular weight of 197.4 with a specific gravity of 1.86 to 25°C. Its boiling point is 50.2°C, with a vapor pressure at 20°C of 244.1 mm Hg. Halothane decomposes in soda lime and in ultraviolet light and will react with metal, as does methoxyflurane. It is a nonflammable, nonexplosive anesthetic agent that should be vaporized in a precision vaporizer for careful administration. The MAC of halothane is 0.8%. It has been used in a large variety of animal species and breeds and has become a popular anesthetic for use in animals (2).

UPTAKE

The MAC for halothane varies among species by as much as 60%. The MAC value for halothane in swine is 1.25 ± 0.04%. This is higher than reported for other mammals (24). A comparison of minimum alveolar concentrations for halothane is shown in Table 7.2. Concurrent medications reduce the halothane MAC requirement. Morphine can reduce the halothane MAC by up to 84%, and alfentanil may reduce requirements up to 48% (25). Xylazine can reduce MAC significantly. In a group of English pointer dogs, halothane MAC was established as 0.92%; after xylazine in the same dogs, MAC was decreased to 0.57% (26). After determination of the xylazine and halothane MAC values, tolazoline, an alpha adrenergic antagonist, was administered. Halothane MAC values significantly increased to 1.24%. Concurrent utilization of nitrous oxide frequently has been used in anesthesia in humans to reduce the MAC requirements to halothane. This is not as effective in animals due to the difference in potency of nitrous oxide in animals as compared to humans. It does, however, reduce the MAC requirements compared to halothane used without nitrous oxide.

There is a difference in the uptake of halothane in young versus older subjects. The fraction of halothane in expired gas divided by the fraction of halothane in inspired gas (FE/FI) indicates that the FE/FI for halothane in the young increases more rapidly than in adults. Myocardial and brain halothane concentrations increase more rapidly in the young, and the early concentrations during anesthetic induction may cause hypotension and bradycardia in the young (27).

CNS EFFECTS

Halothane at 0.8% in dogs decreases the mean rate of cerebrospinal fluid (CSF) production from 0.047 to 0.033 ml/min. This effect persisted throughout 3.5 hours of anesthesia. When halothane concentrations were decreased to less than 0.1%, the control value of CSF production returned within 45 to 50 minutes. In patients at risk from increased intracranial pressure due to increased CSF volume, halothane may be preferred to those anesthetics that increase CSF production, such as enflurane (28). In hemodynamic studies on the distribution of cerebral blood flow in dogs during halothane anesthesia, mean arterial pressure and cardiac output decreased progressively as halothane concentrations increased. Systemic resistance remains relatively constant. Myocardial depression is caused by halothane. At relatively constant mean cerebral blood flow, as mean arterial pressure and cardiac output decreased proportionately, more flow was distributed to specific regions of the brain, such as the hypo-

Table 7.3
Hemodynamic Data Obtained during Halothane-N_2O (66%)-O_2 Anesthesia with Various Concentrations of Halothane

Hemodynamics	Halothane Concentration		
	0.5%	1.0%	1.5%
Mean arterial pressure[a,b]	128.4 ± 6.3	112.0 ± 6.2[c]	90.3 ± 7.4[c]
Central venous pressure[b]	5.5 ± 1.1	6.0 ± 1.4	6.4 ± 1.7
Mean pulmonary arterial pressure[b]	15.9 ± 1.2	15.9 ± 0.9	17.6 ± 1.5
Pulmonary wedge pressure[b]	7.9 ± 0.9	9.2 ± 1.0	10.8 ± 1.0[c]
Sagittal sinus pressure[b]	8.5 ± 0.6	9.9 ± 1.1	11.5 ± 1.0
Heart rate[d]	142.0 ± 9.1	138.1 ± 4.4	132.5 ± 4.4
Stroke volume[e]	9.6 ± 1.0	8.5 ± 1.0	7.6 ± 0.9
Cardiac output[f]	80.9 ± 7.0	69.1 ± 9.8	61.9 ± 7.7[c]
Mean cerebral blood flow[g]	65.9 ± 8.3	67.2 ± 7.4	73.1 ± 11.2
Systemic flow resistance[h]	1.74 ± 0.19	1.91 ± 0.27	1.57 ± 0.17
Cerebral flow resistance[i]	2.24 ± 0.35	1.71 ± 0.23	1.29 ± 0.21[c]

[a] Modified from Chen et al. (29). All values are mean ± SEM.
[b] Pressures in mm Hg.
[c] Compared to 0.5% H:P 0.05.
[d] $Min.^{-1}$.
[e] $Ml.^{-1}$.
[f] $Ml/min.^{-1}$.
[g] $Ml/min^{-1} - 100\ g.^{-1}$.
[h] Mm Hg/ml^{-1}/min/kg.
[i] Mm Hg/ml^{-1}/min/100 g.

thalamus and cervical cord, where neurons related to pressure regulations are located (Table 7.3) (29).

Halothane affects the responses of C fibers and A fiber nociciptive afferents sensitive to mechanical or heat stimuli in monkeys. The responses, however, are greater under halothane anesthesia than during barbiturate anesthesia (30). There is an increase in GABA-transaminase released during halothane anesthesia. The release of both the GABA-transaminase and succinic asemialdehyde dehydrogenase increases with time. This suggests a linkage of anesthetic action to a mitochondrial effect (31). Halothane at 3% is known to depress synaptosomal acetylcholine synthesis by 86% and inhibit adrenal cortical hormone (ACH) release by 50%. It is believed that halothane inhibits the ACH synthesis by directly interfering with the carrier-mediated transport system of choline (32). Complete abolition of the increase in heart rates and a response to somatic nerve stimulation occurs at a halothane end-tidal concentration of approximately 2.2% (33). Spinal cord evoked potentials are less variable during halothane anesthesia than somatosensory cortical evoked potentials (34). Halothane at 0.8% in dogs may increase cerebral blood volume by 11 to 12% and intracranial pressure by 4 to 5 cm of water. This is less than observed during enflurane anesthesia (35). This change in intracranial pressure may in part be due to increased reabsorption of CSF (36). As the concentration of halothane increases, it can markedly reduce central sympathetic and vagal outflows that play a role in peripheral homostatic regulation (37). This may account for the observed changes in heart rate, blood pressure, and cardiac output during halothane anesthesia at this concentration.

CIRCULATION

Naloxone at a dose of 0.05 mg/kg increases the dosage of morpine required for blockade of heart rate responses. The same dose of naloxone does not change morphine values with the combined administration of morphine and halothane. There is an eight-fold increase in the naloxone dosage required to demonstrate antagonistic effect against morphine when it is used in conjunction with halothane (38). Halothane appears to have no direct local effect to cause depression of the carotid sinus baroreceptor function. Its possible action is via CNS inhibition of sympathetic efferents to the carotid sinus (39). Further studies have shown that during 0.75 and 1.5% halothane there is dose-dependent synthetization of baroreceptors of the sinus profusion. At least part of the synthetization appears to be calcium-related (40). At best, halothane appears to exert only a slight direct effect on baroreceptor function. It appears that when carotid sinus pressure is kept constant, the depressive effect of halothane on baroreceptor function is mediated principally via inhibition of the CNS-sympathetic nuclei, thereby reducing baroreceptor nerve activity (41). Even though baroreceptor responses have been affected by halothane, barostatic reflexes do persist; they favor the maintenance of reduced levels of arterial pressure during halothane anesthesia (42).

Coronary colateral blood flow is well maintained during halothane anesthesia at normal heart rates, but tachycardia severely limits blood flow to the colateral subendocardium (43). Halothane probably does not cause direct coronary vasal dilitation. Coronary blood flow drops as halothane concentrations increase until

Table 7.4
Hemodynamics during Halothane Anesthesia in Dogs[a]

	Halothane Concentration		
	0	0.83%	1.6%
Cardiac output, liter/min	2.15	1.76	0.40
Mean arterial pressure mm Hg	92	82	62
Left ventricular (LV) minute work, kgm/min	3.48	2.39	1.53
Heart rate, beats/min	107	101	100
LV change in pressure vs. time, (dP/dt units)	20.0	15.4	10.7
Coronary blood flow, ml/100 g/min	120	81.5	58.4
Myocardial oxygen consumption, ml/100 g/min	12.4	7.31	5.42
Coronary vascular resistance, ml/100 g/min	0.55	0.99	1.01

[a] Modified from Beattie et al. (44).

higher concentrations are reached. Halothane depresses cardiac output, mean arterial pressure, change in pressure with respect to change in time (dp/dt), left ventricular minute work, and myocardial oxygen consumption (Table 7.4).

Halothane does not cause myocardial ischemia even in the presence of severe coronary stenosis (45). Halothane causes a highly significant increase in the electrical impulse threshhold to produce extrasystolies from ischemia areas during halothane anesthesia. Halothane can be beneficial in preventing spontaneously occurring ventricular fibrillation in acute myocardial ischemia (46). The relative reduction in oxygen demand during halothane anesthesia did not reduce myocardial infarct size or salvage myocardium within the area of profusion after coronary ligation in pigs during prolonged anesthesia (47). In dogs, fentanyl usage resulted in a smaller area of infarct size than did halothane. There was greater myocardial blood flow within the infarct area during fentanyl than with halothane (48). Halothane has a greater depressant effect on heart cells than does enflurane (49), leading to the conclusion that, although halothane reduces heart rates and arterial pressure and has a presumed negative inotropic effect, dogs have much greater coronary artery cross profusion than either pigs or man. Halothane administration in the less than ideally profused myocardium should also take into account species variations.

Halothane decreases the stimulation-evoked release of norepinephrine by stimulation of prejunctional inhibitory muscarinic receptors. Halothane may also impair clearance of norepinephrine from the synaptic cleft (50). Halothane and acid-base changes produce cardiac arrhythmias. The action potential duration and effective refractory period of cardiac fiber is shortened during alkalosis and lengthened during acidosis. Action potential duration (APD) and effective refractory period (ERP) are abolished at high levels of halothane anesthesia (51). Less oxidative deamination of norepinephrine occurs in the presence of halothane (52). Halothane does not depress catecholamine-stimulated adenylate cyclase activity in canine myocardial sarcolemmal membranes (53). Halothane depresses contractility in the hypoprofused myocardium to a lesser degree than when normal levels of myocardial perfusion are present. This is probably due to the interaction of two effects, direct depression of halothane on contractile mechanisms and indirect positive inotropic effect (54).

There is an increase in oxygen demand of the myocardium. This has been suspected in several species. In the dog, no significant myocardial changes occurred during the initial 3.5 hours of halothane anesthesia. However, after 4.5 hours, arterial blood pressures increased, coronary sinus blood flow increased, and myocardial oxygen uptake increased 19% (55). After 6 hours anaerobic myocardial metabolism may predispose dogs to myocardial ischemia (56). This may explain partially the detrimental effects of prolonged anesthesia in extended surgical procedures.

The evaluation of heart function during halothane anesthesia can not be complete without an understanding of the role of calcium and related electrolytes. Halothane does not appreciably effect the transport of calcium, but does diminish the amount of calcium within the sarcoplasmic reticulum available for the activation of myocardial contractal activity (57). The negative chronotropic effect of halothane and the dose-dependent depression of dP/dt is consistent with inhibition of slow calcium channels. Negative chronotropic action of halothane interacts in a competitive way with calcium, as indicated by a shift in the dose-response curve in the presence of excess calcium and the specific calcium blocking agent verapamil (58). Verapamil, nifedipine, and diltiazem may be associated with significant hypotension during halothane anesthesia. Caution must be used if halothane is to be administered concurrently with calcium channel blockers (59, 60). There is a clear dissociation between the negative inotropic action of halothane and the lack of change in myocardial intracellular pH. This indicates that intracellular acidosis does not mediate the cardiac-depressing effects of halothane. Halothane does decrease the forward flux of the creatine kinase reaction with a concomitant reduction in the steady-state content of myocardial ATP and phosphocreatine. The negative inotropic action of halothane may be mediated by an abnormality in high energy phosphate metabolism (61).

Halothane slows vagal atrioventricular (AV) conductivity (62). The extent of atrial bundle of His conduction slowing is dose-dependent. Although rates and pressures are commonly reduced with halothane anesthesia, combining halothane and fentanyl can result in a maintenance of contractibility beneficial in patients with compromised myocardial function (63). At 1–2 MAC halothane, left ventricular diastolic pressure volume relationships are not sufficiently altered by halothane. This indicates that left ventricular diastolic compliance does not change with different dosages of halothane (64).

Because halothane has been shown to have significant cardiovascular effects in healthy subjects undergoing elective surgical procedures, it is of interest to determine cardiovascular effects of halothane in chronically anemic animals (Table 7.4). In dogs, halothane demonstrated a progressive dose-dependent reduction in systemic vascular resistance. Control animals showed no change in systemic vascular resistance with increasing halothane concentration. The reduction in systemic vascular resistance in anemic dogs showed an increase in coronary blood flow compared to controls during halothane anesthesia (65) (Table 7.5).

Halothane decreases arrhythmogenic thresholds for epinephrine. The mean arrhythmic dose for epinephrine in the presence of 1.2 MAC of halothane in dogs was found to be 2.15 mcg/kg/min. This threshold was enhanced 13 times by prazosin treatment (66). There was an increase in the arrhythmia dose for epinephrine following D-metoprolol treatment because there was an increase in the threshold in the presence of both $alpha_1$ and $beta_1$ blockade that was much higher with $alpha_1$ blockade. There is evidence that the sensitization by halothane for ventricular arrhythmias is probably due to an $alpha_1$ adrenergic receptor-effective mechanism (66). Halothane concentrations of 0.5, 1.0, 1.5, and 2% showed no significant difference in epinephrine-induced arrhythmias when more than 0.05% halothane was administered. The development of epinephrine-induced ventricular arrhythmias during halothane anesthesia is not dose-related (67). Verapamil increases the minimal arrhythmic dose of epinephrine required during halothane in dogs (68), as does magnesium sulfate (69), quinidine (70), and lidocaine. Aminophylline decreases the amount of epinephrine required to produce arrhythmias in the presence of halothane anesthesia (68). Halothane also increases the defibrillation threshold by 6 or 7 J of energy (71).

RESPIRATORY RESPONSES

Short periods of halothane anesthesia in healthy subjects may appear to affect ventilation only during administration of excessive concentrations of halothane. The influence of spontaneous breathing versus assisted or controlled ventilation, anesthetic concentration influence on cardiac output, and cardiopulmonary conditions can alter pulmonary function during halothane anesthesia. The most complex of the animals in terms of pulmonary response to halothane during general anesthesia is probably the horse in dorsal recumbency, but concern is not limited to this species. In dogs, AV shunts have been shown to be relative to an increase in cardiac output and the levels of hypoxia in awake dogs. There is sufficient shunting during hypoxia. This shunting is even greater during halothane anesthesia up to 21–22% AV shunt. This emphasizes the need to avoid hypoxia during halothane anesthesia (72). Healthy goats show shunting during awake and halothane anesthesia. However, there is a dramatic increase in shunting when pulmonary injury is induced wtih acid aspiration. Patients with respiratory disease or pulmonary edema may be at risk for further deterioration of pulmonary oxygen exchange and development of hypoxemia during halothane anesthesia (73). Ventilation perfusion difficulties have occurred in sheep in the presence of pulmonary shunting during either spontaneous breathing or mechanical ventilation. PaO_2 and inhalation may decrease. Ventilation profusion (VA/Q) and functional residual capacity (FRC) are depressed (74). Halothane does not affect degradation in lung proteins. The inhibition of protein synthesis has a rapid onset, is dose-dependent, and is quickly reversible. It does not appear that there are changes in cellular permeability or decreased availability of amino acids as substrates for protein synthesis as a result of halothane anesthesia (75). Halothane anesthesia has direct inhibitory effect on smooth muscle cells and excitatory neuroelectro-transmission to produce a potent bronchodilation (76). The effect of carbon dioxide on central mechanisms regulating respiratory duration is opposite to that produced by halothane. Respiratory frequency is modified by both the

Table 7.5
Hemodynamic Effects of Halothane in Chronically Anemic Dogs[a]

	Halothane Concentration	Cardiac Output (liter/min)	Coronary Blood Flow (ml/100 g/min)	Myocardial Oxygen Consumption (ml/100 g/min)	Systemic Vascular Resistance (dynes: sec/cm^{-5})
Control dogs	0.75%	2.8 ± 2	151 ± 40	9.4 ± 0.7	2280 ± 180
	1.50%	2.3 ± 2	165 ± 53	6.6 ± 1.0	2430 ± 210
Anemic dogs	0.75%	4.2 ± 0.3[b]	365 ± 45[b]	11.8 ± 1.1[b]	1390 ± 105[b]
	1.50%	3.9 ± 0.4[b]	305 ± 56[b]	10.2 ± 1.8[b]	1210 ± 95[b]

[a] Modified from Miletich et al. (65).
[b] Significantly lower (mean ± SE) than controls.

depth of halothane anesthesia and its relationship to the respiratory response curve of $PaCO_2$ levels (77). In cats, hypoxia depressed ventilation appreciably during halothane administration (78). Halothane can reduce the collateral resistance normally seen during hypocapnia in dogs. The contribution of collateral ventilation to gas exchange is unknown. These changes may act inconjunctionwith hypoxic pulmonary vasoconstriction to adjust ventilation profusion deviations from the ileal and compensate for airway closure (79). Efforts to improve ventilation during halothane anesthesia have included manual assistance to respiration, control volume or pressure, limited mechanical ventilation, or high frequency ventilation technique (80).

Halothane does depress minute ventilation. the ventilatory depression is the consequence of depressed inspiratory neuromuscular output resulting in ultimate decreased inspiratory muscle contractility. Phrenic nerve activity does not significantly change after halothane administration, but the relationship between phrenic nerve activity and $PaCO_2$ increases may be markedly depressed. The decrease in inspiratory muscle contractility is more pronounced during high concentrations of anesthesia (81). It is further understood that halothane depresses the activity of the inspiratory neurons of the solitary tract nucleus and that the depression is dose- and time-dependent. Hypercarbia, hyperoxia, and vagotomy do not block inspiratory neuronal responses to halothane. The depressant effect of halothane on inspiratory neurons is due to direct central action (82).

HEPATIC RESPONSES

Halothane undergoes biotransformation in the liver. For some years, there has been an awareness of the potential for halothane to produce hepatic necrosis. There has been concern as to the role of the hepatic system in halothane metabolism and the potential for halothane to produce allergic or toxic responses of the hepatic system. The alterations in drug disposition observed druing halothane anesthesia are mainly due to inhibition of drug-metabolizing capacity in the liver (83). Further an understanding of the role of the hepatic system and anesthetic responses are discussed in the chapter on hepatic function in this text. Halothane has been shown in ponies to cause at 138% increase in bilirubin excretion, a 16% reduction in plasma bilirubin, and a 46% reduction in biliary bile acid concentration (84). There is evidence that hepatotoxicity from halothane in the hypoxic model is due to toxic in responses during the reductive metabolism of halothane (85). Hypercapnia increases oxygen supply to the liver, but hepatic oxygen consumption also increases during periods of hypercapnia. Thus, increased concentrations of carbon dioxide do not improve hepatic responses during halothane (86). Halothane may inhibit the synthesis of liver proteins. Halothane metabolites in the body are found to be in higher concentration in the liver than in other tissues (88). Thus it can be concluded that active metabolism and halogenation of halothane can occur.

RENAL FUNCTION

During halothane anesthesia, renal function may diminish, only to recover during the postoperative period. Halothane has even been associated with slight improvements in postoperative renal function in surgical patients with pre-existing chronic renal insufficiency (89). Halothane produces significant decreases in aortic pressure with corresponding decreases in renovascular resistance such that renal blood flow is not significantly changed even during acute hemorrhagic hypovolemia. Renal blood flow was not significantly decreased from hypovolemic controls during halothane administration after correction of hypovolemia with blood transfusions. Renal blood flow significantly elevates to above original normal volemic control values. Halothane is perhaps an ideal anesthetic for patients with renal compromise (90). In animals receiving halothane and verapamil, renovascular resistance and mean arterial pressures dropped while renal blood flow remained unchanged (91). This further confirms metabolic changes that take place after halothane anesthesia are primarily reflective of the responses of the hepatic system and not the renal responses.

In terms of the responses of fluids, electrolytes, and blood components, halothane anesthesia at 1% causes up to a 59% decrease in lymph flow within 20 minutes with a return to control level 30 minutes after discontinuing administration of halothane (92). Halothane significantly alters cerebral glucose utilization (93), but there is little difference between halothane and enflurane in the rate of glucose metabolism in heart cells (94). Halothane strongly inhibits gastric acid secretion (95).

HORMONE RESPONSES

Short-term, repeated exposure to halothane at subanesthetic concentrations is probably not associated with any appreciable acute toxicity on male reproductive function (96). It has been postulated that progesterone levels can effect the MAC of halothane in near-term pregnancy. There is now evidence that the decrease in MAC observed in near-term pregnancy is not endorphin-mediated, nor is it due to increased progesterone levels. A decrease in MAC may well be due to more than one of the many complex physiological changes that occur during pregnancy (97). Halothane anesthesia during the late stages of pregnancy should result in compatible acid-base and blood gas values for both the mother and the fetus. Significant higher maternal and fetal lactate was observed during fetal distress compared to nondistressed situations (98). In a study to determine MAC of fetal lambs and pregnant ewes, it was discovered that fetal blood concentration of halothane at MAC was 48 mg/liter, versus 133 mg/liter in the mother. Calculating end-tidal concentrations reveals a 0.33% concentration in the fetal lamb and a 0.69% halothane concentration in the mother (99). In newborn lambs during normoxia, 0.5 and 1 MAC of halothane decreased whole body oxygen consumption, cardiac output, and arterial blood pressure. One-half MAC of halothane had no effect on blood flow to any organ concept muscle. This flow decreased 64%. One MAC halothane decreased blood flow to the brain, heart, kidney, muscle, and gastrointestinal tract. Hypoxia decreased the oxygen consumption about 40%; cardiac output, arterial blood pressure, and heart rate of anesthetized hypoxic animals were no different from those in the previous normoxic condition (100). This leads one to the conclusion that factors influencing the selection of inhalant anesthetics during pregnancy or Caesarean section should focus on rapid recovery more than the pharmacodynamics of the anesthetic agent.

ENFLURANE

Enflurane is 2-chloro-1,1,2-trifluoroethyl-difluoromethyl ether (1). It is a potent, mildly pungent inhalant anesthetic that is easily administered and controlled. It has a molecular weight of 184.5 and a specific gravity at 25°C of 1.52. Its chemical formula is:

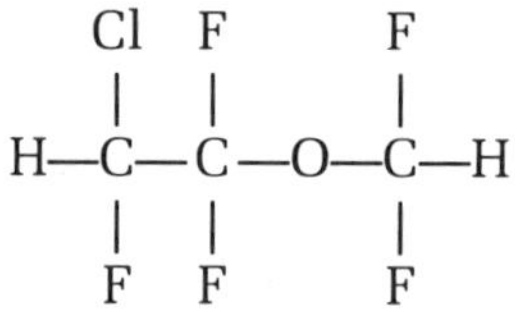

The boiling point is 56.5°C, and it has a vapor pressure at 20°C of 171.8 mm Hg. No preservatives are needed, and it is stable in soda lime and ultraviolet light. It does not react with metal.

Enflurane provides a rapid induction and emergence from anesthesia, moderate level of analgesia, and muscle relaxation sufficient for surgery under many circumstances. Higher concentrations of enflurane can result in inadequate muscle relaxation, and at exceptionally high concentrations, seizure-like activity may be evident if electroencephalograms are recorded. Seizures usually appears in the dog at greater than 3.5% vaporizer-delivered concentration. As with other inhalant anesthetics, concurrent utilization of narcotics and other analgetics decreases the concentration of enflurane required for surgical plane anesthesia. In human subjects, nitrous oxide dramatically reduces the MAC requirements of enflurane.

UPTAKE AND DISTRIBUTION

The relatively low solubility of enflurane in blood and tissues permit a rapid increase in alveolar concentration on induction of anesthesia. Concentrations for inducing anesthesia range from 2 to 4.5% and are reduced to 0.5 to 3% for maintenance. The MAC of enflurane is 1.9%. Reductions in anesthetic concentration for maintenance of anesthesia can usually be accomplished during the first 4 to 10 minutes of the anesthetic procedure.

The uptake of enflurane is not affected by prior administration of aminophylline (101). Higher concentrations of enflurane are known to have potential CNS hyperexcitability or epileptogenic properties. This is seldom observed at concentrations of less than 3.5%, but it does occur at high concentrations. Nitrous oxide has been shown to influence hyperexcitability only partially. There is some evidence of withdrawal hyperexcitability even with combinations of nitrous oxide and enflurane. The changes suggest nitrous oxide and enflurane may have different sites or mechanisms of action (102). In contrast to the seizure-like activity of enflurane in normal subjects, cats with pre-existing epileptic foci, such as in progressive myoclonic epilepsy and photosensitive epilepsy, may be anesthetized with enflurane with a considerable degree of safety (103).

At established MAC levels for enflurane in swine of 1.66%, or with 50% nitrous oxide and 0.82% enflurane, cerebral and total brain blood flow values were the same in controls as during enflurane anesthesia. However, blood flow in the brain stem and the cerebellum exhibited a dose-related increase at 1.5 MAC of enflurane. Vascular resistance in all regions of the brain decreased with enflurane anesthesia. The addition of nitrous oxide to enflurane resulted in a marked increase in cerebral blood flow (104). Narcotics and other analgetics reduce the concentration of enflurane required for surgical plane anesthesia as reflected in MAC values. The MAC of enflurane has been reduced by as much as 65% with the concurrent administration of 15 to 30 μg/kg of fentanyl as a loading dose and maintenance at 0.05 to 0.2 μg/kg/min. Further increases in fentanyl administration did not further reduce the MAC requirements of enflurane (105). It has been shown there is neither evidence of derangement of energy state nor increased anaerobic metabolism in the cerebral cortex during enflurane anesthesia (106).

CARDIOVASCULAR SYSTEM

Enflurane depressed myocardial performance and peripheral circulation. Cardiac output and stroke volume decrease, whereas there is little change in heart rate. Because there is a reduction in cardiac output and a decrease in systemic vascular resistance, arterial blood pressures will decrease accordingly. Cardiac rhythm is normally stable, and the instance of arrhythmias does not appear to be increased appreciably by enflurane, especially in comparison to the response to epinephrine challenge during halothane anesthesia.

It has been shown during induction with enflurane and oxygen that decreased arterial and central venous pressures, coronary flow and cardiac index occurred, but these returned to awake levels on intubation; thus myocardial oxygen extraction occurred during operation with no lactate production. Enflurane and oxygen produced no evidence of myocardial ischemia (107). Enflurane and isoflurane stimulate calcium transport by cardiac sarcoplasmic reticulum (108). Because this implicates enflurane in a modulating intracellular ion flux, it may preserve myocyte integrity during reperfusion by allowing more effective high energy phosphate repletion. Enflurane at 2% depressed myocardial function by as much as 20% (109). Enflurane is a more potent vasodilator than halothane. The reduction in blood pressure during enflurane anesthesia appears to be from potent reduction of systemic vascular resistance by enflurane (110). There is, however, a reduction in left ventricular dynamics by enflurane. Each MAC of enflurane depressed the inotropic state by approximately 20%. This gives a dose-related myocardial depression that contributes further to potential hypotension during enflurane anesthesia (111).

Because enflurane can lead to progressive dose-related increases in myocardial contractility, it is of interest to note the responses in the dog to 2 volumes percent of enflurane, as shown in Table 7.6 comparing responses during enflurane anesthesia to those in control dogs (112).

Enflurane decreased contractile force in dogs at 1 and at 1.25 MAC significantly compared to halothane contractility. The cardiac output at 1.25 and 2 MAC of enflurane was significantly greater than observed with halothane, as was the drop in mean blood pressure. There were no significant differences between halothane and methoxyflurane on body temperature, arterial pCO_2, pO_2, pH, and hematocrit (113). Heart rates in patients anesthetized with enflurane probably increase due to slight enhancement of automaticity associated with the enflurane (114). The systemic vascular resistance decreases may be due to significant biostatic reflexes that modify the cardiovascular depressive effects of enflurane (115). There is not as much depression of oxygen uptake by heart cells during enflurane anesthesia as during halothane (116). Myocardia oxygen consumption drops during induction with enflurane and appears to give a degree of protection against myocardial ischemia during enflurane anesthesia. Coronary blood flow may drop up to 32% due to reduced mean arterial pressure, but coronary resistance does not change (117).

RESPIRATORY SYSTEM

Enflurane is a profound respiratory depressant. It depresses the ventilatory responses to both carbon dioxide and hypoxia. As a result, respiratory acidosis is not unusual. Increased arterial $PaCO_2$ is a respiratory response in animals to enflurane anesthesia. It is predominantly through depression of tidal volume because the frequency of respiration may increase. The increase in respiratory rate is insufficient to compensate for a reduction of tidal volume. Fortunately, oxygen consumption is decreased during enflurane anesthesia. The decreased ventilatory response to hypoxia is similar for halothane, enflurane, or isoflurane (2).

RENAL FUNCTION

Patients with renal insufficiency anesthetized with enflurane do not have significantly greater increases in postoperative serum and organic fluoride levels compared with subjects with normal renal function (118). There is less metabolism of enflurane by the hepatic system than for either halothane or methoxyflurane.

OTHER SYSTEMS

Enflurane leads to inhibition of islet adenylate cyclase activity and to small resultant reductions in islet cyclic AMP content. These effects appear to be of insufficient magnitude to explain completely the ob-

Table 7.6
Ventricular Hemodynamics in Enflurane-Anesthetized Dogs[a]

Hemodynamics	Control	2%	4%
Left ventricle (LV)-systolic pressure, mm Hg	117.0 ± 4.4	−21.8 ± 7.6[b]	−31.5 ± 7.8
LV-end diastolic pressure, mm Hg	9.0 ± 1.4	−19.2 ± 6.3[b]	14.0 ± 3.2[b]
Mean arterial pressure, mm Hg	93.3 ± 7.3	−25.5 ± 6.2[b]	−37.0 ± 6.7[b]
LV-dP/dt_{max}, mm Hg/sec	2810 ± 309	−28.8 ± 7.2[b]	−52.6 ± 9.4[b]
LV-velocity, mm/sec	65.2 ± 5.8	−18.6 ± 3.4[b]	−35.6 ± 3.7[b]
Heart rate, beats/min	86.2 ± 6.1	35.2 ± 12.5[b]	44.4 ± 11.0[b]

[a] Adapted from Zimpfer et al. (112). Mean ± standard deviation. Ventilation controlled and constant.
[b] Significant change $P < 0.01$.

served degree of insulin secretory inhibition by enflurane anesthesia (119). Inhalation of enflurane produces intestinal vascular resistance in a dose-dependent fashion. This is due to both peripheral and CNS sites of action for enflurane (120). Enflurane reduces spontaneous contractile activity in the portal veins, thus affecting responses of the small intestine (121).

PLACENTAL TRANSFER

The administration of enflurane or enflurane and nitrous oxide during pregnancy and birth provides a satisfatory level of anesthesia. There is no difference in blood loss comparing enflurane versus enflurane and nitrous oxide. No biochemical changes indicated maternal or fetal renal dysfunction. The arterial blood gases and pH of newborns after enflurane and oxygen versus enflurane and nitrous oxide were more favorable for the enflurane and oxygen contol patients. There is a reduced serum inorganic fluoridine in umbilical cord blood at levels below those associated with nephrotoxicity (122).

ISOFLURANE ANESTHESIA

Isoflurane is the newest inhalant anesthetic available (2, 123). It is 1-chloro-2,2,2-trifluoroethyl difluoromethyl ether sensitized by Dr. Ross Turrell. It has a molecular weight of 184.5, a specific gravity at 25°C of 1.5, a boiling point of 48.5°C, and a vapor pressure of 239.5 mm Hg at 20°C. It is a stable compound in soda lime or ultraviolet light; it does not react with metal and needs no preservatives. Its chemical formula is:

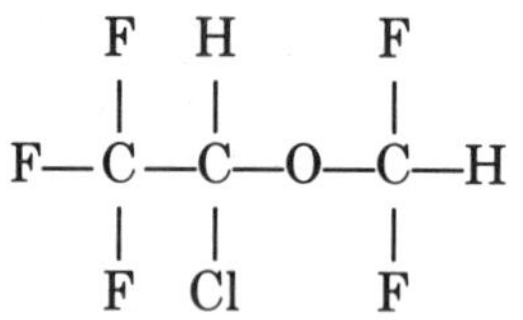

The vapor pressure of isoflurane closely resembles that of halothane so that it can be administered in a halothane-type vaporizer. The MAC of isoflurane lies midway between halothane and enflurane. Many factors may decrease MAC including the administration of nitrous oxide and other depressant drugs, including narcotics and other analgetics.

PHARMACOLOGY OF ISOFLURANE

MAC for isoflurane in of 1.15 humans is one and one-half times that of halothane and two-thirds that of enflurane (123). Isoflurane dilates constricted bronchi and is useful in anesthetic management of patients with chronic obstructive pulmonary disease. Isoflurane has the largest circulatory margin of safety of all potent halogenated agents. It produces the least myocardial depression at a given multiple of MAC. Isoflurane may increase heart rate, particularly in young patients, and occasionally it is associated with tachycardia. It enhances the action of pancuronium and, to a lesser extent, vecuronium or atracurium. Only 0.17% of isoflurane taken up in man appears as urinary metabolites, possibly explaining the minimal or absent hepatotoxicity and nephrotoxicity of isoflurane. Isoflurane provides a greater margin of safety compared to halothane (124). At room temperature, isoflurane concentrations in halothane-type vaporizers are generally greater than dial percentages with low carrier gas flows, but less than dial percentages at higher gas flows for most vaporizers. There is little effect of intermittent positive pressure breathing on vaporizer output at peak inspired circuit pressures less than 12 mm Hg, but halothane-specific vaporizers should be used with caution if isoflurane is used in those vaporizers (125). The MAC of isoflurane in the cat is 1.61%, compared to 1.19% halothane and 2.23% enflurane (126). In rats, isoflurane MAC is 2.4%; it is 1.74% for halothane and 1.25% for diethyl ether (127).

CNS

Cerebral blood fow was significantly lower during administration of isoflurane and nitrous oxide than with either nitrous oxide or halothane and nitrous oxide (128). Isoflurane decreases reabsorption of CSF, whereas enflurane increases absorption. Because decreased reabsorption improves spatial compensation for CSF volume for increased intracranial pressure, isoflurane may offer an advantage over enflurane in patients at risk because of increased intracranial pressure (129). Both halothane and isoflurane reduce blood pressure and intracranial pressures in cats. Halothane produces sufficient significant increases in cerebral blood flow at all dosages, whereas isoflurane causes no significant changes in cerebral blood flow. Both drugs produce dose-related decreases in cerebral vascular resistance, but the changes are greater with halothane (130). Regional blood flow in the cerebral hemispheres and the cortical gray matter shows that isoflurane tends to produce lower blood flow than halothane particularly at the 1.3 MAC concentration. The reverse is true in the posterior fossa structures, the brain stem, and the cerebellum, showing higher blood flows with isoflurane even at 1.7 MAC. Isoflurane may have several advantages over halothane for neurosurgical procedures (131). Isoflurane produces less impairment of the autoregulatory responses to increased blood pressure than halothane. This suggests isoflurane as a desirable volatile agent in head injury (132). Isoflurane's effect on cerebral blood flow during conditions of normocapnia do not occur until isoflurane is administered at levels greater than 1 MAC (133). Halothane is a more potent vasodilator compared to isoflurane (134). Figure 7.1 illustrates the blood flow to the brain compared to cardiac output, heart rate, and mean arterial pressure. Figure 7.2 illustrates the regional blood flow to the brain during halothane and isoflurane anesthesia.

It is believed that the mechanisms of vasodilation of halothane and isoflurane may be similar (135). Isoflurane compared to enflurane in the dog showed little change during enflurane and slight increased cerebral blood flow during isoflurane, by 12% at 0.5 MAC and 15% at 1.5 MAC. The percentage of cardiac output received by the brain increased significantly during isoflurane in enflurane at all concentrations of 0.5 to 1.5 MAC (136). Anesthesia with fentanyl and isoflurane appears to preserve cerebral blood flow to a greater

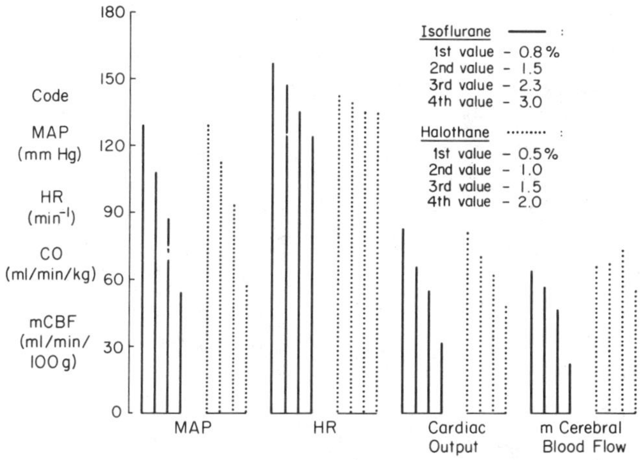

Figure 7.1. Hemodynamic variables during halothane and isoflurane anesthesia in dogs. Modified from Chen et al. (134).

extent than anesthesia with nitrous oxide during severe hypotension. With isoflurane, there appeared to be no change in cerebral blood flow in cortical or subcortical structures when normal tension and hypotensive animals were compared (137).

CARDIOVASCULAR FUNCTION

Myocardial blood flow increases during isoflurane at 1 and 2 MAC in dogs. Isoflurane appears to be a coronary vasodilator with potential beneficial improvement in myocardial blood supply with some concern as to hazardous steal effect on the heart (138). In pigs using 1.5 MAC isoflurane (2.18%), mean aortic pressure decreased during isoflurane anesthesia, whereas cardiac output decreased only above 1.5 MAC and the heart rate remained unchanged. At 1.5 MAC anesthesia, splenic blood flow was increased, as was blood flow to the stomach, small intestine, diaphragm, skeletal muscle, and adipose tissue. Renal/hepatic and cutaneous blood flow remained unaltered (139). In the rat, 1.28% isoflurane depressed myocardial function by 20%. Isoflurane has been shown to modify intracellular calcium transport and protect against calcium-related profusion damage (140). Isoflurane impairs left ventricular systolic performance in a dose-dependent fashion. However, isoflurane in intact dogs does not appear to cause exaggerated or permanent dysfunction of chronically ischemic myocardium (141). Isoflurane at 1.25% delivered concentration shows no deterioration in contractability of the ventricle; on the other hand, there is a negative inotropic effect of 2% isoflurane that may be detrimental (142). The lack of negative inotropic effect of 1.25% isoflurane in the face of significant

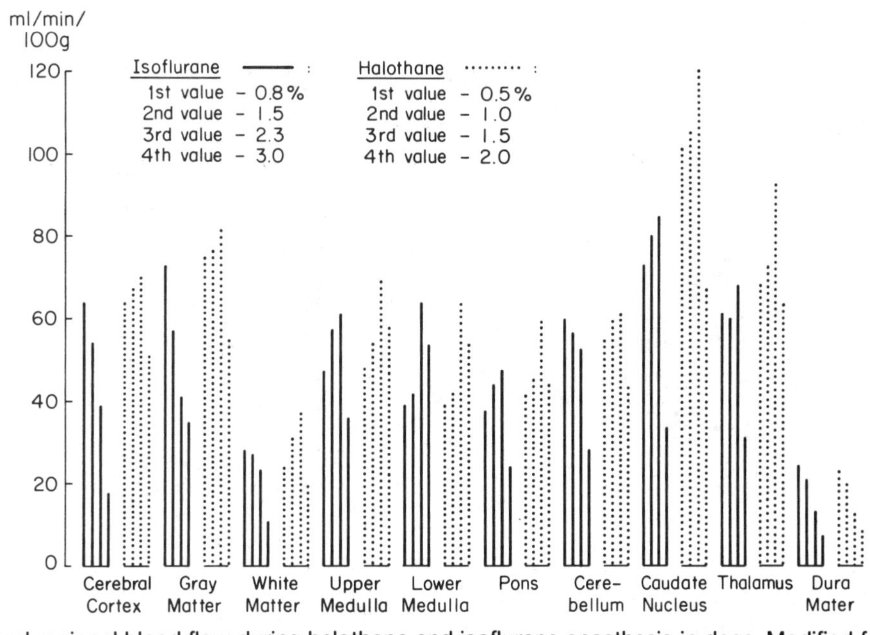

Figure 7.2. Cerebral regional blood flow during halothane and isoflurane anesthesia in dogs. Modified from Chen et al. (134).

decreases in pressure reflects a potential benefit to compromised myocardium (143). Isoflurane causes very little change in cardiac index during anesthesia at concentrations of 1 MAC. Hypertensive animals are more susceptible to cardiovascular depressant effects of isoflurane resulting especially in reduced blood flows to the GI tract and liver (144). Because isoflurane increases coronary flow and, to a lesser extent, capillary microflow, there is an increased coronary venous PO_2 in contrast to unchanged myocardial PaO_2 (145). Isoflurane should be used with caution in animals receiving diltiazem because AV conduction may be prolonged and low concentrations of isoflurane are needed to reduce aortic pressure (146). At 1 MAC and inspired air, myocardial blood profusion in the subendocardial layer shows no principle difference in the ischemic or nonischemic area in dogs with myocardial ischemia. This helps to negate the steal phenomenon (147). Isoflurane alters the distribution of coronary blood flow in the dog with chronic coronary occlusion (148). Isoflurane decreased regional myocardial contraction in a zone of collateral dependent myocardium, at the same time enhancing contraction of a normally profused zone. A pronounced regional myocardial dysfunction may develop when aortic pressure is lowered by isoflurane during underlying coronary artery stenosis (149). There is a greater preservation of coronary reserve during isoflurane anesthesia in the pig than with halothane (150). There is an EEG shift indicating a similar anesthetic depth despite 50% reduction in isoflurane requirements due to the sedative and hypnotic effects of clonidine. The potentiation of isoflurane anesthesia and the improved hemodynamic stablity observed with clonidine may be explained by its inhibitory action on noradrenergic neurons involved in the central control of blood pressure resulting in diminished sympathetic response to afferent stimuli. Its potent depression of nociceptive input at the spinal cord level and its central analgetic properties. Clonidine premedication has been used in the management of patients with fully controlled hypertension (151). The negative inotropic effect of isoflurane is probably competitive inhibition of calcium to influx (152). Fentanyl and isoflurane have been used in patients with myocardial ischemia. This method appears suitable for patients with poor left ventricular function (153). With increasing depth of anesthesia, there is a better preservation of baroreflex responsiveness during isoflurane. It is capable of increasing heart rate in response to isoflurane-induced systemic hypotension. This partial preservation of the baroreflex is responsible for maintaining cardiac output during isoflurane anesthesia (154).

RESPIRATORY RESPONSES

Isoflurane produces respiratory depression. The mechanics of the ventilatory response to a raised $PaCO_2$ during isoflurane is different from halothane. Isoflurane anesthesia is associated with a greater increase in lower airway resistance and subjects increase their driving pressure more than with halothane, but it does not produce a comparable increase in mean inspiratory flow or tidal volume (155). Isoflurane produces an increase in pulmonary shunting in goats after diffused lung injury, but the changes are less than those observed with enflurane or halothane. Ketamine causes no significant decreaess in oxygenation (156). Isoflurane inhibits the oxidative activity of pulmonary alveolar macrophages (157). Isoflurane reduces active changes in flow resistance to collateral ventilation, allowing adjustment in ventilation profusion deviations (158). Isoflurane does not impair arterial oxygenation during one-lung ventilation during thoracotomies (159). Isoflurane does not abolish the vasoconstricture response to hypoxia (160).

METABOLISM, RENAL, AND HEPATIC FUNCTION

There can be an increase in serum fluoride levels after prolonged enflurane or isoflurane anesthesia in obese subjects (161). However, isoflurane is metabolized to such a small extent that any increase in metabolism would be clinically inconsequential (162). Hepatic blood flow during isoflurane anesthesia is not adversely altered by isoflurane. Hepatic blood flow does not decrease during hypotensive conditions. The liver enzyme determinations are inconclusive because there can be a transient increase in serum glutamic oxaloacetic transaminase (SGOT) and serum glutamic pyruvic transaminase (SGPT) without any clinical evidence of hepatic dysfunction postoperatively. Isoflurane-induced hypotension preserves hepatic blood flow and is likely to be safe for the liver (163). Isoflurane anesthesia in ponies does not appear to affect hepatic bile acid transport or biotransformation significantly (164). There is greater protection of the liver during isoflurane anesthesia than halothane (165).

Isoflurane appears to be a very safe anesthetic agent in adults and in pediatrics (166–168). Its usage in high risk patients including those with such myocardial sensitivity as traumatic myocarditis justifies its consideration compared to other anesthetic agents.

References

1. Adriani J: *The Pharmacology of Anesthetic Drugs*, ed 5. Springfield, Charles C Thomas, 1970, p 31–70.
2. Eger EI II: *Enflurane (Ethrane[R]). A Compendium and Reference*, ed 3. Madison, Anaquest, 1985, p 1–3.
3. Suckling CW: Some chemical and physical features in the development of fluothane. *Br J Anaesth* 29:466–472, 1957.
4. Artusio JF Jr, Von Poznak A, Hunt RE, Tiers FM, Alexander M: A clinical evaluation of methoxyflurane in man. *Anesthesiology* 21:512–521, 1960.
5. Von Poznak A: Clinical administration of methoxyflurane. *Clin Anesth* 1:105–120, 1962.

6. Dobkin AB, Nishioka K, Gengaje DB, Kim DS, Ebers W, Israel JS: Ethrane (Compound 347) anesthesia: a clinical and laboratory review of 700 cases. *Anesth Analg* 48:477–494, 1969.
7. Eger EI II: *Isoflurane (Forane). A Compendium and Reference.* Madison, WI, Ohio Medical Products, 1981.
8. Wade JG, Stevens WC: Isoflurane: An anesthetic for the Eighties? *Anesth Analg* 60:666–682, 1981.
9. Eger EI II: Uptake and distribution of inhaled anesthetics. *1971 Annual Refresher Course Lectures ASA*, Atlanta, p 217.
10. Eger EI II: *Anesthetic Uptake and Action*, ed 1. Baltimore, Williams & Wilkins, 1974.
11. Eger EI II: *Nitrous Oxide/N_2O*, ed 1. New York, Elsevier, 1985, pp 81–103.
12. Finck AD: Nitrous oxide analgesia. In Eger EI II (ed): *Nitrous Oxide/N_2O*. New York, Elsevier, 1984, p 43.
13. Steffey EP, Eger EI II: Nitrous oxide in veterinary practice and animal research. In *Nitrous Oxide/N_2O*. New York, Elsevier, 1985, pp 305–311.
14. Dobkin AB, Song Y: The effect of methoxyflurane-nitrous oxide anesthesia on arterial pH, oxygen saturation, $PaCO_2$ and plasma bicarbonate in man. *Anesthesiology* 23:601–604, 1963.
15. Lasiter PS, Garcia J: A methoxyflurane delivery system for steriotoxic surgery. *Brain Res Bull* 13(3):457–460, 1984.
16. Steffey EP, Farver TB, Woliner MJ: Circulatory and respiratory effects of methoxyflurane in dogs: Comparison of halothane. *Am J Vet Res* 45(12):2574–2579, 1984.
17. Canova-Davis E, Waskell L: The identification of the heat-stable microsomal protein required for methoxyflurane metabolism as cytochrome 65. *J Biol Chem* 259(4):2541–2546, 1984.
18. Crandell WB, Pappas SG, MacDonald A: Nephrotoxicity associated with methoxyflurane anesthesia. *Anesthesiology* 27:591, 1966.
19. Mazze RI, Shue GL, Jackson SH: Renal dysfunction associated with methoxyflurane anesthesia: A randomized prospective clinical evaluation. *JAMA* 216:278–288, 1971.
20. Mazze RI, Barry KG: Prevention of functional renal failure during anesthesia and surgery by sustained hydration and mannitol infusion. *Anesth Analg* 46:61, 1967.
21. North WC, Stephen CR: Hepatic and renal effects of methoxyflurane in surgical patients. *Anesthesiology* 26:257, 1965.
22. Paddock RB, Parker JW, Guadagni NP: The effects of methoxyflurane on renal function. *Anesthesiology* 25:707, 1964.
23. Pezzi PJ, Frobese AS, Greenberg SR: Methoxyflurane and renal toxicity. *Lancet* 1:823, 1966.
24. Weiskopf RB, Bogetz MS: Minimum alveolar concentrations (MAC) of halothane and nitrous oxide in swine. *Anesth Analg* 63(5):529–532, 1984.
25. Lake CL, DiFazio CA, Moscicki JC, Engle JS: Reduction in halothane MAC: comparison of morphine and alfentanil. *Anesth Analg* 64(8):807–810, 1985.
26. Tranquilli WJ, Thurmon JC, Corbin JE, Benson GJ, Davis LE: Halothane-sparing effect of xylazine in dogs and subsequent reversal with tolazoline. *J Vet Pharmacol Ther* 7(1):23–28, 1984.
27. Brandom BW, Brandom RB, Cook DR: Uptake and distribution of halothane in infants: in vivo measurements and computer simulations. *Anesth Analg* 62(4):404–410, 1983.
28. Artru AA: Effects of halothane and fentanyl on the rate of CSF production in dogs. *Anesth Analg* 62(6):581–585, 1983.
29. Chen RYZ, Fan FC, Schuessler GB, Chien S: Distribution of cerebral blood flow (CBF) during halothane anesthesia. *Anesthesiology* 57(3):A37, 1982.
30. Campbell NJ, Raja SN, Meyer RA: Halothane sensitizes cutaneous nociceptors in monkeys. *J Neurophysiol* 52(4):762–770, 1984.
31. Cheng SC, Brunner EA, Minieka IA: Induced enzyme release from snyaptosomes by halothane. *Neurochem Res* 9(4):577–585, 1984.
32. Johnson GV, Hartzell CR: Chaline uptake, acetylcholine synthesis and release, and halothane effects in synaptosomes. *Anesth Analg* 64(4):395–399, 1985.
33. Kissin I, Green D: Effect of halothane on cardiac acceleration response to somatic nerve stimulation in dogs. *Anesthesiology* 61(6):708–711, 1984.
34. Land PC, Lai JC: Spinal cord vs. somatosensory-cortical evoked potentials during halothane anesthesia in dogs. *Anesthesiology* 57(3)A318, 1982.
35. Artru AA: Relationship between cerebral blood volume and CSF pressure during anesthesia with halothane or enflurane in dogs. *Anesthesiology* 58(6):533–539, 1983.
36. Artru AA: Effects of halothane and fentanyl anesthesia on resistance to reabsorption of CSF. *J Neurosurg* 60(2):252–256, 1984.
37. Yamamura T, Kimura T, Furukowa K: Effects of halothane, thiamylal, and ketamine on central sympathetic and vagal tone. *Anesth Analg* 62(2):129–134, 1983.
38. Kissin I, Kerr CR, Smith LR: Effect of morphine on the heart rate response to noxious stimulation: interaction with halothane and naloxone. *Pain* 18(4):351–358, 1984.
39. Behnia R, Koushanpour E: Local versus central effect of halothane on carotid sinus baroreceptor function. *Anesthesiology* 61(2):161–168, 1984.
40. Seagard JL, Hopp FA, Bosrjak ZS, Elegbe EO, Kapine JP: Extent and mechanism of halothane sensitization of the carotid sinus baroreceptors. *Anesthesiology* 59(5):432–437, 1983.
41. Koushanpour E, Behnia R, Brunner EA: Halothane: local and central effect on carotid sinus reflex. *Anesthesiology* 55(3):A55, 1981.
42. Price HL, Davidson L: Barostatic reflexes during halothane anesthesia. *Anesthesiology* 55(3):A49, 1981.
43. Sivarajan M, Bashein G: Effect of halothane on coronary collateral circulation. *Anesthesiology* 62(5)588–596, 1985.
44. Beattie C, Todd EP, Wright B, Davis JB: Effects of halothane on coronary blood flow in intact dogs. *Anesthesiology* 55(3):A2, 1981.
45. Buffington CW: Halothane, per se, does not cause ischemic myocardial dysfunction in the presence of coronary stenosis. *Anesthesiology* 63(3A):A20, 1985.
46. Kroll DA: Effects of halothane on ventricular multiple response thresholds: normal vs ischemic myocardium. *Anesthesiology* 61(3A):A35, 1984.
47. Hart AP, Pank JR, Moyers JR, Carter JG, Carter AL, Thompson CS, Wegrzynowicz ES, Tinker JH: Prolonged halothane anesthesia: no reduction in myocardial infarct size in swine. *Anesthesiology* 64(3A):A2, 1984.
48. Mergner GW, Gilman RW, Woolf WA, Patch JH: Effect of halothane and fentanyl on myocardial infarct size and regional blood flow distribution. *Anesthesiology* 57(3):A17, 1982.
49. Miletich DJ, Dinsmore PE, Albrecht RF, Holshouser S: Oxygen uptake by heart cells after halothane or enflurane. *Anesthesiology* 55(3):A1, 1981.
50. Rorie DK, Tyce GM, Mackenzie RA: Evidence that halothane inhibits norepinephrine release from sympathetic nerve endings in dog saphenous vein by stimulation of presynaptic inhibitory muscarinic receptors. *Anesth Analg* 63(12):1059–1064, 1984.
51. Stowe DF, Boznjak ZJ, Zampine JP: Halothane diminishes changes in cardiac fiber action potential duration induced by hypocarbia and hypercarbia. *Anesthesiology* 61(3):245–253, 1984.
52. Lunn JJ, Rorie DK: Halothane-induced changes in the release and disposition of norepinephrine at adrenergic nerve endings in dog saphenous vein. *Anesthesiology* 61(4):377–384, 1984.
53. Bernstein KJ, Verosky M, Trimer L: Halothane inhibition of canine myocardial adenylate cyclase—modulation by endogenous factors. *Anesth Analg* 63(3):285–289, 1984.
54. Kissin I, Thomson CT, Smith LR: Effect of halothane on contractile function of ischemic myocardium. *J Cardiovasc Pharmacol* 5(3):438–442, 1983.

55. Ritter JW, Shigezawa GY, Roe SD Sr, Sullivan SF: Increasing myocardial oxygen demand during prolonged halothane anesthesia in dogs. *Anesth Analg* 62(9):788–792, 1983.
56. Ritter JW, Cumpos J, Roe SD, Law T, Sullivan SF: Prolonged halothane anesthesia causes anaerobic myocardial metabolism. *Anesthesiology* 59(3):A29, 1983.
57. Komai H, Rusy BF: Differences in the myocardial depressant action of thiopental and halothane. *Anesth Analg* 63(3):313–318, 1984.
58. Kampine JP, Boznjak ZJ, Turner LA: Effects of halothane on SA node-role of calcium. *Anesthesiology* 55(3):A58, 1981.
59. Tosone SR, Reves JG, Kissin I, Smith LR, Fournier SE: Hemodynamic responses to nifedipine in dogs anesthetized with halothane. *Anesth Analg* 61(10):903–908, 1983.
60. Kates RA, Zaggy AP, Norfleet EA, Health KR: Comparative cardiovascular effects of verapamil, nifedipine, and diltiazem during halothane anesthesia in swine. *Anesthesiology* 61(1):10–18, 1984.
61. Murray PA, Blanck TJJ, Rogers MC, Jacobus WE: Halothane-induced abnormalities of myocardial high-energy phosphate metabolism. *Anesthesiology* 59(3):A63, 1983.
62. Hantler CB, Felbeck PG, Theisen G, Knight PR: Halothane effects of atrial His-bundle conduction at slow heart rates. *Anesthesiology* 59(3):A62, 1983.
63. Freedman B, Hamm D, Pellon G, Everson C, Knox J, Wechsler A, Christian C: Fentanyl-halothane anesthesia maintains myocardial contractility. *Anesthesiology* 59(3):A35, 1983.
64. Greene ES, Gerson JI: Depth of halothane anesthesia does not alter the left ventricular diastolic pressure-volume relationship. *Anesthesiology* 59(3):A27, 1983.
65. Miletich DJ, Burrera M, Albrecht RF: Cardiovascular effects of halothane in chronically anemic dogs. *Anesthesiology* 59(3):A28, 1983.
66. Maze M, Smith CM: Halothane decreases arrhythmogenic threshold for epinephrine through alpha and beta adrenoceptor mechanisms. *Anesthesiology* 57(3):A16, 1982.
67. Metz S, Maze M: Halothane concentration does not alter the threshold for epinephrine-induced arrhythmias in dogs. *Anesthesiology* 62(4):470–474, 1985.
68. Lina AA, Leon-Ruiz EN, Fouts KE, Dauchot PJ, Anton AH, Sutheimer CA: Influence of verapamil and aminophylline on epinephrine dysrhythmias under halothane anesthesia. *Anesthesiology* 63(3A):A84, 1985.
69. Mayer DB, Feld J, Miletich DJ, Albrecht, RF: The efficacy of magnesium sulfate in the treatment of halothane epinephrine induced cardiac arrhythmias. *Anesthesiology* 63(3A):A86, 1985.
70. Gallagher JD, Kerns D, Moura P, Gessman LJ: Interaction between halothane and quinidine in canine purkinze fibers. *Anesthesiology* 63(3A):A82, 1985.
71. Speck EC, Nemoto EM, Marquez J, Sassano J, Back S, Zapp M: Effect of volatile anesthetics on defibrillation threshold in dogs. *Anesthesiology* 63(3A):A87, 1985.
72. Miller FL, Chen L, Alexander C, Sedrak W, Marshall C, Marshall BE: Halothane, cardiac output, and hypoxic pulmonary vasoconstriction. *Anesthesiology* 61(3A):A482, 1984.
73. Paolin EG, Yazaki S, Winn R, Nadir B, Hildebrandt J: Ethrane and halothane anesthesia increases shunt (Qs/Qt) in goats following acid aspiration. *Anesthesiology* 55(3):A382, 1981.
74. Dueck R, Rathbun M, Greenburg AG: Lung volume and VA/Q distribution response to intravenous versus inhalation anesthesia in sheep. *Anesthesiology* 61(1):55–65, 1984.
75. Rannels DE, Christopherson R, Watkins CA: Reversible inhibition of protein synthesis in lung by halothane. *Biochem J* 210(2):379–387, 1983.
76. Korenaga S, Takeda K, Ito Y: Differential effects of halothane on airway, nerves and muscle. *Anesthesiology* 60(4):309–318, 1984.
77. Nishino T, Honda Y, Yonezawa T: Separate effects of halothane and carbon dioxide on respiratory duration in vagotomized cats. *Br J Anaesth* 55(7):647–654, 1983.
78. vanDissel JT, Berkenbosch A, Olievier CN, de Goede J, Quanjer PH: Effects of halothane on the ventilatory response of hypoxia and hypercapnia in cats. *Anesthesiology* 62(4):448–456, 1985.
79. Alexander CM, Chen L, Ray RJ, Marshall BE: Influence of halothane on pulmonary collateral ventilation. *Anesthesiology* 59(3):A508, 1983.
80. Manabe M, Sawa T, Ikezono E, Colgan FJ: Semi-closed halothane anesthesia by high frequency ventilation. *Anesthesiology* 57(3):A463, 1982.
81. Clerque F, Viires N, Lemesle P, Aubier M, Viars P, Pariente R: Mechanism of halothane-induced ventilatory depression in pentobarbital-anesthetized dogs. *Anesthesiology* 59(3):A494, 1983.
82. Tabatabai M, Kitahata LM, Yuge O, Matsunoto M, Collins JG: Effect of halothane on the activity of the inspiratory neurons of the solitary tract nucleus of the cat. *Anesthesiology* 59(3):A492, 1983.
83. Reilly CS, Wood AJ, Koshakji RP, Wood M: The effect of halothane on drug disposition: Contribution of changes in intrinsic drug metabolizing capability and hepatic blood flow. *Anesthesiology* 63(1):70–76, 1985.
84. Engelking LR, Dodman NH, Hartman G, Valdez H, Spivak W: Effects of halothane anesthesia on equine liver function. *Am J Vet Res* 45(4):607–615, 1984.
85. Plummer JL, Wanwimobruk S, Jenner MA, Hall PD, Cousins MJ: Effects of cimetidine and ranitidine on halothane metabolism and hepatotoxicity in an animal model. *Drug Metabol Dispos* 12(1):106–110, 1984.
86. Thomson IA, Fitch W, Hughes RL, Campbell D: Effect of increased concentrations of carbon dioxide during halothane anaesthesia on liver, blood flow and hepatic oxygen consumption. *Br J Anaesth* 55(12):1231–1237, 1983.
87. Flaim KE, Jefferson LS, McGuire JB, Rannels DE: Effect of halothane on synthesis and secretion of liver proteins. *Mol Pharmacol* 24(2):277–281, 1983.
88. Fiserova-Bergerova V, Kawiecki RW: Effects of exposure concentrations on distribution of halothane metabolites in the body. *Drug Metab Dispos* 12(1):98–105, 1984.
89. Mazze RI, Sievenpiper TS, Stevenson J: Renal effects of enflurane and halothane in patients with abnormal renal function. *Anesthesiology* 59(3):A252, 1983.
90. Priano LL: Effect of halothane on renal hemodynamics during normovolemia and acute hemorrhagic hypovolemia. *Anesthesiology* 59(3):A46, 1983.
91. Hantler CB, Felbeck PG, Tait AR, Knight PR: Renal vascular interactions between halothane and verapamil. *Anesthesiology* 59(3):A45, 1983.
92. Whitwam JG, Pflug JR, Chakrabarti MK, Sapsed S, Gordon G, Jack RD: Effect of halothane on lymph flow. *Br J Anaesth* 56(4):411–414, 1984.
93. Savaki HE, Desban M, Glowinski J, Besson MJ: Local cerebral glucose consumption in the rat. I. Effects of halothane on anesthesia. *J Comp Neurol* 213(1):36–45, 1983.
94. Miletich DJ, Holshouser SJ, Seals CF, Albrecht RF: Differential effects of halothane or enflurane on heart cell utilization of glucose and fatty acids. *Anesthesiology* 57(3):A19, 1982.
95. Stodkilde-Jorgensen H, Sorensen B, Kraglund K, Djurhuus JC: Gastric acid secretion during halothane, chloralose, pentobarbital and etomidate anaesthesia in the pig. *Eur Surg Res* 17(1):33–37, 1985.
96. Cameron AM, Dale O, Haug E, Nilsen OG: Inhalation of enflurane and halothane at subanesthetic concentrations and effects on circulating serum testosteronel luteinizing hormone and follicle-stimulating hormone in the male rat. *Toxicol Lett*

19(3):333–338, 1983.
97. de Rosayro AM, Vogel M, Knight R III: Halothane MAC and pregnancy: Endorphins progesterone, or? *Anesthesiology* 61(3A):A336, 1984.
98. Datta S, Ostheimer GW, Naulty JS, Knapp RM, Weiss JB: General anesthesia for cesarean section: effects of halothane in maternal and fetal acid-base and lactic acid concentration. *Anesthesiology* 55(3):A309, 1981.
99. Gregory GA, Wade JG, Beihl DR, Ong BY, Sitar DS: Fetal anesthetic requirement (MAC) for halothane. *Anesth Analg* 62(1):9–14, 1983.
100. Cameron CB, Gregory GA, Rudolph AM, Heymann M: The cardiovascular and metabolic effects of halothane in normoxic and hypoxic newborn lambs. *Anesthesiology* 62(6):732–737, 1985.
101. Berger JM, Stirt JA, Sullivan SF: Enflurane, halothane, and aminophylline-uptake and pharmacokinetics. *Anesth Analg* 62(8):733–737, 1983.
102. Stevens JE, Oshima E, Mori K: Effects of nitrous oxide in the epileptogenic property of enflurane in cats. *Br J Anaesth* 55(2):145–154, 1983.
103. Oshima E, Urabe N, Shingu K, Mori K: Anticonvulsant actions of enflurane on epilepsy models in cats. *Anesthesiology* 63(1):29–40, 1985.
104. Monohar M, Parks CM: Porcine brain and myocardial perfusion during enflurane anesthesia without nitrous oxide. *J Cardiovasc Pharmacol* 6(6):1092–1101, 1984.
105. Murphy MR, Hug CC Jr: The anesthetic potency of fentanyl in terms of its reduction of enflurane MAC. *Anesthesiology* 55(3):A249, 1981.
106. Seo K, Maekawa T, Taheshita H, Okuda Y: Cerebral energy state and glycolytic metabolism during enflurane anesthesia in the rat. *Acta Anaesthesiol Scand* 28(2):215–219, 1984.
107. Moffitt EA, Imrie DD, Scovil JE, Glenn JJ, Cousins CL, Del Campo C, Kinley CE: Myocardial metabolism and hemodynamic responses with enflurane anesthesia for coronary artery surgery. *Anesthesiology* 59(3):A21, 1983.
108. Blanck T, Thompson M: Enflurane and isoflurane stimulate calcium transport by cardiac sarcoplasmic reticulum. *Anesth Analg* 61:142, 1982.
109. Freedman B, Christian C, Godwin C, Hamm D, Everson C, Wechsler A: Enflurane enhances post-ischemic recovery. *Anesthesiology* 59(3):A22, 1983.
110. Doherty F, Wilkinson PL, Robinson S: Enflurane reduced systemic pressure during cardiopulmonary bypass more effectively than halothane. *Anesthesiology* 55(3):A40, 1981.
111. Christian C, Fagraeus L, Vantright P, Peyton R, Spray T, Pasque M, Pellam G, Wechslar A: Sonomicrometry: Enflurane depresses L.V. dynamics. *Anesthesiology* 55(3):A39, 1981.
112. Zimpfer M, Gilly H, Krosl P, Schlag G, Steinbereithner K: Enflurane-ventricular dynamics in intact, chronically instrumented dogs vs. in isolated heart preparations. *Anesthesiology* 55(3):A5, 1981.
113. Mote PS, Pruett JK, Gramling ZW: Effects of halothane and enflurane on right ventricular performance in hearts of dogs anesthetized with pentobarbital sodium. *Anesthesiology* 58(1):53–60, 1983.
114. Pruett JK, Mote PS, Grover TE, Augeri JM: Enflurane and halothane effects on cardiac purkinje fibers. *Anesthesiology* 55(3):A65, 1981.
115. Henriksson BA, Biber B, Martner J, Pont'en J, Warner O: Cardiovascular studies during controlled baroreflex activation in the dog: I. Effects of enflurane. *Acta Anaesthesiol Scand* 29(1):90–94, 1985.
116. Miletich DJ, Dinsmore PE, Albrecht RF, Holshouser S: Oxygen uptake by heart cells after halothane or enflurane. *Anesthesiology* 55(3):A1, 1981.
117. Moffitt EA, Imrie DD, Scovil JE, Glenn JJ, Cousins CL, Del Campo C, Sullivan JA, Kinley CE: Myocardial metabolism and haemodynamic responses with enflurane anaesthesia for coronary artery surgery. *Can Anaesth Soc J* 31(6):604–610, 1984.
118. Rice SA, Sievenpiper TS, Mazze RI: Liver function and anesthetic metabolism in rats with chronic renal impairment. *Anesthesiology* 60(5):418–421, 1984.
119. Ewart RB, Rusy BF, Bradford MW: Enflurane and adenosine 3′,5′-cyclic monophosphate metabolism in pancreatic islets. *Anesth Analg* 64(1):18–22, 1985.
120. Henriksson BA, Biber B, Lundberg P, Martner J, Pont'en J, Sonander H: Intestinal vascular effects of inhaled and locally administered enflurane in the cat. *Acta Anaesthesiol Scand* 29(3):294–299, 1985.
121. Henriksson BA, Biber B, Lundberg D, Martner J, Pont'en J: Vasodilator responses to enflurane in the small intestine. *Acta Anaesthesiol Scand* 29(3):287–293, 1985.
122. Abbound TK, Shnider SM, Wright RG, Rolbin SH, Craft JB, Henriksen EH, Johnson J, Jones MJ, Hughes SC, Levinson G: Enflurane analgesia in obstetrics. *Anesth Analg* 60(3):133–137, 1981.
123. Eger EI III: The pharmacology of isoflurane. *Br J Anaesth* 56:71S–99S, 1984.
124. Kissin I, Morgan PL, Smith LR: Isoflurane vs halothane: safety margins. *Anesthesiology* 57(3):A370, 1982.
125. Steffey EP, Woliner MJ, Howland D: Accuracy of isoflurane delivery by halothane-specific vaporizers. *Am J Vet Res* 44(6):1072–1078, 1983.
126. Drummond JC, Todd MM, Shapiro AM: Minimal alveolar concentrations for halothane, enflurane and isoflurane in the cat. *J Am Vet Med Assoc* 182(10):1099–1101, 1983.
127. Kissin I, Morgan PL, Smith LR: Anesthetic potencies of isoflurane, halothane, and diethyl ether for various end points of anesthesia. *Anesthesiology* 58(1):88–92, 1983.
128. Drummond JC, Todd MM: The response of the feline cerebral circulation to $PaCO_2$ during anesthesia with isoflurane and halothane and during sedation with nitrous oxide. *Anesthesiology* 62(3):268–273, 1985.
129. Artru AA: Effects of enflurane and isoflurane on resistance to reabsorption of cerebrospinal fluids in dogs. *Anesthesiology* 61(5):529–533, 1984.
130. Todd MM, Drummond JC: A comparison of the cerebrovascular and metabolic effects of halothane and isoflurane in the cat. *Anesthesiology* 60(4):276–282, 1984.
131. Boarini DJ, Kassell NF, Coester HC, Butler M, Sokoll MD: Comparison of systemic and cerebrovascular effects of isoflurane and halothane. *Neurosurgery* 15(3):400–409, 1984.
132. Drummond JC, Tood MM, Shapiro HM: Cerebral blood flow autoregulation in the cat during anesthesia with halothane and isoflurane. *Anesthesiology* 59(3):A305, 1983.
133. Maekawa T, Tommasino C, Shapiro HM, Keifer J: Local cerebral blood flow during isoflurane anesthesia. *Anesthesiology* 59(3):A308, 1983.
134. Chen RYZ, Fan C-C, Carlin RD, Schuessler GB, Chien S: Comparison of regional cerebral blood flow during isoflurane and halothane-induced hypotension. *Anesthesiology* 61(3a):A21, 1984.
135. Drummond JC, Todd MM, Scheller MS: A comparison of the intrinsic vasodilating potencies of halothane and isoflurane in the New Zealand white rabbit. *Anesthesiology* 61(3A):A364, 1984.
136. Goetz AE, Conzer PF, Hobbhahn J, Granetzny T, Peter K, Brendel W: Regional cerebral blood flow with increasing doses of isoflurane and enflurane in a canine model. *Anesthesiology* 63(3A):A41, 1985.
137. Young ML, Smith DS, Keykhah MM, Englebach I, Greenberg J, Reivich M, Harp J: Effects of fentanyl versus isoflurane of

regional cerebral blood flow during severe hypotension. *Anesthesiology* 63(3A):A407, 1985.
138. Gelman S, Fowler KC, Smith LR: Regional blood flow during isoflurane and halothane anesthesia. *Anesth Analg* 63(6):557–565, 1984.
139. Lundeen G, Manohar M, Parks C: Systemic distribution of blood flow in swine while awake and during 1.0 and 1.5 MAC isoflurane anesthesia with or without 50% nitrous oxide. *Anesth Analg* 62(5):499–512, 1983.
140. Freedman B, Christian C, Hamm D, Everson C, Wechsler A: Isoflurane and myocardial protection. *Anesthesiology* 59(3):A25, 1983.
141. Zimpfer M, Gilly H, Mayer N, Steinbereithner K: Effects of isoflurane in global and segmental left ventricular function in intact dogs with chronic myocardial ischemia. *Anesthesiology* 59(3):A32, 1983.
142. Fagraeus L, Christian C, VanTrigt P, Pasque M, Framme J, Neglen P, Pellon G, Wechsler A: Inotropic effects of isoflurane on the hypertrophied left ventricle in dogs. *Anesthesiology* 57(3):A14, 1982.
143. Christian C II, Fagraeus L, Van Tright P III, Pasque M, Pellon G, Frame J, Wechsler A: The effects of isoflurane on global ventricular mechanics. *Anesthesiology* 67(3):A13, 1982.
144. Seyde WC, Longnecker DE: Normotension versus hypertension: does isoflurane influence hemodynamics differently? *Anesthesiology* 63(3A):A13, 1985.
145. Vogel H, Gunther H, Harrison DK, Kessler M, Peter K: The influence of isoflurane and enflurane on tissue oxygenation and microcirculation of the dog myocardium. *Anesthesiology* 61(3A):A5, 1984.
146. Sharvan K, Priebe H-J, Gale J: Effects of diltiazem and isoflurane on cardiovascular function and coronary hemodynamics in dogs. *Anesthesiology* 61(3A):A9, 1984.
147. Ackern KV, Adler M, Bruchner UB, Buell U, Haller M, Ragaller M, Raihel E, Woellner W: Effects of isoflurane on myocardial ischemia in dogs: regional changes of blood flow contractility and metabolism. *Anesthesiology* 61(3A):A32, 1984.
148. Buffington CW, Romson JL, Duttlinger NC: Does isoflurane cause coronary steal. *Anesthesiology* 63(3A):A9, 1985.
149. Priebe H-J, Gale J: Adverse effects of isoflurane on myocardial function in the presence of coronary artery stenosis. *Anesthesiology* 63(3A):A10, 1985.
150. Gilbert M, Roberts SL, Blomberg RW, Tinker JH: Greater coronary reserve in swine anesthetized with isoflurane vs halothane. *Anesthesiology* 63(3A):A15, 1985.
151. Ghigione M, Calvillo O, Quintin L, Iacono C: Anesthesia and hypertension: the effect of clonidine in hemodynamics and isoflurane requirements. *Anesthesiology* 63(3A):A14, 1985.
152. Rusy BF, Hirochika K: Isoproterenol reversal on the negative effect of isoflurane. *Anesthesiology* 63(3A):A101, 1985.
153. Smith JS, Cahalan MK, Benefiel DJ, Lurz FW, Lampe GH, Byrd BJ, Schiller NB, Yee ES, Turley K, Ullyot DJ, Hamilton WK: Fentanyl versus fentanyl and isoflurane in patients with impaired left ventricular function. *Anesthesiology* 63(3A):A18, 1985.
154. Duke PC, Hill K, Trosky S: The effect of isoflurane and isoflurane with nitrous oxide anesthesia in baroreceptor reflex control on heart rate in man. *Anesthesiology* 57(3):A41, 1982.
155. Higgs BD, Carli F: An analysis of the ventilatory response to carbon dioxide with halothane and isoflurane anesthesia. *Anesthesiology* 59(3):A487, 1983.
156. Pavlin EG, Yazaki S, Winn R, Nadir B, Hildebrandt J, Carrico CJ: The effect of isoflurane and ketamine anesthesia on pulmonary shunt (Q_s/Q_t) in goats following acid aspiration. *Anesthesiology* 59(3):A509, 1983.
157. Welch WD: Enflurane and isoflurane inhibit the oxidative activity of pulmonary alveolar macrophages. *Respiration* 47(1):24–29, 1985.
158. Alexander CM, Chen L, Ray R, Marshall BE: The influence of halothane and isoflurane on pulmonary collateral ventilation. *Anesthesiology* 62(2):135–140, 1985.
159. Augustine SD, Benumof JL: Halothane and isoflurane do not impair arterial oxygenation during one lung ventilation in patients undergoing thoracotomy. *Anesthesiology* 61(3A):A484, 1984.
160. Gardoz J-P, Morel Ph, Py P, Gemperle M: Isoflurane and regional pulmonary vascular resistance during labor ventilation hypoxia and collapse in dogs. *Anesthesiology* 63(3A):A531, 1985.
161. Rice SA, Fish KJ: Metabolism and renal function in non-obese and obese rats exposed to enflurane or isoflurane. *Anesthesiology* 61(3A):A264, 1984.
162. Mazze RI: Metabolism of the inhaled anaesthetics: implications of enzyme induction. *Br J Anaesth* 56(Suppl 1):27S–41S, 1984.
163. Lann AM, Herd SF, Mustard RF, Manninen PH, Gelb AW: Hepatic blood flow during isoflurane-induced hypotension in man. *Anesthesiology* 63(3A):A404, 1985.
164. Engelking LR, Dodman NH, Hartman G, Valdez H: Effects of isoflurane anesthesia on equine liver function. *Am J Vet Res* 45(4):616–619, 1984.
165. Gelman S, Fowler KC, Smith LR: Liver circulation and function during isoflurane and halothane anesthesia. *Anesthesiology* 61(6):726–730, 1984.
166. Kingston HGG: Pediatric outpatient anesthesia: a comparison between halothane and isoflurane. *Anesthesiology* 63(3A):A459, 1985.
167. Chinyanga HM, Vandenberghe H, MacLeod S, Soldin S, Endrenyi L: Assessment of immediate post-anaesthetic recovery in young children following intravenous morphine infusions, halothane and isoflurane. *Can Anaesth Soc J* 31(1):28–35, 1984.
168. Wren WS, McShane AJ, McCarthy JG, Lamont BJ, Casey WF, Mannon VM: Isoflurane in paediatric anesthesia. *Anaesthesia* 40:315–323, 1985.

CHAPTER 8

Local and Regional Analgesia

ROMAN T. SKARDA, Dr.Med.Vet., Ph.D., D.A.C.V.A.

What is local or regional analgesia? It may be defined as the reversible loss of pain to a limited body area with minimal effects on the rest of the body.

Due to economical restraints and accepted practice, two techniques are commonly used in horses, dogs, and food animals such as cattle, sheep, goats, and pigs. One technique involves injection of a local analgesic agent into the surgical site, achieving local or infiltration analgesia. A second technique produces regional analgesia after perineural injection of major nerves. With a combination of physical restraint, mild sedation or tranquilization, and local or regional analgesia, many surgical procedures are performed.

Several factors must be considered in the choice of a technique. These factors are:

1. the site, nature, and expected duration of surgery;
2. the species, temperament, and health of the patient;
3. special requirements, such as minimum fetal depression during Caesarean section;
4. the skill and experience of the veterinarian;
5. economics of time and materials.

Local Analgesics

There are many local or regional analgesic drugs; they vary as to potency, toxicity, and cost (Table 8.1) (1–3). Three categories exist based essentially on relative duration of analgesic action. Procaine and 2-chloroprocaine have a relatively short analgesic duration of 30 to 60 minutes. Lidocaine, mepivacaine, and hexylcaine represent agents of intermediate analgesic duration of 90 to 180 minutes. Tetracaine, bupivacaine, dibucaine, and etidocaine are agents with a long duration of analgesia of 180 to 300 minutes (4). The most commonly used local analgesic drugs in veterinary medicine are amide-linked drugs (lidocaine hydrochloride and mepivacaine hydrochloride). These agents, when compared to an esther-linked drug such as procaine hydrochloride, are quicker acting, more persistent in their effect, and spread over a wider field, making a block more certain to be effective (5, 6). Lidocaine hydrochloride solution has become the single agent of choice due to the cost restrictions and limited space in a mobile practice vehicle.

POTENTIATION BY VASOCONSTRICTOR

As a general rule, the addition of a vasoconstrictor to a local analgesic agent, such as epinephrine at a concentration of 1:200,000, allows for increased intensity and prolonged analgesic activity. This concentration may be obtained by adding 0.1 ml of 1:1000 (0.1 mg) epinephrine to 20 ml of local analgesic solution. Although this does reduce the potential toxicity of the local analgesic drug by causing vasoconstriction and thus preventing high blood concentrations (7, 8), epinephrine often causes tissue necrosis along wound edges (9) and increases the risk of cardiac arrhythmia and ventricular fibrillation (10).

POTENTIATION BY HYALURONIDASE

Hyaluronidase (Hylartin Y, Pharmacia Laboratories, Piscataway, New Jersey) has been added to local

Table 8.1
Local Analgesics

Agent (Generic Name)	Trade Name	Chemical Name	Potency (Procaine = 1)	Toxicity (Procaine = 1)	Dosage	Stability	Comments
Procaine	Novocaine (Winthrop Sterns Inc., New York, NY)	Para-aminobenzoic acid ester of diethylaminoethanol	1:1	1:1	1–2% for infiltration and nerve block	Aqueous solutions are heat resistant, decomposed by bacteria	Hydrolyzed by liver and plasma esterase
Chloroprocaine	Nesacaine, (Astra Pharmaceutical Products Inc., Westboro, MA)	Para-amino-2-chlorobenzoic acid ester of B-diethyl amino ethanol	2.4:1	0.5:1	1–2% for infiltration and nerve block	Multiple autoclaving accelerates hydrolysis and impairs potency	Immediate onset of action; 2-hr duration with epinephrine
Lidocaine	Xylocaine (Astra Pharmaceutical Products, Inc., Westboro, MA)	Diethylaminoacet-2,6-xylidide	2:1	0.5%, 1:1; 1%, 1.4:1; 2%, 1.5:1	0.5–2% for infiltration and nerve block; topically, 2–4%	Aqueous solutions are thermostable, multiple autoclaving possible	Excellent penetrability; rate of onset twice as fast as procaine; 2-hr duration with epinephrine
Mepivacaine	Carbocaine (Winthrop Laboratories, New York, NY)	1-Methyl-2′,6′-pipecoloxylidide monohydrochloride	2.5:1	Less toxic than lidocaine	1–2% for infiltration and nerve block	Resistant to acid and alkaline hydrolysis, multiple autoclaving possible	Absence of vasodilator effect makes addition of a vasoconstrictor unnecessary
Tetracaine	Pontocaine (Winthrop Laboratories, New York, NY)	Parabutyl amino benzoyl-dimethyl-amino-ethanol-HCl	12:1	10:1	0.1% for infiltration and nerve block; topically, 0.2%	Crystals and solutions should not be autoclaved	Slow onset of analgesia (5–10 min); 2-hr duration; for eye installation
Hexylcaine	Cyclaine (Merck, Sharpe and Dohme, West Point, PA)	1-Cyclo-hexamino 2-propylbenzoate	1–2:1	2–4:1	0.5–1% for infiltration; 2% for nerve block; 5% topically	Crystals and solutions are thermostable	Recommended for epidural and topical analgesia
Dibucaine	Nupercaine (CIBA Pharmaceutical Products, Summit, NJ)	α-Butyl-oxycinchoninic acid of diethylethylenediamide	20:1	15:1	Topically, 0.1%	Thermostable but precipitation by alkalies	Slowly detoxified
Bupivacaine	Marcaine (Breon Laboratories Inc., New York, NY)	1-Butyl-2′,6 pipecoloxylidide-HCl	8:1	Greater margin of safety than lidocaine	0.25% for infiltration; 0.5% for nerve block; 0.75% for epidural block	Stable compound	Intermediate onset, lasting 4–6 hrs

analgesics at a rate of 150 turbidity reducing units (TRU) per 25 ml to enhance diffusion (11). Increased diffusion results in faster onset of action, but also shortens the duration due to the increased permeability of the tissues.

The combination of hyaluronidase, epinephrine, and procaine hydrochloride solution (1%) will double the area of desensitization and increase five-fold the duration of analgesia (12). New local analgesics with marked penetration have precluded the use of hyaluronidase and epinephrine.

MECHANISM OF ACTION

The primary pharmacological action of local analgesic drugs is the inhibition of the excitation conduction process in peripheral nerves (13). Local analgesic drugs are generally water-soluble acid salts. In solution, they exist in both a charged cationic (+) and uncharged base forms. After deposition into tissue, which has a slightly alkaline pH, the alkaloid base is liberated. The free base of the analgesic then diffuses readily across the nerve sheath, where it is absorbed at the outer lipid membrane of the axon. The amino groups of the drug interact with the polar groups of the cell membrane to prevent the inflow of sodium and subsequent ion flow. With the cell membrane of the nerve cell stabilized in the resting state, phase 0 depolarization and therefore conduction of impulse cannot occur.

The anesthetic base has its greatest lipid solubility when in the nonionized state, which is favored as pH increases. However, alkalinization of local analgesic drugs is not practical because of precipitation of the free base. If tissue is inflamed or infected, tissue pH is low. In acid tissue, poor hydrolysis of the acid salt and liberation of the analgesic base result, precluding effective analgesia in such an area (14). Most recently, the carbonization of the base preparations of lidocaine did not demonstrate the theoretical expectation of increased diffusion and the drug's effect in caudal epidural analgesia in horses (15).

Another important mechanism involves calcium as a membrane-stabilizing agent. Alterations in membrane Ca^{++} may be responsible for deformation or expansion of the cell membrane and thus blockade in the transmission or conduction of nerve impulses (16).

The priority of nerve fibers paralyzed in a mixed nerve trunk after exposure to a sufficient concentration of the analgesic drug depends on the amount of myelination and the size of the nerve involved; the priority is autonomic, sensory, and motor. The sensations disappear in the order of pain, heat and cold, touch, and deep pressure. Recovery of sensation is in the reverse order (13).

All excitable membranes such as exist in heart, brain, and neuromuscular junctions will be affected by local analgesic agents if they achieve a sufficient tissue concentration. Regional analgesia that is properly performed does not result in blood levels of local analgesics that are sufficient to cause systemic effects (17).

PRECAUTIONS

Sharp and sterile needles, sterile syringes in good working condition, and sterile analgesic solution should always be used. The injection sites should be surgically prepared to minimize chances of infection, although the analgesic techniques varies with each procedure and personal preference.

Horse

Although local or regional analgesia can be induced by various techniques, the most commonly used techniques in the horse include surface (topical) analgesia, infiltration analgesia, nerve block (conduction) analgesia, and epidural analgesia.

REGIONAL ANALGESIA OF THE HEAD

The most frequently desensitized nerves of the head are the auriculopalpebral, supraorbital, mental, and infraorbital alveolar. These nerves are branches of the trigeminal (fifth) cranial nerve.

Auriculopalpebral Nerve

The auriculopalpebral nerve is one of the terminal branches of the facial division of the trigeminal nerve. It carries motor fibers to the orbicularis oculi muscles. Blockade of the auriculopalpebral nerve prevents voluntary closure of the eyelids (akinesia), but does not desensitize the eyelids. Desensitization of the auriculopalpebral nerve is most frequently used for examination and treatment of the eye and temporary relief of eyelid spasms. In conjunction with topical analgesia, it is useful for removal of foreign bodies from the cornea and other minor ocular surgery.

Two locations have been suggested to paralyze the palpebral musculature: the most dorsal point on the zygomatic arch (Fig. 8.1, *A*) (18) or the depression caudal to the mandible at the ventral edge of the temporal portion of the zygomatic arch (Fig. 8.1, *B*) (19). In each location, a 2.5-cm, 22-gauge needle is placed subfascially and 5 ml of 2% lidocaine hydrochloride solution are injected in a fan-shaped manner.

Supraorbital Nerve

The supraorbital or frontal nerve is one of the terminal branches of the ophthalmic division of the

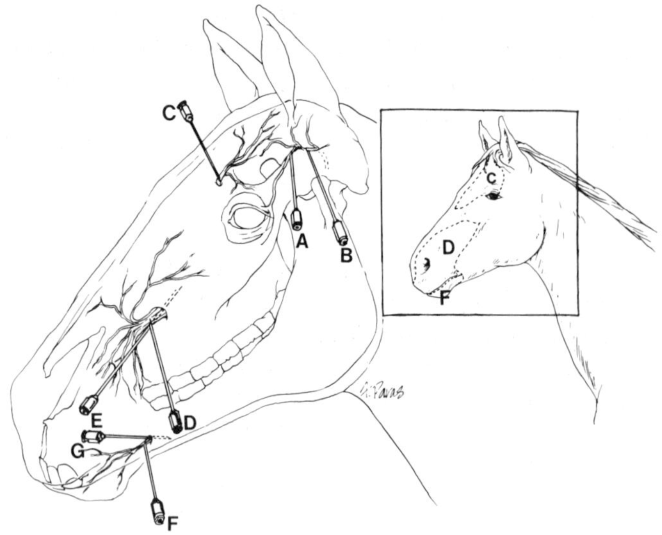

Figure 8.1. Needle placement for nerve blocks on the head: auriculopalpebral (*A* and *B*), supraorbital (or frontal) (*C*), infraorbital (*D*) and (*E*), mental (*F*), and mandibular alveolar (*G*) nerves. Inset, desensitized cutaneous area after C, D, and F blockade.

trigeminal nerve. It emerges from the orbit through the supraorbital foramen and ramifies within the middle portion of the upper eyelid and, in part, within adjacent portions of the forehead (Fig. 8.1, *C*). The supraorbital nerve is most easily desensitized within or around the supraorbital foramen (20, 21). The foramen can be palpated where it perforates the supraorbital process of the frontal bone about 6 cm dorsal to the medial canthus. A 2.5-cm, 22- or 25-gauge needle is inserted into the supraorbital foramen to a depth of 1.0 to 2.0 cm; 2 ml of 2% lidocaine hydrochloride solution are injected into the foramen, 1 ml into the tissues as the needle is slowly withdrawn and 1 ml subcutaneously over the foramen. This procedure desensitizes the middle portion of the upper eyelid and palpebral motor supply from the palpebral branch of the auriculopalpebral nerve.

Infraorbital Nerve

Analgesia of the upper lip and nose is induced by successful blockade of the infraorbital nerve as it emerges from the infraorbital canal (18, 20–23). The infraorbital foramen is located about one-half the distance and 2.5 cm dorsal to a line connecting the nasomaxillary notch and the rostal end of the facial crest. After displacing the flat levator labii superiosis muscle dorsad, a 5-cm, 20-gauge needle is used to make a perineural injection at the bony lip of the infraorbital foramen (Fig. 8.1, *D*). Injection of 5 ml of 2% lidocaine hydrochloride solution induces analgesia of the entire anterior half of the face from the foramen rostrad. If the needle is inserted into the foramen for a depth of up to 3.5 cm and injection is made, local analgesia is provided for extraction of teeth (as far as the first molar), trephination of the maxillary sinus, operations on the roof of the nasal cavity, and the skin almost to the medial canthus of the eye (Fig. 8.1, *E*) (24, 25).

Mental Nerve

Analgesia of the lower lip requires deposition of 5 ml of 2% lidocaine hydrochloride solution with a 2.5-cm, 22-gauge needle over the mental nerve, rostral to the mental foramen (Fig. 8.1, *F*) (18). After displacing the tendon of the pressor labii inferioris muscle dorsad, the lateral border of the mental foramen is easily palpated as a ridge along the horizontal ramus of the mandible in the middle of the interdental space.

Mandibular Alveolar Nerve

If a 7.5-cm, 20-gauge needle is inserted into the mental foramen (Fig. 8.1, G) and is advanced in the mandibular canal as far as possible in a ventromedial direction, the deposition of 10 ml of analgesic will extend the area of analgesia caudad as far as the third premolar (18, 20, 23, 26).

Other techniques (27), which involve desensitizing the maxillary, mandibular, and ophthalmic nerves, are not without dangers and are seldom used.

REGIONAL ANALGESIA OF THE LIMB

Regional analgesia (peripheral nerve blocks) (28–34), intra-articular and intrabursal injections (28, 31 35–38), and local infiltration (ring block) are used as an aid in diagnosis of equine lamenesses and as a means of providing analgesia to a surgery site.

In order to acutely define the lameness problem, a complete lameness examination, including observation of the horse at rest and in motion, use of hoof testers, palpation, and flexions tests, is mandatory. In addition, radiographs are helpful in determining the extent of bony involvement contributing to the lameness. As a general rule, aseptic techniques should be practiced in all injections to prevent infection. Sterile syringes and needles should be used for each injection, along with proper preparation. Intra-articular injections require a 10-minute surgical scrub; clipping the site may or may not be performed. Care must be taken not to traumatize the articular surfaces with the tip of the needle. Subcutaneous injections require an alcohol prep as a minimal preparation. After local analgesics are used, the limb should be rubbed down and wrapped to prevent swelling and inflammation.

In order to gain as much information as possible and properly diagnose the location of the lameness, peripheral nerve blocks and intra-articular injections should be performed on the most distal branches of the nerve trunks and joints first, then the examination should proceed proximally (32).

Digital Nerves

The palmar or plantar digital nerves branch dorsal to the fetlock at the level of the sesamoids forming the three digital nerves, the dorsal or anterior digital, middle digital, and palmar digital. The dorsal or anterior digital nerve supplies sensory fibers to the anterior two-thirds of the hoof. The middle digital nerve is very inconsistent and relatively unimportant. The palmar digital nerve (PDN) is the most consistent as well as the most important clinically, supplying sensory fibers to the posterior one-third of the hoof, including portions, if not all, of the navicular area.

Palmar (or Plantar) Digital Nerve Block. The palmar (or plantar) nerve is desensitized in the palmar region of the pastern joint, medially and/or laterally (Figs. 8.2 and 8.3, *A*). At this site, the palmar nerve is palpated just palmar to the vein and artery, yet dorsal to the flexor tendon. This procedure can be done with the leg in the elevated position or while bearing weight. Using a 2.5-cm, 20- to 25-gauge needle, 2 ml of 2% lidocaine hydrochloride solution are injected subcutaneously just proximal to the collateral cartilages. Then the posterior one-third of the foot including the navicular bursa should be desensitized.

Abaxial (Basilar) Sesamoidean Nerve Block. By palpating the palmar region of the fetlock joint over the abaxial surface of proximal sesamoids, the digital nerve is felt just palmar to the digital artery and vein. Using a 2.5-cm, 22- to 25-gauge needle, 3 ml of the

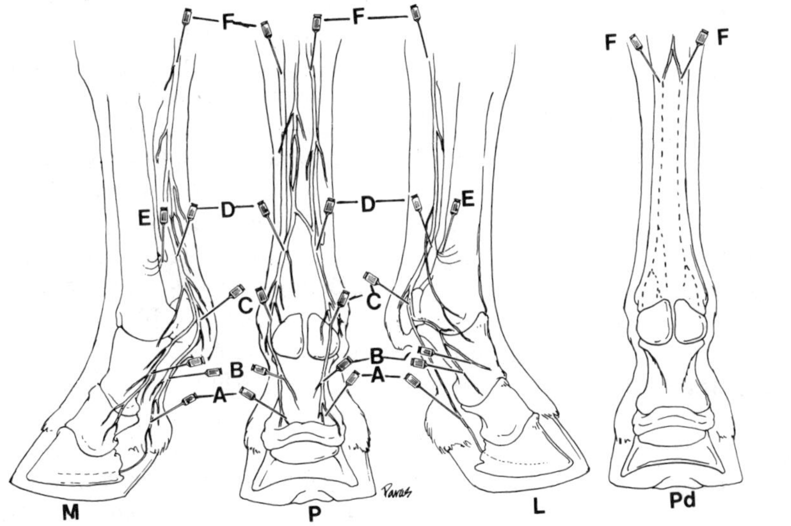

Figure 8.2. Needle placement for nerve blocks on the right forelimb in the horse: palmar digital (*A*), anterior and posterior branches of palmar digital (*B*), abaxial sesamoidean (*C*), palmar (*D*), palmar metacarpal (*E*), and high palmar nerve (*F*); M, medial; P, palmar; L, lateral; and Pd, deep palmar aspect.

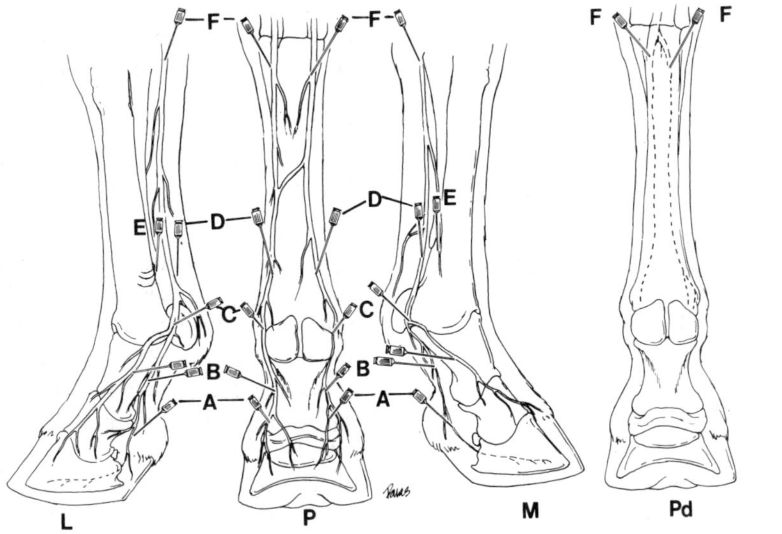

Figure 8.3. Needle placement for nerve blocks on the left hindlimb in the horse: plantar distal (*A*), anterior and posterior branches of plantar digital (*B*), abaxial sesamoidean (*C*), plantar (*D*), plantar metatarsal (*E*), and high plantar nerve (*F*); L, lateral; P, plantar; M, medial; and Pd, deep plantar aspect.

analgesic are injected subcutaneously at that site (Figs. 8.2 and 8.3, *C*). If done successfully, the palmar digital nerve and its dorsal branch, and thus the entire foot, will be desensitized. Partial numbing of the fetlock area may occur.

Intra-articular Coffin Injection

A 5-cm, 20-gauge needle is inserted 1.5 cm proximal to the coronary band at the medial or lateral edge of the extensor tendon and is directed obliquely ventral to the tendon toward the extensor process. After the capsule is penetrated, synovial fluid should appear in the hub of the needle. Injection of 5 to 8 ml of 2% lidocaine hydrochloride solution into the dorsal pouch of the coffin joint capsule is best performed while the limb is weight bearing (Fig. 8.4, *A*). This block desensitizes the coffin joint capsule and navicular bursa. If the horse goes sound after the posterior digital nerve block, then this block can localize a lesion almost exclusively to the navicular bursa.

Midpastern Ring Block

Using a 2.5-cm, 22-gauge needle, 10 to 12 ml of 2% lidocaine hydrochloride solution are placed subcutaneously and deeply around the pastern proximal to the pastern joint. The ring block desensitizes the entire digit distal to the injection, including the coffin and pastern joints.

Intra-articular Pastern Block

To desensitize the pastern joint, 4 to 5 ml of 2% lidocaine hydrochloride solution are injected through a 2.5- to 3.75-cm, 18- to 20-gauge needle that is inserted medial or lateral to the midline on the dorsal aspect of the pastern joint (Fig. 8.4, *B*). The needle is directed from the point of insertion distally and toward the midline.

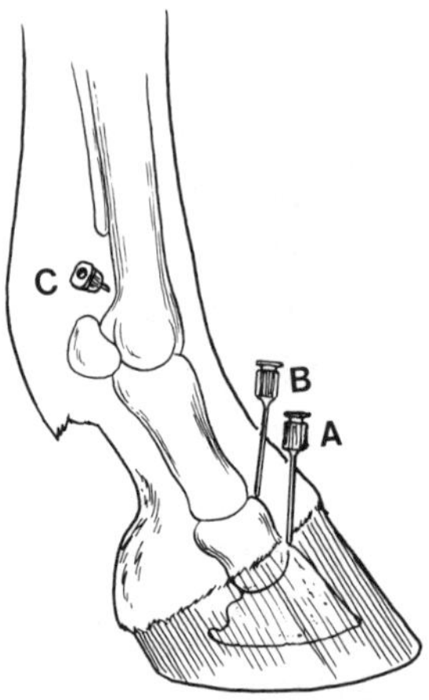

Figure 8.4. Needle placement into coffin joint (*A*), pastern joint (*B*), and volar pouch of fetlock joint capsule (*C*).

Palmar and/or Plantar Nerve Blocks

The palmar or plantar nerves can be desensitized at either a high site (high palmar or high plantar nerve block) or at a low site (low palmar or low plantar nerve block).

Low Palmar or Plantar Nerve Block. The injections for this procedure are performed medially and laterally at the level of the distal enlargements of the metacarpal II and IV and metatarsal II and IV (splints), respectively. The palmar nerves (medial/lateral) are desensitized by injecting the analgesic between the flexor tendon and suspensory ligament (Fig. 8.2 and 8.3, *D*). The palmar metacarpal and metatarsal nerves (medial/lateral) are desensitized by injecting the drug between the suspensory ligament and the splint bone (Fig. 8.2 and 8.3, *E*) (30). Two to three milliliters of 2% lidocaine hydrochloride solution are deposited at each site using a 2.5-cm, 20- to 25-gauge needle while the limb is bearing weight. Successful injections desensitize almost all structures distal to the fetlock and fetlock joint except for the dorsal fetlock joint, which receives sensory fibers from the ulnar and musculocutaneous nerves.

Ring Block Proximal to Fetlock. A 2.5-cm, 20-gauge needle is used; 10 to 12 ml of 2% lidocaine hydrochloride solution are injected subcutaneously proximal to the sesamoids all around the limb. Most structures distal to the injection will be desensitized, including both palmar nerves, both palmar metacarpal nerves, and cutaneous branches of musculocutaneous and dorsal ulnar nerves. The fetlock joint capsule will partially be desensitized.

Intra-articular Fetlock Injection. The fetlock joint and sesamoids are desensitized after injecting 5 to 7 ml of 2% lidocaine hydrochloride solution into the volar pouch between the cannon bone and suspensory ligament. A 2.5- to 3.75-cm, 18- to 20-gauge needle is used for penetration of the skin distal to the splint bone and dorsal to the annular ligament of the fetlock (Fig. 8.4, C).

High Palmar (or Plantar) Nerve Block. This procedure is performed at the level of the proximal quarter of the metacarpus (or metatarsus) proximal to the communicating branch of the medial and lateral palmar (or plantar) nerves (Fig. 8.2 and 8.3, *F*). Five milliliters of 2% lidocaine hydrochloride solution are injected through a 3.75-cm, 22-gauge needle placed subfascillary into the groove between the suspensory ligament and the deep flexor tendon on both the medial and lateral sides (medial and lateral palmar/plantar nerve blocks). The injections desensitize the palmar metacarpal (or plantar metatarsal) region and all of the digit distal to the fetlock. The dorsal metacarpal (or metatarsal) region will still have sensation.

In order to completely desensitize the fetlock joint, three additional nerves in the front foot must be desensitized, the medial and lateral palmar metacarpal nerves as they emerge from under the splint bones and the cutaneous antebrachial nerve where it lies at the medial aspect of the common digital extensor tendon proximal to the fetlock.

In the hindlimb, four additional nerves must be desensitized in order to induce analgesia of the fetlock joint. The medial and lateral plantar metatarsal nerves are desensitized in a fashion similar to the medial and lateral palmar metacarpal nerves of the front limb and in addition the medial and lateral dorsal metatarsal nerves (39).

High Suspensory Block

A 3.75-cm, 22-gauge needle is inserted deep to the proximal palmar aspect of the metacarpus or metatarsus to deposit 5 ml of the analgesic solution to the medial and lateral palmar metacarpal or metatarsal nerves while the limb is elevated. In addition to analgesia of the caudal aspect of the metacarpus or metatarsus and adjacent splint bones, analgesia of the interosseus muscle (suspensory ligament) can be expected.

SELECTED TECHNIQUES IN THE FORELIMB

Intra-articular Carpal Injections

The two most commonly injected carpal joints are the radiocarpal and the intercarpal (Fig. 8.5). The intercarpal and carpometacarpal joints communicate. After the limb is flexed, indentation of the joints can be felt medial or lateral to the extensor carpi radialis tendon (35). A 2.5-cm, 20- to 22-gauge needle is used to deposit 5 to 10 ml of 2% lidocaine hydrochloride solution into each joint.

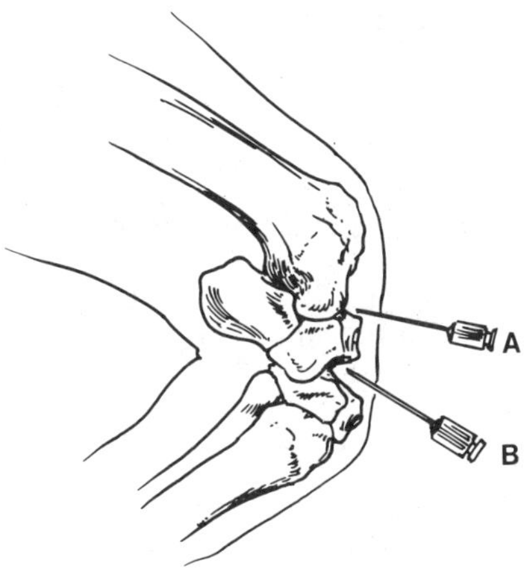

Figure 8.5. Needle placement into the radiocarpal joint (*A*) and intercarpal joint (*B*).

Median, Ulnar, and Musculocutaneous Nerve Blocks

To complete analgesia of the forelimb from the carpus distally, three nerves must be desensitized (31, 32, 34). The median nerve is desensitized on the medial aspect of the forelimb 5 cm ventral to the elbow joint between the posterior border of the radius and the muscular belly of the internal flexor carpi radialis, deep to the posterior superficial pectoral muscle (Fig. 8.6). A 3.75-cm, 20- to 22-gauge needle is used to infiltrate the median nerve with 10 ml of 2% lidocaine hydrochloride solution.

The ulnar nerve is desensitized by using a 2.5-cm, 22- to 25-gauge needle to deposit 5 ml of analgesic solution. The nerve is located 1.5 cm deep beneath the fascia, 10 cm proximal to the accessory carpal bone between the flexor carpi ulnaris and ulnaris lateralis muscles (Fig. 8.7).

The musculocutaneous nerve is desensitized by using a 2.5-cm, 22-gauge needle and 10 ml of the analgesic solution and placing a subcutaneous deposit on the anteromedial aspect of the forelimb halfway between the elbow and carpus (Fig. 8.8). At this site, the musculocutaneous nerve can be easily palpated just cranial to the cephalic vein.

Ring Block Proximal to Carpus

This type of block is performed in order to remove cutaneous sensation remaining in the metacarpus and carpus after desensitization of the median and ulnar nerves. Approximately 15 ml of local analgesic are infiltrated around the limb using a 1.5-cm, 22-gauge needle.

Perineural injection of the analgesic in more proximal portions of the limb are best avoided in order to prevent paralysis of muscular branches and thus collapse of the horse (32).

Intra-articular Elbow Injection

Injection into the elbow joint is relatively difficult. After repeatedly flexing the joint, a depression can be felt between the bony eminence of the lateral condyle of the humerus and the anterior aspect of the lateral ligament of the elbow joint. At that site, a 7.5-cm, 18-gauge needle is inserted in slight caudomedial direction for a distance of 4 to 6 cm (Fig. 8.9, *A*) (40). Up to 10 ml of 2% lidocaine hydrochloride solution is deposited.

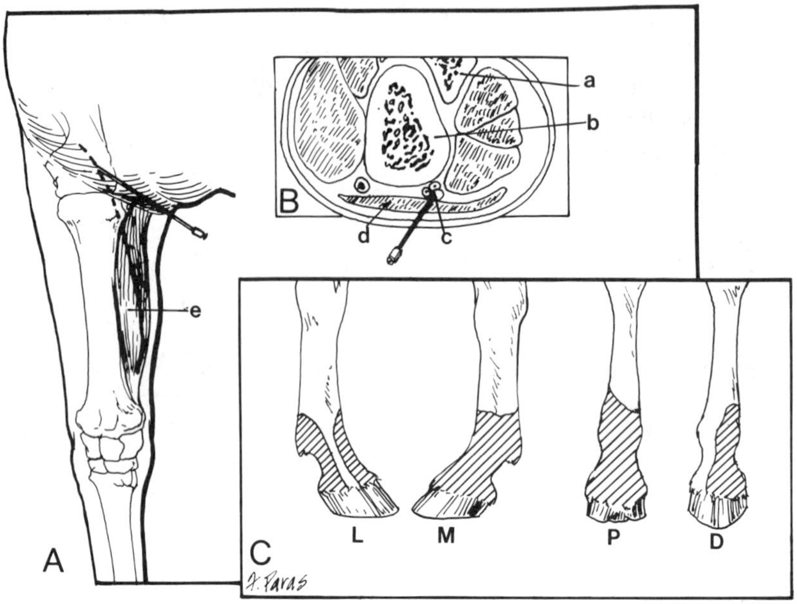

Figure 8.6. Median nerve blocks (right forelimb). *A*, craniomedial aspect; *B*, cross section; *C*, desensitized cutaneous area ; *L*, lateral; *M*, medial; *P*, palmar; *D*, dorsal aspect. *a*, ulna; *b*, radius; *c*, median nerve; *d*, superficial pectoral muscle; *e*, flexor carpi radialis muscle.

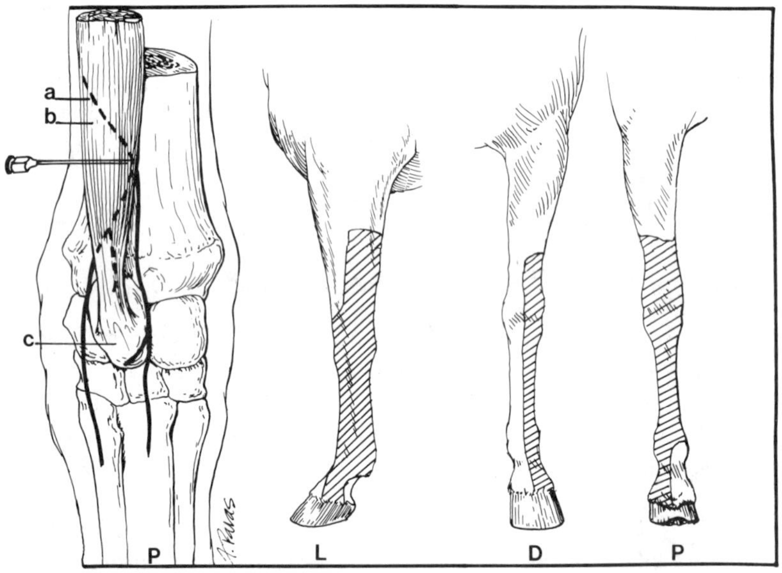

Figure 8.7. Ulnar nerve blocks and desensitized cutaneous area of left forelimb. *P*, palmar; *L*, lateral; *D*, dorsal aspect. *a*, ulnaris laterialis muscle; *b*, ulnaris nerve; *c*, accessory carpal bone.

Bicipital Bursa Injection

A 5-cm, 18-gauge needle is inserted under the brachial biceps tendon from below. Skin penetration is 4 cm ventral and 1.5 cm posterior to the anterior prominence of the lateral tuberosity of the humerus (Fig. 8.9, *B*). To puncture the bursa from that site, the point of the needle is advanced up to 5 cm in a dorsomedial direction along the humerus (36). About 10 to 15 ml of 2% lidocaine hydrochloride solution is required.

Intra-articular Shoulder Injection

The shoulder joint is entered between the prominent projections of the anterior and posterior parts of the lateral tuberosity of the humerus. A 7.5-cm, 16- or 18-gauge needle is inserted approximately 2.5-cm anterior to this point and directed on a horizontal plane in a posteromedial direction at a 45° angle to the body (Fig. 8.9, C) (31). For free flow or aspiration of synovial fluid, the needle must be inserted to a depth of up to 7.5 cm. Frequently, 15 ml or more of 2% lidocaine hydrochloride solution are required.

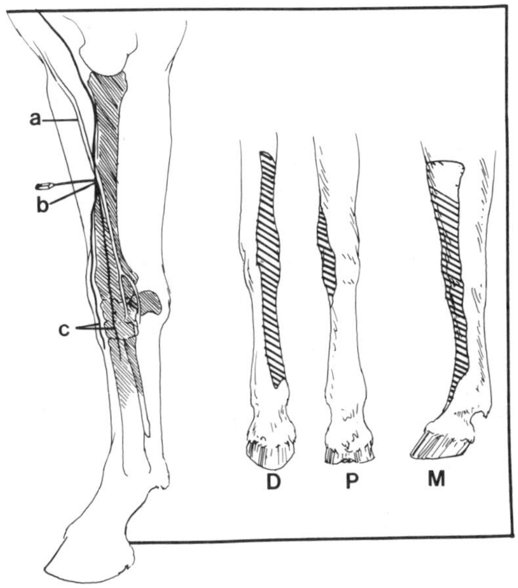

Figure 8.8. Musculocutaneous nerve block and desensitized cutaneous area of right forelimb. *D*, dorsal; *P*, palmar; *M*, medial aspect. *a*, cephalic vein; *b*, musculocutaneous nerve; *c*, medial cutaneous antebrachial nerve.

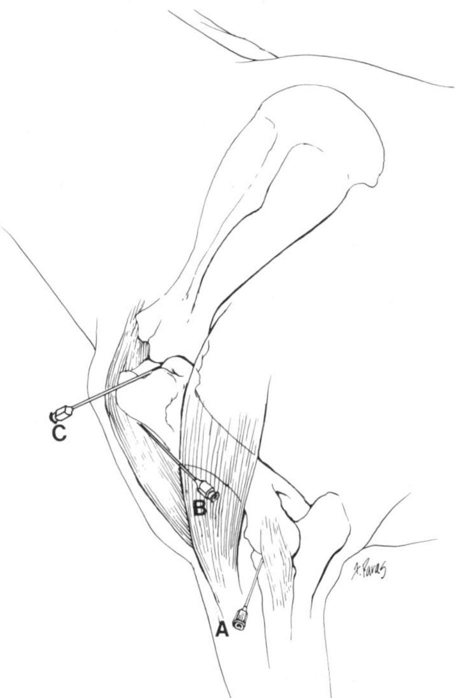

Figure 8.9. Needle placement into elbow joint (*A*), bicipital bursa (*B*), and shoulder joint (*C*).

SELECTED TECHNIQUES IN THE HINDLIMB

Nerve Blocks Proximal to the Tarsus

To induce analgesia of the hindlimb distal to the tarsus, it is necessary to desensitize the tibial, saphenous, superficial peroneal (superficial fibular), and deep peroneal (deep fibular) nerves.

The tibial nerve is desensitized 10 cm proximal to the point of the tarsus between the tendon of the gastrocnemius muscle and deep flexor tendon on the medial aspect of the limb while the limb is partially flexed (31). A 2.5-cm, 22-gauge needle is placed subfascially and 20 ml of a 2% lidocaine hydrochloride solution is deposited around the nerve. Desensitizing the tibial nerve induces analgesia of the posterior metatarsal region and most of the foot, except for the anterolateral region (Fig. 8.10). Complete desensitization requires a ring block of the dorsal metatarsal region (34). The saphenous nerve is desensitized by using a 2.5-cm, 22-gauge needle to deposit 5 ml of 2% lidocaine hydrochloride solution on the dorsal aspect of the median saphenous vein proximal to the tibiotarsal joint (Fig. 8.11). Sensation to the medial aspect of the thigh and part of the metatarsal region will be lost. The superficial and deep peroneal nerves can be simultaneously desensitized by inserting a 3.75-cm, 22-gauge needle between the long and lateral digital extensor muscles at a site 10 cm proximal to the lateral malleolus of the tibia (Fig. 8.12). The tendons of these two muscles can be palpated if the limb is flexed. First, the needle is placed subcutaneously to deposit 10 ml of 2% lidocaine hydrochloride solution around the superficial branch of the nerve. The needle is then advanced an additional 2 to 3 cm to penetrate the deep fascia and to deposit 15 ml of the analgesic around the deep branch. Desensitizing the superficial and deep peroneal nerves provides analgesia to the anteriolateral tarsal and metatarsal regions and to the joint capsule of the tarsus (31).

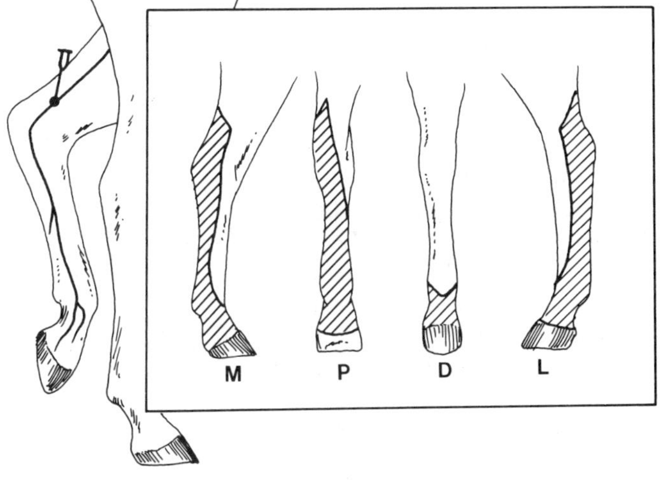

Figure 8.10. Tibial nerve block and desensitized cutaneous area (left rearlimb). *M*, medial; *P*, plantar; *D*, dorsal; *L*, lateral aspect.

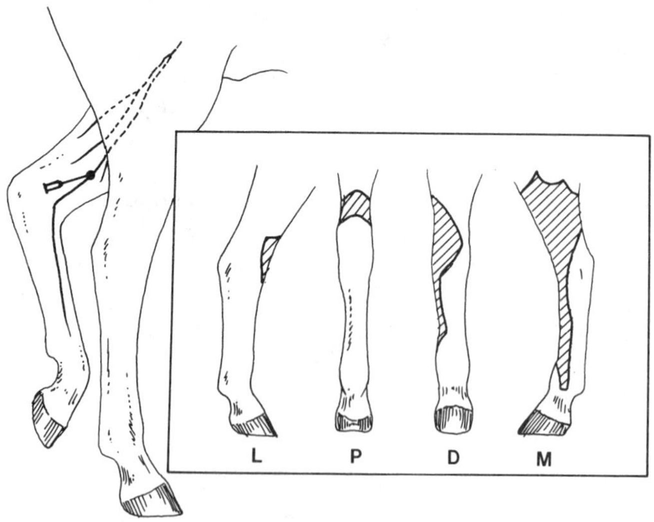

Figure 8.11. Saphenous nerve block and desensitized cutaneous area (left rearlimb). *L*, lateral; *P*, plantar; *D*, dorsal; *M*, medial aspect.

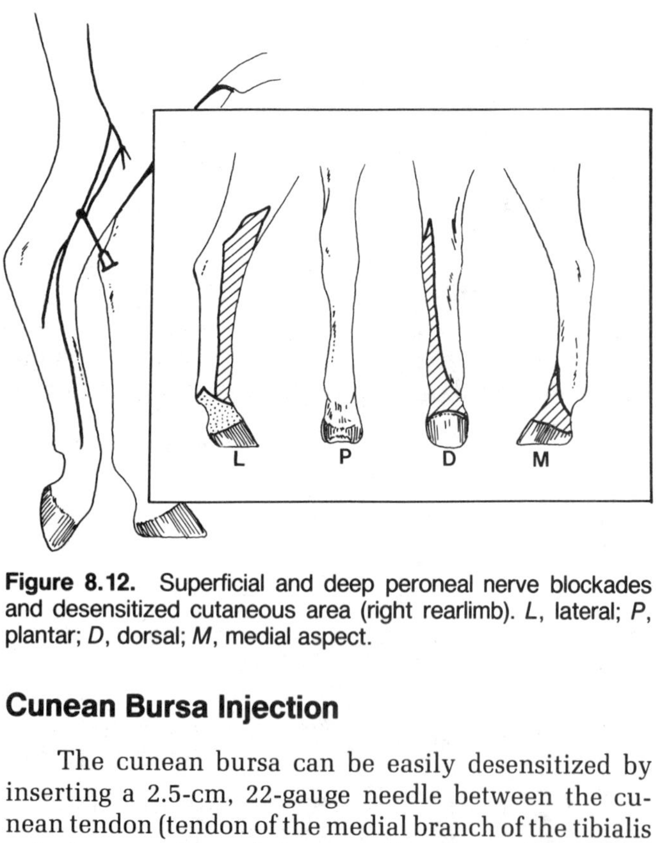

Figure 8.12. Superficial and deep peroneal nerve blockades and desensitized cutaneous area (right rearlimb). *L*, lateral; *P*, plantar; *D*, dorsal; *M*, medial aspect.

Cunean Bursa Injection

The cunean bursa can be easily desensitized by inserting a 2.5-cm, 22-gauge needle between the cunean tendon (tendon of the medial branch of the tibialis anterior muscle) and the tarsal bones on the medial aspect of the tarsus and injecting at least 8 ml of 2% lidocaine hydrochloride solution (Fig. 8.13, *A*). The time required for maximum effect is 20 minutes.

Intra-articular Tarsal Injections

Desensitizing the distal intertarsal and tarsometatarsal joints is helpful in diagnosing early bone spavin, particularly if radiographic osteoarthritis has not developed. The distal intratarsal space is entered by inserting a 2.5-cm, 22-gauge needle at a right angle to the skin ventral to the cunean tendon on the medial aspect of the tarsus (Fig. 8.13, *B*) (8). Approximately 6 ml of 2% lidocaine hydrochloride solution is injected into the joint space under pressure. In an alternative method, a 2.5-cm, 18-gauge needle is used to inject the distal intertarsal joint between the heads of the third metatarsal and fourth tarsal bones. The tarsometatarsal joint is located approximately 2 cm distal to the intertarsal joint and is injected similarly (Fig. 8.10, *C*). If one needle is placed into the distal intratarsal space and a second needle is placed into the tarsometatarsal space, injection of local analgesic into one needle will cause the analgesic to flow from the other, demonstrating communications between the two joints (38, 39).

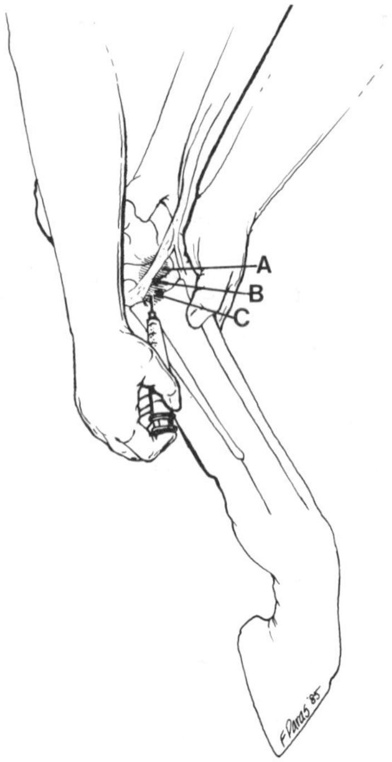

Figure 8.13. Needle placement into cunean bursa (*A*), distal intratarsal space (*B*), and tarsometatarsal space (*C*) of the hock joint.

Intra-articular Stifle Injections

The stifle joint is the largest joint in the hindlimb; it consists of the femoropatellar pouch enclosing the femoropatellar joint and communicating with the medial femorotibial pouch of the femorotibial joint. If the stifle joint is inflamed, the communicating opening can be obstructed, and it requires the injection of local analgesic or medication into each individual compartment (31). The femoropatellar pouch is most easily entered through the space between the middle and medial patellar ligaments (Fig. 8.14, *A*). The lateral femorotibial pouch is entered between the lateral col-

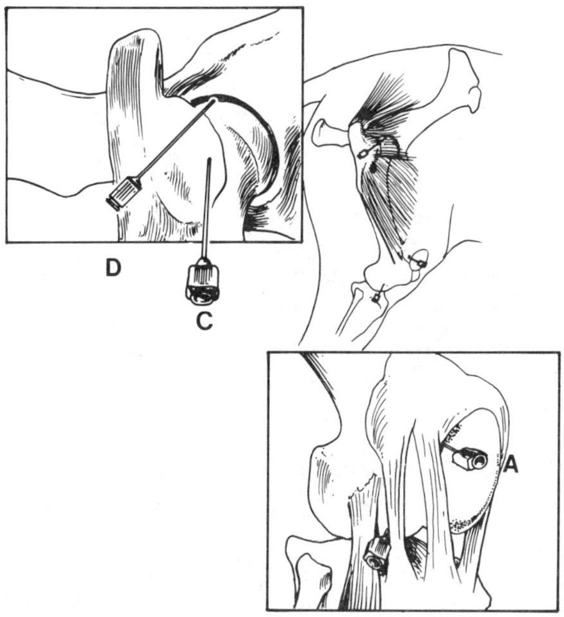

Figure 8.14. Needle placement into femoropatellar pouch (*A*) and lateral femorotibial pouch (*B*) of the stifle joint, trochanteric bursa (*C*), and coxofemoral joint (*D*).

lateral ligament and lateral patellar ligament (Fig. 8.14, *B*). A 5-cm, 18-gauge needle is satisfactory for penetrating the joint capsule and injecting 35 to 50 ml of 2% lidocaine hydrochloride solution into each pouch.

Trochanteric Bursa Block

The trochanteric bursa is located on the lateral aspect of the hip between the anterior crest of the great trochanter of the femur and the middle gluteal muscle. A 7.5-cm, 18-gauge needle is used to penetrate the bursa ventral to the crest (Fig. 8.14, *C*). Continuous suction is applied to a syringe attached to the needle, and synovial fluid is recovered; 10 ml of the analgesic are injected.

Intra-articular Coxofemoral Injection

A 15-cm, 14- to 16-gauge needle is inserted between the anterior and posterior eminences of the great trochanter of the humerus and is advanced in an anteromedial direction along the femoral neck until the joint capsule is penetrated (Fig. 8.14, *D*). After synovia fluid is recovered on aspiration, 20 ml of 2% lidocaine hydrochloride solution are injected. One must wait a minimum of 30 minutes before assessing improvement of the lameness.

When comparing diagnostic intrabursal, intra-articular injections and nerve blocks, it becomes evident that injection of local analgesic drug into a bursa or joint induces analgesia to a more localized area and requires more time (a minimum of 30 minutes) to reach maximal effect than does a perineural injection.

ANALGESIA FOR LAPAROTOMY

Several techniques have been described to produce selective analgesia of the skin, musculature, and peritoneum of the flank region and abdominal wall in the standing horse; these include (*a*) infiltration analgesia, (*b*) paravertebral thoracolumbar analgesia, (*c*) segmental dorso-lumbar epidural analgesia, and (*d*) thoraco-lumbar subarachnoid analgesia. Any of these techniques facilitates exploratory laparotomy, intestinal biopsy, ovariectomy of small granuloma cell tumors, surgical management of uterine torsion, castration of stallions with abdominal cryptorchidism, embryo transfer, and thoracotomy.

Infiltration Analgesia

The easiest and probably the most commonly used technique in equine practice for producing analgesia of the flank is simple infiltration of the incision line (line block) (31). A 2.5-cm, 20-gauge needle is inserted into the skin and subcutaneous tissues at multiple sites; 10 to 15 ml of a 2% lidocaine hydrochloride solution are injected. This is followed by deep infiltration to the peritoneum using a 7.5- to 10-cm 18-gauge needle and 50 to 75 ml of the analgesic in the adult (500 kg) horse. The maximum single infiltrative dose of lidocaine in the horse is 6 g, which is equivalent to 300 ml of a 2% solution (41). The ease of administration and lack of special equipment needed are advantages of the line block when compared to any other technique. Disadvantages include distortion of normal tissue architecture, retardation of healing at the deposition site, and increased costs because of the higher dosages of analgesic that are required.

Paravertebral Thoracolumbar Analgesia

As an alternative to the line block, desensitizing the dorsal and ventral branches of the last thoracic (T18) and first and second lumbar (L1 and L2) spinal nerves produces regional analgesia of the skin, musculature, and peritoneum of the mid-flank region (42).

Three subcutaneous depots with 15 ml of 2% lidocaine hydrochloride solution are made to desensitize the lateral cutaneous branches of dorsal spinal nerves, T18, L1, and L2. The injection sites are between the caudal border of the last rib and distal end of the first lumbar transverse process (for T-18), between the first and second lumbar transverse processes (for L-1), and between the second and third lumbar transverse processes (for L-2), respectively. The injections are made approximately 10 cm from the midline (Fig. 8.15, *A*). The distance between the injection sites ranges from 3 to 6 cm.

To reach the ventral branches of T18, L1, and L2 a 5- to 7.5-cm 18-gauge needle is inserted ventrad at

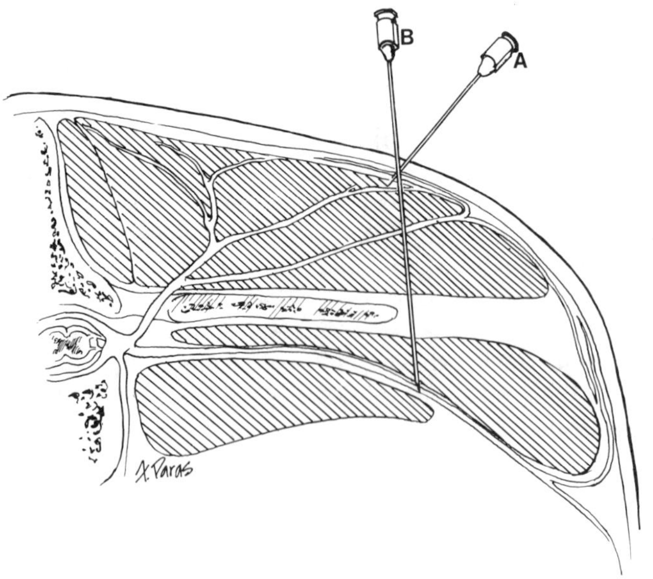

Figure 8.15. Needle placement for paravertebral nerve block in the horse: subcutaneous depot (*A*) and infiltration of ventral branch (*B*).

each site until the peritoneum is punctured (Fig. 8.15, *B*). Loss of resistance to needle insertion and the sound of a slight sucking as air enters the needle are signs that the peritoneum has been entered. The point of the needle should then be withdrawn to a retroperitoneal position, where a second deposit of 15 ml of the analgesic is placed. Selective ipsilateral desensitization of the flank (dermatome T18), caudal flank to the lateral surface of the thigh (dematome L1), and cranial aspect of the thigh to the lateral surface of the stifle (dermatome L2) generally occurs within 10 minutes of injection and may last for up to 2 hours.

The advantages of distal paravertebral lumbar analgesia when compared to local infiltration are the smaller dosages of local analgesic required, the wider and more uniform area of complete analgesia, and the absence of local analgesic from the wound margins. The technique is more difficult to perform, however, especially where the landmarks for injection are not identified or spinal nerves follow a variable course. Also, desensitization of the ventral branch of the third lumbar spinal nerve, which carries motor fibers to the femoral and ischial nerves, must be avoided to maintain pelvic limb function.

Segmental-Dorso-Lumbar Epidural Analgesia

A small dose (3 to 5 ml) of 2% lidocaine hydrochloride solution is injected into a catheter previously placed into the epidural space at the first lumbar (L-1) vertebra to desensitize the adjacent spinal nerves T18 to L2 (43). The technique is technically difficult and requires the use of a unidirectional pointed spinal needle and stiff catheter-stylet unit to catheterize the L-1 epidural space from the lumbosacral epidural space. Although mentioned as a possible technique, it is not recommended because of the frequent occurrence of kinking and misdirection of the catheter with subsequent injection of local analgesic into the lumbosacral epidural space, thereby producing loss of pelvic limb function and excitement in horses.

Segmental Thoracolumbar Subarachnoid Analgesia

In contrast to the epidural placement, subarachnoid catheterization of the thoracolumbar (T18–L1) area from the lumbosacral (L6–S1) intervertebral space is a more practical procedure (43, 44). Palpation of the thoracolumbar and lumbosacral interspaces is the only practicable and reliable guide when attempting to find the proper T18-L1 and L6-S1 interspaces. The thumb of one hand is used to apply vertical pressure to the skin at the highest point of the gluteal region to palpate the depression between the dorsal spinous processes of the sixth lumbar (L-6) and second sacral (S-2) vertebrae. This interspace is approximately defined by the intersection of a line joining the palpable posterior border of the tuber coxae and the midline and 1 to 2 cm caudad of a line drawn between the cranial edge of each tuber sacrale and the dorsal midline. Also, rectal palpation of the ventral lumbosacral eminence may be used to locate the L6–S1 intervertebral space (44). The lumbosacral area is clipped, surgically scrubbed, and disinfected. Approximately 5 ml of 2% lidocaine hydrochloride solution are used to infiltrate the skin at the lumbosacral site to minimize the pain during insertion of a 17.5 cm × 1.4 mm outside diameter (OD) 17-gauge Huber point (Tuohy) needle with stylet (Becton, Dickinson, Rutherford, New Jersey). The point of the needle is advanced along the median plane perpendicular to the spinal cord until it reaches the subarachnoid space (Fig. 8.16, *A*). Penetration of the spinal canal is made with the bevel directed craniad. The stylet is then removed, and the needle is aspirated for cerebrospinal fluid (CSF) to verify the position. An 80-cm Fotmocath polyethylene catheter (Becton, Dickinson) (0.625 mm OD), reinforced with a stainless steel spring guide (USC1, CR Brand Inc., Billerica, Massachusetts) (0.52 mm OD) is passed through the needle and threaded subarachnoidally to the middle position of the thoracic area for about 60 cm. The Huber point needle is withdrawn over the catheter and the spring guide is removed, leaving only the catheter in position. A 23-gauge hypodermic needle and three-way stopcock are attached to the end of the catheter. To place the tip of the catheter at the T18-L1 intervertebral space, the catheter is withdrawn a calculated distance, until the distance between the free end of the catheter and the surface of the skin equals the total length of the catheter (80 cm) minus the sum of the distance be-

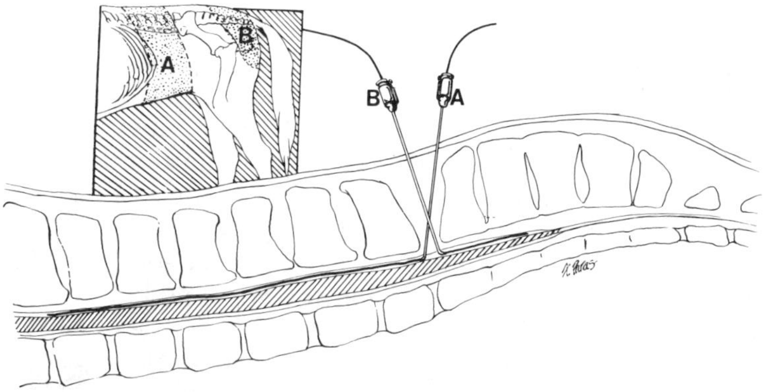

Figure 8.16. Catheterization of the thoracolumbar subarachnoid space (*A*) and sacral subarachnoid space (*B*) in the horse. Inset, desensitized subcutaneous area after segmental (*A*) and caudal (*B*) blockades.

tween the lumbosacral skin surface and subarachnoid puncture site and the distance between the lumbosacral and thoracolumbar intervertebral spaces. The distance between the skin and free subarachnoid space is measured by noting the distance of withdrawal of the spinal needle after introduction of the catheter into the subarachnoid space. The distance between the lumbosacral and T18-L1 intervertebral space is obtained by noting the distance between the skin puncture site and the palpable thoracolumbar (T18-L1) spinal interspace. The T18-L1 interspace is generally located by palpating the depressions between the lumbar spinous processes (L6-L1) and by gradually moving the fingers craniad to the caudal edge of the eighteenth (T-18) thoracic spine.

A small dose (1.5 ml) of 2% lidocaine hydrochloride solution is injected through the catheter using a rate of injection of approximately 0.5 ml/60 seconds. Slow injection allows a more even distribution of the drug within the subarachnoid space and complete desensitization of adjacent spinal nerves before they emerge from the dura mater covering the spinal cord (Fig. 8.16, *B*). Bilateral segmental thoracolumbar (T17-L2) analgesia generally occurs within 5 to 10 minutes of injection and lasts 30 to 60 minutes (Fig. 10–16, *A*). When compared with other field techniques, including infiltration analgesia, paravertebral analgesia, and segmental epidural analgesia, some advantages and disadvantages of segmental subarachnoid analgesia in horses are of considerable importance. The lumbosacral CSF tap is done readily, subarachnoidal passage of a catheter at the thoracolumbar area can be accomplished, and the catheter provides a route for repeated administration of local analgesic drug, making the duration, degree, and area of analgesia more easily controlled. The disadvantages are the potential for traumatizing the conus medullaris; sheering off the catheter, if withdrawn through the needle; curling of the catheter within the subarachnoid space, if the wire guide is recessed from the catheter tip; loss of motor control of the pelvic limbs or hemodynamic disturbances after accidental overdose; and meningitis after septic technique (44).

CAUDAL ANALGESIA

Caudal epidural analgesia, continuous caudal epidural analgesia, and caudal subarachnoid analgesia are techniques to produce analgesia of the tail, rectum, distal colon, bladder, and reproductive organs in the standing horse. Any of these local analgesic techniques will facilitate surgery involving the tail, perineum, anus, rectum, vulva, vagina, urethra (e.g., Caslick's operation, rectovaginal fistula repairs, prolapsed rectum repair, urethrostomy, or tail amputation), and symptomatic relief of painful conditions during obstetric manipulations.

Proper restraint should be used, particularly in fractious horses. The injection site is clipped, shaved, and prepared for aseptic surgery. The skin overlying the site should be desensitized with 1.5 ml of a 2% lidocaine hydrochloride solution using a 1.5-cm, 25-gauge needle. The bleb of analgetic in the subcutaneous tissue minimizes movement during insertion of the spinal needle and also minimizes pain if a stab incision is made through the skin to facilitate passage of the spinal needle.

Caudal Epidural Analgesia

The injection site is the first coccygeal interspace (C_o1-C_o2) (45, 46). This space is located by palpation as the first obvious midline depression caudal to the sacrum. Dorsoventral manipulation of the tail allows the location of the C_o1-C_o2 interspace to be confirmed; it is the first moveable joint caudal to the sacrum. This site is also at the most angular portion of the bend of the tail, at 5 to 7 cm craniad to the beginning of the long tail hairs.

In the standard technique, a 5- to 7.5-cm, 18-gauge spinal needle with fitted stylet is inserted in the center of the intercoccygeal space at an angle of about 30° to the horizontal plane (47, 48) until it strikes the floor of the vertebral canal. The needle is then withdrawn approximately 0.5 cm to avoid injection into the intervertebral disc or ligamentous floor of the canal (Fig. 8.17, *A*). Alternatively, the hub of the needle may be filled with analgesic solution. As the needle is inserted, a slight vacuum in the epidural space will aspirate the solution from the hub (49). Entry into the epidural space is generally identified by a sudden decrease in resistance to passage of the needle. Also, a hissing sound is often heard as air enters the epidural space after removal of the stylet. Lack of resistance to injection of 10 ml of air and no evidence of blood upon aspiration indicates proper position of the tip of the needle in the epidural space. However, if the needle is not in the space, considerable resistance to air or fluid injection is met. The amount of local analgesic injected varies depending upon the local analgesic drug, the size and confirmation of the horse, and the extent of local analgesic desired (Table 8.2). When using a 2% lidocaine hydrochloride solution to achieve standing caudal analgesia in a 500-kg horse, 5 to 7 ml would be needed to desensitize the rectum, vagina, bladder, and urethra. If procaine is used, up to 30 ml of a 2% solution may be required in adult horses. In contrast, only 3 ml of a 5% hexylcaine hydrochloride solution or 5 ml of a 2% mepivacaine hydrochloride solution are needed to achieve similar analgesia of pelvic viscera and genitalia, without loss of hindleg motor control.

The time for maximum effect is 10 to 30 minutes. Desensitization of sensory fibers results in desensitized skin of the tail, the croup as far cranial as the midsacral region, anus, perineum, vulva, and caudal aspect of the thigh. Blockade of motor fibers results in flaccidity of the tail. Uterine motility remains unaffected. Abdominal contractions or straining are abolished, although the abdominal musculature is not paralyzed. Interruption of parasympathetic fibers of the pelvic nerves results in relaxation and dilation of the rectum, bladder, and genitalia. Rectal peristalsis is abolished, the constrictor vulvae muscle is relaxed, and the retractor penis muscle in males is relaxed. If the surgical procedure is to be done standing and the required analgesic dose is unknown, it is best to underdose and wait 20 minutes after injection. After that time, 1.0-ml increments should be given until the desired effect is achieved. The duration of analgesia is dose-related and lasts from 60 to 90 minutes. The needle may be left in place and an injection cap attached so that additional quantities of analgesic can be administered.

Improper injection technique, anatomical abnormalities, or adhesions resulting from previous epidural injections contribute to failure. Inadequate analgesia in the horse is not uncommon; it is manifested mainly as delayed onset time, inadequate intensity, and short duration of analgesia. More serious complications can occur after ataxia of hindlimbs, hindlimb motor blockade, and recumbency are induced in conscious horses by overdosing, particularly if the analgesic drug is readministered before the maximal effect of the drug injection has been reached.

Continuous Caudal Epidural Analgesia

Two methods of continuous caudal epidural injections in horses have been described. In one method, a 10.2-cm, 18-gauge thin-walled Tuohy needle is inserted on the midline into the C_o1-C_o2 interspace while being directed cranially and ventrally at an angle of approximately 45° to the croup (15, 50). After piercing through the interarcuate ligament, the needle is placed in the epidural space. This space is identified by loss of resistance to injection of 10 ml of air. A 91.8-cm, 20-gauge Teflon epidural catheter with stylet (Deseret, Sandy, Utah) is then threaded through the needle and

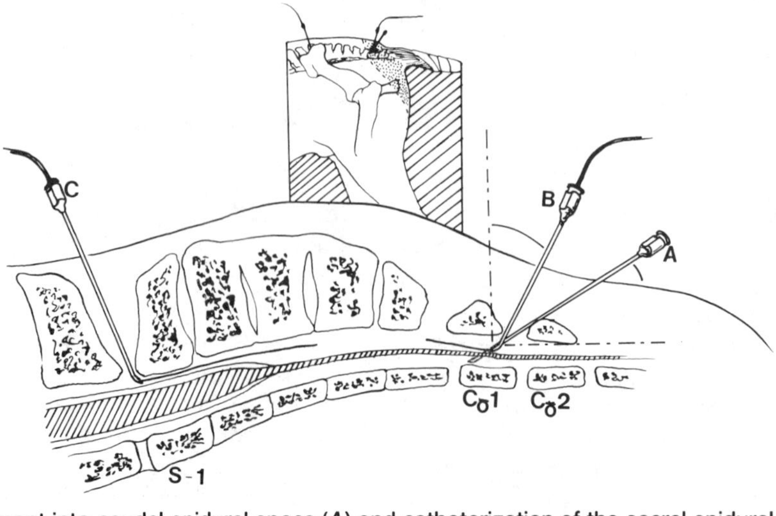

Figure 8.17. Needle placement into caudal epidural space (*A*) and catheterization of the sacral epidural space (technique *B* and *C*).

Table 8.2
Neuroanatomy and Action of Caudal Epidural Analgesia

Nerves	Ventral Branches	Spinal Cord Segment	Sensory	Motor	Parasympathetic	Sympathetic	Action
Caudal		Coccygeal	Most of the tail and skin between anus and tailroot	Coccygeal muscle			
Caudal rectal (hemorrhoidal)		S-5	Anal region, tail folds, tail base	Coccygeus and levator ani externus muscle	Fibers in caudal rectal nerve		Straining in anorectal region due to excessive sympathetic stimulation
Middle rectal	Perineal nerve, caudal scrotal nerves, labial nerves	S-4, S-5	Perineum, posterior croup, scrotum along its caudal aspects, vulva without clitoris		Pelvic nerves, hypogastric plexus		Relaxation of bladder without sphincter, distal colon, rectum, sexual organs
Pudendal	Dorsal nerve of penis, deep perineal nerve	S-4, S-3, S-2	Penis (corpus cavernosum and spongiosum); clitoris and vulva	Perineal muscles fascia of schiorectal fossa, constrictor vulvae muscle		Retractor penis muscle	Prolapse of penis; relaxation of vulva and vagina
Caudal gluteal	Caudal cutaneous femoral nerve	S-2, S-1	Lateral and posterior surface of hip and thigh	Extension of hip			
Cranial gluteal		S-1, L-6, L-5	Lateral aspect of thigh	Flexor and abductors of hip		Splanchnic lumbar nerves (in part)	Relaxation of bladder and sphincter of bladder, distal colon, rectum, sexual organs
Sciatic		S-1, L-6, L-5	Middle to tibial region to foot	Flexor and abductors of hip; flexor of stifle (in part) and extensors of hock and digit			Ataxia, knuckling of hind fetlock

advanced approximate 12 cm in the vertebral canal (Fig. 8.17, *B*). Before injecting the local analgesic, the needle is withdrawn, leaving the catheter in position. The epidural catheter is partially withdrawn a calculated distance until a length of 9.5 cm remains inside the horse. This places the catheter tip approximately at the sacrococcygeal intervertebral space (15). A dose of 4 to 5 ml of 2% lidocaine hydrochloride solution is administered over a period of 1 minute.

In the alternative method, a 19.5-cm, 17-gauge Huber point needle is used to place a catheter with wire guide into the epidural space at the lumbosacral intervertebral junction and to catheterize the caudal portion of the sacral (S-3 to S-5) epidural space (51). The needle with stylet is inserted along the median plane at the lumbosacral intervertebral space perpendicular to the spinal cord and slowly advanced, with the bevel pointed caudad, until the epidural space is identified (Fig. 8.17, C).

Depth of needle penetration ranges from 11 to 14 cm in the adult horse. The catheter is threaded into the epidural space to a length ranging from 10 to 20 cm. After the Huber point needle and wire guide have been removed, a dose of 4 to 5 ml of 2% lidocaine hydrochloride solution is injected at a rate of approximately 1 ml/1 minute. Onset of analgesia is within 15 to 25 minutes and lasts 60 to 90 minutes.

Major advantages of the catheter technique when compared to the needle technique are that the catheter provides a route for deposition of local analgesic solution at the nerve roots of the pudendal and pelvic nerves and that minimal doses of analgesic drug are required and can be given as small fractional doses during surgical procedures while the tail is dorsally reflected for immobilization and surgical exposure. Disadvantages of the catheter technique include potential kinking and curling of the catheter and that radiographs of the catheter are mandatory if the position of the tubing must be known.

Continuous Caudal Subarachnoid Analgesia

The use of a 19.5-cm, 17-gauge directional Huber point needle and 30-cm catheter stylet unit makes it possible to catheterize the sacral subarachnoid space of horses from the lumbosacral intervertebral site (Fig. 8.16, *B*) (51). The lumbosacral interspace is located by palpation of bony landmarks as previously described (44). The needle with stylet is inserted into the midline of the lumbosacral depression perpendicular to the spinal cord or at a 10° angle with the needle tip directed caudad to place the bevel of the needle under the bony arch of the first sacral (S-1) vertebra. The needle is advanced until the subarachnoid space is identified by free flow of spinal flow from the needle hub or by aspiration. The catheter is threaded through the needle and gently advanced into the subarachnoid space to the midsacral region. The third sacral (S-3) space is the approximate end of the subarachnoid space. The catheter tip cannot be advanced beyond this point. The distance between the lumbosacral and caudal subarachnoid space in the horse ranges from 5 to 12 cm. After the needle and wire guide are removed, 1.5 ml of 2% lidocaine hydrochloride solution are injected into the catheter, using an injection rate of approximately 0.5 ml/min (3 minutes). All the roots of the caudal and the last three to four pairs of sacral (S_2–S_5) spinal nerves become desensitized within 10 minutes of injection. Analgesia lasts for 30 to 45 minutes and can be maintained by fractional bolus administration of 0.5 ml of 2% lidocaine hydrochloride solution at 30-minute intervals, or as needed.

Subarachnoid administration of lidocaine hydrochloride requires less drug for a similar degree of caudal analgesia and has a faster onset and a shorter duration than the epidural administration of drug (51). In addition, asymmetric or incomplete analgesia due to septa within the epidural space or inadequate dispersal of the analgesic as a result of escape of drug through patent intervertebral foramina are avoided. The roots of the spinal nerves within the subarachnoid space are not covered by protective dural sheets and are more easily desensitized. The relatively short duration of action reflects the small dose of analgesic drug and the inherent dilution effect of the spinal fluid (52). Technical difficulty, potential trauma to the conus medullaris and nerve fibers by the needle or catheter, and higher frequency of postanalgesic myositis limit the use of subarachnoid analgesia in general practice.

STANDING CASTRATION

Injection of local analgesic drug into the testis (53–55) or spermatic cord (56, 57) is the most commonly used procedure in general equine practice to provide local analgesia for castration in the standing position. Proper restraint of the horse's head and the assistance of a competent handler are required.

A 6.25-cm, 18-gauge needle is quickly inserted perpendicularly through the tensed skin of the scrotum and 20 to 30 ml of 2% lidocaine hydrochloride solution are injected into the center of the testis. The scrotal tissues along the incision site are infiltrated with 5 to 10 ml of the analgesic. These procedures are repeated to desensitize the opposite testis and scrotum. Although lidocaine diffuses quickly (within 90 seconds) (53) from the testis up to the spermatic cord via lymph vessels, 10 minutes are allowed for maximal effect.

For percutaneous analgesia of the spermatic cord, a 2.5-cm, 20-gauge needle is inserted to the cord as close to the external inguinal ring as possible. Twenty milliliters of local analgesia solution are injected with minimal manipulation of the needle to avoid skin puncture and perforation of the spermatic artery and vein. The incision site of the scrotal skin must also be injected.

THERAPEUTIC LOCAL ANALGESIA

Infiltration of sympathetic nerve fibers with local analgesic solution is effective for relief of vasoconstriction and pain. The two common sites, where the equine sympathetic nervous system is desensitized the most effectively, are the cervicothoracic (stellate) ganglion and the paralumbar sympathetic ganglia.

Cervicothoracic (Stellate) Ganglion Block

Blockade of the cervicothoracic ganglion (CTG) is effective in interrupting reflex spasm of the local vasculature and pain in the head, neck, and front leg; therefore, it is indicated and therapeutically recommended for a variety of skin, muscle, nerve, and joint and tendon sheath diseases of that area (58, 59). Acute disorders are responsive to a single blockade, whereas chronic conditions require repeated blockades for good results.

The cranial and paratracheal approach to the CTG is the simplest and safest (58–60). The skin puncture site is approximately 15 cm dorsal to the intermediate tubercle of the humerus in the jugular furrow distal to the jugular vein and carotid artery. This area is surgically scrubbed and infiltrated with 2 to 3 ml of 2% lidocaine hydrochloride solution. A 25-cm, 16-gauge needle is inserted through the desensitized skin and pushed horizontally or 5° dorsomedially until it impinges on the transverse process or body of the seventh cervical vertebra, and 2 to 3 ml of the analgesic are injected. The needle is withdrawn 5 to 10 cm (depending on the thickness and elasticity of the musculus longus colli), and the tip of the needle is redirected more lateral and ventral, thereby bypassing the seventh cervical vertebra and reaching the articulations of the first and second ribs (Fig. 8.18). The needle is then approximately 15 to 17 cm from the surface of the skin (60).

After aspirating to ensure that the needle tip has not entered the thoracic cavity or a vessel, approximately 50 ml of a lidocaine hydrochloride solution are injected. An additional 50 ml of lidocaine are injected during withdrawal of the needle for 6 to 10 cm.

CTG blockade results in increased skin temperature; profuse sweating of the head, particularly at the base of the ear, around the eye, and the rostral aspect of the face, neck, and thoracic limb; Horner's syndrome of ptosis, miosis, and enophthalmos; and laryngeal paresis. These signs are present 10 minutes after injection and last for more than 75 minutes.

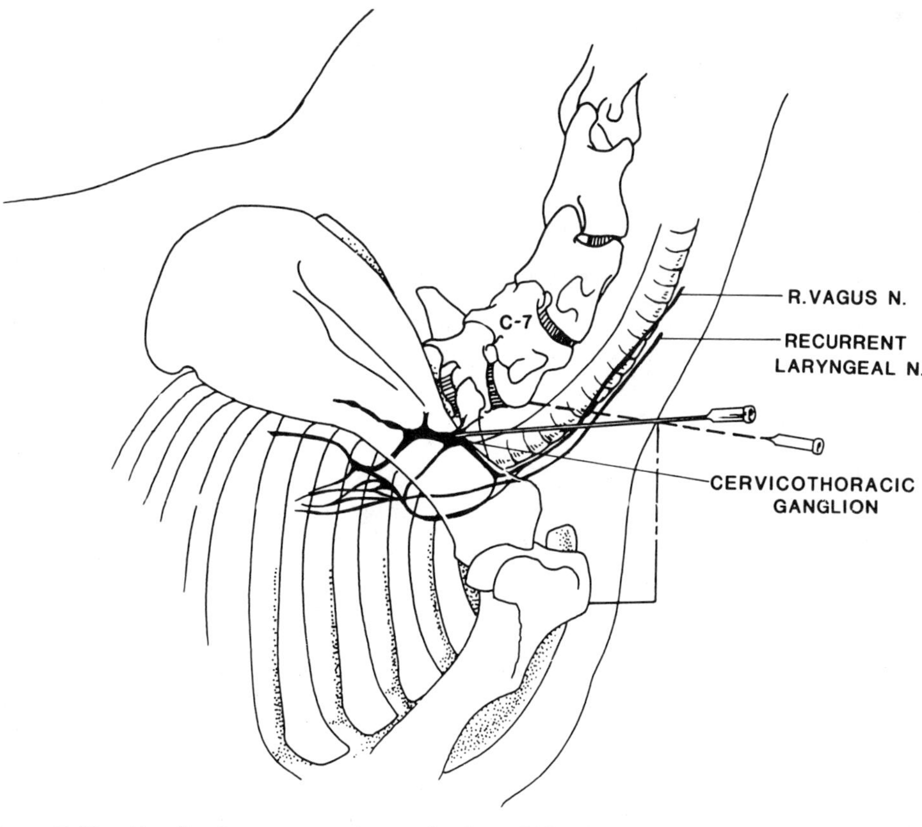

Figure 8.18. Needle placement to the cervicothoracic (stellate) ganglion (right side) in the horse.

Increased skin temperature is related to increased blood flow (vasodilation) to muscle vascular beds. The increase in skin temperature develops despite the cooling effect of profuse sweating. Factors responsible for sweating include increased blood supply and hence increased heat in the area, higher metabolism in the sweat glands, and central stimulation caused by excitement of the horse. Horner's syndrome is caused by interruption of the oculosympathetic pathway at the site of the CTG and/or at the site of the ventral sympathetic roots between the eighth cervical and second thoracic spinal nerves (60).

Transitory brachial plexus and recurrent laryngeal nerve paralysis are potential complications contraindicating bilateral CTG blockade in horses.

Paravertebral Lumbar Sympathetic Ganglion Block

Infiltration of the lumbar sympathetic trunk in horses with local analgesic solution is an effective treatment of myositis, periostitis, coxitis, and paralysis of the fibular and penile nerves (58, 59).

Although any of the interspaces between the first four lumbar vertebrae may be entered, the ideal puncture site is between the transverse processes of the second and third lumbar (L-2 and L-3) vertebrae about 10 cm lateral to their spinous processes (61). This area is aseptically prepared and infiltrated with 2 to 3 ml of 2% lidocaine hydrochloride solution. A 25-cm, 16-gauge needle is inserted through the desensitized skin and advanced until its tip contracts the transverse process of L-2 or L-3. A marker on the needle shaft is used to note the depth of penetration (Fig. 8.19, *A*). The needle is partially withdrawn and then reinserted to walk its tip off the transverse process. The angle between the needle and the vertical is noted after locating the intertransverse ligament (angle alpha). To reach the sympathetic trunk, the needle is withdrawn to the subcutaneous area and inserted at angle alpha and approximately 45° from vertical for the calculated distance, which equals the distance between the marker (skin puncture) and the needle point plus an additional 5 to 8 cm (Fig. 8.19, *B*). Aspiration ensures that neither a blood vessel nor the peritoneum has been punctured, and approximately 100 ml of a 1% lidocaine hydrochloride solution are slowly injected (61). Elevation of skin temperature and profuse sweating over the ipsilateral pelvic limb within 10 minutes are signs of adequate sympathetic blockade. Sensory and motor interruption does not result unless the lumbar somatic nerves have been desensitized. Danger of blood vessel puncture resulting in hematoma, intravascular injection, abdominocentesis, and needle breakage are potential complications.

Ruminants and Swine

Many surgical procedures are performed safely and humanely in ruminants using a combination of physical restraint, mild sedation or tranquilization, and local or regional analgesia. In addition, the standing position of ruminants is optimal for a number of sur-

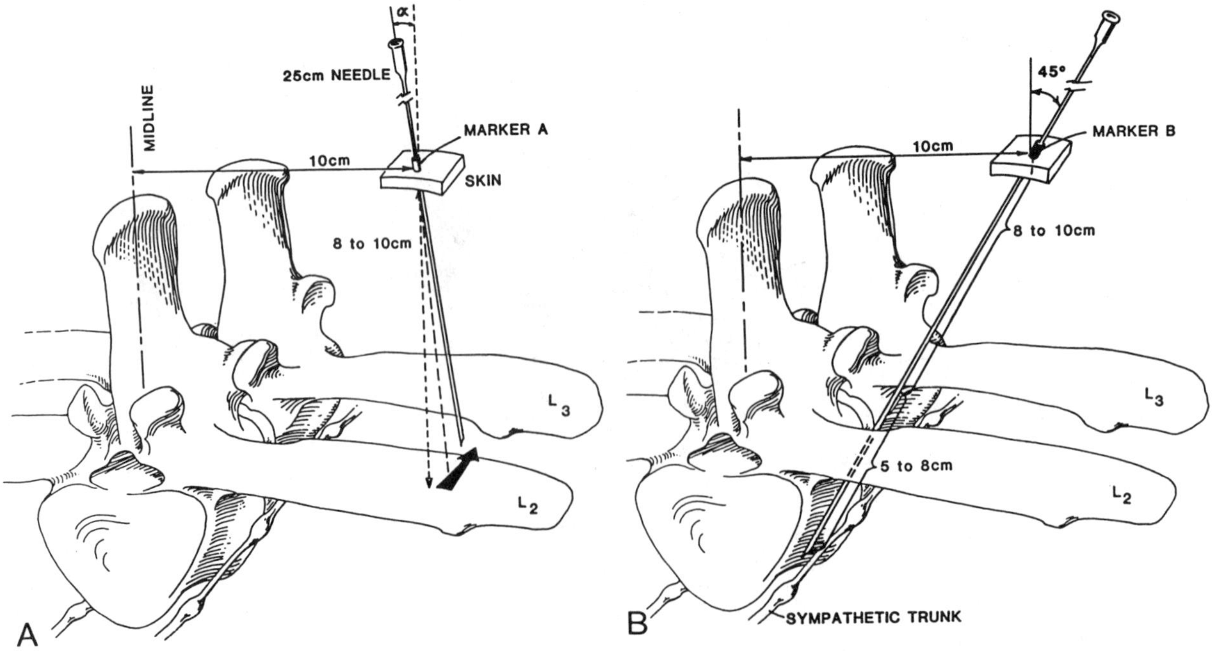

Figure 8.19. Needle placement to the lumbar sympathetic trunk in the horse. Needle tip at transverse process (*A*) and left ganglionic chain (*B*).

gical procedures, reducing the incidence of bloat, salivation, and recumbency-related regurgitation and nerve or muscle damage (62–65).

Local or regional analgesia can be induced by a variety of techniques, but the most commonly used techniques in ruminants include surface (topical) analgesia, infiltration analgesia, nerve block (conduction) analgesia, epidural analgesia, and intravenous regional analgesia. Although there is common use of local analgesics, none has presently been approved by the Food and Drug Administration (FDA) for use in lactating dairy cows. Used as an adjunct to chemical restraint, the most popular techniques are infiltration analgesia, intratesticular injection, and lumbosacral analgesia in swine.

ANALGESIA OF THE EYE AND RELAXATION OF THE GLOBE

Neuroanatomy

Sensory fibers of the ophthalmic division of the trigeminal nerve supply the globe, conjunctiva, nictitans, and most of the eyelids. The extraocular muscles are supplied by motor fibers of the trochlear nerve (superficial oblique muscle), the abducens nerve (lateralis rectus and retractor oculi muscles), and the oculomotorius nerve. Motor fibers of the auriculopalpebral nerve supply the eyelids.

Topical and regional analgesic techniques are used at present to facilitate surgery of the eye and its associated structures. One or two drops of proparacaine hydrochloride (0.5%) solution are instilled in the eye for topical analgesia. Severe epithelial reactions are caused by other ophthalmic analgesic solutions such as xylocaine hydrochloride (4%) or tetracaine hydrochloride. In 30 seconds and for as long as 10 to 15 minutes, pain associated with corneal disease is relieved (66). Particularly when blepharospasm due to superficial irritation of the cornea is relieved, examination of the eye or minor surgery is greatly facilitated. The FDA has approved proparacaine for use in food animals as an analgesic in cauterization of corneal ulcers, removal of foreign bodies and sutures from the cornea, and measurements of intraocular pressure (tonometry) when glaucoma is suspected. Topical analgesics should not be used for treatment of the eye; they are toxic to the corneal epithelium, suppressing mitosis and reducing protective blink reflexes (67).

Analgesia and Akinesia of the Eyelids

Approximately 10 ml of a 2% lidocaine hydrochloride solution are injected subcutaneously on a line about 0.5 cm from the margin of the dorsal and ventral eyelids in adult cattle. Using a 2.5-cm, 22-gauge needle, the analgesic is administered at multiple sites 0.5 cm apart (Fig. 8.20, *A*).

By selectively desensitizing the auriculopalpebral branch of the facial nerve (akinesia), paralysis of the eyelids without analgesia is readily accomplished (68). The nerve block is optimally performed in cattle by injecting 5 to 10 ml of a 2% lidocaine hydrochloride solution through a 2.5-cm, 18- or 20-gauge needle placed subcutaneously anterior to the base of the auricular muscles, where the nerve is sometimes palpable in a notch on the zygomatic arch (Fig. 8.20, *B*). The combination of topical analgesia and auriculopalpebral akinesia is useful for removing foreign bodies from the cornea and conjuncitval sac and for administering bulbar subconjunctival injections.

Analgesia for Enucleation

Either by retrobulbar injection (69) of an analgesic, the Peterson technique (70) or its modification (71), analgesia of the eye and orbit and immobilization of the globe are commonly achieved. When performing these techniques in adult cattle, standing body restraint and moderate sedations or tranquilization are necessary. The head is best secured with a halter or nose grip.

The common use of retrobulbar analgesia is for enucleation or to facilitate surgery and radiation therapy in cattle with squamous cell carcinoma of the cornea. In the presence of deep corneal ulceration and intraocular surgery, retrobulbar injection is contraindicated because of increased risk of vitreous prolapse. Either the upper and lower lids or the lateral and medial canthi are the sites of needle placement for

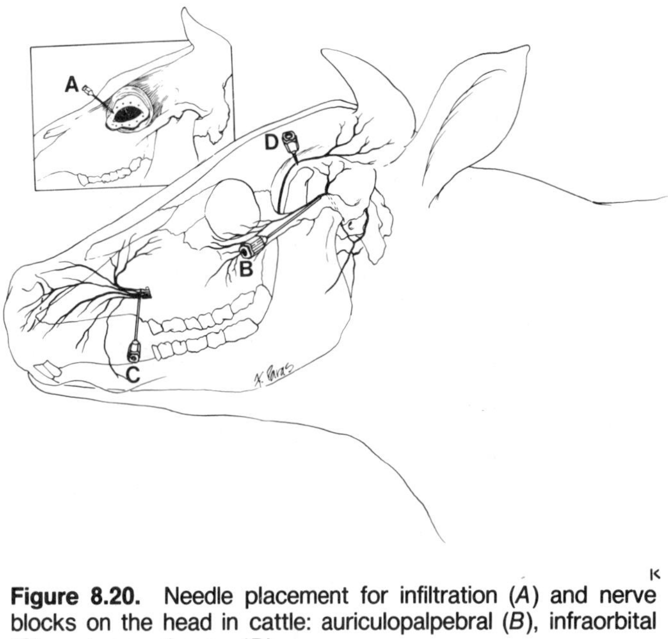

Figure 8.20. Needle placement for infiltration (*A*) and nerve blocks on the head in cattle: auriculopalpebral (*B*), infraorbital (*C*), and cornual nerve (*D*).

retrobulbar injection. In adult cattle, a 7.56- to 12-cm, 18-gauge needle is commonly used. A 3.75-cm, 22-gauge needle may be used in small ruminants. To deflect the globe and protect it from the needle point, the surgeon's index finger is used. When using the medial canthus approach, the needle is inserted in the fornix of the conjunctiva caudal to the nictitans and dorsomedial to the operator's finger (Fig. 8.21). As the needle is inserted in the orbital apex, the medial wall of the bony orbit is felt. In cattle, 10 to 15 ml of a 2% lidocaine hydrochloride solution or equivalent are injected in small increments as the needle is advanced,

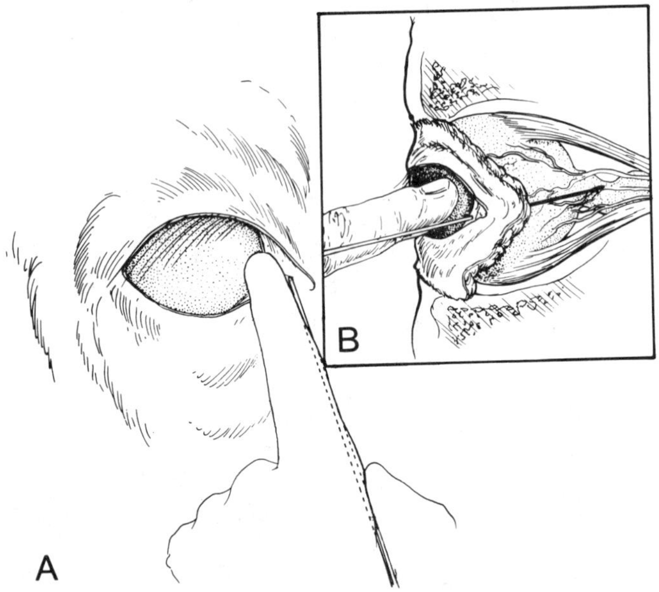

Figure 8.21. Retrobulbar needle placement through the medial canthus (*A*) to the orbital apex (*B*) in cattle.

thereby pushing initial structures from the needle point. The globe will proptose if the analgesic is properly placed within the muscular cone. Corneal analgesia, mydriasis, and proptosis indicate a satisfactory retrobulbar nerve block (72–78).

The notch formed by the supraorbital process cranially, the zygomatic arch ventrally, and the coronoid process of the mandible caudally constitute the site of needle placement for the Peterson eye block (70). Using a 2.5-cm, 22-gauge needle, approximately 5 ml of a 2% lidocaine hydrochloride solution are injected subcutaneously at this site. A 2.5-cm, 14-gauge needle serves as a cannula and is placed through the desensitized skin as far anterior and ventral as possible in the notch (Fig. 8.22). A 10- or 12-cm, 18-gauge straight or slightly curved needle is inserted into the cannula in a horizontal and slightly posterior direction until it strikes the coronoid process of the mandible. Then the needle is gently manipulated off the rostral border of the coronoid process and advanced to the pterygopalatine fossa rostral to the orbitorotundum foramen, which is at a depth of 7.5 to 10 cm. The concavity of a curved needle, if used, is kept caudal to facilitate passage of the needle rostral to the mandibular coronoid process. That the needle has not entered the ventral maxillary artery is ensured by aspiration on the syringe. About 7 to 15 ml of a 2% lidocaine hydrochloride solution are injected to desensitize the oculomotor, trochlear, and abducens nerves, and the three branches of the trigeminal nerve, the ophthalmic, maxillary, and mandibular at the emergence from the foramen orbitorotundum (79). The desensitized cutaneous area of the head, eyes, nose, and lips after ophthalmic, maxillary, and mandibular nerve blockade is shown in Fig. 8.23. It is

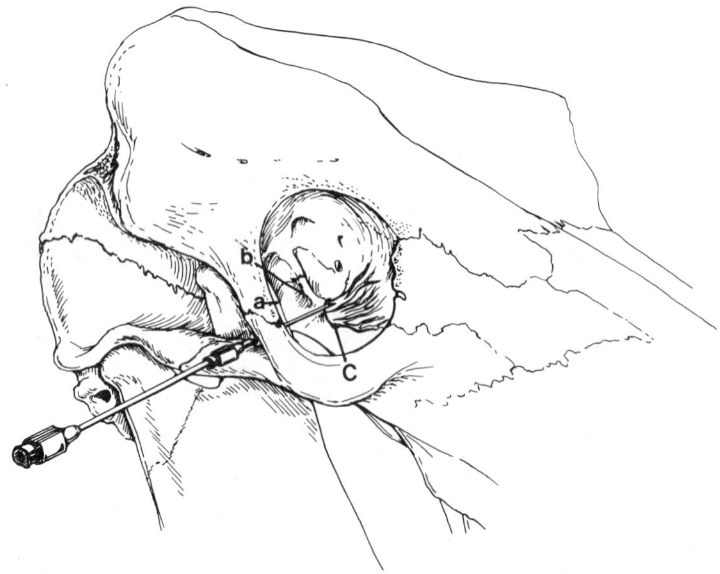

Figure 8.22. Needle placement for Peterson eye block. *a*, coronoid process; *b*, pterygoid crest; and *c*, foramen orbitorotundum.

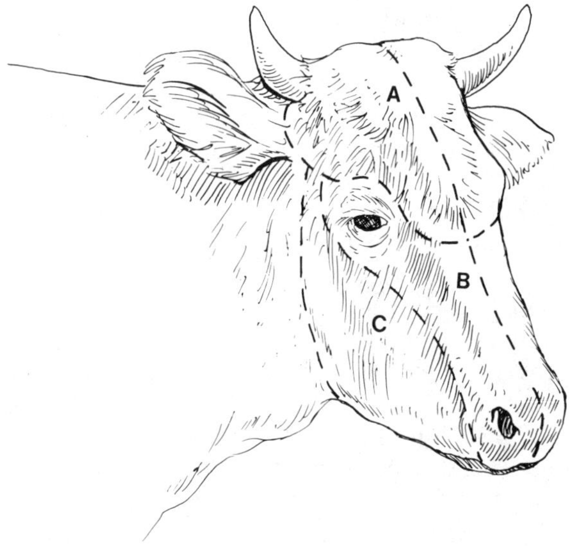

Figure 8.23. Cutaneous areas of the bovine head supplied by sensory fibers from the ophthalmic (*A*), maxillary (*B*), and mandibulary nerve(*C*).

necessary to avoid penetration of the turbinates and injection of local analgesic into the nasopharynx. The needle is withdrawn to the subcutaneous tissue and reinserted caudally and laterally to the zygomatic arch for a distance of approximately 7.5 cm to desensitize the auriculopalpebral nerve with an additional 5 to 10 ml of 2% lidocaine.

It is apparent when comparing the Peterson eye block and retrobulbar injection that the Peterson technique requires more skill to perform correctly but is safer. Adverse effects may result from retrobulbar injections for procedures other than enucleation. These effects may include orbital hemorrhage, direct pressure on the globe, penetration of the globe, damage to the optic nerve, and injection into the optic nerve meninges (72–74).

Both retrobulbar analgesia and Peterson's technique prevent blinking for several hours. If these techniques are used for procedures other than enucleation, sterile saline solution should be frequently applied to the eye during surgery to keep the cornea moist. After orbital replacement of the eye, antibiotic eye ointments should be applied to the cornea. To prevent keratoconjunctivitis, sunlight or wind on the eye must be avoided. Until motor activity of the lid returns, the eye is best medicated with a lubricating agent periodically. Alternatively, the lids may be sutured together.

NASAL ANALGESIA

For repair of nasal lacerations in cattle as well as inserting a nose ring dorsoventrally in a mature, ill-tempered bull, nasal analgesia is required (75). Before nasal analgesia is given, bulls must be restrained and, if unruly, tranquilized. A 3.75-cm, 18-gauge needle is used for perineural injection of the infraorbital nerve as its point of emergence from the infraorbital canal (Fig. 8.20, *C*). Difficult to palpate, the foramen is located rostral to the facial tuberosity on a line extending from the nasomaxillary notch to the second upper premolar. Approximately 20 to 30 ml of a 2% lidocaine hydrochloride solution are injected along this line rostral to the infraorbital foramen and superficial to the maxilla. On the opposite side the injection is repeated.

ANALGESIA OF THE HORN

Analgesic techniques for dehorning cattle (76–78) and goats (79, 80) and for disbudding young kids (81) have been described.

By desensitizing the cornual nerve, which is a branch of the zygomaticotemporal (lacrimal) portions of the ophthalmic division of the trigeminal nerve, analgesia of the horn and base of the horn in cattle is achieved. A 2.5-cm, 20-gauge needle is inserted through the skin approximately 2.5 cm anterior to the base of the horn and lateral to the palpable temporal ridge of the frontal bone. At this site and as the needle is inserted ventromedially close to the frontal bone, 5 to 10 ml of a 2% lidocaine hydrochloride solution are injected subcutaneously (Fig. 8.20, *D*). Needle penetration is from 1.0 cm in small cattle to 2.5 cm in large bulls. If the analgesic agent is placed too deeply in the aponeurosis of the temporal muscle, cornual analgesia will not result. A second injection may be required in adult cattle with well-developed horns posterior to the horn to desensitize the cutaneous branches of the second cervical nerve (82, 83). The Peterson eye block is advocated for analgesia of a fractured horn involving the frontal bone and sinuses (70).

The horns in goats are supplied by the cornual branch of the zygomaticotemporal (lacrimal) and infratrochlear nerves (80, 83). These nerves are best infiltrated with approximately 2.0 to 3.0 ml of a 2% lidocaine hydrochloride solution in the adult goat halfway between the lateral canthus of the eye and the lateral base of the horn (cornual branch of the zygomaticotemporal nerve) and halfway between the medial canthus of the eye and medial base of the horn (cornual branch of the infratrochlear nerve). In order to reach the cornual branch of the zygomaticotemporal nerve, a 2.4-cm, 22-gauge needle is inserted as close as possible to the caudal ridge of the base of the supraorbital process and 1.0- to 1.5-cm deep (Fig. 8.24, *A*). The needle is inserted dorsal and parallel to the dorsomedial margin of the orbit in order to reach the cornual branch of infratrochlear nerve. The analgesic is placed in a line as this nerve is frequently branched (Fig. 8.24, *B*). If the frontal sinus will be entered during horn removal, sedation of the animal is required because these blocks will not desensitize the sinus mucosa and

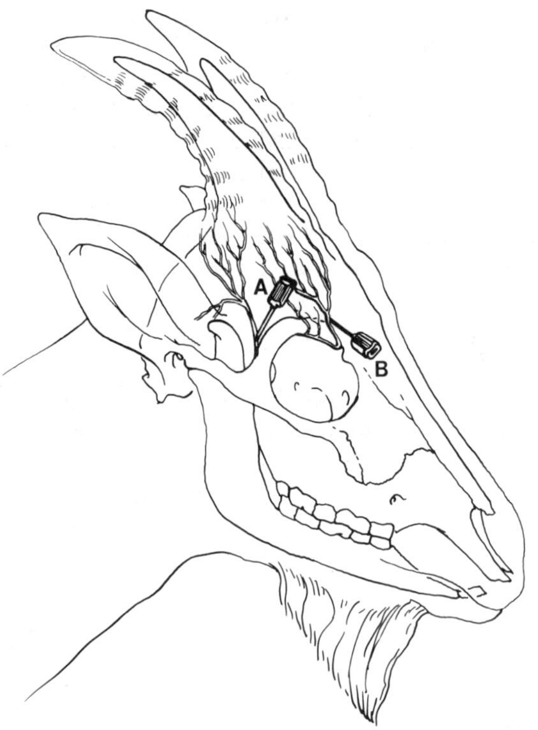

Figure 8.24. Needle placement for desensitizing the cornual branches of the zygomaticotemporal (*A*) and infratrochlear nerve (*B*) in the goat.

periosteum. During disbudding of young kids between 7 and 14 days of age, to alleviate pain a ring block at the horn base is made by injecting no more than 0.5 ml of a 2% lidocaine hydrochloride solution. To minimize adverse reactions, a total dose of 10 mg/kg (0.5 ml of 2% solution/kg) lidocaine must not be exceeded. Apparent signs of toxicity due to overdose include excitation, lateral recumbency, generalized tonic-clonic convulsions, and opisthotonus. Respiratory depression and cardiac arrest can occur after high doses of lidocaine.

ANALGESIA FOR LAPAROTOMY

Introduction to Techniques

At least five techniques for obtaining analgesia of the paralumbar fossa in ruminants have been described, including infiltration analgesia, proximal paravertebral analgesia, distal paravertebral analgesia, segmental dorsolumbar epidural analgesia, and thoracolumbar subarachnoid analgesia. These techniques are used for procedures that include most abdominal surgeries, such as rumenotomy, cecotomy, correction of gastrointestinal displacement, intestinal obstruction and volvulus, Caesarean section, ovariectomy, liver or kidney biopsy, and others (84, 85).

Infiltration Analgesia

The easiest and probably the most commonly used technique in food animal practice is simple infiltration of the incision line (line block). A 2.5-cm, 20-gauge needle, or smaller, is used for multiple subcutaneous injections of 0.5 to 1.0 ml of a 2% lidocaine hydrochloride solution, 1.0 to 2.0 cm apart. If the needle enters the edge of the desensitized skin at an angle of approximately 20° to the horizontal and injection is made slowly and continuously, pain is not felt upon successive injections (Fig. 8.25). A 7.5-cm, 18-gauge needle is inserted through the desensitized skin and used for infiltrating the muscle layers and parietal peritoneum. Depending upon the species and the size of the area to be desensitized, 10 to 100 ml of a 2% lidocaine hydrochloride solution are injected. Whereas in adult goats 10 ml of a 2% lidocaine hydrochloride solution should not be exceeded, adult cattle will safely tolerate 250 ml of a 2% lidocaine hydrochloride solution for the line block. About 10 to 15 minutes are allowed for analgesia to take effect. Diluting a 2% lidocaine solution with equal parts of sterile saline to make a 1% solution is commonly practiced. A 1% solution of lidocaine can also be used cautiously in goats. It has been reported that fetal and newborn lambs are no more sensitive to lidocaine toxicity than are adult sheep (86). It remains advisable to limit dosage in young sheep as in young goats to avoid complications.

Inverted "7" or "L" Block

Basically the inverted "7" or "L" block is a nonspecific regional analgesic technique in which all the nerves entering the surgical field are desensitized. The creation of a wall of analgesia enclosing the incision site occurs when up to 100 ml of a 2% lidocaine

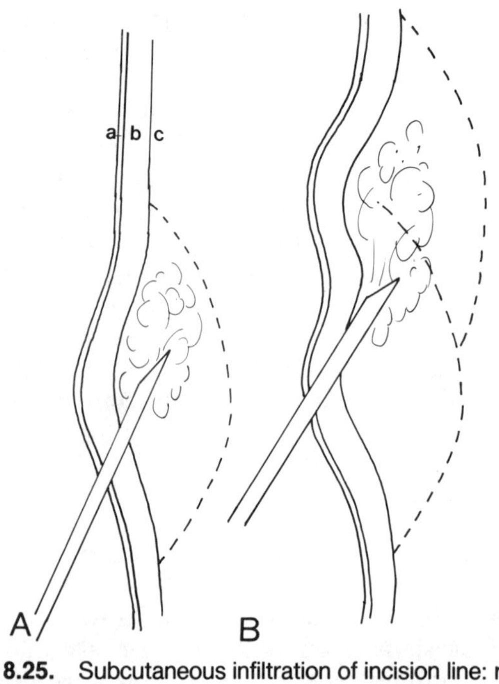

Figure 8.25. Subcutaneous infiltration of incision line: raising a subcutaneous wheal (*A*) and insertion of needle into edge of the wheal (*B*).

hydrochloride solution in cattle are injected into the tissues bordering the dorsocaudal aspect of the last rib and ventrolateral aspect of the lumbar transverse processes (Fig. 8.26). About 10 to 15 minutes are required for the analgesic to take effect.

Compared to the line block, the advantage of the inverted "7" or "L" block is deposition of the analgesic away from the incision site, thus minimizing edema, hematoma, and possible interference with healing. The disadvantages of local infiltration analgesia include incomplete analgesia and muscle relaxation of the deeper layers of the abdominal wall, toxicity after injecting significant amounts of analgesic solution into the peritoneal cavity, and increased cost due to larger doses of analgesics and longer time required.

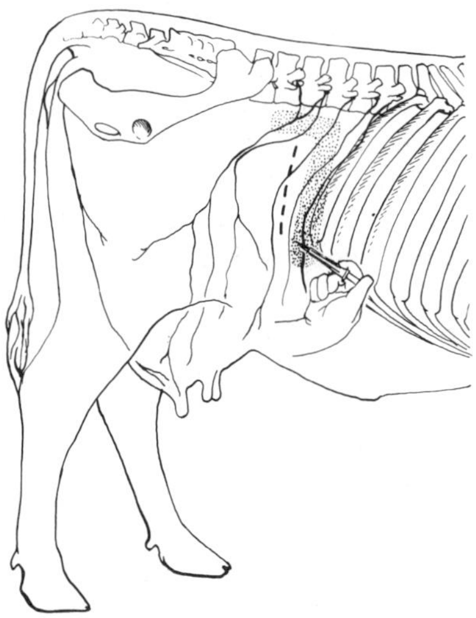

Figure 8.26. Regional analgesia of the bovine flank using inverted "L" infiltration pattern.

Proximal Paravertebral Analgesia

As the dorsal and ventral nerve roots of the last thoracic (T13) and 1lst and 2nd lumbar (L1 and L2) spinal nerves emerge from the intervertebral foramina in this technique, they are desensitized (Fig. 8.27). The technique is also called the Farquharson (87), Hall, or Cambridge technique (88). In addition, if analgesia of the caudal-most part of the paralumbar fossa or ipsilateral fore-teat and mammary gland is desired, the third and fourth lumbar (L3 and L4) spinal nerves are desensitized (89). However, the L3 and L4 blocks result in weakness of the pelvic limb and may cause the animal to lie or fall down. The caudal aspect of the transverse processes of the last thoracic (T-13) and first and second lumbar (L-1 and L-2) vertebrae is the site for needle placement. The skin overlying the spinal column on the side to be desensitized is clipped, surgically scrubbed, and disinfected.

In cattle, the skin at the cranial edges of the transverse processes of L-1, L-2, and L-3 and at a point 2.5 to 5 cm off the dorsal midline is desensitized by injecting 2 to 3 ml of a 2% lidocaine hydrochloride solution using a 2.5-cm, 18-gauge needle. If the T-13 and L-1 transverse processes cannot be palpated, the distance between the more prominent transverse processes of L-2 and L-3 is measured, and the same distance used cranial to L-2 and L-1 to find the sites for desensitizing the nerves L1 and T13, respectively. If using the cranial aspect of the transverse process of L-2, respectively, you will actually be on a line passing through the L-1–L-2 intervertebral foramen and posterior edge of spinous process L-1. To serve as a cannula, a 1.25 cm, 14-gauge needle is used, thus minimizing skin resistance during insertion of a 4.25- to 15-cm, 18-gauge spinal needle.

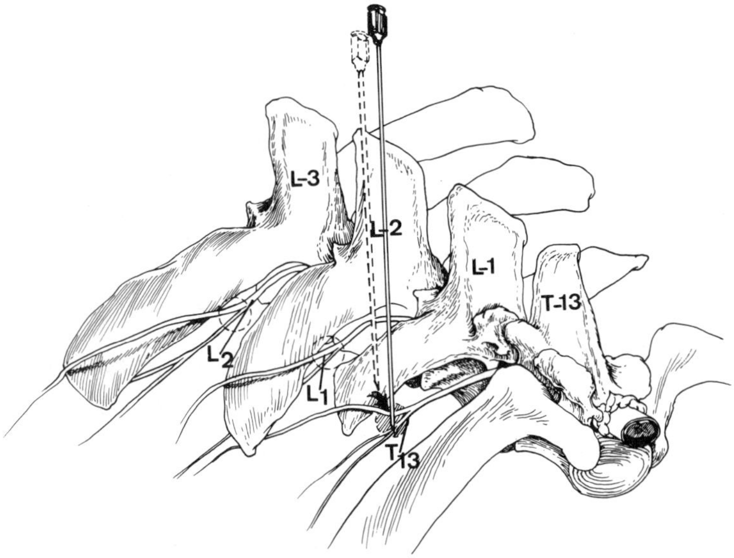

Figure 8.27. Needle placement of proximal paravertebral nerve block in cattle.

The needle is passed ventrally to desensitize T13, until it contacts the transverse process of L-1. The needle point is then walked off the cranial edge of the transverse process and advanced approximately 1.0 cm to pass through the intertransverse fascia. Five to 10 ml of a 2% lidocaine hydrochloride solution are injected with little resistance to desensitize the ventral branch of T13. The needle is withdrawn 1.0 to 2.5 cm to above the fascia and dorsal surface of the transverse process. An additional 5 ml of the analgesic is injected with slight resistance to desensitize the dorsal branch of the nerve.

The needle is inserted just caudal to the transverse processes of L-1 and L-2 to desensitize L1 and L2, and its tip is walked off the caudal edges of the transverse processes to a depth comparable to the previous injection site. L1 and L2 are desensitized similarly to T13.

For sheep and goats, T13, L1, and L2 are desensitized as with cattle, but 2.5 to 3.0 cm off the midline. Using a 5- to 7.5-cm, 18- or 20-gauge needle, approximately 3 ml of a 2% lidocaine hydrochloride solution are injected at each site.

Signs of successful nerve blockade include analgesia of the skin, scoliosis toward the desensitized side due to paralysis of paravertebral muscles, and increased skin temperature due to increased blood flow after paralysis of cutaneous vasomotor nerves. Usually present within 10 minutes after injection, analgesia lasts approximately 90 minutes.

When compared to infiltration analgesia, proximal paravertebra analgesia offers the advantages of small doses of analgesic, a wide and uniform area of analgesia and muscle relaxation, minimal intra-abdominal pressure, increased intestinal tone and motility due to desensitization of sympathetic fibers of rami communicates, and absence of local analgesic from the operative wound margins. The disadvantages of this technique include technical difficulty, arching up of the spine due to paralysis of the back muscles, risk of penetrating vital structures such as the aorta and thoracic longitudinal vein on the left side and the caudal vena cava on the right side, and caudal migration of injection site to femoral nerves with subsequent paresis.

Distal Paravertebral Analgesia (Magda, Cakala, or Cornell Technique)

In this technique (90), the dorsal and ventral rami of the spinal nerves T13, L1, and L2 are desensitized at the distal ends of L-1, L-2, and L-4 (Fig. 8.28).

A 7.5-cm, 18-gauge needle is inserted ventral to the tips of the respective transverse processes in large ruminants where approximately 10 to 20 ml of a 2% lidocaine hydrochloride solution are injected in a fan-shaped infiltration pattern. The needle is completely withdrawn and reinserted dorsal to the transverse process, in a slightly caudal direction, where the cutaneous branch of the dorsal rami is injected with approximately 5 ml of the analgesic. The procedure is repeated for the second and fourth lumbar transverse processes.

When compared to proximal paravertebral analgesia, the advantages of distal paravertebral analgesia include the use of more routine size needles, no risk of penetrating a major blood vessel, lack of scoliosis minimal weakness in the pelvic limb, and minimal ataxia. On the other hand, the disadvantages of the technique are that larger doses of anesthetic are needed and variations in efficiency exist, particularly if the nerves vary in their anatomical pathway.

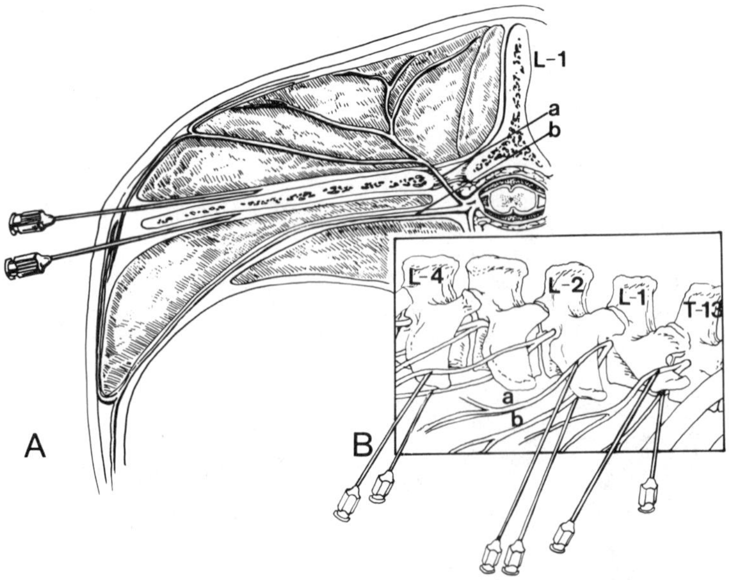

Figure 8.28. Needle placement for distal paravertebral nerve block in cattle to block dorsal (*A*) and ventral (*B*) rami of the spinal nerves.

Segmental Dorsolumbar Epidural Analgesia (Arthur Block)

In this technique (91), local analgesic is injected into the epidural space either between the first and second lumbar (L-1 and L-2) vertebrae or less commonly between the last thoracic (T-13) and first lumbar (L-1) vertebrae to desensitize the nerve roots as they emerge from the dura covering the spinal cord (Fig. 8.29).

During the procedure cattle must be thoroughly restrained. The skin area caudal to the T-13 or L-1 spinous process and contralateral to the flank region to be desensitized is aseptically prepared, and 2.0 to 4.0 ml of local analgesic are injected subcutaneously. Preferably, a 1.25-cm, 14-gauge needle to serve as a cannula for a 11.25-cm, 18-gauge spinal needle is inserted at this site. To reach the epidural space, the spinal needle is inserted for a distance of 8 to 11 cm while being directed ventrally and medially at an angle of 10 to 15° to vertical. Slight resistance during the insertion process is encountered at the interspinous and interarcuate ligaments. If the needle point impinges against the bony arches of T-13 and L-1 or L-1 and L-2, withdrawal and redirection of the needle are necessary. If there is no blood or CSF upon needle aspiration and if no resistance to the injection of air or local analgesic results, the needle can be said to be correctly placed. After piercing through the interarcuate ligament, the needle must not be inserted further and should be removed immediately after injection in order to avoid damage to the spinal cord and meninges. The analgesic dosage will depend upon the size of the cow and the number of nerve roots to be desensitized. Approximately 8 ml of either a 2% lidocaine hydrochloride solution or 5% procaine hydrochloride solution is sufficient to desensitize T13, L1, and L2 in an average 500-kg cow. Analgesia of the entire flank region results 7 to 20 min after injection and lasts for 45 to 120 minutes. By placing the needle tip within the epidural space either across the midline or in the median plane dorsal to the spinal cord, thus injecting the analgesic to the nerve roots on one or both sides, respectively, selective analgesia on one or both sides of the spinal column is achieved (92). The bevel of the spinal needle is directed caudally for limiting the cranial flow of the analgesic.

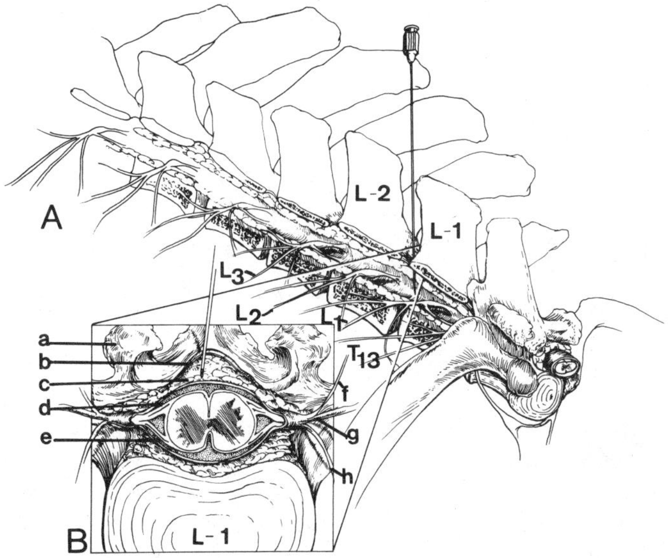

Figure 8.29. *A*, cranial and right lateral aspect of the thoracolumbar vertebra and their associated spinal nerves T-13 to L-3 with needle tip placed at the L-1–L-2 intervertebral space. *B*, cranial view of a transection of the first lumbar vertebra at the location of the intervertebral foramen, showing the relation of the structures inside the spinal canal. *a*, articular process; *b*, interarcuate ligament; *c*, epidural space with fat and connective tissue; *d*, dura mater; *e*, arachnoid membrane; *f*, dorsal branch of L1 vertebral nerve; *g*, ventral branch of L1 vertebral nerve; and *h*, ramus communicans.

When compared to proximal and distal paravertebral analgesia, the advantages of segmental dorsolumbar epidural analgesia are the use of only one injection of a small quantity of analgesic and uniform analgesia and relaxation of the skin, musculature, and peritoneum. The disadvantages of segmental epidural analgesia include difficulty in performing the technique, loss of motor control of the pelvic limbs, and physiological disturbance due to overdose or subarachnoid injection; also, there is potential for trauma to the spinal cord or venous sinuses (93, 94).

Thoracolumbar Subarachnoid Analgesia

Although thoracolumbar subarachnoid analgesia produces the fastest and best controlled surgical analgesia in cattle, special equipment and maintenance of sterility are required (95). A 17.5-cm, 17-gauge Huber point Tuohy needle with stylet and with the bevel directed craniad is inserted aseptically into the subarachnoid space at the lumbosacral (L-6–S-1) intervertebral space (Fig. 8.30). To help minimize pain during the puncture procedure, the skin and thoracolumbar fascia adjacent to the interspinous (L-6–S-1) ligaments are injected with 4.0 to 6.0 ml of a 2% lidocaine hydrochloride solution. After the needle has entered the subarachnoid space, the stylet is removed and 2 to 3 ml of CSF are aspirated. Passed through the needle and advanced approximately 60 cm to the midthoracic area is a Formocath polyethylene catheter 80 to 100 cm long with 0.95 mm OD reinforced with a stainless steel spring guide (0.52 mm OD). First the needle is withdrawn over the catheter, then the spring guide is removed, and a 23-gauge needle and three-way stopcock are attached to the catheter, which is withdrawn a calculated distance to place its tip at T-13–L-1. After removal of 1.0 to 2.0 ml of CSF, 1.5 to 2.0 ml of either a 2% lidocaine hydrochloride solution or 5% procaine hydrochloride solution are injected at a rate of approx-

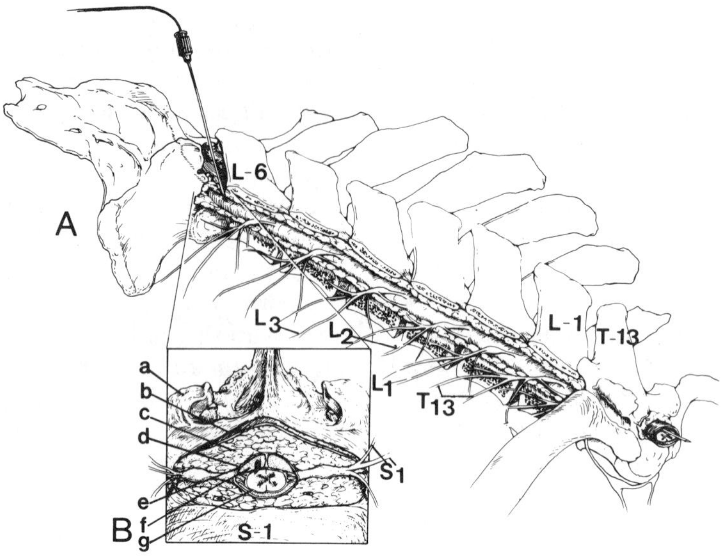

Figure 8.30. *A*, cranial and right lateral aspect of the bovine thoracolumbar and sacral vertebrae and their associated spinal nerves T13 to L3 with needle tip placed at the lumbosacral intervertebral space. *B*, cranial view of a transection of the first sacral vertebra at the location of the intervertebral foramen, showing the relation of the structures inside the spinal canal. *a*, articular process; *b*, interarcuate ligament; *c*, epidural space with fat and connective tissue; *d*, dura mater; *e*, arachnoid membrane; *f*, subarachnoid space with cerebral spinal fluid and needle tip; and *g*, pia mater.

imately 0.5 ml/min. CSF is used to remove the remaining local analgesic from the catheter. Extending from spinal cord segment T-9 to L-3, unilateral or bilateral analgesia is maximal 6 to 10 minutes after injection and lasts for 20 to 80 minutes (95). Surgical analgesia is easily maintained by fractional bolus administration of 0.5 ml of the analgesic at 30-minute intervals or as needed. The duration of analgesia is determined by the decline of the subarachnoid procaine concentration due to absorption of drug into the systemic circulation and not to hydrolysis in CSF (96).

When compared to dorsolumbar epidural analgesia, the advantages of thoracolumbar subarachnoid analgesia include simplicity of needle and catheter placements, minimal dosage, analgesic deposition at nerve roots, rapid onset of analgesia, minimal physiological disturbance, and also that small doses of analgesic can be given for maintenance. Disadvantages of the catheter technique include kinking and curling of the catheter, trauma to the conus medullaris, accidental vascular puncture, precise dosage, and also that catheter positioning may require radiography for confirmation (93, 95–98).

ANALGESIA FOR OBSTETRICAL PROCEDURES AND RELIEF OF RECTAL TENESMUS

Introduction to Techniques

Caudal epidural analgesia, continuous caudal epidural analgesia, sacral paravertebral analgesia, and desensitization of the internal pudendal nerve are techniques commonly used in ruminants to facilitate obstetrical manipulations and surgical procedures involving the tail, perineum, anus, rectum, vulva, prepuce, and skin of the scrotum. Additionally, the techniques are advocated as an adjunct treatment for control of rectal tenesmus associated with irritation of the perineum, anus, rectum, and vagina. The techniques are not effective in pigs.

Caudal Epidural Analgesia

Because this technique is simple, inexpensive, and requires no sophisticated equipment, it is routinely used in the cow, sheep, and goat. A small volume of local analgesic is injected into the epidural space of the spinal canal at either the sacrococcygeal (S-5–C_o-1) space or first intercoccygeal (C_o-1–C_o-2) space. The location is found by elevating and lowering the tail and palpating the depression and movement between the respective vertebrae. The S-5–C-1 interspace has ossified, and thus C_o-1–C_o-2 is the site for needle placement in older cows (99). Success in producing regional analgesia of pelvic viscera and genitalia without losing locomotor functions of the hindlegs will depend upon the cranial flow of local analgesic to desensitize the caudal and last three pairs of sacral nerves in the epidural space as they emerge from the meninges.

A 3.75- to 5-cm, 18-gauge needle is inserted in cattle through the disinfected skin in the center of the C_o-1–C_o-2 joint space, while directing the needle at an almost right angle to the general contour of the croup or ventrocranially at an angle of approximately 10° to vertical. Until it contacts the floor of the vertebral canal, the needle is inserted in a median plane. It is then withdrawn for approximately 0.5 cm to avoid injection into the intervertebral disc or ligamentous floor of the canal (Fig. 8.31). A drop of analgesic at the hub is aspirated into the needle space when the epidural space is reached. Approximately 1.0 ml of a 2% lidocaine hydrochloride solution or equivalent per 100 kg of body weight is injected with minimal resistance. If properly dosed, the area of analgesia extends cranially to the middle of the sacrum and ventrally over the perineum to the inner aspect of the thigh. Then the tail is paralyzed, and the abdominal contractions that exert pressure on the perineal structures are abolished. Uterine motility remains unaffected. Maximal analgesia may require 5 to 20 minutes and can be expected to last 30 to 150 minutes. If epinephrine 1:80,000 (0.125 mg epinephrine per 1 ml) is added to the lidocaine hydrochloride solution, the tone and mobility of the tail can be suppressed for more than 20 minutes (100). If the needle is left in situ, additional amounts of analgesic can be administered simply but should be regulated to keep the cow standing.

The technique for producing caudal epidural analgesia in sheep and goats is similar to that used in

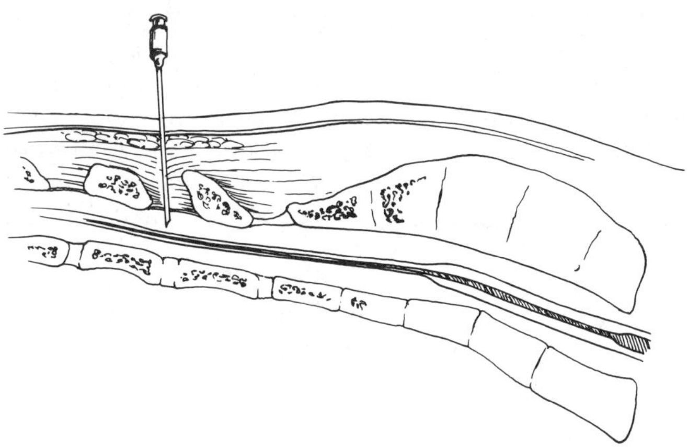

Figure 8.31. Needle placement for caudal epidural analgesia in cattle.

cattle. A 2.5- to 3.75-cm, 18- or 20-gauge needle is inserted epidurally at S-5–C_o-1 or C_o-1–C_o-2 (Fig. 8.32, *A* and *B*). After injecting 0.5 to 1.0 ml of a 2% lidocaine hydrochloride solution per 50 kg of body weight, analgesia of 2 hours' duration without ataxia can be expected (101, 102).

Complications due to caudal epidural analgesia are rare and are usually related to infection rather than trauma to nerves. Infection can result in draining tracts or a permanently immobile tail; however, it can easily be prevented by close adherence to aseptic technique. Trauma to the spinal cord and meninges is nearly impossible because these structures end craniad to the site of injection. Not easily damaged, only the coccygeal nerves and the thin phylum terminale remain in the spinal canal at the site of needle penetration (103).

Continuous Caudal Epidural Analgesia

This technique is used in cattle and sheep with chronic rectal and vaginal prolapse to prevent continuous straining. Continuous caudal epidural analgesia in cattle can be simply achieved after placing a catheter into the epidural space (Fig. 8.33) (104, 105). A 7.5-cm, 16- or 17-gauge thin wall Huber point directional needle or Hustead needle (Monoject-Sherwood, St. Louis, Missouri) is inserted into the epidural space at S-5–C_o-1 or C_o-1–C_o-2. If the puncture procedure is preceded by a subcutaneous wheal made with 2 to 3 ml of a 2% lidocaine hydrochloride solution, pain during insertion is minimal. A stab incision through the anesthetized skin on the midline minimizes resistance to the passage of the somewhat blunt needle. Once through the skin, the needle with stylet in place and bevel directed craniad is directed at approximately 20° to vertical and is advanced until an abrupt reduction in resistance to needle passage is noted, indicating entry into the vertebral canal. The stylet is then removed from the needle. If a test dose of 2 to 3 ml of analgesic is injected without resistance, proper position

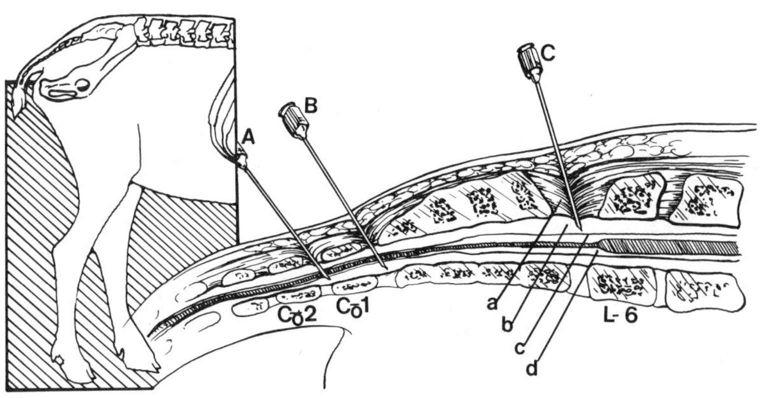

Figure 8.32. Needle placement for caudal epidural analgesia (*A* and *B*) and anterior epidural analgesia (*C*) in the goat. *L-6*, sixth lumbar; *Co1*, first coccygeal; *Co2*, second coccygeal vertebra; *a*, interarcuate ligament; *b*, epidural space; *c*, subarachnoid space; *d*, spinal cord.

of the needle into the vertebral canal is ascertained. A 30-cm long medical grade vinyl tubing (0.036 cm OD) or a commercially available epidural catheter with graduated markings is introduced into the needle and advanced cranially 2.5 to 4 cm beyond the tip of the needle. While the catheter is left in position, the needle is removed from the catheter. A 23-gauge needle and three-way stopcock or catheter adapter are placed on the free end of the catheter. The catheter at the entrance into the skin is secured with adhesive tape that is sutured to the skin. Approximately 5 ml of a 2% lidocaine hydrochloride solution is injected into the catheter at 4- to 6-hour intervals or as needed to abolish straining.

The catheter technique is practical and readily applicable to use in the field. Optimal timing and amounts of repeated analgesic doses, development of tachyphylaxis (acute tolerance to repeated injections), and augmented responses and long-term effects of repeated caudal epidural analgesia have not been reported.

Long-term caudal epidural analgesia can be produced in sheep and goats by using a mixture of equal volumes of 70–95% ethyl or isopropyl alcohol and 2% lidocaine hydrochloride solution as the epidural analgesic. Except that the volume of the alcohol-analgesic mixture must first be determined by a prior epidural injection using only lidocaine (Fig. 8.32, *A*), the technique is similar to the one used for caudal epidural analgesia. Because alcohol causes demyelinization of nerve roots (106), analgesia and paralysis of the tail may last from a few days to 6 months or longer, depending upon the time needed to remyelinate the nerves. The prolonged flaccidity of the tail is of little consequence in sheep with docked tails; however, in cattle the buildup of manure and urine in the perianal area may lead to dermal excoriation and maggot infestation, making alcohol epidural analgesia impracticable.

In sheep and goats, alcohol epidural analgesia is a simple and easy technique to use. Complications may occur. The chronically flaccid tail may become inflamed, necrotic, or purulent. The dosage of alcohol is critical to avoid involving the sciatic nerve roots, resulting in a chronically paralysed animal.

Sacral Paravertebral Analgesia

To induce sacral paravertebral analgesia in female cattle, the third, fourth, and fifth sacral (S3, S4, and S5) spinal nerves are desensitized at the emergence from the sacrum on both sides of the spine (107). In males, S3 supplies motor fibers to the retractor penis muscle and must not be desensitized. The skin of the dorsal sacral area is cleansed and disinfected with the animal in standing restraint. The dorsal sacral foramina S-3, S-4, and S-5 are identified approximately 1.0 to 1.5 cm from the dorsal midline of the vertebral crests. Nerve S5 is at the sacrococcygeal (S-5–C_o-1) junction. Nerves S4 and S3 exit from the S-4 and S-3 foramina, 3 cm and 6 cm cranial to the S-5 foramen in the young adult. A 6.25- to 7.5-cm, 16- or 18-gauge needle, preferably with stylet, is inserted to a depth just beyond where it enters the foramen (Fig. 8.34). Approximately 5 to 10 ml of a 2% lidocaine hydrochloride solution are injected into a 1.0-cm diameter area within each dorsal foramen to desensitize the dorsal and ventral rami of that nerve. Within 10 minutes, analgesia of the anus vulva, and vagina can be expected; it will last for approximately 2 hours. Motor function of the anal sphincter is reduced. Motor function of the tail is maintained. The sphincter of the urinary bladder remains tonic. Sensation to the clitoris is unaffected.

For long-term relief (up to 5 weeks) of rectal te-

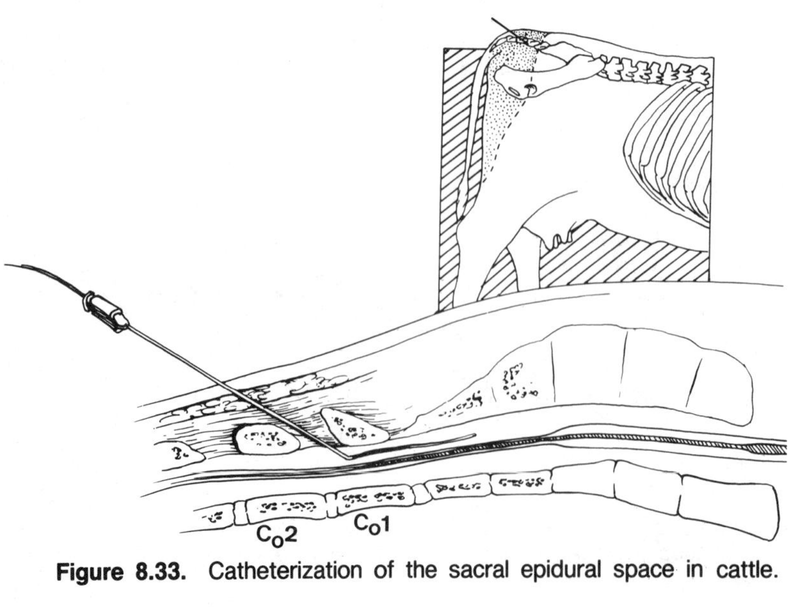

Figure 8.33. Catheterization of the sacral epidural space in cattle.

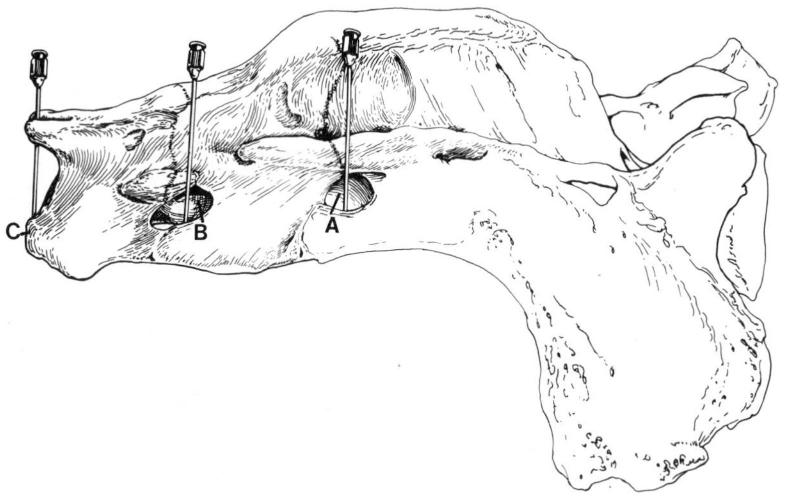

Figure 8.34. Needle placement for sacral paravertebral analgesia in cattle. Third (*A*), fourth (*B*), and fifth (*C*) sacral foramen.

nesmus, 1 to 2 ml of 70 to 95% ethyl or isopropyl alcohol is injected to S3, S4, and S5 without the unfavorable sequelae associated with alcohol epidural analgesia (107). Caudal epidural analgesia with 2% lidocaine greatly facilitates the alcohol paravertebral technique.

By using a 7.5-cm, 18-gauge needle with either lidocaine or lidocaine and alcohol, bilateral sacral (S3, S4, and S5) paravertebral analgesia in sheep is produced similar to that used in cattle.

The advantages of sacral paravertebral analgesia when compared to epidural analgesia are the relief of straining without sciatic nerve dysfunction, thus minimizing the risk of the animal lying down, and maintenance of tail function. The disadvantages are the difficulty of the technique and paraphimosis in bulls if S3 is chronically desensitized with alcohol.

Desensitization of the Internal Pudendal Nerve

This technique is used either in the female (108) for relief of straining due to uterine prolapse or chronic vaginal prolapse or in the male (109) for penile analgesia and relaxation. With cattle restrained in a standing position, the lesser sciatic foramen is located by rectal palpation as a soft circumscribed depression in the sacrosciatic ligament. The internal pudendal nerve is found a finger's width dorsal to the pulsating pudendal artery present in the fossa. The skin over the ischiorectal fossae on both sides is disinfected and desensitized with 2 to 3 ml of a 2% lidocaine hydrochloride solution. A 1.25-cm, 14-gauge needle is inserted at these sites to serve as a cannula for an 8.25-cm, 18-gauge spinal needle. The needle is passed through the cannula for a distance of approximately 5 cm or until it contacts the internal pudendal nerve (Fig. 8.35). After making sure that the needle is medial to the sacrosciatic ligament, 20 to 25 ml of a 2% lidocaine hydrochloride solution are injected around the nerve. The needle is then partially withdrawn and directed 2 to 3 cm caudodorsally, where an additional 10 ml of the analgesic is deposited to desensitize the muscular branches and caudal rectal nerve (middle hemorrhoidal nerve) (109, 110). After replacing the used injection needle with a sterile one, the procedure is repeated on the opposite side. Penile relaxation and cutaneous desensitization over the region of the anus, perineum, posteriomedial thigh, caudal udder to hind teats, vulva, vagina, vestibule, clitoris, and external urethral opening can be expected within 10 to 20 minutes and lasts as long as 2 to 4 hours. If hyaluronidase (150 IU) and epinephrine 1:10,000 are added to the 2% lidocaine hydrochloride solution, less analgesic (25 ml) is required and the duration of analgesia is increased (111).

A lateral approach to the internal pudendal nerve through the gluteal region has been described in sheep (112). The technique is simply to place a finger into the rectum and locate the slit-like sciatic foramen. A 3.75-cm, 18-gauge needle is inserted through the corresponding skin site while advancing its point to the foramen. Three to 5 ml of a 2% lidocaine hydrochloride solution are injected at the foramen. The needle is withdrawn, and the injection site is massaged. With the finger still in the rectum, the procedure is repeated on the other side.

When compared to caudal epidural analgesia, the advantages of internal pudendal nerve desensitization are maintenance of tail tone and sciatic nerve function. Ballooning of the vagina may also aid in retention of the vagina after it is repositioned in the cow with prolapse (108). The disadvantages of the technique are the lack of cervical analgesia and the fact that the injection sites must be identified by rectal palpation. The bull's penis must be protected from injury by

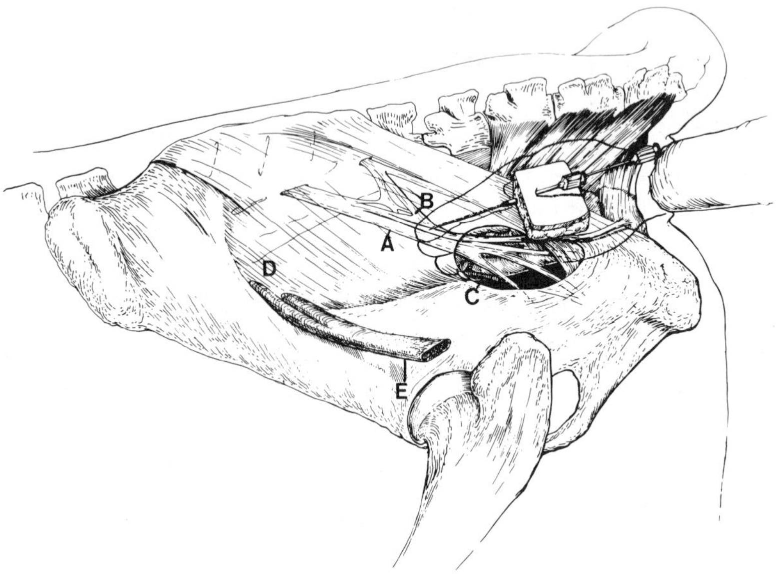

Figure 8.35. Needle placement to the internal pudendal nerve in cattle. The position of the hand palpating the internal pudendal nerve (*A*) on the left side is shown. *B*, caudal rectal nerve; *C*, internal pudendal artery; *D*, sacrosciatic ligament; *E*, sciatic nerve.

replacing it in the prepuce and taping or pursestringing the external preputial orifice.

ANTERIOR EPIDURAL ANALGESIA

Introduction to Techniques

For all procedures caudal to the diaphragm, anterior epidural analgesia is indicated. It is performed either by injecting a small volume of analgesic solution into the epidural space at the lumbosacral (L-6–S-1) junction (lumbosacral epidural analgesia) or by injecting a larger volume of the analgesic into the epidural space at the sacrococcygeal (S-5–C_o-1) or first intercoccygeal (C_o-1–C_o-2) space (high caudal epidural analgesia).

The only practical injection site for producing anterior analgesia is the lumbosacral space in swine. This space also is commonly used in lighter immature cattle, sheep, and goats because the injection sites are usually palpable. The sacrococcygeal or first intercoccygeal space is the injection site of choice in adult cattle for producing anterior analgesia because the technique is relatively simple, and subarachnoid puncture is avoided. Lumbosacral epidural analgesia and high caudal epidural analgesia always result in posterior paralysis. Proper techniques should provide analgesia of the perineal region, the entire inguinal region, the flanks, and the abdominal wall up to the umbilicus.

Various factors have been shown to affect the cranial spread of analgesic solution within the epidural space. They include size and age of the animal, the presence and size of abdominal mass (pregnancy), and other variables that can be controlled by the anesthetist, namely positioning the patient, choosing the site for epidural puncture, orientation of the needle bevel, determining the volume and concentration of the analgesic solution, and speed of injection (93). The area of blockade will increase as the dose of the analgesic is increased. Increasing the volume will improve the segmental spread, whereas increasing the concentration will provide a more rapid onset of analgesia and motor blockade, greater frequency of adequate analgesia, greater depth of motor blockade, and longer duration of analgesia and motor blockade. A faster injection of local analgesic produces a greater area of epidural blockade than does a slower injection. However, the advantage of a larger segmental area of analgesia is offset by the shorter duration, increased occurrence of incomplete analgesia, and the high frequency of patient discomfort upon injection. Because of transient elevation of CSF pressure, rapid injection causes pain.

In the spread of epidural analgesia, gravity has a definite role. The dependent site has a more rapid onset to maximal segmental analgesia, a longer duration of analgesia, and more intense motor blockade than the upper side. Due to preferential escape of the solution toward the paravertebral region, perfect unilateral analgesia can be obtained in sheep and goats. The sitting position of the animal after epidural injection also limits the cephalad spread of analgesia. The volume of the epidural space decreases with increased volume of the dural sack (CSF volume), distension (engorgement) of epidural veins, and increased quantities of fat in obesity. Migration of epidural analgesics is enhanced by transmission of intrathoracic and intraabdominal pressure (pregnancy) and in elderly cattle

(>8 years) with progressively occluded intervertebral foramina (93).

Lumbosacral Epidural Analgesia in Swine

The most commonly used form of regional analgesia in swine is epidural analgesia. The technique is relatively easy to accomplish and greatly facilitates Caesarean section; repair of rectal, uterine, or vaginal prolapses; repair of umbilical, inguinal or scrotal hernias; scirrhous cord; and surgery of the prepuce, penis, or rear limbs (113–116). However, epidural analgesia is contraindicated in patients that are in shock or toxemic because of sympathetic blockade and consequent depression of blood pressure (117). The pig must be properly restrained by using a weighing crate, chute, or hog snare. In some instances, chemical restraint is required. The use of sedatives that might produce ataxia or partial recumbency should be avoided. The site for needle placement is on the midline and caudal to a transverse line between the cranial prominences of the wing of the ilium (iliac crest) on either side, 0.5 to 1.5 cm in pigs weighing 10 to 50 kg and 1.5 to 2.5 cm in pigs weighing 50 kg or more. A vertical line through the patella may be used as a guide to locate the lumbosacral space in large pigs, in which the iliac wings are not palpable (114, 117–119). The site for needle placement is then approximately 2 to 3 cm caudal to the vertical line. Using an angle of 10° caudal to perpendicular (Fig. 8.36), a 6- to 16-cm, 20- or 18-gauge spinal needle with the bevel directed cranially is inserted at the lumbosacral space. A 6- to 8-cm, 20-gauge needle is used for pigs over 100 kg. The tissues over the space are infiltrated with 3 to 5 ml of a 2% lidocaine hydrochloride solution. Especially if the spinal needle must be withdrawn and redirected, a 14-gauge needle can be used as a cannula for support and guidance. The depth of needle penetration depends upon the size and condition of the hog. The needle is inserted 2 to 3.5 cm in pigs weighing 10 to 20 kg. The depth will be 3 to 10 cm in pigs 20 to 100 kg. The penetration may be as deep as 10 to 15 cm in heavy boars and sows. As the needle encounters the interarcuate ligament, it passes through a definite area of resistance. A slight pop is felt as the needle passes into the epidural space. The lumbosacral space is large in the pig (1.5 × 2.5 cm) and allows for a relatively large margin of error (115, 120). A 2% lidocaine hydrochloride solution is slowly injected with little pressure on the syringe plunger after the needle tip is placed into the epidural space.

The dose is calculated either by weight or length of the pig. Analgesia caudal to the umbilicus can be expected after injecting 1.0 ml of a 2% lidocaine hydrochloride solution per 4.5 kg of body weight at a rate of approximately 1 ml/2 to 3 seconds (121). Analgesia should occur within 10 minutes and last approximately 2 hours. A smaller dose, such as 1.0 ml/7.5 kg for pigs up to 50 kg and an additional 1.0 ml for every 10-kg increase in weight, has given similar results (115, 119). The dose should be adjusted to the condition of the patient and the surgical procedure. Regardless of the weight, a total dose of 20 ml must not be exceeded. Four milliliters/100 kg, 6 ml/200 kg, and 8 ml/300 kg of body weight are sufficient for standing castrations; 10 ml/100 kg, 15 ml/200 kg, and 20 ml/300 kg have given satisfactory results for Caesarean sections (120).

Sufficient analgesia of the ventral abdominal wall for laparotomy in sows up to 100 cm in body length has been achieved after injecting 1.0 ml of a 2% lidocaine hydrochloride solution for the first 40 cm (as measured from the external protuberance to the first coccygeal vertebrae) and additional 1.5 ml for every 10-cm increase in length (122). When minimal CNS depression, low morbidity and mortality, and rapid recovery are desired, epidural analgesia is the best choice in swine. If the sow is to nurse pigs or is to be sold for slaughter before other complications develop, a rapid recovery is important. A rapid recovery also allows a specific pathogen-free sow to leave the clinic

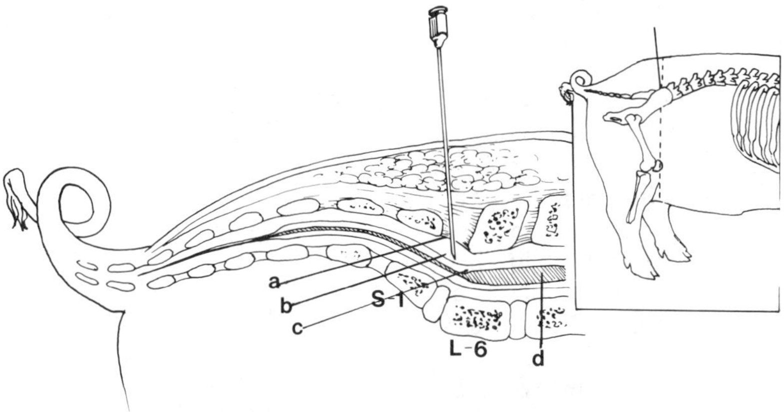

Figure 8.36. Needle placement for lumbosacral epidural analgesia in the pig. *L-6*, sixth lumbar; *S-1*, first sacral vertebra; *a*, interarcuate ligament; *b*, epidural space; *c*, subarachnoid space; *d*, spinal cord.

as soon as the piglets do. Epidural analgesia can also be used in combination with general analgesia (116). It allows a light plane of analgesia with good muscle relaxation in the hindparts. Complications may arise from faulty techniques. They include cardiovascular and respiratory collapse after overdose or subarachnoid injection, meningitis after septic technique, tremors, vomiting, and convulsions after injecting the analgesic into the vertebral venous sinus.

Anterior Epidural and Subarachnoid Analgesia in Small Ruminants

Anterior analgesia is indicated for Caesarean section and udder surgery in small ruminants. The technique may easily be accomplished by injecting a suitable local analgesic into either the epidural space or subarachnoid space at the lumbosacral intervertebral space (123–126). A 6.0- to 7.0-cm, 20-gauge spinal needle is inserted in the midline in adult sheep and goats halfway between the last lumbar (L-7) and first sacral (S-1) vertebrae at approximately 90° to the skin (Fig. 8.32, C). The site for needle placement is usually palpable as a depression on the midline caudal to a line joining the anterior border of the ilium on each side. The technique for epidural injection is similar to the technique used in pigs. A dose of 1 ml of a 2% lidocaine hydrochloride solution per 4.5 kg of body weight will produce posterior paralysis in 2 to 10 minutes. Anterior analgesia extending to three-quarters of the distance from the pubis to the umbilicus can be expected within 3 to 5 minutes; it will last as long as 2 hours.

Subarachnoid injection is done either as a special technique (123, 124) or accidentally, when the needle has passed through the dorsal epidural space, the dura and the arachnoid meninges. The spinal cord and meninges at the lumbo sacral junction in sheep and goats can be traumatized by a needle because these structures extend into the midsacral (S-2–S-3) region (103). Free flow of CSF from the needle hub indicates that the subarachnoid space has been entered. If only one-half the epidural dose (0.5 ml/4.5 kg) is injected at a rate of approximately 1 ml/2 to 3 seconds, serious side effects associated with rapid diffusion of the analgesic through the CSF do not occur. Onset of posterior paralysis is in 1 to 3 minutes. Analgesia may last for 60 to 90 minutes, and it will extend anterior to the last rib. It is not safe to inject the full epidural dose after a puncture hole into the arachnoid membrane has been made. There are complications of major concern, including transient loss of consciousness, flexor spasm, rapid muscular contractions, respiratory paralysis, hypotension, and hypothermia after excessive dose administration (126). Respiratory paralysis is due to desensitization of motor nerves supplying the intercostal muscles and diaphragm. Because of vasodilation from an excessive blockade of sympathetic fibers, hypotension occurs. Hypotension clinically appears as collapse, tachycardia or bradycardia, weak pulse, and shallow, rapid respiration. It is for this reason that anterior analgesia is contraindicated in animals with known cardiovascular disease, bleeding disorders, or low blood pressure (127). The cause of hypothermia is the patient's inability to shiver.

TEAT AND UDDER ANALGESIA OF CATTLE

Anatomy

The udder is supplied primarily from nerve fibers originating from the third and fourth lumbar spinal cord segments, which form the genitofemoral nerve. Caudally the udder is supplied by the mammary branch of the pudendal nerve and distal cutaneous branch of the perineal nerve, which have their origin from the second, third, and fourth sacral spinal cord segments. The skin and some glandular tissue of the forequarters are supplied by the ilioinguinal (L2) and iliohypogastric (L1) nerves (Fig. 8.37) (89, 128). There are no secretory nerves to the udder; the secretion of milk is under hormonal control.

Introduction to Techniques

Most surgical procedures on the teat are generally performed under local analgesia (ring block, inverted "V" block, or teat cistern infusion) with either physical restraint or chemical tranquilization (77, 84, 129). Al-

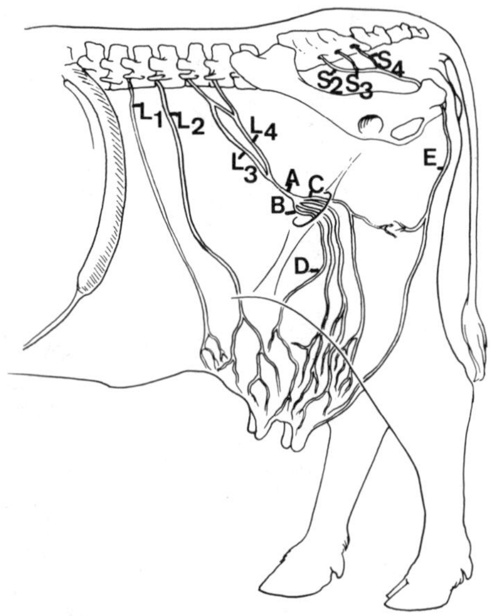

Figure 8.37. Schematic illustration of the nerve supply to the cow's udder. *A*, inguinal nerve; *B*, internal anterior; and *C*, posterior inguinal nerves; *D*, external inguinal nerve; *E*, perineal inguinal nerve. *L1* to *L4*, ventral branches of the first to fourth lumbar vertebral nerves. *S2*, *S3*, *S4*, ventral branches of the second, third, and fourth sacral vertebral nerves.

though standing restraint is advantageous because it prevents udder trauma, sepsis and the safety of the operator must not be compromised. Although the use of a portable tilting hydraulic table offers excellent physical restraint, it generally is not available in field situations; this makes chemical tranquilization with local analgesia the most popular combination.

Using paravertebral analgesia of L1, L2, and L3 or segmental epidural analgesia of these nerves, surgical procedures of the fore udder and foreteats may be performed. Both techniques have been described as difficult and often result in cows lying down.

After desensitizing the perineal nerve in the standing ruminant, surgical procedures of the caudal-most and escutcheon areas of the udder may be performed. Most surgical procedures of the caudal teats and body of the udder, however, require high caudal epidural analgesia or lumbosacral epidural analgesia. Both techniques have been described. High caudal epidural analgesia is the method of choice for major udder surgery if recumbency is desired. A dose of 50 to 150 ml of a 2% lidocaine hydrochloride solution are required to extend the analgesia cranially to L-1 in adult cows. Analgesia should be achieved in 10 to 15 minutes and may last 60 to 90 minutes. There is no indication for preferring lumbosacral epidural analgesia to high caudal epidural analgesia in udder surgery.

Except perhaps for udder amputation, general analgesia is rarely necessary for udder surgery. Complications associated with udder surgery are compartmentalization, bloat, and metabolic disturbances.

Ring Block of the Teat

After the thorough cleansing of the entire teat and teat base, a 1.5-cm, 25-gauge needle is used to infiltrate the skin and muscularis of the teat base around its entire circumference with 4 to 6 ml of a 2% lidocaine hydrochloride solution (Fig. 8.38, *A*). This technique provides adequate analgesia of the teat within 10 minutes for 2 hours, facilitating minor procedures such as laceration repair, wart removal, teat removal in gangrenous mastitis, teat obstruction opening, and fistula and supernumerary teat removal. The technique is simple and inexpensive, and the cow remains standing. However, it does require physical restraint (e.g., holding the nose, using a flank strap, a rope around the legs, or dorsal tail elevation) for asepsis and safety during infiltration.

Inverted "V" Block of the Teat

As an alternative to the ring block, a 1.5-cm, 25-gauge needle and 4 to 6 ml of a 2% lidocaine hydrochloride solution are used to infiltrate the skin and muscularis of the surgical site in an inverted "V" pattern (Fig. 8.38, *B*). Again, combined with adequate physical restraint and chemical tranquilization, the inverted "V" block is a simple technique for repair of lacerations or fistula or wart removal in the standing cow.

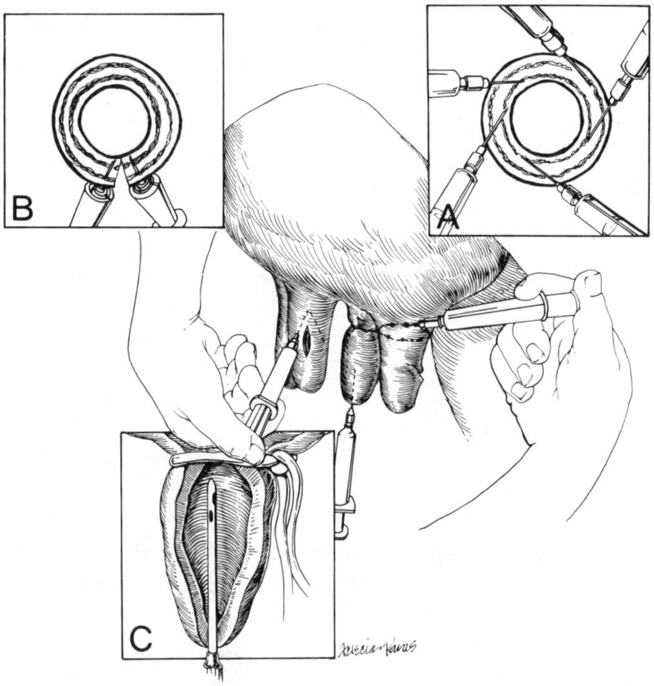

Figure 8.38. Needle placement for bovine ring block (*A*), inverted "V" block (*B*), and teat cistern infusion (*C*).

Teat Cistern Infusion

The teat cistern is infused with local analgesic solution to facilitate removal of teat polyps, open contracted sphincters, or open spider teats in procedures when analgesia of the mucous membrane lining of the cistern only is desired. Adequate physical restraint and chemical tranquilization are required. Before infusing the teat, the cistern is milked out and the orifice is thoroughly cleaned with alcohol. A narrow gauze bandage or suture tape is placed as high up on the teat as possible in order to act as a tourniquet, preventing more milk from entering the teat and diluting the analgesic agent. A teat cannula is introduced, and approximately 10 ml of a 2% lidocaine hydrochloride solution is infused to fill the teat (Fig. 8.38, *C*). The remaining lidocaine is milked out, and after 5 to 10 minutes of exposure the tourniquet is removed. No analgesia is afforded to the muscularis or skin, and aseptic technique is critical.

Perineal Nerve Block

Desensitization of the perineal nerve provides analgesia of the caudal-most udder or escutcheon area (128), thus facilitating repair of lacerations and removal of supernumerary teats or warts in that area. The nerve is readily desensitized by injecting 5 ml of a 2% lidocaine hydrochloride solution into the subcutaneous and subfascial tissues at the ischeal arch, approximately 2 cm lateral to the midline (130). The technique is more technically difficult than local infiltration of the surgical site; however, it does not inhibit wound healing.

ANALGESIA OF THE FOOT

Introduction to Techniques

Analgesia of the foot may be induced by (*a*) infiltrating the tissues around the limb with local analgesic solution (ring block); (*b*) injecting local analgesic solution into an accessible superficial vein in an extremity isolated from circulation by placing a tourniquet on the animal's leg (intravenous regional analgesia); (*c*) desensitizing specific nerves (regional analgesia); and (*d*) using general anesthesia in especially fractious animals or procedures requiring complete immobilization.

Ring Block

Some practitioners prefer to encircle the digit at the junction of the proximal and middle thirds of the metatarsus or metacarpus, infiltrating the analgesic from skin to bone. Approximately 15 ml of a 2% lidocaine hydrochloride solution is injected deep and superficial to the flexor tendons and in a partial circle around medially and laterally to the extensor tendon, using a 2.5-cm, 22-gauge needle. The area between the exterior and posterior injection sites may be divided into thirds; the analgesic may be injected at one-third to two-thirds the distance between them. The ring block has an advantage in that it requires no precise anatomical knowledge of the limb. However, several injection sites are necessary, which increases the risk of inducing pyogenic bacteria. In addition, this technique is often only partially successful.

Intravenous Regional Analgesia

Intravenous regional analgesia (IVRA) is a simple and safe method for producing analgesia of the digit in cattle, small ruminants, and pigs. In cattle, the technique involves placing either an elastic bandage or a tourniquet of stout rubber tubing or an inflatable cuff either above (131, 132) or below (131, 133, 134) the tarsus, above the elbow (135–137), and above (132, 138) or below (134, 139) the carpus. The efficiency of the tourniquet is improved in the pelvic limb by including a roll of bandage in the depression between the tibia and the Achilles tendon (131–133). IVRA is best performed on the leg of an animal that has been cast and restrained in lateral recumbency, but alternatively it can be induced in a raised leg of a sedated animal standing (140). In the thoracic limb, the skin over the prominent plantar metacarpal vein, common dorsal metacarpal vein, or radial vein is prepared aseptically (Fig. 8.39). For injection in the pelvic limb, the cranial branch of the lateral saphenous vein or lateral plantar digital vein may be used (Fig. 8.40). Using a 2.5- to

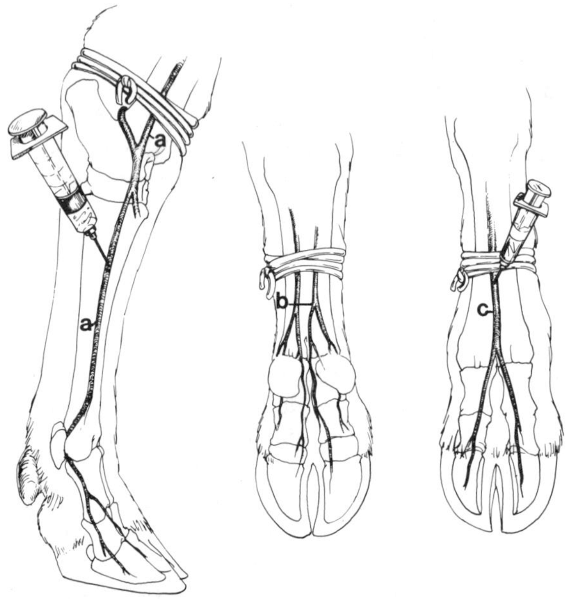

Figure 8.39. Tourniquet and needle placement for IVRA of the bovine forelimb. *a*, dorsal metacarpal vein; *b*, plantar metacarpal vein; and *c*, radial vein.

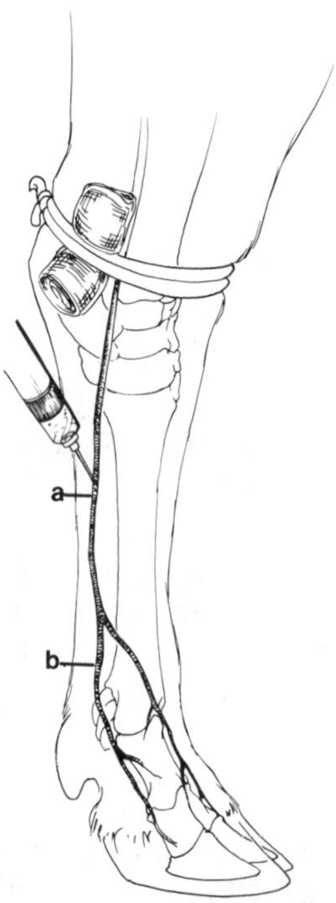

Figure 8.40. Tourniquet and needle placement of IVRA of the bovine rearlimb. *a*, cranial branch of lateral saphenous vein; *b*, lateral plantar digital vein.

3.75-cm, 20- or 22-gauge needle directed either proximally or distally, 10 to 30 ml of a 2% lidocaine hydrochloride solution without epinephrine are injected intravenously as close to the surgical site as possible in adult cattle (131–134, 138, 141). Approximately smaller volumes (3 to 10 ml) of lidocaine are injected in small ruminants and pigs (134).

To prevent hematoma formation, digital pressure and gentle massage are applied to the site of injection. Within 5 to 10 minutes, analgesia of the limb distal to the tourniquet occurs. Once the operation has been completed, the tourniquet is released. Five to 10 minutes after tourniquet removal, sensation and motor function return to the leg and no signs of cardiovascular or CNS toxicity are likely (132, 138, 142, 143). Evidence of partial analgesia may persist for a further 30 minutes or more on return of normal circulation. After early tourniquet removal (<20 min), salivation, tremors, and rapid pulse have occurred in cattle. A large bolus of lidocaine might have been released into the circulation in these animals (136, 137). Toxicity in early tourniquet removal is avoided if the tourniquet is loosened for 10 to 15 seconds and retightened for 2 to 3 minutes and this procedure is repeated several times. If the tourniquet is applied longer than 2 hours, ischemic necrosis, severe lameness, and edema occur (131, 132).

There are advantages of IVRA when compared to ring block or regional nerve block; they include the fact that it is less time-consuming and requires only a single injection site. In addition, the possibility of tissue trauma and contamination of fascial planes or tendon sheaths is lessened because it requires only a single injection site. The amount of bleeding at the surgical site is decreased. The disadvantages of IVRA are hematoma formation and an approximately 7% inexplicable failure rate even if the technique is performed correctly (132, 138).

Regional Analgesia of the Thoracic Limb in Cattle

To produce analgesia distal to the carpus, the musculocutaneous nerve, ulnar nerve, and median nerve must be desensitized (144–146). Local infiltration of skin and subcutis can be used effectively proximal to the carpus, where extensive muscle mass prohibits perineural injection. The musculocutaneous nerve may be desensitized by injecting 5 ml of a 2% lidocaine hydrochloride solution halfway between the elbow and the carpus on the dorsal radius just anterior to the cephalic vein (Fig. 8.41, *A*). The ulnar nerve can occasionally be palpated approximately 10 cm (a hand's breadth) above the accessory carpal bone at the lateral posterior aspect of the thoracic limb in a groove between the flexor carpi ulnaris and the ulnaris lateralis muscle. Approximately 5 ml of 2% lidocaine is injected underneath the superficial fascia at this site (Fig. 8.41, *B*). The median nerve may be palpated approximately 5 cm distal to the elbow anterior to the flexor carpi radialis muscle on the posterior radius. Because the nerve lies deep, it may require a 5-cm, 18- or 20-gauge needle and 10 ml of a 2% lidocaine hydrochloride solution for effective blockade (Fig. 8.41, *C*).

Alternatively, it is possible to produce analgesia from the midmetacarpus distally. At the midmetacarpal area, four nerves are desensitized: the dorsal metacarpal nerve (a superficial branch of the radial nerve), the medial palmar nerve (a continuation of the median nerve), and the dorsal and palmar branches of the ulnar nerve (147). Approximately 5 ml of a 2% lidocaine hydrochloride solution is injected per site through a 1.25-cm, 22-gauge needle. The point of the needle is directed proximally so that if the animal kicks, it will pull the leg away from the needle instead of breaking the needle off. The lateral palmar and dorsal branches of the ulnar nerve are desensitized by

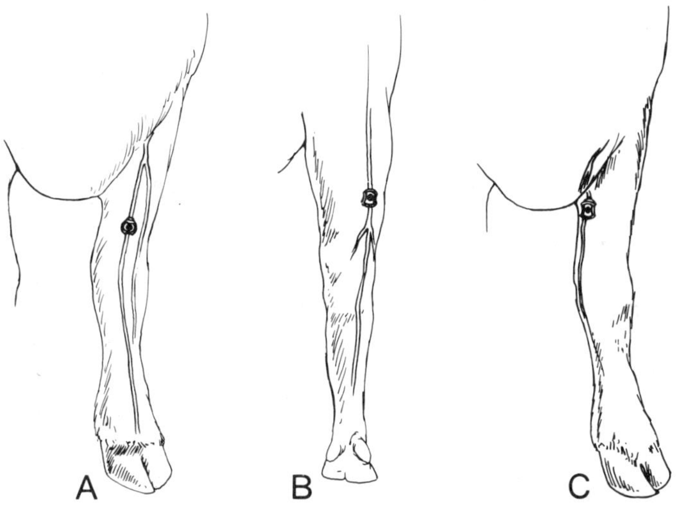

Figure 8.41. Needle placement for desensitizing the musculocutaneous (*A*), ulnar (*B*), and median nerve (*C*) in cattle.

injecting the analgesic anterior and posterior to the suspensory ligament on the lateral aspect of the limb (Fig. 8.42, *A* and *B*). The dorsal metacarpal nerve is desensitized subfascially medial to the medial digital extensor tendon (Fig. 8.42, *C*). The medial palmar nerve is desensitized at the medial aspect of the superficial flexor tendon in the groove between the suspensory ligament and superficial flexor tendon (Fig. 8.42, *D*).

Analgesia of the Interdigital Space of the Thoracic Limb in Cattle

For interdigital analgesia of the front foot, 5 ml of a 2% hydrochloride solution is injected at a depth of 2.5 to 3.5 cm on the dorsal midline of the pastern at a level of the middle of the first phalanx (77). The procedure is repeated on the palmar aspect of the foot (Fig. 8.43). The dorsal and plantar axial digital nerves, if properly infused, should be desensitized adequately for removal of interdigital fibromas ("corns"). Alternatively, it is possible to use a 10-cm, 18-gauge needle directed perpendicularly to the skin on the dorsum of the pastern and to infiltrate the region between the digits from a single injection site using 15 to 20 ml of the analgesic solution.

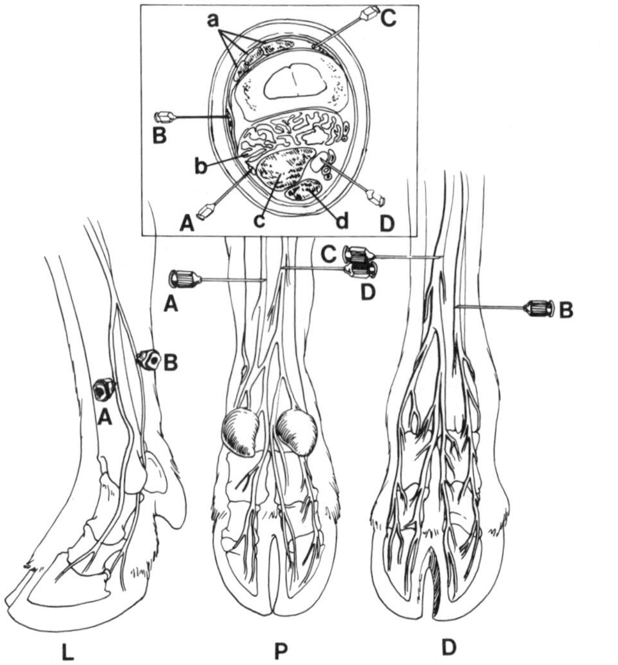

Figure 8.42. Midmetacarpal nerve blocks on left forefoot in cattle: lateral palmar branch of ulnar (*A*), dorsal branch of ulnar (*B*), dorsal metacarpal (*C*), medial palmar nerve (*D*). *L*, lateral; *P*, palmar; *D*, dorsal aspect. *a*, extensor tendons; *b*, interosseus ligament; *c*, deep; *d*, superficial digital flexor tendon.

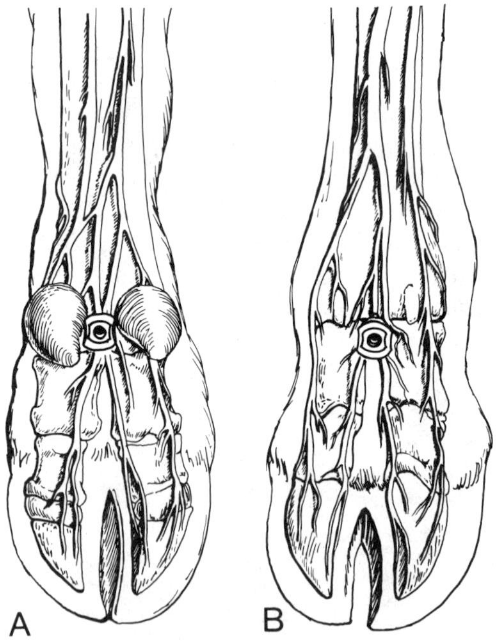

Figure 8.43. Needle placement for desensitizing the axial digital nerves III and IV of the left forefoot in cattle. Palmar (*A*) and dorsal (*B*) aspects.

Regional Analgesia of the Pelvic Limb in Cattle

Proximal to the tarsus, two nerves, the common perineal nerve and tibial nerve, are desensitized (148). Both nerves are continuations of the sciatic nerve (130). A 2.5-cm, 22-gauge needle and approximately 20 ml of a 2% lidocaine hydrochloride solution are used at each site, inducing analgesia in the midtibial area and distally within 10 to 20 minutes. The common peroneal nerve is desensitized at the posteriolateral edge of the tibial epicondyle deep to the aponeuronis of the biceps femoris muscle (Fig. 8.44, *A*). The tibial nerve is desensitized at a point approximately 10 cm above the tuber calcis between the gastrocnemius tendon and the deep digital flexor tendon on the medial aspect of the limb (Fig. 8.44, *B*). As an alternative method, analgesia distal to the tarsus is produced by desensitizing four nerves: the lateral plantar metatarsal nerve, the medial plantar metatarsal nerve (both are continuations of the tibial nerve), and the superficial and deep branches of the peroneal nerve (145–149). A 2.5-cm, 22-gauge needle and approximately 5 ml of a 2% lidocaine hydrochloride solution are used at each site. The lateral and medial plantar metatarsal nerves are desensitized at midmetatarsus between the suspensory ligament and flexor tendon on the lateral and medial aspect of the limb (Fig. 8.45, *A* and *B*). The deep peroneal nerve is desensitized at the junction of the middle and distal thirds of the metatarsal bone by inserting the needle full length deep to the extensor tendon and avoiding the dorsal metatarsal artery (Fig. 8.45, *C*). The superficial peroneal nerve is desensitized subcutaneously on the dorsal surface of the metatarsal bone between its proximal and middle thirds (Fig. 8.45, *D*).

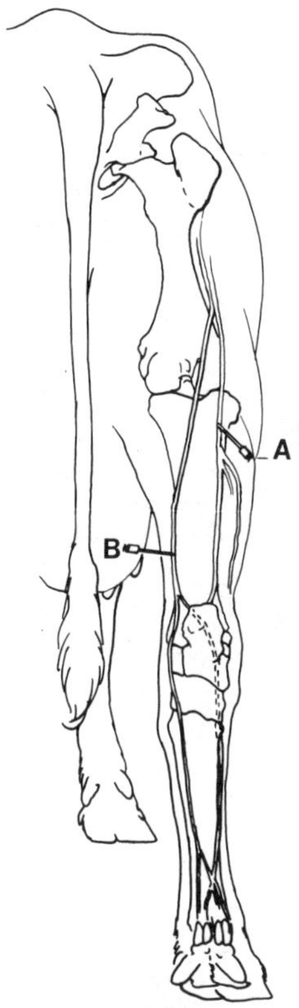

Figure 8.44. Needle placement for desensitizing common peroneal (*A*) and tibial (*B*) nerve in cattle. Caudal aspect.

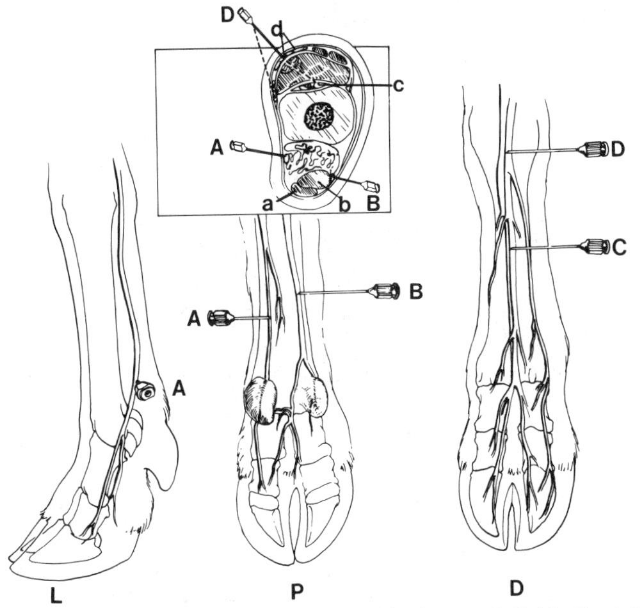

Figure 8.45. Midmetatarsal nerve blocks on left hindfoot in cattle: lateral plantar metatarsal (*A*), medial plantar metatarsal (*B*), deep peroneal (*C*), and superficial peroneal nerves (*D*). *L*, lateral; *P*, plantar; *D*, dorsal aspect. *a*, superficial; *b*, deep flexor digital tendon; *c*, deep peroneal n.; *d*, extensor tendons.

Fewer complications and the animal's ability to walk immediately after surgery are the advantages of regional analgesia of the foot when compared to general analgesia. The most obvious disadvantage of regional analgesia is that it requires a good knowledge of the anatomy of the region. Many injections are needed for each region. Probably due to anastomotic, collateral, or recurrent nerve branches (149), analgesia is often incomplete. Injections into inflamed tissue are often painful and ineffective, and they can cause the spread of infection and absorption of toxins. General anesthesia is the method of choice in fractious animals or for procedures requiring complete immobilization.

Intra-articular Analgesia

Intra-articular analgesia (37) may be considered for diagnostic work in conjunction with examination of joint fluid, but it is seldom rewarding.

ANALGESIA FOR CASTRATION

Castration of food animals is one of the most commonly performed surgical procedures in general practice. The operation may be performed using regional analgesia in either standing or cast position or using general analgesia induced by intravenous or intratesticular injection of a barbiturate. The choice of method to be used largely depends upon the species and the opportunity to observe the animal after castration.

Regional analgesia can be induced by intratesticular injection of a local analgesic solution in all food animals. The scrotum should be cleaned with a detergent antiseptic solution and proper restraint of the animals should be used. One testicle is grasped within the scrotum and the skin is tensed, and the line of incision is subcutaneously infiltrated with 3 to 5 ml of a 2% lidocaine hydrochloride solution. As the skin is pulled on the needle, the analgesic is injected.

A 3.75- to 7.5-cm, 16- or 18-gauge needle is inserted through the skin below the tail of the epididymis in bulls and boars. Using an angle of approximately 30° from the perpendicular without puncturing the side or bottom, the needle is pushed quickly into the center of the testicle. A bull or boar of approximately 200 kg body weight requires 10 to 15 ml of a 2% lidocaine hydrochloride solution injected in each testicle.

A 2.5- to 3.7-cm, 20-gauge needle is used in bull calves, rams, and bucks to allow easy flow of 2 to 10 ml of a 2% lidocaine hydrochloride solution to the center of the testicle and minimize backflow through the needle tract. Because the analgesic quickly passes from the testes up the spermatic cord via the lymph vessels into the blood, overdose must be avoided.

Intratesticular injection of either a short-acting barbiturate (e.g., pentobarbital) or ultrashort-acting thiobarbiturate (e.g., thiamylal or thiopental) is practiced. In large boars in which intravenous injection cannot be done, 1.0 ml of a 32.5% pentobarbital sodium solution (Uthol, Butler Co., Columbus, Ohio) is administered per 7.5 kg of body weight. The dosage is divided between the two testes, with a maximum of 20 ml per testicle for a very large boar (150). The boar is released after the injection; it will assume its normal activity. After a period of 5 to 15 minutes, recumbency may be expected. Castration should be carried out immediately after the boar has reached the stage of light anesthesia, which is usually at 10 to 25 minutes after injection. The testicle first injected is also the first to be removed surgically. Removal of the testes will also remove the source of drug and prevent excessive depth of anesthesia. Recovery normally takes from 20 to 40 minutes, but if poor technique has been used and the boar has been allowed to obtain too great a depth of anesthesia before castration, it may then take several hours.

The dosage of the thiobarbiturate injected intratesticularly also is above that normally estimated to be sufficient for intravenous anesthesia. In a boar of 200 kg estimated body weight, 2 g of thiamylal sodium powder dissolved in 10 to 15 ml of water is injected into one testicle.

In comparing the intratesticular injection of pentobarbital and thiamylal, it is evident that the uptake of thiamylal is more rapid and the recovery is shorter; however, the safety margin is narrower, and castration should be performed rapidly after the thiamylal administration. After the castration is complete, testicular tissue will still contain high concentrations of barbiturates.

Intratesticular Injection of Chem-Cast

Chem-Cast (Bio-Ceutic Laboratories Inc., St. Joseph, Missouri), a sclerosing agent, may be injected into the testes of young bull calves to destroy the testicular tissues painlessly within 60 to 90 days. The solution is injected into the top of the testes in standing calves using a 2.5- to 3.75-cm, 20-gauge needle and aseptic technique (Fig. 8.46). The dosage administered is 1.0 ml per testicle in calves weighing up to 45 kg and 1.5 ml per testicle in calves weighing 46 to 68 kg. Compared to surgical castration and mechanical crushing of the spermatic cord (Burdizzo method), chemical castration can be said to be simple and fast. It does not result in pain, stress, edema, hemorrhage, and unacceptable necrosis, thereby contributing to improved weight gain; further, it reduces the high risk of infection associated with the surgical procedures, and there is no withdrawal time for nontesticular tissues obtained from calves treated with Chem-Cast (151). Chem-Cast is not recommended for use in any animal other than bull calves, nor is it recommended for use in calves weighing more than 70 kg.

Dog

Local analgesic techniques are taught but rarely practiced in the dog because of the preference for using general analgesia. On the other hand, in old dogs or dogs that are considered poor risks with the use of general anesthetics, lumbosacral epidural analgesia, continuous epidural analgesia, and intravenous regional analgesia are distinctly advantageous.

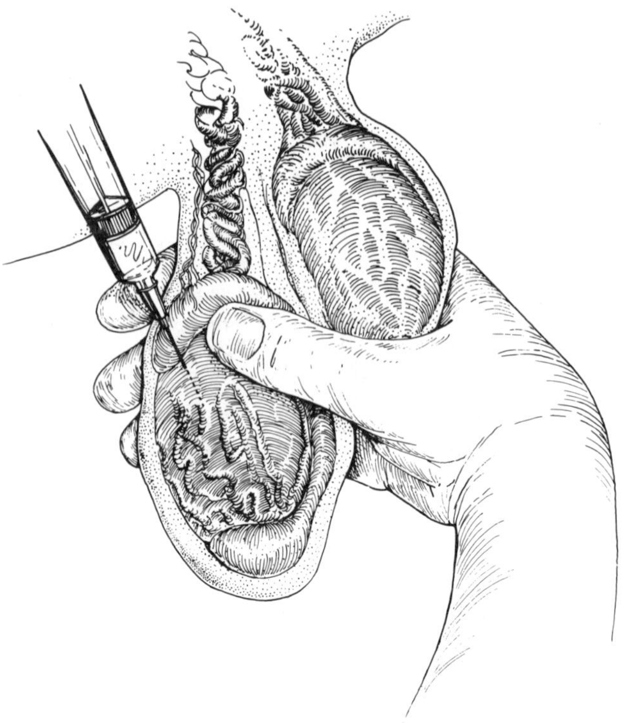

Figure 8.46. Needle placement for intratesticular injection in a bull calf.

EPIDURAL ANALGESIA

When combined with effective sedation, epidural analgesia can be routinely considered in dogs of all ages in postumbilical procedures (152, 158). Abdominal procedures including Caesarean section are less satisfactory and have higher failure rates than pelvic or rear leg procedures (158). Position, failure of sedation, and awareness of surgical manipulation may contribute to the abdominal discomfort. Epidural analgesia is contraindicated in dogs with blood clotting abnormalities or infection. The epidural space is aseptically entered at the lumbosacral space with a 6-cm, 20- or 22-gauge short beveled spinal needle. The space is palpated halfway between the dorsoiliac wings and just caudal to the dorsal spinous process of the seventh lumbar vertebra (152). The spinal needle is placed perpendicular to the skin surface at the midline of the lumbosacral space; with the dog in sternal recumbency, it is pushed ventrally in a slight cranial or caudal angle as needed (Fig. 8.47, *A*). The tip of the needle is inserted to the floor of the spinal canal and then is withdrawn about 5mm. For unilateral surgery and the convenience of the dog, lateral recumbency with the future surgical site ventrad is chosen. A distinct pop is usually felt when the needle is advanced

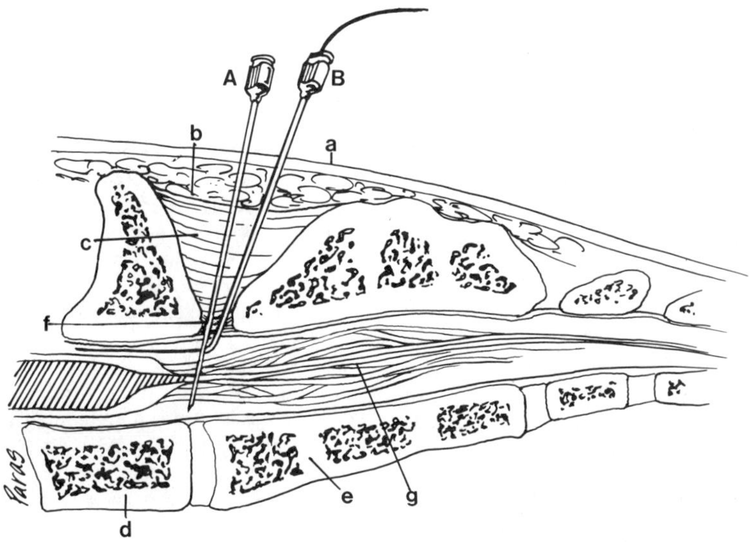

Figure 8.47. Needle placement into lumbosacral epidural space (*A*) and catheterization of epidural space (*B*) in the dog. *a*, skin; *b*, supraspinous ligament; *c*, interspinous ligament; *d*, L-7; *e*, sacrum, *f*, ligamentum interarcuatum (flavum); *g*, cauda equina.

through the ligamentum flavum. After aspiration with a syringe to be sure the needle is not within a venous sinus or the subarachnoid space (spinal fluid compartment), local analgesic solution can be injected with minimal resistance. Proper needle placement can also be checked for by injecting 1 to 2 ml of air without inducing subcutaneous crepitation. The traditional hanging drop technique described for horses and cattle is not useful in dogs.

Selection of drugs and dosage varies depending upon the desired effect. Lidocaine 2% or bupivacaine 0.75% is the agent of choice. As a guide, the dose is 1.0 ml of local analgesic for each 4.5 kg of body weight to produce analgesia as far cranial as the first lumbar (L-1) spinal segment (155, 158). If abdominal analgesia is required up to the fifth thoracic (T-5) spinal segment, the dose must be increased to 1.0 ml of local analgesic per 3.4 kg. It is advisable to dose to effect. One-half of the calculated amount of analgesic solution is injected over a 1-minute period followed by a pause of 30 to 60 seconds to observe relaxation of the anal sphincter and to note respiratory activity. Lidocaine induces early surgical analgesia within 5 to 10 minutes, with maximal effects at 20 minutes lasting 90 to 120 minutes. Bupivacaine is slow in action (latent period 20 to 30 minutes), but induces 5- to 6-hour periods of analgesia (157, 158). Possible complications after epidural overdose or injection into the vertebral sinuses include respiratory paralysis, vomiting, tremors, convulsions, and decreased blood pressure. Advantages of epidural analgesia when compared to general anesthesia are profound muscle relaxation in the desensitized area, less anesthetic equipment, less physiological and pharmacological insult to organ systems, and easier patient monitoring. Disadvantages include more planning, waiting during the prep period for latent periods, possibility of some dogs moving during surgery, and occasional failure with delay while general anesthesia could be instituted.

CONTINUOUS EPIDURAL ANALGESIA

A 7.5-cm, 17-gauge Huber point directional needle (Tuohy needle) is inserted into the epidural space in the dog, as previously described (155). A sterile vinyl catheter is passed through the needle and advanced cranially for a distance up to 2.5 cm beyond the tip of the needle into the vertebral canal. Ease of catheter introduction and failure of aspiration of blood or spinal fluid indicate location within the vertebral canal (Fig. 8.47, *B*). The needle is then carefully withdrawn to prevent cutting the catheter. Once epidural analgesia is established, more local analgesic is injected as needed at one-half the original dose per hour.

An alternative method for long-term pain treatment (up to 23 hours) in the dog is to inject 1.0 mg of morphine hydrochloride in 3 ml of aqueous solution per 10 kg of body weight into the lumbosacral epidural space (159). If a combination of 0.1 mg/kg morphine hydrochloride and 0.7 to 1.0 ml of 0.5% bupivacaine hydrochloride solution/10 cm vertex-coccyx distance is injected epidurally, surgical analgesia caudal to the last rib results and is converted gradually into a phase of postoperative analgesia for 24 hours without affecting motor activities and cardiopulmonary function (159).

INTRAVENOUS REGIONAL ANALGESIA

A rubber tourniquet is placed either around the forearm just proximal to the elbow for thoracic limb surgery (distal to the tourniquet) or proximal to the tarsus for pelvic limb surgery. A 3.75-cm, 22-gauge needle is inserted into any superficial vein distal to the tourniquet and 0.5 ml of a 1% lidocaine hydrochloride solution (without epinephrine) per kg of body weight is injected using light pressure (160). The technique is simple and provides for surgical analgesia in a blood-free area; if the occlusion of blood supply is limited to 2 hours, it is without toxic effects on organs. Irreversible shock occurs after leaving the tourniquet in place for 4 hours. Death due to sepsis and endotoxemia occurs if the tourniquet is removed after 8 to 10 hours.

Conclusion

Sufficient clinical work has been done to establish the usefulness, advantages, and limitations of various local and regional analgesic techniques in horses, ruminants, swine, and dogs. The methods described are safe and provide excellent and reliable analgesia.

References

1. Adriani T: *The Chemistry and Physics of Anesthesia*, ed 2. Springfield, Charles C Thomas Co, 1962.
2. Vickers MD, Wood-Smith GF, Stewart HC: *Drugs in Anesthetic Practice*, ed 5. London, Butterworths, 1978.
3. Booth NH: Local anesthetics. In Jones LM, Booth NH, McDonald LE (eds): *Veterinary Pharmacology and Therapeutics*, ed 4. Ames, Iowa State University Press, 1977, pp 417–436.
4. Covino BG: Ultralong-acting local aneshtetic Agents. *Anesthesiology* 54:263–264, 1981.
5. Link RP, Smith JC: Comparison of some local anesthetics in cattle. *J Am Vet Med Assoc* 129:306–309, 1956.
6. Heavner JE: Local anesthetics. In Steffey EP (ed): *Vet Clin North Am (Large Anim Pract)* 3(1), 1985, pp 209–221.
7. Bonica JJ, Akamatsu TJ, Berges PU, et al: Circulatory effects of peridural block. II. Effects of epinephrine. *Anesthesiology* 34:514–522, 1971.
8. Burfoot MF, Bromage PR: The effects of epinephrine on mepivacaine absorption from the spinal epidural space. *Anesthesiology* 35:488–492, 1971.
9. Owen DW: Local nerve blocks. In *Proc 9th Ann Mtg Am Assoc Eq Pract* 153–156, 1973.
10. Bonica JJ. *Clinical Applications of Diagnostic and Therapeutic Nerve Blocks*. Springfield, Charles C Thomas, 1959.
11. Moore DC: An evaluation of hyaluronidase in local and nerve block analgesia: A review of 519 cases. *Anesthesiology* 11:470–484, 1950.
12. Kirby Ch K, Eckenhoff JE, Looby JP: The use of hyaluronidase with local anesthetic agents in surgery and dentistry. *Ann NY Acad Sci* 52:1166–1170, 1950.
13. Covino BG, Vasallo HG: *Local Anesthetics—Mechanisms of Action and Clinical Use*, ed 1. New York, Grune and Stratton, 1976.
14. Cohen EN, Collis JE, Gunther RE: The role of pH in the development of tachyphylaxis to local anesthetic agent. *Anesthesiology* 29:994–1001, 1968.
15. Schelling CG, Klein LV: Comparison of carbonated lidocaine and lidocaine hydrochloride for caudal epidural analgesia in horses. *Am J Vet Res* 46:1375–1377, 1985.
16. Ritchie JM, Greengard P: On the mode of action of local anesthetics. *Ann Rev Pharmacol* 6:405–408, 1966.
17. Covino BG: Toxicity of Local Anesthetics. *34th Annu Refr Course Lect*, American Society of Anesthesiologists 504:1–7, 1983.
18. Wittman F, Morgenroth H: Untersuchungen über die Leitungsanästhesie des nervus infraorbitalis und des nervus mandibularis bei Zahn-und Kieferoperationen. Festschrift für Eugen Fröhner. Verlag Von Ferdinand Enke, Stuttgart, pp 384–399, 1928.
19. Rubin LF: Auriculopalpebral nerve block as an adjunct to the diagnosis and treatment of ocular inflammation in the horse. *J Am Vet Med Assoc* 144:1387–1388, 1964.
20. Bolz W: Ein weiterer Beitrag zur Leitungsanästhesie am Kopf des Pferdes. *Berl Tierärztl Wschr* 46:529–530, 1930.
21. Manning JP, St Clair LE: Palpebral frontal and zygomatic nerve blocks for examination of the equine eye. *Vet Med* 71:187–189, 1976.
22. Lichtenstern G: Die Verwendung von Tropkakokain in der tierärztlichen Chirurgie mit besonderer Berücksichtigung hinsichtlich seiner Verwendbarkeit in der Augapfelinfiltration beim Pferde. *Münch Tierärztl Wschr* 55:337–359, 1911.
23. Schönberg F: Anatomische Grundlagen für die Leitungsanästhesie der Zahnnerven beim Pferde. *Berl Tierärztl Wschr* 43:1–3, 1927.
24. Eeckhout AV: Un procédé pratique pour obtenir l'anesthésie complète des dents molaires supérieures chez le cheval. *Ann Méd Vét* 66:10–14, 1921.
25. Edwards JF: Regional anaesthesia of the head of the horse: An up-to-date survey. *Vet Rec* 10:973–975, 1930.
26. Bressou C, Cliza S: Contribution a létude de l'anesthésie dentaire chez le cheval et chez le chien. *Rec Méd Vét* 107:129–134, 1931.
27. Skarda RT: Practical regional anesthesia. In Mansmann RA, McAllister ES, Pratt PW (eds): *Equine Medicine and Surgery*, ed 3. Santa Barbara, California, American Veterinary Publications, 1982, vol 1, pp 229–238.
28. Adams OR: *Lameness in Horses*, ed 3. Philadelphia, Lea & Febiger, 1974, pp 91–112.
29. Zeller R: Die Lokalanästhesie bei: der Lahmheitsuntersuchung. *Berl Münch Tierärztl Wschr* 91:166–171, 1978.
30. Gray BW, Engle HN Jr, Rumpf PF, et al: Clinical approach to determine the contribution of the palmar and palmar metacarpal nerves to the innervation of the equine fetlock joint. *Am J Vet Res* 41:940–943, 1980.
31. Wheat JD, Jones K: Selected techniques of regional anesthesia. In Steffey EP (ed): *Vet Clin North Am (Large Anim Pract)* 3(1), 1981, pp 223–246.
32. Worthman RP: Diagnostic anesthetic injections. In Mansmann RA, McAllister ES (eds): *Equine Medicine and Surgery*, ed 3. Santa Barbara, California, American Veterinary Publications, 1982, pp 947–952.
33. Nyrop KA, Coffman JR, DeBowes RM, et al: The role of diagnostic nerve blocks in the equine lameness examination. *Compend Contin Educ* 5(12):669–676, 1983.
34. Colbern GT: The use of diagnostic nerve block procedures on horses. *Compend Contin Educ* 6(10):611–619, 1984.
35. Van Pelt RW: Intra-articular injection of the equine carpus and fetlock. *J Am Vet Med Assoc* 140:1181–1190, 1962.
36. Van Kruiningen HJ: Practical techniques for making injections into joints and bursae of the horse. *J Am Vet Med Assoc* 143:1079–1083, 1963.
37. Tufvesson G: *Local Anesthesia in Veterinary Medicine*. Sodertalje, Sweden, Astra International, 1963.
38. Gabel AA: Treatment of lameness of standardbred race horses due to inflammation of the distal hock. *J Am Vet Med Assoc* 175:1086–1088, 1979.
39. Sack WD: Distal intertarsal and tarsometatarsal joints in the horse. Communication and injection sites. *J Am Vet Med Assoc* 179:355–359, 1981.
40. Westhues M, Fritsch R: *Die Narkose der Tiere*, Band I. Lokalanästhesie. Berlin, Germany, Paul Parey, 1960, pp 49–55.
41. Hall LW: *Wright's Veterinary Anaesthesia and Analgesia*, ed 7.

London, Balliere & Tindall, 1971.
42. Tillmann H: Zur Leitungsanästhesie bei Laparotomien Am Pferd. *Tierärztl Umschau* 4:302–303, 1949.
43. Skarda RT, Muir WW: Segmental epidural and subarachnoid analgesia in horses: A comparative study. *Am J Vet Res* 44:1870–1876, 1983.
44. Skarda RT, Muir WW: Segmental thoracolumbar spinal (subarachnoid) analgesia in conscious horses. *Am J Vet Res* 43:2121–2128, 1982.
45. Pape J, Pitzschk C: Versuche über extradurale Anästhesie beim Pferde. *Arch Wiss Prakt Tierheilkd* 52:558–571, 1925.
46. McLeod WM, Frank ER: A preliminary report regarding epidural analgesia in equines and bovines. *J Am Vet Med Assoc* 72:327–335, 1928.
47. Browne TG: Anaesthesia in veterinary practice. *Vet Rec* 50:1617, 1938.
48. Heinze CD: Equine surgery, variations in technique: Epidural anesthesia. *Mod Vet Pract* 49:39, 1968.
49. Slusher SH: Caudal epidural anesthesia in horses. *VM SAC* 76:1773–1775, 1981.
50. Greene EM, Cooper RC: Continuous caudal epidural anesthesia in the horse. *J Am Vet Med Assoc* 184:971–974, 1984.
51. Skarda RT, Muir WW: Continuous caudal epidural and subarachnoid anesthesia in mares: A Comparative study. *Am J Vet Res*44:2290–2298, 1983.
52. Skarda RT, Muir WW, Ibrahim AL: Plasma mepivacaine concentrations after caudal epidural and subarachnoid injection in the horse: Comparative study. *Am J Vet Res* 45:1967–1971, 1984.
53. Sarparanta L: Die Anwendung der Lokalbetäubung bei den Kastrationen. *Finsh Vet* 33:59–61, 1927.
54. Hudson R: Local anesthesia. *Vet Rec* 2:1053–1054, 1930.
55. Rieger H; Die testikuläre Injektion. *Berl Tierärzte Wschr* 67:107–109, 1954.
56. Matyschtschuk J: Beitrag zur Kastrationen am stehenden Pferd. *Wien Tierärztl Mschr* 36:378–391, 1949.
57. Reed WD: Standing castration. *Proc 14th Ann Mtg Am Assoc Eq Pract* 1968, pp 239–240.
58. Dietz O: Zur Grenzstrangblockade beim Tier. *Arch Exp Veterinärmed* 11:310–330, 349–385, 1958.
59. Heidrich HD, Nöldner H: Ueber die Anwendung der Grenzstrang bzg. Stellatumblockade beim Pferd. *Mh Vet Med* 18:58–61, 1963.
60. Skarda RT, Muir WW, Swanson CR, et al: Cervicothoracic (stellate) ganglion block in conscious horses. *Am J Vet Res* 47(1):21–6, 1986.
61. Skarda RT, Muir WW, Hubbell JA: Paravertebral lumbar sympathetic ganglion block in the horse. *Proc 2nd Intl Vet Anest Congr*. Santa Barbara, California, Veterinary Practice Publishing Co, 1985, p 160.
62. Ames NK, Riebold TW: Anesthesia in cattle. *Proc 11th Annu Conv Am Assoc Bovine Pract* Dez:75–77, 1978.
63. Cox VS, McGrath CJ, Jorgensen SE: The role of the downer cow syndrome. *Am J Vet Res* 43:26–31, 1982.
64. Thurmon JC, Benson, GJ: Anesthesia in ruminants and swine. In *Current Veterinary Therapy, Food Animal Practice*, ed 1. Philadelphia, WB Saunders, 1981, pp 58–89.
65. Trim CM: Sedation and general anesthesia in ruminants. *The Bovine Pract*, No 16, 137–144, 1981.
66. Rubin LF, Gelatt, KN: Analgesia of the eye. In Soma LR (ed): *Veterinary Anesthesia*. Baltimore, Williams & Wilkins Company, 1971, pp 489–499.
67. Cust RE: Anaesthesia and akinesia. In Blogg JR (ed): *The Eye in Veterinary Practice*. North Melbourne, Australia, VS Supplies Limited, 1975, pp 169–178.
68. Maksimovic B: Akinesie des M. orbicularis palpebrum bei Rindern. *Vet Arch* 20:75–78, 1950.
69. Schreiber J: Die anatomischen Grundlagen der Leitungsanästhesie beim Rind. I. Die Leitungsanästhesie der Kopfnerven. *Wien Tierärztl Mschr* 42:129–153, 1955.
70. Peterson DR: Nerve block of the eye and associated structures. *J Am Vet Med Assoc* 118:145–148, 1951.
71. Hare WCD: A regional method for the complete anaesthetization and immbolization of the bovine eye and its associated structures. *Canad J Comp Med and Vet Sci* 21:228–234, 1957.
72. Elmore RG: Food animal regional anesthesia. Bovine blocks: Ocular. *Vet Med Small Anim Clin* 75:1760–1762, 1980.
73. Gabel AA: Practical techniques for bovine anesthesia. *Mod Vet Pract* 45:39–44, 1964.
74. Gibbons WJ: Local anesthesia in bovine practice. *Mod Vet Prac* 40:36–39, 1959.
75. Monke DR: Local nasal anesthesia in the bull. *Vet Med Small Anim Clin* 76:389–393, 1981.
76. Browne TG: The technique of nerve-blocking for dehorning cattle. *Vet Rec* 50:1336–1337, 1938.
77. Elmore RG: *Food Animal Regional Anesthesia*. Edwardsville, Kansas, Veterinary Medicine Publishing Company, 1981.
78. Wheat JD: New landmark for cornual nerve block. *Vet Med* 45:29–30, 1950.
79. Spaulding CE: Procedures for dehorning the dairy goat. *Vet Med Sm Anim Clin* 72:228–230, 1977.
80. Vitums A: Nerve and arterial blood supply to the horns of the goat with reference to the sites of anesthesia for dehorning. *J Am Vet Med Assoc* 125:284–286, 1954.
81. Baker JS: Dehorning goats. *Bov Pract* 2:33–39, 1981.
82. Wallace CE: Cosmetic dehorning. In Amstutz HE (ed): *Bovine Medicine and Surgery*, ed 2, vol II. Santa Barbara, California, American Veterinary Publications, 1980, p 1240.
83. Butler WF: Innervation of the horn region in domestic ruminants. *Vet Rec* 80:480–492, 1967.
84. Gibbons WJ, Catcott EJ, Smithcors JF (eds): *Bov Med and Surg* ed 1. Wheaton, Illinois, American Veterinary Publications, 1970.
85. Oehme FW, Prier JE (eds): *Textbook of Large Anim Surg*. Baltimore, Williams & Wilkins Co, 1974.
86. Morishima HO, Pedersen H, Finster M, et al: Toxicity of lidocaine in adult, newborn, and fetal sheep. *Anesthesiology* 55:57–61, 1981.
87. Farquharson J: Paravertebral lumbar anesthesia in the bovine species. *J Am Vet Med Assoc* 97:54–57, 1940.
88. Hall LW, Clark KW (eds): *Vet Anaesthesia*, ed 8. Eastbourne, England, Bailliere Tindall, 1983.
89. Arnold JP, Kitchell RL: Experimental studies of the innervation of the abdominal wall of cattle. *Am J Vet Res* 18:229–240, 1957.
90. Cakala S: A technique for the paravertebral lumbar block in cattle. *Cornell Vet* 51–64–67, 1961.
91. Arthur GH: Some notes on a preliminary trial of segmental epidural anesthesia of cattle. *Vet Rec* 68:254–256, 1956.
92. Skarda RT, Muir WW: Segmental lumbar epidural analgesia in cattle. *Am J Vet Res* 40:52–57, 1979.
93. Skarda RT: Lumbar epidural and subarachnoid analgesia in cattle, horses, and humans: A comparative study. *Habilitationsschrift*. Switzerland, University of Zurich, 1984.
94. Skarda RT, Muir WW: Hemodynamic effects of unilateral segmental lumbar epidural analgesia in cattle. *Am J Vet Res* 40:645–650, 1979.
95. Skarda RT, Muir WW: Segmental thoracolumbar subarachnoid analgesia in cows. *Am J Vet Res* 42:632–638, 1981.
96. Skarda RT, Muir WW: Effects of segmental subarachnoid analgesia on arterial blood pressure, gas tensions and pH in adult conscious cows. *Am J Vet Res* 42:1747–1750, 1981.
97. Skarda RT, Muir WW: Hemodynamic and respiratory effects of segmental subarachnoid analgesia in adult Holstein cows. *Am J Vet Res* 43:1343–1348, 1982.
98. Skarda RT, Muir WW, Ibrahim AL: Spinal fluid concentration of mepivacaine in horses and procaine in cows after thoraco-

lumbar subarachnoid analgesia. *Am J Vet Res* 46:1020–1024, 1985.

99. Elmore RG: Food animal regional anesthesia. Bovine blocks: Epidural. *Vet Med Sm Anim Clin* 75:1017–1029, 1980.
100. Rülcker C: Lignocaine hydrochloride with and without adrenaline for epidural analgesia in cattle. *Vet Rec* 77:1180–1181, 1965.
101. Bradley WA: Epidural analgesia for tail docking in lambs. *Vet Rec* 79:787–788, 1966.
102. Linzell JL: Some observations on general and regional anesthesia in goats. In Graham-Jones (ed): *Small Animal Anaesthesia*. Proceedings of a symposium organized by the British Small Animal Veterinary Association. Oxford, London, Pergamon Press Ltd, 1964.
103. Hopkins GS: The correlation of anatomy and epidural analgesia in domestic animals. *Cornell Vet* 25:263–270, 1935.
104. Bierschwal CJ: A technique for continuous epidural anesthesia in the bovine. *Vet Med* 55:44–46, 1960.
105. Elmore RG: Food animal regional anesthesia. Bovine blocks: Continuous epidural analgesia. *Vet Med Sm Anim Clin* 75:1174–1176, 1980.
106. Kuzucu EY, Derrick WS, Wilber SA: Control of intractable pain with subarachnoid alcohol block. *J Am Med Assoc* 195:541–544, 1966.
107. Noordsy JL: Sacral paravertebral alcohol nerve block as an aid in controlling chronic rectal tenesmus in cattle. *Vet Med Sm Anim Clin* 77:797–801, 1982.
108. Deshmukh SE, Deshpande KS: Internal pudendal nerve block in cows. *Indian Vet J* 57:73–75, 1980.
109. Larson LL: The internal pudendal (pubic) nerve block for anesthesia of the penis and relaxation of the retractor penis muscle. *J Am Vet Med Assoc* 123:18–27, 1953.
110. Habel RE: A source of error in the bovine pudendal nerve block. *J Am Vet Med Assoc* 128:16–17, 1956.
111. Bhokre AP, Deshpande KS: Experimental study on effect of hyaluronidase in pubic nerve block in bovines. *Indian Vet J* 56:872–874, 1979.
112. McFarlane IS: The lateral approach to pudendal nerve block in the bovine and ovine. *J S Afr Vet Med Assoc* 34:73–76, 1963.
113. Booth NH: Anesthesia in the pig. *Fed Proc* 28(4):1547–1552, 1969.
114. Elmore RG: Food animal regional anesthesia. Porcine blocks: Lumbosacral (epidural). *Vet Med Sm Anim Clin* 76:387–388, 1981.
115. Getty R: Epidural anesthesia in the hog—its technique and applications. In *Sci Proc 100th Annu Mtg Am Vet Med Assoc*. New York, 1966, pp 88–98.
116. Runnels LJ: Practical anesthesia and analgesia for porcine surgery. *Proc Am Assoc Swine Pract* (March):80–87, 1976.
117. Benson GJ, Thurmon JC: Anesthesia of swine under field conditions. *J Am Vet Med Assoc* 174:594–596, 1979.
118. Anderson IL: Anaesthesia in the pig. *Aust Vet J* 49:474–477, 1973.
119. Trim CM: Epidural analgesia in swine. *Vet Anesth* 8:23–25, 1980.
120. Eibl K: Die Lumbalanästhesie in der täglichen Praxis bei Jungbullen und Schweinen. *Münch Tierärztl Wschr* 86:145–148, 1935.
121. Hall LW, Clarke KW (eds): *Vet Anaesth*, ed 8. Eastbourne, England, Bailliere Tindall, 1983.
122. Strande A: Epidural anaesthesia in young pigs, dosage in relation to the length of the vertebral column. *Acta Vet Scand* 9:41–49, 1968.
123. Lebeaux M: Sheep: A model for testing spinal and epidural anesthetic agents. *Lab Anim Sci* 25:629–633, 1975.
124. Nelson DR, Ott RS, Benson GJ, et al: Spinal analgesia and sedation of goats with lignocaine and xylazine. *Vet Rec* 105:278–280, 1979.
125. Grono LR: Spinal anaesthesia in the sheep. *Aust Vet J* 42:58–59, 1966.
126. Hopcroft SC: Technique of epidural anaesthesia in experimental sheep. *Aust Vet J* 43:213–214, 1967.
127. Bradley WA: Epidural analgesia for tail docking in lambs. *Vet Rec* 79:787–788, 1966.
128. St Clair LE: The nerve supply to the bovine mammary gland. *Am J Vet Res* 3:10–16, 1942.
129. Noordsy JL: *Food Anim Surg*. Veterinary Medical Publications, 1978.
130. Getty R: (ed): Sisson and Grossman's *The Anatomy of the Domestic Animals*, ed 5. Philadelphia, WB Saunders, 1975.
131. Estill CT: Intravenous local analgesia of the bovine lower leg. *Vet Med Sm Anim Clin* 72:1499–1502, 1977.
132. Prentice DE, Wyn-Jones G, Jones RS, et al: Intravenous regional anaesthesia of the bovine foot. *Vet Rec* 94:293–295, 1974.
133. Elmore RG: Food animal regional anesthesia. Bovine blocks: Intravenous limb block. *Vet Med Sm Anim Clin* 75:1835–1836, 1980.
134. Knight AP: Intravenous regional anesthesia of the bovine foot. *Bovine Pract* 1(11):14–15, 1980.
135. Kumar R, Monahar M, Tyagi RPS: The fate of intravascularly infused regional anesthesia: A radiologic investigation. *J Am Vet Radiol Soc* 14:87–92, 1973.
136. Manohar M, Kumar R, Tyagi RPS: Studies on the intravenous retrograde regional anaesthesia of the forelimb in buffalo calves. *Br Vet J* 127:401–407, 1971.
137. Tyagi RPS, Kumar R, Manohar M: Studies on intravenous retrograde regional anaesthesia for the forelimbs of ruminants. *Aust Vet J* 49:321–324, 1973.
138. Jones RS, Prentice DE: Some observations of intravenous anaesthesia of the bovine foot. *Assn Vet Anaesth Gr Brit and Irl Proc* 5:13–17, 1974.
139. Fehlings K: Intravenöse regionale Anästhesie an der V. digitalis dorsalis communis III—eine brauchbare Möglichkeit zur Schmerzausschaltung bei Eingriffen an der Vorderzehe des Rindes. *Dtsch Tierärztl Wschr* 87:4–7, 1980.
140. Surborg H: Aspects of treatment of severe claw disease in a large animal practice. *Bovine Pract* No 19 (Nov):227–229, 1984.
141. Weaver AD: Intravenous local anesthesia of the lower limb in cattle. *J Am Vet Med Assoc* 160:55–57, 1972.
142. Antalovsky A: Technik der intravenösen Schmerzausschaltung im distalen Gliedmassenbereich beim Rind. *Vet Med (Prag)* 7:413–420, 1965.
143. Bogan JA, Weaver AD: Lidocaine concentrations associated with intravenous regional anesthesia of the distal limb of cattle. *Am J Vet Res* 39:1672–1673, 1978.
144. Lumb WV, Jones EW (eds): *Veterinary Anesthesia*, ed 2. Philadelphia, Lea & Febiger, 1984.
145. Taylor JA: The applied anatomy of the bovine foot. *Vet Rec* 72:1212–1215, 1960.
146. Westhues M, Fritsch R (eds): *Animal Anesthesia*, vol 1. London, Oliver and Boyd, 1964.
147. Raker CW: Regional analgesia of the bovine foot. *J Am Vet Med Assoc* 128:238–239, 1956.
148. Collin CW: A technique to produce analgesia of the hind digits of cattle. *Vet Rec* 75:833–834, 1963.
149. Jalaluddin AM, Rao SV: Diagnosis of lameness in the ox by means of nerve blocks. *Ind Vet J* 49:1246–1256, 1972.
150. Henry DP: Anaesthesia of boars by intratesticular injection. *Aust Vet J* 44:418–419, 1968.
151. Miller RE: An efficient and safe method of castration for the bovine by the intra-testicular injection of Chem-Cast. *The Bovine Proceedings*. 15 (April):156–159, 1983.
152. Frank ER: Regional anesthesia in the dog and cat. *J Am Vet Med Assoc* 72:336–340, 1927.
153. Riddell WK: Caudal anesthesia in canine surgery. *J Sm Anim Med* 1:159–162, 1952.

154. Bone JK, Peck JG: Epidural anesthesia in dogs. *J Am Vet Med Assoc* 128:236–238, 1956.
155. Klide AM, Soma LR: Epidural analgesia in the dog and cat. *J Am Vet Med Assoc* 153:165–173, 1968.
156. Bradley RL, Withrow SJ, Heath RB, et al: Epidural anaesthesia in the dog. *Vet Surg* 9:153–156, 1980.
157. Alvarez R, Mailhac JM, Chaffaux S: Emploi de la bupivacaine par voie épidurale pour la chirurgie gynécologique de la chienne. *Récueil Méd Vét* 156:291–296, 1980.
158. Heath RB, Broadstone RV, Wright M, et al: Bupivacaine and mepivacaine lumbosacral epidural analgesia in dogs. *Proc 2nd Intl Vet Anes* (abstract). Santa Barbara, California, Veterinary Practice Publishing Company, 1985, p 162.
159. Bonath KH, Saleh AS: Long term pain treatment in the dog by peridural morphines. *Proc 2nd Intl Vet Anes.* Santa Barbara, California, Veterinary Practice Publishing Company, 1985, p 161.
160. Küpper W: Die Intravenöse Regionalanästhesie (Bier) beim Hund. *Zbl Vet Med* (A): 24:287–297, 1977.

CHAPTER

9

Neuromuscular Blocking Agents

LIN V. KLEIN, V.M.D., D.A.C.V.A.

History and Development

The pharmacologic properties of extracts from bark of the creeper plants *Chondodendron tomentosum* and *Strychnos toxifera* were of importance to South American indians prior to the discovery and invasion of the western hemisphere by Europeans in the 15th century, but it was not until the 19th century that the site of action of "ourari" (later corrupted to "curare") was identified as the neuromuscular junction by Claude Bernard. Crude extracts were used in the 19th century in an attempt to control the muscle spasms of patients with rabies and tetanus, but impurities, variations in potency, and presumedly lack of effective methods of control of respiration limited the success of these ventures. The curare extract was purified and its structure determined in the 1930s; it was introduced into the operating room successfully in 1942. When demand for muscle relaxants exceeded the supply available from South America, efforts were directed toward producing a synthetic compound, and gallamine was introduced in 1947 (1). The physiological effects of succinylcholine (SCh) were studied in 1906, but its paralyzing properties went undetected because curarized cats were used in the studies. The relaxant properties of the drug were not described until 1949, and it was introduced into clinical practice in the United States in 1952 (2). Alcuronium, a *Strychnos toxifera* alkaloid, was introduced in 1958 because it had fewer undesirable properties than the older drugs. Pancuronium, introduced in 1964, was designed as a cleaner, more selective blocking agent. More recently, vecuronium and atracurium, which are almost devoid of nonrelaxant properties, have been brought into clinical practice.

Undesirable properties of the older compounds included autonomic effects, histamine release, and minimal metabolic breakdown of the older nondepolarizing agents resulting in long duration of action, as well as muscle pain, K^+ release, and triggering of malignant hyperthermia with succinylcholine. Efforts to produce a family of ideal relaxants continue. The ideal agents would be nondepolarizing, noncumulative after repeated top-up doses, antagonized successfully pharmacologically, have no autonomic effects, and not release histamine. Duration of action would not be prolonged markedly in patients in renal or hepatic failure. Ideally, a family of agents would be available, including an ultrashort-acting agent similar in onset and offset to succinylcholine, an agent of intermediate duration suitable for procedures lasting 20 to 30 minutes, and a longer-acting agent. Vecuronium and atracurium fulfill most of the criteria, but an ultrashort-acting nondepolarizing agent is still not available. Currently, clinical trials in humans are in progress with a new agent, BW B1090U, a nondepolarizer that is hydrolyzed by plasma cholinesterase, has a blockade with a duration of action about twice that of SCh, is virtually noncumulative, and can be antagonized by neostigmine. It is a weak histamine releaser (3, 4).

Use of Neuromuscular Blocking Agents

In sharp contrast to the practice of human anesthesia, neuromuscular blocking agents are not routinely used in veterinary anesthesia. There are some valid reasons for this difference.

Intubation is usually easily accomplished in animal species; difficult intubation may be due to small patient size or peculiar anatomical relationships but are not often due to laryngeal reactivity or excessive muscle tone. Abdominal muscle tone rarely seems to interfere with surgical procedures in animals. Mechanical ventilators are not always available in general practice veterinary surgical facilities. Anesthesia often is given by individuals with limited training, supervised by a veterinarian who is simultaneously doing surgery; there is a desire to keep techniques simple. It is feared that inadequate antagonism of blockade may lead to respiratory insufficiency and, in horses, limb muscle weakness in the recovery period.

With these considerations in mind, there is still a place for relaxant drugs in veterinary anesthesia in managing difficult cases. The newer relaxants with minimal cardiovascular effects can be used to gain immediate control of respiration in animals with cardiovascular compromise who will not tolerate deep levels of anesthesia. Relaxants can also be used to ensure immobility for delicate surgery, such as intraocular, intracranial, and some intrathoracic and orthopedic procedures. There is also a place for the use of neuromuscular blockade in the sedated intensive care unit patient requiring controlled ventilation, such as animals with severe chest or head injuries. There is, in the author's opinion, no justification for the use of neuromuscular blocking agents to immobilize awake animals for surgical procedures or scientific experiments. Regardless of the cost benefit for the former, or the "ideal" conditions provided for the latter, it seems unthinkably inhumane to paralyze awake animals in view of the discomfort and fear experienced by human beings under the same conditions.

Neuromuscular blockings agents have been used in the immobilization and capture of wild animals (5–9). Although this practice should be avoided if possible, there may be certain instances in which no safe alternatives exist. In the case of capture of wild horses (5), SCh was found to be more reliable and safer than etorphine. In the case of immobilization of large reptiles, SCh has been used because of its short duration of action, lasting minutes as opposed to days for injectable anesthetics (10). The drugs should be used only if the animals can be reliably tracked after drug administration and equipment for intubation and ventilation is available.

Mechanism of Action of Neuromuscular Blocking Agents

Although the neuromuscular junction was identified in 1842 as the site of action of the blocking agents, controversy remains today over exact mechanisms. Proponents of the postsynaptic view argue that all of the observable effects of the drugs on neuromuscular function can be explained by their actions at the acetylcholine (ACh) recognition sites at the motor end plate. Others cite numerous studies implicating the motor nerve terminal as an important site of action not only of the nondepolarizing blocking agents but of succinylcholine and neuromuscular facilitatory drugs, such as edrophonium and neostigmine. A detailed discussion of experimental evidence for and against various pre- and postsynaptic mechanisms is beyond the scope of this chapter. Suffice it to say that the agents have been postulated to interact with pre- and postsynaptic ACh recognition sites as well as directly in ion channels. The interested reader is referred to several excellent reviews (11–13).

More important clinically than exact site and mechanism of action are the effects of the blocking agents on responses to peripheral nerve stimulation because this is the method used to monitor blockade quantitatively. Responses vary with stimulus strength and duration, and certain conventions have developed. The stimulus must be supramaximal; that is, sufficient current must be applied to depolarize all of the fibers in the nerve being stimulated so that all of the muscle fibers innervated will contract with every stimulus, unless neuromuscular transmission is blocked. The stimulus should be a monophasic, square wave pulse, and its duration should be short (0.2 msec or less) to avoid direct muscle stimulation or repetitive nerve firing. Biphasic stimulation results in enhanced contractility in muscle fibers. One commercially available stimulator uses a biphasic stimulus and produces greater evoked tension than a monophasic stimulator, but dose responses for gallamine were parallel and similar in magnitude using the two modes of stimulation (14).

Responses to Stimulation at Various Frequencies during Anesthesia in the Absence and Presence of Nondepolarizing Neuromuscular Blockade

RESPONSE TO SINGLE SUPRAMAXIMAL STIMULI AT 0.1 Hz OR LESS

In the absence of blocking agents and after stabilization (upon initiating stimulation, an increment followed by a decrement may occur), successive stimuli yield responses of equal amplitude, either mechanical or electrical. Even when some receptors have been occupied by a blocking agent, there is not enough stress on the system to result in a decrement. It has been estimated that only about 20 to 25% of the end plate ACh receptors are necessary for a maximal single evoked response. This has been called the margin of safety of neuromuscular transmission. It may be more realistic to think of the single twitch as a fairly insensitive indicator of partial receptor blockade, but a useful tool to track deep levels of blockade and to compare drug potencies. An 80 to 90% depression of the single twitch response correlates with adequate surgical relaxation, but clinically significant muscle weakness may be present when twitch response is normal. Effective use of muscle requires sustained contraction in response to short bursts or longer volleys of repetitive nerve impulses. By using repetitive stimuli, partial blockade can be detected when the single twitch is not depressed.

RESPONSE TO STIMULATION AT 2 Hz

It has been observed that if slow repetitive stimulation (2 Hz) is applied in a train of four or five pulses in an awake or anesthetized individual without neuromuscular blockade or disease, there is no decrement or increment within the train of responses. During nondepolarizing blockade, a decrement occurs in the train. As long as at least 10 seconds's rest is allowed between trains, similar tension (or electromyogram (EMG) amplitude) is evoked in each subsequent train. This is called the train-of-four (T_4) response, and the ratio of the tension of the fourth twitch to that of the first is the T_4 fade ratio (T_4FR). A flat response ($T_4FR = 1.0$) requires that about 30% of the ACh receptors be free of blocking agent. This parameter is slightly more sensitive than the single twitch in detecting partial receptor blockade. In a study of D-tubocurarine (dTC) in cats in which twitch, T_4, and 50 Hz responses were compared, it was shown that change in tension of the fourth twitch in the T_4 train was the most sensitive indicator of blockade (15). An advantage of using the T_4FR to assess blockade is that comparison with a baseline twitch amplitude is not necessary.

During dTC blockade with 75 to 80% twitch depression, the T_4FR is zero (that is, the fourth response in the train has disappeared). The third response is lost when the single twitch (or first response in the train) is depressed 80 to 90%. Thus, to maintain adequate relaxation for abdominal, ocular, or limb surgery, increments of the blocking agent can be given until the fourth twitch in the train simply disappears. Additional increments can be given to maintain the block as the fourth twitch reappears. A schematic representation of the idealized relationship of twitch depression to T_4 fade is shown (Fig. 9.1).

Unfortunately, the relationship of twitch to T_4FR is not fixed, but varies with species, muscle type, and the drug being studied as well as the time after instituting blockade. For example, facial nerve-lip muscle system shows very little T_4 (or tetanic) fade in sheep (L.V. Klein, unpublished clinical observations), ponies (16), and horses (17), when compared to the peroneal nerve-digital extensor preparation, especially early in the blockade. Even in the peroneal nerve-digital extensor system, the horse shows very little T_4 fade initially with vecuronium compared to other blocking agents (18). The clinical importance of this lack of T_4 fade is that if the loss of third and fourth twitch is sought as an end point in titrating initial relaxation, overdose may result.

RESPONSE TO TETANIC STIMULATION

Stimulation of rates of 30 to 50 Hz for 5 seconds yields a sustained contraction if only 25% of ACh receptors are available. Sustained tetanus at 100 Hz requires about 50%, and at 200 Hz, 60 to 65% are required (19). In anesthetized animals without neuromuscular blockade or disease, a nearly flat response (sustained contraction) is seen with tetanic stimulation at 30 to 100 Hz, but some individuals may have significant fade during 200-Hz stimulation (20). During nondepolarizing blockade, significant fade is seen with tetanic stimulation so that the response may resemble a single twitch (Fig. 9.2). Fade in response to tetanus is easy to detect by observation and is a sensitive indicator of partial blockade, but if twitch tension is being evaluated during maintenance of blockade, tetanic stimulation should be avoided after tetanus. Significant decurarization occurs in the response to the single twitch, and this phenomenon makes it difficult to assess and maintain the desired degree of block.

RESPONSES TO NERVE STIMULATION DURING SCh BLOCKADE

After administration of a single dose of SCh, muscle contraction occurs and is observed as spontaneous fasciculations or jerks followed by paralysis. The fasciculations have been attributed by postsynapticists to depolarization of the muscle resulting from SCh activation of the ACh receptor at the motor end plate. Presynaptic advocates suggest fasciculations are due to release of ACh in response to depolarization of the motor nerve terminal by activation of presynaptic ACh receptors (12). Initially during paralysis with SCh, there is a flat T_4 response (no fade, Fig. 9.1). Described classically, tetanic responses are weak but sustained, and tetanus does not cause augmentation of subsequent twitch responses. Administration of facilitatory drugs, such as neostigmine or edrophonium, enhances the block at this time. These characteristics define depolarization (or Phase I) block, but the story is not so simple. Depending on the species, anesthetic, and muscle type, the responses vary. For example, in the hal-

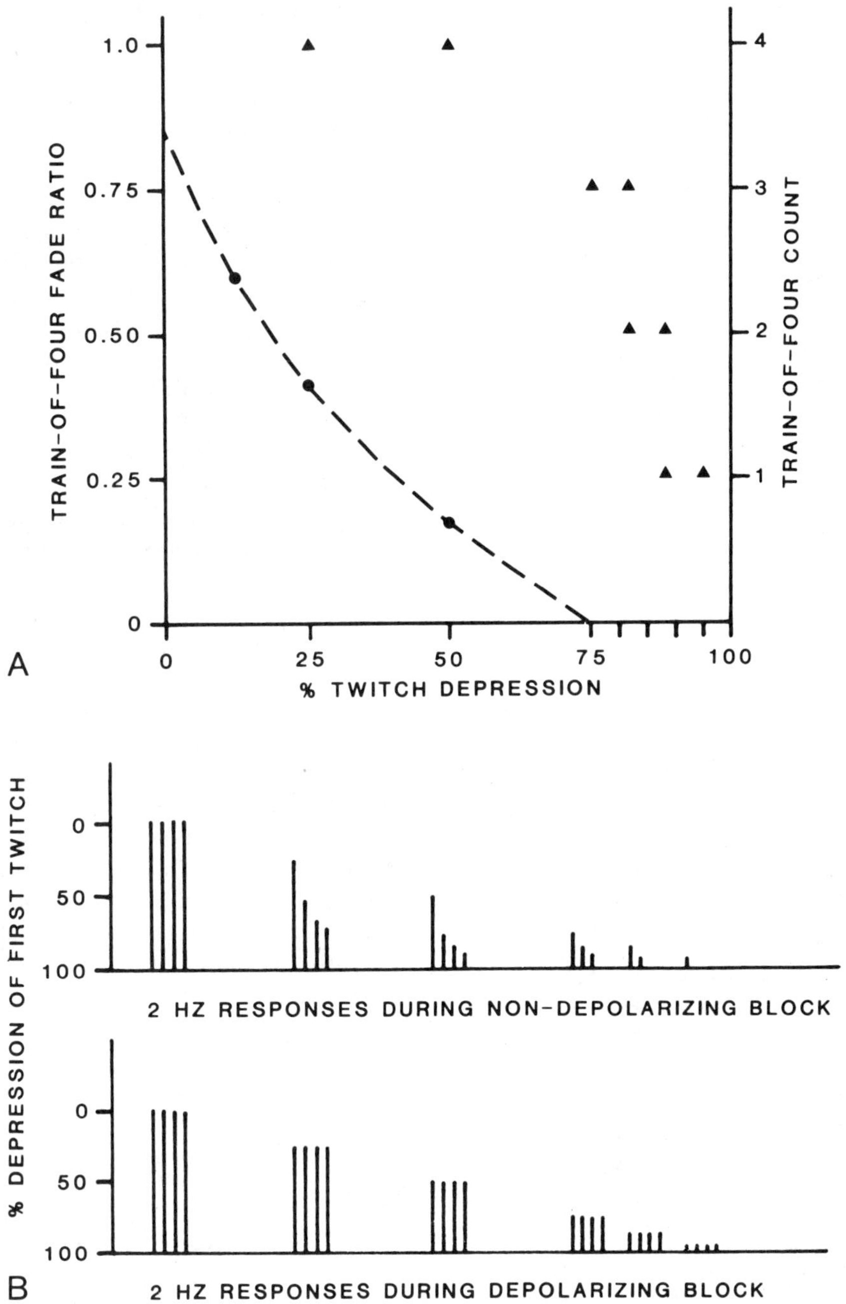

Figure 9.1. *A*, Relationship of train-of-four fade ratio and train-of-four count (2 Hz) to depression of the single twitch during nondepolarizing blockade. *B*, Comparison of train-of-four responses during nondepolarizing and pure depolarizing blockade.

othane-anesthetized horse, a single subparalyzing dose of SCh results in a flat T_4 response, but there may be 80% fade in the response to 5-second 100-Hz stimulation of the peroneal nerve. Neostigmine will enhance the block. In the rat, initial blockade by SCh can be immediately antagonized with neostigmine (21).

In all species studied, repeated doses or prolonged infusion of SCh results in a change in the character of the block. After a period of tachyphylaxis, there is a sudden shift to a block (Phase II) resembling nondepolarizing block. Fade during T_4 and tetanic stimulation becomes prominent, and facilitatory drugs at least partially antagonize the block. In humans, a Phase II block with a T_4FR of less than 0.3 is said to be reversible (22).

Clinical Monitoring of Neuromuscular Function

MECHANICAL RESPONSES

Several inexpensive peripheral nerve stimulators that have the capability to deliver single-twitch, train-

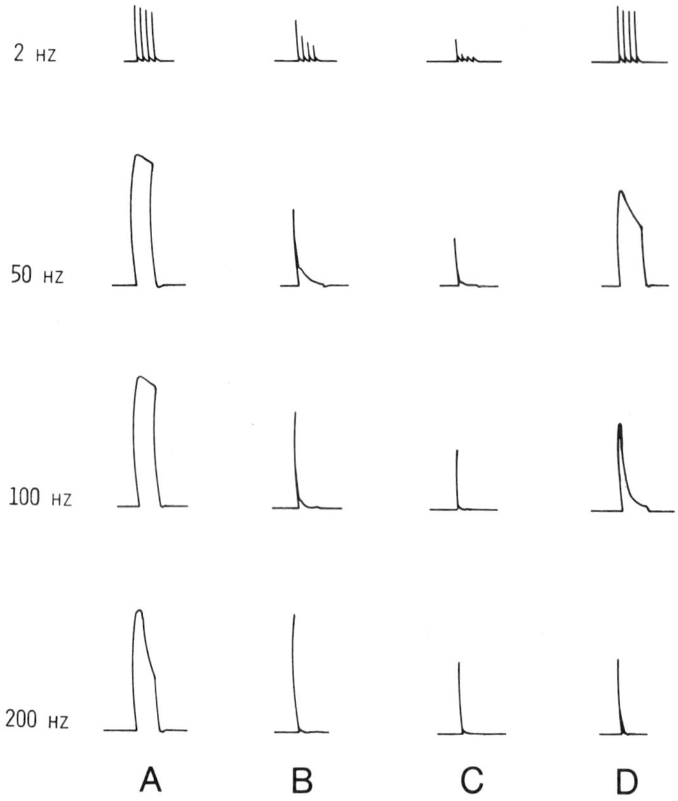

Figure 9.2. Mechanical responses to electrical stimulation of deep peroneal nerve at various frequencies in a halothane-anesthetized horse. Tetanic stimuli were applied for 5 seconds. *A*, Before neuromuscular blockade, tension is well maintained at frequencies up to 100 Hz. *B*, Partial pancuronium-induced blockade: twitch strength (first response at 2 Hz) is depressed approximately 25%, and fade is obvious at 2 Hz. Responses to higher frequency stimulation indicate decreased maximal tension and marked fade. *C*, An additional dose of pancuronium is given. Twitch strength is depressed 60% from control. Third and fourth responses during 2 Hz stimulation have almost disappeared. *D*, Partial recovery: twitch strength and train-of-four are normal, but marked fade is revealed during higher frequency stimulation (213). (reprinted with permission of W.B. Saunders Co.).

of-four (2 Hz) stimuli as well as tetanic stimuli are available (Dupaco, San Marcos, California; J. H. Emerson Co., Cambridge, Massachusetts; and Neuro Technology Inc., Houston, Texas). Sites for stimulation of peripheral motor nerves include the peroneal nerve, which can be palpated as it crosses the shaft of the fibula just distal to the head of that bone, the facial nerve at its location ventral to the eye, and in small animals the ulnar nerve at its superficial location on the medial aspect of the elbow (Fig. 9.3).

Whenever possible, responses to nerve stimulation should be observed in the anesthetized animal before establishing neuromuscular blockade to demonstrate successful electrode placement and to obtain baseline responses for comparison with responses during blockade and reversal.

OBSERVING MECHANICAL RESPONSES

In the experimental situation, evoked isometric tension is recorded, whereas in the clinical situation, strength of contraction is usually evaluated by observation of excursion of the body part. In the author's experience, a 50% depression in twitch strength, as recorded isometrically on a preloaded muscle group, may not be apparent when the twitch response is observed visually in the unloaded muscle group. T_4 fade is more easily observed, but even 60% fade (T_4FR = 0.4) may not be detectable by experienced observers (23). Manual restraint of the limb and palpation of the responses is a somewhat more sensitive method, but the degree of blockade is still underestimated until about 80 to 90% blockade, when the fourth twitch disappears. Far more sensitive, due to the more rigorous test to the system and the inherent capabilities of the eye or hand, is continuous observation and palpation of the response to several seconds of tetanic stimulation. Partial fatiguing or fade in the response is easily detected. To get accurate and consistent evaluation, one must be careful to use a supramaximal stimulus and to evaluate the response over a consistent time period. Five seconds is the conventional period used. It allows enough time for initial fade and stabilization of the response. Tetanic fade during high frequency (≥100 Hz) stimulation is the most sensitive indicator of partial blockade, but in some cases (e.g., facial nerve in herbivores) T_4 and tetanic fade are apparent only after the block has been present for some time. Thus, fade is a poor indicator during onset of blockade; initial tetanic tension is a better parameter.

ELECTROMYOGRAPHIC RESPONSES

Because of the logistic problems encountered in quantitative evaluation of mechanical responses to nerve stimulation in the clinical setting, attempts have been made to use evoked compound action potential to evaluate neuromuscular block. A clinical motor is now available that uses T_4 stimulation at 20-second intervals (NMT 221, Puritan-Bennett, Wilmington, Massachusetts). Provided that preblockade responses have been recorded, the monitor quantitates the percentage of action potential amplitude depression (analgous to percentage of twitch depression). It also quantitates decrement during 2-Hz stimulation (T_4 fade). Although the information provided by this monitor is clearly more reliable than that gained from observation, there are some problems with its use, especially in animals. Electrodes are of the paste-on type, requiring shaving and defatting of the skin for good adherence. If the animal moves or sweats excessively, they may be dislodged. A change in electrode position will make it impossible to compare responses with those

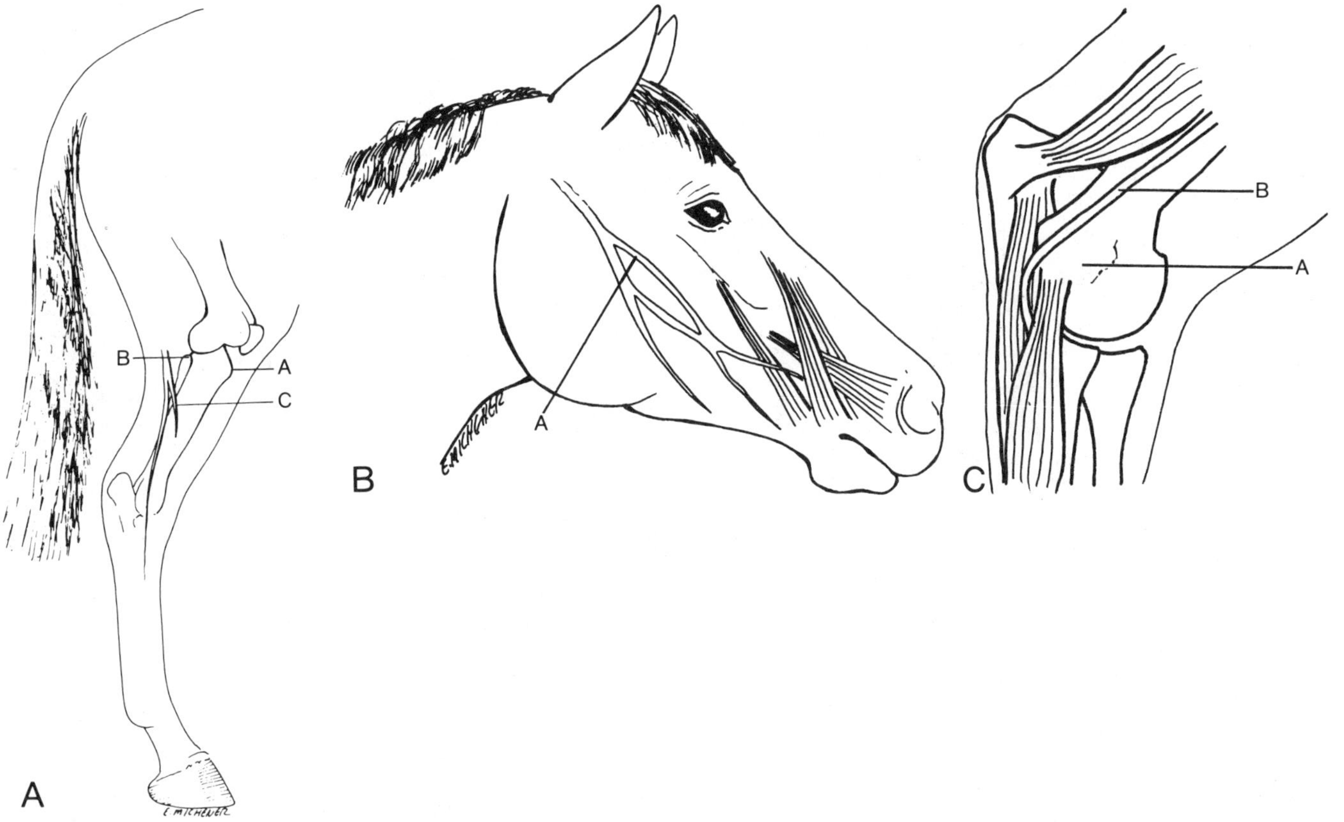

Figure 9.3. *A*, Subcutaneous location of the deep peroneal nerve for stimulation. *A*, Tibial tuberosity; *B*, Head of fibula. Motor branch *C* to digital extensor muscles can be palpated as it crosses shaft of the fibula (213). *B*, Subcutaneous location of facial nerve for stimulation. Placement of negative electrode just ventral to the lateral canthus (*A*) insures that direct stimulation of the levator and zygomaticus muscles does not occur (213). *C*, Medial view of canine elbow showing subcutaneous location of ulnar nerve. *A*, Medial epicondyle of humerus; *B*, ulnar nerve (reprinted with permission of W.B. Saunders Co.).

originally obtained in the baseline state. This is not a serious drawback, because T_4 fade is unaffected by change in electrode position and can be used to estimate degree of blockade. Electrode pads are large and must be placed a minimum of 1.5 to 3 inches apart, precluding their use in smaller individuals. If electrodes could be modified to overcome these problems in small animals, the monitor would be very useful. The following should be kept in mind when using EMG responses. Before recording the baseline amplitude, the response should be observed until it has stabilized, because it may initially increase in amplitude and then drift downward for several minutes. During nondepolarizing blockade, the EMG response consistently underestimates the degree of mechanical weakness, with one study showing an offset in the regression line of 15%. Thus an EMG depression of 60% was associated with an average mechanical twitch depression of 75% (range, 55 to 90%), and an EMG T_4/T_1 ratio of 0.7 predicted a mechanical T_4/T_1 ratio of 0.4 (24–26). If these relationships and their variability are understood, the EMG can be used to establish the desired degree of block and accurately detect a need for top-up doses. The magnitude and duration of effect of these doses can be evaluated with precision. Using the monitor to assess recovery and reversal may not be satisfactory; the author prefers to evaluate mechanical tetanic responses during reversal.

Other Methods of Assessing Degree of Blockade

In some instances, it may be necessary to establish and antagonize neuromuscular blockade without the use of a nerve stimulator, and one must rely on observations of spontaneous or mechanically evoked muscle movements to assess blockade. If shorter-acting drugs are used, such as vecuronium and atracurium, this can probably be done safely. The inability to sustain a muscle contraction is the hallmark of nondepolarizing blockade; as the block develops, eyelid reflexes, anal reflex, spontaneous limb movements, and respiratory efforts to fight the ventilator become incomplete and jerky in nature. If some or all of these parameters are

Table 9.1
Doses of Neuromuscular Blocking Agents in Domestic Species

Species	Dose (μg/kg)	Muscle	% Twitch Depression	Duration (Min)	Duration Criterion	Anesthetic	Reference
				Gallamine			
Calf	400		100%	10–240			198
Sheep	6.0/per min	Rectus abdominis	80 (EMG)[b]	(Steady state)			194
Lamb	400			10–240			198
Horse	793 ± 52	Hindlimb extensor	80	14–40 min	75% dep to 50% recovery	Halothane-O_2	31
Pig	2000–4000			10–20			198, 202
Dog	400	Tibialis	100	26 ± 7[c]	10% recovery of twitch	Halothane	201
				40 ± 11[c]	100% recovery of twitch		
Cat	300–11000						203
	1000		100 (apnea)	10–20	Spontaneous respiration		202
	1200	Gastrocnemius	98 ± 2.6	24 ± 9.4	100% recovery?	Halothane/α-chloralose	204
				Pancuronium			
Calf	43 ± 9[c]	Hindlimb digital extensor	90–99	43 ± 19[c]	To 100% recovery	Halothane-O_2	54
Sheep	5.0 ± 0.61	Hindlimb digital extensor	80	21.0 ± 2.5	To 50% recovery	Halothane-O_2	55
	0.15/per min	Rectus abdominis	80 (EMG)[b]	Steady state		?	194
Horse	82 ± 7.3	Hindlimb extensor	80	20–35 min	To 50% recovery	Halothane-O_2	31
Pony	125 ± 20[c]	Hindlimb digital extensor	90–99	16 min	To 50% recovery	Halothane-O_2	56
Pig	~50		Surgical relaxation			Thiopental N_2O-O_2 or ketamine	199
	10						203
Dog	22 ± 3		90	108 ± 10	Return to 50% control twitch from 3 × ED 90	Halothane	205
Cat	20	Gastrocnemius	80	15 ± 2	100% recovery?[d]	Halothane/α-chloralose	204
	22	Tibialis	88 ± 5	14 ± 2	50% recovery of twitch	Pentobarbital	206
	34	Tibialis	50	8.8 ± 2.3	100% recovery? (not stated)	α-Chloralose/pentobarbital	207
				D-Tubocurarine			
Calf, lamb	60						202
Sheep	44.5 ± 3.2	Hindlimb digital extensor	80	25.2 ± 4.1	85% depression to 50% recovery	Halothane-O_2	55
	0.5/min	Rectus abdominis	80 (EMG)	Steady state			194
Dog	130 ± 19		90	100 ± 19	Return to 50% control twitch from 3 × ED 90	Halothane	205
Cat	200	Gastrocnemius	97 ± 2.7	20 ± 6.2	100% recovery?[d]	Halothane/α-chloralose	204
				Atracurium			
Sheep	~4–7/min (1 hr infusion)	Rectus abdominis	~70–90 (EMG)	~20–30 min	70–90% depression to 95% recovery	Thiopental-N_2O-O_2	195
Horse	70	Hindlimb digital extensor	95–99	~28 min	Maximium depression to 75% recovery	Halothane-O_2	196
Pony	110 ± 10[c]	Hindlimb extensor	98 ± 0.9	~35 min	Maximum depression to 75% recovery	Halothane-O_2	57

Table 9.1—continued

Species	Dose (μg/kg)	Muscle	% Twitch Depression	Duration (Min)	Duration Criterion	Anesthetic	Reference
Dog	125	Gastrocnemius	97 ± 11.5	22 ± 2.8	100% recovery of twitch	α-Chloralose	208
	200	Ulnar nerve—Carpal flexors	100	24.5	100% recovery of twitch	Thiopental-N_2O-O_2	209
Cat	250	Gastrocnemius	99 ± 1.43	29 ± 2.5	100% recovery of twitch	Halothane/chloralose/pentobarbital	208
	125	Gastrocnemius	54 ± 12.9	11 ± 2.2	100% recovery of twitch	Halothane/α-chloralose/pentobarbital	208
				Vecuronium			
Sheep	4.61 ± 0.23	Hindlimb digital extensor	80	13.8 ± 1.7	86% depression to 50% recovery	Halothane-O_2	55
Horse	108 ± 4.5	Hindlimb extensor	80	20–40 min	85% depression to 50% recovery	Halothane-O_2	17
Dog	14 ± 3		90	42 ± 2	Time to 50% recovery of twitch after 3 × ED 90	Halothane	205
Cat	35	Tibialis	88 ± 4	8.3 ± 1.2	90% recovery of twitch	α-Chloralose/pentobarbital	181
	25–40	Tibialis	81 ± 6	9 ± 1	50% recovery of twitch	Pentobarbital	206
	24 ± 3	Tibialis	50	5.0 ± 0.5	25% to 75% recovery of twitch	Isoflurane	210
				Succinycholine			
Horse	330	Hindlimb	100	(Loading dose)		Halothane-O_2	197
	37/min	Hindlimb	100	Steady state		Halothane-O_2	197
Rabbit	500			5–10			198
Ruminants	20			6–8			198, 202
Dog	400	Tibialis	100	22 ± 12[c]	10% recovery of twitch	Halothane	201
	300	Gastrocnemius	100	25 ± 4[d]	50% recovery of twitch	Thiopental N_2O-O_2	211
Cat	75		100			α-Chloralose	212
	100	Front Leg	100	2.9–11.7	100% recovery	Halothane-O_2	200
Pig	2000			2–3 min			202

[a] Mean ± SEM unless noted.
[b] Electromyographic response.
[c] Mean ± SD.
[d] Not stated.

observed at 3 to 5 minutes after incremental drug administration during a stable plane of anesthesia, a desired level of block can be achieved without risk of dangerous overdose leading to a long recovery. In the recovery and reversal stage, similar criteria are used.

Several excellent review articles on monitoring blockade are available (27–29).

Administration of Blocking Agents in the Clinical Situation

Species requirements for the blocking agents are listed in Table 9.1. In general, ketamine and the volatile inhalants enhance the effects of the agents compared to narcotics, barbiturates, and N_2O. Considerable individual variation exists as well. In clinical studies in humans, a standard dose of 0.1 mg/kg dTC produced 0 to 100% block (30). Considerable variation exists in animals also, even under controlled conditions of uniform anesthetic depth and ventilation (31). Certain anesthetics, other drugs, and disease states can further affect sensitivity, and these are discussed in a later section. For these reasons, the author prefers to use an incremental approach to establishing blockade, starting with about one-half of the mean dose to produce 80 to 95% block for the species. (Controlled ventilation should be instituted before drug administration). Further increments can be given at 3- to 5-minute intervals as the response is assessed. This method of administration avoids overdose and minimizes autonomic effects. The end point is a weak twitch or a weak tetanus, loss of fourth response in T_4, or cessation or weakening of spontaneous muscle activity. If the block is to be maintained after signs of recovery from the initial dosage are seen, increments of one-quarter to one-third the original total dose can be given as needed. For most of the agents, recovery rates decrease after multiple top-up doses. This cumulative effect is less obvious with the newer, shorter-acting agents, vecuronium and atracurium, than with older agents.

As shorter-acting, nondepolarizing drugs with little or no cardiovascular effects are developed, less conservative use may be possible, because the only real disadvantages of overdose are prolonged paralysis and heart rate and blood pressure changes.

The duration of action of SCh is short enough that an incremental dosage method is not necessary except in patients suspected of having markedly reduced pseudocholinesterase levels. In normal individuals, duration of SCh action after a single large dose is not likely to exceed even a short anesthetic period.

SCh is the only drug with an onset and recovery time suitably short for "emergency" paralysis for intubation and control of respiration. If SCh is undesirable in an individual because of expected untoward effects (and there are many, discussed in a later section), the alternative is to "overdose" with a nondepolarizing agent to shorten onset time. Vecuronium is probably the best agent to use because of its lack of cardiovascular effects and relatively shorter duration of action (32, 33). The priming principle is advocated by some authors (34–39), that is, giving a very small dose of the agent to the awake patient to "preload" the receptors without compromising airway and respiratory control. This is followed at a fixed interval (3 to 8 minutes, depending on authors) with the remainder of a "normal" paralyzing dose. This method is said to speed onset time and obviate the need for excessive doses for intubation. Priming seems to work better in some hands than others, and there are isolated reports in humans of significant respiratory muscle weakness and pulmonary aspiration after priming doses of nondepolarizers (37, 39). In a recent study, the optimal priming dose and interval for vecuronium was established for humans (40).

Nonrelaxant Properties of Blocking Agents

CARDIOVASCULAR EFFECTS OF NEUROMUSCULAR BLOCKING AGENTS

The newer blocking agents have been synthesized with the intent to minimize or eliminate unwanted cardiovascular effects; indeed, vecuronium is virtually devoid of these effects in clinically useful doses (41–43). Atracurium has little or no effect at autonomic receptor sites, but in some patients, especially with high doses, histamine release may be expected (44–46). This is a relatively rare occurrence compared to the histamine release seen with dTC. In the domestic species, clinically important histamine release and ganglionic blockade occur with dTC and results in severe hypotension in dogs and cats (47, 48) as well as a decrease in pulmonary compliance in dogs (49). In those species, dTC should be avoided. Gallamine and pancuronium are vagolytic; pancuronium releases norepinephrine (50), causing tachycardia, especially in lightly anesthetized individuals. Cardiovascular changes vary depending on the species and anesthetic agent. Gallamine partially blocked vagal-induced bradycardia but did not cause significant tachycardia in anesthetized dogs (51). In awake, unpremedicated dogs given pancuronium and then intubated, tachycardia, hypertension, and ventricular premature contractions occurred. When dogs were premedicated with acetylpromazine or sedative doses or Innovar, pulse rate and blood pressure changes were less and arrhythmias were not observed (52). In halothane-anesthetized dogs, pancuronium caused increases in heart rate and blood pressure, and positive inotropy was observed (53). In halothane-anesthetized calves, pancuronium did not alter heart rate or blood pressure (54). Halothane-anesthetized sheep showed no change in heart rate or blood pressure when dTC, pancuronium, or vecuronium were given (55). In horses, no changes were seen after gallamine, pancuronium, or vecuronium (17, 31). In horses, hypotension did not occur when dTC was used (A.M. Klide, personal communication). In ponies, slight significant increases in heart rate and blood pressure occurred after pancuronium (56), but no changes occurred with atracurium (57). When choosing a neuromuscular blocking agent for a particular patient, cardiovascular effects of the drug should be weighed against the cardiovascular status of the individual. For example, in some patients at risk for development of opioid or surgically induced vagal effects, drugs such as gallamine may offer protection against bradycardia and hypotension compared to vecuronium and even pancuronium (58, 59).

SCh may cause either vagal or sympathomimetic effects, depending on whether muscarinic or sympathetic ganglionic receptors are activated. In awake horses, tachycardia, severe hypertension, and ventricular arrhythmias have been reported after SCh administration (60). In halothane-anesthetized horses, increase or decreases of 10 to 15 mm Hg in blood pressure may be seen. In dogs, hypotension and arrhythmias have been reported (61). In humans, severe bradycardia, conduction disturbances and hypotension have been seen when a second dose of SCh follows the first by about 5 minutes. Thiopental or a small dose of a nondepolarizing agent given just before the SCh is somewhat protective against this occurrence. The bradycardia responds to intravenous atropine but intramuscular atropine in the premedication regime seems to offer no protection (62–66).

PLACENTAL TRANSFER AND NEONATAL EFFECTS OF BLOCKING AGENTS

All of the clinically used neuromuscular blocking agents are large ionized compounds that cross membranes slowly compared to lipophyllic anesthetic drugs. Nevertheless, maternally administered pancuronium, vecuronium, and atracurium have been shown to cross the human placenta. In these studies, umbilical venous levels occasionally reached those that result in up to 50% twitch depression in adult humans, yet neuromuscular blockade was not clinically evident in the newborn infants (67–70). Likewise, when pregnant cats and ferrets were paralyzed with SCh, gallamine, pancuronium, and dTC, fetal twitch strength was unaffected (71). Even when very high doses of blocking agents 30 to 100 times the maternal paralyzing dose were injected into the uterine artery of the pregnant bitch, not all the puppies were clinically weak (72, 73). The reasons for the lack of fetal newborn effects of the drugs are not known, but they may be due partly to differences in sensitivity or protein binding. The results of the animal studies, combined with the continued safe widespread clinical use of neuromuscular blocking agents for Caesarean section in humans, support their safety for that use.

CENTRAL NERVOUS SYSTEM EFFECTS

Encephalographic (EEG) studies in awake, ventilated dogs showed decreased amplitude of high frequency activity and an increased occurrence of slow waves in those dogs given SCh (74). The authors concluded that because these changes mimic certain disease states, SCh may be unsuitable for EEG studies.

SCh injection has been shown to increase cerebrospinal fluid pressure (CSF) in healthy, anesthetized humans, dogs, and cats. The increase was not prevented by controlled ventilation (75–77). Spontaneous purposeful movement is seen occasionally in very lightly anesthetized animals given SCh, and EEG evidence of arousal has been reported (75, 77). These effects are probably due to increased afferent activity from muscle spindles during fasciculations rather than direct central nervous system (CNS) stimulation by the relaxant, and they can be prevented by prior administration of nondepolarizing agents (78). In contrast, pancuronium has been shown to decrease anesthetic requirement. Whether this phenomenon is due to a peripheral or central effect on sensory pathways is not known (79, 80).

INTRAOCULAR PRESSURE

It is known that SCh administration results in an increase in intraocular pressure, theoretically posing a hazard to patients with open eye injuries, although there have been no reports of actual vitreous loss in human patients (81). Because intubation in animal patients is easily accomplished without SCh, it seems best to avoid the drug in these patients. The nondepolarizing agents decrease intraocular pressure and are more suitable for providing muscle relaxation for intraocular procedures (82–85). A review of nonrelaxant actions of blocking agents is available (86).

PROTEIN BINDING, METABOLISM, AND EXCRETION

All of the clinically used neuromuscular blocking agents have been found to bind extensively (70 to 90%) to plasma proteins (87–90). The theoretic significance of protein binding is that disease states lowering plasma proteins and drugs competing for binding sites may lower relaxant requirements. In addition, considerable individual variation in protein binding has been found (90). These considerations provide further arguments for incremental rather than single bolus drug administration to establish blockade. In addition to plasma binding, the agents have been found to bind to mucopolysaccharides in tendons, cartilage, and blood vessel walls during the early redistribution phases.

The kidney is virtually the only route for elimination of gallamine (91–93). Cholestasis does not prolong its action in cats (94). Although significant hepatic metabolism of pancuronium has been documented, the kidney provides the major route for the excretion of the drug and its metabolites. Pancuronium-induced neuromuscular blockade is prolonged in renal failure as well as in biliary obstruction (92–95). Although the major pathway for elimination of dTC is through the kidney, significant amounts are normally excreted in bile, and its action is not prolonged in human patients in renal failure (93). Vecuronium has both hepatic and renal excretion pathways (96). Its duration is only slightly prolonged in human patients with no renal function (97), but clearance is significantly reduced in those with liver disease (98). Among the nondepolarizing agents, atracurium is unique in that its degradation depends on neither renal nor hepatic function. In human patients with no renal function, the action of atracurium was not prolonged (99). At body pH and temperature, the drug is unstable; it breaks down by "Hoffman elimination," i.e., cleavage of the bond between the quaternary nitrogen atoms and the aliphatic portions of the molecule. This destroys the bisquaternary structure and blocking activity. In addition, breakdown by plasma esterases (not dependent on pseudocholinesterase) has been documented (100, 101). The relative importance of these pathways in domestic species is speculative. Some concern has been expressed for the toxicity of the breakdown products of atracurium, laudanosine and monoacrylate (100, 102, 103). In concentrations higher than those achieved after clinical use of atracurium, laudanosine has CNS excitatory effects. When atracurium is used in patients without renal function, laudanosine levels are higher than those found in normal patients (102). The possibility also exists that laudanosine could accumulate in patients in whom infusions of atracurium have been given over long periods. So far, there has been no clinical evidence of laudanosine toxicity. In a study using rats, hydrolysis by plasma carboxylesterase was found to be crucial in determining the duration of action of atracurium, and the authors suggest that this pathway is more important than Hoffman elimination, at least in the rat (100).

SCh is so rapidly destroyed by plasma cholinesterase that under normal circumstances most of the injected dose does not even reach the neuromuscular junction. For this reason, sensitivity varies dramatically with cholinesterase levels. Considerable species differences exist, and numerous drugs, especially organophosphate compounds, lower enzyme levels, prolonging paralysis (104). In humans, an atypical cholinesterase can be inherited that is nearly incapable of hydrolyzing SCh at plasma levels normally expected after injection. In humans with atypical cholinesterase, the action of standard doses of SCh is greatly prolonged (105). This genetic variant has not been documented in domestic animals. Review articles on pharmacokinetics of blocking agents are available (93, 105, 106).

Intrinsic and Extrinsic Factors Affecting Responses to Blocking Agents

In addition to the aforementioned effects of renal or hepatic failure and enzyme deficiency on duration of blockade, a number of intrinsic and extrinsic factors alter dose-response relationships and are responsible for some of the clinically observed variations in sensitivity.

AGE

The very young and very old react to blocking agents differently from other age groups. Human neonates and infants require lower plasma concentrations of dTC than older children and adults to effect blockade, but because neonates and infants have a larger volume of distribution, dose rates for dTC are similar in adults. Clearance of dTC is decreased in neonates and infants, and so decreased recovery rates would be expected after multiple doses (107, 108). Because of the large volume of distribution, dose rates of SCh for infants are higher than for adults (109). In elderly patients, increased sensitivity and increased duration of blocking agents have been attributed to loss of end plate receptors, decreased plasma binding and volume of distribution, and decreased renal perfusion (106). Onset time has also been shown to be longer in older patients, possibly reflecting lower cardiac output and muscle perfusion (110). These studies have been done in humans, but may apply to animals as well.

TEMPERATURE

Development of hypothermia prolongs recovery of muscle strength in paralyzed animals and humans. In one study, EMG responses recovered normally whereas mechanical weakness was prolonged with hypothermia, suggesting that low temperatures affect contractility rather than neuromuscular transmission. Onset time is also delayed in hypothermic patients, possibly because of reduced blood flow to muscle (106–108).

NEUROLOGICAL AND MUSCLE DISEASE

Animals and humans with myasthenia gravis are very sensitive to nondepolarizing neuromuscular blocking agents (111, 112). If these drugs must be used in myasthenic patients, it is probably best to use the newer, shorter-acting agents vecuronium and atracurium at dose rates of ¼ to ½ those for normal patients (113, 114). Other disease states causing abnormalities of neuromuscular transmission, such as botulism, myasthenic syndrome, and amyotrophic lateral sclerosis (115), result in increased sensitivity to blocking agents in humans. Myotonic patients respond normally to nondepolarizing blocking agents, but SCh may cause exaggerated and prolonged fasciculations and spasms, making intubation and ventilation impossible (116). Likewise, facilitatory drugs given to antagonize nondepolarizing blockade may cause prolonged contractures. In halothane-anesthetized horses with myotonia, neostigmine given in incremental doses of 20 μg/kg did not precipitate spasms (L.V. Klein, unpublished clinical observations). A number of conditions result in resistance to nondepolarizing agents. These include upper motor neuron lesions (116), hemiplegia (117), denervation, disuse atrophy (118), and burns (119). In patients with these conditions and those with crush injuries, tetanus, malignant hyperthermia, and closed head injuries, SCh administration is followed by exaggerated fasciculations, contractures, and/or lethal K^+ release. In injured patients, the exaggerated K^+ release may be seen as early as 5 days postinjury; in patients with upper motor neuron lesions, they may persist for up to 6 months (120–130). A review of the pathophysiology of SCh-induced hyperkalemia is available (131).

ANESTHETICS

Although depressant effects on neuromuscular function have been found for narcotics, barbiturates, phenothiazine derivatives, buterophenones, and benzodiazepines (132–138) greater potentiation of neuromuscular blocking agents is seen with volatile inhalants and ketamine (139). Dose requirements for blocking agents are higher with narcotic-N_2O techniques than with volatile inhalants. Isoflurane and enflurane have a greater effect than halothane and methoxyflurane (140–143). Enflurane is interesting in that its effect increases with time of exposure, even when alveolar levels are held constant (142).

ANTIBIOTICS

Several classes of antibiotics have neuromuscular blocking properties, and both pre- and postsynaptic mechanisms have been identified (144–154). The blocking effect has been shown experimentally in a wide variety of species, and there are numerous reports in the human literature of clinically significant respiratory paralysis occurring after antibiotic administration. Most of the reports describe synergism with neuromusuclar blocking agents or anesthetics, but in debilitated patients or those with muscle weakness, antibiotics may act alone to cause paralysis. The characteristics of neomycin blockade were studied in the cat (146). It was found that during almost complete twitch inhibition, tetanus was maintained but was followed by a profound post-tetanic depression. The authors concluded that a patient with antibiotic-induced muscle weakness might be able to respond to a single tetanic stimulus with a sustained muscle contraction and therefore appear to have adequate strength, yet become substantially fatigued in trying to maintain adequate ventilation over a long period of time. Among the aminoglycosides, gentamycin and tobramycin have less neuromuscular effect than neomycin and streptomycin (147), but significant blocking action was found for gentamycin in the cat (150). Acute collapse during tetracycline administration has been seen in horses and cattle, and tetracycline has been shown to decrease ACh release. Neuromuscular blockade (as evidenced by twitch depression) could not be demonstrated after up to 28 mg/kg oxytetracycline in horses unless they were pretreated with magnesium (145). The reason for collapse remains obscure. Blockade by aminoglycosides and tetracyclines can be at least partially antagonized by calcium, but in a study in cattle, tetracycline did not decrease serum-ionized calcium. Polymixin A,B and colistin produce a significant blockade that cannot be antagonized by calcium or neostigmine.

Care should always be taken not to exceed recommended doses of these antibiotics, and it should be remembered that drugs administered into the pleural or peritoneal cavity may gain rapid access to the systemic circulation. Animals with pre-existing muscle weakness due to disease or neuromuscular blocking agents should be monitored carefully during and after administration of these drugs.

ACID-BASE BALANCE

There are numerous conflicting reports of the effects of acute acid-base changes on responses to neuromuscular blocking agents (155–158). The most consistent and clinically important finding has been that respiratory acidosis potentiates nondepolarizing blockade. At $PaCO_2$ levels of about 60 mm Hg and above, blockade cannot be completely antagonized. One study using vecuronium in cats showed that the magnitude of effect varied with muscle type. The soleus and diaphragm were more affected than the tibialis (155). This has obvious clinical implications in that respiratory muscle weakness may go undetected in the clinical situation because muscles normally used for monitoring blockade are likely to be predominantly fast twitch muscles, such as the tibialis.

ELECTROLYTE DISTURBANCES

Hypermagnesemia potentiates the neuromuscular blockade of both SCh and nondepolarizing agents. Clinical weakness unresponsive to neostigmine has been seen in a hypermagnesemic horse given a large dose of $MgSO_4$ for colic who was subsequently paralyzed with gallamine for control of respiration during anesthesia (L.V. Klein, unpublished clinical data). Parturient women treated with magnesium sulfate for preeclamptic hyperreflexia have exaggerated and prolonged responses to both SCh infusions and nondepolarizing blocking agents (159–161). Magnesium blockade or Mg^{++}-nondepolarizing blockade may respond partially to calcium administration, but because Phase II SCh block is augmented by Ca^{++}, it should not be used if a Mg^{++}-SCh block is present (162).

The effects of alterations of Ca^{++}, K^{+}, and Na^{+} are less clearly documented (163). In some instances, hypokalemia will augment the effects of nondepolarizing blocking agents (164), and both hyperkalemia and hypercalcemia may increase relaxant requirements (165).

OTHER DRUGS

Many classes of drugs have been shown to affect neuromuscular transmission. The list seems endless,

Table 9.2
Drugs Shown to Interact with Neuromuscular Blocking Agents

Drug	Effects of Blockade: Depolarizing	Effects of Blockade: Nondepolarizing
Diuretics		
Furosemide, theophylline, thiazides, ethacrynic acid		↑ or ↓
Antiarrhythmics and local anesthetics		
Quinidine, procainamide, propranolol, phenytoin, lidocaine, dysopyramide	↑	↑ ↑
Hypotensive agents		
Nitroglycerine, trimethaphan		May ↑ or prolong
Anticancer drugs		
Azathioprine, cyclophosphamide	↑	↓
Insecticides and anthelmintics		
Carbamates, organophosphates	↑	Chronic exposure may ↑
Echothiophate eyedrops	↑	
Corticosteroids		↓
Epinephrine		↑ or ↓

and the effects of concomitant drug administration to patients receiving blocking agents are not always predictable either in direction or magnitude. Our sickest patients are often those likely to receive blocking agents, and they are the patients most likely to be given a variety of other drugs. Careful monitoring and titration of blocking agents and antagonists is very important in these animals. A partial list of drugs known to interact with blocking agents is shown in Table 9.2. Several review articles on factors affecting the action of neuromuscular blocking agents are available (164, 166, 167).

Other Effects of Neuromuscular Blocking Agents

Release of K^+, enzymes, and myoglobin from muscle occurs after succinylcholine administration, presumedly associated with the initial depolarizing action of the drug. Postoperative muscle pain is common in humans given SCh, and various agents have been used to prevent these untoward effects. Pretreatment with small doses of nondepolarizing agents is effective in preventing SCh-induced fasciculations, but there are conflicting results regarding the incidence of myalgia and release of K^+ and creatine kinase (168–171). Priming or "self-taming" with small doses of SCh prior to the intubation dose in humans reduces the incidence of fasciculations but does not prevent muscle pain (172). Pretreatment with diazepam did not prevent SCh-induced fasciculations in dogs (173), but did reduce the incidence of muscle pain in humans (174).

In susceptible individuals, SCh can trigger malignant hyperthermia. Malignant hyperthermia has been reported in swine, horses, dogs, and a cat (175) and may occur in captured wild animals.

Anaphylactic reactions to neuromuscular blocking agents have been reported and serum from patients who had life-threatening reactions showed cross reactivity to all the clinically used nondepolarizers and SCh (176). Fulminant pulmonary edema and pulmonary hemorrhage after intramuscular SCh have been reported in human infants, probably associated with sympathetic stimulation and pulmonary hypertension (177).

Reversal of Neuromuscular Blockade

The three facilitatory drugs used clinically for pharmacological antagonism of nondepolarizing blockade are edrophonium, neostigmine, and pyridostigmine. The traditionally held view is that they restore neuromuscular function because of their inhibitory action on acetylcholinesterase in the area of the motor end plate. This results in accumulation of ACh, allowing it to compete favorably with the relaxant for the cholinergic receptor. In addition to enzyme inhibition, the facilitatory drugs induce repetitive firing of the motor nerve terminal and enhance ACh release and mobilization. The relative importance of enzyme inhibition versus other proposed mechanisms is not entirely known. It has been suggested that edrophonium may have more presynaptic activity than the other drugs, but in studies using combinations of antagonists, simple additive rather than synergistic effects were found, arguing against different mechanisms of action (178). In the horse, when edrophonium was given after maximum (but not complete) antagonism of nondepolarizing blockade had been achieved with neostigmine, a transient deepening of tetanic fade resulted (20).

The time course of the antagonizing effects of

edrophonium, neostigmine, and pyridostigmine differs, with edrophonium having the most rapid effect (1 to 3 minutes) and, theoretically, the shortest duration of action. The effects of neostigmine are complete in 7 to 10 minutes; pyridostigmine requires about 10 to 15 minutes to work. In the past, the action of edrophonium has been considered to be of too short a duration to be used as an antagonist in the clinical setting, especially when longer acting blocking agents have been used. A study in humans paralyzed with dTC, however, showed that although edrophonium did not always completely restore twitch strength from deep blockade, there was no evidence of recurarization while the patients were monitored for up to 70 minutes (30).

Most instances of incomplete antagonism involve patients with very deep blockade, although enflurane anesthesia (179), other drugs, or disease states may also prevent adequate reversal. It has been stated that the deeper the block, the longer the antagonistic drug takes to work. This is misleading. When results of studies using infusions of blocking agents to produce constant levels of relaxation are examined, it will be seen that the effect of the facilitatory drug is rapid, but that at deeper levels of blockade, the antagonism is incomplete. In the clinical situation, administration of a facilitatory drug may only partially antagonize a very deep blockade. Further improvement occurs over time, representing spontaneous recovery. The rate of this recovery is independent of further doses of antagonist (30, 180).

Recent studies with edrophonium suggest that it is an effective and reliable antagonist, at least when used after the newer, shorter-acting blocking agents (181–184). An advantage of edrophonium over the other two drugs is that its rapid onset allows almost immediate assessment of adequacy of reversal. Some studies indicate edrophonium has fewer and more transient muscarinic effects than neostigmine (181), and edrophonium may have a greater effect on eliminating fade than neostigmine (183). Pyridostigmine may also have less autonomic activity than neostigmine. Its long onset time makes assessment of reversal inconvenient, especially if a titration method is used. Several good reviews of antagonism of blockade are available (178, 185, 186).

Administration of an anticholinesterase drug is usually followed by some manifestation of vagal stimulation, and neostigmine probably has a greater effect in this regard than edrophonium or pyridostigmine. Bradycardia, airway constriction, and secretions can be clinically troublesome. When neostigmine is given rapidly to awake or very lightly anesthetized animals, gastrointestinal stimulation may result in signs suggestive of abdominal discomfort. In halothane-anesthetized horses given neostigmine, bradycardia was not observed, but copious airway secretions were sometimes present. Administration of 11 μg/kg of atropine immediately before the first incremental dose of neostigmine minimized secretions (20). In ponies, 1 mg/kg of edrophonium or 40 μg/kg of neostigmine were used for reversal, and no comment was made about excessive vagal effects (16). In sheep given 10 μg/kg of glycopyrrolate prior to neostigmine reversal, no significant changes in heart rate occurred (55) and secretions were not excessive.

SUGGESTIONS FOR CLINICAL REVERSAL OF NEUROMUSCULAR BLOCKADE

Because of the variations seen in T_4 responses among species, muscle types, and individual nondepolarizing agents and the difficulty in visually recognizing T_4 fade, this parameter may not be the best for assessing reversal in animals. The antagonist should probably be used after blockade even if the T_4 response appears to be flat unless sustained contraction during 5-second 100-Hz stimulation can be demonstrated. For dogs and cats, atropine, 40 μg/kg, or glycopyrrolate, 20 μg/kg, should precede the antagonist drug unless it is thought that a tachycardia would not be tolerated due to the patient's cardiovascular status. If an anticholinergic drug is not used, the antagonist drug should be given very slowly in small increments with the patient under close electrocardiograph observation. In horses, 10 μg/kg and, in ruminants, 20 μg/kg of atropine or equivalent doses of glycopyrrolate seem sufficient to prevent significant vagal activity. If edrophonium is the antagonist, the anticholinergic drug may not be necessary in horses. In dogs and cats, a dose of 22 to 44 μg/kg of atropine has been suggested to prevent vagal effects from neostigmine reversal (187).

The most rational method of antagonist administration is titration while monitoring neuromuscular function. Spontaneous recovery should be allowed to progress so that all four twitches in the T_4 response are visible, otherwise adequate reversal may not be possible. Controlled ventilation should be continued to maintain normocarbia. Train-of-four fade ratio of 0.7 is said to be correlated well with adequate reversal in humans. This may not be true in all species. It is certainly not sufficient evidence of reversal in the horse, which has a psychological need to stand immediately on recovery from anesthesia. In horses and ruminants, good results are obtained giving 10- or 20-μg/kg increments of neostigmine at 6- or 7-minute intervals while monitoring 100 Hz responses until no further reduction in fade is seen. (If edrophonium is used, the interval can be shortened to 3 or 4 minutes.) This method can be applied to dogs and cats as well. In most reports in small animals, however, single large doses of antagonist were used. The potency of edrophonium is approximately 1/20 to 1/10 that of neostigmine, and pyridostigmine is about 1/5 the potency of neostigmine. Until more information from animal studies is available, edrophonium should probably not be used for reversal after large or multiple doses of dTC or gallamine. Incremental administration of antagonist may minimize autonomic effects and will prevent overdose that could result in depolarizing blockade (188). When reversal appears to be maximal, respiratory function should be evaluated. Classically, the diaphragm is described as being more resistant to blockade than the limbs; thus, evidence of reversal of blockade based on limb responses should indicate adequate respiratory function (189). This may not always be true (190, 191), and a method of assessing respiratory function should always be used before an animal is left alone after reversal of blockade. The airway can be occluded somewhere on the inspiratory limb of the breathing circuit or at the endotracheal tube, and respiratory efforts can be observed for sustained muscle contraction. It is helpful to measure negative inspiratory effort. An aneroid gauge on the breathing circuit or endotracheal tube can be used. Depending on depth of anesthesia, −10 to −25 cmH_2O should be generated. The animal should subsequently be monitored for respiratory sufficiency and peripheral muscle function during recovery. A controlled, sustained respiratory effort indicates good function; short, jerky motions with inappropriate head and limb movements indicate blockade is still present. Ability to lift the head and assume sternal and standing posture can also be assessed. Again, short, jerky attempts or fasciculations indicate inadequate reversal.

Reports in the dog of apnea within the first one-half hour after apparent adequate reversal of atracurium have been published (192, 193). The dogs were reintubated, ventilated, and given additional antagonist. Whether these represent cases of true recurarization is not known. In one study in humans, anticholinesterase administration was followed by arousal and respiratory stimulation that appeared to observers to represent adequate muscle function, yet when quantitative responses to nerve stimulation were examined, marked blockade was evident. The patients later became drowsy, and ventilation decreased markedly (30). If clinical weakness in an animal who has received an aminoglycoside or tetracycline antibiotic is present, calcium gluconate, 0.2 mg/kg i.v., may help restore muscle strength.

Fade criteria for predicting reversibility of SCh block have been delineated for human beings. These criteria should not be applied to animals. Depending on the species and anesthetic, SCh block may show significant fade after a single dose, yet a facilitatory drug will enhance rather than reverse the block at this point.

If Phase II block is suspected, very small incremental doses of facilitatory drugs could be given to assess reversibility. If no response occurs, the animal should be ventilated until spontaneous recovery occurs. Administration of neostigmine to human beings in whom Phase II block was suspected but not proven has sometimes resulted in total paralysis requiring hours of ventilatory support.

References

1. Crul JF: Relaxant drugs: From native drugs to the selective agents to today. *Acta Anaesth Scand* 26:409–415, 1982.
2. Durant NN, Katz RL: Suxamethonium.*Br J Anaesth* 54:195–208, 1982.
3. Basta SJ, Savarese JJ, Ali HH, Scott RPF, Gargarian M, Embree PB, Murphy B, Weakly JN, Batson AG: The neuromuscular pharmacology of BW B1090U in anesthetized patients. *Anesthesiology* 63:A318, 1985 (abstract).
4. Savarese JJ, Basta SJ, Ali HH, Scott RPF, Sunder N, Gargarian M, Embree PB, Moss J, Gelb C, Weakly JN, Batson AG: Cardiovascular effects of BW B1090U in patients under nitrous oxide-oxygen-thiopental-fentanyl anesthesia. *Anesthesiology* 63:A319, 1985 (abstract).
5. Borchard RE: Evaluation of chemical restraint methods for potential use in wild, free roaming horses. U.S. Dept. Of The Interior, Bureau of Land Management, Washington, DC, 1981.
6. Harthoorn AM: The use of a neuromuscular blocking agent on domestic cattle. *Vet Rec* 74:395–399, 1962.
7. Heuschele WP: Immobilization of captive wild animals. *Vet Med* Aug:348–351, 1961.
8. Lanphear PR: Tranquilization and immobilization of wild animals. *J Am Vet Med Assoc* 142:1126–1129, 1963.
9. Pistey WR, Wright JF: The immobilization of captive wild animals with succinylcholine. II. *Canad J Comp Med* 25:59–68, 1961.
10. Klide AM, Klein LV: Chemical restraint of three reptilean species. *J Zoo Anim Med* 4:8–11, 1973.
11. Bowman WC: Prejunctional and postjunctional cholinoceptors at the neuromuscular junction. *Anesth Analg* 59:935–943, 1980.
12. Riker WF: Pre-junctional effects of neuromuscular blocking and facilitatory drugs. In Katz RL (ed): *Muscle Relaxants*. New York, American Elsevier, 1975, pp 59–102.
13. Waud BE, Waud DR: Physiology and pharmacology of neuromuscular blocking agents. In Katz RL (ed): *Muscle Relaxants*. New York, American Elsevier, 1975, pp 1–58.
14. Donlon JV, Savarese JJ, Ali HA: Cumulative dose-response curves for gallamine: Effect of altered resting thumb tension and mode of stimulation. *Anesth Analg* 58:377–381, 1979.
15. Lee C, Barnes A, Katz RL: Neuromuscular sensitivity to tubocurarine. *Br J Anaesth* 48:1045–1051, 1976.
16. Hildebrand SV, Howitt GA: Dosage requirement of pancuronium in halothane-anesthetized ponies: A comparison of cumulative and single-dose administration. *Am J Vet Res* 45:2441–2444, 1984.
17. Klein L, Beck E, Hopkins J, Burton B: Characteristics of neuromuscular blockade produced by gallamine, pancuronium and vecuronium (ORG NC-45), and antagonism with neostigmine in anaesthetized horses. Proc Assoc Vet Anaesth Great Britain and Ireland, Cambridge, England. In *Proc 1st Intl Cong Vet Anaesth* (Supplement) 10:173–183, 1982.
18. Klein L, Hopkins J, Rosenberg H: Different relationship of train-of-four to twitch and tetanus for vecuronium, pancuronium and gallamine. *Anesthesiology* 59:A275, 1983.
19. Tassonyi E: A new concept in the measurement of neuromuscular transmission and block. *Anaesthetist* 24:374–377, 1975.

20. Klein L, Hopkins J, Beck E, Burton B: Mechanical responses to peroneal nerve stimulation in halothane-anesthetized horses in the absence of neuromuscular blockade and during partial nondepolarizing blockade. *Am J Vet Res* 44:781–785, 1983.
21. Derkx FHM, Bonta IL, Lagendijk A: Species-dependent effect of neuromuscular blocking agents. *Eur J Pharmacol* 16:105–108, 1971.
22. Lee C: Dose relationships of phase II, tachyphylaxis and train-of-four fade in suxamethonium-induced dual neuromuscular block in man. *Br J Anaesth* 47:841–845, 1975.
23. Donati F, Bevan JC, Bevan DR: Neuromuscular blocking drugs in anesthesia. *Can Anaesth Soc J* 31:324–336, 1984.
24. Kopman AF: The relationship of evoked electromyographic and mechanical responses following atracurium in humans. *Anesthesiology* 63:208–211, 1985.
25. Kopman AF: Correspondence. *Anesthesiology* 64:530–531, 1986.
26. Lee V, Chen J: Caution in making clinical recommendations based on electromyographic measurements (correspondence). *Anesthesiology* 64:529–530, 1986.
27. Ali HH, Savarese JJ: Monitoring of neuromuscular function. *Anesthesiology* 45:216–249, 1976.
28. Lee C, Katz RL: Neuromuscular pharmacology. *Br J Anaesth* 52:173–188, 1980.
29. Viby-Mogensen J: Clinical assessment of neuromuscular transmission. *Br J Anaesth* 54:209–223, 1982.
30. Katz RL: Neuromuscular effects of d-tubocurarine, edrophonium and neostigmine in man. *Anesthesiology* 28:327–336, 1967.
31. Klein L, Hopkins J, Beck E, Burton B: Cumulative dose responses to gallamine, pancuronium, and neostigmine in halothane-anesthetized horses: Neuromuscular and cardiovascular effects. *Am J Vet Res* 44:786–792, 1983.
32. Lennon RL, Olson RA, Gronert GA: Atracurium or vecuronium for rapid sequence endotracheal intubation. *Anesthesiology* 64:510–513, 1986.
33. Bencini A, Newton DEF: Rate of onset of good intubating conditions, respiratory depression and hand muscle paralysis after vecuronium. *Br J Anaesth* 56:959–965, 1984.
34. Doherty WG, Breen PJ, Donati F, Bevan DR: Accelerated onset of pancuronium with divided doses. *Can Anaesth Soc J* 32:1–4, 1985.
35. Foldes F: Rapid tracheal intubation with non-depolarizing neuromuscular blocking drugs: The priming principle (correspondence). *Br J Anaesth* 56:663, 1984.
36. Gergis SD, Sokoll MD, Mehta M, Kemmotsu O, Rudd GD: Intubation conditions after atracurium and suxamethonium. *Br J Anaesth* 55:83S–86S, 1983.
37. Musich J, Walts LF: Pulmonary aspiration after a priming dose of vecuronium. *Anesthesiology* 64:517–519, 1986.
38. Nagashima H, Nguyen HD, Lee S, Kaplan R, Duncalf D, Foldes FF: Facilitation of rapid endotracheal intubation and atracurium. *Anesthesiology* 61:A-289, 1984.
39. Rao TLK, Jacobs HK: Pulmonary function following "pretreatment" dose of pancuronium in volunteers. *Anesth Analg* 59:659–661, 1980.
40. Taboada JA, Rupp SM, Miller RD: Refining the priming principle for vecuronium during rapid-sequence induction of anesthesia. *Anesthesiology* 64:243–247, 1986.
41. Marshall RJ, McGrath JC, Miller RD, Dogherty JR, Lamar JC: Comparison of the cardiovascular actions of ORG NC-45 with those produced by other non-depolarizing neuromuscular blocking agents in experimental animals. *Br J Anaesth* 52:21S–32S, 1980.
42. Fitzal S, Gilly H, Ilias W: Comparative investigations on the cardiovascular effects of ORG NC-45 and pancuronium in dogs. *Br J Anaesth* 55:641–646, 1983.
43. Booij LHDJ, Edwards RP, Sohn YJ, Miller RD: Cardiovascular and neuromuscular effects of ORG NC-45, pancuronium, metocurine, and d-tubocurarine in dogs. *Anesth Analg* 59:26–30, 1980.
44. Fox MA: Atracurium in normal doses may release histamine. *Anesthesiology* 60:386, 1984.
45. Robertson EN, Booij LHDJ, Fragen RJ, Crul JF: Intradermal histamine release by 3 muscle relaxants. *Acta Anaesthesiol Scand* 27:203–205, 1983.
46. Siler JN, Mager JG, Wyche MQ: Atracurium: hypotension, tachycardia and bronchospasm. *Anesthesiology* 62:645–646, 1985.
47. McCullough LS, Reier CE, Delaunois AL, Gardier RW, Hamelberg W: The effects of d-tubocurarine on spontaneous postganglionic sympathetic activity and histamine release. *Anesthesiology* 33:328–334, 1970.
48. Smith G, Proctor DW, Spence AA: A comparison of some cardiovascular effects of tubocurarine and pancuronium in dogs. *Brit J Anaesth* 42:923–927, 1970.
49. Safar P, Bachman L: Compliance of the lungs and thorax in dogs under the influence of muscle relaxants. *Anesthesiology* 17:334–346, 1956.
50. Domenech JS, Garcia RC, Rodriguez JM, Loyola AQ, Oroz JS: Pancuronium bromide: An indirect sympathomimetic agent. *Br J Anaesth* 48:1143–1148, 1976.
51. Hughes R: Haemodynamic effects of tubocurarine, gallamine and suxamethonium in dogs. *Br J Anaesth* 42:928–934, 1970.
52. McGrath CJ, Short CE, Paddleford RR: Pancuronium bromide: An adjunct to the anesthetic management of the dog. *Vet Anesth* 2:14–18, 1975.
53. Reitan JA, Warpinski MA: Cardiovascular effects of pancuronium bromide in mongrel dogs. *Am J Vet Res* 36:1309–1311, 1975.
54. Hildebrand SV, Howitt GA: Neuromuscular and cardiovascular effects of pancuronium bromide in calves anesthetized with halothane. *Am J Vet Res* 45:1549–1552, 1984.
55. Klein L, Sylvina T, Beck E: Neuromuscular blockade with d-tubocurarine, pancuronium and vecuronium in halothane anesthetized sheep. *Proc 2nd Intl Cong Vet Anes* Oct:174, 1985 (abstract).
56. Manley SV, Steffey EP, Howitt GA, Woliner M: Cardiovascular and neuromuscular effects of pancuronium bromide in the pony. *Am J Vet Res* 44:1349–1353, 1983.
57. Hildebrand SV, Howitt GA, Arpin D: Neuromuscular and cardiovascular effects of atracurium in ponies anesthetized with halothane. *Am J Vet Res* 47:1096–1100, 1986.
58. Karhunen U, Nilsson E, Brander P: Comparison of four non-depolarizing neuromuscular blocking drugs in the suppression of the oculocardiac reflex during strabismus surgery in children. *Br J Anaesth* 57:1209–1212, 1985.
59. Starr NJ, Sethna DH, Estafanous FG: Bradycardia and asystole following the rapid administration of sufentanil with vecuronium. *Anesthesiology* 64:521–523, 1986.
60. Zinn RS, Gabel AA, Heath RB: Effects of succinylcholine and promazine on the cardiovascular and respiratory systems of horses. *J Am Vet Med Assoc* 157:1495–1499, 1970.
61. Stevenson DE: A review of some side effects of muscle relaxants in small animals. *J Small Anim Pract* 1:77–83, 1960–61.
62. Magee DA, Sweet PT, Holland AJC: Effect of atropine on bradydysrhythmias induced by succinylcholine following pretreatment with d-tubocurarine. *Can Anaesth Soc J* 29:573–575, 1982.
63. Magee DA, Sweet PT, Holland AJC: Cardiac effects of self-taming of succinylcholine and repeated succinylcholine administration. *Can Anaesth Soc J* 29:577–580, 1982.
64. McIntyre JWR: Succinylcholine-induced bradycardia with reference to methoxyflurane anaesthesia. *Can Anaesth Soc J* 9:408–413, 1962.
65. Schoenstadt DA, Whitcher CE: Observations on the mechanism of succinyldicholine-induced cardiac arrhythmias. *Anesthesiology* 24:358–362, 1963.

66. Stoelting RK, Peterson C: Heart-rate slowing and junctional rhythm following intravenous succinylcholine with and without intramuscular atropine preanesthetic medication. *Anesth Analg* 54:705–709, 1975.
67. Abouleish E, Wingard LB, De La Vega S, Uy N: Pancuronium in caesarean section and its placental transfer. *Br J Anaesth* 52:531–536, 1980.
68. Demetriou M, Depoix JP, Diakite B, Fromentin M, Duvaldestin P: Placental transfer of Org NC-45 in women undergoing caesarean section. *Br J Anaesth* 54:643–645, 1982.
69. Duvaldestin P, Demetriou M, Henzel D, Desmonts JM: The placental transfer of pancuronium and its pharmacokinetics during caesarean section. *Acta Anaesth Scand* 22:327–333, 1978.
70. Flynn PJ, Frank M, Hughes R: Use of atracurium in caesarean section. *Br J Anaesth* 56:599–604, 1984.
71. Evans CA, Waud DR: Do maternally administered neuromuscular blocking agents interfere with fetal neuromuscular transmission? *Anesth Analg* 52:548–552, 1973.
72. Pittinger CB, Morris LE: Placental transmission of d-tubocurarine chloride from maternal to fetal circulation in dogs. *Anesthesiology* 14:238–244, 1953.
73. Pittinger CB, Morris LE: Placental transmission in dogs. *Anesth Analg* 34:107–111, 1955.
74. Knecht CD, Kazmierczak K, Katherman AE: Effects of succinylcholine on the electroencephalogram of dogs. *Am J Vet Res* 41:1435–1440, 1980.
75. Cottrell JE, Hartung J, Giffin JP, Shwiry B: Intracranial and hemodynamic changes after succinylcholine administration in cats. *Anesth Analg* 62:1006–1009, 1983.
76. Halidin M, Wahlin A: Effect of succinylcholine on the intraspinal fluid pressure. *Acta Anaesth Scand* 3:155–161, 1959.
77. Lanier WL, Milde JH, Michenfelder JD: Cerebral stimulation following succinylcholine in dogs. *Anesthesiology* 64:551–559, 1986.
78. Mori K, Iwabuchi K, Fusita M: The effects of depolarizing muscle relaxants on the electroencephalogram and the circulation during halothane anesthesia in man. *Br J Anaesth* 45:604–610, 1973.
79. Forbes AR, Cohen NH, Eger EI: Pancuronium reduces halothane requirement in man. *Anesth Analg* 58:497–499, 1979.
80. Savarese JJ: How may neuromuscular blocking agents affect the state of general anesthesia? *Anesth Analg* 58:449–450, 1979.
81. Jantzen JAH, Hackett GH, Earnshaw G: Succinylcholine and open eye injury. *Anesthesiology* 54:524–525, 1986.
82. Balamoutsos NG, Tsakona H, Kanakoudes PS, Iliadelis E, Georgiades G: Alcuronium and intraocular pressure. *Anesth Analg* 62:521–523, 1983.
83. Bowen DJ, McGrand JC, Palmer RJ: Intraocular pressures after suxamethonium and endotracheal intubation in patients pretreated with pancuronium. *Br J Anaesth* 48:1201–1205, 1976.
84. Konchigeri HN, Lee YE, Venugopal K: Effect of pancuronium on intraocular pressure changes induced by succinylcholine. *Can Anaesth Soc J* 26:479–481, 1979.
85. Sia RL, Rashkovsky OM: Org NC-45 and intraocular pressure during anesthesia. *Acta Anaesth Scand* 25:219–221, 1981.
86. Bowman WC: Non-relaxant properties of neuromuscular blocking drugs. *Br J Anaesth* 54:147–160, 1982.
87. Foldes FF, Deery A: Protein binding of atracurium and other short-acting neuromuscular blocking agents and their interaction with human cholinesterases. *Br J Anaesth* 55:31S–34S, 1983.
88. Ghoneim MM, Pandya H: Binding of tubocurarine to specific serum protein fractions. *Br J Anaesth* 47:853–856, 1975.
89. Skivington MA: Protein binding of three tritiated muscle relaxants. *Brit J Anaesth* 44:1030–1034, 1972.
90. Crankshaw DP, Cohen EN: Uptake, distribution and elimination of skeletal muscle relaxants. In Katz RL (ed): *Muscle Relaxants.* New York, American Elsevier, 1975, pp 125–141.
91. Feldman SA, Cohen EN, Golling RC: The excretion of gallamine in the dog. *Anesthesiology* 30:593–598, 1969.
92. Westra P, Vermeer GA, DeLange AR, Scaf AHJ, Meijer DKF, Wesseling H: Hepatic and renal disposition of pancuronium and gallamine in patients with extrahepatic cholestasis. *Br J Anaesth* 53:331–338, 1981.
93. Wingard LB, Cook DR: Clinical pharmacokinetics of muscle relaxants. *Clin Pharmacokinetics* 2:330–343, 1977.
94. Westra P, Houwertjes MC, DeLange AR, Scaf AHJ, Hindriks FR, Agoston S: Effect of experimental cholestasis on neuromuscular blocking drugs in cats. *Br J Anaesth* 52:747–756, 1980.
95. Somogyi AA, Shanks CA, Triggs EJ: Disposition kinetics of pancuronium bromide in patients with total biliary obstruction. *Br J Anaesth* 49:1103–1108, 1977.
96. Booij LHDJ, Vree TB, Hurkmans F, Reekers-Ketting JJ, Crul JF: Pharmacokinetics and pharmacodynamics of the muscle relaxant drug Org NC-45 and each of its hydroxy metabolites in dogs. *Anaesthetist* 30:329–333, 1981.
97. Fahey MR, Morris RB, Miller RD, Nguyen TL, Upton RA: Pharmacokinetics of Org NC-45 (nocuron) in patients with and without renal failure. *Br J Anaesth* 53:1049–1053, 1981.
98. Lebrault C, Berger JL, D'Hollander AA, Gomeni R, Henzel D, Duvaldestin P: Pharmacokinetics and pharmacodynamics of vecuronium (Org NC-45) in patients with cirrhosis. *Anesthesiology* 62:601–605, 1985.
99. Hunter JM, Jones RS, Utting JE: Use of atracurium in patients with no renal function. *Br J Anaesth* 54:1251–1258, 1982.
100. Nigrovic V, Auen M, Wajskol A: Enzymatic hydrolysis of atracurium in vivo. *Anesthesiology* 62:606–609, 1985.
101. Stenlake JB, Waigh RD, Urwin J, Dewar GH, Coker GG: Atracurium: Conception and inception. *Br J Anaesth* 55:3S–10S, 1983.
102. Fahey MR, Rupp SM, Canfell C, Fisher DM, Miller RD, Sharma M, Castagnoli K, Hennis PJ: Effect of renal failure on laudanosine excretion in man. *Br J Anaesth* 57:1049–1051, 1985.
103. Nigrovic V, Koechel DA: Atracurium—Additional information needed. *Anesthesiology* 60:606–607, 1984.
104. Short CE, Cuneio J, Cupp D: Organophosphate-induced complication during anesthetic management in the horse. *J Am Vet Med Assoc* 159:1319–1327, 1971.
105. Kalow W: The distribution, destruction and elimination of muscle relaxants. *Anesthesiology* 20:505–518, 1959.
106. Miller RD: Pharmacokinetics of competitive muscle relaxants. *Br J Anaesth* 54:161–167, 1982.
107. Fisher DM, O'Keeffe C, Stanski DR, Cronnelly R, Miller RD, Gregory GA: Pharmacokinetics and pharmacodynamics of d-tubocurarine in infants, children, and adults. *Anesthesiology* 57:203–208, 1982.
108. Matteo RS, Lieberman IG, Salanitre E, McDaniel DD, Diaz J: Distribution, elimination, and action of d-tubocurarine in neonates, infants, children, and adults. *Anesth Analg* 63:799–804, 1984.
109. Cook DR: Muscle relaxants in infants and children. *Anesth Analg* 60:335–343, 1981.
110. D'Hollander AA, Nevelsteen M, Barvais L, Baurain M: Effect of age on the establishment of muscle paralysis induced in anaesthetized adult subjects by ORG NC-45. *Acta Anaesth Scand* 27:108–110, 1983.
111. Foldes FF: Myasthenia gravis. In Katz RL (ed): *Muscle Relaxants.* New York, American Elsevier, 1975, pp 345–393.
112. Miller RD, Savarese JJ: Pharmacology of muscle relaxants, their antagonists and monitoring of neuromuscular function. In Miller RD (ed): *Anesthesia.* New York, Churchill Livingstone, 1981, pp 526–527.
113. Baraka A, Dajani A: Atracurium in myasthenics undergoing thymectomy. *Anesth Analg* 63:1127–1130, 1984.
114. Buzello W, Noeldge G, Krieg N, Brobmann GF: Vecuronium for muscle relaxation in patients with myasthenia gravis. *Anesthe-*

siology 64:507–509, 1986.
115. Rosenbaum KJ, Neigh JL, Strobel GE: Sensitivity to nondepolarizing muscle relaxants in amyotrophic lateral sclerosis: Report of two cases. *Anesthesiology* 35:638–641, 1971.
116. Miller RD, Savarese JJ: Pharmacology of muscle relaxants, their antagonists and monitoring of neuromuscular function. In Miller RD (ed): *Anesthesia*. New York, Churchill Livingstone, 1981, pp 527–528.
117. Moorthy SS, Hilgenberg JC: Resistance to nondepolarizing muscle relaxants in paretic upper extremities of patients with residual hemiplegia. *Anesth Analg* 59:624–627, 1980.
118. Waud BE, Amaki Y, Waud DR: Disuse and d-tubocurarine sensitivity in isolated muscles. *Anesth Analg* 64:1178–1182, 1985.
119. Martyn JAJ, Goudsouzian NG, Matteo RS, Liu LMP, Szyfelbein SK, Kaplan RF: Metocurine requirements and plasma concentrations in burned paediatric patients. *Br J Anaesth* 55:263–267, 1983.
120. Baraka A: Suxamethonium-induced muscle contracture following traumatic denervation in man. *Br J Anaesth* 50:195–199, 1978.
121. Cooperman LH, Strobel GE, Kennell EM: Massive hyperkalemia after administration of succinycholine. *Anesthesiology* 32:161–164, 1970.
122. Gronert GA, Lambert EH, Theye RA: The response of denervated skeletal muscle to succinylcholine. *Anesthesiology* 39:13–22, 1973.
123. Kendig JJ, Bunker JP, Endow S: Succinylcholine-induced hyperkalemia: Effects of succinylcholine on resting potentials and electrolyte distributions in normal and denervated muscle. *Anesthesiology* 36:132–141, 1972.
124. Kopriva C, Ratliff J, Fletcher JR, Van Tassel P, Stout R: Serum potassium changes after succinylcholine in patients with acute massive muscle trauma. *Anesthesiology* 34:246–249, 1971.
125. Lee C, Yang E, Katz RL: Focal contracture following injection of succinylcholine in patients with peripheral nerve injury. *Canad Anaesth Soc J* 24:475–478, 1977.
126. Mazze RI, Escue HM, Houston JB: Hyperkalemia and cardiovascular collapse following administration of succinylcholine to the traumatized patient. *Anesthesiology* 31:540–547, 1969.
127. Stevenson PH, Birch AA: Succinylcholine-induced hyperkalemia in a patient with a closed head injury. *Anesthesiology* 51:89–90, 1979.
128. Stone WA, Beach TP, Hamelberg W: Succinylcholine—Danger in the spinal cord injured patient. *Anesthesiology* 32:168–169, 1970.
129. Tolmie JD, Joyce TH, Mitchell GD: Succinylcholine danger in the burned patient. *Anesthesiology* 28:467–470, 1967.
130. Roth F, Wuthrich H: The clinical importance of hyperkalaemia following suxamethonium administration. *Brit J Anaesth* 41:311–316, 1969.
131. Gronert GA, Theye RA: Pathophysiology of hyperkalemia induced by succinylcholine. *Anesthesiology* 43:89–99, 1975.
132. Boros M, Chaudhry IA, Nagashima H, Duncalf RM, Sherman EH, Foldes FF: Myoneural effects of pethidine and droperidol. *Br J Anaesth* 56:195–202, 1984.
133. Driessen JJ, Vree TB, Van Egmond J, Booij LHDJ, Crul JF: Interaction of midazolam with two non-depolarizing neuromuscular blocking drugs in the rat in vivo sciatic nerve-tibialis anterior muscle preparation. *Br J Anaesth* 57:1089–1094, 1985.
134. Duke PC, Johns CH, Pinsky C, Goertzen P: The effect of morphine on human neuromuscular transmission. *Canad Anaesth Soc J* 26:201–205, 1979.
135. Gudnason HV, Edgar EE: Influence of morphine on muscle relaxants in anesthetized dogs. *Southern Med J* 62:1394–1397, 1969.
136. Kotkin S, Lear E, Chiron AE, Pallin IM, Dickler D: Preliminary studies on the muscle relaxing properties of chlorpromazine. *Anesthesiology* 17:494–499, 1956.
137. Seyama I, Narahashi T: Mechanism of blockade of neuromuscular transmission by pentobarbital. *J Pharmacol Exp Ther* 192:95–104, 1975.
138. Torda TA, Gage PW: Postsynaptic effect of IV anaesthetic agents at the neuromuscular junction. *Br J Anaesth* 49:771–776, 1977.
139. Miller RD: Factors affecting the action of muscle relaxants. In Katz RL (ed): *Muscle Relaxants*. New York, American Elsevier, 1975, p 185.
140. Lebowitz MH, Blitt CD, Walts LF: Depression of twitch response to stimulation of the ulnar nerve during ethrane anesthesia in man. *Anesthesiology* 33:52–57, 1970.
141. Miller RD, Eger EI, Way WL, Stevens WC, Dolan WM: Comparative neuromuscular effects of forane and halothane alone and in combination with d-tubocurarine in man. *Anesthesiology* 35:38–42, 1971.
142. Stanski DR, Ham J, Miller RD, Sheiner LB: Time dependent increase in sensitivity to dTC during enflurane anesthesia. *Anesthesiology* 51:S269, 1979.
143. Waud BE, Waud DR, Phil D: Effects of volatile anesthetics on directly and indirectly stimulated skeletal muscle. *Anesthesiology* 50:103–110, 1979.
144. Adams HR: Acute adverse effects of antibiotics. *J Am Vet Med Assoc* 166:983–987, 1975.
145. Bowen JM, McMullan WC: Influence of induced hypermagnesemia and hypocalcemia on neuromuscular blocking property of oxytetracycline in the horse. *Amer J Vet Res* 36:1025–1028, 1975.
146. Lee C, Chen D, Barnes A, Katz RL: Neuromuscular block by neomycin in the cat. *Canad Anaesth Soc J* 23:527–533, 1976.
147. Lippmann M, Yang E, Au E, Lee C: Neuromuscular blocking effects of tobramycin gentamicin and cefazolin. *Anesth Analg* 61:767–770, 1982.
148. Mathew BP, Teske RH, Robinson JA, Adams HR: Neuromuscular blocking effects of certain antibacterial agents in pigs and lambs. *J Vet Pharmacol Ther* 1:171–175, 1978.
149. Pittinger C, Adamson R: Antibiotic blockade of neuromuscular function. *Annu Rev Pharmacol* 12:169–184, 1972.
150. Potter JM, Edeson RO, Campbell RJ, Forbes AM: Potentiation by gentamicin of non-depolarizing neuromuscular block in the cat. *Anaesth Intens Care* 8:20–25, 1980.
151. Singh YN, Marshall IG, Harvey AL: Some effects of the aminoglycoside antibiotic amikacin on neuromuscular and autonomic transmission. *Br J Anaesth* 50:109–117, 1978.
152. Singh YN, Marshall IG, Harvey AL: Depression of transmitter release and postjunctional sensitivity during neuromuscular block produced by antibiotics. *Br J Anaesth* 51:1027–1033, 1979.
153. Singh YN, Marshall IG, Harvey AL: Pre- and postjunctional blocking effects of aminoglycoside, polymyxin, tetracycline and lincosamide antibiotics. *Br J Anaesth* 54:1295–1306, 1982.
154. Sokoll MD, Gergis SD: Antibiotics and neuromuscular function. *Anesthesiology* 55:148–159, 1981.
155. Funk DI, Crul JF, Pol FM: Effects of changes in acid-base balance on neuromuscular blockade produced by ORG NC-45. *Acta Anaesth Scand* 24:119–124, 1980.
156. Hughes OP R: The influence of changes in acid-base balance on neuromuscular blockade in cats. *Brit J Anaesth* 42:658–668, 1970.
157. Miller RD, Van Nyhuis LS, Eger EI, Way WL: The effect of acid-base balance on neostigmine antagonism of d-tubocurarine-induced neuromuscular blockade. *Anesthesiology* 42:377–383, 1975.
158. Wirtavuori K, Salmenpera M, Tammisto T: Effect of hypocarbia and hypercarbia on the antagonism of pancuronium-induced neuromuscular blockade with neostigmine in man. *Br J Anaesth* 54:57–61, 1982.
159. Ghoneim MM, Long JP: The interaction between magnesium and other neuromuscular blocking agents. *Anesthesiology*

32:23–27, 1970.
160. Giesecke AH, Morris RE, Dalton MD, Stephen CR: Of magnesium, muscle relaxants, toxemic parturients and cats. *Anesth Analg* 47:689–695, 1968.
161. Sinatra RS, Philip BK, Naulty JS, Ostheimer GW: Prolonged neuromuscular blockade with vecuronium in a patient treated with magnesium sulfate. *Anesth Analg* 64:1220–1222, 1985.
162. Miller RD, Savarese JJ: Pharmacology of muscle relaxants, their antagonists and monitoring of neuromuscular function. In Miller RD (ed): *Anesthesia*. New York, Churchill Livingstone, 1981, p 525.
163. Miller RD: Factors affecting the action of muscle relaxants. In Katz RL (ed): *Muscle Relaxants*. New York, American Elsevier, 1975, pp 176–177.
164. Ham J: Factors affecting administration of nondepolarizing neuromuscular blocking agents. *ASA Ref Course Outline* 61(8):61–78, 1980.
165. Waud BE, Waud DR: Interaction of calcium and potassium with neuromuscular blocking agents. *Br J Anaesth* 52:863–866, 1980.
166. Foldes FF: Factors which alter the effects of muscle relaxants. *Anesthesiology* 20:464–504, 1959.
167. Standaert FG: Interactions among neuromuscular blocking agents and other drugs. In Hershey SG (ed): *Refresher Courses in Anesthesiology*. The American Society of Anesthesiologists, Inc, 1978, pp 111–123.
168. Erkola O, Salmenpera A, Kuoppamaki R: Five non-depolarizing muscle relaxants in precurarization. *Acta Anaesth Scand* 27:427–432, 1983.
169. Ferres CJ, Mirakhur RK, Craig HJL, Browne ES, Clarke RSJ: Pretreatment with vecuronium as a prophylactic against post-suxamethonium muscle pain. *Br J Anaesth* 55:735–741, 1983.
170. Masey SA, Glazebrook CW, Goat VA: Suxamethonium: A new look at pretreatment. *Br J Anaesth* 55:729–733, 1983.
171. Stoelting RK, Peterson C: Adverse effects of increased succinylcholine dose following d-tubocurarine pretreatment. *Anesth Analg* 54:282–396, 1975.
172. Brodsky JB, Brock-Utne JG: Does "self-taming" with succinylcholine prevent postoperative myalgia? *Anesthesiology* 50:265–267, 1979.
173. Raffe MR, Crimi AJ, Ruff J: Effect of diazepam pretreatment on succinylcholine-induced muscle fasciculation in the dog. *Am J Vet Res* 43:510–512, 1982.
174. Verma RS, Chatterji S, Mathur N: Diazepam and succinylcholine-induced muscle pains. *Anesth Analg* 57:295–297, 1978.
175. Klein L, Rosenberg H: Malignant hyperthermia in animals other than swine. In Britt BA (ed): *Malignant Hyperthermia*. Hughia, Mass, Kluner Acad Pub, 1987, in press.
176. Harle DG, Baldo BA, Fisher MM: Cross-reactivity of methocurine, atracurium, vecuronium and fazadinium with IgE antibodies from patients unexposed to these drugs but allergic to other myoneural blocking drugs. *Br J Anaesth* 57:1073–1076, 1985.
177. Cook DR, Westman HR, Rosenfeld L, Hendershot RJ: Pulmonary edema in infants: Possible association with intramuscular succinylcholine. *Anesth Analg* 60:220–223, 1981.
178. Cronnelly R: Muscle relaxant antagonists. *Seminars in Anesth* 4:31–40, 1985.
179. Delisle S, Bevan DR: Impaired neostigmine antagonism of pancuronium during enflurane anaesthesia in man. *Br J Anaesth* 54:441–445, 1982.
180. Miller RD, Van Nyhuis LS, Eger EI, Vitez TS, Way WL: Comparative times to peak effect and durations of action of neostigmine and pyridostigmine. *Anesthesiology* 41:27–33, 1974.
181. Baird WLM, Bowman WC, Kerr WJ: Some actions of ORG NC-45 and of edrophonium in the anaesthetized cat and in man. *Br J Anaesth* 54:375–385, 1982.
182. Ferguson A, Egerszegi P, Bevan DR, Chir B: Neostigmine, pyridostigmine, and edrophonium as antagonists of pancuronium. *Anesthesiology* 53:390–394, 1980.
183. Jones RM, Pearce AC, Williams JP: Recovery characteristics following antagonism of atracurium with neostigmine or edrophonium. *Br J Anaesth* 56:453–457, 1984.
184. Kopman AF: Edrophonium antagonism of pancuronium-induced neuromuscular blockade in man: A reappraisal. *Anesthesiology* 51:139–142, 1979.
185. Cronnelly R, Morris RB: Antagonism of neuromuscular blockade. *Br J Anaesth* 54:183–194, 1982.
186. Miller RD: Antagonism of neuromuscular blockade. *Anesthesiology* 44:318–329, 1976.
187. Levy WI: Muscle relaxants in anesthesia for dogs and cats. *JAAHA* 8:379–384, 1972.
188. Payne JP, Hughes R, Azawi SA: Neuromuscular blockade by neostigmine in anaesthetized man. *Br J Anaesth* 52:69–76, 1980.
189. Waud BE, Waud DR: The margin of safety of neuromuscular transmission in the muscle of the diaphragm. *Anesthesiology* 37:417–422, 1972.
190. Alderson AM, Maclagan J: The action of decamethonium and tubocurarine on the respiratory and limb muscles of the cat. *J Physiol* 173:38–56, 1964.
191. Li TH, Jacobs BR, Aviado M, Schmidt CF: Early respiratory depression by curare and curare potassium antagonism. *J Pharmacol Exp Ther* 104:149–161, 1952.
192. Jones RS, Clutton RE: Clinical observations on the use of the muscle relaxant atracurium in the dog. *J Small Anim Pract* 25:473–477, 1984.
193. Hall LW, Kellagher REB, Watkins SB: Respiratory problems after atropine and neostigmine in dogs. *Br J Anaesth* 57:1046, 1985.
194. Cass N, Brown WA, Ng KC, Lampard DG: Dosage patterns of non-depolarizing neuromuscular blockers in the sheep. *Anaesth Intens Care* 8:13–15, 1980.
195. Lampard DG, Brown WA, Cass NM, Ng KC: Computer-controlled muscle paralysis with atracurium in the sheep. *Anaesth Intens Care* 14:7–11, 1986.
196. Hildebrand SV, Arpin D: Neuromuscular and cardiovascular effects of atracurium in healthy adult horses anesthetized with halothane. *Proc 2nd Intl Cong Vet Anes*. Sacramento, CA, The Veterinary Practice Publishing Co, 1985, p 175.
197. Benson GJ, Hartsfield SM, Smetzer DL, Thurmon JC: Physiologic effects of succinylcholine chloride in mechanically ventilated horses anesthetized with halothane in oxygen. *Am J Vet Res* 40:1411–1416, 1979.
198. Green CJ: Muscle Relaxants. In: *Animal Anaesthesia*. London, Laboratory Animals Ltd, 1979, p 49.
199. Denny HR, Lucke JN: Anaesthetic and surgical technique for bilateral adrenalectomy in stress sensitive pigs. *Res Vet Sci* 23:372–377, 1977.
200. Reynolds WT: Use of suxamethonium in cats fitted with dichlorvos flea collars. *Aust Vet J* 62:106–107, 1985.
201. Evans AT, Anderson LK, Eyster GE, Sawyer DC: Cardiovascular effects of gallamine triethiodide and succinylcholine chloride during halothane anesthesia in the dog. *Am J Vet Res* 38:329–331, 1977.
202. Hall LW, Clarke KW: *Veterinary Anaesthesia*, ed 8. Bailliere Tindall, London, pp 115–140, 1983.
203. Lumb WV, Jones EW: *Veterinary Anesthesia*, ed 2. Lee & Febiger, Philadelphia, pp 333–356, 1984.
204. Hughes R, Chapple DJ: Effects of non-depolarizing neuromuscular blocking agents on peripheral autonomic mechanisms in cats. *Br J Anaesth* 48:59–68, 1976.
205. Booij LHDJ, Edwards RP, Sohn YJ, Miller RD: Comparative cardiovascular and neuromuscular effects of ORG NC45, pancuronium, metocurine and d-tubocurarine. *Anesth Anagl*, (Cleve) 19:26–30, 1980.

206. Durant NN, Houwertjes MC, Crul JF: Comparison of the neuromuscular blocking properties of ORG NC45 and pancuronium in the rat, cat and rhesus monkey. *Br J Anaesth* 52:723–730, 1980.
207. Durant NN, Marshall IG, Savage DS, et al: The neuromuscular and autonomic blocking activities of pancuronium analogues, in the cat. *J Pharm Pharmacol* 31:831–836, 1979.
208. Hughes R, Chapple DJ: The pharmacology of atracurium, a new competitive neuromuscular blocking agent. *Br J Anesth* 53:31–44, 1981.
209. Jones RS, Hunter JM, Utting JE: Neuromuscular blocking action of atracurium in the dog and its reversal by neostigmine. *Res Vet Sci* 34:173–176, 1983.
210. Lee C, Tran BK, Durant N, Nguyen NB: Vecuronium, isoflurane and hypotensive anesthesia in the cat. *Anesthesiology* 59:A271, 1983.
211. Jones RS, Heckmann R, Wuersch W: Observations on the duration of action of suxamethonium in the dog. *Br Vet J* 134:521–523, 1978.
212. Marshall IG: Comparison of atracurium and vecuronium in the cat. Presented at the International Symposium on Relaxants Boston, August 24–25, 1983.
213. Klein L: Neuromuscular blocking agents in equine anesthesia. *Vet Clin NA Lg Anim Pract* 3:135–161, 1981.

CHAPTER

10

Drug Interactions

CHARLES J. McGRATH, D.V.M., D.A.C.V.A.

The intent of this book is to provide the veterinary clinician with an appreciation of the scope and practice of veterinary anesthesia. In keeping with this goal, it is hoped that the information on drug interactions in this chapter will enhance the clinician's awareness of the complexities of multiple drug usage in our patients.

What Are Drug Interactions?

Drug interaction is two or more drugs acting together to produce effects that may or may not result from any one of the drugs given alone. Because most anesthetic patients are given more than one drug during the anesthetic or perianesthetic period, the probability of drug interaction in our patients is essentially 100%. In a recent survey in our small animal clinic, it was found that dogs were given 3.9 drugs on the average during the perianesthetic/anesthetic periods. This survey did not include antimicrobials, dewormers, vaccines, or intravenous fluids given either before, during, or after the anesthetic period. To understand the rationale for multiple drug usage during anesthesia, a brief statement regarding the author's approach to anesthesia is in order.

WHAT IS ANESTHESIA?

Anesthesia is an artificial state that is chemically induced and to some extent resembles sleep from which the patient is not arousable. During anesthesia, mental, sensory, motor, and autonomic reflex functions are attenuated or altered. The concurrent attenuation or alteration of these four components is, in fact, the anesthetic state. The effects of anesthetic drugs on these four functions vary greatly between classes of drugs and vary to a lesser extent between drugs in the same class. For example, thiopental (a sedative-hypnotic drug) predominantly alters the mental component, producing unconsciousness. However, the sensory, motor, and reflex components are not attenuated to the same degree as would occur during a comparable level of unconsciousness produced by halothane. At the other end of the spectrum, succinylcholine attenuates the motor component without affecting the mental, sensory, or reflex components of anesthesia. With the four-component concept of the anesthetic state in mind, the optimal anesthetic state might best be produced by using a multiple drug approach specifically to attenuate these individual components to achieve an appropriate anesthetic state for a particular patient.

DRUG INTERACTIONS—GOOD OR BAD?

The term drug interaction does not imply either good or bad effects. Whether or not the specific interaction is good or bad, beneficial or detrimental, depends on the effect desired by the clinician and the health status of the patient. As an example, the somnolence produced by a neuroleptanalgesic combination such as acepromazine and morphine would be desirable in an intractable dog, but it might prove detrimental to a postoperative patient given the combination to alleviate postoperative pain. The clinician uses these well-planned drug interactions to create an optimal and safe anesthetic procedure.

Selection of an anesthetic regime consisting of multiple drugs constitutes "balanced anesthesia." The proper selection will create an anesthetic state in which the mental, sensory, motor, and reflex components are attenuated and the risk to the patient is minimized. The clinician must, however, be wary of interactions with drugs given for purposes other than creating balanced anesthesia.

Types, Sites, and Mechanisms of Drug Interaction

There are probably three basic types of drug interactions; these are physical or chemical, pharmacokinetic, and pharmacodynamic interactions.

PHYSICAL OR CHEMICAL INTERACTIONS

These are most frequently encountered outside the patient and typically result from intentional or unintentional mixing of drugs in solution. Of the list of approximately 40 drugs used in veterinary anesthesia practice, one author (1) suggests that less than 10% are known to be compatible when combined. Probably 10 to 20% of the possible combinations are known to be incompatible, and the vast majority of all possible two-drug combinations from this list are of unknown compatibility (1, 2).

Fewer drug incompatibilities in solution will occur if saline or dextrose 5% in water is in use as the intravenous solution to which the medication is added. Whole blood, dextrose, and Ringer's lactate are not ideal solutions to which to add medications. Specifically, either thiopental or thiamylal sodium is more compatible in saline or 5% dextrose in water than in Ringer's lactate.

The addition of sodium bicarbonate to solutions increases incompatibility to a number of medications, including levarterenol bitartrate, meperidine HCl, morphine sulfate, phenothiazine, oxytetetracycline, and tetracycline. The addition of calcium to solutions increases incompatibility of sodium bicarbonate and antihistamines. Even heparin is incompatible with such medications as meperidine and morphine. Succinyl choline is incompatible with ultrashort barbiturates, and glycopyrrolate is incompatible with acetylpromazine.

It is not uncommon to encounter "favorite cocktails" among veterinary clinicians. Acepromazine added to a vial containing ketamine is one frequently encountered example. More recently, ketamine combined in the same syringe with diazepam (Valium) has become popular. Although precipitation does not appear to occur with either of these two combinations, the compatibility of these drugs in solution is essentially unknown. The lack of precipitation with the latter combination is quite surprising in view of the manufacturer's recommendations regarding the addition of diazepam to intravenous solutions or methods of injection into an intravenous administration set or catheter. In our experience, the solution becomes cloudy in the intravenous tubing immediately after the addition of diazepam.

Precipitation is only one of several possible chemical or physical interactions. The pH of one drug may alter the absorption, availability, or effect of the second drug. Physical and chemical incompatibility is probably most often encountered when calcium or bicarbonate ions are contained in the solution. Some general guidelines for minimizing these interactions include:

1. The number of drugs added to a solution should be limited as much as possible.
2. Addition of a drug to a solution should be based on knowledge of compatibility rather than assumption.
3. Proper labels should be applied to indicate drug additives and their concentrations.
4. Solutions with a precipitate or unexpected color change should be discarded.
5. Whole blood, plasma, and other blood substitutes should not be used as diluents for any drug. A separate intravenous fluid administration set and catheter should be used so that unintentional addition of drug to whole blood does not occur.

Strict avoidance of drug mixtures or drug combinations in solution and careful attention to administration technique when injecting drugs into an intravenous line should minimize the risk of physical or chemical drug interactions.

In addition to the potential for physical or chemical interactions, the author believes that the use of drug mixtures or cocktails poses another threat to the patient in that it permits the clinician to use multiple drugs without first establishing the need for more than one drug or the need for that particular drug combination.

PHARMACOKINETIC INTERACTIONS

Absorption, distribution, biotransformation, and excretion are all components of pharmacokinetics. In essence, pharmacokinetics are influenced by all processes, both active and passive, drug movement from the time and site of drug administration to the ultimate elimination from the body (3, 4).

Absorption

If the absorption of one drug is altered by giving a second drug, then a pharmacokinetic interaction has occurred. Slowing of absorption of local anesthetics by the addition of a vasoconstrictor such as epinephrine is an example of pharmacokinetic interaction that is intentionally used both to prolong the local anesthetic effect at the desired site and to reduce the risk of toxicity by slowing absorption of the local anesthetic. Slow transition from thiopental induction to methoxyflurane maintenance is in part due to a pharmacokinetic interaction of thiopental (reduced spontaneous ventilation) and methoxyflurane (a resultant slower rise in alveolar concentration).

Distribution

The two most commonly encountered interactions that affect distribution are hemodynamic alterations and competition for protein binding sites. Drugs that alter cerebral blood flow may influence the effect (either rapidity, magnitude, or both) of concurrently or subsequently administered drugs. Thiopental causes a reduction in cerebral blood flow by direct vasomotor action and may further retard the onset of effect of methoxyflurane. Halothane causes a vasodilation in skeletal muscle, and any resultant increase in muscle blood flow would speed the onset of neuromuscular blockade produced by muscle relaxants.

Several drugs that are given during the perianesthetic and anesthetic periods are highly protein bound. Displacement from binding sites results in an increase effect because more free or unbound drug is available to exert its effect. Phenylbutazone will reduce the number of protein sites to which thiopental normally binds. The resultant effect of thiopental may in this instance reflect a relative or even absolute overdose.

Because most drugs are bound to albumins, we need to give greater consideration to this protein fraction than to globulins or total plasma protein concentration. It also seems reasonable to expect that drugs that are highly bound to albumin will be affected to a greater degree than those that are bound only slightly or moderately. For example, we would expect hypoalbuminemia to result in a more pronounced effect from thiamylal (65 to 80% bound) than from phenobarbital (20% bound).

Of the drugs considered thus far in this section, large amounts of protein binding occur with digitoxin (up to 97%), steroids (at least 90% with cortisol), thiobarbiturates (65 to 80%), chloramphenicol (60%), and furosemide ("large amount") (3, 4). Moderate amounts of meperidine (40%), pentobarbital (35%), tetracycline (25 to 30%), and digoxin (25%) are bound to protein, and lesser amounts of tetracycline (20 to 25%), phenobarbital (20%), and procainamide (15%) are bound.

Biotransformation

Phenobarbital pretreatment causing hepatic microsomal enzyme induction and more rapid biotransformation of subsequently administered barbiturates is one classic example of interactions that enhance biotransformation. Because the enzyme induction process involves de novo synthesis of protein, enhancement of biotransformation by this process usually occurs over a period of several days.

Hepatic microsomal enzymes can also be inhibited. For example, chloramphenicol can inhibit enzymatic biotransformation of pentobarbital and other barbiturates, which is reflected as prolonged sleep time. This mechanism may often involve inhibition of protein synthesis, and the time course (from a few hours to a few days) over which it occurs therefore is dependent on the turnover rate of the particular enzyme in question.

A third mechanism of drug interaction that influences biotransformation involves competition between two concurrently administered drugs for the same biotransformation process. The ester-type local anesthetic procaine competes with succinylcholine in the biotransformation process involving plasma cholinesterases. Concurrent use of procaine and succinylcholine would be expected to prolong the effects of both drugs in proportion to the relative doses used and the patient's plasma cholinesterase levels.

Excretion

When the process of excretion is considered, the urinary system and especially the kidneys come to mind. However, biliary excretion may be an important consideration with some drugs. Prolonged action of a drug may occur if the drug or active metabolite is excreted via the bile and subsequently absorbed from the intestinal tract. This enterohepatic circulation appears to be clinically important only when a pharmacologically active compound (parent drug or metabolite) is involved. Drugs that undergo biotransformation to an inactive form do not influence duration of drug effect by this mechanism.

Renal excretion can be impaired by hemodynamic alterations produced by concurrently administered drugs. Any drug that reduces renal blood flow has the potential to decrease renal excretion in proportion to the reduction in glomerular filtration rate.

Table 10.1
Acid-Base Alterations and Effects on Drug Activity

Drug	Effect of Decreased pH	Effect of Increased pH
Atropine	Inhibition	Potentiation
Barbiturates (All)	Potentiation	Inhibition
Diazepam	Inhibition	
Lidocaine	Inhibition	Potentiation
Narcotic analgesics	Inhibition	Potentiation
Fentanyl		
Meperidine		
Morphine		
Oxymorphone		
Vasopressors	Inhibition	Potentiation
Epinephrine		
Isoproterenol		
Levarterenol		

Acid-base alterations that influence the proportion of ionized versus nonionized drugs may alter renal excretion (5). Several drugs used in anesthesia are potentially enhanced or inhibited by alterations in acid-base balance (Table 10.1). By varying the ratio of nonionized:ionized forms, acid-base changes may produce any or all of the following results: (*a*) variation in the amount of drug absorbed from the injection site; (*b*) alteration of the amount of drug that reaches the effector organ; and (*c*) varied renal excretion, as the urine becomes acidic or alkaline. An increase in the ionized portion of drug in plasma will generally retard renal excretion of that drug. As with biliary excretion, this mechanism is clinically important only if the parent drug or an active metabolite is excreted by the kidney.

PHARMACODYNAMIC INTERACTIONS

Pharmacodynamic interactions alter the effect of drugs at specific or nonspecific receptors. Several examples of this type of interaction are well known. Two such examples are apparent in the "reversal" of neuromuscular blockade produced by a nondepolarizing muscle relaxant.

When the cholinesterase inhibitor neostigmine is given to reverse neuromuscular blockade produced by pancuronium, for example, acetylcholine concentration at the neuromuscular junction and at muscarinic sites increases (a pharmacokinetic effect involving enzyme inhibition). Acetylcholine then competitively displaces pancuronium from acetylcholine receptors at the neuromuscular junction (a pharmacodynamic interaction between endogenous acetylcholine and pancuronium), and muscle relaxation is reversed. Atropine is usually given to competitively antagonize the effects of neostigmine (actually acetylcholine) at muscarinic receptors sites in the heart, exocrine glands, and smooth muscle (another pharmacodynamic interaction between atropine and acetylcholine).

Similarly, there is competition for opiate receptors between morphine and naloxone. The agonist morphine reversibly and competitively binds to receptors producing analgesia. The antagonist naloxone, which does not produce analgesia, competes with morphine for these receptor sites. The receptor affinity of naloxone is much greater than that of morphine, thereby reversing analgesia and other opiate effects.

Both receptor affinity and receptor specificity are important considerations in pharmacodynamic interactions. Acetylcholine receptor specificity in different tissues varies considerably among drugs. Most muscle relaxants are highly specific for acetylcholine receptors at the neuromuscular junction, whereas atropine is more specifically involved with receptors at the muscarinic sites mentioned previously.

Nonanesthetic-related medications also have an effect on anesthetic management. Two classic examples are the antibiotics and the anhelminthics. The organophosphate products greatly reduce pseudocholinesterase levels, which are necessary for reversal of succinylcholine. The needed level of pseudocholinesterase may not be adequate for at least 14 days after drug is discontinued.

The concurrent usage of tetracycline and methoxyflurane in geriatric patients with pre-existing renal dysfunction has resulted in serious complications and some deaths. Neomycin and related antibiotics may greatly enhance the muscle-relaxing characteristics of the anesthetics and muscle relaxants. Total loss of respiratory capability in animals under halothane anesthesia with concurrent high concentrations of neomycin have occurred.

In summary, drug interactions are commonly used to the advantage of the clinician in producing balanced anesthesia with a multiplicity of drugs. The four components of the anesthetic state (mental, sensory, motor, and reflex) can be attenuated by judicious use of a variety of drugs to achieve anesthesia. However, other physical, chemical, pharmacokinetic, or pharmacodynamic interactions may pose a threat to the patient.

References

1. McGrath CJ, McGrath DH: Pharmacology. In Sattler FP, Knowles RP, Whittick WG (eds): *Veterinary Critical Care*. Philadelphia, Lea & Febiger, 1981, p 298.
2. Martin EW: *Hazards of Medication*. Philadelphia, JB Lippincott, 1971.
3. Fingl E, Woodbury DM: General principles. In Goodman LS, Gilman A (eds): *The Pharmacological Basis of Therapeutic*, ed 5. New York, Macmillan, 1975, p 1.
4. Baggot DJ: Mechanisms of drug action. In Booth NH, McDonald LE: *Veterinary Pharmacology and Therapeutics*, ed 5. Ames, Iowa State University Press, 1982, p 23.
5. Eltherington LG: Drug interactions in Anesthesia. In American Society of Anesthesiologists Refresher Course No 212, Atlanta, Georgia, 1983.

CHAPTER 11

Dissociative Anesthesia

CHARLES E. SHORT, D.V.M., M.S., D.A.C.V.A.

The dissociative anesthetics are a group of related chemical compounds that are capable of producing a state of anesthesia during which the patient has an apparent dissociation from its environment. These chemical compounds are commonly referred to as the cyclohexamines. They are capable of producing immobilization, analgesia, and depression. There is variation among the animal species relative to the degree of response, the characteristics of response of the central nervous system (CNS), and the outward signs of this anesthetic state, so often referred to as dissociative anesthesia. It would appear that the dissociate state is caused by the interruption of CNS impulses and the differential depression of various areas of the brain (1). Oculogyric activity, tearing, and nystagmus are common (2, 3). This state of anesthesia is characterized by active ocular, oral, laryngeal, and swallowing reflexes. The eyes usually remain open with dilatation of the pupils. A number of animals will have noticeable salivation, and muscle tone may become more pronounced (4). This muscle tone in a few individuals will include extensor rigidity, tonic spasticity, and evidence of CNS stimulation. There occasionally will be strong evidence of convulsions (5, 6). The respiratory pattern is apneustic.

The original dissociative anesthetics were phencyclidine and cyclohexylamine. Phencyclidine was predominantly used in subhuman primates. Its early application revolutionized the chemical restraint and handling procedures in various research laboratories. The drug could be administered by intramuscular injection in subhuman primates with a wide margin of safety, and the tolerance to repeat dosages was encouraging. The use of phencyclidine in our laboratories in the domestic cat produced analgesia, but there were prolonged recovery and postanesthetic effects that resembled hallucination, confusion, and occasional spastic responses. It became evident that the utilization of phencyclidine or cyclohexylamine in human subjects or in a wide range of animal subjects was not desirable.

Because of its use as an abused drug, it became evident that phencyclidine could produce hallucinations with major contributing complications in human subjects. Veterinarians frequently became involved in treatment of these early drug abuse cases because patient history upon admission to medical hospitals frequently included the use of an animal tranquilizer. The author was consulted on three human drug abuse-overdose cases during the 1960s. The patients were young adults with an over-response to injections of phencyclidine. In addition to their hallucinations, there was muscle rigidity, apneustic respiration, loss of body temperature, and renal dysfunction. Supportive care including rehydration and re-establishment of renal function was crucial. As a result of the drug abuse potential of phencyclidine, it was withdrawn from the veterinary market, and the development of other dissociative agents that are of greater potential in animal anesthesia, further discussion of phencyclidine and cyclohexamine is not justified.

Ketamine Hydrochloride

Ketamine hydrochloride is a member of the dissociative anesthesia family of compounds. Ketamine has become popular for use alone or in combination with a variety of drugs in many species since its development in 1963. This was a successful attempt to produce a phencyclidine-like product with a shorter recovery period, fewer postanesthetic psychotomimetic effects, and fewer undesirable CNS responses during the anesthetic period (7). Ketamine is produced as a white crystalline compound with a melting point of 259°C. It is chemically 2-(O)-chlorophenyl)-2-methyl amino cycloxexanone hydrochloride. Ketamine is a clear, odorless, and colorless solution soluble in water. It is supplied as a 10% aqueous solution with a pH of 3.7. Because of the low pH, the compound is slightly irritating to tissues; animals show some evidence of a slightly painful response to injections when the drug is administered by the intramuscular route. The drug is not known, however, to cause excess tissue reactions, such as profound swelling or necrosis at the injection site, as can be observed with ultrashort-acting barbiturates. The drug has a high lipid solubility and is absorbed quickly after administration. Plasma levels will usually drop quickly at first due to distribution of the drug to other body tissues. This is usually followed by a slow drop in plasma levels over the next 4 to 8 hours with an estimated plasma half-life of 2 hours.

Ketamine hydrochloride has become the most popular dissociative cyclohexamine anesthetic. Its popularity stems from several characteristics. It is easy to use, being administered by either intramuscular or intravenous routes. It has a relatively large margin of safety, especially when compared with the barbiturates or inhalant anesthetics, and it is compatible with other drugs used to produce tranquilization or sedation. It may be used as part of an injectable anesthetic regime or as a means of inducing anesthesia prior to general anesthesia with supplemental volatile anesthetic agents. Ketamine enjoys this popularity in spite of the occasional emergence delerium and the lack of a direct antagonist to reverse the effects of prolonged anesthesia due to a relative overdose of ketamine or more profound depression than expected for the dosage of anesthetic administered. Ketamine usage may be associated with several undesirable side effects; however, the patient even in high-risk circumstances seldom dies.

ANESTHETIC ACTION AND EFFECT ON THE CNS

Ketamine produces profound and reversible effects on the CNS. The drug produces a loss of sensory perception or response and a state of unconsciousness. There is a coma-like condition, often referred to as cataleptoid anesthesia, which differs markedly from the classic signs of anesthesia produced by volatile and gaseous anesthetic agents. Neither does it resemble the deep hypnotic or narcosis state induced by the barbiturates. Even the fact that the eyes remain open with corneal and light reflexes suggests the mechanisms involved in dissociative anesthesia are different from those of inhalant anesthetics. Ketamine appears to alter the reactivity of the CNS to various sensory impulses without blocking the sensory input at spinal or brain stem levels. The input may reach cortical receiving areas, but it fails to be perceived because of depression or disorganization of the associated areas during periods of anesthesia (7, 8). Depressant effects of ketamine have been determined in the central nucleus of the thalamus (9), the neocorticothalamic axis (10), and the nociceptive cells in the medial medullary reticular formation (11). Electroencephalographic (EEG) activation of the hippocampus is seen at the time of onset of thalamocortical depression (10, 12). Seizure discharges are likely to be seen in the hippocampus in the cat at dosages of 25 to 40 mg/kg (13). Because the seizure threshold for dissociative anesthetics used without potent sedatives or other drugs to control CNS activity may be reached in the cat, one would anticipate a very small dosage would be required to cause similar seizure activity as demonstrated on the EEG in the horse. Considerations of safety for both subject and investigator make it inappropriate to evaluate the potential electroencephalographic seizure thresholds of dissociative anesthetic agents in horses.

Ketamine has induced seizures in other species. In dogs, several patients not known to be epileptic have had seizure activity. Seizure activity may occur during the more pronounced effective period of ketamine in the dog or as much as 24 hours later as observed in our laboratories (14). Ketamine seizures have occurred in the dog when the drug has been used alone or in combination with tranquilizers, including diazepam and acetylpromazine, the sedative xylazine, or the barbiturate thiamylal sodium (15–18). It is apparent that ketamine is less likely to produce seizure activity in cats, subhuman primates, and young children than in the dog, the horse, teenaged or adult human subjects, or other species. Even though early evidence in rats indicated ketamine was effective in antagonizing electrically induced seizures, its utilization in animals with a history of epilepsy should be avoided or used with caution.

Ketamine has been shown to increase cerebral blood flow and intracranial pressure (19). There is evidence that anesthetic action of ketamine requires the function of the cerebral cortex, including failure of ketamine to induce anesthesia in cases of massive injury (20–22). As a result, utilization of ketamine in patients with cerebral trauma or intracranial masses requires caution and careful management.

A number of studies have been made to determine the mechanism of ketamine activity in the brain. Ketamine causes dopamine-related behavioral patterns. Its effect is antagonized when brain dopamine is depleted. It is reasonable to postulate that at least part of ketamine's action is to increase the release of dopamine in the brain (23–25). It has also been shown that there is an increased amount of serotonin during ketamine-induced anesthesia and the norepinephrine levels increase during the recovery period, especially in recoveries associated with some degree of excitement (26). In cats anesthetized with ketamine, serotonin appeared to mediate catalepsy and respiratory irregularity. Ketamine was also shown to have dopamine receptor involvement in muscle twitching (27). Ketamine-induced anesthesia appears to be related to an imbalance of muscarinic-nicotinic cholinergic activity with muscle jerking and emergence delerium apparently related to muscarinic and ketamine-induced catalepsy. In contrast, dopaminergic and nicotinic cholinoceptive receptors were mediated by ketamine-induced anesthesia (28).

In reality, the mechanisms of action in the brain of ketamine-induced responses remains complex. Because the outward symptoms of CNS response to ketamine vary among the animal species, even determination of the actual mechanisms of ketamine response in the CNS of one species does not assure that these mechanisms are correct in other species. One can reach a similar conclusion if one can carefully evaluate the responses to ketamine anesthesia in neonatal adult patients. With the variation in responses to dissociative anesthesia produced by ketamine hydrochloride, it was only reasonable to predict that tranquilizers, sedatives, and other medications would be used in conjunction with ketamine to provide a more balanced state of anesthesia. These drug combinations, including most commonly ketamine combined with xylazine, diazepam, or acetypromazine, have resulted in a reduction in undesirable CNS responses, an improvement in the degree of muscle relaxation achieved, and a reduction in the recovery delerium that appeared to be associated with the use of ketamine as a sole agent.

The extent of analgesia that can be anticipated with ketamine alone will vary according to the innervation of the affected sites. There is a greater extent of somatic analgesia than for the visceral areas. This has been demonstrated in humans, in whom analgesia was more effective for surgery involving the extremities than for abdominal procedures (29). Further evidence of this phenomenon is demonstrated during such abdominal procedures as ovariohysterectomies in the cat where a complete absence of response is observed during the incision of the abdominal wall. The animal then may show signs of responsiveness incuding mild vocalization during the manipulations of the genital tract. Further evidence of somatic analgesia has been demonstrated in various burn units with repeated application for debridement of damaged tissue and multiple skin grafts. The need for an anesthetic for the treatment of severe burns was one of the primary objectives in the original development of ketamine anesthesia in humans. Thus, better somatic than visceral analgesia should be expected.

CARDIOVASCULAR RESPONSES TO KETAMINE ANESTHESIA

During the early evaluation of ketamine as an anesthetic in cats, dogs, and subhuman primates, the lack of a major reduction in blood pressure was noted. Heart rates tended to be increased. There was less sensitivity to norepinephrine or epinephrine for the production of cardiac arrhythmias. There was a rise in blood pressure, perhaps caused by an increased myocardial contractual force, increased heart rate, and an increase in cardiac output. It was found that total peripheral resistance remained unchanged or perhaps dropped slightly after the injection of ketamine in intact anesthetized dogs. It appeared that the increase in cardiovascular activity was more pronounced in the dog than in the cat.

Because these early impressions showed either a stimulation of cardiovascular function or at least less depression of cardiac function than generally expected from other anesthetic agents, a number of investigations into cardiovascular responses were completed. Consider the variation in CNS response to ketamine in different species or the effect other agents used in conjunction with ketamine may have on the overall cardiovascular function during the anesthetic period. The cardiovascular responses to ketamine in the clinically normal patient include an increase in heart rate, cardiac output, and arterial pressure (7). This may be an indirect effect due to a combination of inhibitory effects on the parasympathetic innervation of the heart and a stimulatory sympathomimetic effect on the heart. As a result, one seldom sees hypotension in a normal animal. It has been shown that intravenous ketamine at 2, 4, 6, and 8 mg/kg i.v. in the cat produces little change in central autonomic response, whereas sodium thiamylal at 3, 6, 9, and 12 mg/kg i.v. reduced sympathetic tone by 10% with little effect on vagal tone. Halothane depresses both sympathetic and vagal tone (30). Ketamine appeared to have positive chronotropic and inotropic effects, as demonstrated by the release of catecholamines from peripheral tissue stores, stimulation of CNS sympathetic efferent discharge, interference with cardiac vagal tone, increases in calcium influx, and perhaps inhibitions of calcium sequestration by the sarcoplasmic reticulum (31). Ketamine has been demonstrated to produce positive and chronotropic and inotropic effects on isolated hearts and heart tissue preparations as well (32). Hemodynamic measurements of healthy cats receiving 22 mg/kg of ketamine were studied for heart rate, systemic and pulmonary blood pressure, peripheral vascular resistance, cardiac output, indirect assessment of cardiac contractibility (d.p./d.t.: change in pressure relative to time), and myocardial oxygen consumption as determined by rate pressure product. The results illustrated in Table 11.1 show an increase in heart rate, ventricular pressure, and aortic pressure, but no change in left ventricular contractibility. Cardiac output and left ventricular and diastolic pressure increased after ketamine administration, giving support to the conclusion there is either little effect or an increase in activity of the cardiovascular system in healthy cats.

An increase in heart rate of 18% while stroke volume fell 27% during ketamine administration has been reported (33). There was a concurrent drop of 18% in oxygen uptake in the next hour of anesthesia and surgery, with cardiac output displaying a transient decrease. During the second hour, oxygen uptake returned to the awake state. A small percentage of critically ill human patients showed reduced blood pressures, blood flow, and myocardial performance related to hypovolemia in associated medical conditions (34).

Ketamine and thiopenthal were studied in hypovolemic swine to further characterize the potential sympathetic stimulation that might exist in moderate hypovolemia. These swine with 30% of estimated blood volume removed showed an increase in plasma epinephrine/norepinephrine and renin activity when anesthetized with ketamine but not with thiopenthal. Both anesthetics depress systemic vascular resistance, mean systemic arterial blood pressure, heart rate, and cardiac output. Ketamine decreased stroke volume, but neither anesthetic affected oxygen consumption. After treatment of the hypovolemia with blood transfusions, all animals responded. The cardiac output was greater in the animals given ketamine than in those receiving thiopenthal wtihin 30 minutes. Ninety minutes after the infusion, no differences existed among the treatment groups (35). Further studies during the hypocapnic state in ketamine-anesthetized swine to evaluate organ blood flow during ketamine anesthesia showed there was no change in the fraction of cardiac output received by the brain, heart, and splanchnic organs, but there was an increase in the perfusion of the kidneys and liver compared to control. Blood flow to the brain, heart and splanchnic organs decreased, kidney and skeletal muscle blood flow was unaltered, and hepatic arterial blood flow increased from the awake state (36). In rabbits, a significant drop in mean arterial blood pressure with 6 and 18 mg/kg of ketamine i.v. has been observed. There was an increase in heart rate, but cardiac output and blood flow to tissues was not changed by ketamine. There was an increased blood flow to the cerebral hemispheres with a concurrent vasodilation in the cerebral hemispheres (37). It can be concluded that ketamine anesthesia is no more likely to cause cardiovascular depression than other anesthetic agents; it has on numerous occasions been used in the presence of cardiac arrhythmias without being detrimental. Ketamine should be used with caution, and appropriate monitoring of cardiac function is desirable in patients with traumatized myocardium, uncontrolled cardiac arrhythmias, and valvular insufficiency or cardiac disease.

RESPIRATORY RESPONSES

The respiratory responses to ketamine in the cat are quite characteristic. Respiratory rate increases, tidal volume decreases, and there is an apneustic pattern of breathing produced after intramuscular or intravenous ketamine administration. Most pulmonary function tests remain within normal limits. Higher doses are more likely to produce respiratory depression, hypoxemia, and hypercarbia. Rather typical responses of the respiratory system to administration of ketamine in the cat are shown in Table 11.2. Although minute volumes did not change significantly, decreased respiratory rate and apneustic breathing patterns caused elevation in end-tidal CO_2. The apneustic pattern of breathing produced an increase in functional residual capacity (FRC). The utilization of xylazine or

Table 11.1
Hemodynamic Measurements in Cats Receiving 22 mg/kg of Ketamine[a]

Time	Control	5 Minutes	15 Minutes	30 Minutes	45 Minutes
$\dot{V}$ Max	3.72 ± 1.02	3.41 ± 0.55	4.0 ± 0.45	4.10 ± 0.68	5.38 ± 0.90
Heart rate (beats/minute)	171.7 ± 8.31	160.0 ± 6.8	180.0 ± 7.3	181.7 ± 10.5	198.0 ± 12.8
LVEDP (mm Hg)	4.2 ± 3.0	5.7 ± 2.5	5.2 ± 2.4	5.0 ± 1.5	3.4 ± 12.8
LV systolic (mm Hg)	119.5 ± 17.3	127.8 ± 12.3	135.7 ± 8.2	137.5 ± 12.0	134.4 ± 11.0
Arterial blood pressure, systolic (mm Hg)	117.2 ± 16.5	124.7 ± 10.2	130.8 ± 7.2	138.0 ± 11.9	126.6 ± 10.6
Mean arterial blood pressure (mm Hg)	95.6 ± 13.0	103.7 ± 7.6	111.7 ± 6.9	113.2 ± 11.7	102.6 ± 8.7
Diastolic blood pressure (mm Hg)	85.0 ± 11.5	93.2 ± 6.2	100.2 ± 6.0	100.7 ± 11.7	90.8 ± 7.7
Cardiac output (ml/kg)	157.0 ± 16.0	162.0 ± 14.0	182.0 ± 18.0	176.0 ± 17.0	181.0 ± 16.0

[a] Adapted from Muir (31).

Table 11.2
Respiratory Measurements during 22 mg/kg of i.v. Ketamine in Cats[a]

RR Breaths/min	16.6 ± 1.8
V_T ml	102.9 ± 18.3
$\dot{V}_M$ lit/min	1.5 ± 0.3
$\dot{V}$ lit/min	7.2 ± 1.1
(CO_2)ET%	6.7 ± 0.4
V_{DP}/VT	0.5 ± 0.1
FRC ml	217.7 ± 36.2
FRC/wt ml/kg	51.1 ± 6.7
P_{TP} cm H_2O	4.1 ± 0.7
$C_{dyn} = V_T/P_{TP}$ cc/cm H_2O	28.2 ± 4.6
$R_{tot} = \Delta P/\Delta F$ cm H_2O/lit/sec	0.3 ± 0.1
IOP Control (−cm/H_2O)	22.3 ± 3.7

[a] Adapted from Muir (31). Values reported as mean ± SEM. Air flow (V) and tidal volume (V_T) were recorded using a pneumotachygraph transducer system attached to a cuffed endotracheal tube inserted into the trachea after orotracheal intubation. Transpulmonary pressure (P_{TP}) was measured as the pressure difference between the thoracic esophagus and the open airway using an esophageal balloon. Total respiratory system resistance, R($P_{TP/V}$), dynamic compliance (C_{dyn}), respiratory rate (RR), and minute ventilation (V_M) were calculated from the recording of P_{TP}, V, and V_T. Functional residual capacity was measured using nitrogen washout techniques. Inspiratory occlusion pressure (IOP), a measurement of drug-induced respiratory center depression, was determined by occluding the inspiratory value and recording the negative pressure developed during inspiration. The percent end tidal carbon dioxide concentration (CO_2ET%) was recorded and used to calculate the physiological dead space (V_{PD}) using the Bohr equation. This value is expressed relative to tidal volume (V_{PD}/V_T). Pulmonary function variables were recorded and compared 15 minutes after induction with the anesthetic.

other medications in conjunction with ketamine may also cause a slight increase in $PaCO_2$, a slight decrease in arterial pH, and as much as a 10% decrease in PaO_2 (38–43). This not only occurs in the cat, but in other animals, including horses, sheep, and calves. In contrast, respiratory rates and tidal volume increased in dogs given ketamine (44, 45).

Laryngeal and pharyngeal reflexes are reasonably maintained during ketamine-induced anesthesia in all species. Regurgitation may occur, and, although there is some protection against regurgitation, there may not be adequate swallowing reflexes to avoid aspiration (7). Ketamine frequently produces salivation, but this can be controlled by administration of anticholinergics (7).

Cats receiving very high doses of 40 and 80 mg/kg of ketamine continue an apneustic breathing pattern characterized by prolonged inspiratory duration and relatively short expiratory time. In spite of the high dosage of ketamine administered in this group of cats, the ventilatory response to increased CO_2 was similar to unanesthetized cats to produce an increase in mean inspiratory air flow. Thus, the ventilatory response to increased CO_2 remains high for ketamine compared to the normal change in CO_2 response curve as seen with narcotics and general anesthetics (46). Our studies have indicated that the typical respiratory response in the cat will reveal a drop in pH and PaO_2 and an increase in $PaCO_2$ within 5 minutes of the administration of ketamine with a return to normal values in healty cats between 40 to 60 minutes after the administration of ketamine.

HEPATIC RESPONSES

In both human and canine studies, there was no evidence of hepatic dysfunction after ketamine anesthesia. In dogs, high dose administration of ketamine (40 mg/kg i.m. daily for 6 weeks, produced transient increases in hepatic enzymes (12). Ketamine is metabolized by the body with a distribution of drug not only to organs, but to body fat, liver, and kidneys. Metabolism is very rapid, with very little unchanged drug excreted in most animal species after i.v. administration. Four metabolic products were isolated from monkey urine by the Research Laboratories at Parke-Davis. They included the primary amine produced by N-demethylation, referred to as Metabolite 1, and the partially unsaturated cyclohexanone-derivative, referred to as Metabolite 2. Acid hydrolysis of urine yielded a third metabolite. This was isolated and identified as an immediate oxidation product with a hydroxy group in the alpha carbon of the cyclohexanone ring, Metabolite 3. A fourth metabolite was identified as the beta-hydroxy derivative Metabolite 4. Perhaps there are other metabolites of unknown chemical structure.

It has been clinically observed that animals with hepatic dysfunction do not metabolize ketamine as rapidly as normal animals and that animals with renal dysfunction or obstruction to urinary flow have prolonged sleep time after the administration of ketamine. Animals with renal failure have been shown to continue in the anesthetized state until the re-establishment of urinary function and urinary output. This emphasizes the need for supportive care in prolonged responses to ketamine anesthesia, as well as the need for fluid and electrolyte balance in these individuals to assure normal recovery patterns.

Recovery from ketamine has sometimes been associated with emergence reactions. There is less reaction when the patient is kept quiet and there is no excessive noise or activity. The concurrent use of xylazine or acetylpromazine with ketamine has helped to minimize side effects; studies using diazepam show reduced violent reactions during recovery situations. The recovery pattern in some individuals resembles what might be described as an hallucinogenic response, although it is difficult to determine whether animals experience true hallucinogenic responses as have been reported in humans. Attempts have been made to determine an antagonist to reverse ketamine anesthesia and induce a more rapid recovery. Efforts that stimulate the CNS may in some instances increase the likelihood of adverse reactions. Use of yohimbine, which stimulates seretonin release, has been shown to shorten the time until righting reflexes are regained after ketamine-induced anesthesia, but this is not a predictable response (47). Naloxone, a narcotic antagonist, may reduce the duration in some species, but has not gained wide acceptance (48). Presently, the primary mechanism for improving recovery response is supportive care.

USE OF KETAMINE IN OBSTETRICS

Ketamine has been shown to cross the placental barrier. The maternal effects of ketamine consist of increases in mean arterial pressure, cardiac output (slight and transitory) and uterine tone, but uterine blood flow remained constant (49). A comparison of thiopentone and ketamine in newborns after elective Caesarean section showed ketamine to be a good alternate barbiturate as induction agent for Caesarean section (50). Ketamine has not been widely used in obstetrical anesthesia, but its responses appear to be no worse than those of barbiturates.

CLINICAL APPLICATIONS OF KETAMINE

Ketamine has been a useful drug for chemical restraint, induction of anesthesia, or production of surgical anesthesia alone or in combination with other medications in a large number of species, including laboratory animals and wildlife. The use of ketamine in laboratory animals and wildlife will not be discussed here because it is covered in chapters concerning those specific topics. Initially, ketamine was used as a dissociative anesthetic in veterinary practice in the cat. Dosage recommendation was of 10 to 45 mg/kg of body weight by i.m. injection. As a result, during the early usage of ketamine in veterinary practice, prolonged recoveries, hypothermia, and emergence delerium occurred in a relatively high number of cats. The results improved dramatically when the dosage was limited to 10 to 30 mg/kg of body weight. At this dosage level, the predominant undesirable response to ketamine anesthesia was lack of adequate relaxation, inadequate visceral analgesia for some procedures, and some prolonged recoveries.

Concurrent medications of preketamine medications in cats have resulted in better muscle relaxation, reduction in salivation, more complete analgesia, and fewer undesirable reactions during the recovery pattern. Ketamine has been used in the cat in conjunction with narcotics, tranquilizers, sedatives, and anticholinergics. Either glycopyrrolate or atropine may be used to reduce salivation. Utilization of the anticholinergic does not appreciably increase the heart rate in the cat above that observed with ketamine alone. The utlization of acetylpromazine or diazepam as a preanesthetic prior to ketamine in the cat results in a smoother induction, improved muscle relaxation, and fewer complications in recovery. It also provides an opportunity to reduce the level of ketamine administration required to produce chemical restraint, light anesthesia, induction of anesthesia prior to inhalants, or surgical plane anesthesia. In conjunction with these tranquilizers, 5 to 15 mg/kg of i.m. ketamine is usually adequate to achieve chemical restraint or general anesthesia in a dose-related response. Intravenous doses of 2 to 5 mg/kg of ketamine result in shorter term effects usually lasting no more than 10 to 15 minutes before the return of righting reflex.

Xylazine has been a useful agent to improve muscle relaxation, the degree of visceral analgesia, and recovery (51). Xylazine is usually administered at 0.2 to 0.5 mg/kg i.m. 10 to 15 minutes before ketamine induction in small animals (52–54) and 1.1 mg/kg i.v. in horses. Unless anticholinergics are used, xylazine may cause bradycardia or atrioventricular conduction heart block. The administration of ketamine usually corrects bradycardia. The premedication in conjunction with 15 mg/kg i.m. ketamine has been satisfactory as surgical anesthesia for minor procedures. It does not seem that there are important advantages to using narcotics in conjunction with ketamine anesthesia in cats. Ketamine as an inducing agent has been very effective in the cat prior to inhalant anesthesia of methoxyflurane, halothane, isoflurane, or nitrous oxide. The predominant anesthetic effect after intramuscular use of ketamine is observed during the first 45 to 60 minutes of the procedure. This will influence the concentration of inhalant anesthetic required. After intravenous administration of ketamine, anesthetic effects will last only a short time, usually no more than 5 to 20 minutes, with the balance of anesthesia due to the inhalants administered. After ketamine induction in the cat, laryngeal responses will remain slightly to moderately active at the time of intubation. These laryngeal responses are not always sufficiently active to avoid aspiration in instances of regurgitation.

Ketamine has become a popular drug for use in horses, either for short surgical procedures or as an inducing agent. In contrast to utilization of ketamine in the cat, where responses can be controlled to assure appropriate levels of dissociative anesthesia, ketamine should not be administered as a sole agent in the horse. The most commonly used medication prior to the use of ketamine in the horse is xylazine, usually at a dosage level of 1.1 mg/kg i.v. 4 to 5 minutes prior to the administration of ketamine at a dosage rate of 2.2 mg/kg i.v. (14). Guaifenesin at 55 mg/kg of body weight i.v. has been administered in conjunction with xylazine/ketamine to produce a greater degree of relaxation (55). Diazepam at 0.22 mg/kg has also been used to reduce the muscle fasciculations and improve the quality of combined anesthesia.

Adequate sedation and tranquilization by xylazine or other potent tranquilizers and sedatives must be evident if one is to expect satisfactory results from the intravenous administration of ketamine. With insufficient tranquilization, the horse may not be induced with 2.2 mg/kg i.v. ketamine, or the horse may become recumbent but have profound muscle rigidity, muscle fasciculations, and active eye responses with sinus tachycardia, reduced tidal volume, and apneustic respiratory patterns. Intubation is difficult because of failure of the combination to produce adequate relaxation of masseter muscles.

When adequate tranquilization and sedation have been accomplished with xylazine or xylazine combinations as preanesthetics, more complete relaxation is obtained, surgical plane anesthesia that lasts from 15 to 20 minutes from the initial injection can be accomplished, or anesthetic induction before inhalant anesthesia can be satisfactorily accomplished. Inductions of the horse with a combination of preketamine administration of guaifenesin until there is muscle relaxation followed by 2.2 mg/kg of i.v. ketamine have been used. These horses have outwardly shown symptoms of muscle relaxation and unconsciousness. Unfortunately, guaifenesin is not a potent CNS depressant; although it may control the muscle fasciculation and rigidity associated with dissociative anesthetics without premedication in the horse, the CNS might undergo similar responses if ketamine alone were administered. As a result, the use of guaifenesin and ketamine without sedation in the horse is strongly discouraged because of its potential inhumane application. Xylazine and ketamine have been used in our hospital for induction of horses with equine colic requiring surgical correction for the past 9 years. Our experiences have shown this to be a safe induction in horses showing physical, clinical, pathological, and physiological signs of shock, debilitation, and toxemia.

Ketamine anesthesia in the horse from a single injection will have a duration of 15 to 20 minutes. A smooth recovery pattern usually occurs within 20 to 35 minutes after induction of anesthesia. Anesthesia may be prolonged by several methods, including using the xylazine/ketamine combination for induction of anesthesia prior to inhalant anesthesia. If this method is used, one should be aware that a period of inadequate surgical plane anesthesia may occur 15 to 20 minutes after the administration of ketamine unless inhalant anesthetic concentrations are adjusted accordingly. The redistribution of ketamine in the horse occurs with a characteristic rapid arousal during this time period after intravenous administration. One should further anticipate that bradycardia or heart block may occur during the next 3 to 10 minutes because the effects of xylazine with its potential bradycardia or heart block exists along with the cardiac-depressing effects of halothane without the cardiac-stimulating effect of ketamine. Although this problem is rare, responses are quite severe in the horse. The use of additional xylazine at this time to control the level of anesthesia should be avoided because supplemental administration of xylazine during halothane maintenance may be associated with severe bradycardia or cardiac arrest.

Deliberate prolongation of anesthesia with xylazine and ketamine to produce up to 1 hour of anesthesia has been accomplished after the induction of anesthesia with xylazine and ketamine. One-half of the initial dosage is repeated at approximately 10 and 20 minutes after the initial induction of anesthesia. This study was completed in 10 horses with a mean sternal recumbency of 55 minutes. The horses stood successfully on their first attempt 60 minutes after initial induction. Respiration initially increased after anesthetic induction, then gradually decreased during the 50-minute period postinduction. Arterial oxygen decreased significantly from the usual preanesthetic values of 80 to 100 mm Hg PaO_2 to 77 mm Hg within 10 minutes after induction and to 57 mm Hg 30 minutes after the induction with xylazine/ketamine maintenance. The arterial CO_2 levels increased from a preinduction value of 37 mm Hg $PaCO_2$ to 40 mm Hg within 10 minutes and 43 mm Hg at 30 minutes of anesthesia.

The heart rate showed a slight decrease from preanesthetic levels to the level during anesthetic maintenance with xylazine/ketamine; mean blood pressure was 109/55 immediately after induction of anesthesia, which increased to 130/93 within 10 minutes and to 131/95 after the second supplemental dose of xylazine/ketamine. This study, conducted in our laboratories in cooperation with Dr. John Lowe and associates, demonstrated an effective method of deliberately prolonging xylazine/ketamine anesthesia in the horse. It indicated that, although there were drops in oxygen levels, slight increases in carbon dioxide, and slight increases in blood pressure, it could be used as a method of field anesthesia in healthy horses.

Horses have been maintained on injectable anesthesia with supplemental administration of guaifenesin and barbiturate medication after xylazine/ketamine induction. This has been a successful procedure, but the speed of administration of the guaifenesin barbiturate and the dosage level administered are crucial factors in the safety of this procedure. Because the animals are usually not receiving supplemental oxygen, this combination of medication can reduce oxygen availability, increases in carbon dioxide levels may occur, and the potential for reduction in minute respiratory volume exists.

Ketamine has been used alone in cattle, but more

frequently it follows xylazine. Ketamine used alone in cattle is administered at the rate of 2 to 5 mg/kg i.v., as high as 11 mg/kg i.m. or i.v. in calves (56–60).

Sheep and goats are very sensitive to the administration of xylazine. We have successfully used a level of 0.04 to 0.06 mg/kg i.v. prior to 2.2 to 4.4 mg/kg of i.v. ketamine in sheep and goats. This has resulted in satisfactory induction of anesthesia that lasts for periods of 10 to 15 minutes. Other investigations indicated xylazine levels of 0.22 mg/kg before ketamine administration of 5 to 22 mg/kg i.v. (61–63). Higher dosage levels will prolong the anesthetic period and recovery time. Deliberate prolongation of anesthesia time can be achieved in sheep and goats; 4 usually requires 1 to 3 mg/kg i.v. as supplemental injections (64, 65).

Ketamine has been used in swine (66–70). The degree of relaxation is not as desired unless preanesthetics such as xylazine are administered. These combinations show promise for field anesthesia in swine.

It can be concluded that ketamine is an effective dissociative agent in a number of species. The combination of ketamine with other medications may be used effectively to produce anesthesia by injectable technique or as an inducing agent prior to inhalant anesthesia. When ketamine is to be used as an anesthetic agent, one should be aware of the characteristics of the drug, the responses of various species and individual animals with their existing physiological characteristics, and the role that the dissociative agent has in anesthetic management. The margin of safety with ketamine is high, but because there are few methods by which to dramatically affect the recovery patterns of ketamine anesthesia, careful attention to hydration, body temperature, ventilation, and renal function are suggested.

Telazol

The parenteral anesthetic agent, Telazol, was developed as an agent useful for anesthesia or chemical restraint in a variety of animal species. The compound is composed of two ingredients in equal amounts of weight; these are tiletamine hydrochloride, an arylcycloalkylamine, and zolazepam hydrochloride, a pyrazolodiazepinone. Tiletamine hydrochloride has a molecular formula of $C_{12}H_{17}NOS$-HCl and is designated chemically as 2-(ethylamino)-2-(2-thienyl) cyclohexanone-HCl.

When administered alone, tiletamine hydrochloride produces profound analgesia and cataleptoid anesthesia that, in some animals, can be accompanied by convulsive seizures and clonic muscular reactions (cats) (71).

The other ingredient, zolazepam hydrochloride, is a nonphenothiazine, pyrazolodiazepinone with minor tranquilizing properties. Chemically, it is 4-(0-fluorophenyl)-6,8-dihydro-1,3,8-trimethylpyrazolo-3,4-3e 1,4 diazepin-7 (IH)-one monohydrochloride.

Zolazepam hydrochloride is combined with tiletamine hydrochloride to reduce convulsive and clonic muscle reactions and to provide better muscle relaxation. The ultimate results of administration of the combination of drugs provides a state of anesthesia similar to ketamine and a tranquilizer. An intramuscular injection of tiletamine hydrochloride in cats and horses was accompanied by convulsive seizures and clonic muscular reactions during the deep surgical anesthetic state. Because these physiological reactions were considered detrimental, zolazepam hydrochloride was combined with tiletamine hydrochloride and administered intramuscularly. The combination caused muscle relaxation and a dissociative anesthetic state in dogs, cats, and many wild animal species. Its use in the horse needs further study. Potential adverse effects in the horse have been minimized by xylazine premedication.

Telazol can be classified as a general anesthetic. There will be a better understanding of the responses observed if it is related to such other dissociative anesthetics as ketamine and phencyclidine. Tiletamine is more potent than ketamine, but not as profound as phencyclidine. The patient's eyes are usually open even during profound surgical anesthesia with telazol. In addition, many reflexes are not abolished. Anesthetized animals respond to corneal and palpebral stimuli; laryngeal, pharyngeal, pedal, and pinnal reflexes may also persist. A common occurrence in most animals receiving telazol is salivation. Should salivation be objectionable, atropine sulfate or glycopyrrolate should be considered for control.

ROUTES OF ADMINISTRATION

Telazol is effective whether administered intramuscularly or intravenously. Anesthetic doses are the same for either intramuscular or intravenous routes of administration. Time for attainment of surgical anesthesia does vary with route of administration and usually is reached within 30 to 90 seconds after intravenous dosing and within 5 to 12 minutes after intramuscular dosing.

Dosage varies with the physical condition of the animal and duration of the surgical procedure. Starting doses for either intramuscular or intravenous administration depend upon effect desired. The dosage range in the cat is 2 to 15 mg/kg, and in the dog, it is 2 to 13 mg/kg. Low dosages of telazol may be used to produce a measurable tranquil state of light anesthesia, thus permitting or expediting procedures not requiring complete anesthesia. This state has been referred to as chemical restraint; it is desirable when working with fractious, dangerous species of animals.

Telazol can be utilized as an induction agent prior to intubation and transfer to volatile anesthesia. Intubation is not difficult even though pharyngeal and laryngeal reflexes are functional.

METABOLIC DISPOSITION OF TILETAMINE HYDROCHLORIDE IN LABORATORY ANIMALS

In cats, only 5 to 10% of the dose of tiletamine hydrochloride was detected in urine. None appeared in the feces; however, some drug was found in bile. Plasma half-life in cats was 2 to 4 hours; in rhesus monkeys, 1 to 1.5 hours; and in rats, 30 to 40 minutes. Tissue half-life appeared to be considerably longer than plasma half-life in both the cat and rat. The unchanged drug and two metabolites were isolated from monkey urine. These metabolites were identified as 2-(ethylamino)-2-(2-thienyl)cyclohexanol (Metabolite 1) and 2-amino-2-(2-thienyl)cyclohexanol (Metabolite 2). In addition to these, another metabolite was isolated in cat urine, 2-amino-2-(2-thienyl)cyclohexanone (Metabolite 3) (72).

METABOLIC DISPOSITION OF ZOLAZEPAM IN LABORATORY ANIMALS

The major metabolite in cats was 8-demethyl 1-6-hydroxy-zolazepam (Metabolite 5). The 8-demethyl-zolazepam (Metabolite 1) and 1,8-didemethyl-zolazepam (Metabolite 3) metabolites were found after single doses, but the concentration of these metabolites decreased with repeated dosing. In male and female rats, 6-hydroxy-zolazepam (Metabolite 4) was produced. The principal sex-related difference in rats was the presence of 1-demethyl-zolazepam (Metabolite 2) in the urine of female rats only. In beagle dogs, Metabolite 2 was found in the urine together with a hydroxylated derivative of Metabolite 2 (Metabolite 6), which was not found in the urine of rat or monkey (72).

PLACENTAL TRANSFER AND PLASMA LEVELS OF ZOLAZEPAM HYDROCHLORIDE IN LABORATORY ANIMALS

A study in normal beagle dogs showed that peak plasma levels were observed 1.5 to 2 hours after dosing with zolazepam hydrochloride, 50 mg/kg by mouth. Plasma half-life was 4 to 5 hours, somewhat longer than in the rat (3 hours) and considerably longer than in the monkey (1 hour). Peak urinary excretion occurred in the first 8-hour collection period after dosing, with lesser amounts appearing in the 8- to 24-hour period. Total recovery in urine represented 2.9 to 8.7% of the dose as unchanged zolazepam hydrochloride; approximately 1% of the dose was recovered in the feces.

CARDIOVASCULAR EFFECTS IN DOGS

A marked persistent tachycardia occurred within 2 minutes after 10 and 20 mg/kg of telazol i.m. Stroke volume was decreased proportionately at the lower dose, accompanied by little or no change in net cardiac output, suggesting that the decreased stroke output was principally a result of decreased filling time. At the higher dose, however, the relationship between stroke output and rate was disproportionate, with a resultant substantial (maximum 29%) decrease in net output. Further, contractility and mean blood pressure were decreased by the higher dose of telazol, indicating that decreased function was a result of direct myocardial depression. Ventricular function appeared to be adequately maintained, with no sign of left ventricular failure, as evidenced by essentially normal left ventricular and diastolic pressures through the period of study.

PULMONARY EFFECTS IN DOGS

Pulmonary function was substantially altered during the first 15 minutes after i.m. administration of 20 mg/kg of telazol; respiratory rate doubled, and tidal volume decreased to less than one-half of control values. The effective ventilatory volume was approximately one-third of control by 15 minutes, and dynamic pulmonary resistance had increased from 8 to 21 cm H_2O/liter/second. Some signs of respiratory difficulty accompanied the measured parameters. There was also evidence of hypoxemia and cyanosis in some of the animals. Arterial pO_2 levels decreased during the first 15 minutes, but returned to normal within 35 minutes after dosing.

CARDIOVASCULAR EFFECTS IN CATS

Telazol was rapidly absorbed after intramuscular injection. A slight lowering of the blood pressure by 10% was seen during the first hour after injection; this was followed by a return to control levels. Heart rate may change, but electrocardiogram patterns were unaffected by telazol.

RESPIRATORY EFFECTS IN CATS

Arterial blood pO_2 can drop after 20 mg/kg and after 10 mg/kg. This has been seen 3 minutes after injection, with recovery by the 15- or 35-minute sampling time. The cause of hypoxemia is probably decreased tidal volume.

Elevated blood pO_2 may be typically seen 35 to 65 minutes after injection. This was the consequence of the effect of decreased body temperature upon the oxygen-hemoglobin dissociation curve; the animals have a greater response by this time, and tidal volume may increase.

EFFECTS ON EPINEPHRINE-INDUCED ARRHYTHMIAS

Sensitization potentials of telazol and halothane to catecholamine-induced arrhythmias have been studied in dogs and cats. Under halothane anesthesia (1.25 to 1.5% in a 95/5 mixture of O_2/CO_2), all of the animals tested developed severe ventricular arrhythmias after 1 mg/kg of epinephrine i.v., and fibrillation occurred in the majority of dogs and one-third of the cats after epinephrine challenge.

During telazol anesthesia, some arrhythmias occurred in dogs after 3 to 100 mg/kg of epinephrine. Fibrillation did not occur in any of the telazol-anesthetized animals with epinephrine doses as high as 100 mg/kg. Phenathizine tranquilizers such as acetylpromazine to control tachycardia should not be used concurrently with telazol.

EFFECTS OF TELAZOL ON RECTAL TEMPERATURE IN DOGS AND CATS

Body temperature is depressed by the administration of anesthetic telazol. Therefore, it is prudent to monitor body temperature and supply supplemental heat as indicated for the well being of anesthetized and recovering patients.

CONCLUSIONS OF LABORATORY STUDIES

Telazol in Dogs

Initial, single i.m. doses of 15 or 30 mg/kg of telazol resulted in smooth, rapid induction of cataleptoid anesthesia in young laboratory dogs with little or no aberrant clinical or laboratory findings other than transient increase in pulse rates and transient decrease in body temperature. Dogs survived daily injections of telazol at doses of 15 mg/kg for 14 days or 30 mg/kg for 8 days, but developed persistent elevation of alkaline phosphatase and transaminases, anorexia, weight loss, depression, and fatigue after a few days. These effects are slowly reversible after cessation of dosing. Telazol produced little clinically evident trauma at injection sites, but did induce a slight to moderate myositis histologically. Repeated injections of telazol given during a single day induce clinical and laboratory reactions similar to those seen with daily constant dose injections. Tolerance to the induction or maintenance of surgical anesthesia tends to develop on an unpredictable basis after a few doses of telazol when given either during a single day or on consecutive days.

Telazol in Cats

In a preliminary study conducted to obtain dosage data in domestic cats as a basis for designing toxicological studies,it was learned that without prior exposure to telazol, dosages of 100 mg/kg and above were fatal in 1 to 2 hours; cats with prior experience with telazol survived dosages as high as 150 mg/kg; and dosages of 12, 36, and 60 mg/kg of telazol were well tolerated at daily intervals for 7 consecutive days, with evidence of a shortening of recovery time with succeeding doses.

In a toxicological study, 24 cats were randomly divided into 4 groups of 6 cats each. One group received 24 mg/kg of telazol i.m. on alternate days for 7 anesthetic episodes; a second group received 36 mg/kg of telazol i.m. plus additional doses, as needed, to maintain surgical anesthesia for 8 hours on study days 1, 5, 9, and 13; a third group received 72 mg/kg of telazol i.m. on alternate days for 7 anesthetic episodes; and a control group was given 0.24 ml/kg of physiological saline solution i.m. on alternate days for 7 injections. Hematological, biochemical, and urinary studies were performed on each cat.

Cats used for the 24, 36, and 72 mg/kg of telazol dosage regimens did not have hematological, biochemical, or urinary findings that were significantly different from those of control cats. Likewise, bone marrow data were not significantly different between the treated and control cats. The most consistent gross and microscopic lesion at time of necropsy was at the injection site, where there was a minimum to moderate hemorrhage, necrosis, and resolution by endomesial proliferation. Because the same injection site was used for all injections of telazol at high doses (usually 7 within a 2-week period), it is reasonable to assume that injection site reaction would not be of significance for a single clinical dose (6 to 12 mg/kg).

Three further conclusions regarding the toxicity of telazol in domestic cats were drawn. First, the only toxic effects observed at 2.0 to 12.5 times higher than the intended clinical dosage were a dose-related lesion at the injection site and elevations of serum glutamic oxaloacetic transaminase (SGOT). The lesions at the injection sites were observed after 7 injections of the drug had been made in 14 days at the same site, the quadriceps femoris muscle; muscle lesions were not detected on physical examination. Clinically significant increases in SGOT occurred after 4 cats received 12.5 times the recommended dose of telazol and remained in surgical anesthesia in excess of 24 hours. Second, the effects of telazol when given at the intended clinical doses of 3.0 to 12.0 mg/kg were not considered to be significantly more toxic than intramuscular injections of physiological saline solution. Third, telazol is a safe anesthetic for cats with a wide margin of safety.

Telazol has been used in a wide range of diagnostic and surgical procedures in dogs, cats, and wild animal species. Midrange dosages are more likely to be associated with favorable responses, as with other dissociative anesthetic agents. Low dosage administration followed by painful procedures can result in elevated heart rate and blood pressure, body movement, and other signs of inadequate anesthesia, whereas high doses may result in symptoms of respiratory depression, prolonged sleep, and other symptoms of excessive anesthesia. As with all anesthetics, telazol should be administered with appropriate attention to the condition of the animal, the procedure to be performed, and the dosage needed. There is a greater extent of somatic analgesia than visceral analgesia, and many of the characteristics of ketamine anesthesia may be observed.

Telazol was developed in the Research Laboratories of Parke Davis and Company, Ann Arbor, Michigan. It is approved for use in veterinary medicine. The efforts of Doctors D.A. McCarthy, C.C. Beck, and James Mosier (all deceased) and their coworkers in the development of this product are recognized. Much of the data for these studies was determined by the author.

References

1. Snell LD, Mueller ZL, Gannon RL, Silverman PB, Johnson KM: A comparison between classes of drugs having phencyclidine-like behavioral properties on dopamine efflux *in vitro* and dopamine metabolism *in vivo*. *J Pharmacol Exp Therap* 231:261–269, 1984.
2. Green CJ, Knight J, Precious S, Simpkin S: Ketamine alone and combined with diazepam or xylazine in laboratory animals: A 10 year experience. *Lab Anim* 15:163–170, 1981.
3. Arnett BD, Brightman AL II, Musselman EE: Effect of atropine sulfate on tear production in cats when used with ketamine hydrochloride and acetylpromazine maleate. *J Am Vet Med Assoc* 185:214–215, 1984.
4. Maleque MA, Warnick JE, Albuquerque EX: The mechanism and site of action of ketamine on skeletal muscle. *J Pharmacol Exp Therap* 219:638–645, 1981.
5. Jaspar N, Mazzarelli M, Tessier C, Milic-Emili J: Effect of ketamine on control of breathing in cats. *J Appl Physiol* 55:851–859, 1983.
6. Arnbjerg J: Clinical manifestations of overdose of ketamine-xylazine in the cat. *Nord Vet Med* 31:155–161, 1979.
7. Wright M: Pharmacologic effects of ketamine and its use in veterinary medicine. *J Am Vet Med Assoc* 180(12):1462–1470, 1982.
8. Sparks DL, Corssen G, Sides J: Ketamine-induced anesthesia: Neural mechanisms in the rhesus monkey. *Anesth Analg (Cleve)* 52:288–297, 1973.
9. Massopust LC, Wolin LR, Albin MS: Electrophysiologic and behavioral responses to ketamine hydrochloride in the rhesus monkey. *Anesth Analg (Cleve)* 51:329–341, 1972.
10. Miyasaka M, Domino EF: Neuronal mechanisms of ketamine-induced anesthesia. *Int J Neuropharmacol* 7:557–573, 1968.
11. Ohtani J, Kikuchi H, Kitahata LM: Effects of ketamine on nociceptive cells in the medial medullary reticular formation of the cat. *Anesthesiology* 51:414–417, 1979.
12. Corssen G, Miyasaka M, Domino EF: Changing concepts in pain control during surgery: Dissociative anesthesia with CI 581. *Anesth Analg (Cleve)* 47:746–758, 1968.
13. Winters W, Ferrer-Allado T, Guzman-Flores C: The cataleptic state induced by ketamine: A review of the neuropharmacology of anesthesia. *Neuropharmacology* 11:303–315, 1972.
14. Kaka JS, Klavano PA, Hayton WL: Pharmacokinetics of ketamine in the horse. *Am J Vet Res* 40:978–981, 1979.
15. Kaplan B: Ketamine HCl anesthesia in dogs: Observation of 3 cases. *VM SAC* 67:631–634, 1972.
16. Humphrey WJ: Ketamine HCl as a general anesthetic in dogs. *Mod Vet Pract* 52:38–39, 1971.
17. Reid JS, Frank RJ: Prevention of undesirable side reactions of ketamine anesthetic in cats. *J Am Anim Hosp Assoc* 8:115–119, 1972.
18. Beck CC: Evaluation of Vetalar (ketamine HCl): A unique feline anesthetic. *VM SAC* 66:993–997, 1971.
19. Shaprio HM, Wyte SR, Harris AB: Ketamine anesthesia in patients with intracranial pathology. *Br J Anaesth* 44:1200–1204, 1972.
20. Drury WL, Clark LC: Ketamine failure in acute brain injury: A case report. *Anesth Analg (Cleve)* 49:859–861, 1970.
21. Janis KM, Wright W: Failure to produce analgesia with ketamine in two patients with cortical diseases. *Anesthesiology* 36:405–406, 1972.
22. Corssen G: Discussion remark, Ketamine. In Gemperle M, Kreuscher H, Langrehr D (ed): *Neue Ergebnisse in Forschung und Klinik*. Berlin, Springer Verlag, 1973, pp 269–270.
23. McCarthy DA, Chen G, Kaump DH: General anesthetic and other pharmacological properties of 2-(0-chlorophenyl)-2-methylamino cyclohexanone HCl(CI-581). *J New Drugs* 5:21–33, 1965.
24. Chen G, Ensor CR, Bohner B: The neuropharmacology of 2-(0-chlorophenyl)-2-methylaminocyclohexanone hydrochloride. *J Pharmacol* 152:332–339,1966.
25. Myslobodsky MS, Golovchinsky V, Mintz M: Ketamine: Convulsant or anticonvulsant? *Pharmacol Biochem Behav* 14:27–33, 1981.
26. Ylitalo P, Saarnivaara L, Ahtee L: The effect of ketamine anaesthesia on the content of monoamines and their metabolites in the cat brain. *Acta Anaesthesiol Scand* 20:216–220, 1976.
27. Hatch RC: Prevention of ketamine catalepsy and enhancement of ketamine anesthesia in cats pretreated with methiothepin. *Pharmacol Res Commun* 5:311–319, 1973.
28. Hatch RC: Ketamine catalepsy and anesthesia in dogs pretreated with antiserotonergic or antidopaminergic neuroleptics or with anticholinergic agents. *Pharmacol Res Commun* 6:289–299, 1974.
29. Azar I, Ozomek E: The use of ketamine for abdominal tubal ligation. *Anesth Analg (Cleve)* 52:39–42, 1973.
30. Yamamura T, Kimura T, Furukawa K: Effects of halothane, thiamylal and ketamine on central sympathetic and vagal tone. *Anesth Analg* 62(2):129–34, 1983.
31. Muir WW: Cyclohemanone drug mixtures: The pharmacology of ketamine and ketamine drug combinations. *Proceedings 2nd Intl Cong Vet Anes* (5), Veterinary Practice Publishing Co., Santa Barbara, Calif, 1985.
32. Adams JR, Parker JL, Mathew BP: The influence of ketamine on inotropic and chronotropic responsiveness of heart muscle. *J Pharmacol Exp Therap* 201:171–183, 1977.
33. Tokics L, Brismar B, Hedenstierna G, Lundh R: Oxygen uptake and central circulation during ketamine anaesthesia. *Acta Anaesthesiol Scand* 27(4):317–322, 1983.
34. Lippmann M, Appel PL, Mok MS, Shoemaker WC: Sequential cardiorespiratory patterns of anesthetic induction with ketamine in critically ill patients. *Crit Care Med* 11(9):730–734, 1983.
35. Weiskopf RB, Bogetz MS, Roizin, Reid IA: Cardiovascular and

metabolic sequalae of inducing anesthesia with ketamine or thiopental in hypovolemic swine. *Anesthesiology* 60(3):214–219, 1984.
36. Tranquilli WJ, Thurmon JC, Benson GJ: Organ blood flow and distribution of cardiac output in hypocapnic ketamine-anesthetized swine. *Am J Vet Res* 44(8):1578–1582, 1983.
37. Dhasmana KM, Saxena PR, Prakash O, Van der Zee HT: A study on the influence of ketamine on systemic and regional haemodynamics in conscious rabbits. *Arch Int Pharmacodyn Ther* 269(2):323–334, 1984.
38. Aouad JI, Wright EM, Shaner TW: Anesthesia evaluation of ketamine and xylazine in calves. *Bovine Pract* 2:22–31, 1981.
39. Muir WW, Skarda R, Milne DW: Evaluation of xylazine and ketamine hydrochloride for anesthesia in horses. *Am J Vet Res* 38:195–201, 1977.
40. Buyniski JP, Christie GJ: Ketaset Plus: A new combination anesthetic for cats. *VM SAC* 72:559–567,1977.
41. Ellis RG, Lowe JE, Schwark WS: Intravenously administered xylazine and ketamine HCl for anesthesia in horses. *J Equine Med Surg* 1:259–265, 1977.
42. Waterman A, Livingston A: Some physiological effects of ketamine in sheep. *Res Vet Sci* 25:225–233, 1978.
43. Thurmon JC, Kumar A, Cawley AJ: Changes in acid base status of sheep anaesthetized with a combination of atropine sulphate, acepromazine and ketamine hydrochloride. *Aust Vet J* 51:484–487, 1975.
44. Traber DL, Wilson RD, Priano LL: A detailed study of the cardiopulmonary response to ketamine and its blockade by atropine. *South Med J* 63:1077–1081, 1970.
45. Kelly RW, Wilson RD, Traber DL: Effects of two new dissociative anesthetic agents, ketamine and CL-1848C, on the respiratory response to carbon dioxide. *Anesth Anal (Cleve)* 50:262–269, 1971.
46. Jaspar N, Magzarelli M, Tessier C, Milie-Emili J: Effect of ketamine on control of breathing in cats. *J Appl Physiol* 55(3):851–859, 1983.
47. Hatch RC, Ruch T: Experiments on antagonism of ketamine anesthesia in cats given adrenergic, serotonergic, and cholinergic stimulants alone and in combination. *Am J Vet Res* 35:35–39, 1974.
48. Kraynack LL, Gintautas J, Kraynack BJ: Antagonism of ketamine induced narcosis by naloxone. *Anesthesiology* 53:S69, 1980.
49. Craft JB Jr, Coaldrake LA, Gonekura ML, Dao SD, Co EG, Roizin MF, Mozel P, Gilman R, Shokes L, Trevor AJ: Ketamine, catecholamines and uterine tone in pregnant ewes. *Am J Obstet Gynecol* 146(4):429–434, 1983.
50. Bernstein K, Gisselsson L, Jacobsson L, Ohrlander S: Influence of two different anaesthetic agents on the newborn and the correlation between foetal oxygenation and induction delivery time in elective caesarean section. *Scand Acta Anaesthesiol* 29(2):157–160, 1985.
51. Faulk RH: Xylazine and ketamine synergism for ultrashort anesthesia in cats. *Feline Pract* (8)15–17, 1978.
52. Stephenson JC, Blevins DI, Christie GJ: Safety of Rompun/Ketoset combination in dogs: A two-year study. *VM SAC* 73:303–306, 1978.
53. Kirkpatrick RM: Use of xylazine and ketamine as a combination anesthetic. *Canine Pract* 5:53–57, 1978.
54. Clark DM, Martin RA, Short CE: Cardiopulmonary responses to xylazine/ketamine anesthesia in the dog. *JAAHA* 18:815–821, 1982.
55. Muir WW, Skarda RT, Sheehan W: Evaluation of xylazine, guaifenesin, and ketamine hydrochloride for restrain in horses. *Am J Vet Res* 39:1274–1278, 1978.
56. Pezzoli G, de Bue M: Use of ketamine in general anesthesia of cattle. *Bovine Pract* 11:88, 1976.
57. Tadmor A, Marcus S, Eting E: The use of ketamine hydrochloride for endotracheal intubation in cattle. *Aust Vet J* 55:537–538, 1979.
58. Kumar A, Singh H: Ketamine and xylazine anaesthesia in bovine paediatric surgery. *Indian Vet J* 56:219–222, 1979.
59. Fuentes VO, Tellez E: Ketamine dissociative analgesia in the cow. *Vet Rec* 94:482, 1974.
60. Fuentes VO, Tellez E: Midline caesarian section in a cow using ketamine anesthesia. *Vet Rec* 99:338, 1976.
61. Kumar A, Thurmon JC, Dorner JL: Hematologic and biochemical findings in sheep given ketamine hydrochloride. *J Am Vet Med Assoc* 165:284–287, 1974.
62. Thurmon JC, Kumar A, Link RP: Evaluation of ketamine hydrochloride as an anesthetic in sheep. *J Am Vet Med Assoc* 162:293–297, 1973.
63. Taylor P, Hopkins L, Young M: Ketamine anaesthesia in the pregnant sheep. *Vet Rec* 90:35–36, 1972.
64. Kumar A, Thurmon JC, Hardenbrook HJ: Clinical studies of ketamine HCl and xylazine HCl in domestic goats. *VM SAC* 71:1707–1713, 1976.
65. Keller GL, Bauman DH: Ketamine and xylazine anesthesia in the goat. *VM SAC* 73:443–444,1978.
66. Thurmon JC, Nelson DR, Christie GJ: Ketamine anesthesia in swine. *J Am Vet Med Assoc* 160:1325–1330, 1972.
67. Benson GJ, Thurmon JC: Anesthesia of swine under field conditions. *J Am Vet Med Assoc* 174:594–596, 1979.
68. Gray KN, Raulston GL, Flow BL: Repeated immobilization of miniature swine with an acepromazine-ketamine combination. *Southwest Vet* 31:27–30, 1978.
69. Kyle OC, Novak S, Bolooki H: General anesthesia in pigs. *Lab Anim Sci* 29:123–124, 1979.
70. Roberts FW: Anaesthesia in pigs. *Anaesthesia* 26:445–449, 1971.
71. Massopust LC, Wolin LR, Abbin MS: The effects of a new phencyclidine derivative and diazepinone derivative on the electroencephalographic and behavioral responses in the cat. *J Life Sci* 3:1–10, 1973.
72. Baukema J, Overholm RA, Glazko AJ: Metabolism of Flupyrazopon (CI-716) in laboratory animals. Paper presented to *Am Soc Pharmacol Exp Ther*, Aug. 1973.

SECTION 2

Special Clinical Considerations

CHAPTER 12

Clinical Considerations and Complications

PART 1

Anesthetic Considerations of the Ophthalmic Patient

THOMAS J. KERN, D.V.M., D.A.C.V.D., A.C.V.O.

Introduction

Anesthesia, whether local, regional, or general, is necessary for the humane performance of certain ophthalmic diagnostic techniques and all ophthalmic surgical procedures. The fulfillment of anesthesia's objectives of analgesia and immobilization are of paramount importance to the ophthalmic surgeon because many techniques cannot be safely or effectively performed on animals that are mobile or uncooperative.

Certain general aspects of ocular surgery may pose inconvenience or problems for anesthesiologists. Procedures are confined to the head, orbit, or globe, thus impairing access to the endotracheal tube and its connections. Unnatural or extreme positioning of the head and neck to facilitate optimal exposure of the surgical field may potentially cause airway obstruction. Accessory surgical instrumentation such as operating microscopes, ophthalmic cryosurgical or thermosurgical units, cautery units, special focused light sources, and television cameras may provide additional barriers to both anesthesiologist and surgeon for access to the patient and preservation of a sterile surgical field. The opportunity to monitor anesthetic depth by ocular or palpebral reflexes is lost. Lastly, the pre-, peri-, and intraoperative administration of potent ophthalmic drugs with systemic side effects (e.g., autonomic agents, anti-inflammatory agents, antibiotics) may increase the likelihood of problematic drug interactions with and even without the added influences of anesthetic agents.

Specific anesthetic considerations are important for different ophthalmic surgical and diagnostic procedures (1). Surgery of the orbit, eyelids, lacrimal system, cornea, and conjunctiva and intraocular surgery as well as certain radiological and electrophysiological techniques each merit special consideration (2).

Ophthalmic Surgery

ORBIT

Enucleation or evisceration of the globe, exenteration of the orbit, and orbital exploration, performed for several indications in all species, present special anesthetic management considerations of blood loss, excessive globe traction, and the effects of concurrently administered medications. These surgical procedures hold the greatest potential of all ophthalmic procedures for significant hemorrhage. Although seldom life-threatening, blood loss may be of special concern in very small animals such as neonates, cats, birds, and laboratory animals. Fluid replacements may be necessary. Orbital hemorrhage may be expulsive or prolonged, especially in horses and ruminants, in which large orbital blood vessels may be difficult to locate and ligate.

Excessive traction on the globe during surgery may activate the oculocardiac reflex, resulting in bradycardia or cardiac arrest. This is not as likely to occur if anticholinergics have been administered. Medications administered to a patient for the treatment of glaucoma, ocular or orbital inflammation, or infection (e.g., antibiotics, corticosteroids, or nonsteroidal anti-inflammatory agents) may exert significant effects on the animal's preanesthetic, metabolic, or autonomic status.

EYELIDS AND LACRIMAL SYSTEM

Indications for eyelid surgery include correction of congenital and acquired structural and functional defects, repair of traumatic injuries, treatment of neoplasms and post-therapy reconstruction, and manipulations to "bandage" the cornea. General anesthesia is desirable and frequently used in small animal practices. In horses and ruminants, tranquilization and local or regional anesthesia is usually more practical and desirable. The use of analgetics in conjunction with these procedures should be considered if there is evidence of postsurgical pain.

Minor manipulations and surgery of the lacrimal excretory system, such as nasolacrimal cannulation and flushing or imperforate puncta repair, are readily accomplished under topical anesthesia. Tranquilization and even anesthesia may be required for uncooperative cats and horses. Parotid duct transposition, performed most frequently in the dog, is completed with general anesthesia. Most of these procedures are not considered to produce high risk to the patient, nor do they normally occur in high risk patients.

CORNEA AND CONJUNCTIVA

Diagnostic procedures such as corneal and conjunctival scrapings for exfoliative cytological examination and conjunctival snip biopsies are easily performed under topical anesthesia. Horses usually require tranquilization or chemical restraint.

Corneal surgery is performed to repair injuries as well as to remove pigmentation, congenital anomalies (e.g., dermoids), neoplasms (e.g., squamous cell carcinoma), and foreign bodies. General anesthesia should be considered to ensure freedom from pain and adequate relaxation to avoid movement of the animal for delicate surgical manipulations performed with the aid of magnification. Lubricating ointments frequently used in the eyes during anesthesia should not be instilled into the conjunctival sac before surgery that risks or intends perforation of the anterior chamber. The oily ointment base may cause intractable uveitis if accidentally introduced into the eye.

Conjunctival surgery is most often performed to provide temporary bandaging of corneal ulceration or repaired lacerations as well as to remove neoplasms such as squamous cell carcinoma. For these, general anesthesia is usually indicated. Anesthetic technique is usually routine unless preanesthetic evaluation reveals other contributing factors.

INTRAOCULAR SURGERY

Surgery of this class of ophthalmic procedures includes extra- and intracapsular lens extraction and management of its postoperative complications, iridectomy and iridocyclectomy, evisceration of the globe with silicone prosthesis implantation, and glaucoma filtering procedures. Lens removal in animals poses several challenges for both anesthesiology and surgery (3).

Ophthalmic premedication for surgery is extensive, with medications used for at least 24 hours preoperatively to accomplish several imporant objectives (4, 5). Maximal mydriasis to facilitate lens extraction is achieved with topical anticholinergics such as 1% atropine or methylscopolamine (q.i.d.), as well as with topical sympathomimetics such as 2.5% or 10% phenylephrine (NeoSynephrine, Sterling-Winthrop) (q.i.d.). Combined use of drugs from these two classes results in better, more sustained mydriasis pre- and postoperatively. Potential side effects include intoxication and tachycardia with atropine or hypertension with phenylephrine. Although preoperative antibiotic prophylaxis is controversial, many surgeons recommend topical, oral, parenteral, or subconjunctival administration of broad-spectrum antibiotics. Chloramphenicol, bacitracin-neomycin-polymixin (topical only), gentamicin, ampicillin, and others are used. Antibiotic therapy can increase the extent of muscle relaxation during anesthesia and may prolong recovery. Treatment and/or prevention of iatrogenic anterior uveitis is accomplished with use of intensive topical (q.i.d.+) and oral or parenteral corticosteroids. Corticosteroids may reduce systemic blood pressure due to vasodilation unless adequate hydration is present. Nonsteroidal anti-inflammatory agents, including aspirin, flunixin meglumine (Banamine, Schering), or phenylbutazone, are frequently administered for 1 to 2 days before lensectomy. These medications, especially phenylbutazone, may influence protein binding and the duration of barbiturate anesthesia.

Mannitol (2 g/kg i.v.) or glycerin (1 to 1.5 g/kg p.o.) may be administered immediately preoperatively to dehydrate the vitreous and to reduce aqueous production, promoting desirable hypotony and minimizing risk of vitreous loss. The dehydration, electrolyte imbalances, and hemodynamic alterations induced by these drugs may pose management problems for the attending anesthesiologist. Cardiac arrhythmias may develop due to these alterations. Electrocardiographic evaluations of the animal prior to induction of anesthesia is desirable. The presence of arrhythmias should be addressed prior to anesthesia, and anesthetic agents that can be used in the presence of cardiac sensitivities should be selected.

Preoperative intraocular pressure elevations may require management with one or several medications. Oral carbonic anhydrase-inhibiting diuretics, such as dichlorphenamide (Daranide, Merck, Sharp, and Dohme), methazolamide (Neptazane, Lederle), and acetazolarnide (Diamox, Lederle), promote acidosis, hypokalemia, and dehydration. Inhalant anesthetics with supplemental oxygen should improve function in these patients. Topically applied 0.25 or 0.5% timolol maleate (Timoptic, Merck, Sharp, and Dohme), a beta-adrenergic blocking agent, reduces aqueous production and may pose problems for animals with certain respiratory disorders, heart block, or heart failure. Heart rates may drop during anesthesia, and preanesthetic agents such as xylazine should be avoided. The concentration of anesthetic agents administered must be carefully monitored. Topical miotic drugs (direct-acting pilocarpine or indirect-acting demecarium bromide (Humorsol, Merck, Sharp, and Dohme) or echothiophate (Phospholine Iodide, Ayerst)) are effective in increasing facility of aqueous outflow. Even topical use of the indirect-acting miotics, which are related to organophosphates, may deplete cholinesterases necessary for normal metabolism of muscle-paralyzing agents such as succinylcholine. If muscle relaxants are to be used, nondepolarizing agents such as gallamine or pancuronium should be used. The nondepolarizing agents can be reversed with an antagonist.

Animals requiring lens removal are frequently geriatric, with attendant age-related major organ dysfunction or marginal compensation. This frequently includes congestive heart failure, obesity, and renal and hepatic failure. It is not unusual for dogs with cataracts to also be diabetic with added complications to anesthesia.

Intraoperative use of autonomic drugs instilled into the anterior chamber may be necessary to facilitate surgery or to avert disaster (1–4). Acetylcholine chloride 1:100 (Miochol, Cooper Vision) may be used to cause miosis and to limit or prevent vitreous loss. Bradycardia may result. Dilute (1:1000 to 1:100,000) epinephrine may be used in small amounts by intracameral injection or in larger amounts incorporated into the ocular irrigating solution to control hemorrhage, maintain mydriasis, and minimize fibrin formation. If the myocardium has been sensitized to catecholamines by gaseous anesthetics such as halothane, cardiac arrhythmia or even arrest may ensue after epinephrine use. Systemic hypertension and major cardiac arrhythmias including multiple premature ventricular contractions or ventricular tachycardia or fibrillation may result. Pretreatment with intravenous lidocaine prior to use of epinephrine can prevent these problems. Surgery is often prolonged, requiring 1 to 3 hours for completion.

Absolute immobilization of the patient's eye is necessary to successfully perform these technically exacting procedures. Use of succinylcholine is contraindicated because the transient extraocular muscle contractions it stimulates greatly increase intraocular pressure. Nondepolarizing muscle relaxants (such as pancuronium bromide) do not have the same dangerous effect. Because the eye is so responsive to pain, more than 1 times the minimal alveolar concentration (MAC) of anesthesia is almost always required. As the concentration of anesthetic is increased, cardiopulmonary depression will be influenced.

Globe manipulation, such as traction, external pressure, or duction, may stimulate the oculocardiac reflex. This is more likely to occur if anesthesia is inadequate for complete analgesia, anticholinergics have not been used, or there is pre-existing heart block.

Recovery from anesthesia must be smooth. Vomiting, excitement, and the attendant risk of self-trauma must be avoided to preserve a good postoperative result. Postsurgical medications may be used during recovery periods. Tranquilizers may be used to control excitement but have little effect on pain. Early administration of medication after anesthesia may result in excess depression of function.

Iridectomy and iridocyclectomy may be occasionally performed for biopsy or for en bloc uveal neoplasm removal. Pre-, intra-, and postoperative anesthetic considerations are similar to those for lensectomy.

Evisceration of the globe with silicone prosthesis implantation is performed as a cosmetic alternative to enucleation. The only special considerations are increased risk of oculocardiac reflex induction due to excessively traumatic manipulation of the globe during complete removal of the uvea, lens, vitreous, and retina and excessive hemorrhage from uveal remnants.

Surgery for the control of glaucoma includes filtering procedures, which require sclerectomy and iris incarceration in the wound, as well as cyclocryotherapy, which utilizes a liquid nitrogen or nitrous oxide-activated cryoprobe to effect ciliary epithelial cryodestruction by its scleral application over the ciliary body. Filtering procedures require vigilance by the anesthesiologist similar to that for lensectomy. Cyclocryotherapy requires general anesthesia for relatively shorter periods (30 to 60 minutes) than filtering procedures or lensectomy and does not require an ocular incision.

Diagnostic Procedures

SKULL RADIOGRAPHY

Highest quality skull radiographs, whether plain or special studies (e.g., zygomatic sialography, cranial sinus venography, or orbitography), require an absolute immobilization of the patient best achieved through general anesthesia. Anesthetic management will be influenced by other abnormal functions that may exist at the time of anesthesia.

ELECTRORETINOGRAPHY AND VISUAL EVOKED POTENTIAL MEASUREMENT

These procedures may be performed with the patient awake, tranquilized, or under general anesthesia. The choice depends upon the electrophysiological apparatus in use, the preference of the electroretinographer, the degree of sophistication of ocular responses required, and the patient's health status. Anesthetic and tranquilizing agents do alter some parameters of electrophysiological measurements, such as amplitudes, latency, and implicit times, so a standard anesthetic protocol is desirable to keep these alterations constant and the measurements made reliable (5, 6). Monitoring of the patient during electroretinography is difficult due to the darkness in the room and the lack of use of ocular responses to determine depth of anesthesia. This may contribute to anesthetic complications.

ULTRASONOGRAPHY

Both A- and B-scan ultrasonography are useful in imaging the globe and orbit. In small animals, this procedure may be performed under topical anesthesia with manual restraint. In large animals, tranquilization, auriculopalpebral nerve block, and topical anesthesia may be necessary for diagnostic quality results, operator safety, and instrument safety.

The selection of anesthetics and techniques for ophthalmic diagnostic and surgical procedures is influenced by the need to provide a painless experience while not excessively interfering with the physical requirements to complete the procedures. One must be aware in accomplishing these objectives that other organ systems may be adversely affected. Monitoring and timely assessment of responses with correction of undesirable cardiovascular, pulmonary, and neurological responses are required.

References

1. Brunson DB: Anesthesia in ophthalmic surgery. *Vet Clin North Amer Ophthalmol* 10(2):481–496, 1980.
2. Havener WH: *Ocular Pharmacology*, ed 5. St. Louis, CV Mosby Co, 1983, pp 72–119.
3. Gwin RM: The canine lens. In Gelatt KN (ed): *Veterinary Ophthalmology*. Philadelphia, Lea and Febiger, 1981, pp 450–463.
4. Henkind P, Walsh JB, Berger AW (eds): *Physician's Desk Reference for Ophthalmology*, ed 13. Oradell, NJ, Medical Economics Co, 1985.
5. Gelatt KN: *Veterinary Ophthalmic Pharmacology and Therapeutics*, ed 2. Bonner Springs, KS, Veterinary Medical Publishing Inc, 1978.
6. Raitta C, Karhunen U, Seppalainen AH, Naukkarinen M: Changes in the electroretinogram and visual evoked potentials during general anesthesia. *AV Graefes Arch Klin Exp Ophthalmol* 211(2):139–144, 1979.

PART 2

Special Considerations for Veterinary Neuroanesthesia

ALAN VAN POZNAK, M.D., D.A.B.A., F.A.C.A.

Introduction

Neurosurgical anesthesia for veterinary practice has several important similarities and differences from human neurosurgical anesthesia. Veterinary clinical practitioners will probably be more concerned with anesthesia for spinal rather than intracranial surgery. Researchers will need to be aware of problems in both spinal and intracranial areas because animal models are frequently used to develop better methods of treatment in humans. The student who has yet to make his choice of a career must be aware of problems that confront the practitioner and the researcher.

Spinal surgery is frequently performed for herniated discs and spinal stenosis. Anesthesia management is similar to that for other cases in that there must be meticulous attention to the airway and to ventilation. A point of particular importance is that of proper positioning of the patient. Because these operations are done with the patients in prone or sternal recumbent position, it is extremely important to be sure that there is no excessive pressure on the abdominal viscera. This is to prevent excessive bleeding. Normally, the blood returns from the lower or hind extremities mainly through the iliac veins and the inferior vena cava. If there is undue pressure on the abdominal viscera, then the blood cannot return through its usual channel but instead must seek an alternative pathway through the vertebral venous plexus. When surgery is performed on the spine and there is augmented flow through the vertebral venous plexus, then bleeding may become very difficult to control. It is important to position the patient in such a way that the lower part of the body is suspended by a properly positioned frame or by rolled towels or blankets placed in such a way that there is no undue pressure on the abdominal viscera. Endotracheal intubation and management, principally with an inhalation agent, is probably the technique of choice, although intravenous agents might alternatively be used.

In addition to the cardiopulmonary problems previously mentioned, there are certain special respiratory considerations. Patients in the prone position have somewhat restricted respiratory activity because the weight of the body is resting on the thorax and abdomen, thus limiting thoracic and diaphragmatic muscle motion. Proper positioning and support of the patient may help to minimize this problem, but respiratory assistance or control may be required in order to secure adequate respiratory gas exchange.

Operations in the region of the cervical spinal cord present certain additional special problems. The respiratory and vasomotor centers are located high in the cervical cord and can be affected during surgical manipulation. For this reason it is important to monitor both cardiovascular and respiratory function closely during surgery in this region.

It is desirable to minimize excessive bleeding for several reasons. Bleeding not only makes it more difficult for the surgeon to see what he is doing, but blood loss is a threat to life. There are two types of bleeding: venous and arterial. Venous bleeding can be controlled by proper positioning of the patient. If the body is tilted so that the head and neck are raised above the level of the heart, the venous pressure will become progressively less with further elevation. However, one must be careful not to elevate the area so high that significant negative venous pressure develops and poses a threat of venous air embolism. Arterial bleeding may be lessened by lowering the arterial pressure to some extent. There are several factors that enter into control of arterial pressure. The first of these is the depth of inhalation anesthetic used, the second is the position of the table as previously mentioned, the third is a consideration of the relative blood volume in the patient, and the fourth is the use of deliberate hypotension-inducing drugs such as trimethaphan or nitroprusside. If the first three factors are carefully controlled, it is rarely necessary to resort to the use of deliberate hypotension-inducing drugs. If these drugs are required, only small doses will be needed. The problems of toxicity normally associated with the large amounts of these drugs will be avoided (1).

In cases of spinal column trauma, great care should be taken to assure that the patient is transported and positioned very carefully so that additional trauma to the spinal cord does not occur as a result of excessive motion of damaged bony parts.

The considerations of the animal patient undergoing diagnostic procedures for spinal lesions are discussed in the chapter by Riedesel. After the diagnosis of spinal lesions and the decision for surgery, certain clinical considerations are important in addition to an understanding of the basic concepts of neuroanesthesia.

Recent or chronic use of steroids for control of inflammation and swelling may contribute to hypotension during anesthesia for spinal surgery. One should give appropriate consideration to other adjunct medications that may be used to control pain, swelling, or inflammation.

There are physical considerations that influence the response during neurological procedures for spinal problems. The animals are normally positioned to provide a stable, nonmoving surgical site. This may interfere with the ability of the patient to have the desired tidal volume. Thus there can be accumulation of carbon dioxide to the extent of hypercarbia and respiratory acidosis. Mechanical ventilation must be used with discretion because movements of the chest must be coordinated with the surgeon's efforts and the pressure generated by intermittent positive pressure breathing may contribute to an increase in hemorrhage at the operative site.

Manipulation of the spinal cord or spinal nerves or removing disc or other materials may initiate cardiac arrhythmias. Although this is not a common occurrence, its potential should be realized.

Surgical procedures to correct spinal disc problems at C-5–C-6 may be associated with dramatic cardiac disturbances. Stimulation in this area may result in sinus tachycardia or sudden severe bradycardia with hypotension and potential arrest. This has been observed in dogs with careful monitoring. Although the physiology of this crisis is not thoroughly understood, one can theorize that it is a neurological feedback to over-stimulation of the parasympathetic nervous system.

Due to the anatomical relation of the spine and other tissues and organs, the anesthesiologist should be alert to the potential hemorrhage from the surgery. There is also the potential for pneumothorax, especially for thoracic disc procedures.

Excessive depression from too much anesthesia may be associated with spinal surgery. One frequently observes an area of hyperalgesia near and cranial to the spinal lesion. The utilization of standard anesthetic technique to control this sensitivity may be associated with profound concentration of anesthetics.

The use of cautery during spinal surgery results in movement unless the patient has received paralytic agents. One should not attempt to eliminate all responses to electrical cautery, especially in the spinal area with anesthetics alone. This will result in excess depression of the patient. Unless the spinal injury is acute, some patients will be presented with fluid and electrolyte imbalance. The dog with these problems is not physically able to always maintain appropriate fluid intake. Some dogs with spinal lesions will have urinary incontinence, but others will have overdistended urinary bladders and some uremia if appropriate hospital care has not been provided.

Fortunately, recovery after spinal surgery in small animals can be controlled adequately. This is not always the case with large animals recovering from spinal lesions after diagnostic or corrective procedures.

Anesthesia for Intracranial Procedures

There are several important considerations for anesthesia for intracranial surgery. The brain receives a relatively large percentage of the cardiac output, (12–15%) although its weight is a much lower percent of the total body mass. In providing anesthesia for intracranial work, one must preserve insofar as possible an appropriate flow of blood to the brain, but at the same time one must minimize blood loss in order to preserve life and also to prevent shed blood from obscuring the neurosurgeon's vision.

Cerebral blood flow (CBF) is normally about 50 ml/100 g of brain tissue/1 minute. The CBF can be reduced considerably without damage to the brain, but when it becomes as low as 18 to 20 ml/100 g of brain tissue/1 minute, the flow is dangerously low. Temporary or permanent brain damage may develop if flows drop to 12 to 14 ml/100 g of brain tissue/1 minute. Two essential substances are supplied by this flow. One is oxygen, the delivery of which varies from 1.3 to 1.74 μM/g/min. The other is glucose, the cerebral metabolic consumption of which varies from 4.8 to 6.5 mg/100 g/1 min. These flows and consumptions vary in different parts of the brain and in general can be said to be greater in areas of gray matter than they are in areas of white matter (2, 3).

It is important that blood be delivered to the brain in a constant fashion. Blood flows through the arterial supply in accordance with certain rules of hydrodynamics.

Poiseuille's law of hydrodynamics states that

$$P = \frac{8L}{\pi r^4 FV}$$

where P is the pressure gradient, F is the flow rate, V is the viscosity, L is the length, and r to the fourth is the radius of the tube. Poiseuille's law is said to be true for newtonian fluids. Blood is not a newtonian fluid because it contains particles and also because its viscosity varies with the flow rate as well as with changes of hematocrit, plasma proteins, and water content. The pulsatile nature of arterial flow also results in deviations from Poiseuille's law. Blood flow in vessels may be laminar or turbulent. Turbulence develops when the Reynolds number exceeds two thousand. At this Reynolds number, a murmur may be heard over a vessel carrying blood under these conditions. The Reynolds number is given by the equation

$$R = \frac{UDP}{V}$$

where U is the linear velocity, D is the cross sectional area, P is the density, and V is the viscosity.

There are many factors that affect the CBF (4, 5). It is directly related to the perfusion pressure across the brain and inversely related to cerebral vascular resistance. Perfusion pressure may be defined as the difference between mean arterial pressure and intracranial pressure. Changes in perfusion pressure do not normally result in changes of cerebral blood flow because of the factor called autoregulation. Autoregulation usually exists between mean arterial blood pressures of 50 to 150 mm Hg. The mechanism of autoregulation is not entirely clear, but it appears to be a responsiveness of the smooth muscles within the arterial system to the pressure of the blood flowing through the arteries. There are many factors that can lessen or abolish autoregulation. Many general anesthetics and vasoactive drugs may impair autoregulation.

All anesthetics affect CBF and metabolism (4, 6). Of the intravenous agents, barbiturates produce a suppression of electrophysiological activity. There is usually a reduction in CBF and metabolic rate. This has led to the development of deliberately induced barbiturate coma for the treatment of the traumatized brain in the hope that it could be allowed to rest metabolically while attempting to repair itself (7). This form of treatment has been shown to be effective in dogs when the barbiturate coma is induced prior to hypoxic insult. It is less effective or not effective when the insult precedes the induction of the barbiturate coma. The intravenous agents fentanyl and droperidol have likewise been shown to reduce CBF (6, 8). Some researchers have found a reduction in cerebral metabolic consumption of oxygen, but others have found that there has not been a significant lowering of cerebral metabolic rate (CMRO2). The intravenous agent ketamine had produced variable results on cerebral blood flow; some studies showed a decrease and others an increase (9, 10). Some studies have shown an increase in oxygen consumption and others have shown no change (11).

Nitrous oxide is the most widely used inhalation agent in man. It is frequently used as a component of the so-called balanced anesthetic technique. It is also used as a diluent for the potent inhalation anesthetics such as halothane, enflurane, and isoflurane. When it is administered in a concentration of 70% to humans, nitrous oxide provides analgesia and amnesia. There may be an increase in intracranial pressure that may be due to an increase in CBF (12). This increase in intracranial pressure may be particularly marked in the presence of intracranial disorders. Variable results have been reported for the effect of nitrous oxide on CBF. Earlier studies have shown that 70% nitrous oxide has little effect on CBF but reduced CMRO2 by as much as 23% (13). More recent studies in the rat have shown no significant difference in CMRO2 or CBF in animals inhaling either 70% nitrous oxide or 70% nitrogen. In animals its use should be in conjunction with potent inhalant agents to assure adequate levels of anesthesia.

Halothane has been shown to depress cerebral function and metabolism, reducing CMRO2 by as much as 75% in some experiments (14). However, halothane produces considerable impairment of autoregulation and augmentation of CBF, especially if carbon dioxide levels are allowed to rise. Enflurane is a potent inhalation anesthetic based on the methyl ethyl ether skeleton. It has advantages over halothane in providing a more stable heart rhythm and probably has less tendency to produce liver damage. Because it can produce activation of the electroencephalogram to a point of frank seizure activity, its use in neuroanesthesia has been limited (15). However, I have found from personal experience that enflurane and nitrous oxide used after a thiopental induction produce excellent clinical anesthesia even in patients whose presenting symptomatology included seizures. Much of the early work on enflurane was done in dogs where no preanesthetic medication or thiopental induction had been given. High concentrations of enflurane were used, and the animals were hyperventilated to a PCO_2 as low as 20. In such a setting, seizures were frequently observed. However, it is to be remembered that the dog is more prone to seizures under anesthesia than the human, that high dosages of enflurane were used, and that extreme hyperventilation was used far beyond that amount that is employed in clinical practice. These differences in techniques may account for the differences in results (16).

Isoflurane is an isomer of enflurane. It produces many of the desirable effects of enflurane in that it is a complete inhalation anesthetic, nonflammable, chemically stable, and with a low solubility in blood so the anesthetic level may be adjusted rapidly. It has an even more favorable effect on heart rhythm than enflurane in that epinephrine arrhythmias are more difficult to provoke. In addition, isoflurane is the least metabolized potent inhalation anesthetic, being metabolized about 0.2%, compared to 2% for enflurane and at least 20% for methoxyflurane. For all these reasons, isoflurane has rapidly become an inhalation agent of choice in neurosurgical anesthesia. Anesthesia with isoflurane at a level between 0.6 and 1.1 minimum alveolar concentration (MAC) did not alter CBF, but an increase in CBF was seen when the concentration of isoflurane was brought to 1.6 or 1.7 MAC. A decrease in CMRO2 has been demonstrated for isoflurane. If hyperventilation is performed, the increase in intracranial pressure that may be caused by isoflurane can be very effectively controlled or abolished. Isoflurane has minimal effects on tissue and organ systems. In my opinion, it is the inhalation agent of choice for neurosurgical procedures (17, 18).

Factors Affecting Cerebral Vascular Resistance

Blood flow is related to the fourth power of the vessel radius. Relatively small changes in vascular diameter can therefore have great effect on the blood flow rate. Several factors can effect arterial diameter and cerebral vascular resistance.

The most important cerebral vasodilating agent is carbon dioxide (19). CBF varies between 0.95 and 1.75 ml/min/100 g of brain tissue for every 1 mm Hg change in the partial pressure of carbon dioxide. This is of great practical importance because CBF can be easily altered by changing the arterial carbon dioxide level. Carbon dioxide is a normal product of metabolism. Functional activity of the nerve cells will result in production of carbon dioxide which in turn exerts a vasodilating influence causing lactate and hydrogen ion to be cleared from the extracellular space. In the practice of neurosurgical anesthesia, accumulation of carbon dioxide is usually to be avoided because the increase in brain volume caused by carbon dioxide accumulation can result in a very great increase in intracranial pressure if the cranium is closed at the time of the carbon dioxide accumulation.

When the cranium is open, accumulation of carbon dioxide may cause herniation of the brain through the craniotomy wound. Conversely, reduction of arterial carbon dioxide level causes cerebral vasoconstriction and reduction in the total brain bulk. This results in a slack brain that is more easily manipulated by the neurosurgeon. This in turn causes less petechial hemorrhage in the cortex and less postoperative edema. The importance of judicious hyperventilation cannot be overemphasized. However, there are times when CBF may be compromised because of the vascular lesions, such as carotid stenosis. In such cases, CBF has been reduced because of coexisting carotid disease. Hyperventilation with additional decrease in CBF may be harmful in such situations.

Hydrogen ion concentration is also of importance. Acidosis produces mild cerebral vascular dilation, and alkalosis produced mild vasoconstriction. Severe metabolic acidosis, as in diabetes, may produce a CBF 20% greater than normal even though arterial carbon dioxide has been reduced through hyperventilation.

Oxygen does not have much effect on cerebral vascular resistance until PaO_2 has been reduced to about 50 mm Hg and arterial oxygen saturation is down to 40 or 50%. If inspired oxygen concentration is reduced to 8% in the presence of constant arterial PCO_2 levels, CBF will increase by 36%. Because hypoxia is the most primitive danger confronting the organism, it is not unreasonable to expect that extreme hyperventilation with lowering of arterial CO_2 levels will produce hypoxia. This has been the concern of some investigators. If extreme vasoconstriction is produced by hyperventilation, even though the $PaCO_2$ is very low, any resulting hypoxia will quickly induce vasodilation that will increase regional CBF and offset the effects of the low $PaCO_2$ (20, 21).

Intracranial pressure also affects CBF. A rise in intracranial pressure reduces cerebral perfusion pressure and will probably result in a compensatory vasodilation. There is usually little change in CBF until intracranial pressure reaches 35 mm Hg.

Body temperature also affects CBF. Hypothermia reduces the rate of cerebral oxygen consumption that in turn reduces the amount of carbon dioxide produced by the tissues. If body temperature is elevated, CBF does not increase until a temperature of about 39.4°C is reached. At a temperature of 42°C, CBF may be increased 30 to 50% above normal.

Neurogenic factors can also affect cerebral circulation (22, 23). Nerve fibers have been found along the blood vessels, but their functional significance is as yet unclear. Norepinephrine appears to produce vasoconstriction that can be abolished by alpha-adrenergic blocking agents. Responses to carbon dioxide may be affected by activity in the sympathetic and parasympathetic nerves. The neurogenic effects, however, seem to be minor in comparison with the effect of carbon dioxide (24–27).

Other factors that can affect CBF and cerebral metabolic rate of oxygen consumption include arterial hypertension, which does not seem to be of practical importance in many hypertensive patients. Cerebral vascular resistance may become significantly elevated in advanced hypertension so that the lower limit of autoregulation may be raised. In normotensive patients, the critical closing pressure of pial arteries is about 20 mm Hg. In hypertensive patients, it may be near 40 mm Hg. Another disease state that can disturb CBF and metabolism is subarachnoid hemorrhage. Vasospasm is frequently found after subarachnoid hemorrhage. Ischemic infarction may occur if CBF is reduced below critical thresholds. Intracranial hypertension may also adversely affect CBF as well as hydrocephalus if the cerebral spinal fluid pressure reaches 20 to 25 mm Hg. Head injury can produce alterations in CBF that vary widely depending upon the degree and extent of head injury. Autoregulation may be disturbed, and cerebral edema, compression of the circulation, and further reduction of CBF may occur (28, 29).

Several practical considerations emerge from consideration of the above factors. The task of the neuroanesthesiologist is to provide maximum safety for his patient and optimum operating conditions for the surgeon. The safety of the patient is secured through close monitoring and careful attention to anesthetic detail. While the patient is kept safe, asleep, and comfortable, the surgeon must be provided with an operative field that does not bleed excessively. He must also be provided with sufficient room to work within the cranium. The control of excessive bleeding has been mentioned previously. It consists of providing sufficient anesthetic depth, sufficient tilt of the table, consideration of the relative blood volume to the patient, and the use of hypotension-inducing drugs. These four factors will provide adequate control of the arterial blood pressure. The venous blood pressure is controlled by the positioning of the patient. As the head is raised higher than the rest of the body, the venous pressure progressively decreases. If the head is raised too high, the threat of venous air embolism arises. In practice, the anesthesiologist should observe the operative field to see that a small amount of blood comes out from veins when they are opened. This will indicate a small amount of positive pressure within the venous channels and a fairly certain protection against the danger of entrainment of atmospheric air. Controlled ventilation with positive end-expiratory pressure also guards against the entry of atmospheric air into the venous system because it tends to raise the pressure within the venous channels (30).

Providing sufficient room for the neurosurgeon to work within the cranium is accomplished in several ways. Hyperventilation is effective in reducing the size of the cerebral vasculature and in turn decreasing the total bulk of the brain. The administration of hypertonic solution such as 20% mannitol in a dose of 1 g/kg will draw water from the brain cells into the vascular space. This water will eventually be excreted by the kidney. Additional room within the cranial cavity can also be secured by drainage of cerebrospinal fluid through a lumbar puncture needle or catheter. The use of induced arterial hypotension also helps to reduce brain bulk and allows the neurosurgeon to retract the brain more easily (31).

I prefer to induce anesthesia with thiopental and intubate after the administration of succinylcholine. Although the claim has been made that succinylcholine may increase intracranial pressure, I do not believe this to be of any practical importance. After intubation, the patient should be hyperventilated promptly on a mixture of isoflurane, oxygen, and perhaps nitrous oxide. Nitrous oxide is useful because of its rapid effect. After equilibration of the isofluorane, the nitrous oxide is no longer necessary and may be discontinued, especially in cases where air embolism is thought to be a threat. With sufficient hyperventilation, it is usually not necessary to administer muscle relaxants. Prior to intubation, the cardiovascular response may be attenuated by the intravenous administration of lidocaine, 1.5 mg/kg, or a narcotic such as fentanyl in a dose of approximately 1 μg/kg.

Monitoring during the procedure should include careful clinical observation of the patient plus electrocardiogram, blood pressure and temperature measurement, and, if possible, some means of determining the level of carbon dioxide, either by an indwelling arterial line for measurement of arterial blood gases or an end-tidal carbon dioxide-measuring device. In practice, I have found that the Siemens 900B ventilator with end-tidal carbon dioxide measurement provides a very satisfactory ventilator with an adjustable positive end-expiratory pressure plus breath-to-breath carbon dioxide analysis. In this way we have been able to spare the patient the possible complications of arterial puncture and the expense of multiple blood gas determinations.

Toward the termination of the procedure, the end-expiratory carbon dioxide level is allowed to return toward normal levels by progressively decreasing the hyperventilation. Patients are left intubated until they begin spontaneous movements of their extremities. I have found this is a reliable clinical indication of the ability to maintain airway reflexes. There are, however, two exceptions to this rule. If the patient has an anatomical abnormality of the airway that either existed prior to surgery or was caused by surgery, the patient may not be able to maintain an open airway even though it can move its extremities. The other exception is posterior fossa disease involving the 9th and 10th cranial nerves. Since these nerves specifically control the airway reflexes, it is possible that a patient may be unable to swallow or cough effectively if the 9th and 10th cranial nerves are damaged. The danger of aspiration of secretions into the tracheobronchial tree is then present, even though the patient may be able to move his extremities satisfactorily.

Postoperative pain medication should be judiciously administered to a patient who has had an intracranial procedure. Intracranial disease plus surgical manipulation may produce depression of vital respiratory and cardiovascular functions. Addition of excessive doses of narcotics may produce serious or fatal consequences. Therefore, pain medication should be titrated carefully according to the needs of the individual patient. Patients in pain should not be denied narcotics but should be given them in titrated intravenous doses until the desired degree of comfort has been secured. Patients who have had spinal surgery often require large doses of narcotics to control their postoperative pain because the amount of muscle and bone surgery done may involve several levels of the vertebral column.

Titration of intravenous narcotics to produce an adequate expiratory pause is the safest and best method I know for securing adequate postoperative analgesia. The normal respiratory pattern consists of a pause at the end of expiration before the next inspiration occurs. In the presence of pain, this expiratory pause shortens or disappears. The normal expiratory pause can be restored by incremental titration of narcotic. At this point the patient is usually reasonably comfortable. Observation of the pattern of respiration will guide even the relatively inexperienced practitioner to a point of optimum titration. Excessive amounts of narcotics will cause too long an expiratory pause between breaths. If this should occur, back titration with very small increments of naloxone may be performed. By following this very simple method of intravenous titration of narcotics, postoperative comfort can be secured (32).

References

1. Michenfelder JD: Cyanide release from sodium nitioprusside in the dog. *Anesthesiology* 46:196–201, 1977.
2. Kety SS, Schmidt CF: The nitrous oxide method for the quantitative determinations of cerebral blood flow in man: theory, procedure and normal values. *J Clin Invest* 27:478–483, 1948.
3. Himmich HE: *Brain Metabolism and Cerebral Disorder.* Baltimore, Williams and Wilkins, 1951.
4. Heiss ND: Effects of drugs on cerebral blood flow in man. *Ann Neurol* 25:95–116, 1979.
5. Kety SS, Sheukin HA, Schmidt CF: The effects of increased intracranial pressure on cerebral circulatory functions in man. *J Clin Invest* 27:493–499, 1948.
6. Michenfelder JD, Theye RA: Effects of fentanyl, droperidol and innovar on canine cerebral metabolism and blood flow. *Br J Anaesth* 43:630–636, 1971.
7. Bendtsen AO, Sorenson PM, Rosenorn J: Additional reduction of CBF-$CMRO_2$ during halothane/nitrous oxide anesthesia by thiopental loading. *J Cer Blood Flow Metab* V (Suppl):409–410, 1981.
8. Artru AA: Effects of halothane and fentanyl on the rate of CSF production in dogs. *Anesth Analg* 62:581–585, 1983.
9. Takeshita H, Okuta Y, Sari A: The effects of ketamine on cerebral circulation and metabolism in man. *Anesthesiology* 36:69–75, 1972.
10. Dawson B, Michenfelder JD, Theye RA: Effects of ketamine on canine cerebral blood flow and metabolism. Modification by prior administration of thiopental. *Anesth Analg (Cleve)* 50:443–447, 1971.
11. Lassen N: Cerebral blood flow and oxygen consumption in man. *Physiol Rev* 39:183–238, 1959.
12. Henriksen HT, Jorgensen PB: The effect of nitrous oxide on intracranial pressure in patients with intracranial disorders. *Br J Anaesth* 45:486–492, 1973.
13. Smith AL, Wollman H: Cerebral blood flow and metabolism. *Anesthesiology* 29:113–118, 1968.
14. Theye RA, Michenfelder JD: The effect of halothane on canine cerebral metabolism. *Anesthesiology* 29:113–118, 1968.
15. Michenfelder JD, Cucchiara RF: Canine cerebral oxygen consumption during enflurane anesthesia and its modification during induced seizures. *Anesthesiology* 40:575–580, 1974.
16. Artru AA, Nugent M, Michenfelder JD: Enflurane causes a prolonged and reversible increase in the rate of CSF production in the dog. *Anesthesiology* 57:779–784, 1978.
17. Cucchiara RF, Theye RA, Michenfelder JD: The effects of isoflurane on canine cerebral metabolism and blood flow. *Anesthesiology* 40:571–574, 1974.
18. Schettini A, Mahig J: Comparative intracranial dynamic responses in dogs to three halogenated anesthetic, abstracted. Scientific Papers, *Ann Mtg Amer Soc Anesthesiologists* 123–124, 1973.
19. Raichle ME, Stone HL: Cerebral blood flow autoregulation and graded hypercapnia. *Eur Neurol* 6:1–5, 1971.
20. Turner J, Lambertsen CJ, Owens SG: Effect of .08 and .8 atmospheres of inspired PO_2 upon cerebral neurodynamics of a constant alveolar PCO_2 of 43 mm Hg. *Fed Proc* 16:310, 1957.
21. Cohen PJ, Alexander SC, Smith TC: Effects of hypoxia and normoraphia on cerebral blood flow and metabolism in conscious man. *J Appl Physiol* 23:183–189, 1967.
22. Stone HL, Raichle ME, Hernandez M: Sympathetic innervation and carbon dioxide sensitivity. In Langfitt T, McHenry LC, Reivich M, et al. (eds): *Cerebral Circulation and Metabolism.* New York, Springer-Verlag, 1975, pp 428–430.
23. James JM, Miller RA, Purres MJ: Observations on the extrinsic neural control of cerebral blood flow in the baboon. *Circ Res* 25:77–93, 1969.
24. Reivich N: Arterial pCO_2 and cerebral neurodynamics. *Am J Physiol* 206:25–35, 1964.
25. Schmidt CF: The influences of cerebral blood flow on respiration. *Am J Physiol* 84:202–259, 1928.
26. Kety SS, Schmidt CF: The effects of altered arterial tensions of carbon dioxide and oxygen on cerebral blood flow and cerebral oxygen consumption of normal young men. *J Clin Invest* 27:484–492, 1948.
27. Davis JN, Carlsson A: The effect of hypoxia on monoamine synthesis, levels and metabolism in rat brain. *J Neurochem* 21:783–790, 1973.
28. Emeroldsen EM, Jensen FT: Autoregulation and CO_2 responses of cerebral blood flow in patients with acute severe head injury. *J Neurosurg* 48:689–703, 1978.
29. Siesjo BK: *Brain Energy Metabolism.* New York, John Wiley and

Sons, 1978, p 607.
30. Voorhies RM, Fraser RAR, Van Poznak A: Prevention of air embolism with positive end expiratory pressure. *Neurosurgery* 12:503–506, 1983.
31. Lofgren J, Von Essen C, Zewtnow NN: The pressure-volume curve of the cerebrospinal fluid space in dogs. *Acta Neurol Scand* 49:557–574, 1973.
32. Van Poznak A: Role of respiratory patterns in the treatment of pain and anxiety. In Luczun ME (ed): *Postanesthesia Nursing*. Rockville, Aspen Systems Corporation, 1984, 66–69.

PART 3

Cardiac Anesthesia

N. SYDNEY MOISE, D.V.M., M.S., D.A.C.V.I.M., AND
CHARLES E. SHORT, D.V.M., M.S., D.A.C.V.A.

Anesthesia of the veterinary patient with cardiac disease demands (*a*) knowledge of the hemodynamic alterations induced by various congenital and acquired diseases of the heart; (*b*) ability to recognize, differentiate, and treat supraventricular and ventricular arrhythmias; (*c*) understanding of cardiac drugs and their interaction with anesthetic agents; and (*d*) knowledge of diagnostic, therapeutic, and surgical procedures performed on cardiac patients for which tranquilization or anesthesia is required. Most veterinary patients with cardiac diseases that require anesthesia are dogs and cats; these patients will be emphasized in this chapter. Animals with disease of the heart may be anesthetized for evaluation of their disease (e.g., angiography), surgical correction of a defect (e.g., ligation of a patent ductus arteriosus), or for noncardiac therapy or surgery (e.g., dental work or correction of medial patellar luxation). This chapter will discuss the evaluation of the dog and cat with heart disease so that the degree of hemodynamic compromise can be adequately assessed before anesthesia. Cardiac diagnostic procedures and their associated risks and cardiac monitoring will be discussed. The therapy of important arrhythmias and drug interaction will be given. Discussion of specific cardiac diseases will precede specific anesthetic recommendations. Additionally, common noncardiac diseases that frequently affect the cardiovascular system will be presented.

History and Examination of the Cardiac Patient

The importance of signalment, history, and physical examination cannot be overemphasized. The specific cardiac disease alone may not dictate the seriousness of the animal's condition and the anesthetic risk. For example, anesthetizing an asymptomatic 3-month-old puppy for a thoracotomy and ligation of a patent ductus arteriosus is not likely to be as risky as anesthetizing a 13-year-old dog that has significant congestive heart failure secondary to severe mitral insufficiency for repair of a femoral fracture. The duration and severity of such clinical signs of cardiac disease as coughing, dyspnea, weakness, syncope, abdominal swelling, or exercise intolerance are keys in evaluating risk.

A careful, complete, systematic physical examination is paramount in the preanesthetic assessment of the cardiac patient. Vital signs (temperature, respiration, heart rate, and body weight) should be recorded. The animal's general appearance is judged as to body condition (e.g., debilitated, thin, normal, obese) and attitude (e.g., alert and responsive, depressed, comatose).

The animal's respiratory pattern is important in the evaluation of the cardiac patient. Normal breathing is subtle and easy. Tachypnea indicates rapid breathing. This pattern may be seen in the excited animal or the animal with disease. Dyspnea indicates a labored difficult breathing. Dyspnea may be primarily inspiratory, expiratory, or both. Inspiratory dyspnea is evidenced by deliberate, prolonged inspirations that may be accompanied by marked abdominal lift or movement of the diaphragm. Inspiratory dyspnea indicates restriction to air filling the lungs and is seen with pleural effusion or pulmonary edema. Pure expiratory dyspnea is characterized by effortless inspiration, but forced expirations. Expiratory dyspnea is seen with airway obstruction. Dynamic compression of the airways occurs with changes in intrapleural pressures during expirations. Bronchial diseases are typically associated with forced expirations; however, bronchoconstriction and reactive airways can exist in some animals with pulmonary edema secondary to cardiac disease. In these animals, mixed dyspnea (inspiratory plus expiratory) is observed. Simply observing the respiration of an animal may reveal difficulty not yet appreciated by the owner.

Mucous membrane color is judged as pink, pale, purple, or blue. Although pink mucous membranes are ideal, this does not guarantee normal oxygenation or circulation. The visual detection of cyanosis requires at least 5 g of deoxygenated hemoglobin per 100 ml of blood (1). In the anemic animal, cyanosis can be more difficult to recognize from visual inspection. Pale mucous membranes do not always indicate anemia. Marked peripheral vasoconstriction results in a pale to white mucous membrane color. This degree of vasoconstriction is seen in conditions with low cardiac output and cardiogenic shock, such as severe heartworm disease or cardiomyopathy. Capillary refill time is the time needed for a return of mucous membrane color after blanching with the finger the mucous membranes of the animal's gums. Normal capillary refill time is less than 2 seconds. This test, although frequently done, is not always reliable in indicating capillary circulation. It is also difficult to judge in anemic animals.

The jugular veins are examined for distension or pulsations. Breathing that causes movement of the thoracic inlet should not be confused with the presence of jugular pulses. Pulsations, if present, will be seen at the midpoint of the neck. Jugular pulses indicate an elevation in the venous pressure, and situations associated with venous congestion should be considered. Diseases that cause right heart failure, such as heartworm disease, tricuspid insufficiency, or dilated cardiomyopathy, are included in a differential diagnosis. The presence of a jugular pulse may be a warning of pericardial effusion, exclusive of right heart disease. If the pulsations observed are irregular and not associated with every heart beat, the etiology may be an arrhythmia that causes the ventricle to contract when the tricuspid valve is open. Examples of the latter include third degree heart block, ventricular tachycardia, or artificial pacemaker rhythm.

The femoral arterial pulses are evaluated for rate, strength, regularity, symmetry, and association with ventricular systole. The pulse rate should be judged as acceptable, too slow, or too rapid. Weak femoral arterial pulses are indicative of poor forward cardiac output. Pulses that are bounding may indicate an increased cardiac output (e.g., hyperthyroidism) or a wide pulse pressure (pulse pressure equals systolic pressure-diastolic pressure) (e.g., patent ductus arteriosus or aortic insufficiency). Irregular pulses may be normal if associated with a sinus arrhythmia. The pulse rate will speed up with inspiration and slow with expiration. This change corresponds to decreases and increases in vagal tone caused by breathing. Left and right femoral pulses should be equal. Discrepancy in this finding may indicate thromboembolism, and this is most frequently seen in cats with cardiomyopathy. Absence of both pulses is most commonly seen with feline thromboembolism. Each femoral arterial pulse should be briefly preceded by the heart beat. This can be assessed by simultaneous palpation of the cardiac apex or cardiac auscultation. The absence of a femoral pulse when ventricular systole occurs is termed a pulse deficit. Pulse deficits are detected in arrhythimas that do not allow adequate diastolic filling of the heart for a preload capable of providing an adequate stroke volume to be detected in a femoral pulse. Arrhythmias frequently associated with pulse deficits include ventricular or atrial tachycardia, ventricular or atrial premature complexes, and atrial fibrillation or flutter.

After palpating the femoral pulses, the examiner can slide the hands down the back legs and palpate for any swelling, indicating peripheral edema, and judge peripheral limb temperature. The front legs are also palpated. Cool to cold extremities, when compared to the trunk and abdomen, may indicate poor cardiac output.

The abdomen is palpated to determine the presence or absence of hepatomegaly or ascites, both signs of passive venous congestion. The thoracic cage is palpated and percussed. Percussion can be valuable in the determination of pleural fluid. The thorax with normally inflated lungs is resonant, but a line of demarcation detected bilaterally between resonant and dull sounds indicates pleural fluid. This finding may indicate the need for radiographs or thoracocentesis before anesthetic induction or it may be reason to anticipate more resistance when ventilating the anesthetized animal.

Auscultation of the lungs and heart is crucial in the evaluation of the cardiac patient. Auscultation of entire lung fields should reveal bronchial breath sounds near the tracheobronchial bifurcation, very soft vesicular sounds, or quiet sounds peripherally. Bronchial sounds are heard primarily during expiration, whereas vesicular sounds are heard primarily during inspiration. Normal variations should be known. Young puppies and kittens and some cats can have increased bronchovesicular sounds that may be interpreted as harsh lung sounds or dry rales. Also, dogs that are panting will have similar increases in lung sounds. Rales are abnormal lung sounds. Crackles, fine to coarse bubbling sounds similar to the sound generated by rubbing hair between your fingers near your ears, may indicate edema fluid. These sounds may originate from fluid movement in or around airways or as a result of airways snapping open. Rhondi are coarser louder sounds generated by the narrowing of larger bronchial airways that are partially obstructed by bronchospasm or secretions. They are better heard on expiration because of dynamic compression. In large bronchi, they are low pitched, sonorous, and almost continuous. In small bronchi they are high pitched, sibilant, or squeaky. When the sounds are squeaky, they may be described as wheezing. It is important to remember that a noisy airway at any level of the tracheobronchial tree is an obstructed airway and needs to be investigated. When ausculting the thorax, if lung sounds are heard dorsally but not ventrally, pleural fluid, lung consolidation, or mass lesion should be suspected.

Auscultation of the heart in the patient with cardiac disease is an essential diagnostic step. All valves must be carefully ausculted. A common mistake is not to listen to the heart far enough cranially; because of this error, a patent ductus arteriosus can be missed. In addition to describing the location of a cardiac murmur (apex versus base, aortic, pulmonic, or mitral tricuspid), the loudness or intensity of the murmur is graded. The intensity of a murmur does not always correlate with the severity of the disease. For example, a dog with significant mitral regurgitation may not have as loud a murmur as a dog with a small regurgitative stream that squirts blood through a small hole made by inadequately meeting mitral leaflets. Cardiac murmurs are graded on a scale of 1 to 6. A Grade 1 murmur is a murmur that is difficult to find, very soft, and heard only over a localized area. A Grade 2 murmur is a murmur that is easy to find but heard only in a localized area. If a murmur is very easy to find, loud, and radiates locally, it is classified as a Grade 3. A Grade 4 murmur is very loud and radiates over both sides of the thorax. If a murmur is very loud, radiates to both sides of the thorax, and a thrill is palpated, the murmur is a Grade 5. A Grade 6 murmur is a very loud, widely radiating murmur that can be felt and heard even when the stephoscope is not touching the skin. Heart murmurs are classified as to their time and duration. A murmur is systolic if it occurs during ventricular systole and diastolic if it occurs during ventricular diastole. The murmur may be early, mid, or late systolic or diastolic. If the murmur continues throughout systole or diastole, it is holosystolic or holodiastolic. A murmur that goes beyond systole or diastole has the prefix "trans" or "pan" added. The quality of a murmur also can be assessed to include low or high frequency, crescendo, decrescendo, crescendo-decrescendo, or plateau shape. The complete description of a cardiac murmur is required in the communication of cardiac disease.

Diagnostic Procedures before Anesthesia of the Cardiac Patient

Based on the history and physical examination, the appropriate diagnostic test should be evaluated for an individual patient before anesthesia. Diagnostics may include blood work, electrocardiography, radiography, phonocardiography, or echocardiography. Laboratory data that may be specifically helpful in the animal with heart disease include a complete blood count, liver and kidney function, electrolytes, and blood gases. The presence of anemia in a dog with inadequate circulation due to cardiac disease merits special attention. In the presence of normal hydration, polycythemia should be an indicator of a possible right-to-left shunt. Elevation in the white blood cell count with a neutrophilia and a left shift may indicate concurrent endocarditis. Hepatic congestion will increase liver enzymes, and poor cardiac output will elevate the blood urea nitrogen. If azotemia is present, it is imperative that a differentiation be made as to a renal or prerenal origin. Determination of electrolytes is essential in the evaluation of the critically ill cardiac patient. Hypokalemia is a common reason for the lack of conversion of ventricular tachycardia to a normal sinus rhythm with antiarrhythmics. Blood gas abnormalities are frequent in the critically ill patient with cardiac complications. Metabolic acidosis certainly contributes to the ventricular arrhythmias seen in dogs with gastric torsion-volvulus. Electrolytes and blood gas determinations may be required during the anesthetic period.

Electrocardiograms are recorded to assess cardiac enlargement or rhythm. The ECG is better at the latter. An arrhythmia, suspected from the physical examination, should be confirmed and evaluated by the ECG. Commonly encountered conduction disturbances will be discussed below.

Electrocardiographic monitoring is commonly continued during anesthesia of the cardiac patient. Thoracic radiographs are usually taken before the cardiac patient is anesthetized. The cardiac silhouette is studied for evidence of right or left heart enlargement. The pulmonary arteries and veins are evaluated for engorgement. The pulmonary parenchyma is examined for evidence of cardiogenic edema. Pleural fluid, hepatomegaly, and vena caval enlargement are sought as extracardiac signs of congestive heart failure.

Echocardiography is an exciting noninvasive diagnostic tool that is becoming more and more available to the veterinarian in the evaluation of cardiac patients (2, 3). Echocardiography is an ultrasound examination of the heart. High frequency sound waves are directed toward the heart with a hand-held transducer. The transducer contains a crystal that has piezoelectric properties. That is, the crystal has the ability to change electrical impulses into ultrasound waves and vice versa. As the sound waves encounter the border between structures of different acoustic impedence, called an acoustic interface, some sound waves are reflected back and others continue to travel forward. The acoustic impedence is the resistance that influences the speed that sound waves travel through a media. Sound waves that are reflected back to the transducer are converted back to electrical impulses and processed so that an image of dots reflected back at certain distances from the transducer are displayed on an oscilloscope monitor. Because the ultrasound waves are constantly sent and received, the heart can be seen beating. There are currently three types of echocardiography: M-mode echocardiography, two-dimensional echocardiography, and Doppler echocardiography. M-mode echocardiography uses essentially a single beam of ultrasound to image a very small, icepick portion of the heart. Two-dimensional echocardiography uses many ultrasound beams to image a slice of the heart, giving an image similar to a tomogram. Doppler echocardiography is used for the evaluation of blood flow as ultrasound waves are reflected from circulating red blood cells. This technique allows, for example, determination of pressure gradients across stenotic valves, degrees of valvular regurgitation, and cardiac output. Doppler echocardiography is relatively new, and its use in veterinary medicine is limited. M-mode echocardiography has been used for about 10 years and two-dimensional examinations for about 5 years in our profession. With M-mode or two-dimensional echocardiography, a much more detailed evaluation of cardiac size, structure, and function can be achieved than by other noninvasive diagnostic tools available to the veterinarian. The thickness of the myocardial wall, the diameter of cardiac chambers, and the systolic and diastolic motion of the walls and valves can be visualized. Two-dimensional echocardiography is preferred because a more complete spatial orientation of the heart is seen than with M-mode echocardiography. Diagnoses can be made without endangering the compromised animal. To familiarize the reader with the possible diagnostic capabilities of echocardiography, examples are shown in Figures 12.1 to 12.7.

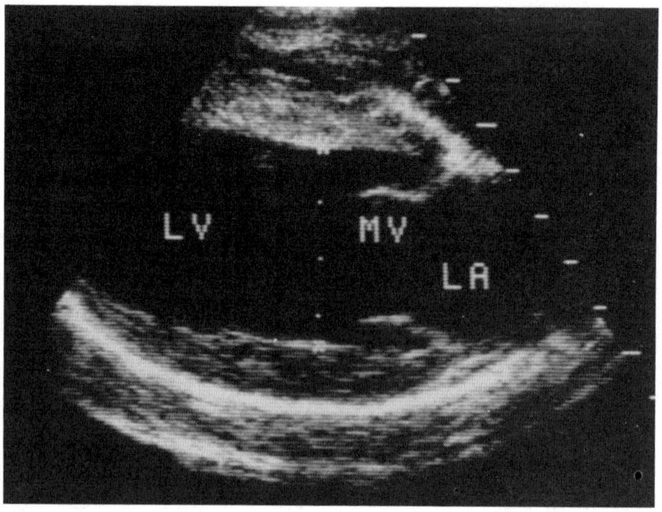

Figure 12.1. Long-axis two-dimensional echocardiogram recorded from a normal dog showing the structures of the left heart. LV, left ventricular chamber; MV, mitral valve orifice; LA, left atrium.

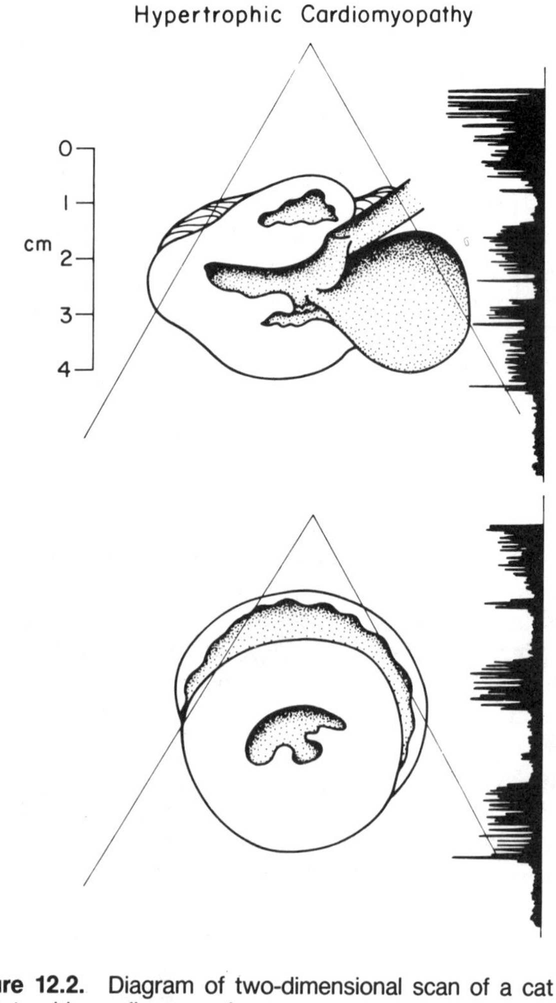

Figure 12.2. Diagram of two-dimensional scan of a cat with hypertrophic cardiomyopathy.

Arrhythmias Commonly Encountered in the Cardiac Patient

The dog or cat with cardiac disease may have an arrhythmia before anesthesia or arrhythmias may occur during anesthesia. Occasionally, an arrhythmia that was present in the awake animal disappears once the animal is anesthetized. It is vital that the anesthesiologist be able to recognize abnormal conduction and know when treatment is necessary and when it is not.

To accurately interpret an electrocardiogram (ECG) consistently, a systematic evaluation of the recording must be done (4). Rhythm analysis, rather than enlargement patterns, is the major concern of the anesthesiologist; therefore, these will be emphasized. The reader is referred to electrocardiography texts for a more detailed discussion (4). The following questions should be answered for every ECG:

1. What is the ventricular heart rate?
2. Is the rate within normal limits for the species or is a bradycardia or tachycardia present?
3. Is the rhythm regular or irregular?
4. Are there P waves?
5. Are all the P waves and the QRS complexes related?

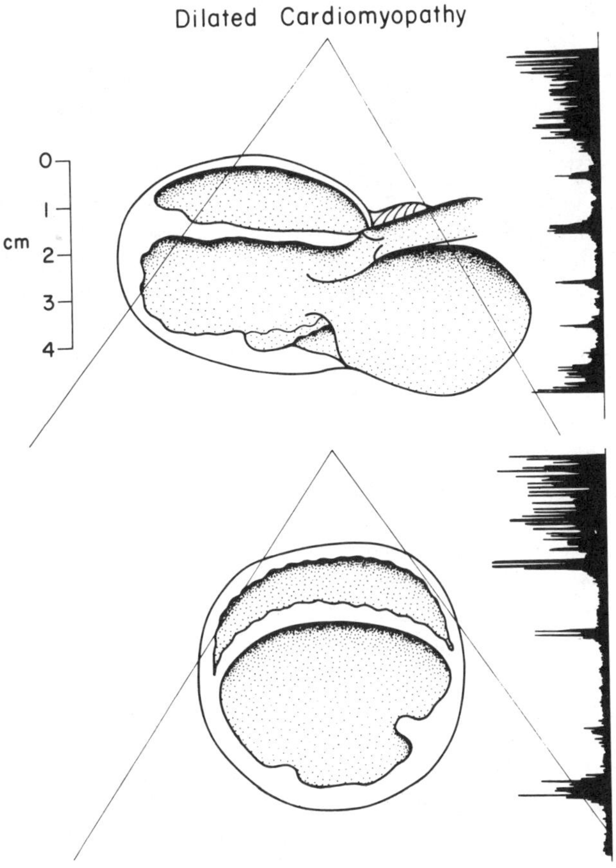

Figure 12.3. Diagram of two-dimensional scan of a cat with dilated cardiomyopathy.

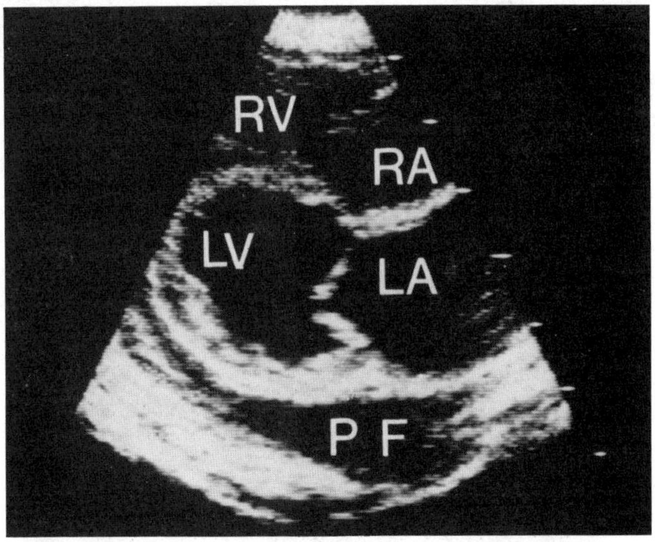

Figure 12.5. Long-axis two-dimensional echocardiogram recorded from a cat with dilated cardiomyopathy. RV, right ventricle; RA, right atrium; LV, left ventricle; LA, left atrium; PF, pleural fluid.

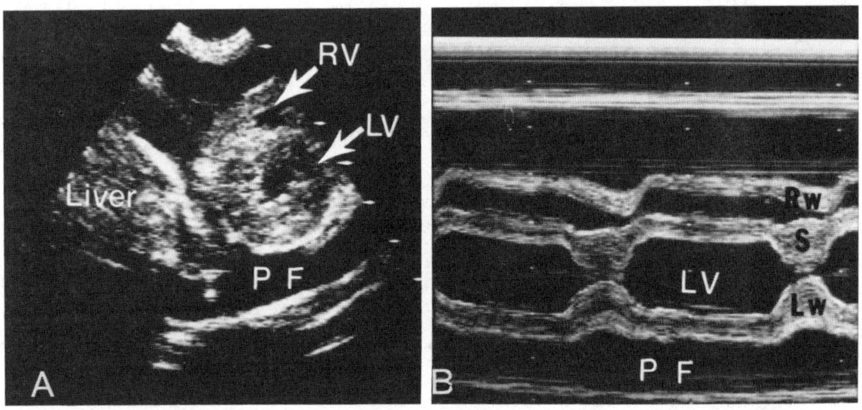

Figure 12.4. *A*, Short-axis two-dimensional echocardiogram recorded from a cat with hyperthyroidism and secondary hypertrophy of the heart and congestive heart failure. *B*, M-mode echocardiogram recorded at the ventricular apex of the cat seen in *A*. RV, right ventricle; LV, left ventricle; PF, pleural fluid; S, interventricular septum; Lw, left ventricular wall; Rw, right ventricular wall.

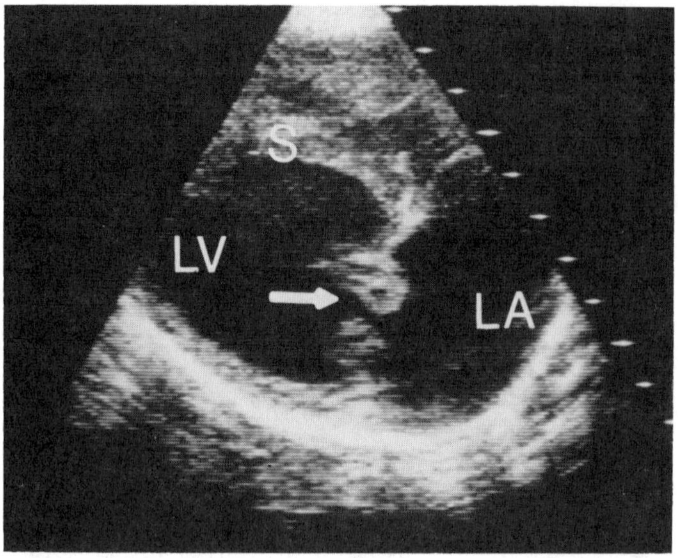

Figure 12.6. Long-axis two-dimensional echocardiogram recorded from a dog with mitral insufficiency secondary to valvular endocardiosis. Large lesions are seen on the valve leaflets (*arrow*). S, interventricular septum; LV, left ventricle; LA, left atrium.

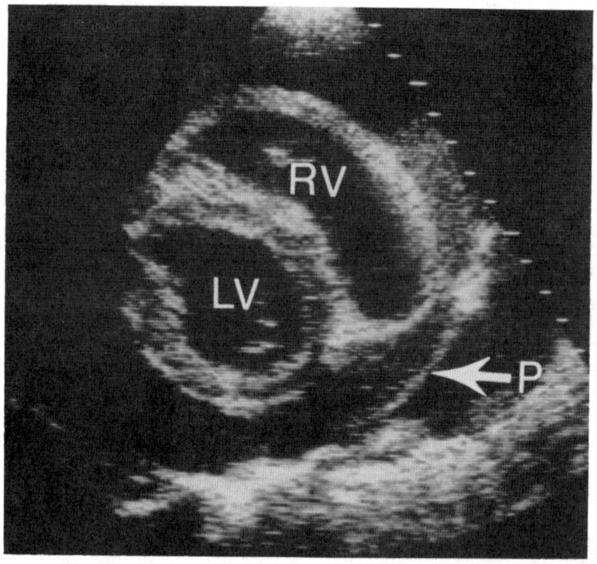

Figure 12.7. Short-axis two-dimensional echocardiogram recorded from a dog with pericardial and pleural fluid. The pericardium (*P*) is seen. RV, right ventricle; LV, left ventricle.

6. Do all the QRS complexes and P waves look alike?
7. Are the QRS complexes wide or narrow?
8. Is the amplitude of the wave normal and do the time intervals represent a normal response?
9. What is the diagnosis?
10. Is therapy necessary?
11. What therapy is indicated?

Bradyarrhythmias include sinus bradycardia, sinus arrest, sinoatrial block, atrial standstill (hyperkalemia), or atrioventricular blocks. Sinus bradycardia or sinus arrest may be seen in healthy dogs with a high vagal tone and are not of concern. Brachycephalic breeds commonly have upper airway disease and slow heart rates. Sinus bradycardia can be induced by increases in vagal tone caused by disease of the respiratory, gastrointestinal, urogenital, or central nervous systems. The sinus bradycardia may be so severe that vagolytic or sympathomimetic therapy is required. This is particularly true of the animal experiencing severe bradycardia secondary to cranial trauma. Bradycardia also may be induced by anesthetic agents (Fig. 12.8).

Atrial standstill (hyperkalemia) is most frequently encountered in cats with urethral obstruction or dogs with hypoadrenocorticism. The cat with urethral obstruction and hyperkalemia may need tranquilization to pass a urinary catheter or general anesthesia for an emergency perineal urethrostomy. The degree of hyperkalemia can be estimated from the electrocardiogram. Mild elevations (serum potassium greater than 5.5 meq/liter but less than 6.5 meq/liter) result in large peaked T waves. With a serum potassium between 6.5 and 8.5 meq/liter, the heart rate slows, R wave and P wave amplitude is decreased, QRS and P-R intervals are prolonged, S-T segment is depressed, and the Q-T interval is increased. The P wave disappears with serum potassium concentrations of more than 8.5 meq/liter, and a sinoventricular rhythm results. The rhythm is not ventricular tachycardia and not an idioventricular rhythm (Fig. 12.9). The sinus node still fires with hyperkalemia, but intraventricular conduction disturbance is present. With serum potassium concentrations of 10 meq/liter or more, the QRS complex becomes very wide and eventually ventricular flutter or fibrillation and finally ventricular asystole result. Before tranquilizers or anesthetics are given, the heart must be stabilized when the serum potassium is elevated. Usually, the seriously ill cat does not require chemical restraint for the passage of a urinary catheter

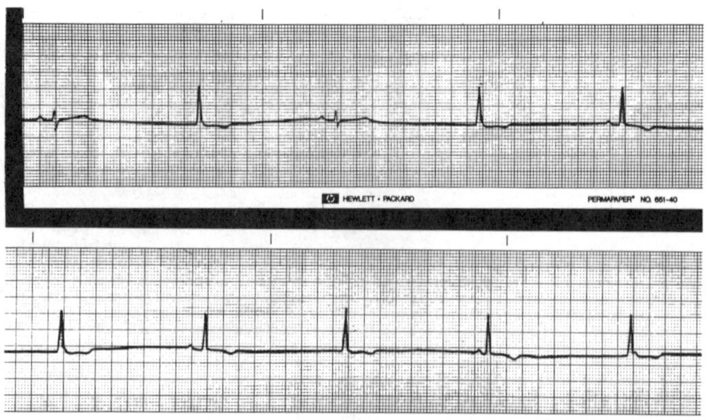

Figure 12.8. Electrocardiogram recorded from a cat given xylazine (0.5 mg/kg i.m.). A profound sinus bradycardia with escape beats is seen. Atropine sulfate was administered, and the severity of the bradycardia lessened (50 mm/sec, 1 cm = 1 mV).

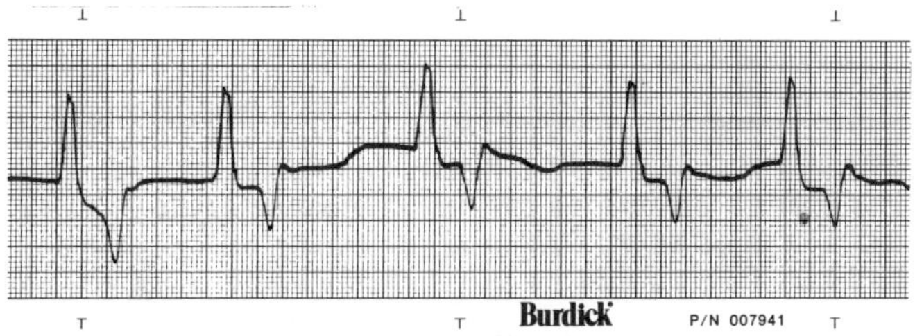

Figure 12.9. Sinoventricular rhythm in a cat with urethral obstruction. The serum potassium was 11.5 mEq/liter. The cat was treated with intravenous 5% dextrose, sodium bicarbonate, 1 unit of intravenous regular insulin, and an additional 2 g of dextrose as a 20% solution given over 60 min. Simultaneously with the above, a urinary catheter was passed, and the cat was unobstructed. Perineal urethrostomy was performed 4 days later (50 mm/sec, 1 cm = 1 mV).

and placement of an intravenous line. In some difficult cases when a urinary catheter cannot be passed and cystocentesis with a 23- to 25-gauge needle is required, emergency perineal urethrostomy may need to be performed to keep the bladder decompressed if a catheter cannot be passed after cystocentesis. In addition to treating the underlying cause, the following therapy can be given to decrease the serum potassium concentration. The fluid of choice is 5% dextrose and water. The dextrose will stimulate endogenous insulin secretion, and together the dextrose and insulin cause the movement of potassium into the cell. Cats with urethral obstruction frequently have a metabolic acidosis. Sodium bicarbonate (1 to 2 meq/kg) is administered intravenously for the acidosis, but it also forces the extracellular potassium into the intracellular compartment. For severe hyperkalemia, intravenous regular insulin (0.5 units/kg) is administered with intravenous dextrose (2 g of dextrose/unit of insulin). Concentrated dextrose solutions can be administered to meet this dextrose requirement, but to avoid nausea and vomiting, the dextrose solution should be diluted (approximately 20% solution) and administered slowly. The use of insulin in these cats is controversial. Some advocate the prompt relief of severe hyperkalemia with intravenous dextrose and sodium bicarbonate alone. In emergency situations where cardiac arrest is impending, calcium gluconate as a 10% intravenous solution (0.5 to 1 ml/kg) can be given slowly. Calcium gluconate does not decrease the potassium concentration, but it does directly antagonize the cardiotoxic effects.

Persistent atrial standstill (silent atrium) is an uncommon arrhythmia; it is seen in English springer spaniels, although occasionally other breeds are affected (4). There are no P waves because the atria are degenerated. Junctional or ventricular escape rhythms pace the heart. Dogs are usually presented for syncope or weakness. Permanent pacemaker implantation is the required therapy; this will be discussed below.

Atrioventricular blocks are classified as first, second, or third degree (4). First degree block is characterized by a prolonged P-R interval, and all P waves are followed by a QRS complex because atrioventricular conduction is complete, although delayed. Second degree heart block also may be characterized by prolongation of the P-R interval, but not all atrial depolarizations are transmitted to the ventricles. Therefore, there will be P waves without an accompanying QRS complex. The number of nonconducted P waves will vary from few to many, and this determines the clinical signs and seriousness of the disease. Escape beats from the atrioventricular junction or ventricle may occur, and these must not be confused with ventricular premature complexes. Third degree heart block also is known as complete heart block. The sinoatrial node is firing and depolarizing the atria, but none of the P waves are conducted to the ventricles. An escape rhythm most commonly from the ventricle, saves the heart from asystole. One should not suppress a ventricular escape rhythm with antiarrhythmic drugs. These may be mistaken for ventricular premature beats or ventricular tachycardia. The therapeutic management of high grade second and third degree heart block will be discussed in the section on pacemaker therapy.

Tachyarrhythmias include sinus tachycardia, atrial tachycardia, atrial flutter, atrial fibrillation, arteriovenous (A-V) junctional tachycardia, and ventricular tachycardia. Sinus tachycardia is commonly encountered in the normal anxious dog or cat. It also is seen in situations demanding augmented cardiac output, such as shock, heat stroke, hyperthyroidism, anemia, fever, infection, or hypoxia. Dogs or cats in congestive heart failure may have a sinus tachycardia. Sinus tachycardia may be so rapid that P waves are not seen; instead, they are superimposed on the preceding T waves. Sinus tachycardia must be differentiated from atrial tachycardia. Atrial tachycardia is a rapid regular rhythm that originates from an ectopic focus in the atria other than the sinoatrial node. The P waves have a different configuration than those originating from the sinus node. One premature beat from such a focus is called an atrial premature contraction (APC). These premature beats may appear in pairs or they may alternate every other depolarization with a normal sinus beat. The later arrhythmia is termed "atrial bigeminy." Atrial tachycardia usually occurs when there are diseased atria. Frequently, the tachycardia is paroxysmal, and at times conduction through the A-V node is physiologically blocked because of the number of impulses with which it is presented. Performing a vagal maneuver such as carotid artery massage or ocular pressure may convert atrial tachycardia back to a normal sinus rhythm, but with sinus tachycardia no response or only a brief response is observed. Digoxin is the therapy of choice for atrial tachycardia. Propranolol may also be used. Occasional APCs need not be treated unless more than 20 occur per minute.

Atrial fibrillation is most commonly observed in the dog and horse. It is rare in the cat. A critical mass of tissue must be present for atrial fibrillation to be maintained. Atrial fibrillation is seen in dogs with diseased and dilated atria because of cardiomyopathy or severe mitral insufficiency. Occasionally, a large breed dog presented for gastric torsion-volvulus will have atrial fibrillation secondary to electrolyte and blood gas disturbances. After correction of these abnormalities, the arrhythmia resolves. The horse differs from the dog because atrial fibrillation can occur without cardiac disease. Atrial fibrillation is characterized by the absence of P waves, rapid irregular ventricular rate, and fine undulations of the baseline. Coarse undulations may be called fibrillation-flutter waves; larger regular undulations of the baseline are known as flutter waves (Fig. 12.10) (4). Therapy with quinidine sulfate frequently converts atrial fibrillation to a normal sinus rhythm in the horse, but this is very rare in the dog. An occasional dog will convert with digoxin. Therapy for atrial fibrillation in the dog is aimed at controlling the ventricular response rate. The rapid heart rate in atrial fibrillation is detrimental because of the decreased diastolic filling time. Oral digitalization will slow atrioventricular conduction and decrease the heart rate. Rates of more than 250 beats/minute can be dangerous in large breed dogs. In these cases, an oral loading dose of digoxin or intravenous digoxin may be necessary. Alternatively or in addition to the digoxin, oral or intravenous propranolol may be needed. Frequently, low doses of propranolol given orally work within 1 to 2 hours to decrease the heart rate. Calcium channel blockers such as verapamil also have been reported to help decrease the tachycardia of atrial fibrillation (4).

Atrioventricular junctional rhythms frequently have a negative P wave and the QRS complex is normal in configuration as depolarization of the ventricle follows normal conduction pathways. Therapy for tachyarrhythmias of junctional origin is the same as for atrial tachycardia or atrial fibrillation (4).

Ventricular arrhythmias are commonly encountered by the anesthesiologist. Ventricular premature complexes may occur singularly, in pairs, or in runs of four or more (ventricular tachycardia) (Fig. 12.11). When ventricular premature complexes alternate every other beat with abnormal sinus complex, the rhythm is termed "ventricular bigeminy" (Fig. 12.12). Sustained ventricular tachycardia has a rate of greater than 100 beats/minute. Most commonly, the rate is above 130/minute. If the rate is between 60 and 100, it is termed an "idioventricular rhythm" (4). Classically, a ventricular premature complex (VPC) is characterized by a wide and bizarre configuration. Most of the time if such a complex is seen, it is probably of ventricular origin, although this is not always true. The abnormal shape of a VPC occurs because it is originating from a ventricular ectopic foci and depolarizing the ventricle through the myocardium instead of through normal specialized conduction pathways. If VPCs look alike, they probably come from the same ventricular foci; if they change in shape, however, this indicates different sites of origin. In the latter situation, the VPCs

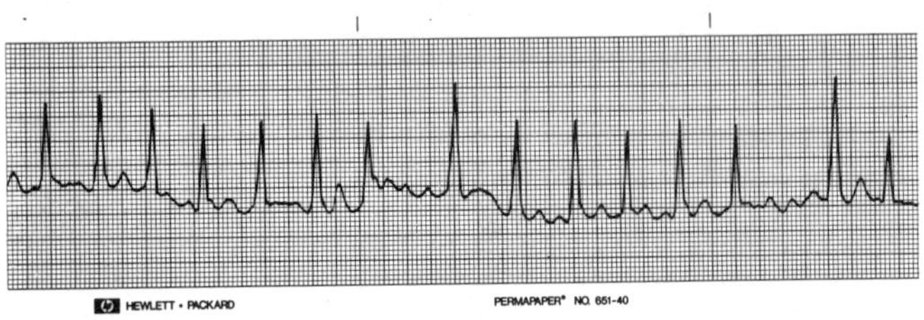

Figure 12.10. ECG recorded from a great Dane with a gastric torsion volvulus. The dog also had dilated cardiomyopathy. The ECG reveals atrial fibrillation-flutter (50 mm/sec, 1 cm = 1 mV).

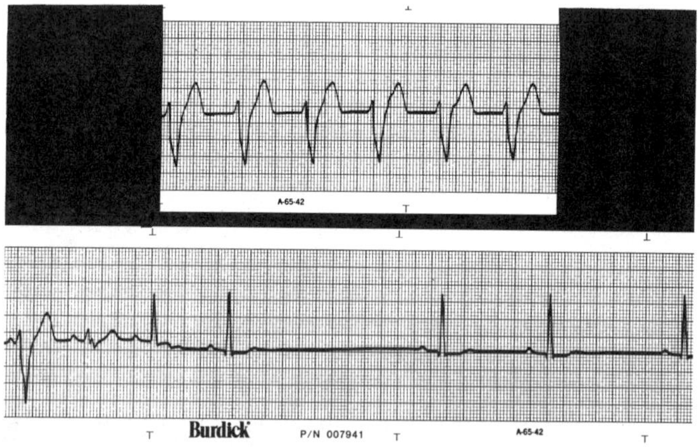

Figure 12.11. Unifocal ventricular tachycardia (rate 160) in a dog with traumatic myocarditis 36 hours after being struck by an automobile. Intravenous lidocaine (2 mg/kg i.v. bolus) converted the dog to a sinus rhythm. Continuous strip recording. Note fusion beat (second complex from left) on bottom tracing (50 mm/sec, 1 cm = 1 mV).

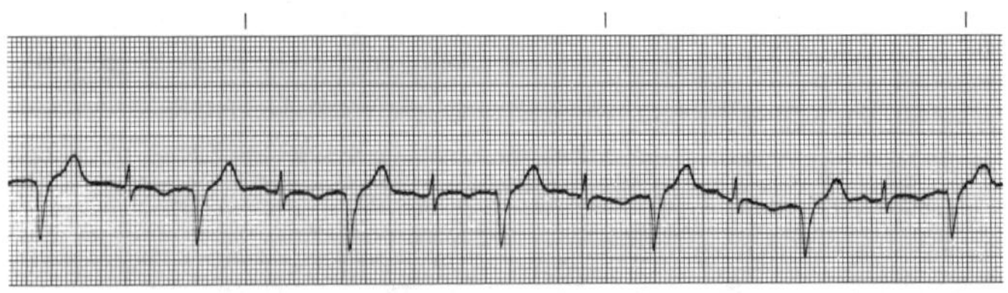

Figure 12.12. ECG recorded from a cat with bilateral renal cyst. The cat was to undergo surgery for removal of the cyst when ventricular bigeminy was identified before any preanesthetic medications were given. Low-dose propranolol and lidocaine did not convert the rhythm; however, when the cat was premedicated with atropine, a normal sinus rhythm resulted. During surgery, no arrhythmias were recorded, but once the cat was fully recovered, the ventricular bigeminy returned (50 mm/sec, 1 cm = 1 mV).

are termed "multifocal." Multifocal VPCs or ventricular tachycardia is of greater concern than beats of unifocal origin (Fig. 12.13). Occasionally, supraventricular premature complexes or rhythms can have a wide and bizarre configuration due to aberrant conduction. Aberrant conduction implies that the normal pathway was still partially refractory to depolarization when confronted with an electrical stimulus and the abnormal complex reflects altered conduction (5). A supraventricular rhythm of sinus or atrial origin can be confused with an ectopic ventricular rhythm if a right or left bundle branch block exists. In Figure 12.14, a sinus tachycardia in a dog with pre-existing right bundle branch block could be confused with ventricular tachycardia. The key in differentiating this arrhythmia from a ventricular arrhythmia is the presence of consistently related P and QRS waves. In Figure 12.14, every wide and bizarre QRS complex is preceded by a P wave with a consistent P-R interval. Although P waves will be seen with ventricular tachycardia, the P waves and QRS complexes are not related. The P waves are still present with ventricular tachycardia because the atria are not depolarized by a depolarization wave originating in the ventricle. Instead, these complexes stop within the A-V node. Because the atria and, therefore, S-A node are not affected by depolarization, it continues to fire. However, with supraventricular complexes, the atria and S-A node depolarize and can be refractory to stimulus, thus resetting the S-A node.

The question of when to treat ventricular arrhythmias is an important one because the indiscriminant use of antiarrhythmias is to be discouraged. Antiarrhythmic drugs can be arrhythmogenic themselves. Ventricular arrhythmias can cause serious circulatory deficits. The complete cardiovascular examination is important in assessing the detrimental effects of the arrhythmia (Fig. 12.15). The following guidelines are given for the treatment of VPCs or ventricular tachycardia (4, 6): (*a*) before using antiarrhythmic drugs, identify the possible underlying cause and correct it (e.g., hypoxia or excessive inhalant anesthetic); (*b*) treat if there are more than 20 to 30 VPCs per minute; (*c*) treat multifocal VPCs; and (*d*) treat if the R on T phenomenon is present (VPCs occurring on top of preceding T wave are occurring during the vulnerable period that subjects the heart to a high probability of ventricular fibrillation). In Figure 12.16, a flow chart is given for the acute treatment of ventricular tachycardia. Drugs for the treatment of supraventricular and ventricular arrhythmias are listed in Table 12.1.

In addition to arrhythmias, signs of hypoxia are important for the anesthesiologist to recognize. Hypoxia may cause large T waves (greater than 25% of the R wave) (4) (Fig. 12.17), changes in the T wave configuration, S-T segment depression or elevation (Figs. 12.18 and 12.19), or cardiac arrhythmias. If these alterations in the T wave occur during anesthesia, oxygen delivery should be evaluated.

Drugs Used in the Cardiac Patient

Drugs that affect the cardiovascular system, such as diuretics, positive inotropes, vasodilators, and antiarrhythmics, may change the usual response expected to anesthetic drugs (6–8). These drugs are commonly used in dogs and cats in the treatment of congestive heart failure and arrhythmias. An understanding of the mechanism of action is important so that possible interactions between anesthetics and preanesthetics can be avoided.

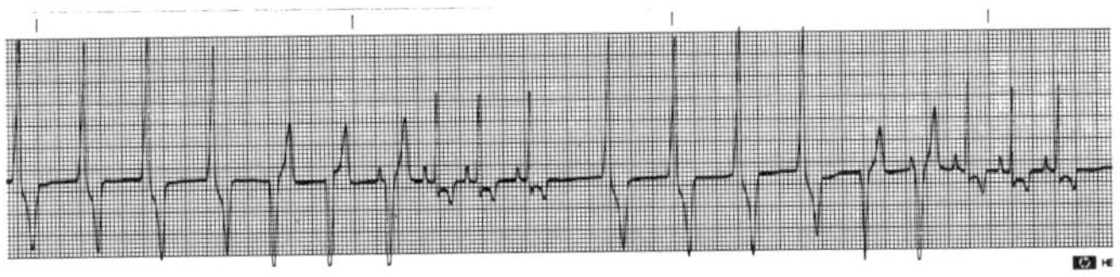

Figure 12.13. ECG recorded from a 13-year-old collie-mixed dog that was to undergo repair of a ruptured cruciate. Multifocal ventricular tachycardia is present. Occasionally, the sinus rhythm captures the heart. There is also S-T segment depression. This is a serious arrhythmia and needs therapy. The elective surgery was not performed (25 mm/sec, 1 cm = 1 mV).

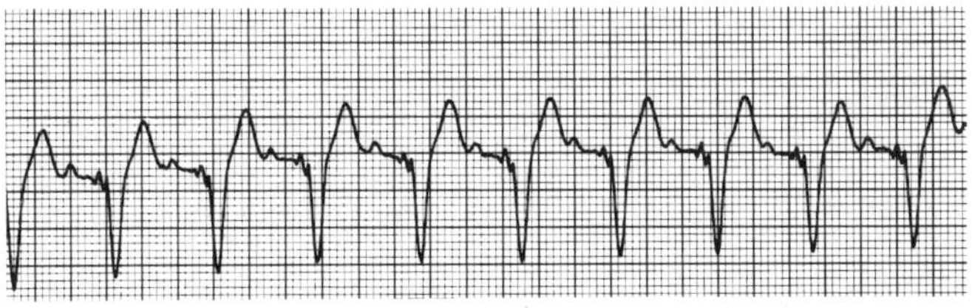

Figure 12.14. ECG recorded from a dog with urethral obstruction secondary to a urethral transitional cell carcinoma. The dog needed surgery to remove the obstructing tumor. This dog does not have ventricular tachycardia; instead, it has a sinus tachycardia with a right bundle-branch block. Note that every bizarre complex is associated with a preceding P wave (50 mm/sec, 1 cm = 1 mV).

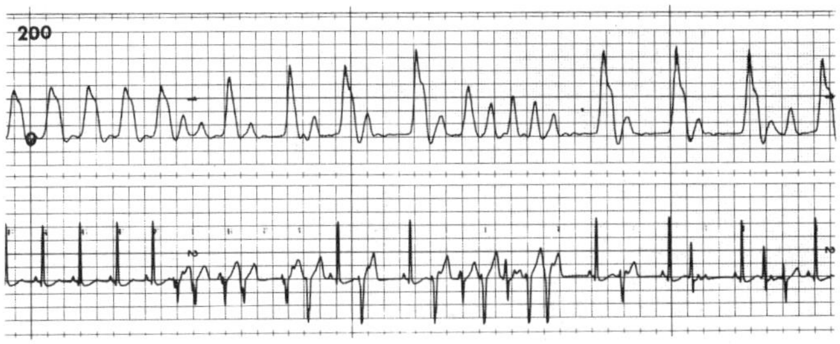

Figure 12.15. Continuous left ventricular pressure tracing and ECG in a dog. The catheter induced multifocal ventricular premature complexes. Note the poor pulse pressure generated by the premature beats. On physical examination, this would be detected as pulse deficits (25 mm/sec, 1 cm = 1 mV). Units are in mm Hg.

ELIMINATE UNDERLYING CAUSES IF POSSIBLE

(e.g., hypoxia, fluid imbalance, electrolyte imbalance, acidosis, alkalosis)

Unsuccessful

Lidocaine hydrochloride 2%,[a] i.v. bolus 1 mg/kg slowly up to maximum dosage of 8 mg/kg.

Successful

Continue to monitor.

Unsuccessful

(Are there electrolyte, fluid, or blood gas abnormalities?) (Reassess the animal's physical status) Procainamide[b] i.v. 6 to 8 mg/kg *slowly* over 5 minutes.

Successful

Maintain on lidocaine drip, 40 to 80 μg/kg/min. For a drip rate of 50 μg/kg/min, take 50 cc of fluid out of 1000 ml of Lactated Ringers solution (LRS), add 50 cc of 2% lidocaine, and drip at maintenance fluid rate (65 ml/kg/day). (Constant rate infusion formula: body weight (kg) × dose μg/kg/min) × 0.36 = total dose to give i.v. over 6 hours.

Unsuccessful

(Are there electrolyte, fluid, or blood gas abnormalities?) (Reassess the animal's physical status.) Quinidin gluconate,[b] 6 to 20 mg/kg i.m. of q6 hours.

Successful

Maintain on procainamide drip, 25 to 40 μg/kg/min, *or* give procainamide 6 to 20 mg/kg q4–6 hours i.m.

Unsuccessful

(Are there electrolyte, fluid, or blood gas abnormalities?) (Reassess the animal's physical status.) Try combination[c] of lidocaine and procainamide (low end of dosage range for each) or procainamide and quinidine (low end of dosage range for each).

Successful

Maintain on quinidine 6 to 20 mg/kg i.m. q6 hours.

Unsuccessful

(Are there electrolyte, fluid, or blood gas abnormalities?) (Reassess the animal's physical status.) Could arrhythmia be sympathetic-induced? Propranolol, 0.2 to 1.0 mg/kg orally t.i.d. or 0.04 to 0.06 mg/kg i.v. slowly. (Valium response test may help indicate success of propranolol therapy 2.5 to 5 mg i.v., but this is controversial.) Try combination of propranolol with lidocaine, procainamide, or quinidine at low end of dosage range.

Successful

Maintain on combination therapy.

Unsuccessful

(Are there electrolyte, fluid, or blood gas abnormalities?) (Reassess the animal's physical status.) Experimental drugs.

Successful

Maintain on lowest dose of oral propranolol or combination therapy and reduce stress.

Unsuccessful

Maintain animal's circulatory system, avoid stress, correct underlying cause. If arrhythmia worsens while on antiarrhythmic, stop drug as it may be arrhythmogenic.

Successful

Maintain on experimental drug.

Ventricular tachycardia in a cat: propranolol, 2.5 to 5 mg b.i.d.-t.i.d. orally or 0.04 mg/kg slowly i.v., or lidocaine HCl, 0.25 to 1 mg/kg i.v. over 5 minutes.

* Therapy given is for the immediate and short term treatment of ventricular tachycardia. Once stable, oral antiarrhythmics are begun when indicated.

[a] Toxicity: CNS signs (ear twitching, depression, nervousness, nausea, seizures).

[b] Toxicity: Hypotensive if given too rapidly i.v.; vomiting, depression, diarrhea.

[c] Toxicity: Be cautious when drugs are used in combination. Assess renal and hepatic function.

Figure 12.16. Flow chart for acute therapy of ventricular tachycardia in the dog. Therapy is given for the immediate and short-term treatment of ventricular tachycardia. Once the animal is stable, oral antiarrhythmics are begun when indicated.

Table 12.1
Drugs Used in the Therapy of Cardiac Arrhythmias[a]

Generic Name	Commonly Used Preparations	Indications	Adverse Effects	Approximate Dosage[b]
Atropine	Atropine sulfate USP, 0.4 mg/ml	Sinus bradycardia, sinoatrial arrest, incomplete AV block	Sinus tachycardia; ectopic complexes; ocular, gastrointestinal, and pulmonary side effects; paradoxic vagomimetic effects	0.01–0.02 mg/kg i.v., i.m.; 0.02–0.04 mg/kg s.c. (dog and cat)
Digitoxin	Crystodigin, 0.2 mg/ml; 0.1, 0.2 mg tablets; Foxalin, 0.1, 0.25, 0.5 mg	Supraventricular premature complexes, supraventricular tachycardia, atrial flutter/fibrillation	Anorexia, depression, vomiting, diarrhea, AV block, ectopia, junctional tachycardia	Oral maintenance: 0.04 to 0.1 mg/kg divided b.i.d. to t.i.d. Rapid i.v. digitalization; 0.01 to 0.03 mg/kg; administer ½ of calculated dose i.v., wait 30 to 60 min and administer ¼ of dose, wait 30 to 60 min
Digoxin	Lanoxin elixir 0.05 mg/ml; 0.125, 0.25, 0.5 mg tablets; Cardoxin elixirs, 0.05, 0.15 mg/ml	Supraventricular premature complexes, supraventricular tachycardia, atrial flutter/fibrillation	Anorexia, depression, vomiting, diarrhea, AV block, ectopia, junctional tachycardia	Oral maintenance: 0.01 to 0.02 mg/kg divided b.i.d. Rapid i.v. digitalization: 0.01 to 0.02 mg/kg i.v. as per digitoxin. Rapid oral digitalization: 0.02 to 0.06 mg/kg divided b.i.d. for one day. Cat: 0.007 to 0.015 mg/kg divided b.i.d.
Glycopyrrolate	Robinul injection, 0.2 mg/ml	Sinus bradycardia, sinoatrial arrest	Sinus tachycardia, ectopic complexes; ocular, gastrointestinal, and pulmonary side effects; paradoxic vagomimetic effects	0.005 to 0.01 mg/kg i.v., i.m.; 0.01 to 0.02 mg/kg s.c. (dog and cat)
Isopropamide	Darbid, 5 mg tablets	Incomplete AV block, sinoatrial arrest	As per atropine, keratoconjunctivitis sicca	2.5 to 5 mg b.i.d.-t.i.d.
Isoproterenol	Isuprel HCl injection 0.2 mg/ml; 1 and 5 ml ampuls; Proternol, 20, 40 mg tablets; Isuprel glossets, 10 mg	Sinoatrial arrest, sinus bradycardia, complete AV block	CNS stimulation, ectopic complexes, tachycardia, emesis	0.4 mg in 250 ml D5W, drip slowly to effect; Proternol, 10 to 20 mg q4–6 hours; Isuprel glossets, 5 to 10 mg sublingual or per rectum q4–6 hours
Lidocaine HCl	Xylocaine (without epinephrine) 2% (20 mg/ml)	Ventricular premature complexes, ventricular tachycardia	CNS excitation, seizures, tremors, emesis, other rhythm disturbances	2 to 4 mg/kg i.v. slowly, repeat to maximum of 8 mg/kg. For the cat: 0.25 to 1 mg/kg i.v. over 5 min. Constant-rate infusion (CRI)[c] for the dog: 24 to 75 μg/kg/min
Procainamide	Pronestyl injection of 100 or 500 mg/ml, 250 and 500 mg tablets; Procan sustained release (SR) 250, 500 mg	Ventricular premature complexes, ventricular tachycardia	Weakness, hypotension, decreased contractility, anorexia, vomiting, diarrhea, widening of QRS and QT interval, AV block	6 to 8 mg/kg i.v. over 5 min; CRI: 25 to 40 μg/kg/min, 6 to 20 mg/kg i.m. q4–6 hours (see text). Tablets 8 to 20 mg/kg q6 hours; Procan SR, 8 to 20 mg/kg q6–8 hours
Propranolol HCl	Inderal 1 mg/ml vials, 10, 20, 80 mg tablets	Supraventricular premature complexes and tachyarrhythmias, atrial fibrillation, ventricular premature complexes	Decreased contractility, bronchoconstriction, loss of compensatory mechanisms	0.04 to 0.06 mg/kg i.v. slowly; 0.2 to 1.0 mg/kg orally t.i.d. (dog and cat)

Table 12.1—continued

Generic Name	Commonly Used Preparations	Indications	Adverse Effects	Approximate Dosage[b]
Quinidine sulfate, gluconate, polygalacturonate	Quinidine gluconate USP injection 80 mg/ml; Quinidine sulfate tablets USP 200 mg; Quinidex (sustained release) tablets, 300 mg; Quinaglute Dura-tabs (quinidine gluconate), 324 mg; Cardioquin tablets (quinidine polygalacturonate) 275 mg	Ventricular premature complexes, ventricular tachycardia, acute atrial fibrillation, refractory supraventricular tachycardias	Weakness, hypotension, decreased contractility, anorexia, vomiting, diarrhea, widening of QRS and QT interval, AV block, drug interaction with digoxin, urine retention	6 to 20 mg/kg i.m., q6 hours, 6 to 16 mg/kg orally q6 hours, Quinaglute Dura-tabs (quinidine gluconate) and Cardioquin tablets) (quinidine polygalacturonate), 8 to 20 mg/kg orally q6–8 hours

[a] With permission from Bonagura JD, Muir WW: Antiarrhythmic therapy. In Tilley LP (ed): *Essentials of Canine and Feline Electrocardiography*. Philadelphia, Lea & Febiger, 1985, p 298.

[b] All dosages are for the dog unless otherwise noted.

[c] Formula for CRI: Body weight (in kg) × dose in (μg/kg/min) × 0.36 = total dose in mg to administer intravenously over 6 hours (e.g., 20 kg dog, 50 μg/kg/min infusion; (20) (50) (0.36) = 360 mg over 6 hours).

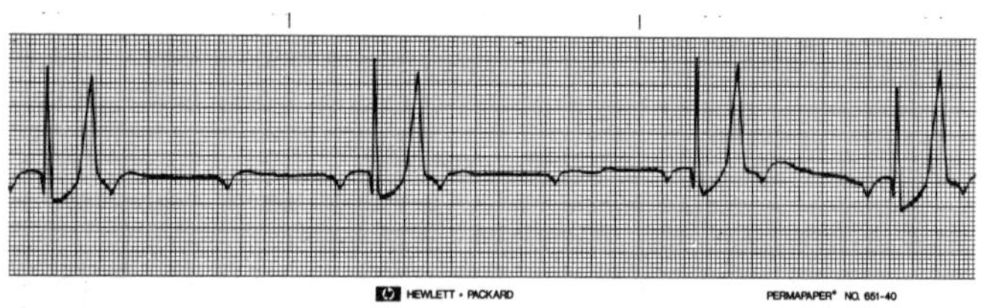

Figure 12.17. ECG recorded from a dog given Innovar. The dog experienced apnea and became hypoxic. Negative P waves indicate an origin in the AV junction or low in the atria. Not all P waves are conducted. The S-T segment is depressed, and the T waves are very large (50 mm/sec, 1 cm = 1 mV).

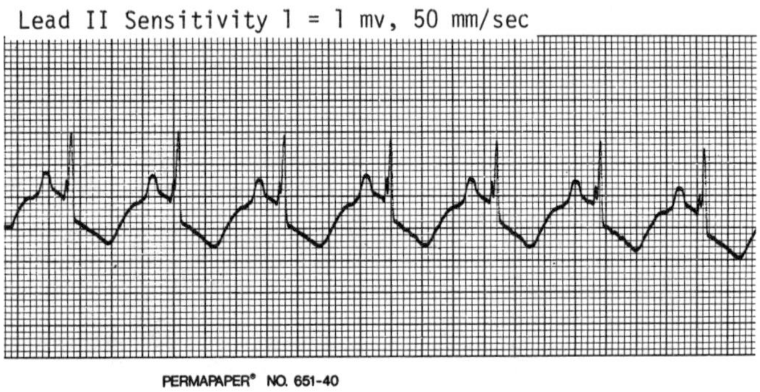

Figure 12.18. ECG recorded from a 4-week-old kitten with a patent ductus arteriosus. In addition to left heart enlargement, profound S-T segment depression is evident, indicating myocardial hypoxia (50 mm/sec, 1 cm = 1 mV).

Furosemide is the most commonly used diuretic in animals for congestive heart failure. Furosemide is a powerful naturietic that causes volume contraction because of the obligatory loss of water that follows the loss of sodium. The amount of chloride and potassium excreted in the urine also is increased. Furosemide causes systemic venodilation. If excessive loss of fluid occurs, the animal may become dehydrated and hypotensive. Because of the diuretic and venodilatory effects of furosemide, preload is reduced and congestion relieved. Before dogs and cats are anesthetized, it is ideal to have congestion controlled; furosemide is a mainstay in achieving this goal. The amount of fluids administered intravenously during anesthesia to an animal with cardiac abnormalities must be closely monitored. Even though furosemide can often be given intravenously during anesthesia or postanesthesia to correct miscalculations of fluid therapy resulting in exacerbation of congestion (e.g., pulmonary edema), overhydration is best avoided.

Digitalis is used as a positive inotrope in congestive heart failure and as therapy for supraventricular arrhythmias. Digoxin is the most commonly used preparation of digitalis, although digitoxin can be used as well. Digoxin inhibits NaK ATPase so that more calcium is available for contraction, thereby shifting the Frank-Starling curve up and to the left, indicating enhanced myocardial strength. For a given end-diastolic pressure, an increased amount of cardiac work can be performed in the digitalized animal. The increased work performed would tend to increase the amount of myocardial oxygen used, but this effect is offset by the decrease in heart rate accompanying digitalization. With proper digoxin dosages, vagal tone is increased, sympathetic tone is decreased, and conduction through the atrioventricular node is slowed. These changes result in a decreased use of oxygen by the myocardium. If an animal is digitalized, the medication should be continued in the perianesthetic period. However, if clinical signs of digitalis toxicity, such as vomiting, depression, or anorexia, are present the drug should be stopped and this complication resolved if possible before anesthesia. Digitalis toxicity can in-

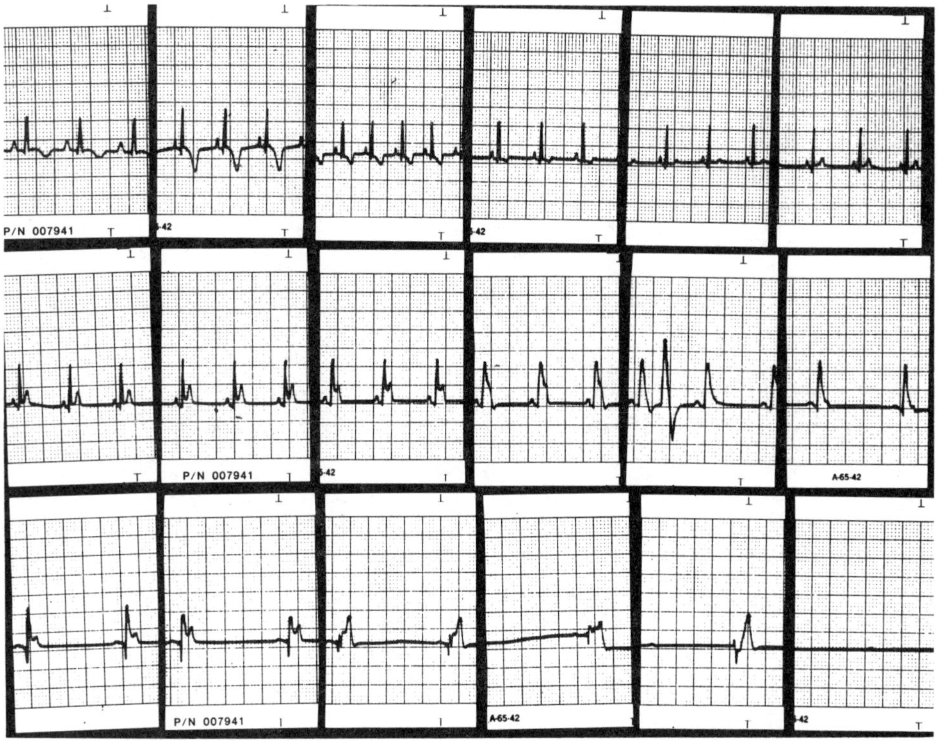

Figure 12.19. Portions of a continuous electrocardiogram recorded from a dying dog. Frames read from left to right. Note changes in T wave and S-T segment indicating hypoxia (25 mm/sec, 1 cm = 1 mV).

duce any arrhythmia; therefore, if new arrhythmias develop or if there is a worsening of an arrhythmia already present, the drug should be suspected as the cause. Digitalis toxicity is more likely with hypokalemia, so attention to proper electrolyte and fluid therapy in the perianesthetic period is necessary. Digoxin is eliminated primarily through the kidney.

Propranolol is a negative inotrope and negative chronotrope that is used in the treatment of subaortic stenosis, hypertrophic cardiomyopathy, hyperthyroidism, and supraventricular arrhythmias. Propranolol is a nonselective (beta 1 and beta 2) beta-adrenergic blocker. It also has the ability to stabilize membranes, making them less susceptible to generating arrhythmias. Propranolol will decrease cardiac output, contractility, and arterial blood pressure, but peripheral vascular resistance is increased. Propranolol can have detrimental effects if improperly given; these include depression, hypotension, bradycardia, exacerbation of congestive heart failure, or bronchospasm. The dosage of propranolol does not necessarily correlate with signs of toxicity. Because of its beta-adrenergic blocking properties, the sympathetic nervous system will not be able to respond to stress normally; this may be an asset or a detriment depending on the individual patient. This response alteration should be recalled in monitoring heart rate and blood pressure. Isoproterenol competitively eliminates some of the adverse effects of propranolol. Although many undesirable effects occur with the use of propranolol, abrupt cessation of the drug in the cardiac patient is not recommened just before anesthesia.

Calcium channel blockers such as verapamil are being used with increasing frequency in the treatment of supraventricular tachycardia, subaortic stenosis, and hypertrophic cardiomyopathy. Verapamil decreases calcium transport in conduction tissue with slow channels. These are the sinoatrial and atrioventricular nodes. Verapamil also causes peripheral vasodilation, coronary arterial dilation, and negative inotropy. In the above diseases, these affects are desirable. If used in excess, verapamil could result in bradycardia, hypotension, and aggravation of congestive heart failure. Both propranolol and verapamil are cleared through the liver. Many of the effects of verapamil can be tempered with calcium. This is important in the anesthetized animal receiving this medication, which appears to cause a worsening of cardiac function.

Vasodilator therapy is now advocated in the therapy of congestive heart failure. The rationale for the use of vasodilators revolves around the concepts of preload and afterload. Preload is related to the myocardial wall tension at end diastole and is related to end diastolic volume. Preload determines the stretch of the myocardial fibers relating to the Frank-Starling law. Within physiological limits, the more myocardial stretch (the longer the myocardial fibers) just before systole, the more contraction that will occur. The normal heart, again within physiological limits, can rid itself of the blood volume (preload) it is presented.

However, the diseased heart may not have the inherent contractile strength to unload itself of this same volume of blood. When this occurs, congestion results. Afterload is the wall tension that exists after the onset of contraction. Left heart afterload is related to the myocardial wall thickness, distensibility of the aorta, and peripheral vascular resistance. Peripheral vascular resistance is primarily governed by the vascular tone of arterioles (degree of vasoconstriction). The greater the afterload, the more work the heart must do to unload its volume of blood. In congestive heart failure, the sympathetic tone and renin-angiotensin system are enhanced; these changes cause arterial vasoconstriction, thus increasing afterload. If afterload is excessive, a diseased heart may not be able to rid itself of a certain volume, and congestion occurs. If preload and afterload can be decreased, the diseased heart will not work as hard or use as much oxygen, and congestion will resolve.

Preload is reduced with drugs that decrease blood volume or cause dilation of venous capacitance vessels. Afterload is reduced with drugs that cause systemic vasodilation. Furosemide is a preload reliever because it decreases volume and causes some venodilation. Nitroglycerin ointment is commonly used in veterinary medicine for its potent venodilatory effects. Some arterial dilation also occurs. Nitroprusside is used only intravenously and is both a preload and afterload reliever. Because this drug is so powerful and has a short half-life, it is appropriate for the treatment of acute congestive heart failure and not chronic therapy. With careful monitoring, this drug may be useful in situations of severe congestion that develop during anesthesia. Prazosin is an alpha-adrenergic blocking agent that decreases preload and afterload because it dilates veins and arterioles. Hydralazine primarily dilates arterioles and, therefore, decreases afterload. Animals on chronic therapy with hydralazine frequently have elevations in aldosterone and may need additional diuretic therapy. Captopril, an angiotensin-converting enzyme inhibitor, is both a preload and afterload reliever. The formation of angiotensin II is stopped, as is the formation of aldosterone. By decreasing angiotensin concentration, vasodilation occurs; by decreasing aldosterone, fluid retention is suppressed. Vasodilators may assist in the preparation for anesthesia of the cardiac patient with congestion. With the vasodilators, serious complications can result from improper use or unexpected side effects. Hypotension with reflex tachycardia, anorexia, weakness, or gastrointestinal disturbances may occur. The side effects of these drugs must be balanced with the benefit for each individual animal.

The cardiac patient with ventricular arrhythmias may have been treated with antiarrhythmic therapy. Therapy should not be stopped before anesthesia. The animal should be examined for adverse effects; if there are none, therapy should not disrupted.

Common Congenital Defects of the Dog and Cat

Congenital cardiac defects may be grouped as those causing right-to-left shunts, left-to-right shunts, valvular insufficiency, obstruction to outflow, or any combination of the above (9–11). Right-to-left shunts result in underperfusion of the lungs and cyanosis. Left-to-right shunts and valvular insufficiencies cause overperfusion of the lungs and congestive heart failure. Obstruction to outflow induces myocardial hypertrophy. The anesthesiologist needs a knowledge of the diagnostic procedures likely to be performed under anesthesia, pathophysiology of specific anomalies, and surgical procedures for correction or palliation of the defect.

Noninvasive diagnostic procedures such as electrocardiography, echocardiography, and radiography are done while the animal is awake. Occasionally, tranquilization is necessary. Invasive diagnostics such as selective angiography, pressure determinations, and oximetry require general anesthesia. Each of these procedures involves catheterization of the heart and, with angiography, the rapid injection of contrast material. In the diseased heart, catheters and contrast material can precipitate arrhythmias (most frequently, ventricular tachycardia) during anesthesia. If the arrhythmia is due to the catheter tip irritating the endocardium, simply backing the catheter out a few milliliters will frequently alleviate the problem. Arrhythmias induced after a bolus of contrast material can usually be handled by backing the catheter out a few millimeters, turning the anesthetic gas off, and bagging the animal with 100% oxygen. If after 30 to 60 seconds the arrhythmia persist, intravenous boluses of lidocaine are advised. Although ventricular arrhythmias are most common with catheterization, some defects are more prone to atrial arrhythmias (e.g., congenital tricuspid insuficiency and atrial flutter).

The most common right-to-left shunt in dogs and cats is tetralogy of Fallot. This complex anomaly includes a pulmonic stenosis, ventricular septal defect (VSD), overriding aorta, and right ventricular hypertrophy. The right ventricular hypertrophy is a secondary response to the pulmonic stenosis. Hemodynamically, the left and right ventricular pressures are nearly equal (Fig. 12.20). High pressures of the right ventricle, positioning of the aorta over the right ventricle, and narrowed pulmonic valve favor the blood flow into the aorta and systemic circulation instead of the pulmonic valve and the lungs. A kitten or puppy presenting with

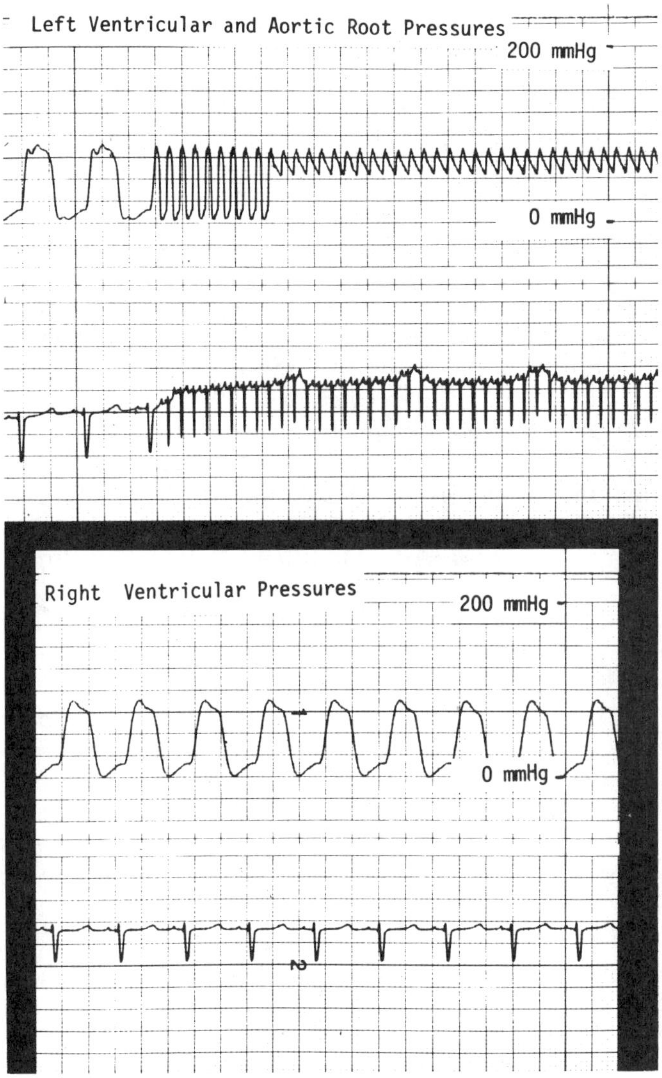

Figure 12.20. Pressure recordings from the left and right ventricles in a cat with tetralogy of Fallot. The ventricular pressures are equal. *Top frame* shows pressure from left ventricle to aortic root.

cyanosis most commonly is afflicted with this defect. Some animals will have syncopal episodes, especially during defecation. Severe dyspnea occurs with stress. The severity of the right-to-left shunt dictates the degree of shunting and cyanosis. Low-grade systolic murmurs over the pulmonic valve or the right hemithorax may be ausculted. The pulmonic stenosis and VSD are responsible for the cardiac murmurs. Electrocardiographic (right axis shift, deep S waves in Leads I, II, III, aVF, CV_6LL, and CV_6LU) and radiographic evidence of right ventricular hypertrophy is associated with the respiratory distress. Echocardiography reveals the ventricular septal defect, right ventricular obstruction, overriding aorta, and poststenotic dilation of the pulmonary trunk. Nonselective angiography demonstrates simultaneous filling of the aorta and pulmonary trunk. Dilated bronchoesophageal arteries are detected. Hypoperfusion of the lung parenchyma may be seen. Corrective surgery necessitates open heart surgery with hypothermia or heart bypass, and it is usually not attempted. Palliative surgery to create a left-to-right shunt and increase pulmonary perfusion can be performed with general anesthesia. The Blalock-Taussig operation involves the anastomosis of the left subclavian artery to the pulmonary artery. Direct shunts from the ascending or descending aorta (Pott's operation) to the pulmonary artery also increases pulmonary blood supply. Despite the use of these procedures, the prognosis is guarded.

Other congenital defects with right-to-left shunting, and, therefore, cyanosis include defects usually associated with left-to-right shunting, but because of pulmonary hypertension (Eisenmenger's syndrome), right-sided pressures are elevated, such as right to left (VSD), patent ductus arteriosus (PDA), and atrial septal defect (ASD). Truncus arteriosus is occasionally seen in cats with cyanosis. Very severe pulmonic stenosis may cause cyanosis. Rare congenital defects that may be associated with cyanosis are double outlet right ventricle, aortic atresia, or pulmonic atresia.

One of the predominant concerns in the anesthetic management of animals with right-to-left shunts is associated cyanosis. This is usually a result of altered pulmonary circulation. The compensatory mechanisms of the cyanosis may increase sympathetic tone with associated tachycardia. This may in turn increase cardiac output and oxygen delivery. Before proceeding with premedication, careful monitoring of the patient in the preinduction phase should be done, including examination by stethoscope and ECG. Analysis of blood gases and pH is beneficial; however, even when equipment is available, physical restraint of the patient to obtain blood samples may cause undue distress, especially if cyanosis is severe. Premedication should be selected relative to the extent of deterioration of the patient. In the patient showing considerable depression, premedication with a belladonna drug as the sole preanesthetic may be indicated. The use of glycopyrrolate versus atropine sulfate is less likely to produce undesirable heart rates or to excite cardiac dysrhythmias.

In animals not showing depression, low dose administration of mild tranquilizers such as diazepam, 0.025 to 0.05 mg/kg or acepromazine may be used to reduce excitement. If narcotics are to be used as part of the induction regimen or preanesthetic medication, administration of oxygen by face mask should be incorporated to avoid further deterioration in available oxygen. Anesthetic maintenance is best achieved by administering inhalant anesthetic by mask to complete induction. Some form of injectable is usually indicated for induction of anesthesia in these cases because the inhalant technique in animals with right-to-left shunting is usually slow. The uptake of the anesthetic from the pulmonary circulation will delay obtaining adequate concentrations to cause rapid central nervous system (CNS) depression and anesthesia. If injectable barbiturates are used to reduce induction time, caution must be used in the rate of administration and the total dose administered. As soon as possible, intubation should be accomplished and assisted or controlled ventilation utilized in any patient with inadequate spontaneous respiration to correct cyanosis.

The inhalant anesthetic regimen can be accomplished through the utilization of isoflurane or halothane. Methoxyflurane can be safely used if uptake is appropriate. Methoxyflurane compared to other agents must be justified in view of the need to control ventilation from the early onset of anesthesia. Isoflurane is less likely to be associated with cardiac arrhythmias, whereas halothane is more likely to cause some reduction in blood pressure and cardiac output. Either can be used effectively provided there is aggressive cardiovascular monitoring, tempered by good judgement, technical proficiency, and an analysis of the risk factors involved. During the procedure, arterial pressure monitoring is of great value. Central venous pressure measurements can be quite beneficial due to the increases in right side pressures. Careful attention should be paid to the administration of fluids to avoid fluid overload.

Nitrous oxide should be avoided in most circumstances due to the potential contribution to cyanosis concurrent with pulmonary circulation. Ketamine at low doses may be utilized in lieu of narcotics in these cases to initiate anesthetic induction. It does not depress the cardiac action excessively. Supplementation with oxygen should be incorporated early in the procedure as the animal starts to relax.

During assisted breathing in these patients, airway pressures should receive careful attention. Normally anticipate from 20 to 50% lower airway pressure than in normal subjects to reduce the incidence of pulmonary edema, damage to the alveoli, or further increases in pulmonary pressures. As a general rule, even with lower pressures and assisted breathing, utilization of high oxygen content in the anesthetic regimen will compensate for the lower oxygenation capabilities seen in the awake subject.

Left-to-right shunting congenital heart defects are more common. In the dog, the most common defect is a PDA; in the cat, a VSD is more common. Other anomalies that cause overcirculation to the lungs include ASD, common atrioventricular canal, truncus arteriosus, and aortic pulmonic window. Because left pressures are greater than right pressures, excessive blood is shunted to the lungs. The size of the defect determines the resistance of flow and the degree of shunting. Clinical signs relate to the degree of shunting and range from asymptomatic to severe dyspnea due to congestive heart failure.

A PDA is observed more frequently in poodles, collies, Shetland sheepdogs, and pomeranians. The severity of the defect determines the degree of shunting that may be observed. The cardiac murmur is usually loud and has a point of maximum intensity over the left thorax at the third intercostal space between the aortic and pulmonic valves. The murmur is continuous, occurring during systole and diastole, although it does not wax and wane in intensity. It is loudest in middle to late systole. Classically, the murmur of a PDA is described as "machinery" because it sounds like a washing machine in operation. Auscultation of the lungs may reveal moist crackles. The femoral pulses are bounding with a quick rise and fall. If right heart failure is present in addition to left heart failure, ascites, hepatomegaly, pleural effusion, and jugular vein distension or pulses may be detected. The ECG reveals a marked left ventricular enlargement pattern (tall R waves in I, II, III, aVF, CV_6LL, and CV_6LU), although the mean electrical axis is usually normal because right heart enlargement also is present. Some dogs develop atrial fibrillation with marked atrial enlargement. Atrial premature contractions or VPCs also may be present. Radiographs reveal generalized cardiomegaly, with enlargement of both pulmonary arteries and veins demonstrating overcirculation to the lungs. In the dorsoventral projection, three bulges may be seen because of the enlarged pulmonary trunk, aortic aneurysm, and dilated left auricle. Pulmonary edema usually is observed. Echocardiographically, chamber enlargement and some reduction in cardiac function are detected. If noninvasive diagnostics are inconclusive and angiography is required, selective catheterization and injection of contrast into the aortic root or left ventricle is required to demonstrate the PDA. If left and right heart failure are present, end diastolic ventricular pressures may be elevated. A wide pulse pressure is present in the aorta. Oxygen saturation and content will be elevated in the pulmonary trunk.

Ventricular septal defects in dogs and cats are usually high, and the signs of heart failure depend on the degree of left to right shunting. The murmur is systolic and loudest on the right at the third intercostal space. If volume overload is present, the femoral pulses may be bounding. Physical examination findings of heart failure may be present. The degree of cardiomegaly varies, and the ECG may be normal or indicate left or right heart enlargement. Likewise, radiographs reveal cardiomegaly with significant shunting of blood and engorged pulmonary vessels and pulmonary edema. The defect is usually identified with an echocardiogram. If angiography is needed, selective catheterization of the left ventricle is required. Cardiac pressures may be normal. Oximetry reveals elevated oxygen saturation and content in the right ventricle near the defect and in the pulmonary artery.

Animals with any of the above anomalies may be anesthetized for diagnostic procedures; however, usually only the animals with a PDA undergo corrective surgery, because open heart surgery is required for the other defects. Palliative surgery such as banding of the pulmonary artery may be done in an animal with a large VSD. By banding the pulmonary artery, right ventricular pressures are increased so that less blood is shunted from left to right. The best preparation for anesthesia of an animal with a left-to-right shunt is to medically control the heart failure. The aggressiveness of therapy depends on the individual degree of failure. Cage rest and a low salt diet are the best means to stabilize the compromised patient. Diuretics, vasodilators, antiarrhythmics, and positive inotropes are in the pharmacological armamentarium for control of congestive heart failure. Drug combinations and dosages must be titrated to the individual. From 1 to 10 days will be required to stabilize the animal. If after 10 days and various drug therapies congestion cannot be controlled, it may be necessary to proceed with correction of the underlying problem (ligation of the PDA) before the animal will improve. In this situation there is of course increased risk.

The extent of preanesthetic medication in patients with left-to-right shunts must be based on the findings of the preinduction physical examination. Utilization of belladonna products should be judged according to the observed heart rate. In many cases, belladonna products are administered after the induction of anesthesia to control heart rates as needed in lieu of premedication because there is usually a higher heart rate in these cases prior to anesthesia. In this group of patients, excessive pulmonary blood flow is present.

A left-to-right shunt does not significantly affect the induction time. As a result, a variety of approaches may be used to induce anesthesia, depending on the condition of the patient. Injectable barbiturates may be used with caution to induce anesthesia. The dosages should be as low as possible, and rapid intubation and oxygen support should be administered immediately after the induction. The utilization of such neuroleptanalgesia as acepromazine-oxymorphone technique has been safely used. It too should be supported by supplemental oxygenation and intubation as soon as possible. In the event induction is incomplete with neuroleptanalgesia, oxygen and inhalant anesthetic by face mask to complete the induction is desirable. Nitrous oxide has been utilized as part of the induction regimen and included for maintenance until thoracotomy. Its benefit is highly debatable in animal subjects due to the lack of potency of nitrous oxide as well as the reduction in oxygen concentration that results with its concurrent usage.

Inhalant anesthetic techniques utilizing isoflurane or halothane have been very effective in these patients. Mask induction followed by maintenance on the agents is anticipated. Deep levels of anesthesia can increase hypoxemia by depressing cardiac output. Deep levels may also reduce systemic vascular resistance. The latter may be beneficial to reduce pulmonary blood flow with left-to-right shunts; it is not advisable in right-to-left shunts. Early assistance in respiration can be quite beneficial to reduce the possibility of hypoxemia in these cases.

The utilization of muscle relaxants to control spontaneous attempts at respiration during surgical correction of PDA is indicated. The reversible muscle relaxants such as pancuronium are preferred over succinylcholine. A special consideration during the surgical correction of the PDA is the reduction in respiratory volume during the procedure. Careful attention should be paid to the surgical manipulations to avoid inflation of the lung at inconvenient times during the surgical procedure. This requires careful coordination of the efforts of the anesthesiologist and the surgeon.

During the ligation of the patent ductus, cardiac arrhythmias and alterations in circulation and blood pressure may occur. It is preferable that the ductus to be partially ligated with a pause in the procedure for determination of stability of the patient at intervals until the ligation is complete. Cardiac medications should be available for the control of responses, especially medications to increase or decrease sensitivity of the heart for maintenance heart rate in control of ventricular arrhythmias as the procedure is completed.

After the completion of the surgical correction of the patent ductus, the top lung is placed in normal position. Care should be taken to gradually reinflate the lung using several breaths to bring the lung to full inflation. After the chest closure is under way, a full volume breath is indicated to fill the lung and chest cavity, driving off air within the chest cavity. From an anesthesiologist's point of view, a chest tube for removal of entrapped air in the thoracic cavity during the final stages of closure and during early recovery is beneficial for maintenance of a negative pressure within the thoracic cavity. Mild to severe pneumothorax or pneumohemothorax after procedures for correction of PDA will not be seen with nearly the frequency as in more severe procedures of the thorax.

Animals with congenital valvular insufficiencies (atrioventricular or semilunar) are volume overloaded. These animals are not anesthetized for surgical correction but may need invasive diagnostic studies or noncardiac surgery. Their heart failure should be controlled before anesthesia, as discussed above.

The anesthetic regimen of valvular insufficiency should avoid bradycardia even to the point that an elevated heart rate is more desirable to help maintain adequate cardiac output and profusion of tissues. The fluid administration should be adequate for reasonable volume status in order to maintain adequate preload to compensate for regurgitation and to maintain as close to normal cardiac output as possible. If systemic vascular resistance is elevated, vasodilation may be helpful. As a result, premedication with alpha-blocking agents such as acetylpromazine may be beneficial. Induction of anesthesia should be done with caution, and inhalant anesthetic maintenance should be utilized. The utilization of inhalant anesthetic regimens at lower concentrations to avoid depression of cardiac function will be helpful. It is encouraging that blood flow to tissues observed with isoflurane anesthesia increases its potential for use in these cases. Halothane may be used if isoflurane is not available. With mitral regurgitation, increases in pulmonary resistance are not uncommon. If caution is not used during assisted breathing and excessive pressures and rates are utilized, damage to the alveoli may occur. This may be sufficiently severe to produce pulmonary edema. The administration of excess fluids can further contribute to pulmonary edema.

Monitoring of arterial and central venous pressure is beneficial. It is preferable to avoid nitrous oxide in animal patients with valvular insufficiency, even though it may be beneficial in maintaining heart rates. This advantage is offset by the reduction in oxygen.

Aortic and pulmonic stenosis are common congenital anomalies. Aortic stenosis is most prevalent in German shepherds, Newfoundlands, and golden retrievers. Aortic stenosis is most frequently subvalvular (SAS) in dogs. Aortic stenosis is seen in cats. Usually dogs with SAS are asymptomatic, although ventricular arrhythmias may be present. If the mitral valve is also abnormal (cleft), mitral regurgitation results, and signs of congestive heart failure develop. The murmur of aortic stenosis is a harsh crescendo-decrescendo and is heard loudest at the fourth intercostal space on the left over the aortic valve. However, the murmur may radiate to the right side and be very loud in this location. The murmur also may radiate up the carotids. The femoral pulse of a dog with aortic stenosis may be weak. The intensity of the murmur and strength of the pulse frequently varies with the sympathetic tone in the dog with this defect. Because of the left ventricular outflow obstruction, left ventricular hypertrophy develops. The hypertrophy may be so great and the intraventricular pressure so high that perfusion of the myocardium is restricted and ischemia results. Coronary blood flow occurs during diastole, and flow through the vessels is limited if intramyocardial pressures exceed the aortic diastolic pressure that propels the blood through the vessels. The ECG may reveal left heart enlargement, S-T segment elevation or depression, or large T waves. Ventricular premature complexes or ventricular tachcyardia may be documented. Left heart enlargement is seen radiographically, and poststenotic dilation of the ascending aorta also may be detected. The two-dimensional echocardiogram may reveal the band of subvalvular stenosis. The pressure gradient across the stenotic area determines the severity of the lesion (Fig. 12.21). Gradients of more than 75 mm Hg are considered marked. Left ventricular pressures will be high. Palliative surgery using conduits to shunt the blood and avoid the stenosis have been proposed, but most animals are treated medically with negative inotropes and coronary dilators (e.g., propranolol or verapamil). Dogs with aortic stenosis may live a normal life or die suddenly. These dogs are frequently presented for noncardiac surgery.

Pulmonic stenosis is most common in wirehaired terriers, English bulldogs, and Boston terriers. Pulmonic stenosis in dogs is primarily valvular with secondary infundibular hypertrophy. The dogs are usually asymptomatic. The murmur of pulmonic stenosis is loudest over the third left intercostal space and is crescendo-decrescendo. Right heart failure rarely occurs. Exercise intolerance may be noted in severe cases. Right ventricular pressures are elevated because of the outflow obstruction, and right heart enlargement is detected on the ECG and radiographs. A poststenotic dilation of the pulmonic trunk is appreciated radiographically and echocardiographically. The pressure gradient determines the need for surgical intervention. Gradients across the valve of 75 mm Hg or more are considered severe, and valvulectomy or the patch graph technique are recommended. Pressure gradients between 50 and 75 mm Hg are indicative of moderate stenosis, and surgical intervention is questionable. If the gradient is less than 50 mm Hg, a mild stenosis is present; therapy is not necessary. Medical therapy before anesthesia includes positive inotropes, diuretics, and vasodilators.

Anesthesia in patients with pressure overload due to conditions such as pulmonic stenosis must be handled with caution. Monitoring of fluid administration is needed to avoid further compensation in these patients. The degree of pulmonic stenosis will influence the amount of fluid that can be administered to the individual patient. Anesthetic management should be planned to include inhalant anesthetic technique. Hypotensive agents such as halothane anesthesia will reduce pressures. Xylazine is normally avoided in the preanesthetic regimen because this family of drugs

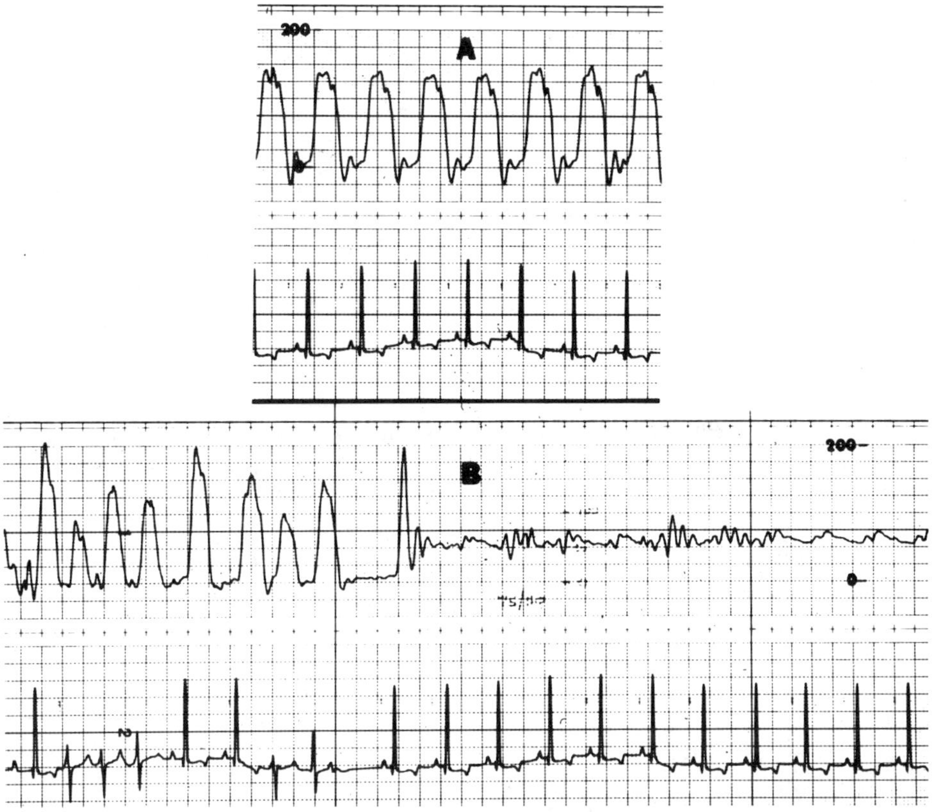

Figure 12.21. Simultaneous pressure and electrocardiogram recordings from a German shepherd with subaortic stenosis. The left ventricular systolic pressure is elevated (*A*); when the catheter is pulled from the left ventricle to the aortic root (*B*), a pressure gradient of 65 mm Hg is detected.

may be associated with hypertension during the first few minutes after injection, which may increase afterload and then may cause associated hypotension.

Acquired Cardiac Diseases of the Dog and Cat

Mitral insufficiency, tricuspid insufficiency, heartworm disease, hypertrophic cardiomyopathy, and dilated cardiomyopathy are acquired cardiac diseases that occur frequently in the dog and cat (12–14).

Small breed older dogs are most frequently afflicted with valvular endocardiosis that results in valvular insufficiency and regurgitation of blood back into the atria. Although the mitral valve is most commonly involved, the tricuspid valve also is affected. The disease progresses slowly. Because older dogs are in need of veterinary care and the disease process spans several years, the need for anesthesia in these animals frequently occurs. Clinical signs of heart failure vary with the degree of valvular insufficiency. A systolic murmur of variable quality (whooping to harsh) is ausculted over the left fifth intercostal space if mitral regurgitation is present and over the right third to fourth intercostal space with tricuspid regurgitation. Electrocardiography usually reveals left heart enlargement and may reveal right heart enlargement. Cardiomegaly corresponding to the affected atrioventricular valve is seen on radiographs. Enlarged pulmonary arteries and pulmonary edema are present with left heart failure; pleural fluid, enlarged caudal vena cava, hepatomegaly, or ascites are observed with severe tricuspid insufficiency. Usually forward cardiac output and myocardial contractility are maintained until late in the disease process. Numerous compensatory mechanisms are involved in maintaining adequate blood flow to the body, including activation of the renin-angiotensin-aldosterone system that is responsible for fluid retention and volume expansion. Increased sympathetic tone and angiotensin are responsible for increased vascular tone. The animal with atrioventricular insufficiency is in a volume overloaded state and may have a high sympathetic tone. Each of these factors are considered in managing the anesthesia of these patients. Drug intervention (diuretic, vasodilator, or digoxin) will complicate this, although hopefully improving the condition of the animal. All medications and dosages should be reviewed before administering an anesthetic.

Animals with acquired mitral and tricuspid insufficiency are usually aged patients. In addition to the cardiac disease, other complications associated with age must be considered, including hepatic and renal function. The agent selected, therefore, needs to assure cardiovascular dynamics and improved respiration, as well as a reduction in renal and hepatic toxicity. Isoflurane is a drug of choice in many of these patients because of its reduction in potential toxicity in the geriatric patient. All patients with severe mitral or tricuspid insufficiency must be considered as high risk. There is a threatening low cardiac output potential as well as pulmonary venous hypertension.

Efforts should be made to maintain a normal to slightly increased heart rate in the patient. Afterload reduction is useful in improving cardiac output in animals with myocardial insufficiency when adequate preload is present. Supplemental medication with vasodilators and/or positive inotropic drugs may be beneficial in these cases.

Occasionally, anesthesia must be given to a dog with heartworm disease, although it is better to avoid this. Infected dogs without clinical evidence of heartworms other than a positive test usually do not have difficulty because pulmonary hypertension does not exist or is minimal. However, when pulmonary hypertension is present, alteration in anesthetic delivery may occur. Patients with pulmonary hypertension should be treated with a regimen similar to patients with mitral insufficiency.

Hypertrophic cardiomyopathy (HCM) is common in cats but rare in dogs. Usually cats with this type of cardiomyopathy are longer lived after diagnosis than cats with dilated cardiomyopathy. Hemodynamically, HCM is a problem of ventricular compliance (diastolic filling problem) with fairly normal systolic function. Myocardial oxygen perfusion may be impaired for reasons that have been discussed under SAS. Clinical signs may vary from asymptomatic to severe dyspnea. As many of 50% of those cats affected will present with thromboembolism. Dyspnea is the result of pulmonary edema, and thromboembolism is caused by a thrombus originating in the left atrium or ventricle becoming dislodged and passing to the iliac trifurcation. Thromboembolism also may occur in only one hind limb or a forelimb. Anesthesia is not recommended for cats in acute failure or with thromboembolism, although sedation may be helpful to calm the anxious cat. Acepromazine is most commonly used for this purpose. In the older literature, embolectomy is recommended for cats with thromboembolism, but this is no longer the case. These cats should be treated medically with heparin, aspirin, and time. Surgery is not indicated. All cats with HCM should indefinitely be treated with aspirin. Cats with HCM may have a systolic murmur or gallop rhythm. Pulse quality and signs of failure vary with the individual animal. ECGs of cats with HCM may be normal, indicate left ventricular enlargement, or show cardiac arrhythmias. Radiographs usually show cardiomegaly and possibly pulmonary artery enlargement with pulmonary edema. Echocardiography easily provides the diagnosis of HCM, and anesthesia is not needed; however, if this diagnostic tool is not available, then nonselective angiography may be needed to confirm the diagnosis. Cats with a diagnosis of HCM may need anesthesia for noncardiac surgery.

Both dogs and cats may be affected with dilated cardiomyopathy (DCM). This is a severe disease of the myocardium. Large breed dogs (e.g., doberman pinschers, Irish wolfhounds, or great Danes) and Siamese and Burmese cats most commonly are affected. Systolic (pump) function exists with DCM. Contractility is severely reduced. Cardiac output is reduced, and this is appreciated on the physical examination. Thromboembolism is seen in approximately one-half of affected cats. ECGs frequently reveal atrial fibrillation and left atrial and ventricular enlargement in dogs. Left ventricular enlargement may be revealed in cats by electrocardiography. Cats frequently have bradycardia. Radiographs reveal generalized cardiomegaly in dogs and cats. Dogs usually have pulmonary edema and possibly pleural effusion. Cats with DCM more commonly have pleural effusion instead of pulmonary edema. The dilated poorly contracting heart is evidenced by echocardiography; anesthesia is not necessary, although angiography may be needed if echocardiography is not available. All animals with dilated cardiomyopathy are high risk patients with a poor to grave prognosis. Medical therapy before anesthesia includes positive inotropes, diuretics, and vasodilators.

During the anesthetic management of hypertrophic cardiomyopathy, efforts should be made to avoid excitement of the patient and the release of endogenous catecholamines that may further precipitate severe reduction in cardiac output. Anesthetic management should be designed to avoid tachycardia, which limits left ventricular filling. Anesthesia must be induced rapidly either using an ultrashort barbiturate with caution or using intravenous narcotics or dissociatives with maintenance with halothane or isoflurane in concentrations that do not decrease preload, but also may diminish contractility. Halothane may produce beneficial reduction in contractility, but it is more likely to be associated with arrhythmias and potential sensitivity to catecholamines in cases of excitement. These factors influence the choice of halothane or isoflurane anesthesia. It is important to maintain sinus rhythm because the atrial contribution to ventricular filling is vital. If preload is reduced or tachycardia occurs during anesthesia, the obstruction will worsen and stroke volume will be severely reduced in hypertrophic cardiac myopathy. In cardiac dilation, changes may preclude anesthetic procedures that cause further reduction in cardiac output.

Premedication of these patients should be light. Induction is best accomplished with an agent that does not decrease heart rate or contractility, and the animal should be maintained with medications that, in addition to maintaining heart rate and cardiac contractibility, avoid decreases in preload. Excessive loads of vasodilators such as the alpha-blocking agents should not be used.

Rapid induction with ultrashort barbiturates may result in cardiac arrest. Ketamine may be considered because it causes little to no depression of cardiac activity. Mask induction can be beneficial. Careful attention can be given to physiological responses as anesthetic induction progresses and adverse responses can be avoided.

The concurrent usage of nitrous oxide to reduce cardiac depression from anesthetic agents can be beneficial; caution must be used if concurrent respiratory abnormalities exist. Halothane is more likely to reduce cardiac function than methoxyflurane. Additional review of the cardiac response to anesthetics discussed in this text on inhalant anesthetics is suggested.

Monitoring of anesthetic depth to avoid severe depression of arrest is necessary. The patient with dilated cardiomyopathy in arrest does not respond well to cardiopulmonary resuscitation.

Anesthesia for Pacemaker Implantation

Currently, epicardial pacemakers are the most frequently used permanent pacemakers in dogs, although some permanent endocardial lead pacemakers are being implanted. Epicardial lead placement requires a thoracotomy and general anesthesia (15–16). Before anesthesia for the placement of the permanent pacemaker, an endocardial lead positioned in the right ventricle and attached to a temporary pacemaker is required. This section will discuss the preparation of the animal for anesthesia and pacemaker implantation.

If the normal automatic pacemaker of the heart fails to initiate depolarization or if the depolarization wave is unable to fully activate the heart and trigger cardiac contraction, an artificial pacemaker may be indicated. The most frequent reason for artificial cardiac pacing in dogs is a bradycardia (heart rate less than 40 to 60 beats per minute). Reasons for such a severe bradycardia include high grade second degree heart block, third degree heart block, persistent atrial standstill, or sick sinus syndrome (Fig. 12.22). With

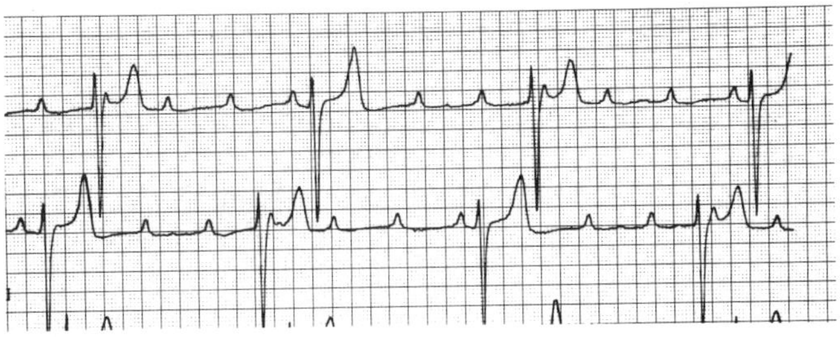

Figure 12.22. Lead II of a dog with third degree heart block and a ventricular escape rhythm (50 mm/sec, 1 cm = 1 mV).

severe bradycardia, a dog may be weak or have episodes of syncope because of poor cardiac output. An animal experiencing syncope will generally collapse suddenly for a few seconds and then recover. Occasionally, dogs with severe bradycardia will have signs of congestive heart failure such as coughing, dyspnea exercise intolerance, or weakness. The heart failure may only be due to an extremely slow heart rate, but more frequently these dogs also have concurrent cardiac pathology such as an insufficient valve.

Sick sinus syndrome is seen in miniature schnauzers and occasionally in dachshunds. Sick sinus syndrome may be characterized by severe sinus bradycardia or a mixture of sinus bradycardia and supraventricular tachycardia. The latter is termed the bradycardia-tachycardia syndrome.

Medical therapy with agents to increase the S-A node discharge rate or to increase the conduction velocity through the A-V node is frequently unsuccessful in dogs with pathological lesions in their conduction system. However, parasympatholytic agents such as atropine sulfate (0.02 to 0.04 mg/kg intramuscularly or intravenously) or glycopyrrolate (0.011 mg/kg) or sympathomimetic agents such as isoproterenol HCL (approximately 0.01 to 0.02 mg/kg/minute intravenously) may be administered in an attempt to increase the heart rate. If these medical maneuvers are successful, pacemaker implantation is delayed and medical management is given with oral isopropamide tablets (2.5 to 5 mg, twice to three times daily), propantheline bromide (3.75 to 7.5 mg twice to three times daily), or isoproterenol tablets (10 to 20 mg every 4 to 6 hours). Although some dogs may respond to these drugs, the side effects may not be tolerated; medical therapy is then abandoned. In the symptomatic dog with a medically unresponsive bradycardia, pacemaker implantation is the next option.

Before a permanent pacemaker is implanted in a dog, a temporary pacemaker that is external to the body is used. Permanent pacemaker implantation requires general anesthesia; therefore, it is mandatory that the abnormal heart rhythm be controlled with a temporary pacemaker first. A temporary pacemaker consists of the pulse generator (power source and electronics) and a pacemaker lead (lead wire and an electrode). The pacemaker generator is powered by an ordinary alkaline or mercury battery. The lead wire is bipolar with both an anode (positive) and cathode (negative) pole. These two poles are on the wire tip, and this part is placed into the heart. The portion of the wire that is external to the body and attaches to the pacemaker power source separates into two ends (cathode and anode).

To pass the pacemaker lead of the temporary pacer into the heart, most dogs require some sedation. The principle consideration in dogs for placement of a temporary pacemaker is to avoid an anesthetic regimen that may adversely reduce heart rate. Utilization of agents such as xylazine, heavy concentrations of halothane, or rapid administration of high concentrations of ultrashort barbiturates may result in cardiac arrest. The materials and equipment for placement of a temporary pacemaker should be available and ready for use prior to the administration of medications. The utilization of belladonna products is not likely to improve heart rate. The procedures should utilize approaches that also provide supplemental oxygenation because these procedures are frequently done in animals with both impaired cardiovascular function and inadequate oxygen capability. Morphine (0.2 to 0.4 mg/kg, intramuscularly) has been used for this purpose. Morphine does have the potential for slowing the heart. Narcotics are reversible. Many narcotics may produce rapid respiratory patterns. Diazepam (0.1 to 0.25 mg/kg, intravenously) does not produce excessive depression or major undesirable effects. The pacemaker wire is passed intravenously through a percutaneously placed large diameter (14-gauge) catheter into the external jugular vein to the right ventricle. From the right ventricle, the heart can be paced. The electrode tip of the pacemaker wire is positioned within the right ventricle by fluoroscopic monitoring. Alternatively, the location of the electrode tip may be identified by intracardiac ECG (Fig. 12.23). To pass the wire by the latter method, the two external ends of the pacemaker wire are attached to the exploring lead of the ECG. The other limb leads are attached in the usual manner. The ECG is turned to display the V lead. This selection is available on most machines. The ECG recorded is generated from the tip of the pacemaker wire. As the wire is advanced through the catheter toward the heart and into the right atrium and right ventricle, the complexes seen on the ECG change. The appearance of the complex identifies the wire's location (Fig. 12.24). Once the wire tip is correctly positioned, the pacer can stimulate ventricular contractions. The wire is sutured to the skin, and antibacterial ointment is applied to the exit port on the skin. The neck is then carefully wrapped, and the temporary pacemaker is secured to the dog (Fig. 12.25). Elizabethan collars may be necessary to prevent the dog from chewing the wire.

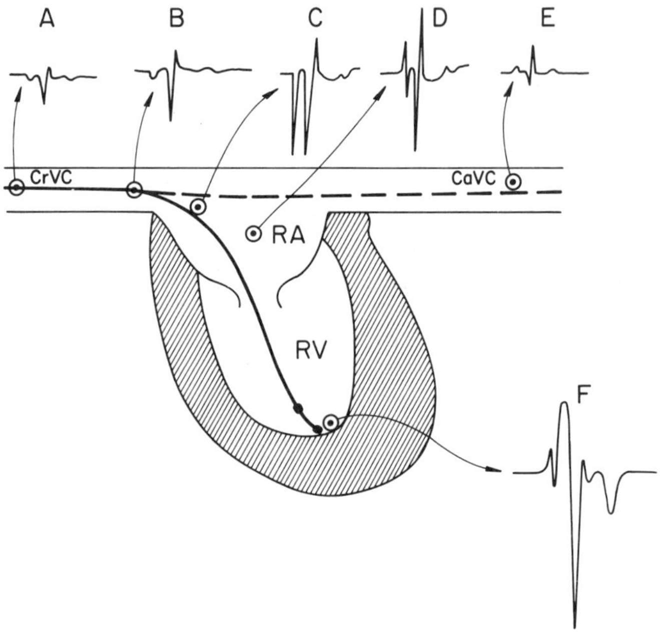

Figure 12.23. Diagram of the heart showing the intracardiac ECG recorded as the temporary pacemaker wire is paced from the cranial vena cava (CrVC) to the right atrium (RA) and into the right ventricle (RV). Electrocardiogram *A* shows a negative P wave and a large negative deflection for ventricular depolarization because the electrical activity of the heart is moving away from the electrode at this point. As the wire is advanced into the right atrium, the P wave becomes very large. Midway through the ventricle, if the wire is heading toward the caudal vena cava (CaVC), the P wave and QRS complex become biphasic. If the wire passes out of the heart and into the caudal vena cava, the P-QRS-T complex looks similar to a peripheral lead II. If the wire has been successfully passed into the right ventricle, the P waves appear large and positive and the depolarization of the ventricle is depicted as a large negative complex resembling a ventricular complex.

The temporary pacemaker has controls for adjusting the heart rate, voltage, and mode of pacing. The heart rate is adjusted to a physiological level compatible with the species and breed. Most dogs should have pacemaker rates of approximately 100 to 120 beats/minute. However, caution should be used in turning the heart rate up too high above the escape rhythm rate until the temporary wire is well secured. Excessively driving the heart may suppress any escape focus that may be needed should the wire lose contact with the endocardium. By setting the heart rate at a lower rate, overdrive suppression is less likely to occur (Fig. 12.26). The voltage is adjusted to the lowest level that assures ventricular capture. The mode of pacing can be either fixed (asynchronous) or demand (synchronous). Ideally, the pacemaker should always be placed on demand. A demand pacemaker senses beats of an underlying rhythm. In this mode the pacer will only fire when the heart rate is below a predetermined level; it is not competitive with any underlying rhythm. For example, if a dog's own ventricular heart rate happens to increase to 110 beats/minute and the pacemaker

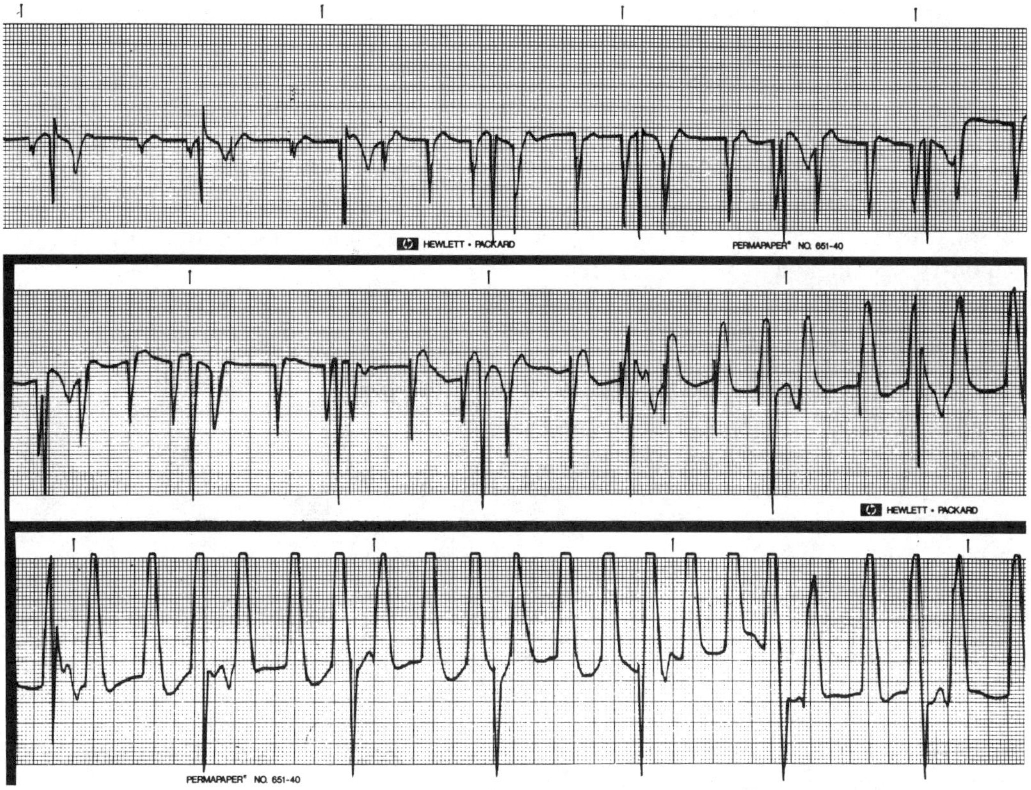

Figure 12.24. Continuous intracardiac ECG recorded from a dog with third degree heart block. In the *top* strip, the endocardial wire is in the cranial vena cava and advanced into the right atrium. In the *middle* strip, the wire is passed from the right atrium into the right ventricle, and in the *bottom* strip, the wire is in the right ventricle. In the *bottom* strip the complexes are so huge they will not fit on the paper. Note the number of atrial depolarizations relative to the number of ventricular depolarizations (three compared to one). This dog had an escape rhythm of 40 beats/min and a sinus rate (nonconducted P waves) of 120 beats/min (25 mm/sec, 1 cm = 1 mV).

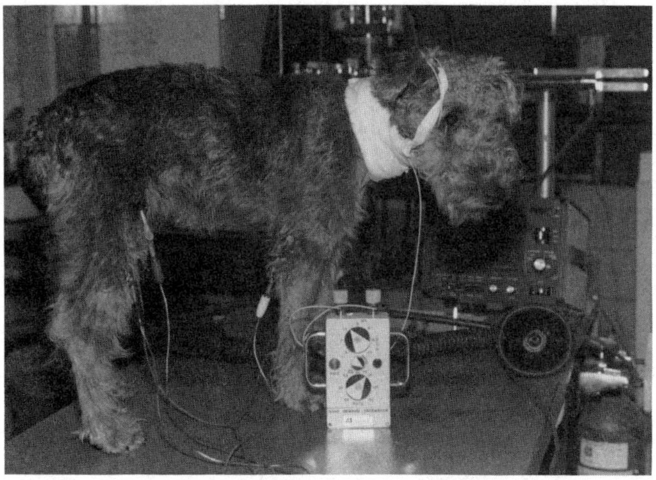

Figure 12.25. Dog with temporary pacemaker in place ready for anesthesia for permanent implantation.

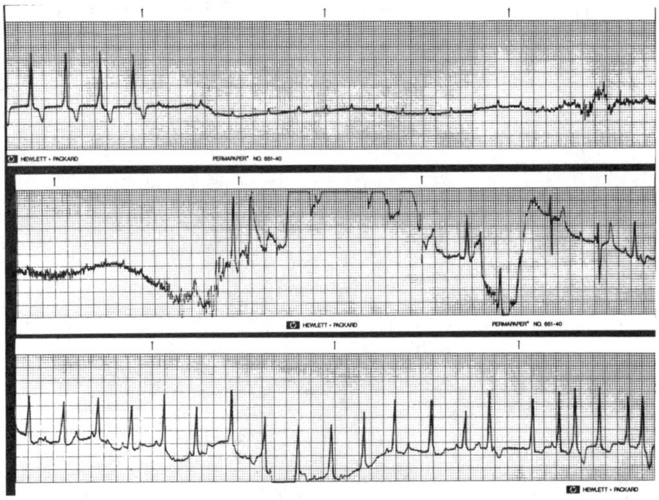

Figure 12.26. Continues lead II ECG recorded from dog shown in Figure 12.22 after a temporary pacemaker had been placed. The pacemaker rate was set at 115 beats/min. The artifacts of the pacemaker spike are not easily seen. Because the heart is depolarized from the right endocardium, the complexes are positive in lead II (compare with complexes generated from left apex with epicardial lead in Fig. 12.28). The endocardial lead was tenuously positioned against the right ventricular endocardium. The dog turned its head, and contact was lost. The dog was in complete heart block, and no escape beats rescued the heart from ventricular asystole. The dog fainted (movement artifact in middle frame) until the wire was manipulated to again contact the endocardium and resume pacing. The catheter did cause some irritation, as seen by ventricular premature complexes (three beats in bottom strip). The pacemaker rate was turned down to 60 to avoid overdrive suppression of the escape focus (25 mm/sec, 1 cm = 1 mV).

rate is set for 100 beats/minute, the pacer will sense the normal rate and it will not fire. However, if the pacemaker is set on a fixed rate, it will fire (competitively) regardless of the dog's own variable heart rate. This latter situation can be dangerous if the pacemaker fires an impulse during the vulnerable period of a normal preceding beat precipitating ventricular fibrillation and possible death.

Once the temporary pacemaker has been secured and tested, the dog is anesthetized and prepared for surgery. If the dog is admitted in congestive heart failure, the dog's response to temporary pacing is evaluated before a permanent implantation is performed (Figs. 12.27 and 12.28).

In patients with permanent pacemakers, one should be aware that the anticholinergic agents are usually not indicated due to the heart rates being controlled by the pacemaker. Utilization of products that influence vascular resistance, such as the alpha-blocking tranquilizers including acetylpromazine, or products that may change vascular responses for increases in blood pressures, such as xylazine, should be used with caution.

Preanesthetics such as diazepam and low concentrations of medications such as butorphanol or oxymorphone may be more appropriately utilized as premedicants. Induction of additional inhalant anesthetics may be accomplished by mask. Careful monitoring of fluid administration should be done to maintain appropriate fluid volume. Neither hypovolemia or hypervolemia should be tolerated if possible to maintain appropriate preload and afterload to the heart.

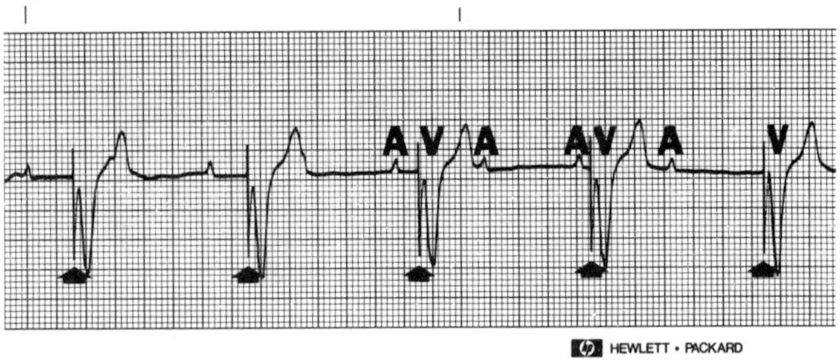

Figure 12.28. Lead II ECG recorded from a dog with a permanent epicardial pacemaker. The heart rate was set at 100 beats/min. *Arrows* point to spike artifact of pacemaker. Because the impulse is originating from the left apex (point of lead attachment), the ventricular complex is negative. A, atrial depolarization; PCV, ventricular depolarization (50 mm/sec, 1 cm = 1 mV).

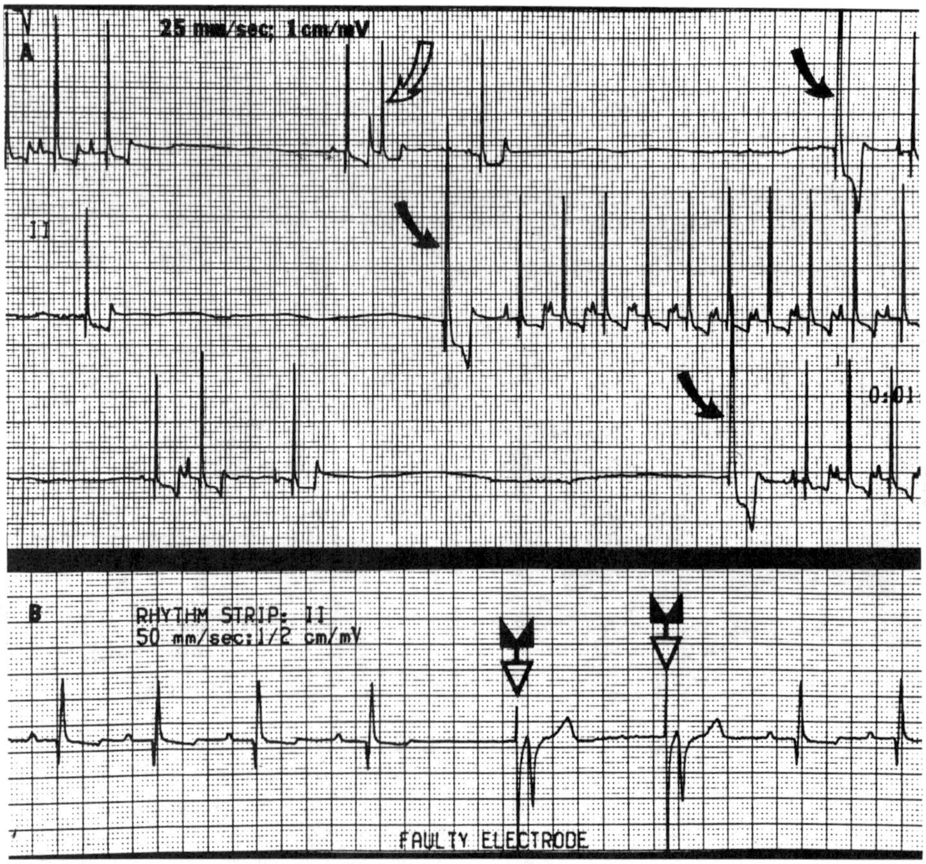

Figure 12.27. ECG recorded from a miniature schnauzer with syncope secondary to sick sinus syndrome. *A*, the dog's preoperative ECG with long periods of sinus arrest followed by an escape beat. *B*, the dog after permanent pacemaker implantation. The demand pacemaker only fires when the dog has long periods of sinus arrest.

Even in simple procedures, supplemental oxygen should be utilized during the periods of depression in cases requiring either temporary or permanent pacemakers. An anesthetic regimen should be selected that provides an opportunity for either rapid reversal of the procedure or fast spontaneous recoveries. Preanesthetic agents that provide prolonged sedation may result in undesirable cardiovascular responses.

Most anesthesia in acquired heart disease in veterinary medicine is for the completion of surgical or diagnostic procedures in cardiac patients for other than cardiac surgery. Unfortunately for the risk involved, some of these procedures require extensive anesthetic preparation, such as the geriatric patient with heart disease who requires surgery for ophthalmic procedures. It is not unusual for these cases to also have cancerous masses. The tissue handling, potential blood loss, and potential stress to the patient can have adverse effects. Extensive efforts should be made in the anesthetic regimen in this type of patient to maintain as near stable conditions as possible during the entire anesthetic period.

Anesthesia in patients with congenital disease for which surgical correction will probably be limited to PDA due to its relative simplicity of surgical correction. The characteristics of the anesthetic agents and adjunctive medication affecting the autonomic nervous system should be well understood before attempting management of patients with either acquired or congenital heart disease. The equipment and medications appropriate for cardiovascular patients should be assembled in a readily available and organized fashion. Monitoring equipment should be available for careful attention to the ECG responses and, when possible, to blood pressure. These procedures should be well monitored by personnel devoting full attention to the anesthetic regimen during anesthesia of the cardiac patient for either cardiac or noncardiac surgery. Loss of life or detrimental conditions that may occur are more likely to be avoided when there is early detection so that appropriate action can be taken immediately to reduce the incidence of further complications.

References

1. Shapiro BA, Harrison RA, Walton JR: *Clinical Application of Blood Gases*, ed 2. Chicago, Year Book Medical Publishers Inc, 1977, pp 72–94
2. Bonagura JD: M-mode echocardiography basic principles. *Vet Clin N Amer [Small Anim Pract]* 13(2):299–319, 1983.
3. Bonagura JD, O'Grady MR, Herring DS: Echocardiography principles of interpretation. *Vet Clin N Amer [Small Anim Pract]* 15(6):1177–1194, 1985.
4. Tilley LP: *Essentials of Canine and Feline Electrocardiography*, ed 2. Philadelphia, Lea and Febiger, 1985.
5. Chung EK: *Principles of Cardiac Arrhythmias*. Baltimore, Williams and Wilkins Company, 1983, pp 473–487.
6. Bonagura JD, Muir WW: Antiarrhythmic therapy. In Tilley L (ed): *Essentials of Canine and Feline Electrocardiography*, ed 2. Philadelphia, Lea and Febiger, 1985, pp 281–316.
7. Hug CC, Kaplan JA: Pharmacology—cardiac drugs. In Kaplan JA (ed): *Cardiac Anesthesia*. New York, Grune and Straton, 1979, pp 39–70.
8. Kittleson M: Drugs used in the management of heart failure. In Kirk RW (ed): *Current Veterinary Therapy VIII*. Philadelphia, WB Saunders Company, 1983, pp 285–296.
9. Bland JW, Williams WH: Anesthesia for treatment of congenital heart defects. In Kaplan JA (ed): *Cardiac Anesthesia*. New York, Grune and Straton, 1979, pp 281–346.
10. Netter FH: *The CIBA Collection of Medical Illustrations—Heart*, vol 5. Summit, NJ, CIBA, 1969, pp 133–164.
11. Thomas WP: Congenital heart disease. In Kirk RW (ed): *Current Veterinary Therapy VIII*. Philadelphia, WB Saunders Company, 1983, pp 301–310.
12. Harpster NK: Feline cardiomyopathy. *Vet Clin N Amer [Small Anim Pract]* 7(2):355–372, 1977.
13. Keene B, Bonagura JD: Valvular heart disease. In Kirk RW (ed): *Current Veterinary Therapy VIII*. Philadelphia, WB Saunders Company, 1983, pp 311–320.
14. Wood GL: Canine myocardial disease. In Kirk RW (ed): *Current Veterinary Therapy VIII*. Philadelphia, WB Saunders Company, 1983, pp 321–328.
15. Zipes DP, Duffin EC: Cardiac pacemakers. In Braunwald E (ed): *Heart Disease: A Textbook of Cardiovascular Medicine*. Philadelphia, WB Saunders Company, 1984, pp 744–773.
16. Klement P, Del-Nido PJ, Wilson GJ: The use of cardiac pacemakers in veterinary practice. *Comp Cont Educ Pract Vet* 6(10):893–902, 1984.

PART 4

Clinical Considerations of Complications of the Pulmonary System

URS SCHATZMANN, Prof. Dr.Med.Vet.

Introduction

In the cells of a living mammal, O_2 must be available with only short interruptions and in a sufficient amount. The organism is not able to store it; its uptake therefore must be in correspondence to its consumption. During the metabolism of nutritive material, CO_2 is produced by decarboxylation processes and must be immediately eliminated. The external respiration and therefore the elimination rate of CO_2 is mainly related to the pH of the tissues and the circulating blood.

The aim of external respiration in the lungs is the uptake of O_2 and the elimination of CO_2; this is provided by mechanical alterations in the tissues of lung and thorax and followed by diffusion of gases through the alveolar membranes. O_2 and CO_2 are transported by the blood. Therefore, normal respiration is strongly correlated with the circulation, and both systems are modulated by regulatory mechanisms. In a sound organism, these functions are equilibrated and can be modified according to different alterations. When one of these processes is disturbed, however, a normal function can no longer be provided. Within certain limits, compensation by one mechanism or more is possible. Whenever these limits are exceeded, disturbances in oxygenation of the tissues or in the pH regulation are inevitable (1).

Under pathological conditions, one or more factors of the intrapulmonary gas exchange can be disturbed. The sequel is an uneven ventilation or perfusion of the gas-exchange system in the lungs, followed by a disturbance of O_2 uptake and CO_2 elimination. It is therefore of primary importance that pathological conditions be recognized before sedation or anesthesia is induced. The management of the patient has always to be adapted to the circumstances. The anesthetist has to be in close contact with the animal and has to be aware of the problems of lung physiology and pathophysiology (2).

During most anesthetic procedures, the function of the respiration is altered. Not only general anesthetics but also sedative agents and neuroleptanalgesic mixtures depress the activity of the respiratory centers by decreasing the sensitivity against an increasing CO_2 partial pressure in the blood. The consequence is a decrease in the respiratory minute volume. The energy requirements and therefore the oxygen demand of the tissues in a sound animal are markedly decreased during general anesthesia. Difficulties can be expected when pre-existing problems of adequate oxygenation are present or develop as a sequel of mismanagement before or during anesthesia. Whenever the alveolar ventilation under anesthesia is insufficient to deliver enough O_2 to the tissues, the body is hypoventilated. When room air is inhaled, the O_2 partial pressure in the alveoli becomes insufficient, and more unsaturated hemoglobin leaves the lungs (hypoxemia). Simultaneously, the alveolar CO_2 pressure increases and the elimination of this gas is inhibited (hypercapnia). The increase of the arterial CO_2 pressure leads, according to the Henderson-Hasselbach's equation, to a decrease in pH (respiratory acidosis, Fig. 12.29). The characteristics of a hypoventilation during anesthesia are, under room air ventilation, hypoexmia, hypercapnia and respiratory acidosis. If high concentrations of oxygen are administered, only CO_2-retention and respiratory acidosis are present in most cases.

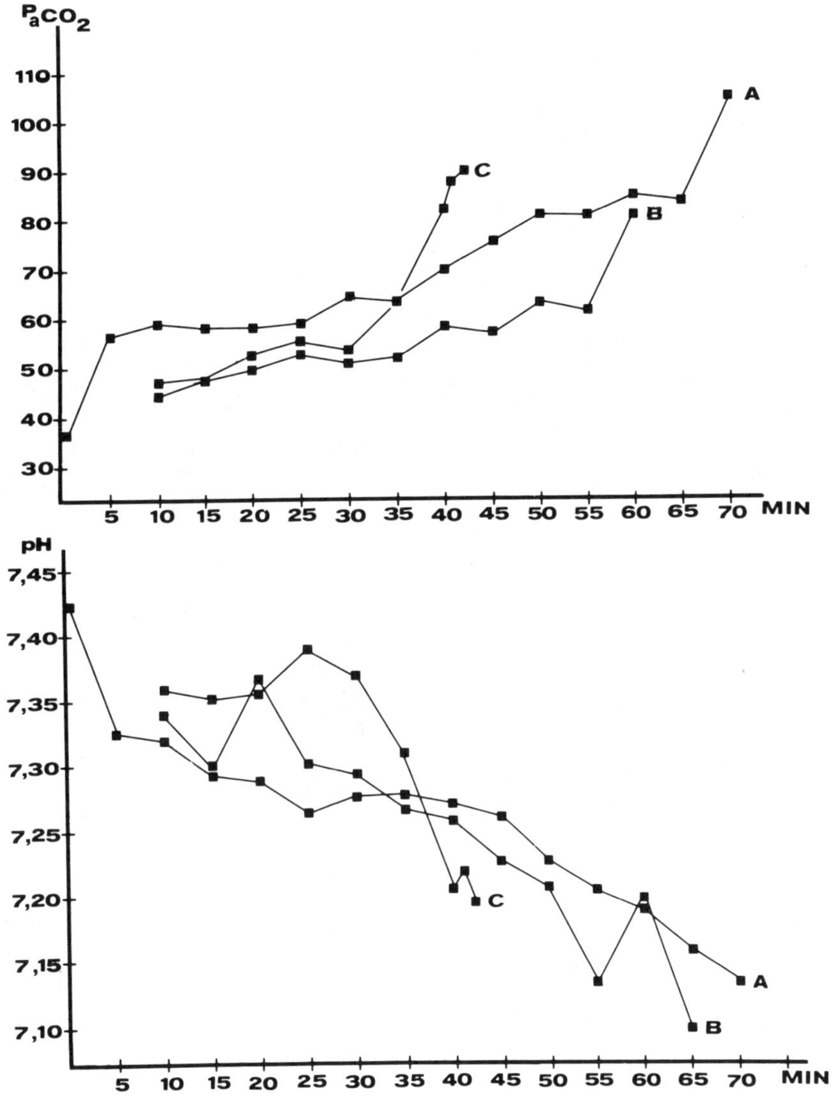

Figure 12.29. Alterations in arterial carbon dioxide pressure and pH of three adult horses under halothane anesthesia in lateral recumbency (spontaneous ventilation).

General Causative Factors

VENTILATION DISTURBANCES

Most correctly administered anesthetic procedures in sound small and large animals provoke a partial blockade of respiratory centers because of a nonselective action in the brain. Barbiturates, opiates, and inhalation anesthetics are especially known for their unwanted side effects on respiration. In Figure 12.30, arterial oxygen pressures of five sound German shepherd dogs under pentobarbitone anesthesia are graphically shown. Other factors must also be considered, including disturbances of the neuromuscular transmission to the respiratory muscles (lesion in the medulla, infections, blockade with muscle relaxants, and spinal anesthesia). All restrictions of free movement of the thorax (e.g., elbow of the surgeon resting on the thorax (small animals), increased pressure of full intestines on the diaphragm (large animals), pleural effusions, pneumothorax, neoplasms within the thorax, and adipositas) provoke in lateral and dorsal recumbency a decrease of normal ventilation. The lung itself, when not extended enough, can be a factor restricting normal ventilation. This mainly in cases of interstitial pneumonias, atelectases, and indurations. Obstructions in the upper airways caused by endotracheal tubes, respiratory tubes, and valves may aggravate respiratory difficulty. When a large inhalation anesthesia machine is attached to a very small patient, dead volume ven-

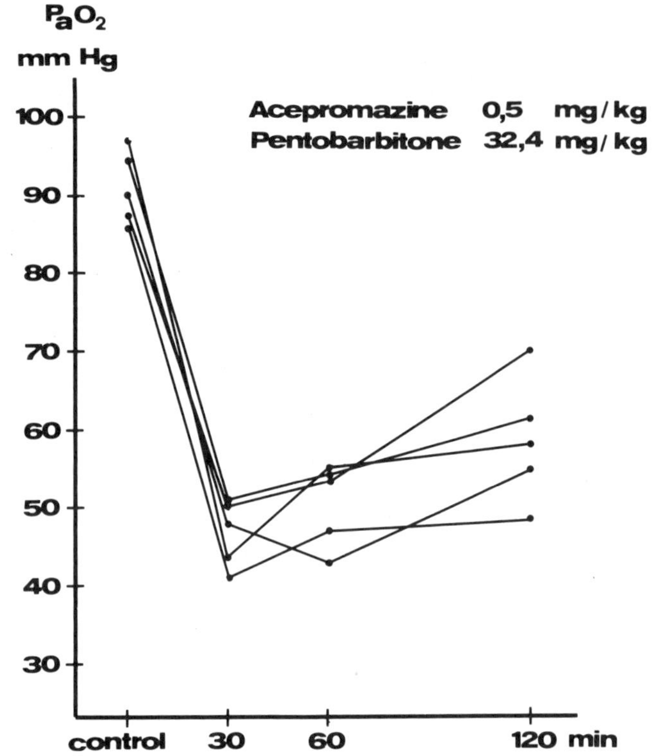

Figure 12.30. Alterations in arterial oxygen partial pressure during pentobarbitone anesthesia in five sound German shepherd dogs.

tilation with all symptoms of hypoventilation occurs (rebreathing of exhaled air).

DIFFUSION DISTURBANCES

For a normal exchange of O_2 and CO_2 between alveolus and blood vessel, a difference in partial pressure is necessary. Although the alveolocapillary membrane is enlarged in cases of bronchopneumonia, lung fibrosis, and some tumors, the diffusion disturbances play a minor role under clinical circumstances and are seldom causative factors for the occurrence of hypoxemia.

PERFUSION DISTURBANCES

The circulation within the lungs is a low pressure system. Modulated by different reflex mechanisms, perfusion of upper- and lower-lying lung parts can be altered according to the demand. It is known that well ventilated areas can be better, while nonventilated regions may be less, perfused. Pathological conditions of lung perfusion mainly occur as a sequel of heart disease (increased venous pressure in cases of heart failure or insufficiencies) leading to pulmonary edema. In large animals, gravity seems to be a major factor in that upper lung parts are less perfused and lower parts are better perfused just because the low blood pressure is unable to perfuse lung parts with 30 to 40 cm higher pressure. It has also to be assumed that adequate perfusion of the lower-lying areas in these species is inhibited (3–6).

VENTILATION/PERFUSION DISTURBANCES

The distribution of inhaled air to the different lung regions is also uneven under physiological conditions. Some alveoli are overventilated; others are underventilated. Regulatory and reflex mechanisms allow modification of perfusion and ventilation according to the needs in a certain lung area whenever the animal lives under physiological conditions. These control mechanisms are disturbed by anesthetics, by pathological conditions, and, mainly in large animals, by nonphysiological lateral or dorsal recumbency (3–6). Theoretically, two forms of extreme disturbances in distribution of blood and air within the lungs can be differentiated. The first is a decrease of ventilation in relation to perfusion. Whenever a large area of the lung is overperfused but underventilated, venous admixture to arterialized blood is increased (shunting), leading to hypoxemia. The symptoms are comparable to those of a right-to-left shunt in the heart. The partial pressure of CO_2 in arterial blood may remain within normal limits because of hyperventilation in normal perfused lung areas. The O_2 partial pressure, however, cannot be increased by hyperventilation (oxygen dissociation curve). Therefore, arterial hypoxemia is inevitable (7). The second disturbance is an increase of ventilation in relation to perfusion. Whenever a (mostly upper lying) part of the lungs is overventilated but underperfused, clinical disturbances under physiological conditions are rare, because lung perfusion can be modified and diverted to better ventilated parts.

Under clinical conditions these two extreme forms are generally present simultaneously with more or less pronounced symptoms. They are of major importance in large animals. Whenever horses are brought to lateral recumbency, an immediate hypoxemia occurs. In Fig. 12.31, it is graphically shown that in contrast to small animals, the arterial CO_2 pressures remain unchanged. A pure ventilation disturbance, provoked by the anesthetic, can therefore be excluded. It was shown that alveolar-arterial oxygen pressure differences increase from an average of 16 mm Hg in the standing to 54 mm Hg in the laterally recumbent horse (Table 12.2). These increased differences lead to arterial hypoxemia as long as the horse is recumbent and disappear only after a standing position is achieved (Fig. 12.32). It can also be demonstrated that the right-to-left intrapulmomary shunt increases from 5% in the standing and awake horse to 15% under halothane anesthesia. As causative factors, different problems have to be considered, including uneven distribution

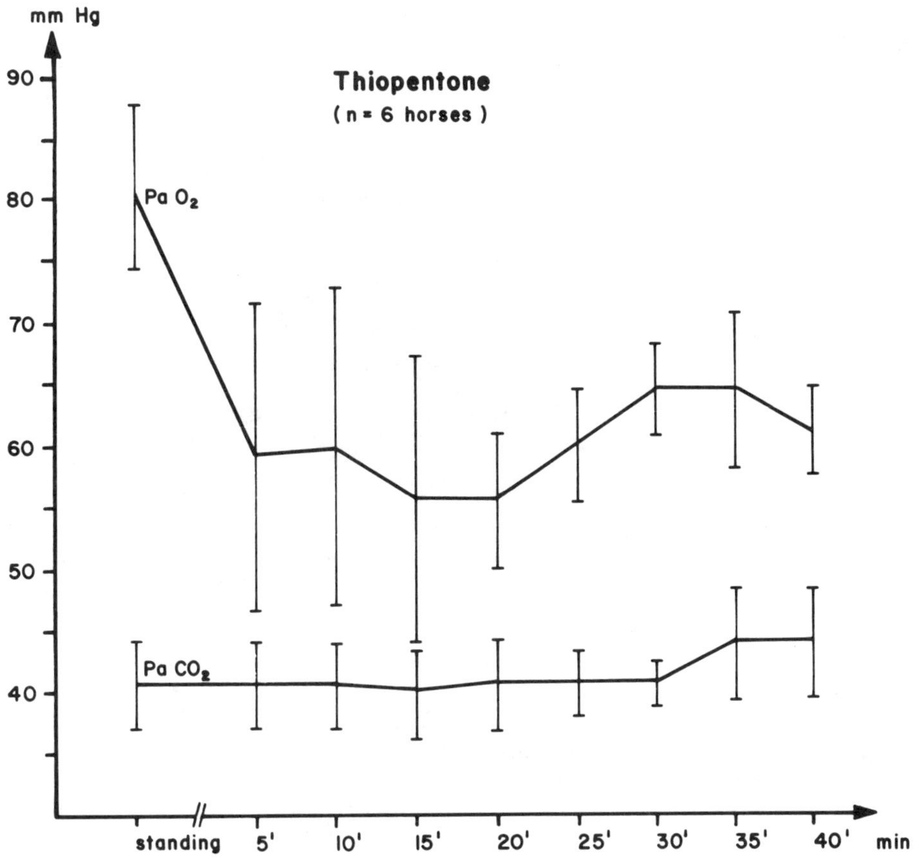

Figure 12.31. Mean alterations in arterial oxygen and carbon dioxide pressures during injection anesthesia with thiopentone (with standard deviations). Note that carbon dioxide pressure remains unchanged.

Table 12.2
Alveolar-Arterial Oxygen Pressure Differences ($\Delta P_{(A\text{-}a)} O_2$) in Standing and Lateral Position (with Standard Deviations)

Standing $\bar{x}$ = 16 (9) mm Hg		Lateral Recumbency, $\bar{x}$ = 54 (12) mm Hg	
Sound 7–20	Pneumopathy 20–35	Sound 42–50	Pneumopathy 50–75

of blood flow due to different gravity pressures; different distribution of ventilation (ventilation of the lowermost lung is more reduced than the blood flow to it); and reduction of lung volume of the lower lung due to recumbency.

The different disturbances in different lung areas after different time intervals are not yet clearly defined. Major difficulties arise because blood flow and distribution of ventilation may change by gravity or depth of anesthesia and/or control mechanisms during the course of anesthesia. However, it is generally agreed that the function of the lowermost and uppermost lung parts in the recumbent large animal are highly disturbed and that the lowermost areas lose their function within 20 minutes because of alveolar collapse, regional pulmonary congestion, and/or interstitial edema. It is further agreed that the disturbances in oxygenation cannot be controlled by increasing respiratory pressures (assisted or controlled ventilation, intermittent positive pressure ventilation (IPPV), positive end expiratory pressure (PEEP) (8, 9).

Clinical Considerations

Most agents used for sedative premedication and general anesthesia also may provoke functional disturbances within the lungs in sound animals. These disturbances are, in small animals, mainly restricted to hypoventilation. The occurrence of ventilation/perfusion inequalities in large animals, however, seems to occur without the depressive action of anesthetics, mainly based upon the nonphysiological lateral or dorsal position and represents a pathological condition within the lungs (10–12). Because the problems of small and large animals in terms of diagnosis and therapeutic consequences are different, they are separately discussed.

LUNG PROBLEMS IN THE HORSE

In the average horse population presented for surgical intervention, lung problems are frequently diag-

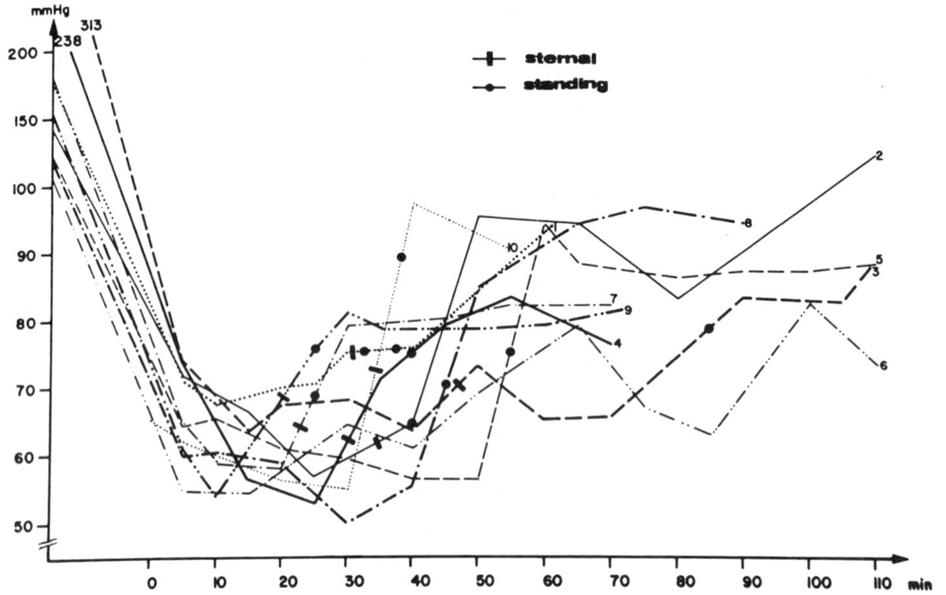

Figure 12.32. Oxygen partial pressures in 10 adult horses during recovery without application of oxygen.

nosed. According to diagnostic experience, more than 50% of all horses suffer from subacute or chronic lung disease. In order of the frequency of occurrence, the following diagnoses have to be mentioned.

Chronic Bronchitis/Bronchiolitis

This is a very often diagnosed disease, often occurring after a viral infection. The diagnosis is based upon a chronic, mostly nonproductive cough and/or increased vesicular breathing, with vesicular noise mainly during expiration. Dyspnea eventually is present during work.

Spastic Bronchitis and Bronchial Asthma

These are characterized by acute bronchospasms, mostly combined with a pre-existing bronchitis, and asthmatic wheezes. A typical finding is an attack of expiratory dyspnea.

Chronic Alveolar Lung Emphysema

The disease occurs as a sequel of chronic bronchitis. There are mixed, mainly expiratory dyspnea; ineffective forceless cough; wheezes and rales, and increased lung margins.

Acute Bronchitis/Bronchiolitis

This mainly occurs with viral infections (myxovirus influenza A equine 2). Clinically dominant are an expiratory dyspnea, frequent cough, and increased vesicular noises. There often is nasal discharge when secondary infections are present.

Acute or Chronic Pneumonias

Pneumonia is mostly caused by specific infections. There are fever and often heavy nasal discharge, with areas of dullness during percussion and often dyspnea. In horses with allergic lung diseases, interstitial pneumonias are common.

Other Lung Problems

Although there are other problems, such as lung edema, lung abscesses, or pleuritis, horses with these diseases are very seldom presented for surgery.

Pneumothorax

Wounds with opening of the thoracic cavity are common in the horse. If a communication between the interpleural space and the external atmosphere occurs, room air is entering between the thorax and lung surface. The lung collapses to its minimal volume followed by a mechanically based respiratory insufficiency by restriction of the number of ventilated alveoli. Horses with pneumothorax present with an extreme dyspnea and in a critical state of health. Immediate surgical intervention is necessary. As a further complication, a horse with pneumothorax often is found in a state of shock.

CLINICAL DIAGNOSIS IN RELATION TO GENERAL ANESTHESIA

Clinical Examination

A chronic lung disease, although an important factor for anesthetic problems, can often not be diagnosed during a superficial clinical examination. The horse has therefore to be preoperatively examined in a quiet area for alterations in normal breathing. A respiratory rate above 12/minute is suspicious for lung disease. The type of respiration (increased abdominal force at the end of expiration) requires special attention. Eventually, the horse has to be worked and checked for spontaneous coughing, dyspnea, and nasal discharge. A slight increase in body temperature above normal may be an indication of the existence of an acute, subacute, or even chronic lung problem. By auscultation and percussion of the lung, nonphysiological sounds are detected.

Laboratory Examinations

Lung Function Tests. The diagnosis of the function of a diseased lung before general anesthesia is generally not possible. Lung function tests are performed only in specialized laboratories and are generally not available for preoperative diagnostic purposes.

Hematological Examinations. Hematological examinations (red and white blood count, white cell differentiation, and blood chemistry) are performed in every clinic. These examinations may give further diagnostic criteria, but are of limited value when the lung function must be evaluated. The cell count and the cell differentiation, however, are important in the preoperative examination of a horse with lung disease. In cases of anemia, the oxygenation of the tissues can be further reduced by the decreased capacity of oxygen transportation. The white blood picture is important because acute, subacute, and many chronic infections may provoke secondary anemias. Acute bacterial infections provoke leukocytosis with neutrophilia. More chronic lung problems (bronchitis/bronchiolitis) even with dyspnea generally do not influence the composition of leucocytes in peripheral blood in a significant matter, although the total white cell count seems to give some indication of the activity of a bronchitis/bronchiolitis. Horses with asthmoid bronchitis (chronic obstructive pulmonary disease, COPD) or pulmonary emphysema often have an increased total leukocyte count.

Blood-Gas Analysis (PaO_2, $PaCO_2$, pH, and HCO_3^-). Blood-gas determinations of arterial blood have become a very valuable tool in the functional diagnosis of equine lung disease in daily practice. They allow determination of both the momentary status and also the effect of a medication or a therapeutic manipulation. However, blood-gas analysis remains an auxiliary method and will never replace a thorough clinical examination (10–12).

In Table 12.3, the effects of different lung symptoms in the standing, awake horse on arterial O_2 and CO_2 pressures are listed. It can be demonstrated that even slight symptoms of bronchitis/bronchiolitis influence oxygenation and can be detected preoperatively.

Table 12.3
Oxygen and Carbon Dioxide Partial Pressures (mm Hg) in Sound Horses and Horses with Chronic Respiratory Diseases, According to Meister et al. (1976) (12)

	Group I[a]	Group II[b]	Group III[c]	Group IV[d]
x̄ (mm Hg) $PaO_2 \pm$ SD	95	88	79	64
	4	5	4	11
x̄ (mm Hg) $PaCO_2 \pm$ SD	35	37	39	41
	5	4	5	7
Number of horses	16	38	16	13

[a] Sound horses.
[b] Horses with moderate lung symptoms (increased vesicular sounds).
[c] Horses with pathological lung symptoms (increased respiratory rate, slight dyspnea, harsh bronchial tones, rales, wheezes, mainly allergic etiology).
[d] Horses with heavy dyspnea (status asthmaticus), mainly allergic etiology, suspicion of lung emphysema.

In horses with chronic lung diseases, a combination of the disturbances described above can be demonstrated (ventilation-diffusion, ventilation/perfusion, or perfusion disturbances). Horses with allergic lung diseases (COPD) suffer from bronchospasms, thickening of the bronchioles, and irreversibly damaged alveoli with spastic contracted bronchi, often blocked by secretions and with a reduced number of capillaries. According to the predominance of the alterations, the CO_2 partial pressure can be increased, normal or decreased (partial or global insufficiency). Hypoxemia, however, is always present.

Radiological Examinations. Radiographs of good quality can, under certain circumstances, be used for preoperative evaluation of the lungs (Fig. 12.33). However, the diagnostic value in relation to lung function is restricted in large animals.

RESPIRATORY PROBLEMS IN THE SOUND HORSE DURING ANESTHESIA

Even a sound awake horse never remains in complete lateral recumbency for more than 15 minutes. This fact may be explained partially by ventilation perfusion disorders occurring as soon as lateral recumbency is achieved. The increased alveolar-arterial pressure differences of oxygen ($\Delta P_{(A\text{-}a)}O_2$) lead to an immediate hypoxemia when room air is inhaled. The corresponding CO_2 partial pressures remain generally unchanged (Fig. 12.31). It can be assumed that the hypoxemia occurring under room air ventilation in the adult horse stimulates respiratory centers. The simultaneous occurrence of hypercapnia is therefore prevented. The anesthetics chloral hydrate, thiopentone, and halothane/room air seem to play only a minor role in the occurrence of this problem (Table 12.4). When a sufficient oxygenation of the blood is provided by in-

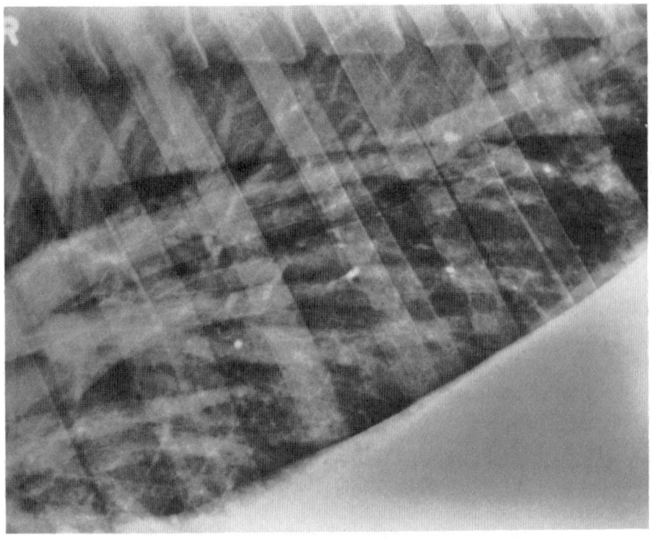

Figure 12.33. X-Ray of the lungs of an adult horse showing signs of COPD (increased filling of blood vessels and thickening of bronchial and bronchiolar walls). Courtesy of Prof. Dr. G. Ueltschi, Klinik für Nutztiere und Pferde der Universität Bern.

creasing the O_2 partial pressure in inspiratory air, hypoxemia does not occur in most cases. Hypercapnia and respiratory acidosis seem to appear always and only when oxygenation of the circulating blood is sufficient. Mainly in heavy horses and in horses with chronic lung disease, despite an application of 100% oxygen, arterial hypoxemia may occur. Oxygen pressures below 50 mm Hg may provoke anesthetic death, as demonstrated in Table 12.4; presumably this is caused by hypoxia.

RESPIRATORY PROBLEMS IN THE HORSE WITH PRE-EXISTING LUNG DISEASE DURING GENERAL ANESTHESIA

It was demonstrated above that sound horses develop heavy disturbances in lung function whenever they are placed in lateral recumbency. Tables 12.2 and 12.3 show that in standing horses with even slight lung problems higher alveolar-arterial O_2 pressure differences ($\Delta P_{(A-a)}O_2$) and therefore lower arterial O_2 pressures are measured. The sedative premedication with all substances used in routine practice including xylazine and detomidine provokes a further decrease in O_2 partial pressure (Table 12.5) eventually caused by a perfusion disturbance in the lung circulation. When these horses are placed in lateral or dorsal recumbency, the partial pressure of O_2 is further reduced and can without further oxygenation provoke dangerous degrees of hypoxemia. Horses with acute respiratory insufficiency with acute or subacute pneumonias are high risk cases. The most dangerous hypoxias can to a certain degree be prevented by the horse itself by hyperventilation when anesthesia remains in a very superficial stage. In deep anesthesia of long duration (more than 30 minutes), problems are inevitable. Anesthetic deaths occurred in our material when O_2 partial pressures below 50 mm Hg were measured. By experience we found that horses with chronic and long-lasting lung problems, such as COPD and lung emphysema, seemed to be more resistant to hypoxemia than animals with acute or subacute lung diseases.

PROBLEMS DURING RECOVERY

Sufficient oxygenation of arterial blood can generally be maintained by application of high percentage O_2 mixtures in inspiratory air with an inhalation anesthesia machine. A hypoxic crisis is, however, inevitable when the horse is disconnected from the apparatus and is breathing room air with an O_2 percentage of about 20%. Figure 12.32 and Table 12.6 show the extent of postoperative hypoxemia after routine surgery. Oxygen pressures generally increase when sternal position is achieved. Normal values are measures only in the standing animal. By insufflation of oxygen (15 liter/minute) in the nasopharynx, hypoxia can be prevented in nearly all cases. An insufflation of O_2 into the lower airways (bronchi) will not produce higher arterial O_2 pressures than application in the nostrils. Because of mechanical damage, insufflation should therefore not be performed in the trachea.

MONITORING OF THE HORSE WITH LUNG DISEASE

The immediate analysis of O_2 and CO_2 pressures in arterial blood is most helpful and provides perhaps the only valuable parameter for preoperative evaluation and for intraoperative and postoperative monitoring (12). Horses with a suspicion of lung insufficiency of a certain degree, in addition to clinical examination, should also be checked for hypoxemia by arterial blood-gas analysis. In those horses, arterial blood has to be withdrawn before sedative premedication. For this purpose the right carotid artery can be punctured in the standing horse (Fig. 12.34). In lateral recumbency, the facial artery also can be cannulated for determinations of arterial blood pressure (Fig. 12.35). The correct monitoring of general anesthesia requires O_2 and CO_2 determinations at regular intervals of every 30 minutes in addition to a close and careful clinical observation of the patient. When horses are breathing pure O_2, CO_2 partial pressures can be approximately measured by capnography in expiratory air (Fig. 12.37). Determinations of arterial blood pressures throughout anesthesia are most helpful.

Table 12.4
Mean Oxygen and Carbon Dioxide Partial Pressures (mm Hg) in Arterial Blood under Different Anesthetic Procedures in Adult Horses. Lateral Recumbency (with Standard Deviations).

Anesthetic	No. of Horses	PaO_2 Duration of Anesthesia			$PaCO_2$
		10 min	20 min	30 min	
Chloral hydrate	24	60 (7)	58 (8)	58 (9)	39 (2.6)
Thiopentone	6	59 (13)	56 (5)	64 (3)	41 (1.1)
Halothane/O_2	6	351 (69)	339 (95)	324 (136)	61 (13.9)
Halothane/O_2/N_2O (1:1)	6	141 (64)	142 (64)	129 (48)	63 (5.6)
Halothane/room air	4	46	44	38[a]	33 (3.9)

[a] One horse died.

Table 12.5
Effect of Sedative Premedication on Arterial Oxygen and Carbon Dioxide Pressure in the Horse (with Standard Deviations, n = 6 Adult Horses).

		PaO_2	$PaCO_2$
Acepromazine, 10 mg/100 kg body weight	Before	92.6 (1.5)	32.4 (4.4)
	After	77.1 (2.8)	32.9 (5.3)
Propiopromazine, 10 mg/100 kg body weight	Before	92.1 (1.5)	35.4 (2.4)
	After	77.7 (6.1)	35.5 (2.3)
Xylazine, 80 mg/100 kg body weight	Before	93.6 (1.8)	35.1 (1.9)
	After	75.3 (5.3)	38.7 (2.2)
Detomidine, 100 μg/kg body weight	Before	96.0 (6.3)	35.1 (2.8)
	After	42.2 (4.4)	35.8 (2.6)

ANESTHETIC PRINCIPLES AND MEASURES IN THE HORSE WITH LUNG DISEASE

General Principles

When there are pre-existing lung problems, all measures should be taken to limit anesthesia time as much as possible. The surgical preparation of the operation site should be performed in the standing animal.

Horses with symptoms of acute infections with increased body temperature should only be anesthetized in emergency cases when surgical intervention cannot be postponed. Although a sufficient gas exchange within the lungs generally is possible with appropriate methods, the anesthetic risk in these cases is increased. It further has to be considered that, whenever tracheal tubes and anesthesia machines are used, they become contaminated, and the infection may be transferred to other sound horses. Horses with severe chronic dyspnea (COPD) can be pretreated with 2 mg/100 kg of atropine to alleviate the symptoms and to provide better oxygenation. When elective surgery is possible, these horses should be pretreated with corticosteroids and/or dustfree environmental conditions (without hay). When clinical and laboratory results of the preoperative examination indicate an important respiratory insufficiency, maximum oxygenation before, during, and after anesthesia should be ensured.

Starvation

In horses with lung problems, preanesthetic starvation is even more essential than in sound animals. A starved horse seems to require less anesthetic for an optimal surgical stage. In addition, the presence of intestines on the diaphragm is decreased, leading to an increase in functional residual capacity (FRC) of up to 30%. Food should therefore be withheld for 12 to 18 hours whenever elective surgery is planned.

Sedative Premedication

Because all available substances used for tranquilization or sedation in the horse provoke a decrease in arterial O_2 pressure of about 15 mm Hg (Table 12.5) and a pooling of red blood cells in the spleen, the lowest possible dose should be administered (14, 15). The sedation should prevent possible excitations during the induction period. Excitations and agitations lead to increased O_2 consumption and CO_2 production and may aggravate symptoms of a pre-existing respiratory insufficiency. Horses with respiratory insufficiency have to be artificially oxygenated before, during, and after anesthesia up to the moment when they are standing again. Before and after endotracheal intubation, an O_2-carrying catheter is placed through the nostrils in the nasopharynx (Fig. 12.36). O_2 is administered with a flow of about 15 liters/minute.

Methods of General Anesthesia

As a rule, only medications with a fast distribution and elimination rate should be used. Therefore, chloral hydrate or its combinations with barbiturates should be avoided.

When a sufficient oxygenation of the patient is provided, all accepted methods for inducing and maintaining general anesthesia are possible. An endotracheal tube is generally necessary and allows mainte-

Table 12.6
Mean Arterial Oxygen Pressures (PaO_2, mm Hg) during the Recovery Period with and without Applications of 15 liters/min Oxygen.

		End of Inhalation Anesthesia	Lateral Recumbency	Sternal Recumbency	Standing
Without oxygen	x̄	182	69	71	88
	SD	67	7	9	7
	min/max	125/327	58/78	57/81	81/101
Oxygen in nasopharynx	x̄	242	174	134	95[a]
	SD	37	51	46	10
	min/max	195/290	121/281	95/217	82/105
Oxygen in trachea	x̄	186	146	144	98[a]
	SD	66	42	23	3
	min/max	93/287	86/189	118/159	95/101

[a] Without oxygen application.

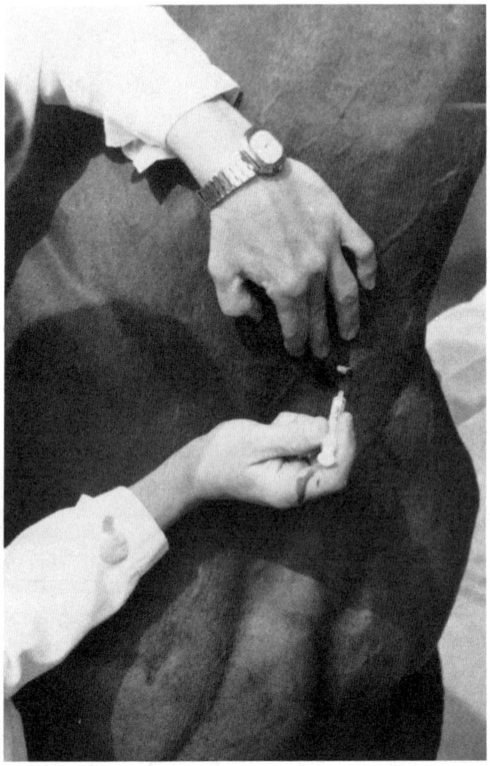

Figure 12.34. Arterial puncture of the carotid artery in the standing horse.

nance of a sufficient respiratory volume, spontaneous breathing or attachment to oxygen source as needed. Injection anesthesias of more than 30 minutes should be avoided because of an often-prolonged recovery period, even with additional oxygenation. Short anesthesias are possible with ketamine or with an ultrashort-acting barbiturate with or without guaifenesin when O_2 is offered. For surgery of more than 30 minutes, inhalation anesthesia is required. An admixture of nitrous oxide requires regular measurement of arterial blood gases (PaO_2). Because most anesthetics, such as halothane, depress spontaneous respiration and arterial blood pressure according to the level in the

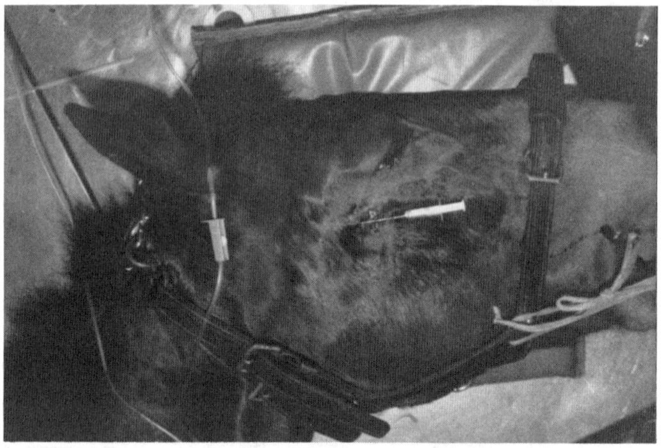

Figure 12.35. Cannulation of the facial artery for determination of arterial blood gases and for invasive blood pressure monitoring.

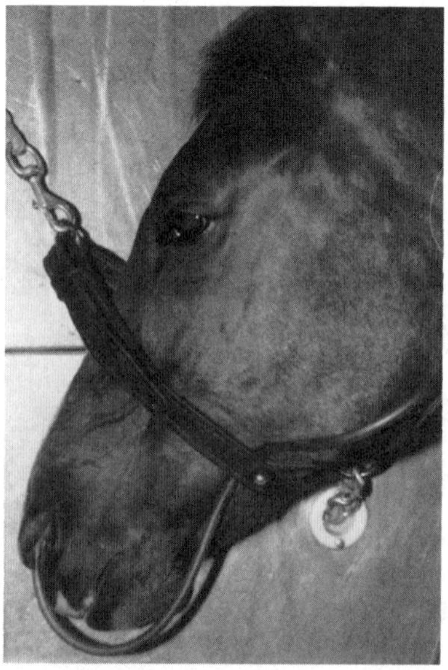

Figure 12.36. Application of oxygen through a catheter in the nasopharynx before induction of anesthesia and during recovery (flow, 15 liters/min).

blood, anesthesia should be as superficial as possible (16).

When ventilation disturbances are present or occur during anesthesia, as diagnosed by a diminished respiratory volume or by an increase in CO_2 pressure above 50 mm Hg, IPPV becomes necessary. For assisted or controlled ventilation, an especially designed respirator is ideal, although not mandatory (17). A sufficient respiratory volume can be achieved by manual compression of the respiratory bag or by intermittent insufflation with O_2 through the endotracheal tube without an anesthesia machine. The aim of IPPV is the maintenance of a physiological CO_2 pressure in arterial blood, whereas O_2 uptake cannot be increased by this procedure because of the various reasons described above. Whenever circulatory problems (shock) are present, ventilation should be assisted because a fully controlled ventilation leads to a further decrease in cardiac output and may aggravate the symptoms. In cases of pneumothorax, IPPV is indicated as soon as anesthesia is induced and has to be extended to the moment when the wound is closed (18).

The arterial blood pressure has to be supported to provide an adequate perfusion. Infusions of lactated Ringer's solution or plasma expanders are used when hypotension is measured or detected by clinical observation and palpation of the peripheral pulse. Infusions of a solution of dopamine have had good results in clinical practice. In Figure 12.37, the capnogram during dopamine infusion is shown. It demonstrates that CO_2 elimination is markedly increased, presumably as a sequel to better peripheral perfusion.

POSITIONING OF A HORSE WITH LUNG DISEASE

Horses with lung disease and respiratory insufficiency should be positioned on the left side whenever the surgery interference allows. The function of the larger and uppermost right lung is less impaired by the weight of the animal in this position. The limbs of these horses should not be fixed together with hobbles; spontaneous ventilation has proved to be significantly impaired by this procedure. The lowest impairment is obtained when the horse is in an oblique lateral/dorsal position with the limbs fixed apart from each other a normal distance (Fig. 12.38).

Horses with lung problems should remain on the same side during anesthesia and postoperative recovery. During lateral recumbency, the lowermost lung parts become afunctional and cannot be ventilated when suddenly lying uppermost. In dorsal recumbency, gas exchange is disturbed even more than in lateral position. Horses affected with lung diseases should therefore only be positioned on the back when absolutely necessary (19).

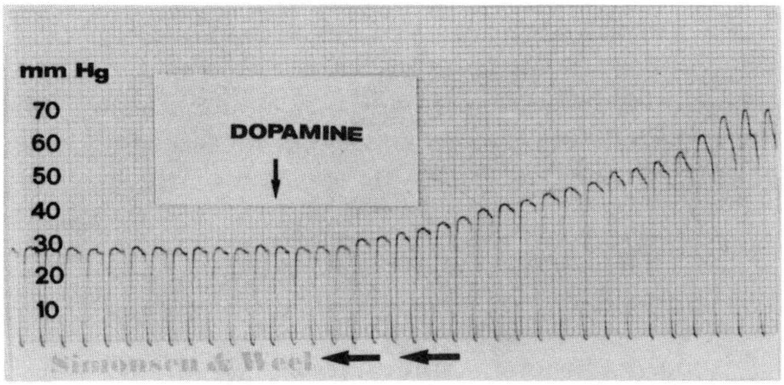

Figure 12.37. Capnogram during infusion of dopamine under controlled ventilation. Note that CO_2 elimination is increased by increasing peripheral perfusion.

CONCLUSIONS

It has been demonstrated that all large animals develop lung problems as soon as they are placed in lateral or dorsal recumbency. Thus every patient potentially suffers from a lung disease. In manifest lung diseases as diagnosed by clinical and laboratory examinations (blood gasses), these primary problems have to be considered. These horses have to be oxygenated before, during, and after general anesthesia. Although very severe hypoxemias occasionally are observed, anesthetic deaths based on chronic lung diseases seldom are, whereas horses with more acute disturbances seem to be more sensible to oxygen lack. By thorough clinical examination, close supervision, and appropriate therapy, most fatal problems can be avoided.

Lung Disease and General Anesthesia in Small Animals

In contrast to the more often-occurring apparent lung diseases in large animals, problems related to

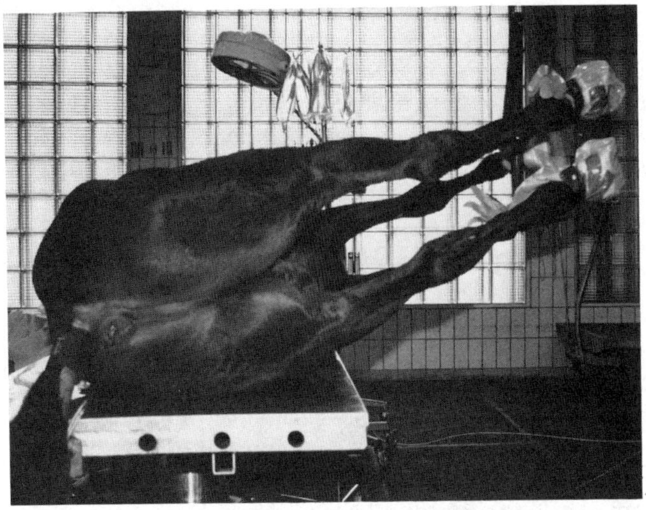

Figure 12.38. Positioning of the horse in lateral recumbency.

general anesthesia are more seldom seen in dogs and cats (13). In addition, the ventilation/perfusion disorders commonly occurring in recumbent large animals are not of clinical importance in these species. Also, most lung diseases in cats and dogs are diagnosed only when clinical symptoms are very severe, such as in chronic inflammatory or neoplastic diseases. These animals then are presented in a very bad state of health and very rarely appear for surgery. They often are enthanized before a clinical diagnosis can be confirmed.

In principle, induction of general anesthesia in small animals may be associated with hypoxemia. Anesthesia maintained with unsuitable methods provokes hypoxemia even in normal animals. The origin is in most cases a ventilation disturbance caused by depression of respiratory centers. In Figure 12.30, the arterial oxygen partial pressures of five sound dogs during pentobarbitone anesthesia are graphically shown. With a pre-existing lung problem, anesthetic deaths can be expected. Pre-existing disturbances and diseases in the respirtory tract have therefore to be detected in these animals by a thorough clinical, hematological, and, if necessary, radiological examination.

VENTILATORY DISTURBANCES

Dogs with brachicephalic skulls have a predisposition for obstructions in the upper airway. Stenosis is generally increased during general anesthesia, leading to a diminished respiratory volume. Toy and miniature breeds often develop symptoms of a tracheal stenosis or a tracheal collapse. During anesthesia of very fat animals, normal expansion of the thorax is impeded, leading to respiratory depression and hypoxemia. Pneumothorax, pleural effusion, neoplasm, pulmonary collapse, and diaphragmatic hernia have in common that normal respiratory movements and therefore sufficient expansion of the lungs are mechanically impeded or disturbed, causing ventilatory insufficiency. Although in the awake animal these disturbances may be compensated for by increased respiratory work, acute insufficiencies can appear under the influence of general anesthesia in lateral or dorsal recumbency.

MIXED DISTURBANCES

Here most problems not primarily based on hypoventilation are considered. Of clinical importance are diseases with a restriction of diffusion, disturbances of ventilation/perfusion, and perfusion problems of the lungs. In many diseases a combination of these factors can be found, as with pneumonias of various origins, aspiration pneumonia, chronic bronchitis, bronchiectasis, and lung emphysema. All these diseases show as main symptoms a more or less frequent cough and, most important for general anesthesia, a more or less pronounced dyspnea. Blood gas analyses show that the cause of dyspnea may be hypoxemia.

Although the pulmonary edema is in most cases more a secondary symptom of a primary disturbance in heart function or of an overdosage with parenteral administered fluids, the gas exchange within the lungs is disturbed. Therefore, lung edema has to be considered as a pulmonary complication.

DIAGNOSIS IN RELATION TO GENERAL ANESTHESIA

A thorough clinical examination and the recognition of the disturbance is, as in large animals and in other diseases, the basic condition for a successful outcome of general anesthesia. According to these findings, special measures have to be taken; these are discussed later in this chapter. Special attention is required in animals with primary heart disease and with signs of dyspnea. Hematological examinations (white and red blood count and differentiation of white cells) will give valuable information about the presence of acute or chronic infection. Acutely infected animals should only be anesthetized when surgery cannot be postponed because of the danger of transmission of the disease to other animals by endotracheal tubes and anesthesia machines. A hematological examination also gives information about the presence of anemia. In contrast to large animals, arterial blood-gas determinations in the awake animal are generally not possible. Judgment of respiratory insufficiency is therefore mainly based upon clinical examination and experience. However, additional information can be obtained by radiographic examination of the chest.

THERAPEUTIC MEASURES IN SMALL ANIMALS WITH LUNG DISEASE

In cases of obvious respiratory insufficiency, O_2 partial pressure in inspiratory air should be increased during the whole anesthetic procedure. Oxygen should be administered by face mask before sedative medication to ensure an optimal saturation of hemoglobin and to overcome an hypoxic crisis during the induction phase. It is important to avoid any agitation or excitation generally concomitant with an increased O_2 consumption.

SEDATION AND INDUCTION OF ANESTHESIA

Sedative premedication with a phenothiazine derivative (Acepromazine) should be avoided in severe cases because of an alpha-sympathicolytic action on the circulatory system with decreased venous return and pooling of blood in peripheral vessels. Whether opiates can be administered is not clear. These substances provoke severe respiratory depression by partial blockade of regulatory mechanisms and should only be administered under additional oxygenation. Although these drugs improve the clinical appearance of a respiratory insufficiency, they only mask the clinical symptoms without any improvement of respiratory function.

An ideal sedative premedication and induction agent should provide a fast transition from the awake animal to a state that allows endotracheal intubation or eventually an application of tight face mask. Animals with pre-existing and diagnosed respiratory disease should always be endotracheally intubated.

In the dog, we suggest induction of general anesthesia without sedative premedication with an ultrashort-acting barbiturate after atropinization (e.g., 5 to 10 mg/kg thiopentone i.v. to effect). In the cat, intravenous anesthesia induction with alphaxalone/alphadolone (Saffan) and eventually with a small dose of acepromazine has proved to be safe and reliable. In countries where this is unavailable, ketamine is frequently substituted.

MAINTENANCE OF ANESTHESIA

Whenever possible, small animals with respiratory insufficiency should be anesthetized with an inhalation anesthetic such as halothane or isoflurane. Inhalation anesthesia with these gases allows fast induction, control of anesthetic depth, and recovery. In addition, optimal oxygenation is guaranteed by O_2 as a carrier gas. Admixture of nitrous oxide should never exceed 50% in inspiratory air. In cases of severe lung or heart problems, pure O_2 with the anesthetic is advised. No further nitrous oxide should be administered when there is a suspicion of gas-filled areas in the gut or the thorax. Nitrous oxide diffuses very rapidly in these spaces, leading to an increase in volume and therefore to a further disturbance of ventilation.

The anesthetic gases should be offered through a semi-open or semi-closed anesthesia machine suitable to the size of the patient. Endotracheal intubation is mandatory because maintenance of an adequate respiratory volume by external means (IPPV) is only possible when an airtight communication with the lungs exists. After endotracheal intubation, the anesthetist has to control the exact position of the tip of the tube. When introduced too deeply into a main bronchus, very dangerous complications occur when functional disturbances pre-exist. The cause of this crisis is not easily detectable during the surgical procedure. For this reason, both lungs have to be auscultated after intubation to ensure ventilation of the whole lung.

Animals with severe respiratory insufficiencies require IPPV during anesthesia with a respirator or by manual squeezing of the respiratory bag. A peripherally acting muscle relaxant may improve gas exchange by complete relaxation of the respiratory muscles.

When gas exchange is impeded by pulmonary edema, the treatment has to provide adequate oxygenation and removal of CO_2. Artificial ventilation with PEEP seems to be the best therapy during anesthesia according to experience and the available literature. Animals with a pre-existing or intraoperatively diagnosed lung edema must therefore be artificially ventilated. By this procedure transudation is impeded by the increased pressure within the bronchioalveolar system. Treatment of the primary cause (heart insufficiency) is also necessary by strophantine or heart glycosides.

MONITORING

In addition to a constant and close supervision of the patient according to anesthetic rules, the anesthetist has to control the respiratory volume with an especially designed volume meter incorporated in the circle system (Fig. 12.39) or by judging the ventilated volume according to the movements of the respiratory bag. For routine use, a capnograph can be used to control CO_2 pressures in expiratory air. It allows a noninvasive control of ventilation during spontaneous and controlled ventilation. In animals with respiratory insufficiency, blood-gas measurements from arterial blood are also indicated (12).

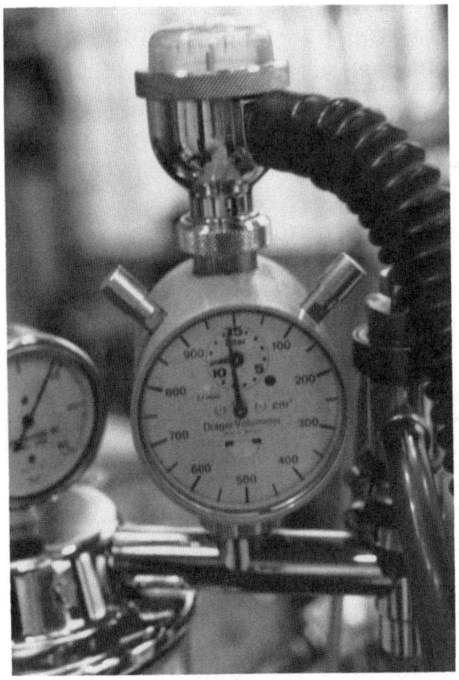

Figure 12.39. Volumeter incorporated in the anesthetic system.

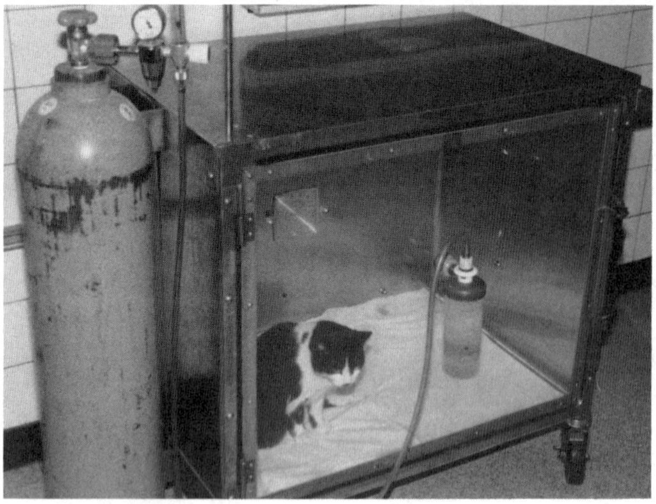

Figure 12.40. Oxygen cage, allowing an increase of oxygen pressure in inspiratory air during recovery.

POSTOPERATIVE MEASURES

As in large animals, a hypoxic crisis may occur immediately after disconnection of the animal from the anesthesia machine or after extubation. All measures must aim to provide sufficient ventilation and oxygenation from the moment of disconnection from the apparatus until the animal is fully awake (9).

Although oxygen can be administered through a catheter in the endotracheal tube or through a face mask, a specially designed oxygen cage is of advantage (Fig. 12.40). The animals remain in this environment with a high inspiratory oxygen pressure, controlled humidity, and an increased temperature until recovery is complete.

CONCLUSIONS

Small animals suffering from pulmonary diseases of a light or moderate degree generally seem to tolerate appropriately performed general anesthesia better than large animals. However, special attention is required when severe disturbances of pulmonary function are diagnosed preoperatively. All measures must be taken to ensure additional oxygenation before, during, and after anesthesia. In addition, lung function must be ameliorated by increasing the respiratory volumes by controlled ventilation through IPPV.

References

1. Ducket J, Schatzmann U, Ammann E: Die postnarkotische Hypoxämie und ihre Theraie beim Pferd. *Pherdeheilkunde* 1:95–98, 1985.
2. Dudziak R: *Lehrbuch der Anaesthesiologie*. Stuttgart, Schattauer Verlag, 1980.
3. Gillespie JR, Tyler WS, Hall LW: Cardiopulmonary dysfunction in anesthetized, laterally recumbent horses. *Am J Vet Res* 30:61–72, 1969.
4. Hall LW: General anesthesia. In *The Veterinary Clinics of North America*, ed 3. Philadelphia, WB Saunders Co, 1981, pp 3–17.
5. Hall LW: Oxygenation of pulmonary vein blood in conscious and anesthetized ponies. *Equine Vet J* 11:71–75, 1979.
6. Hall LW, Clarke K: *Veterinary Anaesthesia*. London, Bailliere Tindall, 1983, pp 203–244.
7. Hall LW, Gillespie JR, Tyler WS: Alveolar-arterial oxygen tension differences in anesthetized horses. *Br J Anaesth* 40:560–568, 1968.
8. Hall LW, Trim CM: Positive end-expiratory pressure in anaesthetized spontaneously breathing horses. *Br J Anaesth* 47:819–824, 1975.
9. Lutz H: Das Lungenoedem. In Frey R, et al (eds): *Lehrbuch der Anaesthesiologie, Reanimation and Intensivpflege*. New York, Springer Verlag, 1972, p 484.
10. McDonnell WN: The effect of anaesthesia on pulmonary gas exchange and arterial oxygenation in the horse. Ph.D. thesis, Cambridge, England, 1974.
11. McDonnell WN, Hall LW, Jeffcott LB: Radiographic evidence of impaired pulmonary function in laterally recumbent anesthetized horses. *Equine Vet J* 11:24–32, 1979.
12. Meister U, Gerber H, Tschudi P: Die arterielle Blutgasanalyse in der Diagnostik und Ueberwachung chronisch lungenkranker Pferde. *Schweiz Arch Tierheilk* 118:99–104, 1976.
13. Pamock PW, Archibald J: Diseases of the respiratory system. In Carcock EJ (ed): *Canine Medicine*. Santa Barbara, California, American Veterinary Publications, 1968, pp 561–584.
14. Rohr W: Wirkung und Nebenwirkung einiger Kombinationen gängiger Beruhigungsmittel zur Ruhigstellung des Pferdes. *Diss Med Vet Bern* 1981.
15. Rohr W, Schatzmann U, Hyss H, Tschudi P: Detomidine (Domosedan®) ein neues Sedativum und Analgetikum für Pferde Tierheilkunde. In press, 1986.
16. Schatzmann U: Respiration of the horse under anesthesia. Proc. 1st Int. Congress Vet. Anaesthesia, Cambridge, England, 1982.
17. Schatzmann U: Untersuchung zur Anwendbarkeit eines nichtdepolarisierenden Muskelrelaxans (Alloferin®) beim Pferd unter besonderer Berucksichtigung der kontrollierten Beatmung nach Blutgasanalysen. *Habilitationsschrift Vet Med*, Bern University, 1976.
18. Spörri H, Stuenzi H: *Pathophysiologie der haustiere*. Berlin, Paul Parey, 1969, pp 169–214.
19. Stolk P: Pulmonary blood flow in lateraly recumbent horses. Ph.D. thesis, Cambridge, England, 1979.

PART 5

Pathophysiological Changes of the Hepatic System

NICHOLAS H. DODMAN, B.V.M.S., M.R.C.V.S., D.A.C.V.A.
LARRY R. ENGELKING, Ph.D., and M. SAWKAT ANWER, Ph.D.

Introduction

The liver is the largest gland in the body. Apart from its central role in the metabolism of fat, protein, and carbohydrate, the liver is the primary site of detoxification of various exogenous and endogenous substances such as bilirubin and drugs. Bile, the exocrine secretion of the liver, provides a route of excretion for cholesterol, bilirubin, and metabolized or unmetabolized drugs, among other substances. Bile also assists in digestion and absorption of fat by providing bile acids and phospholipids to the duodenum and partially neutralizes acidic chyme from the stomach. Because of its location and ability to efficiently extract a wide variety of compounds from blood, the liver plays a central role in removing toxic materials before their entry into the systemic circulation. Substances entering the enteric lymphatic system, however, will bypass the liver.

The effects of hepatic dysfunction are widespread and involve practically all other organ systems of the body. Clinical signs of liver disease, however, are often not apparent until the disturbance is fairly well advanced because of a large hepatic functional reserve. Animals with liver disease often fail to thrive as a result of depressed metabolic functions, and digestive disturbances sometimes result from impaired biliary secretion. Hematological and hemodynamic imbalances occur in seriously affected animals, and toxic compounds can accumulate in blood, resulting in neurological sequelae. Cardiopulmonary disturbances can occur secondary to hepatic dysfunction, and renal failure may also be precipitated. Even endocrine function is affected in liver disease, as hormones such as insulin and corticosteroids fail to be deactivated at the normal rate.

The anesthesiologist is sometimes faced with the difficult task of having to anesthetize a patient with compromised hepatic function. The degree of risk will depend on the severity of the disturbance. Even after careful consideration of the patient's clinical history and a thorough physical examination, it is often difficult to diagnose the type or degree of liver dysfunction with accuracy. Liver function tests are invaluable in this respect and often help to establish the nature and extent of the disease process. Once hepatic dysfunction has been confirmed, the risks of anesthetizing such a patient should be weighed against the possible benefits of surgery.

Preanesthetic Evaluation

CLINICAL HISTORY

Standards of practice are constantly rising in veterinary medicine; it is now considered inappropriate to omit careful preanesthetic evaluation of patients scheduled for anesthesia. One important aspect of this evaluation is obtaining a comprehensive clinical history of the patient because this can provide valuable information regarding the functional status of major organ systems. Jaundice is a sign frequently associated with hepatic disease, but it often remains unidentified by owners. However, they may notice progressive enlargement of the abdomen after the development of ascites, and occasionally signs of a hemorrhagic diathesis, such as petechiation, hemorrhagic enteritis, or hematuria, may be reported. Such other nonspecific signs as polydipsia and polyuria frequently accompany hepatic disturbances. Where there is biliary tract obstruction, acholic feces or the orange-tinted urine characteristic of bilirubinuria may become apparent. In extreme cases, neurological disturbances related to hepatic encephalopathy may be noticed with these signs being the primary cause of the animal's referral.

It is important to obtain information from the owner regarding medications administered to the animal in the immediate past. This can be useful in assessing the liver's metabolizing ability and is essential if drug interactions are to be avoided. Some drugs affect the ability of the liver to metabolize anesthetic agents. Treatment with phenobarbital, for example, induces hepatic microsomal enzymes and facilitates drug metabolism. Conversely, the detoxifying ability of the liver is decreased by prior administration of chloramphenicol. The interactions of drugs are numerous and defy description here, but it should be noted that concurrent medications can and do affect the action of anesthetic agents. Anesthetic agents themselves can reduce the ability of the liver to remove foreign compounds from the blood by decreasing hepatic blood flow, hepatic oxygen uptake, or bile flow. Even local anesthetics are known to decrease hepatic excretion of certain drugs because they decrease uptake of bile salts and thus decrease bile flow (1). When appropriate, concurrent medications should be withdrawn prior to anesthesia in order to minimize the likelihood of drug interactions.

CLINICAL EXAMINATION

Clinical signs of liver disease are not always easy to detect unless the disease is fairly advanced. In acute severe liver disease, the most obvious signs are often jaundice, hepatomegaly, and anterior abdominal pain. None, however, is a specific or sensitive indicator of liver disease.

Jaundice (or icterus) develops when bilirubin accumulates in plasma and tissues and can usually be detected when the plasma level exceeds 2 to 3 mg/dl. Notable species differences occur in the frequency with which icterus is observed in association with liver disease (2). In sheep and cattle dying of terminal hepatic failure, there usually is a significant elevation in plasma bilirubin, but the value may not be high enough to produce clinical icterus (3, 4). This may be due to a substantial reserve capacity of the liver to excrete bilirubin or to the adaptation of extra hepatic mechanisms for bilirubin excretion and/or degradation. Clinical icterus in ruminants is most frequently associated with hemolytic anemia, in which acute overproduction of bilirubin exceeds the excretory capacity (2). The significance of icterus in the horse is often difficult to evaluate. The sclera and visible mucous membrances of most normal horses do not appear icteric. In 10 to 15% of normal horses, however, a slight but definite yellow discoloration of the sclera and/or oral mucous membranes can be detected (5). Scleral icterus of a moderate degree may also be observed in horses with a variety of illnesses that do not appear to involve the liver directly (2). This is because a reduction of food intake in the horse produces a rapid rise in the plasma bilirubin concentration (6–11). In both hemolytic anemia and hepatic failure in the horse, the degree of icterus is usually much greater than that seen under conditions associated with reduced food intake (2). Severe icterus in this species is almost invariably present in acute hepatic necrosis (5, 12). The dog and cat appear to be intermediate between ruminants and the horse in the development of clinical icterus. Hemolytic disease, hepatocellular dysfunction, and extrahepatic bile duct obstruction are usually associated with icterus in these species (2). In experimental extrahepatic bile duct obstruction in the dog, plasma bilirubin increases immediately after the surgical procedure and clinical icterus is observed within 1 to 3 days. After 2 to 3 weeks, however, the plasma bilirubin of some dogs begins to decline, and clinical icterus may disappear. This may be related to the adaption of extrahepatic mechanisms of bilirubin excretion, particularly in the kidney. The canine kidney is capable of adapting so that the rate of renal conjugation and excretion of bilirubin equals the rate of formation. In cats with complete extra hepatic bile duct obstruction, no such decrease is observed, and persistent hyperbilirubinemia and icterus are characteristic (2).

In chronic liver disease with cirrhosis, the size of the liver is often reduced, and ascites may sometimes be confirmed by palpation of an ascitic thrill transmitted through the abdomen on percussion. Other signs of chronic liver disease include the development of an accessory portal circulation and, in some cases, evidence of neurological disturbances or coagulopathy. Whatever the pattern of clinical signs in an individual patient, it is often difficult to diagnose liver disease with certainty without reference to hepatic function tests and other ancillary aids to diagnosis.

HEPATIC FUNCTION TESTING

Subtle disturbances of hepatic function may only be detected by biochemical screening. This approach should be adopted in cases where liver function may be compromised.

Tests of Substrate Metabolism

Tests of carbohydrate metabolism are not particularly useful as indicators of hepatic function because they lack specificity and sensitivity. The galactose tolerance test is probably the most specific test of carbohydrate metabolism because nearly all galactose is initially metabolized by the liver. It can provide some useful information not supplied by other forms of testing, but the results should not be interpreted in isolation. A substantial portion of the liver must be nonfunctional before tests of carbohydrate metabolism are significantly affected.

Hepatic function tests related to protein metabolism have proven to be quite useful. The liver produces most of the plasma proteins, including albumin, alpha and beta globulins, fibrinogen, and prothrombin. Gamma globulins are the exception because they are synthesized by plasma cells. One simple way of evaluating liver function in terms of synthetic ability is to measure the plasma albumin concentration or, slightly less specifically, total serum protein (or solids). It should be remembered that only about 10% of serum albumin is synthesized daily in most species, and a substantial time lapse is required for reduced synthesis to become apparent. Hypoalbuminemia is not specific for liver disease. Low levels of serum albumin are found in certain types of nephrosis, chronic cardiac disease, enteropathies, pancreatic deficiency, and whenever there is a dietary deficiency of protein. Hypoalbuminemia accompanied by hypergammaglobulinemia as demonstrated by a low albumin:globulin ratio is more indicative of hepatic disease.

Coagulopathies may be associated with advanced liver disease (13). These coagulopathies may result from either: (*a*) decreased synthesis of clotting factors, (*b*) primary fibrinolysis, (*c*) disseminated intravascular coagulation, or (*d*) circulating anticoagulants. Blood clotting abnormalities caused by decreased synthesis of clotting factors are a common complication of hepatic disease in both humans and animals (14). Measurement of the activated clotting time prothrombin time or partial thromboplastin time can help determine the nature and extent of coagulation defects.

Tests of Hepatic Excretory Function

Bilirubin, the principle degradation product of heme, is the most common endogenous compound used for liver function evaluation. It is esterified almost exclusively by the liver and subsequently excreted in bile mainly as glucuronide, glucoside, or xyloside derivatives (15). Because impaired biliary excretion with reflux of hepatic metabolites into plasma occurs in many forms of hepatobiliary disease and accumulation of bilirubin in plasma and tissues causes obvious clinical signs such as jaundice and dark urine, determination of serum bilirubin became one of the earliest of the standard liver function tests.

The concept that serum can contain various forms of bilirubin was introduced by van den Bergh and Muller (16), who discovered the indirect- and direct-reacting bilirubins, later tentatively identified as unconjugated bilirubin and as bilirubin esterified with one or two glucuronic acid moieties (conjugated bilirubin), respectively (17–19). The conjugated hyperbilirubinemias are associated with hepatobiliary disease. Unconjugated hyperbilirubinemias occur not only as a result of hepatobiliary disorders, but also because of overproduction of bilirubin, deficient hepatic uptake, or deficient conjugation of bilirubin (20). It should be remembered that the plasma bilirubin level is the algebraic sum of input into plasma from hepatic and extrahepatic sources, removal of bilirubin from plasma, and return of either unconjugated or conjugated bilirubin from hepatocytes to plasma. Only the second and third processes rely exclusively on normal hepatic function; therefore, the specificity of the bilirubin assay is limited. This limitation can generally be overcome by use of the ratio of direct to total bilirubin (from the van den Bergh reaction), bearing in mind that excretion is the limiting step in bilirubin transport from blood to bile (except possibly in the horse) (6–11). Increased bilirubin production, which will occur during hemolytic crises, should decrease the direct to total ratio, whereas hepatic dysfunction should increase it. Biliary obstruction prior to inevitable hepatocellular damage should greatly increase the direct/total ratio to 50 or 60%.

Urinary bile pigments can be used to aid in the diagnosis of liver disease; for example, conjugated bilirubin appears in urine during extrahepatic biliary obstruction. In this instance, no urobilinogen is found in urine because bilirubin is unable to reach the intestine where urobilinogen is formed. Bilirubin conjugates are not normally found in urine of the horse, sheep, pig, or cat (21). Dogs, however, have a low renal threshold for unconjugated bilirubin and are able to conjugate heme to bilirubin in the kidney and excrete it in urine. Urine suspected of containing conjugated bilirubin can be field-tested in a bottle. After vigorous shaking, the presence of a greenish-yellow foam is indicative of bilirubinuria (21). Occasionally, false-positive results may occur associated with high levels of urinary urobilinogen.

Hemolytic crises are associated with urinary urobilinogen without bilirubinuria. Hepatitis and other forms of hepatocellular pathology will result in the presence of both urobilinogen and conjugated bilirubin in urine. The reason for this is that altered hepatocytes are unable to re-extract urobilinogen from portal blood, and they are also unable to adequately excrete conjugated bilirubin into bile (Fig. 12.41).

Tests for Liver Cell Membrane Integrity

One of the most effective means of securing meaningful information to aid in the diagnosis of hepatobiliary disease is to assay plasma levels of enzymes known

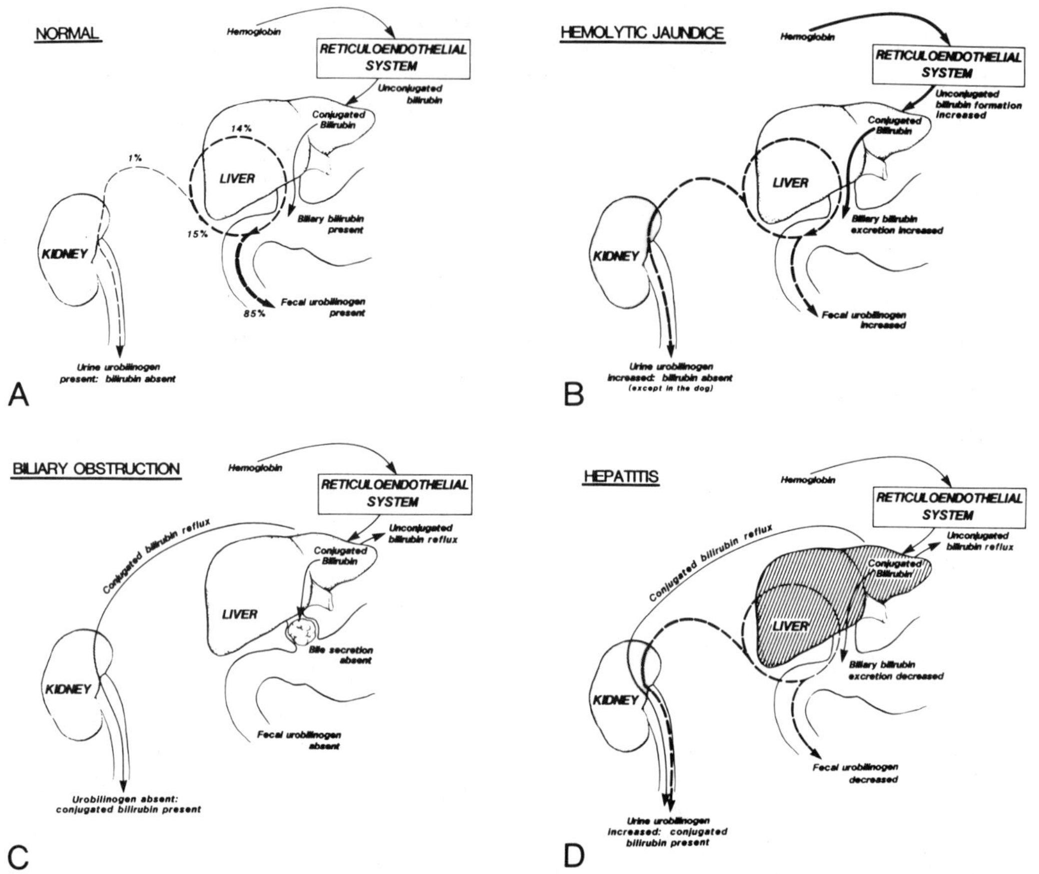

Figure 12.41. Hemoglobin-bilirubin-urobilinogen cycle. (*Dotted arrows*, urobilinogen; *solid arrows*, bilirubin.) As conjugated bilirubin reaches the terminal ileum and large intestine, some deconjugation takes place by bacterial enzymes and the pigment is subsequently reduced by fecal flora to a group of colorless tetrapyrolic compounds known as urobilinogens. From 10 to 20% of urobilinogen is reabsorbed in the terminal ileum and large intestine and normally extracted (95%) from portal blood by the liver. Urobilinogen is excreted into bile unchanged; it returns to the intestine, thereby completing the enterohepatic urobilinogen cycle. Because the liver extracts approximately 95% of urobilinogen from portal blood, normally there are mere traces that pass by the liver to enter the peripheral circulation. What little is there is quickly handled by the kidneys, where it passively diffuses across the glomerulus and renal tubular cells to appear in urine. In the dog, renal secretion of urobilinogen is enhanced significantly by acidification of urine. The colorless urobilinogen is oxidized by light to the highly colored urobilin, which imparts color to urine. In cases of complete biliary obstruction, urobilinogen is not present in urine, yet conjugated bilirubin is. In cases of hemolytic jaundice, unconjugated bilirubin production and therefore urobilinogen production are increased, thus increasing the amount of urobilinogen in urine. In cases of hepatitis or hepatocellular pathology, both urinary conjugated bilirubin and urobilinogen would be expected to increase.

to exist in hepatocytes or biliary ductular cells. Many injuries, including those from infection and toxins, result in damage to liver cell membranes with resulting loss of cytoplasmic or mitochondrial constituents. Determination of increases in the level of these leaking compounds within the plasma compartment is, therefore, indicative of a loss of cell membrane integrity. An enzyme to be used in the diagnosis of hepatocellular injury should be limited to and in high concentration in the liver. Because most enzymes present in hepatocytes are also present in other tissues, they are generally used in combination with other types of liver function tests in order to achieve the specificity required for diagnosis of liver disease.

Numerous reports can be found in the literature of normal and abnormal levels of enzymes known to leak from hepatocytes as a result of injury. However, reported values vary widely between and within species (Table 12.7). In addition, serum enzymes suspected of originating from liver cells should be evaluated with an understanding that elevations observed may be occurring by processes other than liver cell necrosis (Table 12.8).

Apart from the considerations regarding serum enzyme activity listed in Tables 12.7 and 12.8, the most common cause of increased serum enzyme levels is cell death in which alterations in the cell membrane will cause irreversible loss of cell constituents. Enzymes that are known to increase in concentration in blood after hepatic necrosis are generally divided into two groups, those that are liver-specific and those that are found in other tissues in addition to the liver.

Table 12.7
Reasons for Variations in Reported Serum Enzyme Levels Used in the Diagnosis of Liver Disease

1. Methods for measuring serum enzyme levels vary between laboratories.
2. Normal values vary between species.
3. Normal values depend upon numerous physical and biochemical variables known to affect enzyme activity. Each clinical and/or research laboratory should determine their "normal range" before interpreting values obtained from animals suspected of having liver disease.
4. Age can affect the results. For example, young animals may normally have serum alkaline phosphatase levels two to three times higher than adult animals due to an increased rate of bone metabolism associated with growth.
5. Time of assay after sample collection may affect the results. Several serum enzymes used to diagnose acute liver damage have biological half-lives of only a few hours.
6. Temperature variations may greatly affect enzyme biological activity.
7. The method or site of blood collection may affect results. Hemolysis may elevate serum levels of enzymes known to be present in erythrocytes as well as the cytosol of hepatocytes.
8. The degree of increase in serum enzyme levels depends in large part on the stage and severity of the insult. Enzymes are generally elevated most in acute, extensive liver cell damage and elevated least in chronic conditions when the number of liver cells being destroyed at any one time is low.

Enzymes that are liver-specific are present in high concentrations in hepatic tissue primarily. They include the following three enzymes. Alanine aminotransferase (ALT) is found in primates, dogs, cats, and other small animal species. Use of serum ALT should be confined to small animals and primates because large animals possess little hepatic ALT activity. Second, sorbitol dehydrogenase (SDH), glutamate dehydrogenase (GLDH), and arginase are found in high concentrations in the liver of dogs and most large animals. Levels rise and fall rapidly, in contrast to transaminases, which have a longer half-life. Third, gamma-glutamyltransferase (GGT) is found primarily in biliary tissue and, therefore, is a good indicator of intra- or extrahepatic cholestosis, particularly in ruminants.

Enzymes that are in high concentrations in other tissues in addition to the liver include aspartate aminotransferase (AST), lactate dehydrogenase (LDH), isocitrate dehydrogenase (ICD), and alkaline phosphatase (SAP). Although these enzymes are not liver-specific, they are nonetheless useful diagnostically as a screening test for liver necrosis. If all other tissues known to contain these enzymes are free of pathology, their specificity increases. However, a diagnosis of hepatic necrosis should not be made on the basis of elevation in the serum levels of these nonspecific enzymes alone. They are useful when used in conjunction with other more specific enzymes as well as other nonenzymatic liver function tests.

Table 12.8
Processes Other Than Liver Cell Necrosis That May Elevate Serum Enzymes Used in the Diagnosis of Liver Disease

1. There may be an increased need for a reaction catalyzed by a given enzyme. In this case, an increased enzyme production and/or turnover could lead to increased plasma levels in the absence of cellular necrosis. Prolonged fasting elevates intracellular and serum levels of enzymes needed for gluconeogenesis. Some of these enzymes are used in the assessment of liver disease.
2. Cytoplasmic enzymes such as sorbitol dehydrogenase and creatine phosphokinase are subject to rapid release from cells after a relative minor insult to the plasma membrane. Hauling large animals long distances can cause significant physiological elevations in plasma levels of creatine phosphokinase, and animals with transient gastrointestinal disorders may develop high levels of sorbitol dehydrogenase (22). The animal suffering from chronic liver failure might have only modest elevations of sorbitol dehydrogenase, if any. In contrast, enzymes that are bound in mitochondria require greater insult to the cell before they will be detected in serum.
3. Liver damage may occur in association with or as a result of damage in other organs which themselves elevate serum enzyme levels.
4. There may be a failure to remove enzymes from the circulation in the absence of liver disease. Therefore, inhibitory effects on the reticuloendothelial system or other components of the enzyme degradative and/or excretory mechanism may result in elevated serum enzyme levels unrelated to increased entry (i.e., necrosis) or metabolic need (i.e., fasting). A clinically relevant example of this phenomenon can occur in horses when septicemia leads to macrophage blockage and elevation of serum enzyme levels (22).
5. Liver cell regeneration reflecting an increased production of intracellular enzymes frequently follows acute liver damage.
6. Drug-induced enzyme induction or drug-induced hepatic disease may also elevate serum enzyme levels.

If disturbed liver function is suspected but not confirmed after liver enzyme analysis, other more elaborate tests can be performed including isoenzyme analysis, bile acid analysis, and/or plasma clearance of dyes that are principally removed and excreted by the liver. Prominent among the dyes used clinically are bromosulphalein (BSP) and indocyanine green (ICG). The methodology for using organic anion clearance data for the detection of hepatic dysfunction can be found in recently published works (11, 23–34).

Ancillary Aids to Diagnosis

Ancillary aids to diagnosis such as radiography are useful occasionally. Hepatomegaly caused by inflammation or neoplasia can often be confirmed by plain film radiography, as can the reduction in liver size associated with cirrhosis. Positive contrast radiography is particularly helpful in confirming portal vascular anomalies. The latter procedure, as well as aiding in diagnosis, also helps determine the feasibility of surgery.

The liver biopsy is a more definitive method of

confirming and differentiating various types of liver disease. It is normally performed using a local analgesic technique. False-negative results are possible if an unrepresentative sample is obtained. This is quite possible if lesions are discrete and localized. One of the major complications of liver biopsy is hemorrhage, but fortunately this complication is thought to be relatively uncommon (35, 36).

Options Available for Patient Management

Once it has been determined that a patient has some degree of liver dysfunction, there are several options available to the veterinarian. These are the following:

1. Cancel anesthesia and surgery indefinitely. This is only possible in the case of a purely elective procedure.
2. Perform surgery under local or regional analgesia. Unfortunately, local or regional techniques are not often a practical alternative to general anesthesia in many species.
3. Treat the patient medically until the disease condition improves or resolves. This should be the course of action when the liver disease is ameliorative or the surgical procedure can be delayed.
4. Proceed with anesthesia and surgery in the face of hepatic dysfunction if the disease process is intractable or in the case of a surgical emergency. If this is the case anesthetic agents should be selected with a knowledge of their pharmacokinetics and activity and how these are affected by liver dysfunction. No agent should be used that relies heavily on hepatic metabolism or excretion for its inactivation. Agents that have minimal effects on hepatic blood flow and oxygenation should be selected. Hepatotoxic agents should be avoided at all times. Anesthetic techniques that cause minimal physiological disturbance should be used.

Preanesthetic Preparation

Animals that have been losing fluid and electrolytes from the gastrointestinal tract as a result of vomiting or diarrhea may require plasma volume augmentation as a preoperative measure to restore hemodynamic stability. Because the plasma albumin level is often subnormal in animals with liver disease, care should be taken to avoid superimposed dilutional hypoalbuminemia that may result from injudicious use of crystalloid solutions. Plasma or dextran infusions in conjunction with isotonic electrolyte solutions are invaluable in this situation. Electrolyte depletion is relatively uncommon in animals with hepatic disease; however, a deficiency in total body potassium similar to that seen in man may be encountered (37). It is prudent to ensure that crystalloid solutions used contain at least 4 to 8 meq of potassium/liter to avoid superimposed iatrogenic hypokalemia.

A proportion of patients with liver disease will have low hemoglobin values that result from either nutritional deficiencies, coagulation abnormalities, or gastrointestinal hemorrhage. Transfusion with fresh blood will help restore hematocrit and hemoglobin levels to a more acceptable range. A hemoglobin of 8 g/dl is regarded as the minimum acceptable level prior to surgery and anesthesia. This corresponds to a hematocrit of about 25%, providing the mean corpuscular hemoglobin content is within the normal range. Transfusion with whole blood will also help restore plasma albumin deficiencies; if the blood is fresh, missing clotting factors will also be supplied. Vitamin K_1 is essential in the formation of prothrombin. Daily injections of vitamin K_1 can help correct coagulation problems if they are secondary to impaired vitamin K absorption.

Advanced liver disease is often associated with ascites, which may cause restrictive lung defects as a result of lung compression (38). This type of defect can cause pulmonary arteriovenous shunting with subsequent hypoxemia. Ascitic fluid should be removed by paracentesis shortly before anesthesia to decrease forward pressure on the diaphragm. It should be remembered that this procedure may precipitate cardiovascular collapse unless it is performed correctly. It is important to drain ascitic fluid in a slow, controlled fashion while monitoring such cardiovascular parameters as heart rate and rhythm, pulse quality, the color of mucous membranes, and capillary refill time. Central venous pressure is also a useful measurement under these circumstances. If cardiovascular function deteriorates, aggressive intravenous fluid replacement therapy should be instituted, preferably with a colloidal solution that will be retained within the vascular compartment.

Occasionally, patients with hepatic disease present showing signs of hepatic encephalopathy; however, the disease must be fairly severe before this syndrome appears. Hepatic encephalopathy is currently thought to result from either hyperammonemia, overproduction of false neurotransmitters such as octopamine within the brain, or increased absorption and decreased catabolism of true inhibitory neurotransmitters such as gamma aminobutyric acid (GABA). The common factor is defective handling of the breakdown products of protein metabolism. Clinical signs of hepatic encephalopathy may be ameliorated preoperatively by reducing dietary protein or by judicious use of oral antibiotics that are effective against gram-negative enteric bacteria. In most instances, animals with hepatic encephalopathy are not suitable candidates for surgery. There is, however, at least one reasonably common condition that sometimes lends itself to surgical correction and often presents as hepatic encephalopathy. This condition is portocaval shunt, one of the congenital portal vascular anomalies.

Systemic antibiotics are indicated preoperatively when there is bacterial hepatitis or cholangitis or when proliferation of hepatic bacterial flora is suspected. It is best to chose antibiotics that are metabolized or excreted by the liver.

Premedication

The purpose of premedication is to calm or sedate a nervous or anxious patient before anesthesia and in some instances to minimize side effects of other agents used during anesthesia. It may be necessary to administer sedative premedication to an animal that has hepatic dysfunction. When this occasion arises, it should be remembered that all central depressants have an exaggerated response in patients with hepatic disease (39). Some or all of the following factors may be involved:

1. Increased cerebral sensitivity. It has recently been postulated that there may be an increase in the number of central GABA receptors during chronic liver failure as evidenced by an increased sensitivity of the brain to drugs that mimic the action of GABA, such as benzodiazepines and barbiturates (40).

2. Decreased rate of metabolism. The ability of the liver to metabolize and inactivate drugs is often diminished with hepatic dysfunction.

3. Decreased volume of distribution. When the plasma albumin level is low, the volume of distribution of drugs that bind to albumin is reduced accordingly. A decrease in the volume of distribution can lead to drug overdose, but it should also be noted that as the unbound fraction of drug increases, there is also increased hepatic clearance.

4. Decreased hepatic blood flow. This can occur with, for example, cirrhosis and portocaval shunt. The effects of a decrease in hepatic blood flow are not uniform and depend on the hepatic extraction efficiency of the drug under consideration. The clearance of drugs with a high hepatic extraction efficiency is affected most severely by reductions in hepatic blood flow.

5. Decreased extraction efficiency. Interaction of drugs and hepatic microsomes, known as intrinsic factor, is an important factor in drug clearance. Although various mixed function oxidase enzymes are reduced in advanced liver disease, this does not necessarily imply a decrease in drug clearance.

It can be seen that it is not always possible to predict the precise effects of liver disease on the pharmacokinetic profile of drugs. What is apparent is that it is best to avoid drugs that are extensively cleared or metabolized by the liver. If this is not possible, the veterinarian should be prepared to adjust the dosage and monitor possible side effects that result from overdose toxicity.

The major classes of drugs used for preoperative medication are sedatives, narcotic analgesics, and anticholinergics. Individual agents will be discussed according to this classification in terms of their suitability for premedication in animals with disordered hepatic function.

Sedatives

ACEPROMAZINE

Acepromazine is currently the most widely used phenothiazine tranquilizer. It has the advantage of producing mild to moderate sedation that has a ceiling of activity. There are, however, several considerations regarding the administration of acepromazine to patients with hepatic dysfunction.

First, acepromazine causes alpha adrenergic blockade and consequently lowers systemic vascular resistance and blood pressure. Lowering arterial pressure will tend to decrease hepatic arterial flow and reduce hepatic oxygenation. This effect may be offset by an increase in portal venous flow resulting from a decrease in splanchic vascular resistance. Also, acepromazine has hypothermic activity. The central nervous system (CNS) depressant effects of most drugs are enhanced and hepatic metabolism is prolonged during hypothermia. This is particularly undesirable in patients with hepatic disease.

Acepromazine has weak anticholinesterase activity due to inhibition of plasma cholinesterase (41). The diseased liver may have a reduced ability to synthesize cholinesterase, and premedication with acepromazine may further decrease cholinesterase activity. This would tend to prolong the action of drugs such as procaine or succinylcholine, which are hydrolyzed by plasma cholinesterase.

Acepromazine lowers the convulsive threshold. In animals with hepatic encephalopathy that manifests as seizure activity, acepromazine is best avoided. Finally, phenothiazines have been shown to produce hepatic injury in humans (42). In rare instances, jaundice has developed after a single dose of a phenothiazine tranquilizer (43). The mechanism is thought to be a result of sensitivity to the drug, and the jaundice produced is attributed to cholestasis (44).

Considering the pharmacological actions of acepromazine, it appears that it would be better to avoid it in patients with moderate to severe liver disease. In mild or compensated liver disease, it may be possible to administer low levels of acepromazine (0.05 mg/kg i.m.) without serious untoward effects.

DROPERIDOL, LENPERONE, AND AZAPERONE

These three butyrophenone tranquilizers are often used in the chemical restraint of animals. (For a full description of their uses, refer to Chapter 3.) They have properties similar to those of the phenothiazines, but they tend to be more potent sedatives and have a more potent antiemetic action. Butyrophenones also block alpha-adrenergic antagonists and have hypothermic activity, but they are less potent than the phenothiazines in this respect. Ventilatory depression is not a feature of butyrophenone sedation. Experimental work indicates that droperidol may actually stimulate ventilation in dogs (45). There are points in favor of butyrophenones when compared with phenothiazines in patients with liver disease. These include less respiratory depression and greater stability of systemic blood pressure and body temperature. The more potent antiemetic action of butyrophenones is also beneficial in animals that are vomiting. As a group, these drugs are generally considered to be less toxic than the phenothiazines (41), and studies indicate that hepatic injury in man is less likely than with phenothiazines (44). The same precautions apply to the injudicious use of these potent CNS depressants as apply to phenothiazines. Basically, they should be used with great care in patients with hepatic disorders and should be avoided when liver disease is severe.

XYLAZINE

Xylazine is known to cause considerable physiological depression in a number of animal species (46, 47). Xylazine reduced cardiac output to 37.3% of the control value in one study in dogs, and the arterial partial pressure of oxygen was found to fall significantly (48). In addition, this drug can produce profound CNS depression, marked hyperglycemia, and emesis. We are of the opinion that xylazine is not a suitable premedicant for patients with liver disease.

DIAZEPAM

Although diazepam is not usually classified as a sedative, it can produce soporific and sedative effects in dogs and small ruminants (49, 50). The sedation produced by diazepam is often minimal or unapparent in small animals and horses, but the central depressant action may be enhanced to useful levels in the presence of liver disease. Diazepam offers several advantages over often more commonly used sedative premedicants for use in patients with hepatic disease. These include mild, dose-related CNS depression, little cardiopulmonary depression, anticonvulsant action that increases seizure threshold and muscle relaxation.

Diazepam is metabolized in the liver by a series of biotransformational pathways. Some of the intermediate compounds formed, such as N-desmethyldiazepam and oxazepam, are pharmacologically active and may account for the long duration of action of this drug. Despite the fact that diazepam has been associated with cholestatic jaundice in man (51, 52), it is considered safe to use as a premedicant in patients with compensated liver disease (53).

Narcotic Analgesics

Members of this group of compounds, including those based on the antagonist structure, will be considered together because of similarities of action. Narcotic analgesics or agonist-antagonists commonly used in veterinary anesthesia include morphine, meperidine, oxymorphone, fentanyl, pentazocine, and butorphanol. Studies involving several narcotic analgesics indicate that these agents have little or no adverse effect on the liver (54, 55). Narcotic effects of these drugs may be enhanced in patients with hepatic dysfunction due to increased cerebral sensitivity and an increase in the unbound drug fraction (55). The cardiovascular system is reasonably stable after opiate/opioid premedication, with the exact response varying slightly between drugs and species. Caution should be exercised if morphine is to be given to dogs with hepatic disease because of histamine release. In this species, histamine release causes spasm of the hepatic vein with resultant hepatic congestion. It may be better to avoid morphine in dogs under these circumstances or to use small doses administered intramuscularly. Ventilatory depression occurs in all species after narcotic premedication, but the degree does not appear to be unacceptable judging from reports on the use of several different narcotic analgesics in dogs and horses (56–59). One of the gastrointestinal effects of morphine-related drugs is to increase tone in smooth muscle, including the sphincter of Oddi, an observation that may have significance in obstructive biliary disease. Under these circumstances, agonist-antagonist compounds may be the analgesics of choice (55). Narcotic analgesics are metabolized in the liver at different rates, and their action may be prolonged when hepatic function is reduced. Fortunately, their effects can be antagonized by specific antagonists, such as naloxone. One other fact that should be contemplated before administering morphine to an animal with liver disease is that there can be a significant reduction in urine output as a result of ADH release. This tends to delay renal excretion of other drugs given simultaneously.

Neuroleptanalgesic Combinations

Various combinations of neuroleptic agents and centrally acting analgesic drugs are used for the chemical restraint of a number of species. Innovar Vet is frequently used in small animal anesthesia, and xylazine or acepromazine in combination with morphine, demerol, pentazocine, or butorphanol is used for standing restraint and analgesia in horses. When contemplating such combinations for use in patients with hepatic disease, it is necessary to consider the properties of each agent individually and to make selections accordingly. Innovar Vet, the combination of a butyrophenone and a narcotic analgesic, seems to be a reasonable choice for patients with hepatic disease. The potentially enhanced effects of such a combination, under these circumstances, may necessitate modifying the dose or titrating the combination to effect. In either case, the narcotic antagonist naloxone must be readily available.

Anticholinergic Agents

Atropine is hydrolyzed in plasma and liver by an hepatically synthesized esterase. Its actions, which are peripheral rather than central, may be prolonged in hepatic disease, but such prolongation is usually of little consequence. Scopolamine is a closely related compound that has significant central actions as well as peripheral anticholinergic effects. Scopolamine differs from atropine in another important respect; it is almost entirely hydrolyzed by the liver (60). It would appear from the above considerations that atropine is more suitable than scopolamine for premedication in patients with liver disease.

Induction of Anesthesia

INJECTABLE AGENTS

Barbiturates

Thiobarbiturates. Controversy has existed for years regarding the role of hepatic metabolism in recovery from thiobarbiturate anesthesia. Recent evidence indicates that at least in humans it is unlikely that hepatic metabolism influences the termination of activity of these drugs (61). Despite this evidence, animal experiments have shown a prolongation of the action of thiopental in the presence of hepatic dysfunction (62). The explanation for this may be increased cerebral sensitivity to central depressants, which is known to occur in hepatic disease, and perhaps reduced protein binding, which results from hypoalbuminemia. It is our opinion that thiobarbiturates should be used with extreme caution in patients with mild to moderate degrees of hepatic dysfunction because of attendant risks of overdosage and prolonged recovery. These drugs are contraindicated in severe cases of liver disease in which clinical signs are obvious.

Methohexital. Methohexital is metabolized faster than thiobarbiturates in many species of animals, and there is convincing evidence for a more rapid recovery than occurs with thiopental (63). Arterial levels fall as a result of redistribution to muscle and fat, but hepatic metabolism is so rapid that it too makes a substantial contribution to recovery. Although the action of methohexital will be prolonged in liver disease, the drug should act for a shorter period of time than an equivalent dose of thiopentonal or thiamylal under the same conditions. The precautions that apply to the use of methohexital in patients with reduced hepatic function also apply to thiobarbiturates.

Dissociative Agents—Ketamine

Induction of anesthesia with ketamine can be satisfactorily achieved after premedication with a substantial dose of a sedative drug to prevent undesirable extrapyramidal side effects. As previously discussed in the section on preanesthetic medication, large doses of sedatives are not appropriate where there is a significant degree of liver dysfunction. This factor alone limits the usefulness of ketamine as an anesthetic for animals with hepatic disease. Recovery from the effects of small doses of ketamine is thought to be largely a result of drug redistribution. The majority of an injected dose of ketamine is metabolized in the liver of most species, and the metabolites are excreted in urine. The situation is different in the cat, where 87% of the administered dose is excreted unchanged in urine (64). In species in which hepatic metabolism is largely responsible for clearance of drugs from the circulation, it may be anticipated that recovery from effects of large doses of ketamine will be prolonged. Therefore, ketamine should probably not be used in animals bordering on hepatic failure. Ketamine should also be avoided in animals showing signs of hepatic encephalopathy because the central stimulant action may precipitate seizures. If ketamine is to be used in patients with hepatic disease, it should be reserved for those with mild disturbances and administered at a substantially reduced dosage.

INHALATIONAL INDUCTION

The interaction of inhalational agents with the liver is discussed in detail in the following section. Inhalation induction with an appropriate agent is a relatively safe technique for patients with hepatic dysfunction. It is the method of choice in patients with decompensated liver disease because the depth of anesthesia can be titrated easily depending on the response of the animal. Most if not all inhalation anesthetics undergo some hepatic metabolism, but their primary route of elimination is through the respiratory tract. An inspired oxygen fraction (FIO_2) of at least 0.3 is necessary at all times during induction, and up to 0.5 may be advisable in extremely debilitated patients in order to ensure adequate oxygenation. The administration of oxygen by face mask for a few minutes prior to induction with injectable agents (preoxygenation) is a technique that is useful in patients with a variety of diseases, including hepatobiliary dysfunction. When inhalational induction is used, preoxygenation is implicit in the technique.

Maintenance of Anesthesia

GENERAL POINTS

When a patient with hepatic dysfunction is to be anesthetized, inhalational maintenance of anesthesia is generally preferred to maintenance by continuous or intermittent injection techniques. The level of CNS depression can be controlled more readily with inhalation anesthetics, and risk of cumulacy associated with injectable agents is avoided. The use of an endotracheal tube and anesthetic circuit ensures that the airway is protected, and positive pressure ventilation can be initiated without delay should it become necessary. Oxygen enrichment of inspired air, although not exclusive to inhalational maintenance of anesthesia, is normal practice with this technique. The essence of any good anesthetic technique is to maintain anesthesia at the lightest level compatible with the surgery being performed. If this is ensured by careful monitoring, physiological depression can be minimized. In patients with hepatic dysfunction, liver blood flow and oxygenation should be maintained at optimal levels.

The liver requires an adequate supply of oxygenated blood in order to perform its vital functions. Under normal circumstances, it receives blood from the portal vein (approximately 20% cardiac output) with the remainder derived from the hepatic artery (approximately 7% of cardiac output). Although portal venous blood is poorly oxygenated, it is responsible for about 50% of the oxygen supply to the liver because of its relatively high flow rate. Because vasomotor control to the liver is minimal, a reduction in hepatic blood flow is usually caused by decreased portal venous pressure or hepatic arterial pressure. The former will occur with increased splanchnic vascular resistance, and the latter will occur with decreased systemic vascular resistance (65). Increased hepatic venous pressure compounds both these effects on hepatic blood flow. Anesthetic agents and techniques cause complex direct and indirect effects on hepatic perfusion; in general, however, it is reduced during anesthesia.

Blood gases should be kept within clinically acceptable limits in order to minimize the effects of anesthesia on hepatic blood flow and oxygenation. This can be achieved by avoiding drugs that cause significant ventilatory depression or by the judicious use of positive pressure ventilation. Hypocarbia produced by hyperventilation has been shown to cause a significant decrease in portal blood flow (PBF) and a small decrease in hepatic arterial blood flow (HABF) in anesthetized dogs (66). Hughes (66) showed that adding carbon dioxide to restore normocarbia reverses the changes in PBF but causes a decrease in HABF. The restoration of PBF was ascribed to the direct effects of carbon dioxide in reducing splanchnic vascular resistance. The initial fall in HABF was thought to be due to the effects of positive pressure ventilation in increasing hepatic venous pressure, and the subsequent fall was considered to be the result of carbon dioxide increasing sinusoidal pressure. In the same trial it was demonstrated that hypoxia causes a transient decrease in PBF and a significant but transient fall in HABF. The author suggested that the fall in HABF was caused by the stress response to hypoxia affecting the hepatic artery.

Techniques or agents that reduce cardiac output and increase systemic vascular resistance will cause a reduction in hepatic blood flow. A fall in cardiac output directly reduces HABF, and increased systemic vascular resistance reduces PBF. Many anesthetic techniques are associated with a fall in cardiac output. Under normal conditions, portal blood flow is strongly dependent on cardiac output (67). Any decrease in PBF is usually accompanied by an increase in HABF. It has been suggested that this is a compensatory mechanism maintaining oxygen supply to the liver—a form of hepatic autoregulation. This autoregulation is lost during deep anesthesia. Most inhalational anesthetic agents cause a dose-dependent reduction in hepatic blood flow. Some agents, however, produce more profound reductions than others and should be avoided when choosing a technique of anesthesia for the patient with reduced liver function.

INHALATIONAL AGENTS

Halothane

The primary circulatory effect of halothane is to produce a concentration-related fall in arterial blood pressure that is largely related to a fall in cardiac output (68). HABF is also decreased during halothane anesthesia, a reduction which correlates well with changes in cardiac output and mean arterial pressure in the dog (69). PBF is reduced by halothane; this effect appears to be proportional to the drop in cardiac output (69). To minimize reductions in HABF and PBF and thus maintain hepatic oxygenation, the inspired halothane concentration should be kept as low as possible to avoid undue depression of cardiac output and mean arterial pressure.

Respiration is depressed under halothane anesthesia with arterial carbon dioxide normally increased in relation to the depth of anesthesia (70). Arterial oxygenation, however, is rarely depressed providing that the inspired gas mixture contains at least 30% oxygen. Modest increases in arterial carbon dioxide have been shown to increase PBF and decrease HABF with a resultant increase in liver blood flow (66). As a result of this work, it was postulated that hypercarbia may be beneficial to the liver by increasing blood flow without changing oxygen consumption.

Although at one time all inhalational anesthetics except trichloroethylene were considered to be metabolically inert, it is now evident that all of these agents with the possible exception of nitrous oxide are at least partially biotransformed in the liver. Evidence exists to show that halothane undergoes metabolism catalyzed by enzymes of the mixed function oxidase system (cytochrome P-450) bound to the endoplasmic reticulum (71–78). These enzymes are most highly concentrated in hepatocytes (79). Approximately 20% of the administered dose of halothane is oxidized to the nontoxic end product trifluoroacetic acid under normal aerobic conditions (75, 80). When anaerobic conditions prevail, particularly when these enzyme systems have been induced by phenobarbital, halothane can be reduced to free radicals that bind to microsomal phospholipids and proteins and promote hepatocyte lipid peroxidation (81).

Halothane, like phenobarbital, induces hepatic enzymes of the cytochrome P-450 system by increasing cytochrome P-450 synthesis and possibly turnover (82). Earlier studies of bilirubin formation have shown a precursor heme pool exists within hepatocytes that may freely exchange with heme of cytochrome P-450 (83). Little is known of the identity and intracellular localization of the free heme pool, but it might be viewed as a pool of relatively small size and rapid rate of turnover into which newly synthesized heme is fed and out of which heme is drawn for synthesis of hemoprotein or degradation to bile pigments (bilirubin). It is possible that acute induction of microsomal enzymes with resultant stimulation of heme turnover could in part account for the enhanced bilirubin excretion observed in ponies under halothane anesthesia (15) (Fig. 12.42).

Both hypoxia and liver enzyme induction are normally required for the development of "halothane associated hepatitis" (HAH) in the rat model (84). This is apparently not true in all species. Recently, a guinea pig model has been described in which liver damage occurs in about 60% of animals exposed to 1% halothane in 21% oxygen for 4 hours (85). Whatever its role in HAH in a particular species, hypoxia must be avoided during anesthesia for all the usual reasons, including the fact that hepatic hypoxia per se can cause centrilobular hepatic necrosis.

Genetic factors have been implicated in the genesis of halothane-associated lver injury, as have immunological mechanisms. The latter were predicated on rather empiric phenomena of higher attack rates after a second administration of halothane (86). Halothane hepatitis is a rare condition in humans with an incidence of serious hepatic damage ranging from 1:6,000 to 1:110,000 (87). It may also be rare in animal species, but the exact incidence remains unknown. Recently, a case of hepatic necrosis was reported in a dog after halothane anesthesia (88), but the evidence in this case was not conclusive. We observed a case of severe hepatic dysfunction after halothane anesthesia in a horse, but again it was impossible to rule out other causes.

Despite its equivocal potential for causing hepatitis, halothane is not necessarily contraindicated in the presence of liver disease. It should, however, be used at low concentrations because of its effects on liver blood flow. In the unlikely event of having to anesthetize a patient who has previously experienced hepatitis after halothane anesthesia, halothane should be avoided due to potential for a hypersensitivity reaction (89).

Methoxyflurane

Methoxyflurane has effects on the cardiovascular system that are similar to those of halothane (90, 91). Despite this, methoxyflurane anesthesia is associated with an even more marked reduction in hepatic blood flow than halothane in humans (92). Respiration is depressed slightly more by methoxyflurane than it is by halothane, and it may be necessary to control ventilation in order to avoid respiratory acidosis (90, 91).

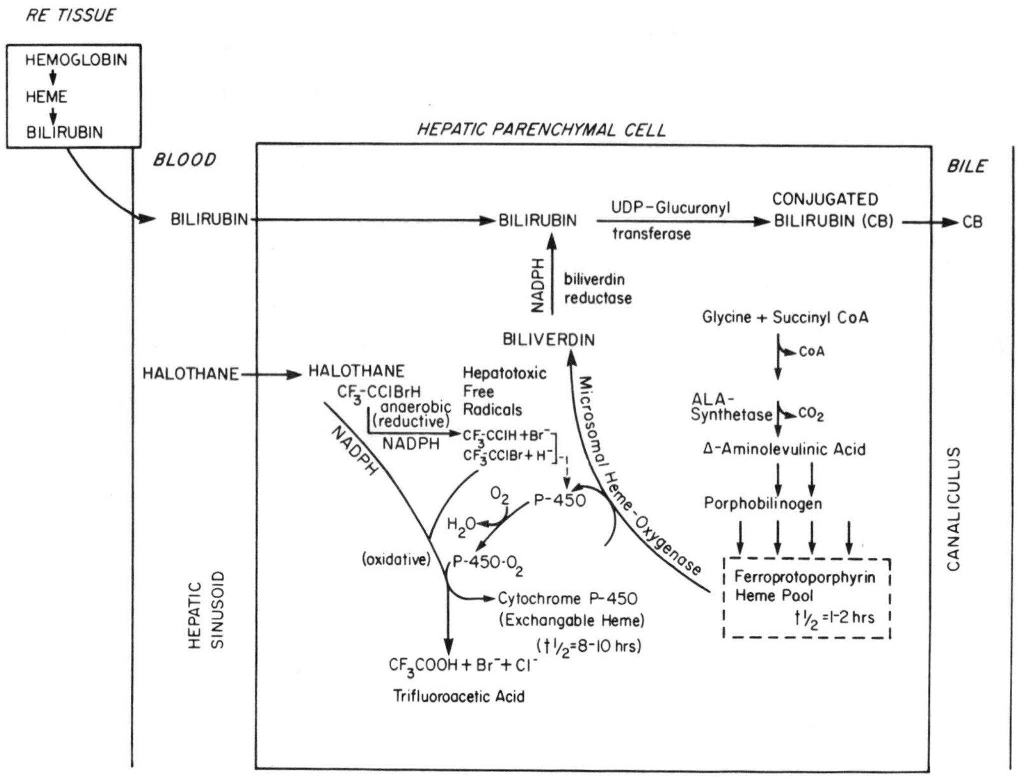

Figure 12.42. Proposed scheme of hepatic halothane degradation in ponies and its potential influence on the enhancement of hepatic bilirubin production. RE, reticuloendothelial, NADPH, reduced form of nicotinamide adenine dinucleotide phosphate; UDP, uridine 5-diphosphate; CoA, coenzyme A, ALA, aminolevulinic acid; t½, half-life (15).

In keeping with the usual principles, the inspired concentration should be kept as low as possible to minimize both circulatory and respiratory effects of this anesthetic.

Like halothane, methoxyflurane undergoes significant biotransformation in the liver with the formation of oxalic acid, free fluoride, and chloride ions (93). The degree of biotransformation is greater than that for halothane, and hepatic degradation accounts for up to 50% of methoxyflurane uptake from the lungs (94). There have been several cases of methoxyflurane-associated hepatotoxicity reported in both humans and animals (95–97); however, postoperative renal dysfunction (attributable to free fluoride ions) appears to be more classically associated with methoxyflurane toxicity in humans (98). Possible mechanisms for the generation of postoperative hepatic dysfunction are similar to those for halothane-associated hepatitis (95). It has also been suggested that cross sensitization may occur with halothane (91). Until further information becomes available, it would be prudent to avoid methoxyflurane in patients who have previously experienced postoperative hepatitis after exposure to methoxyflurane or halothane anesthesia. If methoxyflurane is used in patients with hepatic dysfunction, it should be used at minimal concentrations to avoid depression of arterial blood pressure, alveolar ventilation, and hepatic blood flow.

Isoflurane

This agent is a potent volatile anesthetic agent that has physical properties similar to those of its isomer, enflurane (99–101). It is one of the most widely used anesthetics in human medicine. Isoflurane has been reported to lower arterial blood pressure in a dose-related fashion. The reduction in blood pressure is similar to that seen with halothane; unlike halothane, however, hypotension is largely related to a fall in peripheral resistance. Portal blood flow has been found to decrease during isoflurane anesthesia, but not as dramatically as with halothane, and hepatic arterial blood flow has been found to increase (69). Increased hepatic arterial flow tends to preserve hepatic oxygen supply during isoflurane anesthesia, a characteristic that favors its use in patients with hepatic disease. Ventilation is depressed more with isoflurane than with halothane, yet carbon dioxide levels during spontaneous ventilation remain at or near normal values in the clinical situation (100).

Isoflurane is subject to little or no biotransformation in humans; the average recovery in exhaled air is

95% (101). Miniature swine have no measurable hepatic uptake of isoflurane at various subanesthetic concentrations (94). The significance of volatile anesthetic metabolism lies in the association between metabolism and liver or kidney toxicosis (102). The minimal metabolism of isoflurane suggests that this anesthetic probably is neither hepatotoxic nor nephrotoxic, and data from animal studies to date support this hypothesis (103). Biotransformation, if it occurs, is only minimal, and no reductive metabolites have been demonstrated (104). Pretreatment of rats with phenobarbital (to induce liver enzymes) and 1 MAC isoflurane anesthesia for 2 hours under hypoxic conditions do not produce hepatic necrosis. Under similar circumstances, 1 MAC halothane anesthesia causes measurable hepatotoxicity (105). Also, in rats pretreated with phenobarbital, a sham abdominal operation under isoflurane anesthesia does not produce hepatic necrosis, while the same operation under halothane anesthesia does (106). Recent studies on the effects of isoflurane anesthesia in ponies indicate that although isoflurane enhances biliary bilirubin excretion, its effects on hepatic bilirubin formation and/or clearance are modest (107). In addition, bile acid excretion and bile formation are not significantly affected. These results indicate that the heme-containing cytochrome P-450 pool may be affected less by isoflurane than by halothane, an hypothesis that is consistent with current knowledge regarding the minimal metabolism of isoflurane.

Liver enzyme analysis and hepatic function tests indicate that there appears to be fewer deleterious effects on the liver with isoflurane than with either methoxyflurane or halothane. Methoxyflurane and halothane anesthesia result in elevated AST levels and significant reductions in postoperative BSP clearance (108). Isoflurane, on the other hand, appears to leave hepatic function virtually intact (108).

From the forgoing discussion, isoflurane appears to be the agent of choice for patients with hepatic disease or patients who have experienced jaundice after administration of other anesthetic agents. Nonetheless, in keeping with good anesthetic practice, the level of anesthesia should be maintained in a light plane and the inspired gas mixture should have an FIO_2 of at least 0.3. This is particularly important in patients with decompensated liver disease where considerations other than direct or indirect hepatotoxicity assume great importance.

Nitrous Oxide

Nitrous oxide is useful in patients with hepatic disease because it reduces the requirement of the more potent volatile anesthetics, such as halothane, while causing minimal physiological depression. Nitrous oxide may have a slight negative inotropic and chronotropic effect on the heart and is thought to produce alpha-adrenoreceptor stimulation of the peripheral circulation (91). Arterial blood pressure appears to be maintained, and there is a moderate reduction in hepatic blood flow (109).

Ventilatory parameters are unaffected by nitrous oxide. The only serious respiratory problem reported to date is arterial hypoxia, which occurs if the FIO_2 is inadequate. Diffusion hypoxia may complicate recovery from nitrous oxide anesthesia if the inspired gas is not enriched with oxygen for the first 5 to 10 minutes after discontinuation.

There is no evidence of biotransformation of nitrous oxide by the liver, but centrilobular hepatic cell degeneration attributable to nitrous oxide has been shown to occur in the hypoxic rat model (104). This is an interesting observation that opens the door to new speculations regarding the mechanism of hepatotoxicity of all anesthetics. From a clinical perspective, it reinforces the importance of avoiding hepatic hypoxia. This is particularly important in patients with preexisting hepatic disease.

MUSCLE RELAXANTS

Nondepolarizing Agents

For reasons that are not entirely clear, patients with liver disease may be resistant to nondepolarizing muscle relaxant drugs (65). Because large doses may have to be given to obtain the desired effect, problems may be encountered in reversing the effects of these agents at the end of surgery. Vecuronium is mainly cleared from plasma by hepatic uptake and biliary elimination. This agent should, therefore, be avoided in patients with disturbed liver function (110). Pancuronium and gallamine are respectively largely or exclusively excreted in urine and may be satisfactory for patients with hepatic dysfunction providing renal function is not impaired. Atracurium is a new muscle relaxant that has a short duration of action terminated largely by temperature and pH-dependent Hoffman elimination. For this reason, it is the logical choice for patients with liver disease. Its action has been reported to be remarkably unaffected by hepatic failure (110).

Depolarizing Relaxants

Succinylcholine is the only member of this group of compounds that has been used to any extent in veterinary practice. It is metabolized by plasma cholinesterase, and its action may be prolonged in patients with liver disease when plasma levels of this hepatically synthesized enzyme are low. It is recommended that succinylcholine be avoided in patients with liver disease.

Mephenesin-like "Centrally-Acting" Muscle Relaxants

Guaifenesin is the most commonly used compound in this group. It is frequently used in equine anesthesia, but has also been recommended for other species (111, 112). Guaifenesin produces little cardiopulmonary depression; however, its action is terminated by hepatic metabolism and may be prolonged where there is disturbed hepatic function. Because cardiovascular and ventilatory function are little affected by this relaxant drug, the prolonged duration of action may not be too serious a problem.

Monitoring and Supportive Therapy

Monitoring and recording the vital functions of the patient should be the major activity of the anesthetist during anesthesia. The disequilibrating effects of the patient's disease, the surgery, and the anesthetic agents can then be counteracted by "titrated management"(113). Patients with hepatic dysfunction should have the following parameters monitored at frequent intervals: heart rate and rhythm, blood pressure, respiratory rate and depth, body temperature, and, where possible, blood gases. It may also be useful to monitor blood glucose, hematocrit, total serum solids, and urine output, depending on the severity of liver damage.

Supportive therapy should be directed at normalizing any imbalance detected. The cardiovascular system may be supported by appropriate use of vasoactive drugs as well as blood volume replacement therapy. An indwelling wide-bore intravenous catheter should be placed prior to anesthesia to facilitate such therapy. It is recommended that an isotonic crystalloid solution be administered at a rate of 5 to 10 ml/kg/hour throughout the anesthesia period to keep the intravenous line patent, meet maintenance requirements, and offset plasma volume discrepancies that result from "third spacing" or minor blood loss. Faster rates of infusion may be indicated as circumstances dictate.

When crystalloid solutions are used for plasma volume replacement, care should be taken to avoid inducing a dilutational hypoalbuminemia. This can be prevented by monitoring the total serum protein level and changing to colloidal fluid administration when total serum protein levels approach 3.5 g/dl.

Ventilatory function is best monitored by serial blood gas analysis of arterial blood samples. When this is impractical, a Wright's respirometer may be used to determine the minute ventilatory volume. Respiratory rate and character should also be evaluated. If ventilation is inadequate, it may be necessary to institute intermittent positive pressure ventilation. Controlled ventilation is always indicated when neuromuscular blocking agents are used.

It is important to maintain body temperature within normal limits due to the detrimental effects of hypothermia on the biotransformation of drugs. Body core temperature should be monitored at regular intervals using a properly placed rectal probe or esophageal probe. A circulating hot water blanket is an effective device for minimizing surface cooling, and pulmonary cooling can be avoided by humidification of inspired gas (114).

Recovery

Recovery from anesthesia should be supervised and intensively monitored in patients with significant hepatic disturbance. A primary concern is that the stress of anesthesia and surgery, coupled with the increased half-life of many anesthetic agents, may prolong recovery and create a setting for the gradual physiological deterioration of the animal. A prolonged recovery may be inevitable in some cases; however, physiological deterioration during this period may be circumvented by appropriate therapy. Recovery should be monitored carefully, and supportive therapy should be provided in much the same way as during the maintenance phase of anesthesia. Oxygen, intravenous fluids, and heat should be supplied until patients can support their own vital functions. It may be necessary to administer glucose intravenously in seriously debilitated patients. The requirement for carbohydrate therapy is best determined by monitoring the blood glucose level. Analgesia should be provided as necessary and can improve recovery by making it less unpleasant and stressful and therefore less physiologically taxing for the patient. Local or regional analgesic techniques are preferred for postoperative pain relief, but it may be necessary to resort to the judicious use of narcotic analgesics either alone or in combination with modest doses of appropriate tranquilizers.

References

1. Anwer MS, Hegner D: Sodium chloride dependency of dibucaine—and procaine—induced choleresis in isolated perfused rat livers. *J Pharmacol Exp Ther* 225:284–290, 1982.
2. Tennant BC, Hornbuckle WE: Diseases of the liver. In *Veterinary Gastroenterology*, ed 1. Philadelphia, Lea & Febiger, 1980.
3. Hjerpe CA, Tennant BC, Crenshaw GL, Baker NF: Ovine fascioliasis in California. *J Am Vet Med Assoc* 159:1266, 1971.
4. Finn JP, Tennant B: Hepatic encephalopathy in cattle. *Cornell Vet* 64:136, 1974.

5. Tennant B, Baldwin B, Evans CD, Keneko JJ: Diseases of the equine liver. *Proc Am Assoc Equine Pract*, 21st Annual Meeting, Boston, 1975, p 410.
6. Gronwall R: Effects of fasting on hepatic function in ponies. *Am J Vet Res* 36:145–148, 1975.6.
7. Gronwall R, Mia AS: Fasting hyperbilirubinemia in horses. *Am J Dig Dis* 17:473–476, 1972.
8. Engelking LR, Gronwall R: Effects of fasting on hepatic bile acid clearance. *Proc Soc Exp Biol Med* 161:123–127, 1979.
9. Gronwall R, Engelking LR, Noonan N: Direct measurement of biliary bilirubin excretion in ponies during fasting. *Am J Vet Res* 41:124–126, 1980.
10. Gronwall R, Engelking LR: Effect of glucose administration on equine fasting hyperbilirubinemia. *Am J Vet Res* 43:801–803, 1982.
11. Engelking LR, Anwer MS, Lofstedt J: Hepatobiliary transport of indocyannie green and sullfobromophthalein in fed and fasted horses. *Am J Vet Res*, 46(11):2278–84, 1985.
12. Thomsett LR: Acute hepatic failure in the horse. *Equine Vet J* 3:15, 1971.
13. Strombeck DR, Krum S, Rogers Q: Coagulopathy and encephalopathy in a dog with acute hepatic necrosis. *J Am Vet Med Assoc* 169:813–816, 1976.
14. Badylak SF, Dodds J, Van Fleet JF: Plasma coagulation factor abnormalities in dogs with naturally occurring hepatic disease. *Am J Vet Res* 44:2336–2340, 1983.
15. Engelking LR, Dodman NH, Hartman G, Valdez H, Spivak W: Effects of halothane anesthesia on equine liver function. *Am J Vet Res* 45:607–615, 1984.
16. Hijmans van den Bergh A, Muller P: Ueber eine direkte und indirekte Diazoreaktion auf Bilirubin. *Biochem Z* 77:90–103, 1916.
17. Talafant E: Properties and composition of bile pigment giving a direct diazo reaction. *Nature* 2:312, 1956.
18. Schmid R: The identification of "direct reacting" bilirubin as bilirubin glucuronide. *J Biol Chem* 229:881–888, 1957.
19. Billing B, Cole P, Lathe G: The excretion of bilirubin as a diglucuronide giving the direct van den Bergh reaction. *Biochem J* 229:881–888, 1957.
20. Van Hootegam P, Fevery J, Blanchkaert N: Serum bilirubins in hepatobiliary disease: comparison with other liver function tests and changes in the postobstructive period. *Hepatology* 5:112–117, 1985.
21. Cornelius CE: Liver function. In *Clinical Biochemistry of Domestic Animals*, ed 3. New York, Academic Press, 1980.
22. Coffman JR: *Equine Clinical Chemistry and Pathophysiology.* Bonner Springs, KA, Veterinary Medicine Publishing Company, 1981.
23. Paumgartner G: The handling of indocyanine green by the liver. *Schweiz Med Wochenschr* (suppl) 105:1–30, 1975.
24. Gronwall R, Cornelius CE: Maximal biliary excretion of sullfobromophthalein sodium in sheep. *Am J Dig Dis* 15:37–47, 1970.
25. Center SA, Bunch SE, Baldwin BH, Hornbuckle WE, Tennant BC: Comparison of sulfobromophthalein and indocyanine green clearances in the dog. *Am J Vet Res* 44:722–726, 1983.
26. Center SA, Bunch SE, Baldwin BH, Hornbuckle WE, Tennant BC: Comparison of sulfobromophthalein and indocyanine green clearances in the cat. *Am J Vet Res* 44:727–730, 1983.
27. Anwer MS, Engelking LR, Gronwall R, et al: Plasma bile acid elevation following CCl_4 induced liver damage in dogs, sheep, calves and ponies. *Res Vet Sci* 20:127–130, 1976.
28. Anwer MS, Gronwall R, Engelking LR, et al: Bile acid kinetics and bile secretion in the pony. *Am J Physiol* 229:592–597, 1975.
29. Engelking LR, Gronwall R, Anwer MS: Effect of bile acid on hepatic excretion and storage of bilirubin in ponies. *Am J Vet Res* 37:47–50, 1976.
30. Engelking LR, Gronwall R, Anwer MS: Effect of dehydrocholic, chenodeoxycholic, and taurocholic acids on the excretion of bilirubin. *Am J Vet Res* 41:355–361, 1980.
31. Engelking LR, Gronwall R: Bile acid clearance in sheep with hereditary hyperbilirubinemia. *Am J Vet Res* 40:1277–1280, 1979.
32. Engelking LR, Barnes S, Dasher CA, Naftel DC, Hirschowitz BI: Radiolabeled bile acid clearance in control subjects and patients with liver disease. *Clin Sci* 57:499–508, 1979.
33. Jones MB, Weinstock S, Kovetz R: Clinical value of serum bile acid levels in chronic hepatitis. *Digest Dis Sci* 26:978–983, 1981.
34. Mannes GA, Stellard F, Paumgartner G: Increased bile acids in cirrhosis with normal transaminases. *Digestion* 25:217–221, 1982.
35. McGill DB: Predicting hemorrhage after liver biopsy. *Digestive Diseases and Sciences* 26:385–387, 1981.
36. Feldman EC, Ettinger SJ: Percutaneous transthoracic liver biopsy in the dog: a review of 75 cases. *Calif Vet* 13:17–22, 1977.
37. Casey TH, Summerskill WHJ, Orvis AL: Body and serum potassium in liver disease. *Gastroenterology* 48:198–207, 1965.
38. Borland LM, Roule M, Cooke DR: Anesthesia for pediatric orthotopic liver transplantation. *Anesth Analg* 64:117–24, 1985.
39. Ettinger SJ: *Textbook of Veterinary Internal Medicine: Diseases of the Dog and Cat*, ed 2. Philadelphia, WB Saunders Co, 1983, Vol 2, p 1424.
40. Jones AE, Schafer DF, Ferenci P, Pappas SC: The neurobiology of hepatic encephalopathy. *Hepatology* 4:1235–1242, 1985.
41. Booth NH, McDonald LE: *Veterinary Pharmacology and Therapeutics*, ed 5. Ames, IA, Iowa State University Press, 1982, pp 321–337.
42. Ebert MH, Shader RI: Hepatic effects. In Shader RI, DiMascio A (eds): *Psychotropic Drug Side Effects: Clinical and Theoretical Considerations.* Baltimore, Williams and Wilkins, 1970, pp 175–197.
43. Zarowitz H, Friedman IS: Jaundice following small amounts of chlorpromazine. *NY J Med* 57:1922, 1957.
44. Zimmerman HJ: *Hepatotoxicity: The Adverse Effects of Drugs and Other Chemicals on the Liver.* New York, Appleton-Century-Crofts, 1978, pp 398–404.
45. Glen JB: Neuroleptanalgesia with "Thalamonal Vet" in the dog. *Assoc Vet Anesth Gr Britain and Ireland, Proceedings* 1:38–48, 1970.
46. Clarke KW, Hall LW: "Xylazine"—A new sedative for horses and cattle. *Vet Rec* 85:512–516, 1969.
47. Klide AM, Calderwood HW, Soma LR: Cardiopulmonary effects of xylazine in dogs. *Am J Vet Res* 36:931–935, 1975.
48. McDonell W, Van Gorder J: Cardiopulmonary effects of xylazine/ketamine in dogs. In *Proceedings of American College of Veterinary Anesthesiologists Scientific Meeting*, Las Vegas, Oct 21, 1982, p 28.
49. Hall LW: Prolonged anaesthesia. *J Sm An Pract* 17(10):661–668, 1976.
50. Hall LW, Clarke KW: *Veterinary Anaesthesia:* London, Balliere Tindall, 1983, p 273.
51. Fors B, Nilsson F: Hepatitis probably induced by diazepam medication. *Laekartidningen* 65:4528, 1968.
52. Stacher G: Intrahepatische Cholestase nach einer hochdosierten Kombinationstherapie mit Diazepam and Barbituren bei Tetanus-Patienten. *Wien Klin Wochenschr* 22:401, 1973.
53. Strunin L: Anesthesia for patients with diminished hepatic function. In Gray TC, Nunn JF, Utting JE (eds): *General Anaesthesia*, ed 4. London, Butterworths, 1980, pp 779–795.
54. Zimmerman HJ: *Hepatotoxicity: The Adverse Effects of Drugs and Other Chemicals on the Liver.* New York, Appleton-Century-Crofts, 1978, p 546.
55. White PF: Selection of narcotic and administration technique in class I and II patients. *35th Annual Refresher Course Lectures*

and Clinical Update Program 505:1–7, 1984.
56. Trim CM: Cardiopulmonary effects of butorphanol tartrate in dogs. *Am J Vet Res* 44:329–331, 1983.
57. Muir WW, Skarda RT, Sheehan WC: Hemodynamic and respiratory effects of xylazine-morphine sulfate in horses. *Am J Vet Res* 40:1417–1420, 1979.
58. Robertson JT, Muir WW: A new analgesic drug combination in the horse. *Am J Vet Res* 44:1667–1669, 1983.
59. Short CE, Greenwald W, Bendick F: Oxygen, carbon dioxide, and pH responses in arterial blood of dogs given analgesic, neurolept analgesic, and ataractic agents. *J Am Vet Med Assoc* 156:1406–1414, 1970.
60. Cullumbine H: Cholinergic blocking drugs. In *Drill's Pharmacology in Medicine*, ed 4. New York, McGraw-Hill Co, 1971, pp 608–625.
61. Burch PG, Stanski DR: The role of metabolism and protein binding in thiopental anesthesia. *Anesthesiology* 58:146–152, 1983.
62. Dundee JW, Clarke RSJ: Non-inhalational anaesthetics. In Gray TC, Nunn JF, Utting J (eds): *General Anaesthesia*, ed 4. London, Butterworths, 1980, pp 217–255.
63. Hall LW, Clarke KW: *Veterinary Anaesthesia*, ed 8. London, Bailliere Tindall, 1984, p 308.
64. Lumb WV, Jones EW: *Veterinary Anesthesia*, ed 2. Philadelphia, Lea & Febiger, 1984, p 308.
65. Strunin L: Anesthesia for patients with diminished hepatic function. In Gray TC, Nunn JF, Utting JE (eds): *General Anesthesia*, ed 4. London, Butterworths, 1980, pp 779–795.
66. Hughes RL: Liver blood flow and blood gases in the greyhound. *Association of Veterinary Anaesthetists of Great Britain and Ireland*, Proceedings No. 8 (1978–1979), pp 55–58.
67. Bulkey GB, Kvietys PR, Perry MA, Granger DN: Effects of cardiac tamponade on colonic hemodynamics and oxygen uptake. *Am J Physiol* 244:G604–612, 1983.
68. Prys-Roberts C, Gersh BJ, Baker AB, Reuben SR: The effects of halothane on the interactions between myocardial contractility, aortic impedance and left ventricular performance. *Br J Anaesth* 44:634–649, 1972.
69. Gelman S, Fowler KC, Smith LR: Liver circulation and function during isoflurane and halothane anesthesia. *Anesthesiology* 61:726–730, 1984.
70. Merkel G, Eger EI: A study of halothane and halopropane anesthesia including method for determining equipotency. *Anesthesiology* 24:346, 1963.
71. Conn HO: Halothane-associated hepatitis: a disease of medical progress. *ISR J Med Sci* 10:404–415, 1974.
72. Van Dyke RA, Gandolfi AJ: Anaerobic release of fluoride from halothane: relationship to the binding of halothane metabolites to hepatic cellular constituents. *Drug Metab Dispos* 4:40–44, 1976.
73. Benumof JL, Bookstein JJ, Saidman LJ: Diminished hepatic arterial flow during halothane administration. *Anesthesiology* 45:545–551, 1976.
74. McLain GE, Sipes IG, Brown BR: An animal model of halothane hepatotoxicity: roles of enzyme induction and hypoxia. *Anesthesiology* 51:321–326, 1979.
75. Kubic VL, Anders MW: Mechanism of the microsomal reduction of carbon tetrachloride and halothane. *Chem Biol Interact* 34:201–297, 1981.
76. Van Dyke RA, Wood CL: In vitro studies on irreversible binding of halothane metabolite to microsomes. *Drug Metab Dispos* 3:51–57, 1975.
77. Van Dyke RA, Wood DL: Binding of radioactivity from ^{14}C-labeled halothane in isolated perfused rat livers. *Anesthesiology* 38:328–332, 1973.
78. Brown BR Jr, Sagalyn AM: Hepatic microsomal enzyme induction by inhalation anesthetics: mechanisms in the rat. *Anesthesiology* 40:152–161, 1974.
79. Benson GJ, Brock KA: Halothane-associated hepatitis and methoxyflurane-related nephropathy: a review. *J Vet Pharmacol Ther* 3:187–196, 1980.
80. Cousins MJ, Sharp JH, Gourlay GK: Hepatotoxicity and halothane metabolism in an animal model with application for human toxicity. *Anaesth Intensive Care* 7:9–24, 1979.
81. Brown BR: Hepatic microsomal lipoperoxidation and inhalation anesthetics: a biochemical and morphologic study in the rat. *Anesthesiology* 36:458–465, 1972.
82. Van Dyke RA, Chenweth MB, Poznak A. Metabolism of volatile anesthetics. I. Conversion in vivo of several anesthetics to CO_2 and chloride. *Biochem Pharmacol* 13:1239–1248, 1964.
83. Schmid R: Synthesis and degradation of microsomal hemoproteins. *Drug Metab Dispos* 1:256–258, 1973.
84. Cousins MK: Mechanisms and evaluation of hepatotoxicity. In *1984 ASA Annual Refresher Course Lectures*, 204:1–7, 1984.
85. Lunam CA, Hall P de la M, Cousins MJ: Halothane hepatitis in a guinea pig model in the absence of enzyme induction and hypoxia. *Clinc Exp Pharmacol Physiol* 9:469–470, 1982.
86. Brown BR: Anesthetic hepatotoxicity. *ASA Annual Refresher Course Lectures*, 138A:1–4, 1981.
87. Cahalan MK: Post-operative hepatic dysfunction. In *1982 ASA Annual Refresher Course Lectures*, 133:1–3, 1982.
88. Meuten DJ, Pecquet-Goad ME: Hepatic necrosis associated with use of halothane in a dog. *J Am Vet Med Assoc* 184:478–480, 1984.
89. Cahalan MK: Do anesthetics cause hepatotoxicity? In *1983 ASA Annual Refresher Course Lectures*, 209:1–4, 1983.
90. Steffey EP, Farver TB, Wolinjer MJ: Circulatory and respiratory effects of methoxyflurane in dogs: comparison of halothane. *Am J Vet Res* 45:2574–2579, 1984.
91. Black GW: Cardiovascular, respiratory and hepatic effects of inhalational anesthesia. In Gray TC, Nunn JF, Utting JE (eds): *General Anaesthesia*. London, Butterworths, 1980, pp 159–187.
92. Price HL, Pauca AL: Effects of anesthesia on the peripheral circulation. *Clin Anesth* 3:73, 1969.
93. Halsey MJ: Biotransformation of anaesthetics in relation to toxicity. In Gray TC, Nunn JF, Utting JE (eds): *General Anaesthesia*. London, Butterworths, 1980, pp 141–158.
94. Halsey MJ, Sawyer DC, Eger EI: Hepatic metabolism of halothane, methoxyflurane, cyclopropane, Ethrane, and Forane in miniature swine. *Anesthesiology* 35:43–47, 1971.
95. Zimmerman HJ: *Hepatotoxicity: The Adverse Effects of Drugs and Other Chemicals on the Liver*. New York, Appleton-Century-Crofts, 1978, pp 387–388.
96. Ndiritu CG, Weigel J: Hepatorenal injury in a dog associated with methoxyflurane: a case report. *Vet Med/Small Animal Clin* 71:545–550, 1977.
97. Douglas TA, Jennings S, Longstreeth J, Weaver AD: Methoxyflurane anesthesia in horses and cattle. *Vet Rec* 76:615–623, 1964.
98. Benson GJ, Brock KA: Halothane-associated hepatitis and methoxyflurane-related nephropathy: a review. *J Vet Pharmacol Therap* 3:187–196, 1980.
99. Vitcha JF: A history of Forane. *Anesthesiology* 35:4–7, 1971.
100. Eger EI II: *Isoflurane (Forane): A Compendium and Reference*. Madison, Ohio, Medical Products, 1981.
101. Eger EI II: Isoflurane: A review. *Anesthesiology* 55:559–576, 1981.
102. Cohen EN, Van Dyke: *Metabolism of Volatile Anesthetics: Implications of Toxicity*. Reading, MA, Addison-Wesley, 1977.
103. Byles PH, Dobkin AB, Ferguson JH: Forane (compound 469). II Biochemical effects of repeated administration to animals, response to bleeding, and compatability with epinephrine. *Can Anaesth Soc J* 18:387–396, 1971.
104. Fassoulaki A, Eger ER II, Johnson BH, Ferrell LD, Smuckler EA, Harper MH, Eger RR, Cahalan MK: Nitrous oxide, too, is hepa-

totoxic in rats. *Anesth Analg* 63:1076–1080, 1984.
105. Harper MH, Collins P, Johnson B: Hepatic injury following halothane, enflurane, and isoflurane anesthesia in rats. *Anesthesiology* 56:14–17, 1982.
106. Harper MH, Collins P, Johnson B: Decrease in hepatic blood flow may cause hepatic injury during halothane anesthesia. *Anesth Analg (Cleve)* 60:253–254, 1981.
107. Engelking LR, Dodman H, Hartman G, Valdez H: Effects of isoflurane anesthesia on equine liver function. *Am J Vet Res* 45:616–619, 1984.
108. Stevens WC, Eger EI II, Joas TA: Comparative toxicity of isoflurane, halothane, fluroxene and diethyl ether in human volunteers. *Can Anaesth Soc J* 20:327, 1973.
109. Thompson IA, Hughes RL, Fitch W, Campbell D: Effect of nitrous oxide on liver haemodynamics and oxygen consumption in the greyhound. *Anaesthesia* 37:548–553, 1982.
110. Savarese JJ: Do the newer muscle relaxants offer any advantage over the old? *1984 ASA Annual Refresher Course Lectures* 221:1–6, 1984.
111. Thurmon JC, Tranquilli WJ, Benson GJ: Glyceral guaiacolate, ketamine and xylazine; balanced anesthesia by intravenous infusion in swine. *Proceedings of ACVA Scientific Meeting*, October 12, 1984, p 21.
112. Benson GJ, Thurmon JC, Tranquili WJ: Intravenous infusion of glycral guaiacolare, ketamine and xylazine in dogs: cardiopulmonary responses. *Proceedings of ACVA Scientific Meeting*, October 12, 1984, p 21.
113. Winter PM, Miller JN: Anesthesiology. *Scientific American* 252(4):124–131, 1985.
114. Dodman NH, Brito-Babapulle LAP: The role of humidification in anaesthesia. *Association of Veterinary Anaesthetist of Great Britain and Ireland, Proceedings No. 8* (1978–1979), pp 141–152.

PART 6

Anesthesia and the Kidney: Special Considerations

G. JOHN BENSON, D.V.M., M.S., D.A.C.V.A., and J. C. THURMON, D.V.M., M.S., D.A.C.V.A.

Anatomy and Physiology

The kidneys are paired organs making up about 0.3% (cow) to 1.3% (cat) of total body weight (1). Structurally, they consist of three anatomical zones, the cortex, outer medulla, and inner medulla. They are located retroperitoneally on either side of the vertebral column against the dorsal body wall (2, 3). The kidney's primary contribution to maintaining homeostasis is by filtration, reabsorption, and secretion. These processes are integrated to accomplish the functions of regulation and composition of body fluids, detoxification and secretion of nonessential materials, participation in extrarenal regulatory mechanisms, and endocrine function (3).

Although the kidneys comprise approximately 0.4% of total body mass, they receive 20 to 25% of cardiac output; thus, the kidneys receive more blood per gram of tissue than other organs, including heart, brain, liver, and exercising skeletal muscle (4). The kidney has the highest oxygen consumption per gram of tissue of any major organ (6 ml/100 g/min). Its blood flow is much greater than that required to provide oxygen and metabolic substrates (2, 4). Whereas 25% of the oxygen consumed is required to maintain basal function, 75% is used primarily for the purpose of active sodium ion reabsorption. Because blood flow determines filtration rate and, therefore, the amount of sodium presented for reabsorption, oxygen consumption is proportional to and determined by blood flow (2–4). As a result, the kidney is unique in that the arterial-venous oxygen difference is constant and low (i.e., 1 to 2 ml/100 ml).

From the large blood flow, the renal glomeruli filter nearly 50 to 60 times the plasma volume daily (2). This glomerular filtrate has the same crystalloid concentration as plasma and is extensively reabsorbed by the renal tubules. Although water reabsorption varies to regulate plasma volume, nearly all the sodium and chloride presented to the tubules is reabsorbed. Potassium and hydrogen ions may be actively secreted. In addition, tubular cells manufacture ammonia, which removes hydrogen ions in the urine as ammonium ions. Thus, the kidney controls plasma osmolality and acid-base balance (2, 3).

Renal regulation of hydrogen ion concentration occurs principally by alteration of bicarbonate concentration in the extracellular fluid. This is accomplished through hydrogen ion secretion, sodium ion reabsorption, bicarbonate ion excretion, and ammonia secretion. Hydrogen ion secretion into tubular fluid occurs in the epithelial cells of the proximal tubules, distal tubules, and collecting ducts. Carbon dioxide in the presence of carbonic anhydrase combines with water to form carbonic acid in the tubular epithelial cells that dissociates into hydrogen ions and bicarbonate ions. Hydrogen ions are excreted into the lumen of the renal tubule in exchange for sodium ions. These hydrogen ions combine with filtered bicarbonate ions in the renal tubules to form carbonic acid, which disassociates into carbon dioxide and water. Essentially all of the carbon dioxide diffuses into the paratubular tissue; the water is secreted in the urine. As a result, if sufficient hydrogen ions are available, nearly all of the bicarbonate ions in the glomerular filtrate are removed from the tubules. When pH is above 7.40, the ratio of bicarbonate ions filtered into the tubules to hydrogen ions secreted increases; thus, more bicarbonate ions enter the tubules than hydrogen ions. Because bicarbonate ions cannot be reabsorbed without first reacting with hydrogen ions, the excess bicarbonate ions pass into the urine, and alkalosis is relieved (5).

In acidosis, the ratio of carbon dioxide to bicarbonate ions in extracellular fluid increases. As a result, the rate of hydrogen ion secretion exceeds the rate of bicarbonate filtration; thus excess hydrogen ions are excreted into the urine, relieving acidosis. The excess hydrogen ions entering the renal tubules are buffered by filtered phosphate and secreted ammonia ions (5).

If plasma glucose concentration does not exceed the proximal renal tubules' capacity for reabsorption, it will not appear in the urine. Normally, urine is protein-free (1). The kidney is the only route of elimination of protein metabolites, especially urea and creatinine. Lastly, urine is the major source of excretion of water-soluble drugs and their conjugates. Although most drug metabolism occurs in the liver, renal tissue has microsomal oxidase enzyme systems that allow some drug metabolism to occur in the kidney (6).

The functional unit of the kidney is the nephron. Nephrons are classified as either superficial or juxtamedullary according to location and length of their tubular structure (Fig. 12.43). Although both types originate in the cortex, approximately 85% are superficial and have short loops of Henle. Of the nephrons, 15% are located in the juxtamedullary area and have long loops of Henle that dip deep into the renal papilla. The glomeruli and proximal and distal convoluted tubules are confined to the cortical portion of the kidney. These structures receive approximately 80% of the renal blood flow. Henle's loop and the major portion of each collecting duct are located in the renal medulla. These structures receive blood from the vasa recta, which are derived from the efferent arterioles of the juxtamedullary nephron (2, 3, 5, 7).

Glomerular filtrate flows from the glomerular capsule into the proximal tubule consisting of a convoluted segment (pars convoluta) and a straight segment (pars recta). Fluids exit the pars recta and enters the thin segment of the loop of Henle. The thin segment descends, reverses direction, and terminates at the thick segment of Henle's loop (2). The thick segment of the loop of Henle ascends and terminates in the distal tubule in contact with the glomerulus (from which it originates) and with its associated afferent and efferent arterioles. These three structures comprise the juxtamedullary glomerular apparatus (2). The distal convoluted tubule enters the collecting duct, which terminates in a papilla, delivering urine to the renal pelvis. Juxtamedullary nephrons are characterized by larger glomeruli and longer proximal tubules and longer loops of Henle that extend deep into the medulla. Thus, the renal medulla consists of the long loops of Henle derived from the juxtamedullary nephrons, the collecting ducts, and the vasa recta (2, 3, 5, 7).

The renal arteries arise from the aorta and give rise to several interlobular arteries. These divide to form the arcuate arteries located between the renal cortex and medulla. The arcuate arteries send numerous parallel branches toward the renal surface, giving rise to the glomerular afferent arterioles that terminate in the glomerulus. Glomerular capillaries coalesce to form glomerular efferent arterioles. These branch to form the peritubular network. In the juxtamedullary region, the efferent arterioles divide. One division forms the peritubular network that surrounds the loop of Henle and collecting ducts in the outer medulla. The others form bundles of vessels (vasa recta) that penetrate deeply into the medulla before further branching and forming a capillary network around the thin loop of Henle in the inner medulla. The vasa recta makes no contact with the proximal tubules (2, 3, 7, 8) (Fig. 12.43).

The glomerular efferent and afferent arterioles are

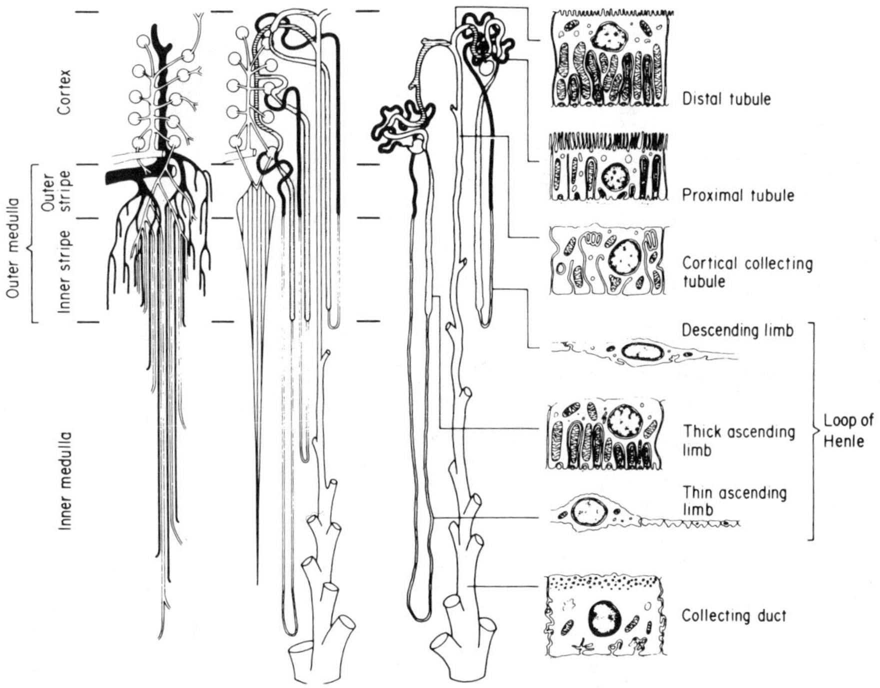

Figure 12.43. "Vascular and tubular structures of the kidney. *Left panel:* Arrangement of the blood vessels. Arteries are shown in white, veins in solid black. The largest artery shown, the arcuate artery, runs parallel to the surface of the kidney near the junction of the cortex and outer medulla. The interlobular artery branches off the arcuate artery and runs toward the surface of the kidney. Afferent arterioles branch from the interlobular artery and enter glomeruli, shown as spheres. Efferent arterioles leave the glomeruli. Efferent arterioles from the glomeruli closest to the medulla form descending vasa recta, which are blood vessels that run straight into the medulla. The venous drainage follows the arterial supply. *Middle panel:* Relationship between the tubules and the arteries, arterioles, and glomeruli. *Right panel:* Two nephrons. The one closest to the surface is a superficial nephron. This type, which represents the majority of the nephrons in each kidney, has a relatively short loop of Henle, with a descending limb that turns precisely at the junction of the inner and outer medullary zones. Superficial nephrons have no thin ascending limbs. The longer tubule is a juxtamedullary nephron. The descending limb runs into the inner medulla some distance before turning. The thin ascending limb runs parallel to the descending limb and changes morphology abruptly at the margin of inner and outer zones of the medulla. Thick ascending limbs from juxtamedullary and superficial nephrons are indistinguishable from each other. The figures on the far right show the major ultrastructural features of each nephron segment." Reproduced with permission from Marsh DJ: *Renal Physiology*, ed 1. Copyright 1983 by Raven Press, New York.

the most important control areas of renal blood flow and have the greatest resistance in the renal vascular tree. Normally, glomerular blood flow is controlled so that approximately 20% of glomerular plasma is filtered into the tubules. Capillary hydrostatic pressure is the major force favoring glomerular filtration (2). It is dependent on cardiac output, systemic arterial blood pressure, and the vascular tone of the afferent and efferent arterioles. This filtration pressure is opposed by plasma osmotic pressure and the capsular or tubular hydrostatic pressure (2). In addition, the glomerular filtration rate (GFR) is dependent not only on the filtration pressure but upon glomerular permeability (10 to 100 times greater than that of other capillaries) and upon total glomerular surface area (2).

Unlike the arterioles of other organs, the afferent and efferent arterioles present low resistance. As a result, there is always some blood flow in all renal capillaries rather than the vasomotion (i.e., intermittent opening and closing of capillaries) that occurs in other body tissues (2, 3). In addition to extrinsic neural and hormonal regulation, the kidney is equipped with an intrinsic mechanism that automatically regulates renal blood flow (RBF). This autoregulation maintains RBF and GFR relatively constantly over an arterial blood pressure range variously reported to be 60 to 160 to 80–180 mm Hg (2–4, 8, 9). This autoregulation occurs within the kidney itself and is mediated by changing arteriolar tone, especially in the afferent arterioles, by mechanisms that have not been fully elucidated. Each nephron controls its own GFR. In addition, autoregulation is influenced by several extrarenal factors. Central blood volume affects RBF and consequently GFR, probably by atrial stretch receptors. Hypovolemia, sodium depletion, and states of low cardiac output induce renin release and angiotensin synthesis leading to decreased RBF and GFR (2).

Autoregulation is of importance because it protects glomerular capillaries from large increases in pressure occurring during hypertensive episodes and maintains glomerular filtration and renal tubular function during periods of modest hypotension. RBF is pressure-dependent outside the range of mean arterial pressure associated with autoregulation (3).

Neural regulation of RBF results from sympathetic vasoconstrictor fibers arising from thoracolumbar spinal segments passing through the celiac and renal plexuses (3, 8). There is no sympathetic dilator innervation of the kidney. Parasympathetic fibers innervate the arterioles, probably passing via the renal hilum; however, their function is unknown (2, 3). At rest in a neutral thermal environment, RBF is autoregulated, and there is little sympathetic influence. During minimal or moderate stress, RBF decreases slightly whereas GFR is maintained, suggesting efferent arteriolar constriction. Severe stress such as that caused by hypoxia, strenuous exercise, pain, hemorrhage, or general anesthesia induces large decreases in both RBF and GFR. These responses are thought to be mediated by sympathetic activity (2–4). Alpha and beta adrenergic receptors are found in the arterioles, with the former greatly outnumbering the latter. At all dose levels, epinephrine and norepinephrine induce arteriolar constriction. Dopamine is present in high concentration in the renal cortex. In low doses (1 to 3 μg/kg/min), dopamine induces vasodilation mediated by specific receptors located in the renal arterioles. When given in high doses (i.e., greater than 10 μg/kg/min) dopamine induces vasoconstriction via alpha adrenergic receptor stimulation. In spite of this information, the physiological role of dopamine in regulation of renal hemodynamics has not been fully elucidated (2–4). Sympathetic nervous stimulation induces renal vascular constriction and markedly decreases RBF even when mean arterial pressure is within the range associated with autoregulation (3, 8).

Renin is released from the juxtaglomerular cells in response to sympathetic nervous stimulation, decreased renal perfusion pressure, and decreased sodium delivery to the distal convoluted tubules. Renin and alpha 2 globulin in plasma react to form angiotensin I. In the lung, angiotensin I is converted to angiotensin II, which is a potent pressor and renal vessel constrictor (2–4, 6). Furthermore, angiotensin II induces the release of aldosterone from the adrenal cortex. The net effects of angiotensin II are similar to those induced by epinephrine infusion. Small amounts decrease RBF without altering GFR; larger concentrations decrease both RBF and GFR. Thus, decreased renal blood flow occurring during hemorrhagic hypotension results from increased circulating concentrations of catecholamines, angiotensin, and aldosterone (2–4, 8). Prostaglandins PGE_2 and PGI_2 are produced in the renal medulla (8). Their release is stimulated by increased concentration of angiotensin II and increased sympathetic activity. The prostaglandins are vasodilators that tend to offset the decrease in RBF induced by the renin-angiotensin system. Prostaglandins regulate intrarenal blood flow by increasing flow to the outer cortical nephrons and decrease medullary flow. This results in increased sodium excretion independent of GFR and diuresis. At the present time, there is no evidence that other vasoactive hormones in physiological concentration (e.g., vasopressin or serotonin) affect total RBF or regulate intrarenal distribution of blood flow (2–4, 6–9).

The renal tubules function to decrease the quantity of glomerular filtrate and alter its composition through reabsorption and excretion. The proximal convoluted tubule and loop of Henle are a direct continuation of Bowman's capsule of the glomerulus. In the proximal convoluted tubule, most of the filtered sodium, chloride, potassium, bicarbonate, protein, and water are reabsorbed into the peritubular capillaries (2, 4–6). Glucose is actively reabsorbed in the proximal convoluted tubule (10). Parathormone promotes reabsorption of calcium and excretion of phosphate by the proximal convoluted tubules (6). Urea is passively reabsorbed in the proximal tubules and collecting ducts, especially when urine flow is decreased. Organic anions are poorly filtered at the glomerulus because they are protein-bound. They are secreted in the proximal tubules. In addition to endogenous substances, these include penicillins, cephalosporins, diuretics, and salicylates. Organic cations are also secreted in the proximal tubules and include catecholamines, atropine, and morphine. The net result is that, although 60 to 70% of the glomerular filtrate is reabsorbed in the proximal tubules, only minor changes in composition occur due to concurrent passive reabsorption of water (2, 3, 7, 10).

The loop of Henle and the vasa recta function through the well-known countercurrent mechanism. This mechanism is most efficient in the juxtamedullary nephron, which reabsorbs a further 15 to 20% of solute and water from the nephron. In addition, a major osmotic mechanism is established in the renal medulla to allow further reabsorption of water from the collecting ducts. The descending portion of the loop of Henle has no known active transport mechanism. Because the interstitial concentration of sodium, chloride, and urea increases as the loop of Henle extends deeper into the medulla, there is a progressive movement of water out of the loop and into the surrounding interstitium and hence into the vasa recta. This medullary osmotic gradient is created by active reabsorption of sodium and chloride by both the ascending segment of the thin loop and the thick segment of the loop of Henle and by reabsorption of urea by the collecting ducts. The distal tubule is a functional extension of the thick ascending limb. Active salt transport (i.e., reabsorption of sodium and excretion of potassium and hydrogen) continues under the regulation of aldosterone. Because permeability to water is low, tubular fluid becomes progressively more dilute. Vasopressin increases water permeability of the distal portion of the distal tubule, resulting in passive reabsorption of water and conservation of body fluid. The collecting duct is poorly permeable to electrolytes and water, but active transport mechanisms exist for active reabsorption of salts. However, the duct can become freely permeable to water in the presence of vasopressin, allowing the composition of the residual filtrate to be adjusted to yield urine of appropriate volume and composition compatible with homeostasis (1–3, 5).

Effects of Anesthetics on Renal Function

After general anesthesia, all measures of urinary function are temporarily depressed, including RBF, GFR, urinary flow rate, and electrolyte excretion (2, 9, 11–22). Similar changes are observed after spinal or epidural anesthesia, with the magnitude of change proportional to the degree of sympathetic blockade. Generally, spinal or epidural anesthesia induces one-third to one-half the decrease in renal function of general anesthesia (3). A number of factors contribute to the generalized decrease in renal function associated with anesthesia and surgery. They include physical status of the patient, especially cardiovascular and renal systems; pre- and intraoperative blood volume; type and duration of surgical procedure; fluid and electrolyte balance; depth of anesthesia; and anesthetic agents (2, 3). In general, alterations in renal function associated with anesthesia and surgery are completely reversible (3). After short, uncomplicated procedures, RBF and GFR return to normal within a few hours. Where surgery is extensive and anesthesia is prolonged, secondary endocrine effects may be manifested by impaired ability to excrete water or concentrate urine. These effects may persist for several days (23, 24). The alteration in renal function induced by anesthetic agents is due to indirect effects on the circulatory, sympathetic nervous, and endocrine systems and direct effects upon tubular transport mechanisms (e.g., sodium and para-aminohippurate (PAH)). Thus, measurements of RBF based upon PAH clearance in anesthetized patients may be invalid (2, 4). In general, the indirect effects of anesthetic agents upon renal function are thought to be more important than are direct effects.

Anesthesia and surgery may induce major disturbances in the circulation, resulting in equally major alteration in renal hemodynamics and tubular function. Renal blood flow may be decreased subsequent to hypotension, renal vasoconstriction, or a combination of both. Because all anesthetics directly depress the myocardium, arterial blood pressure is proportional to depth of anesthesia and dependent on peripheral vasocular tone (3). During ether anesthesia, blood pressure is maintained by increased concentration of circulating catecholamines. This increase in catecholamines induces a marked increase in renal vascular resistance, resulting in decreased RBF and GFR (3). Halothane, enflurane, isoflurane, methoxyflurane, and thiopental anesthesia are not accompanied by increased catecholamine response (3, 25). However, a moderate increase in renal vascular resistance and decreased RBF and GFR occur in response to vascular hypotension induced by myocardial depression and peripheral vasodilation (2, 3).

It appears that circulating catecholamines induce a marked decrease in cortical perfusion and redistribution of intrarenal blood flow. This redistribution may be prevented by alpha blockade but not by prophylactic administration of mannitol. Therefore, administration of anesthetics or anesthetic adjuncts having alpha adrenergic blocking activity (e.g., acetylpromazine) will tend to preserve renal hemodynamics (26, 27).

Hemorrhagic shock induces a decrease in RBF and altered distribution of cortical blood flow at a mean arterial pressure of 70 mm Hg in dogs. Systemic vasoconstriction that involves the kidney is induced by increased sympathetic tone to maintain arterial blood pressure. Thus, renal blood flow is severely decreased at blood pressures normally within the range of autoregulation (60 to 160 mm Hg to 80 to 180 mm Hg) (2, 28, 29).

Indirect Sympathetic Nervous Effects

Glomerular filtration rate is maintained by regulation of RBF. During mild to moderate stress, RBF is decreased, but filtration fraction (GFR/RBF) increases such that GFR remains constant, suggesting efferent renal arteriolar constriction. Severe stress (i.e., general anesthesia, pain, severe exercise, and hemorrhage) decreases RBF and GFR through increased sympathetic nervous activity. It appears that the decrease in RBF and GFR induced by general anesthesia is a result of increased sympathetic tone (2, 3, 30). In contrast, spinal or epidural anesthesia induces minimal alteration in renal function if systemic blood pressure is maintained (2, 9, 21, 22). In the perioperative period, renal function is influenced by endocrine activity. Vasopressin is the most important regulator of urine volume. Renin, angiotensin, aldosterone, epinephrine, and norepinephrine regulate electrolyte excretion and RBF (5). It is widely accepted that general anesthetic agents and opioid receptor agonists induce vasopressin release. This effect and the decreased GFR associated with the volatile inhalation anesthetics are a major cause of decreased urine production and increased urine concentration that may follow anesthesia (31).

Vasopressin release induced by preoperative withholding of water may be preventd by preoperative intravenous administration of crystalloid solutions (32). However, vasopressin release by anxiety, pain, or anesthetic induction may still occur (2). In addition, hemodynamic alterations induced by hemorrhage and intermittent positive pressure ventilation (IPPV), even though arterial CO_2 is decreased, may cause vasopressin release via reflex baroreceptor mechanisms (33).

Renin release during anesthesia and surgery may be stimulated by sodium depletion, increased circulating catecholamines, increased sympathetic tone, and decreased RBF. It has been demonstrated that renin concentration in peripheral blood increases with surgical stimulation but not with anesthetic drug administration (2, 3, 9, 34).

Aldosterone is produced in the zona glomerulosa of the adrenal cortex and is responsible for moment-to-moment control of sodium excretion (2, 7). It is not known whether or not anesthetics act directly on the adrenal gland to cause aldosterone release (3). Anesthetics probably act indirectly by (*a*) inducing vasopressin release that subsequently stimulates ACTH release; (*b*) stimulating the sympathetic nervous system, inducing renal vasoconstriction leading to renin and ultimately angiotensin II formation; and (*c*) inducing peripheral vasodilation that via bioreceptor reflexes leads to activation of the renin-angiotensin system (3, 9). In summary, it is not possible to separate the effects upon renal function of anesthesia per se from those of anxiety, pain, surgical stimulation, or blood loss. Nevertheless, the renal effects of anesthesia appear to be dose-related and ameliorated by adequate replacement of extracellular fluids (2). It is not known whether the effects of anesthesia are greater in the diseased kidney than in normal kidneys, although this would appear to be a logical assumption (2).

Evaluation of Renal Function

Renal function is evaluated preoperatively by laboratory tests that reflect GFR and renal tubular function. Because these tests are not sensitive measurements, significant renal disease may exist despite normal laboratory values (8, 10, 35). In addition, trends are more valuable than single tests for evaluation of renal function. Evaluation of renal function should not be time-consuming for the veterinarian or veterinary assistants and should be accomplished with minimal cost (8, 10, 35). Urine-specific gravity is the only part of urinalysis that directly relates to kidney function. Although a urine low specific gravity is not diagnostic of renal dysfunction, it indicates that renal or extrarenal disease may exist (10). Renal tubular dysfunction is established when the kidneys do not excrete appropriately concentrated urine in the face of a physiological stimulus that elicits vasopressin release (8). Other portions of the urinalysis, such as casts and proteinuria, may indicate that renal damage has occurred but do not provide information on renal functional capacity (10).

Blood urea nitrogen (BUN) concentration varies with GFR. However, BUN may be a potentially misleading indicator of renal function because of the influence of diet, other illnesses, or intravascular fluid volume (10). Diets high in protein or gastrointestinal bleeding result in increased BUN despite a normal GFR (35). Other causes for increased BUN in the presence of normal GFR include increased protein catabolism during a febrile disease and dehydration (10). Dehydration causes increased BUN through increased urea absorption due to slow movement of filtrate through renal tubules. When this occurs, serum creatinine concentration remains normal (8, 10). A low protein diet, pregnancy, or hepatic dysfunction may result in normal BUN concentration even though GFR is reduced (8, 10).

Serum creatinine concentration is a specific indicator of GFR. Unlike BUN concentration, serum creatinine is not influenced by protein metabolism nor by the rate of fluid flow through the renal tubules (8, 10, 35). In general, serum creatinine levels are proportional to GFR. Creatinine is a product of skeletal muscle metabolism, the release of which into the circulation is believed to be relatively constant (8, 10, 35). Thus, creatinine serum concentration varies with body composition (muscle mass) and physical activities. In most domestic species, measurement of serum creatinine and BUN is a rough estimate of GFR (10). Although creatinine is the better indicator of GFR, its nonrenal elimination increases progressively as degree of azotemia increases. Therefore, serum creatinine may not be proportional to renal creatinine clearance (10). Thus, BUN may correlate more directly with symptoms of uremia than does serum creatinine. Because BUN and serum creatinine can be determined relatively simply, they are logical methods for assessing renal function (10). Normal values for BUN and serum creatinine and ability to concentrate urine are evidence that renal dysfunction is not an imminent threat to life (10). Unless there is specific reason to question renal function (i.e., proteinuria or casts), clinical analysis is discontinued at this point. In the absence of proteinuria or casts, it is recognized that normal BUN, serum creatinine, and urine concentrating ability may be present with loss of up to two-thirds of renal parenchyma (10). Conversely, abnormal levels of BUN or serum creatinine are indicative of prerenal, primary renal, or postrenal abnormalities. When azotemia is severe, little if any additional relevant clinical information is derived from application of more sensitive tests (10). Additional tests to evaluate renal function are indicated when BUN, serum creatinine or urine specific gravity are normal or equivocal, but it is of importance to establish that adequate renal reserve exists (10).

Pathophysiology of Renal Failure

Renal failure may be categorized as acute or chronic. Acute renal failure is defined as a relatively abrupt and severe decrease in renal function that is potentially reversible in a patient previously normal. Acute renal failure has been further cateogorized as prerenal, parenchymal, or postrenal. The term "prerenal" implies that the decreased renal function is induced by dehydration or impared renal perfusion resulting from cardiovascular dysfunction and is reversible upon correction of the systemic abnormality (36). However, prerenal dysfunction probably represents a state of impaired perfusion that if prolonged will progress to structural damage and parenchymal dysfunction (36). Parenchymal or primary renal failure may be induced by a variety of nephrotoxins (e.g., heavy metals, oxalates, aminoglycoside antibiotics, sulfonamides, hemoglobin, or myoglobin nephropathy), immunological processes, infectious diseases, and ischemia (10). Ischemic renal failure may be caused by major venous or arterial occlusion or relative renal ischemia, which may produce acute renal tissue necrosis (36). The mechanism by which all these etiologies induce renal damage has not been definitively established. Possible mechanisms include renal vasoconstriction, tubular blockade with intraluminal debris, and interstitial edema and total reabsorption (passive backflow) of glomerular filtrate (33, 36, 37).

The most reliable indication of acute renal failure is a progressive rise in BUN and serum creatinine (6). Although most animals with acute renal failure have anuria or severe oliguria, nonoliguria or polyuria may occur (10). The normal or increased urine output that sometimes occurs with acute renal failure may result from a failure of the animal to secrete vasopressin (6, 10). In addition, those nephrons that are functional may produce a reasonable volume of urine in an effort to excrete the solute load presented to them. Nevertheless, retention of substances occurs because functional nephrons cannot excrete the total load required to maintain homeostasis (6).

Chronic renal failure implies that the dysfunction is not reversible and usually is due to some inherent disease of the kidneys themselves. It is often the consequences of slow insidious destruction of renal parenchyma. Clinical signs of disease may not develop for years after the onset because of the kidney's reserve capacity. Thus, definitive determination of etiology is difficult (6). In chronic renal failure, the number of functional nephrons is gradually reduced, followed by a consequent decrease in GFR. Because solute load is undiminished, the remaining functioning nephrons are in a state of diuresis. This results in polyuria, inability to concentrate urine, and decreased ability of the distal tubules to conserve cations, acidify urine, or form ammonia (6, 10). Water and electrolyte imbalances and metabolic acidosis account for most of the clinical manifestations of chronic renal failure (6, 10). Retention of substances such as urea and phosphates have only limited clinical effects until advanced renal failure has developed (6). Common causes of chronic renal failure include immunological destruction of renal tissue, urinary tract infection, urinary tract obstruction, congenital lesions, and hypertension (6).

Clinical Picture of Renal Failure

The clinical and biochemical features of acute and chronic renal failure are similar, although the time course of development may vary (6). Azotemia and increased serum phosphate concentration occur with severe renal failure of any duration (10). With a sudden onset of renal failure, concentration of these and other blood components normally excreted by the kidney may increase progressively from day to day. In contrast, chronic renal failure may result in a stable level of function with concentration of retained elements remaining relatively constant until further functional alterations occur (10). Hyperkalemia is a common feature of anuric renal failure and has major clinical significance. During anuria, hyperkalemia is the result of release of intracellular potassium in association with body cell injury and death, intracellular to extracellular shift that occurs with acidosis, and continued dietary intake of potassium. Death from renal failure is the result of cardiac arrest induced by hyperkalemia (10).

Water overload with development of edema may result from the inability to control water excretion in renal failure. This does not usually occur in domestic animals because of normal water loss via the skin and lungs, adipsia, and vomiting (10). However, fluid restriction may lead to dehydration in patients still capable of excreting some urine in an attempt to rid the body of a high solute load and in those incapable of concentrating urine because of insufficient renal tubular function (10). In anuric patients, administration of parenteral fluids may result in overhydration. In addition, hypertension may result from retention of sodium and, concomitantly, water. In renal failure, normal urinary excretion of hydrogen ions does not occur. This results in retention of hydrogen ions and decreased pH (6, 8, 35). Because the kidney is unable to metabolize parathormone, phosphate is retained, limiting the kidney's ability to excrete hydrogen ions and increasing urinary loss of bicarbonate, which results in a metabolic acidosis (6, 10). Plasma calcium concentration is often normal but may be decreased with renal failure. Because of acidosis, renal tubular reabsorption of calcium ions is decreased. In addition, decreased absorption of calcium from the gut occurs due to deficiency of vitamin D resulting from insufficient renal conversion of precursors to active vitamin D (6). Secondary hyperparathyroidism occurs in an attempt to mobilize calcium from the bone (10).

Similar to potassium, magnesium excretion is impaired although plasma concentration may be normal (35). Cardiac dysrhythmias and insufficiency, commonly occurring in animals with renal failure, are the result of alterations in the relationship of sodium, calcium, hydroxyl, potassium, magnesium, and hydrogen ions (6). In addition to electrolyte disturbances, various metabolites, including urea, creatinine, amines, and urochromogen, are retained in the plasma. Amines are thought to cause lassitude and nausea characteristic of acute renal failure (6). Alterations in blood components caused by acute anuric failure are a direct result of anuria. Thus, identical alterations will be seen with anuria of extrarenal origin (10). Urethral obstruction commonly occurs in dogs, cats, and ruminants; traumatic rupture of the urinary bladder is common in dogs. In cats with an obstructed urethra, azotemia is accompanied by metabolic acidosis, mild hyponatremia, hyperkalemia, hypermagnesemia, hypocalcemia, hyperphosphotemia, hyperglycemia, and hyperproteinemia (10). Rupture of the urinary bladder in the dog is characterized by hyperkalemia, marked hyponatremia, hypochloremia, hyperphosphotemia, and metabolic acidosis, which may be respiratory-compensated (10). Rupture of the urinary bladder secondary to trauma or urolithiasis is common in cattle and small ruminants. Hyponatremia and hypochloremia occur during uroperitoneum in ruminants. Unlike nonruminant species, hyperkalemia and acidosis are not constant features. Either acidosis or alkalosis occurs, and hypokalemia may be present (38). Because urea can be recycled to usable protein via the rumen, azotemia may not be present if the animal continues to eat and has normal ruminal microflora. Furthermore, serum urea values greater than 300 mg/dl have been reported in normal cattle. Therefore, azotemia is not a reliable indicator of renal disease in ruminants (38). Nevertheless, renal failure in cattle has been associated with increased BUN and serum creatinine, hypochloremia, hypokalemia, hypocalcemia, hyponatremia, hyperphosphotemia, hypermagnesmia, and metabolic alkalosis (38).

A common feature of renal failure is anemia resulting from insufficient synthesis of erythropoietin (6, 8, 35). A contributing factor to the anemia is gastrointestinal bleeding. Patients compensate for anemia associated with renal failure by increasing cardiac output and through increased production of 2,3-diphosphoglycerate (2,3 DPG) (6, 8, 35). In cases where blood volume is normal, blood viscosity is decreased as a result of decreased red blood cell mass. In addition, metabolic acidosis shifts the oxygen-hemoglobin dissociation curve to the right (6, 8, 35). In patients with renal failure, blood transfusion has no long-term benefit and may, in fact, temporarily increase depression of bone marrow function (6). Further, blood transfusion will increase the load of potassium, sodium, water, and hemoglobin, which may have adverse effects upon the patient and renal function. Bleeding diathesis, prolonged partial prothromboplastin time, and high plasma fibrinogen concentration have been associated with uremia in cattle (35, 39, 40). Features of renal failure are given in Table 12.9.

Acute Postoperative Renal Failure

In humans, acute renal failure (ARF) in surgical patients is a highly lethal complication having a mortality rate ranging from 40 to 90% for nonoliguric and anuric forms, respectively (37). In clinical practice, more than 80% of ARF is due to acute tubular necrosis. This is predominately vascular in origin and as such is termed "vasomotor nephropathy" (33). A reduction in RBF of more than 50 to 75% induces sustained afferent arteriolar constriction and cortical ischemia (33). In addition, renin-angiotensin activation occurs, which

Table 12.9
A Summary of Clinical Conditions Associated with Renal Failure

Anemia
Hypertension
Increased cardiac output
Coagulopathy due to decreased platelet adhesiveness
Nausea
Vomiting
Diarrhea
Decreased resistance to systemic infection
Hepatitis
Hyperparathyroidism
Altered intravascular fluid volume as a result of inability to concentrate urine
Congestive heart failure, cardiomegaly, or myocarditis
Hyperkalemia
Metabolic acidosis (ruminants may be alkalotic)

further decreases RBF. As a result, glomerular permeability decreases with tubular backleak and obstruction of renal tubules (33). Once the syndrome is fully established, GFR remains low even after restoration of RBF. Volatile inhalation anesthetics, vasodilators, and osmotic diuretics such as mannitol may provide a degree of glomerular protection if present at the time of glomerular insult (33). Although postoperative ARF is a significant problem in human medicine, the incidence in veterinary surgical patients has not been fully established. Animal models are not considered to be good analogues of human renal disease and appear to have little to offer regarding the pathogenesis of vasomotor nephropathy in people (36). Neverthless, it seems logical that this syndrome could occur under the correct circumstances.

The two primary causes of vasomotor nephropathy are ischemia and nephrotoxins. In postischemic vasomotor nephropathy, the primary insult is shock, which may lead directly to renal failure. In most cases, the initial ischemia is exacerbated by secondary and/or iatrogenic insults that lead to the persistence of ARF in spite of improved renal circulation (33, 37).

Nephrotoxic vasomotor nephropathy may be induced by a variety of endogenous and exogenous substances with nephrotoxic properties (33). Renal effects of toxins are dose-related and synergistic. Toxicity of most nephrotoxins is enhanced by furosemide (33). The combination of an aminoglycoside (e.g., gentamicin), cephalothin, and possibly other cephalosporins is four times as toxic as when aminoglycosides are used alone (33, 37). In addition, toxicity is enhanced by advanced age, dehydration, heme pigments, and chronic renal failure. Tetracycline-derived antibiotics, although not directly nephrotoxic, increase protein catabolism and urea generation (33, 37). Other causes of postoperative renal failure may include acute interstitial nephritis induced by hypersensitization to penicillin or sulfonamides; acute glomerulonephritis associated with *Streptococcus*, *Staphylococcus*, or gram-negative bacterial endocarditis and pyogenic abscessation; and renal vascular injury, especially with septic emboli associated with bacterial endocarditis and acute or chronic renal failure (33, 37). Some commonly occurring nephrotoxins are given in Table 12.10.

Table 12.10
Nephrotoxins of Significance in Anesthetized Patients

Endogenous
Heme pigments
Myoglobin—trauma, seizures, heat, and myositis
Hemoglobin—blood transfusion, sepsis, postparturition
Bilirubin—cholangitis, cirrhosis
Exogenous
Anesthetic agents
Methoxyflurane (?)
Antibiotics
Aminoglycosides—streptomycin, gentamycin, neomycin, lincomycin
Amphotericin B—cephalosporins, vancomycin
Iodinated radiographic dyes

Nonsteroidal anti-inflammatory drugs, such as aspirin, phenylbutazone, and flunixin meglumine, inhibit prostaglandin, further enhancing nephrotoxicity of such toxic agents as antibiotics and heme pigments by depleting intravascular fluid volume and thus increasing transit time through the nephron (33, 37).

METHOXYFLURANE-RELATED NEPHROPATHY

Among the anesthetic agents, only methoxyflurane causes nephrotoxicity (3). In 1966, a syndrome of polyuric vasopressin-resistant renal insufficiency related to methoxyflurane anesthesia was described in humans (41). This syndrome may occur on initial or repeated exposure to methoxyflurane. It is characterized as a nephrogenic diabetes insipidus that is unresponsive to fluid administration of vasopressin, thus indicating a renal tissue lesion (41). Urine osmolality approaches that of serum. Polyuria results in a negative fluid and abnormal electrolyte balance in untreated patients. Serum sodium, osmolality, and BUN are increased (41). Severity of the syndrome is proportional to the total dose of methoxyflurane (i.e., MAC hours) (42). The condition is aggravated by obesity because more of the fat-soluble agent is retained and metabolized, by prolonged administration of methoxyflurane, and by the concurrent administration of nephrotoxic drugs, especially tetracycline and gentamycin (33, 37). Because of the methoxyflurane molecule has two sites that are attacked by the cytochrome P-450 enzyme, it is the most highly metabolized inhalation anesthetic in use in veterinary practice (43). Metabolism at either site results in the release of free fluoride ions. Several experiments have demonstrated inorganic fluoride ion to be the cause of renal toxicity after methoxyflurane anesthesia. The syndrome is dose-related, enhanced by liver enzyme induction, and attenuated by enzyme inhibition. It can be induced in animals not exposed to methoxyflurane by intravenous injection of inorganic fluoride (44, 45). Oxalic acid may contribute to the severity of the syndrome or it may prevent recovery, but it is not the major cause of altered renal function (42, 44).

Although methoxyflurane-induced renal toxicity occurs in humans, it is not commonly recognized in animals. However, a physiological and histological renal tubular lesion identical to that in humans has been produced in rats (46). The nephrotoxicity induced is proportional to the dose of methoxyflurane and appears to be caused by the inorganic fluoride ion released by methoxyflurane metabolism. Severity of the syndrome is markedly aggravated by gentamycin

(45). In the dog, increased serum fluoride concentration and transient polyuria and polydipsia have been reported to follow methoxyflurane anesthesia (47). Methoxyflurane anesthesia in excess of 5 MAC hours has produced a transient polyuria with urine osmolality that returns to normal within 3 days (48). In a separate report, maximum serum fluoride concentration after 4 hours of methoxyflurane anesthesia was 116.2 μmol/liter in nontreated dogs and 194 μmol/liter in dogs treated with tetracycline and anesthetized with methoxyflurane (49). Although serum fluoride concentration exceeded that which induced nephrotoxicity in humans (80 to 175 μmol/liter), nephrotoxicity was not substantiated in these dogs (49). In a study at the University of Illinois, serum fluoride concentration in dogs after 75 minutes of methoxyflurane anesthesia was 153 μmol/liter (50). Intravenous administration of sodium fluoride has been shown to cause a syndrome similar to that occurring in humans after methoxyflurane anesthesia. Although the severity of the lesion was proportionate to serum fluoride concentration, the threshold for toxicity (206 μmol/liter) was three to four times that required in humans (50 to 60 μmol/liter) (42, 51). Brunson, Stowe, and McGrath administered 6 MAC hours of methoxyflurane anesthesia to dogs. All dogs had increased serum and urine fluoride concentration postanesthesia. Of 8 dogs, 6 achieved serum fluoride concentrations comparable to those reported to cause nephrotoxicity in humans. Two of these had serum fluoride concentrations as high as those reported to induce nephropathy in dogs injected with sodium fluoride (52). Because fluoride concentrations were comparable to those associated with nephropathy in humans but renal dysfunction did not occur, it appears that dogs are more resistant to the renal effects of fluoride than are humans (52). Although this evidence appears to indicate that the dog may be more resistant to the acute effects of fluoride ions, methoxyflurane nephropathy could still occur under the appropriate conditions of dose and anesthetic biotransformation.

Chronic Renal Disease

Preoperative Assessment

It is necessary to establish the patient's state of hydration, electrolyte and acid-base status, hemoglobin concentration, concurrent drug therapy, and current treatment for renal failure (6). Signs of dehydration or water overload, serum plasma concentration of 5.5 meq/liter or more, or serious acid-base derangements are indications for further medical management and postponement of elective surgical procedures (6, 8, 35). The anemic patient should not be transfused unless anemia induces exercise intolerance (6, 53).

SPECIAL ANESTHETIC CONSIDERATIONS

Because patients with chronic renal disease, in general, are underweight, they are more prone to pressure injury and peripheral nerve damage. Thus, extra care should be taken in positioning and padding (6). The patient's weight should be ascertained for precise calculation of drug doses and allowance should be made for any edema (e.g., ascites or water overload).

Chronic renal disease adversely affects the cardiovascular system. As a result of chronic activation of the renin-angiotensin system, hypertension commonly occurs, which can lead to cardiomegaly and heart failure. In addition, cardiac output is increased in an effort to maintain tissue oxygenation because the oxygen-carrying capacity of the blood is decreased by anemia (6, 8, 35). As a result of increased myocardial work, cardiac reserve is decreased, and these patients are at increased risk of myocardial insufficiency and failure. Increased tissue blood flow is important in offsetting effects of anemia. Thus, the decreases in cardiac output induced by volatile anesthetics and IPPV must be minimized (8, 27, 35).

The most serious electrolyte abnormality associated with chronic renal disease is hyperkalemia. Hyperkalemia adversely affects cardiovascular function by inducing abnormal electrical conduction and dysrhythmias; therefore, it is recommended that elective surgery not be performed if serum potassium concentration exceeds 5.5 meq/liter (6, 8, 35). When surgery cannot be delayed, therapeutic measures should be taken to decrease serum potassium concentration. These include glucose-insulin infusion (0.5 units of regular insulin/kg and 2 g of dextrose/unit of insulin) and/or judicious use of hyperventilation (6, 8, 35). When metabolic acidosis accompanies hyperkalemia, sodium bicarbonate is indicated (8). In addition, intravenous calcium is effective in promoting normal cardiac electrical conductivity and myocardial contractility (35, 54). As a result of the foregoing (i.e., decreased cardiac reserve and decreased oxygen-carrying capacity of blood), excessive cardiopulmonary depression by anesthetics and anesthetic adjuvants must be avoided. It appears that atropine may not be beneficial because it induces tachycardia, increasing myocardial oxygen consumption in the face of increased cardiac output and anemia (6, 53). Furthermore, atropine may increase the incidence of dysrhythmias through overdrive syndrome (55).

Anesthesia is associated with a generalized decrease in renal function, primarily mediated via effects upon the cardiovascular system and endocrine effects (i.e., vasopressin, renin-angiotensin, aldosterone, and catecholamines) (2, 3, 56). Perioperative vasopressin, renin-angiotensin, and aldosterone secretion can be minimized by adequate fluid loading with 0.9% saline or balanced electrolyte solution prior to preanesthetic medication and induction of anesthesia. Use of normal saline or balanced electrolyte solutions rather than low sodium solutions (e.g., half-strength saline dextrose in water) helps to prevent hyponatremia, aldosterone secretion, oliguria, and hypokalemia alkalosis (33). Ideally, the patient should be in a mild state of diuresis prior to induction of anesthesia. This may be accomplished by preoperative hydration with 10 to 20 ml/kg of intravenous balanced salt solution. After induction, fluid loading may be ineffective in overcoming these endocrine effects, and renal function will further deteriorate (33, 35, 54, 56). In addition, intraoperative maintenance of renal function is dependent upon avoidance of events that induce renal vasoconstriction, such as stressful rough induction, pain, or hemorrhage; minimizing cardiovascular depression; and maintenance of adequate intravascular fluid volume (35). Urinary output should be maintained between 0.5 to 1 ml/kg/hr in the operative and postoperative periods. This is best achieved by 3 to 5 ml/kg/hr of balanced salt solution administered intravenously (35).

Regardless of the status of hydration or circulating blood volume, patients with chronic renal disease frequently respond to anesthesia as though they were hypovolemic. Likelihood and severity of hypotension upon induction of anesthesia may be increased if sympathetic nervous function is decreased by uremia or agents having sympatholytic activity, such as acetylpromazine (35).

Because patients with renal disease are often nauseated, vomiting or regurgitation with subsequent aspiration may occur upon induction. For this reason, rapid and efficient intubation should be performed to prevent aspiration and ensure a patent airway. Lastly, because of the increased susceptibility to infection of patients with renal disease, all precautions to ensure sterile surgical and anesthetic technique should be taken (8, 35, 54).

Chronic Renal Disease

Almost all the commonly employed anesthetic techniques have been used successfully in patients with chronic renal disease (6). However, it is prudent to avoid drugs that are primarily excreted in the urine in active form (e.g., ketamine in cats) or agents having metabolites with nephrotoxic potential (e.g., fluoride ion from methoxyflurane metabolism) (6, 56). The major problem associated with drug administration in patients with chronic renal disease is related to altered volume of distribution, which can result in prolonged half-life and prolonged activity. This is best avoided by using precisely calculated, modest drug doses to avoid relative overdose of individual patients (6). All the common analgesics, tranquilizers, and sedatives are metabolized by the liver and excreted in the urine. Because of altered volumes of distribution and hepatic dysfunction (frequently accompanying renal disease), half-life of removal of these drugs from the plasma may be increased, leading to prolonged drug action (6). Because it is usually the nonactive metabolites that are excreted in the urine, impaired renal excretion per se is unlikely to prolong drug activity (6). Nevertheless, it is prudent to anticipate prolonged action of drugs in patients with chronic renal disease. There is evidence that the blood-brain barrier in patients with chronic renal disease may not be intact in the presence of uremia; thus, the incidence of excessive drug effect as reflected by central nervous depression is increased (35, 57). Exaggerated central nervous system and ventilatory depression has been reported to occur after small doses of opiates (58). A similar increased response to the barbiturates may be observed (35, 53). In addition to alterations in the blood-brain barrier, this may be due to decreased protein binding as a result of acidosis and/or alterations in the protein molecules' ability to bind barbiturate in uremic patients (35, 59). Phenothiazine and butyrophenone tranquilizers may induce hypotension and block dopamine receptors (33). Their use in patients with renal disease should be avoided when the use of dopamine is anticipated for purposes of maintaining renal function.

Induction of Anesthesia

Good anesthetic induction technique and judicious dosing are more important than actual choice of induction agent(s). Induction should be smooth, rapid, and as physiological as possible to avoid either excessive cardiopulmonary depression or a stress response and attendant adverse effects upon renal function (6).

Induction of anesthesia and intubation of the trachea can be safely accomplished with the intravenous injection of an ultrashort-acting barbiturate regardless of the severity of renal disease (35). Other induction techniques are acceptable and have been successfully used (e.g., ketamine-diazepam, etomidate, alphaxalone-alphadolone, and neuroleptanalgesic combinations) (29, 56).

Optimally, anesthesia should be maintained with an inhalation agent(s) in oxygen. However, methoxyflurane should probably be avoided in all but the most minor procedures of short duration (6, 8, 33, 35, 37, 56). Potent volatile anesthetics are indicated because they induce muscle relaxation, thereby decreasing the requirement for specific muscle relaxants, and decrease the incidence of hypertension that may be induced by surgical manipulation (8, 35). However, excessive depression of cardiac output must be avoided if renal function is to be preserved. If the patient is anemic, decreased tissue perfusion that may accompany cardiovascular depression jeopardizes tissue oxygen delivery (6, 8, 35, 53, 56). In addition, severe anemia (often accompanying renal disease) may decrease blood-gas parturition coefficients of inhalation agents by as much as 20% (60). As a result, induction may occur more rapidly than expected, increasing the possibility of excessive cardiovascular depression.

Although the use of inhalation anesthetics provides safe anesthesia in patients with renal disease, concurrent use of opiates decreases inhalation agent requirements, thereby enhancing cardiovascular function. Thus, it would appear that the optimal anesthetic technique is a combination of opiates, such as oxymorphone, fentanyl, or sufentanil, and inhalation agents in oxygen, such as halothane or isoflurane with or without nitrous oxide (8, 35, 56). Opiate anesthetic techniques in the absense of a volatile agent are ineffective in the control of intraoperative hypertension induced by surgical manipulation (35). Lastly, prolonged central nervous and respiratory depression may occur in patients receiving opiates, necessitating vigilant postoperative management that may entail repeated administration of opiate antagonists such as naloxone (8).

Management of Ventilation during Anesthesia

Anesthetic-induced respiratory depression results in hypoventilation, characterized by retention of carbon dioxide and respiratory acidosis. Respiratory acidosis results in movement of potassium from the intracellular to the extracellular compartment, accentuating hyperkalemia and thus adversely affecting myocardial performance. Furthermore, respiratory acidosis can induce release of vasopressin and activation of the renin-angiotensin system, further compromising renal function. Conversely, hyperventilation will result in respiratory alkalosis. Although this can be beneficial by promoting transfer of potassium from the extracellular to the intracellular compartment, decreasing hyperkalemia, hyperventilation may be detrimental. Hyperventilation will decrease cardiac output and tissue perfusion, which is especially undesirable in anemic patients. Respiratory alkalosis shifts the oxyhemoglobin disassociation curve to the left, further decreasing tissue oxygen availability. Thus, one should strive to achieve and maintain normocapnia through appropriately controlled ventilation.

Muscle relaxants may be used to enhance anesthetic-induced muscle relaxation, thereby decreasing anesthetic requirement. Succinylcholine may be given to patients with chronic renal disease if serum potassium concentration is not elevated (8, 35). Because its administration has been shown to be associated with an acute increase of serum potassium of 0.5 to 1 meq/liter, succinylcholine should not be given to patients whose preoperative serum potassium concentration is in or above the high normal range (4.5 to 5.5 meq/liter) (6, 8, 35).

Of the nondepolarizing muscle relaxants, pancuronium is the most commonly used in veterinary medicine. Although its duration of action may be slightly prolonged in patients with renal disease due to delayed renal excretion, it has been safely used (5). Atracurium and vecuronium are two short-acting, nondepolarizing muscle relaxants. Because these agents are rapidly and extensively metabolized by the liver, renal excretion is of only secondary importance to termination of action. Thus, these agents would appear to be the best muscle relaxants for use in patients with chronic renal disease.

Although regional anesthetic techniques (e.g., epidural) may be used in selected cases (56), "there is no convincing evidence that regional anesthesia is safer than general anesthesia and the choice should probably be based on other considerations" (54). Appropriate intraoperative monitoring of cardiopulmonary function includes heart rate and rhythm through electrocardiogram (ECG), arterial blood pressure, central venous pressure, and arterial blood gases. The only intraoperative method of monitoring renal function is through urinary output, which is determined by urinary bladder catheterization. Urinary output should be maintained between 0.5 and 1.0 ml/kg/hr through judicious administration of a balanced salt solution (3 to 5 ml/kg/hr). Overzealous administration of fluids can result in overhydration and subsequent pulmonary edema and thus should be avoided (8, 33, 35).

Treatment of Intraoperative Oliguria

If urine flow suddenly ceases or dramatically decreases, mechanical obstruction of the urinary catheter must be excluded as a cause (32). If not contraindicated by concurrent problems, such as congestive heart failure or pulmonary edema, a fluid challenge of 4 to 8 ml/kg of 0.9% saline may be administered empirically even if intravascular volume is thought to be adequate (33). A subsequent increase in urine production is indicative of hypovolemia, and fluid administration rate should be increased. If oliguria (less than 0.5 ml/kg/hr) persists in spite of a patent urinary outflow tract, adequate hydration, and hemodynamic stability, early acute renal failure exists. Urine flow may be restored at this stage by administration of mannitol (0.25 to 0.5 mg/kg). Mannitol should be used cautiously because excessive use may induce pulmonary edema, water intoxication, and hyponatremia in patients not responding with diuresis (33). Furosemide should only be used when intravascular volume is known to be adequate or excessive. This drug enhances all renal insults (including nephrotoxicity of other substances) and further worsens hypovolemia if that is the cause of oliguria (33). Furosemide (1 to 2 mg/kg) may be used to promote diuresis in patients suffering from pulmonary edema (8). As a result of the foregoing, the use of diuretics in the perioperative period is controversial. In oliguric patients that are adequately hydrated, dopamine should be infused at a rate of 2 to 8 μg/kg/min to promote renal perfusion and urine production. This dose should maximize dopaminergic and beta adrenergic effects while avoiding the progressive alpha adrenergic effects and associated increases in renal vascular resistance that occur with higher doses (33).

In summary, it is generally accepted that all anesthetic techniques decrease GFR. Some anesthetics decrease RBF. There is presently no evidence that either of these factors per se is detrimental in terms of producing acute renal insults. As a result of decreased GFR, all anesthetics decrease urinary output. As with GFR and RBF, decreased urinary output per se has not been proven to be detrimental. Normal to increased urinary output should not be expected during surgical anesthesia. Maintenance of adequate intravascular volume and renal tissue perfusion will ensure renal homeostasis in spite of decreased urinary output. The kidney should be allowed to function rather than have its function manipulated with diuretics and other drugs (9). In patients with pre-existing renal disease presented for anesthesia, however, greater care must be taken to preserve cardiovascular function in order to meet the needs of the kidney and preserve its functional integrity.

References

1. Macfarlane WV: Water and electrolytes in domestic animals. In Phillis JW (ed): *Veterinary Physiology*. Philadelphia, WB Saunders, 1976, p 463.
2. Cousins MJ, Skowronski G, Plummer JL: Anaesthesia and the kidney. *Anaesth Intens Care* 11:292–320, 1983.
3. Mazze RI: Renal physiology and the effects of anesthesia. In Miller RD (ed): *Anesthesia*, ed 2. New York, Churchill-Livingstone, 1986, p 1223.
4. Bastron RD: Renal haemodynamics and the effects of anaesthesia. In Prys-Roberts C (ed): *The Circulation in Anaesthesia: Applied Physiology and Pharmacology*. Oxford, Blackwell Scientific Publications, 1980, p 227.
5. Guyton AC: *Textbook of Medical Physiology*, ed 5. Philadelphia, WB Saunders, 1976, p 485.
6. Strunin L, Pettingale KW: Renal disease. In Vickers MD (ed): *Medicine for the Anaesthetist*, ed 2. Oxford, Blackwell Scientific Publications, 1982, p 137.
7. Marsh DJ: *Renal Physiology*. New York, Raven Press, 1983, p 36.
8. Stoelting RK, Miller RD: Renal disease. In Stoelting RK and Miller RD (ed): *Basics of Anesthesia*. New York, Churchill-Livingstone, 1984, p 305.
9. Priano LL: The effects of anesthesia on renal blood flow and function. In ASA Annual Refresher Course Lectures. Park Ridge, IL, American Society of Anesthesiologists, 1984, p 240.
10. Finco DR: Kidney function. In Kaneko JJ (ed): *Clinical Biochemistry of Domestic Animals*, ed 3. New York, Academic Press, 1980, p 337.
11. Theye RA, Maher FT: The effects of halothane on canine renal function and oxygen consumption. *Anesthesiology* 35:54–60, 1971.
12. Vatner FF, Smith NT: Effects of halothane on left ventricular function and distribution of regional blood flow in dogs and primates. *Circ Res* 34:155–167, 1974.
13. Hill GE, Lunn JK, Hodges MR, Stanley TH, Sentker CR, Johansen R, Hatt J: N_2O modification of halothane-altered renal function in the dog. *Anesth Analg* 56:690–695, 1977.
14. Bastron RD, Perkins FM, Pyne JL: Autoregulation of renal blood flow during halothane anesthesia. *Anesthesiology* 46:142–144, 1977.
15. Bastron RD, Pyne JL, Inagaki M: Halothane-induced renal vasodilation. *Anesthesiology* 50:126–131, 1979.
16. Tranquilli WJ, Manohar M, Parks CM, Thurmon JC, Theodorakis MC, Benson GJ: Systemic and regional blood flow distribution in unanesthetized swine and swine anesthetized with halothane + nitrous oxide, halothane and enflurane. *Anesthesiology* 56:369–379, 1982.
17. Priano LL: Effect of halothane on renal hemodynamics during normovolemia and acute hemorrhagic hypovolemia. *Anesthesiology* 59:A46, 1983.
18. Theye RA, Michenfelder JD: Individual organ contributions to the decrease in whole-body VO_2 with isoflurane. *Anesthesiology* 42:35–40, 1975.
19. Priano LL: Alteration of renal hemodynamics by thiopental, diazepam and ketamine in conscious dogs. *Anesth Analg* 61:853–862, 1982.
20. Priano LL, Vatner SF: Morphine effects on cardiac output and regional blood flow distribution in conscious dogs. *Anesthesiology* 55:236–243, 1981.
21. Kennedy WF, Sawyer TK, Gerbershagen HU, Cutler RE, Allen GD, Bonica JJ: Systemic cardiovascular and renal hemodynamic alterations during peridural anesthesia in normal man. *Anesthesiology* 31:414–421, 1969.
22. Silvarajan M, Amory DW, Lindbloom LE: Systemic and regional blood flow during epidural anesthesia without epinephrine in the Rhesus monkey. *Anesthesiology* 45:300–310, 1976.
23. Gullick HD, Raisz LG: Changes in renal concentrating ability associated with major surgical procedures. *N Engl J Med* 262:1309–1314, 1960.
24. Hayes MA, Goldenberg IS: Renal effects of anesthesia and operations mediated by endocrines. *Anesthesiology* 24:487–499, 1963.
25. Mazze RI, Cousins MJ, Barr GA: Renal effects and metabolism of isoflurane in man. *Anesthesiology* 40:536–542, 1974.
26. Gorman HM, Craythorne NWB: The effects of a new neurolepanalgesic agent (Innovar) on renal function in man. *Acta Anesth Scand Suppl* 24:111, 1966.
27. Helperin BD, Feeley TW: The effects of anesthesia and surgery on renal function. *International Anesthesia Clinics* 22:157–168, 1984.
28. Rosen SM, Truniger BP, Kreik HR: Intrarenal distribution of blood flow in the transplanted dog kidney: Effect of denervation and rejection. *J Clin Invest* 46:1239–1253, 1967.
29. Priano LL: Renal hemodynamic alterations following administration of thiopental, diazepam or ketamine to conscious hypovolemic dogs. *Advan Shock Res* 9:173–188, 1983.

30. Berne RM: Hemodynamics and sodium excretion of denervated kidneys in anesthetized and unanesthetized dogs. *Am J Physiol* 171:148–158, 1952.
31. Bastron RD, Deutsch F: Anesthesia and the kidney. New York, Grune and Stratton, 1976.
32. Barry KG, Mazze RI, Schwartz FD: Prevention of surgical oliguria and renal hemodynamic depression by sustained hydration. *N Engl J Med* 270:1371–1377, 1964.
33. Sladen R: Can we prevent postoperative renal failure intraoperatively? ASA Annual Refresher Course Lectures, Park Ridge, IL. American Society of Anesthesiology, 1982, p 211.
34. Slawson KB: Anaesthesia for the patient in renal failure. *Br J Anaesth* 44:277–282, 1972.
35. Hilgenberg JC: Renal disease. In Stoetting RK, Dierdorf FF (ed): *Anesthesia and Coexisting Disease*. New York, Churchill-Livingstone, 1983, p 379.
36. Tonnesen AS: Pathophysiology of renal insufficiency as a foundation for therapy. ASA Annual Refresher Course Lectures, Park Ridge, IL. American Society of Anesthesiologists, 1984, p 239.
37. Cullen DJ: Acute renal failure: Pathophysiology and prevention. In Miller RD (ed): *Anesthesia*, ed 2. New York, Churchill-Livingstone, 1986, p 2229.
38. Brobst DF, Parish SM, Torbeck RL, Frost OL, Braken FK: Azotemia in cattle. *J Am Vet Med Assoc* 173:481–485, 1978.
39. Divers TJ, Crowell WA, Duncan JR, Whitlock RH: Acute renal disorders in cattle: Retrospective study of 22 cases. *J Am Vet Med Assoc* 181:694–699, 1982.
40. Tulleners EP, Deem DA, Donawick WJ, Whitlock RH: Indications for unilateral bovine nephrectomy: Report of four cases. *J Am Vet Med Assoc* 179:696–700, 1981.
41. Crandell WB, Pappas SG, MacDonald A: Nephrotoxicity associated with methoxyflurane. *Anesthesiology* 27:591–607, 1966.
42. Cousins MJ, Mazze RI: Methoxyflurane nephrotoxicity—A study of dose responses in man. *JAMA* 225:1611–1616, 1973.
43. Benson GJ, Brock KA: Halothane-associated hepatitis and methoxyflurane related nephropathy: a review. *J Vet Pharmacol Therap* 3:187–196, 1980.
44. Cousins MJ, Mazze RI, Kosek JC, Hitt BA, Love FV: The etiology of methoxyflurane nephrotoxicity. *J Pharmacol Exp Therap* 190:530–541, 1974.
45. Barr GA, Mazze RI, Cousins MJ, Kosek JC: An animal model for combined methoxyflurane and gentamycin toxicity. *Br J Anaesth* 45:306–311, 1973.
46. Mazze RI, Cousins MJ, Kosek JC: Dose related methoxyflurane nephrotoxicity in rats: a biochemical and pathological condition. *Anesthesiology* 36:571–587, 1972.
47. Pedersoli WM: Serum fluoride concentration, renal and hepatic function results in dogs with methoxyflurane anesthesia. *Am J Vet Res* 38:949–953, 1977.
48. Stubbs S, Fuerg H, Wade JG: The penthrane controversy. High output renal failure following methoxyflurane (penthrane), anesthesia in the dog. In *Scientific Proceeding of Anesthesia and the Kidney*. Department of Anesthesia, Department of Pharmacology and Therapeutics, University of Manatoba, Winnepeg, Manatoba, Canada, Nov 12–14, 1971.
49. Stoelting RK, Gibbs PS: Effects of tetracycline therapy on renal function after methoxyflurane anesthesia. *Anaesth Analg* 52:431–436, 1973.
50. Brock KA: Hemodynamic and renal effects of mannitol in dogs anesthetized with methoxyflurane in oxygen. Masters thesis, University of Illinois, 1980.
51. Frascino JA, Vanamee P, Rosen PP: Effects of inorganic fluoride on the renal mechanism: possible nephrotoxicity in man. *J Lab Clin Med* 79:192–203, 1972.
52. Brunson DB, Stowe CM, McGrath CJ: Serum and urine inorganic fluoride concentration and urine oxalate concentrations following methoxyflurane anesthesia in the dog. *Am J Vet Res* 40:197–203, 1979.
53. Muller MC: Anesthesia for the patient with renal dysfunction. *Internat Anesth Clin* 2:169–187, 1984.
54. Bastron RD: Anesthesia for the patient with renal disease. In ASA Annual Refresher Course Lectures, Park Ridge, IL, American Society of Anesthesiologists, 1983, p 111.
55. Muir WW: Effects of atropine on cardiac rate and rhythm of dogs. *J Am Vet Med Assoc* 172:917–921, 1978.
56. Klide AM: Anesthesia for urogenital surgery. In Stone E (ed): *Veterinary Clinics of North America*. Philadelphia, WB Saunders, 1984, p 15.
57. Freeman RB, Sheff MF, Maher JF, Schreiner GE: The blood-cerebrospinal fluid barrier in uremia. *Ann Intern Med* 56:233–249, 1962.
58. Don HF, Dieppa RA, Taylor P: Narcotic analgesics in anuric patients. *Anesthesiology* 42:745–747, 1975.
59. Wood M: Plasma drug binding: Implications for anesthesiologists. *Anesth Analg* 65:786–804, 1986.
60. Ellis DE, Stoelting RK: Individual variations in fluroxene, halothane and methoxyflurane blood-gas partition coefficient, and the effects of anemia. *Anesthesiology* 42:748–750, 1975.

PART 7

Pathophysiological Changes in the Endocrine System

MARK E. PETERSON, D.V.M., D.A.C.V.I.M.

Dogs and cats with underlying endocrine disease are frequently encountered as surgical candidates. The management of animals with disorders of the thyroid gland (hyper- and hypothyroidism), adrenal cortex (adrenal insufficiency and hyperadrenocorticism), adrenal medulla (pheochromocytoma), or endocrine pancreas (diabetes mellitus and insulin-secreting tumor) requires preoperative planning to prevent serious complications during the operative and postoperative periods. This chapter will discuss the anesthetic and medical management of these animals in the perioperative period.

Thyroid Gland

FELINE HYPERTHYROIDISM

Hyperthyroidism is a multisystemic disorder resulting from overproduction of the thyroid hormones, thyroxine (T4) and triiodothyronine (T3). Functional thyroid adenoma (adenomatous hyperplasia) involving one or both thyroid lobes is the major cause of hyperthyroidism in the cat (1, 2). Diagnosis is confirmed by demonstrating elevated circulating thyroid hormone concentrations. Surgical thyroidectomy is a highly effective treatment for feline hyperthyroidism but can be associated with significant morbidity and mortality (2, 3). Although thyroidectomy in itself is a relatively simple procedure, hyperthyroidism is a systemic illness that affects all body systems; resultant cardiovascular, hepatic, and gastrointestinal dysfunctions greatly increase the anesthetic and surgical risk in cats with hyperthyroidism. All cats should therefore be prepared for surgery by administration of an antithyroid drug, propranolol (Inderal, Ayerst Laboratories), or both to mitigate the metabolic and cardiac derangements caused by thyroid hormone excess. In addition, judicious use of anesthesia and intensive intraoperative and postoperative monitoring are necessary for a successful outcome. The medical management of a hyperthyroid cat before and during an extrathyroidal anesthetic procedure is similar to that used for thyroidectomy.

Preoperative Assessment and Management

An adequate data base is essential in the preoperative evaluation of the hyperthyroid cat and should include a complete blood count, serum chemistry profile, electrocardiogram, and serum thyroid hormone determinations. Chest radiographs and echocardiography may also be indicated if thyrotoxic-induced hypertrophic cardiomyopathy or congestive heart failure is suspected (4).

Use of an antithyroid drug is the method of choice for the preoperative preparation of a hyperthyroid cat. Methimazole (Tapazole, Eli Lilly and Co.) and propylthiouracil (PTU) are the two antithyroid drugs available for use in the United States. After administration, these drugs are actively concentrated by the thyroid gland, where they act to inhibit the synthesis of the thyroid hormones. Because methimazole is better tolerated and safer than PTU, it is the antithyroid drug of choice in the preoperative management of cats with hyperthyroidism (2). Methimazole should be administered at a dose of 15 mg/day; although single daily doses may be adequate in some cats, divided doses administered every 8 to 12 hours usually provide a more reliable response. Serious reactions that develop in less than 5% of cats treated with methimazole include agranulocytosis (severe leukopenia with a total granulocyte count below 250/mm^3) and severe thrombocytopenia (platelet count below 75,000/mm^3) (5). To evaluate the efficacy of methimazole treatment and screen for adverse hematological effects, serum thyroid hormone concentrations and complete blood and platelet counts should be monitored at 2-week intervals. In most hyperthyroid cats treated with a daily methimazole dose of 15 mg, serum T4 concentrations fall to normal or low values within 2 weeks of treatment (2, 5). If little or no decrease in serum T4 concentrations occurs during this initial period, the methimazole dose should be increased to 20 to 25 mg/day after assurances by the owner that the medication was administered as directed. After antithyroid drug treatment has maintained euthyroidism for 2 to 3 weeks, most systemic dysfunctions associated with hyperthyroidism will have improved or resolved, and the anesthetic and surgical complications will be greatly minimized. The last dose of methimazole should be administered on the morning of surgery. If serious hematological reactions develop, drug administration should be discontinued and supportive therapy instituted; these adverse reactions should resolve within 5 days after the methimazole is withdrawn (2, 5).

In hyperthyroid cats that can not tolerate antithyroid drug treatment, alternate preoperative preparation with propranolol should be used (2). Although propranolol, a beta-adrenergic blocker, does not lower elevated serum thyroid hormone concentrations, this drug blocks many of the cardiovascular and neuromuscular effects of thyroid hormone excess and controls the tachycardia and hyperexcitability associated with feline hyperthyroidism. Propranolol should be administered for 7 to 14 days before surgery at a dosage of 2.5 to 5.0 mg t.i.d., as required to decrease resting heart rate to within normal range and control hyperexcitability.

Prior to surgery, cats that have developed congestive heart failure secondary to chronic thyroid hormone excess should be stabilized with digoxin and furosemide, in addition to methimazole (6). Oxygen therapy and thoracocentesis might be required in severe or acute cases. Propranolol should be used with extreme caution in these cases. Propranolol should be used with extreme caution in these cats, however, because the drug depresses myocardial function.

Anesthetic and Intraoperative Management

Anesthetic management of the hyperthyroid cat should include the judicious use of agents that have minimal cardiac arrhythmic effects. A variety of anesthetic agents and techniques can be used for the hyperthyroid cat, and none has advantages that exclude use of all others, especially if the hyperthyroid state has been controlled with methimazole prior to surgery.

Premedication with acetylpromazine is useful because this drug reduces autonomic manifestations of hyperthyroidism and may prevent arrhythmias induced by the thiobarbiturates and inhalation agents (7, 8). Use of xylazine (Rompum, Haver-Lockhard, Miles Laboratories) for premedication is contraindicated because it potentiates the development of cardiac arrhythmias induced by barbiturate or inhalation anesthesia (7). Atropine should also be omitted because it stimulates adrenergic activity and may induce tachycardia and arrhythmias (8, 9). If an anticholinergic agent is used, glycopyrrolate (Robinul-V, A.H. Robins Co.) is the drug of choice because it has minimal effects on cardiac rate and rhythm (10). Because hyperthyroid cats are particularly susceptible to catecholamine-induced arrhythmias, anesthetic agents that stimulate sympathoadrenal activity, such as ketamine, should be avoided. Thiobarbiturates are acceptable induction agents because they possess antithyroid activity and do not stimulate catecholamine secretion (8, 11). Althesin (Saffan, Glaxo Laboratories) can also be used as the induction agent because it is relatively safe and may prevent the development of catecholamine-induced arrhythmias in the cat (12, 13); unfortunately, however, althesin is not available for use in the United States. Many inhalation agents are acceptable for maintaining anesthesia in cats with hyperthyroidism. Methoxyflurane inhibits catecholamine secretion (14) but exerts a direct negative inotropic effect on the myocardium (15); therefore, it must be used with caution should beta-adrenergic blocking agents be required, because the combination may precipitate congestive heart failure. Halothane, with or without nitrous oxide, may also be used as the primary anesthetic agent. If available, enflurane or isoflurane are preferred over methoxyflurane and halothane because they sensitize the heart to catecholamine-induced arrhythmias to a lesser extent (16–18).

During the anesthetic period, continuous monitoring of the anesthetic level and electrocardiogram is essential. Ventricular arrhythmias are common, especially in cats not rendered euthyroid prior to surgery (3). If arrhythmias develop, the anesthetic concentration should be lowered and the cat ventilated with a higher concentration of oxygen. If the arrhythmia persists, small doses (0.1 mg) of intravenous propranolol usually restore normal sinus rhythm.

Postoperative Management

Careful monitoring of vital functions should be continued during the immediate postoperative period. Hypothermia is a common problem during the recovery period. After nonthyroidal surgery, methimazole should be reinstituted as soon as oral intake is possible. Complications associated with thyroidectomy may include hypoparathyroidism, Horner's syndrome, and vocal cord paralysis (2, 3). The most serious complication is hypocalcemia, which develops after the parathyroid glands are injured, devascularized, or inadvertently removed. Because only one parathyroid gland is required for maintenance of normocalcemia, hypoparathyroidism develops only in cats treated with bilateral thyroidectomy. After bilateral thyroidectomy, the serum calcium concentration should be monitored on a daily basis until it has stabilized within the normal range. In most cats with iatrogenic hypoparathyroidism, clinical signs associated with hypocalcemia will develop within 1 to 3 days of surgery. Although mild hypocalcemia (6.5 to 7.5 mg/dl) is common, laboratory evidence of hypocalcemia alone does not require treatment; however, if accompanying signs of muscle tremors, tetany, or convulsions develop, therapy with vitamin D and calcium is indicated (19, 20).

After hemithyroidectomy for unilateral thyroid lobe involvement, serum thyroid hormone concentrations fall to subnormal levels for 2 to 3 months postoperatively; however, thyroxine supplementation is rarely required during this period. If total thyroidectomy has been performed; L-thyroxine (0.1 mg/day) should be started 24 to 48 hours after surgery (2). Although thyroxine supplementation at this low dosage can be safely continued indefinitely, the low serum concentrations of T4 and T3 that develop 24 to 48 hours after bilateral thyroidectomy may spontaneously increase to within normal range weeks to months postoperatively; thyroxine administration can then be discontinued. It can be difficult to remove all abnormal thyroid tissue while concurrently preserving parathyroid function. Small remnants of thyroid tissue that remain attached to the capsule may regenerate and produce normal amounts of circulating T4 and T3. In some cats, such regeneration of residual adenomatous thyroid tissue continues until recurrent hyperthyroidism develops. Therefore, all cats treated with surgical thyroidectomy should have serum thyroid hormone concentrations monitored at 6- to 12-month intervals to ensure that relapse does not occur.

HYPOTHYROIDISM

Hypothyroidism, resulting from lymphocytic thyroiditis or idiopathic atrophy of the thyroid gland, is a relatively common disorder in the dog. Although naturally occurring feline hypothyroidism is extremely rare, iatrogenic hypothyroidism has recently become a well-recognized disease of the cat because of the increased use of thyroidectomy and radioactive iodine (^{131}I) for treatment of hyperthyroidism (2, 3).

The prevalence of morbidity during anesthetic procedures in the unrecognized or untreated animal with hypothyroidism is unknown. Anesthesia and surgery in the untreated hypothyroid dog or cat, however, may be associated with several potential complications, including hypothermia, cardiovascular and respiratory depression, and prolonged recovery time.

Preoperative Management

If possible, surgery should be postponed in the dog or cat with untreated hypothyroidism until replacement therapy with synthetic L-thyroxine (20 μg/kg/day) has been administered for at least 2 weeks. Once a euthyroid state has been re-established, the anesthetic and surgical risk decreases to that of an animal without thyroid disease.

If emergency surgery is required in the dog and cat with severe untreated hypothyroidism, rapid preoperative repletion of the peripheral thyroid hormone pool is desirable. This can be best accomplished by administration of a single intravenous dose of L-thyroxine (20 to 40 μg/kg). Alternatively, by virtue of its rapid onset of action, L-triiodothyronine (T3) can be given orally using a dosage of 4 to 6 μg/kg three to four times daily. With either regime, an initial effect is usually achieved after several hours.

Anesthetic, Intraoperative, and Postoperative Management

Animals with mild, unrecognized hypothyroidism usually tolerate anesthesia and surgery well but may have prolonged anesthetic recovery periods (21). In the dog or cat with moderate to severe hypothyroidism that requires emergency surgery, reduced preanesthetic and anesthetic drug doses are usually needed. In addition, close monitoring of body temperature, cardiopulmonary function, and hematological status is essential because hypothermia, hypotension, hypoventilation, and bleeding diathesis may develop during the operative and postoperative periods (22). Respiratory support, shock therapy, and body warming may be necessary if complications arise. Postoperatively, oral replacement therapy with L-thyroxine should be initiated as soon as the animal can tolerate oral medication.

Adrenal Cortex

ADRENOCORTICAL INSUFFICIENCY

Animals with adrenocortical insufficiency or limited adrenocortical reserve require careful preoperative and postoperative management, even if well controlled with maintenance corticosteroid therapy prior to surgery. Normally, cortisol production increases by five- to ten-fold during periods of severe stress, such as major surgery. In animals with limited adrenal reserve that undergo anesthesia and operation, this normal cortisol response does not occur; if increased glucocorticoid supplementation is not administered during the perioperative period, adrenocortical crisis may develop (23, 24). Because glucocorticoid excess may delay healing and increase infection rates, however, glucocorticoid supplementation should only be given in adequate and necessary doses during the perioperative period (23).

There are three major causes for adrenocortical insufficiency or limited adrenocortical reserve in the dog and cat. These include naturally occurring primary or secondary hypoadrenocorticism (25), iatrogenic secondary hypoadrenocorticism resulting from administration of pharmacological doses of glucocorticoids or progestogens (i.e., megesterol acetate or medroxyprogesterone acetate) (25, 26), and decreased adrenocortical reserve secondary to treatment of pituitary-dependent hyperadrenocorticism with the adrenocorticolytic drug (o,p′-DDD), (1,1 dichloro-2(O-chlorophenyl)-2-(p-chlorophenyl)ethane also known as mitotane (27).

Preoperative Assessment and Management

A complete history helps determine the need for perioperative steroid supplementation in dogs and cats that have recently received glucocorticoid or progestagen agents. Many factors, including the dosage, duration, and frequency of treatment and time interval between the last dose of glucocorticoid or progestagen and operation, influence the need for steroid coverage during surgery. If feasible, an adrenocorticotropic hormone (ACTH) stimulation test is a reliable means of evaluating the functional ability of the adrenal cortex to secrete cortisol and respond to the stress associated with anesthesia and surgery. If the cortisol response to ACTH stimulation is subnormal, glucocorticoid supplementation is indicated. In an emergency situation, it is reasonable to provide steroid coverage if the animal has recently received supraphysiological doses of glucocorticoids or progestagens for longer than 1 week.

In animals with naturally occurring primary adrenocortical insufficiency (Addison's disease), blood urea nitrogen and serum electrolytes should be determined before surgery to ensure adequate corticosteroid replacement therapy. If azotemia, hyponatremia, or hyperkalemia are detected, operation should be deferred until these abnormalities have been corrected.

In dogs with pituitary-dependent hyperadrenocorticism, o,p′-DDD treatment must decrease adrenocortical reserve below normal in order to maintain circulating cortisol concentrations within normal resting range (27). Therefore, all dogs adequately controlled with o,p′-DDD treatment will require glucocorticoid supplementation during the perioperative period. Although normal secretion of aldosterone is usually maintained during o,p′-DDD treatment, about 5% of dogs will develop complete hypoadrenocorticism, characterized by undetectable basal and post-ACTH stimulated cortisol concentrations and electrolyte changes of hyperkalemia and hyponatremia. Therefore, in the preoperative assessment of dogs treated with o,p′-DDD, both serum electrolytes and the cortisol response to exogenous ACTH stimulation should be evaluated. Hypocortisolism, hyponatremia, and hyperkalemia should all be corrected with corticosteroid replacement therapy before surgery.

Operative and Postoperative Management

The aim of operative preparation in the dog and cat with adrenocortical insufficiency or limited adrenocortical reserve is to provide the glucocorticoid supplementation necessary to prevent circulatory collapse and adrenal crisis during or after surgery. In general, the extent of the surgical procedure (major versus minor) determines the duration of glucocorticoid and supportive treatment. With adequate preparation, elective surgery should carry no more risk for these animals than for animals with normal adrenocortical function.

For major surgical procedures, an appropriate regimen for increased steroid coverage is to administer soluble hydrocortisone (4 to 5 mg/kg), dexamethasone (0.1 to 0.2 mg/kg), or prednisolone sodium succinate (1.0 to 2.0 mg/kg) intravenously either 1 hour before surgery or at the time of induction of anesthesia (28). Upon completion of the operation, one should again administer the preoperative dose of soluble glucocorticoid preparation intravenously or intramuscularly. On the first postoperative day, glucocorticoid supplementation should be continued at approximately five times maintenance dosage as prednisone (0.5 mg/kg b.i.d.), prednisolone (0.5 mg/kg b.i.d.), cortisone acetate (2.5 mg/kg b.i.d.), or dexamethasone (0.1 mg/kg s.i.d.). Once the animal is eating, the medication can be given orally rather than parenterally. Unless postoperative complications arise, the glucocorticoid dosage can be decreased to normal maintenance levels of prednisone (0.2 mg/kg s.i.d.), prednisolone (0.2 mg/kg s.i.d.), or cortisone acetate (0.5 mg/kg b.i.d.) by the third postoperative day. Should fever or other complications occur or persist, however, the glucocorticoid supplementation should be maintained at or be increased to a dosage of five times the maintenance dose until such problems subside.

For minor elective surgery or short diagnostic procedures that require anesthesia, an appropriate schedule for increased glucocorticoid substitution therapy is to administer hydrocortisone, dexamethasone, or prednisolone sodium succinate intravenously prior to induction of anesthesia, using the same dosages listed above for major surgical procedures. After recovery from anesthesia, the preoperative dose of glucocorticoid should again be injected intravenously or intramuscularly. Maintenance glucocorticoid therapy, if required, can usually be resumed on the first postoperative day.

HYPERADRENOCORTICISM

Spontaneous canine hyperadrenocorticism results from the excessive production of cortisol by the adrenal cortex. The two major causes of this disorder include excessive pituitary ACTH secretion with resultant bilateral adrenocortical hyperplasia (pituitary-dependent hyperadrenocorticism) and unilateral cortisol-secreting tumors of the adrenal cortex (27). The cause of hyperadrenocorticism determines treatment. Unilateral adrenalectomy is the treatment of choice for adrenal tumors. With surgical excision, the prognosis for dogs with adrenal adenomas is excellent; although surgical cure is rare with adrenocortical carcinomas, operation may help reduce tumor mass and the degree of cortisol oversecretion. Pituitary-dependent hyperadrenocorticism can be effectively treated with either bilateral adrenalectomy or hypophysectomy; however, because of the technical difficulty of these operations and the need for lifelong hormone replacement therapy, medical management with o,p′-DDD is usually preferred for this disorder (27).

Dogs with hyperadrenocorticism may have multiple metabolic derangements that increase anesthetic and surgical risks, including hyperglycemia, serum electrolyte abnormalities, and acid-base disturbances. The hypertension associated with chronic cortisol excess, as well as coexisting atrioventricular valvular insufficiency, may produce left ventricular hypertrophy and congestive heart failure. Weakness of the muscles of respiration, thoracic fat deposition, and increased diaphragmatic abdominal pressure resulting from hepatomegaly and intraabdominal fat accumulation all contribute to the respiratory distress or hyperventilation found in many dogs with hyperadrenocorticism. Finally, the marked catabolic effects of cortisol excess may result in severe muscle wasting and thinning of the skin. The tissues may have poor tensile strength, tear easily, retain sutures poorly, heal slowly, and become infected. All of these factors should be considered in the anesthetic and surgical management of dogs with hyperadrenocorticism.

Preoperative Assessment and Management

An adequate data base is essential in the preoperative evaluation of dogs with hyperadrenocorticism and should include a complete blood count, serum chemistry profile, electrocardiogram, and chest radiograph. If an adrenal tumor is suspected, abdominal radiographs may help localize an adrenal mass, especially when unilateral calcification in the area of an adrenal gland can be visualized (27).

Preoperative management may require correction of fluid and electrolyte imbalances, stabilization of diabetes mellitus, and treatment of congestive heart failure. In dogs with severe, advanced hyperadrenocorticism, use of either o,p′-DDD or inhibitors of adrenocortical secretion (i.e., metyrapone or aminoglutethimide) to reduce cortisol secretion before surgery should be considered (23, 27).

Anesthetic and Intraoperative Management

A variety of anesthetic agents and techniques can be used for dogs with hyperadrenocorticism, and none has advantages that exclude use of all others (23). Both the thiobarbiturates and etomidate (Amidate, Pitman-Moore Inc.) decrease circulating cortisol concentrations and are acceptable induction agents (29, 30). After induction, anesthesia may be maintained with a variety of inhalation agents according to the preference of the anesthesiologist (23, 29).

Dogs with hyperadrenocorticism may have multiple metabolic disturbances that require careful induction and monitoring of the anesthetic level. Capillary refill time, rectal temperature, heart and lung sounds by esophageal stethoscope, electrocardiogram, and blood pressure should all be monitored continuously during surgery, if possible, An intravenous catheter should also be inserted to provide fluid and glucocorticoid supplementation during the perioperative period.

Use of either adrenalectomy or hypophysectomy for treatment of hyperadrenocorticism will cause a precipitous drop in circulating cortisol concentrations. Glucocorticoid therapy should therefore begin in the immediate preoperative period and continue into the postoperative period, as outlined for major surgical procedures in the section on adrenocortical insufficiency.

Postoperative Management

Possible postoperative complications after adrenalectomy or hypophysectomy include fluid and electrolyte imbalances, hemorrhage from the excision site, infection, poor wound healing, and thromboembolism. Pancreatitis secondary to surgical retraction during adrenalectomy may also develop during the first 24 to 72 hours after surgery.

After either adrenalectomy or hypophysectomy, postoperative adrenocortical insufficiency will also occur unless large doses of glucocorticoids are continued after surgery. During the first postoperative day, glucocorticoid supplementation should be continued using prednisone (0.5 mg/kg b.i.d.), prednisolone (0.5 mg/

kg b.i.d.), or cortisone acetate (2.5 mg/kg b.i.d.). The glucocorticoid should be tapered to a maintenance dosage of prednisone (0.2 mg/kg s.i.d.), prednisolone (0.2 mg/kg s.i.d.). or cortisone (0.5 mg/kg b.i.d.) over the next 1 to 2 weeks.

In dogs from which a unilateral adrenal tumor was removed, glucocorticoid supplementation should be continued at maintenance dosage until the remaining contralateral adrenal gland is functioning normally based on the results of ACTH stimulation testing. After bilateral adrenalectomy for treatment of pituitary-dependent adrenocortical hyperplasia, both glucocorticoid and mineralocorticoid replacement therapy will be necessary for the remainder of the dog's life. In dogs in which hypophysectomy is used as treatment for pituitary-dependent hyperadrenocorticism, life-long replacement therapy with glucocorticoids and L-thyroxine is required; in addition, treatment with analogues of antidiuretic hormone (e.g., pitressin tannate in oil) may also be necessary if diabetes insipidus develops during the postoperative period.

Adrenal Medulla

PHEOCHROMOCYTOMA

In the dog, pheochromocytoma is a rare endocrine tumor that arises from the adrenal medulla (31). Hypertension and tachycardia, the classical features of pheochromocytoma, result from the excessive production of catecholamines by the tumor. The clinical manifestations of pheochromocytoma are quite variable and may include restlessness, dyspnea, weakness, polyuria, or anorexia (30). The preoperative diagnosis of pheochromocytoma is based upon biochemical demonstration of excessive catecholamine release, most often with measurements of urinary catecholamines and their metabolites (29, 31–33).

Surgery is the treatment of choice for dogs with pheochromocytoma. Without adequate preoperative preparation and careful monitoring during the operative and postoperative periods, however, a spectrum of potentially serious complications may arise, including refractory hypotension, ventricular arrhythmia, and death.

Preoperative Management

The goal of preoperative preparation in dogs with pheochromocytoma is to normalize the elevated blood pressure levels with alpha- and beta-adrenergic blocking agents. Phenoxybenzamine (Dibenzyline, Smith Kline and French) is the drug of choice for alpha-adrenergic blockade (31–33). Starting with an oral dose of 0.2 to 0.4 mg/kg b.i.d., the dosage of phenoxybenzamine should be gradually increased over several days until the hypertension and associated clinical signs have resolved. A total daily dosage of 1.5 to 3.0 mg/kg is sufficient to normalize blood pressure in most dogs. Preoperative preparation with beta-blocking agents, such as propranolol (0.15 to 0.5 mg/kg p.o. t.i.d.), is indicated for control of tachycardia, cardiac arrhythmias, or hypertension which persists despite alpha-adrenergic blockade. Beta-adrenergic blocking agents should never be given, however, until adequate alpha-adrenergic blockade has been established, because severe hypertension may result from the unopposed alpha-adrenergic effect of the secreted catecholamines (31–33).

Anesthetic and Intraoperative Management

Anesthetic management of the dog undergoing surgery for removal of a pheochromocytoma involves use of agents that do not sensitize the myocardium to the effect of catecholamines and promote cardiac arrhythmias. Atropine should be avoided because it stimulates adrenergic activity and may induce tachycardia and arrhythmias (9); if an anticholinergic agent is used, glycopyrrolate is the drug of choice because it has minimal effects on cardiac rate and rhythm (10). Thiobarbiturates are acceptable induction agents because they do not stimulate catecholamine secretion (11); they do have the disadvantage of being arrhythmogenic, however. Alternatively, induction with the narcotic-tranquilizer combination of fentanyl and droperidol (Innovar Vet, Pitman-Moore Inc.) may be preferred; fentanyl has alpha-adrenergic blocking effects, and droperidol antagonizes the pressor effects of catecholamines and prevents arrhythmias (32–34). Of the inhalation maintenance agents, methoxyflurane, enflurane, or isoflurane are preferred over halothane because they sensitize the heart to catecholamine-induced arrhythmias to a lesser extent (17, 18, 32, 33).

The three major concerns during surgery are cardiac arrhythmias, hypertensive crisis, and maintenance of normal intravascular volume. Prior to induction, intra-arterial and jugular catheters are inserted for measuring arterial blood pressure and central venous pressure (CVP), and continuous electrocardiographic monitoring should be initiated. Arrhythmias that develop during surgery usually respond to small intravenous doses of propranolol (0.03 to 0.1 mg/kg). If propranolol fails to control arrhythmias, administration of lidocaine as an intravenous bolus (2 to 3 mg/kg) and appropriate maintenance infusion (40 to 80 μg/kg/min) may be required. If acute hypertension develops during induction or surgery, intravenous boluses of the short-acting alpha-adrenergic blocker phentolamine (Regitine, CIBA Pharmaceutical Co.) in doses of 0.02 to 1.0 mg/kg should be administered (31–33). An alternate approach for maintenance of normal blood pressure is the continuous infusion of sodium nitroprusside (1 to 5 μg/kg/min) during the intraoperative period (32, 33). Throughout surgery, liberal replacement of estimated blood loss with intravenous isotonic fluids is indicated. A precipitous fall in blood pressure should be anticipated at the time of tumor resection. If hypotension develops, rapid infusion of isotonic fluids as necessary to maintain a normal systolic blood pressure is indicated; careful monitoring of the CVP is essential in determining the maximal rate of infusion.

Postoperative Management

Close monitoring is mandatory during the immediate postoperative period. The hypotension that commonly develops after pheochromocytoma removal may persist into the early postoperative period and requires continued vigorous fluid expansion. Mild, transient hypertension is not uncommon during the first 24 hours after surgery and usually requires no treatment. Postoperatively, markedly elevated blood pressure measurements suggest residual pheochromocytoma tissue. Even if blood pressure is normal, urinary concentrations of catecholamines and their metabolites should be re-evaluated several days after surgery to ensure that tumor resection was complete. If catecholamine concentrations are still elevated, a second surgical exploration or medical treatment with phenoxybenzamine should be considered.

Endocrine Pancreas

DIABETES MELLITUS

In the anesthetic and surgical management of the diabetic dog or cat, one must be prepared to treat a broad spectrum of problems ranging from hypoglycemia to severe ketoacidosis and dehydration. The goal of diabetic management is not to achieve perfect metabolic homeostasis but rather to avoid profound body fluid, electrolyte, acid-base, and carbohydrate abnormalities during the perioperative period. The ideal therapeutic goals should include prevention of hypoglycemia, prevention of ketoacidosis, control of severe hyperglycemia and glycosuria, maintenance of normal fluid and electrolyte balance and resumption of oral alimentation as soon as possible.

Preoperative Assessment and Management

If possible, the diabetic dog or cat should be admitted to the hospital 1 day prior to elective surgery to allow time for careful evaluation of overall metabolic status and for metabolic stabilization. Essential preoperative laboratory evaluation should include a complete blood count, fasting blood glucose, serum electrolytes, blood urea nitrogen and creatinine, and complete urinalysis.

Most dogs or cats with previously diagnosed diabetes mellitus will be on a regimen consisting of an intermediate-acting (e.g., NPH) or long-acting (e.g., PZI) insulin given once or twice a day. If severe hyperglycemia (blood glucose greater than 300 mg/dl) or ketoacidosis are detected preoperatively, supplemental regular insulin should be administered subcutaneously at 6-hour intervals to help correct these metabolic abnormalities before surgery. Appropriate treatment with intravenous fluids and electrolytes should also be administered during the preoperative period when needed (35).

Occasionally, dogs or cats with newly diagnosed or poorly controlled ketoacidotic diabetes mellitus require emergency operation. Unless immediate surgery is necessary to sustain life, treatment with intravenous fluids and regular insulin (given by low-dose continuous intravenous infusion, low-dose hourly intramuscular injection, or subcutaneous administration every 4 to 6 hours) should be initiated prior to surgery (36). In general, the fluid, electrolyte, and acid-base abnormalities associated with diabetic ketoacidosis can be corrected during 6 to 8 hours of vigorous therapy. Once hydration has been re-established, blood glucose concentration has decreased to less than 300 mg/dl, and serum bicarbonate (or total CO_2) concentration has risen to greater than 18 meq/liter, it is reasonably safe to proceed with the operation.

Anesthetic and Intraoperative Management

The choice of preanesthetic and anesthetic agents has little impact on intraoperative blood glucose management. Although commonly used anesthetic agents may affect glucose metabolism, their direct contribution to altered blood glucose concentrations is relatively modest, especially when compared to the hyperglycemic effects associated with the stress of surgery (37–39).

A number of different regimens have been advocated in the management of the insulin-dependent diabetic during surgery (29). These methods include avoiding both intravenous glucose and insulin during surgery, using intravenous glucose but no insulin during surgery, using intravenous glucose with one-third to one-half of the usual dose of insulin given subcutaneously before surgery, using intravenous glucose with the usual dose of insulin given subcutaneously before surgery, and using intravenous glucose mixed with regular insulin infused continuously during surgery. Although all of the above regimens may be effective, we have found the method outlined in Table 12.11 to

Table 12.11
Insulin Management on the Day of Surgery

1. Administer 50% of usual morning dose of insulin subcutaneously 1 hour preoperatively.
2. Start infusion of 5% glucose solution 1 hour preoperatively.
3. Determine blood glucose concentrations at 1-hour intervals during surgery and recovery. Adjust rate of glucose infusion or administer regular insulin subcutaneously as needed.
4. Monitor blood glucose concentrations every 6 hours until next morning.
5. Administer regular insulin subcutaneously every 6 hours to maintain blood glucose concentrations between 150 and 250 mg/dl.

be both convenient and reliable. With this regimen, the animal receives the normal dose(s) of insulin and is fed as usual on the day before surgery. No food is given after midnight. If possible, the operation is scheduled for the early morning because this allows for closer observation after surgery. Approximately 1 hour before induction of anesthesia, an infusion of a 5% glucose solution is started and one-half of the usual morning dose of insulin is given subcutaneously. If the blood glucose concentration is greater than 300 mg/dl on the morning of surgery, a supplemental dose of regular insulin (0.25–0.5 I.U./kg s.c.) should also be administered prior to operation.

During surgery, the blood glucose concentration should be monitored at hourly intervals. Use of glucose oxidase-impregnated test strips, such as Chemstrip bG or Dextrostix, provides a rapid and convenient means of determining approximate blood glucose concentrations. Because the stress associated with anesthesia and surgery usually raises the blood glucose concentration, the development of hypoglycemia is relatively uncommon; however, if the blood glucose value falls below 100 mg/dl, the rate of the glucose infusion should be increased. If severe hyperglycemia (blood glucose concentrations greater than 300 mg/dl) develops, the rate of the glucose infusion should be decreased or additional regular insulin should be given subcutaneously or both.

Postoperative Management

Guidelines for managing the diabetic dog or cat during the postoperative period must be individualized, depending on when oral intake can be resumed. The intravenous glucose infusion should be continued and regular insulin should be given subcutaneously at 6-hour intervals as needed to maintain blood glucose concentrations below 250 mg/dl until oral feeding is feasible (29). In most cases, the diabetic can be returned to the routine schedule of insulin administration and feeding by the first to second day after surgery. Utilization of medication such as isoflurane for anesthesia provides a rapid recovery and early return to normal habits compared to other anesthetic regimes.

PANCREATIC INSULIN-SECRETING TUMORS

Insulin-secreting islet cell tumor of the pancreas, which produces clinical signs related to hypoglycemia, is a well-recognized endocrine neoplasm of the dog. Diagnosis is based on the biochemical demonstration of fasting hypoglycemia in conjunction with relative or absolute elevations in circulating insulin concentrations (40–42). Although most insulin-secreting islet cell tumors in the dog are malignant, surgical excision is the treatment of choice for these tumors because it offers the best chance for long-term control of both hypoglycemia and associated neurological signs. Successful perioperative management of insulin-secreting pancreatic tumors requires control of hypoglycemia and treatment of complications that develop during the postoperative period.

Preoperative Management

Once the diagnosis of insulin-secreting tumor of the pancreas is established, it is important to avoid further episodes of hypoglycemia before surgery. In some dogs, this can be accomplished with frequent feedings. Others require a continuous infusion of a 5 to 20% glucose solution, adjusted as needed to maintain normal blood glucose concentrations. Adjunctive therapy with diazoxide or glucocorticoids also provides a useful means for controlling hypoglycemia during the preoperative period.

Diazoxide (Proglycem, Schering Corp.) acts to directly inhibit both pancreatic insulin secretion and glucose uptake by tissues and is effective in raising blood glucose concentrations in 50 to 75% of dogs with insulin-secreting tumors of the pancreas (40–42). The initial dosage of diazoxide is 10 mg/kg/day in divided doses; this dosage can be increased to 40 mg/kg/day as needed to control hypoglycemia. The most common adverse effects of diazoxide include anorexia and vomiting.

Glucocorticoid therapy is also useful in maintaining normoglycemia in dogs with islet cell tumors. These agents raise the blood glucose concentration by increasing hepatic glucose production and decreasing glucose uptake by tissues (40). Prednisone, administered at daily doses of 0.25 to 1.0 mg/kg, will control hypoglycemia in most dogs with insulin-secreting tumors of the pancreas. Preoperative administration of large doses of glucocorticoids, however, should probably be reserved for those dogs in which hypoglycemia persists despite use of other means to maintain normoglycemia, because they may delay healing and increase infection rates during the postoperative period (43).

Anesthetic and Intraoperative Management

A rational anesthetic plan for dogs with insulin-secreting pancreatic tumors is to use anesthetic agents that decrease the cerebral demand for its major substrate, glucose. Induction of anesthesia can be safely accomplished with the thiobarbiturates, which are agents that decrease cerebral glucose metabolism (44). Anesthesia can be maintained with a variety of inhalation agents; however, halothane or enflurane may be the agents of choice because both appear to decrease the cerebral metabolism of glucose (44).

Because anesthesia obliterates the characteristic central nervous signs of hypoglycemia, it is of utmost importance to recognize and treat hypoglycemia during the operative period. The safest means to maintain normoglycemia during the perioperative fasting period is to start a 5 to 20% glucose infusion the evening before surgery and continue the infusion throughout the procedure (44, 45). Blood glucose concentrations should be monitored immediately prior to induction of anesthesia and every 30 minutes thereafter until the dog has recovered from anesthesia. Use of glucose oxidase-impregnated test strips (e.g., Chemstrip bG or Dextrostix) provides a convenient and rapid means of determining blood glucose concentrations; however, the results may be inaccurate in the very low ranges. If hypoglycemia develops during surgery, it should be corrected immediately by increasing the infusion rate or concentration of the glucose solution.

Postoperative Management

During the immediate 12- to 24-hour postoperative period, blood glucose concentrations should be monitored at frequent intervals. The glucose infusion should be discontinued once blood glucose stabilizes at concentrations above 100 mg/dl. Of those dogs in which tumor resection is successful, the blood glucose concentration usually rises into the hyperglycemic range by 1 to 2 days after surgery. Such hyperglycemia appears to result from transient suppression of normal pancreatic beta cell function by the excessive levels of insulin previously secreted by the islet cell tumor. Because hyperglycemia is usually transient and resolves within 3 to 5 days, exogenous insulin treatment is not required unless severe hyperglycemia persists or ketoacidosis develops.

Persistent hypoglycemia is expected in dogs with surgically unresectible metastasis. Despite resection of all identifiably tumor masses, hypoglycemia may also persist in other dogs because of residual neoplastic tissue that was not detected at surgery. In these dogs with postoperative hypoglycemia, medical therapy with diazoxide or glucocorticoids should be initiated, as described above.

Prolonged hypoglycemia can cause focal or pseudolaminar necrosis of the cerebral cortex, which may result in acquired epilepsy. If focal or generalized convulsions persist into the postoperative period despite correction of hypoglycemia, acquired epilepsy should be suspected and treatment with anticonvulsant agents should be initiated.

Iatrogenic pancreatitis can develop as a sequella to surgical removal of islet cell tumors. Therefore, during the first 48 to 72 hours after surgery, oral food and water should be withheld and isotonic fluids should be administered intravenously. Serum amylase and lipase concentrations should be determined on a daily basis during this period.

References

1. Peterson ME, Kintzer PP, Cavanagh PG, Fox PR, Ferguson DC, Johnson GF, Becker DV: Feline hyperthyroidism: pretreatment clinical and laboratory evaluation of 131 cases. *J Am Vet Med Assoc* 183:103–110, 1983.
2. Peterson ME, Turrel JM: Feline hyperthyroidism. In Kirk RW (ed): *Current Veterinary Therapy IX*. Philadelphia, WB Saunders, 9:1026–1032, 1986.
3. Birchard SJ, Peterson ME, Jacobson A: Surgical treatment of feline hyperthyroidism: results of 85 cases. *J Am Anim Hosp Assoc* 20:705–709, 1984.
4. Liu Si-Kwang, Peterson ME, Fox PR: Hypertrophic hyperthyroidism in the cat. *J Am Vet Med Assoc* 185:52–57, 1984.
5. Peterson ME, Kintzer PP, Hurvitz AI: Evaluation of methimazole for the treatment of feline hyperthyroidism. *Proceedings of the American College of Veterinary Internal Medicine*, 1985, p 128.
6. Bond BR, Fox PR: Advances in feline cardiomyopathy. *Vet Clin North Am (Small Anim Prac)* 14:1021–1038, 1984.
7. Muir WW, Werner LL, Hamlin RL: Effects of xylazine and acetylpromazine upon induced ventricular fibrillation in dogs anesthetized with thiamylal and halothane. *Am J Vet Res* 36:1299–1303, 1975.
8. Stehling LC: Anesthetic management of the patient with hyperthyroidism. *Anesthesiology* 41:585–595, 1974.
9. Muir WW: Effects of atropine on cardiac rate and rhythm in dogs. *J Am Vet Med Assoc* 172:917–920, 1978.
10. Short CE, Miller RL: Comparative evaluation of the anticholinergic agent glycopyrrolate as a preanesthetic agent. *Vet Med Small Anim Clin* 73:1269–1273, 1978.
11. Joyce JT, Roizen MF, Eger EI: Effect of thiopental induction on sympathetic activity. *Anesthesiology* 59:19–22, 1983.
12. Dodds MG, Twissell DJ: Effects of althesin (CT 1341) on circulating responses to adrenaline and on halothane-adrenaline cardiac dysrhythmias in the cat. *Postgrad Med J* 48:(Suppl 2) 17–24, 1972.
13. Evans JM, Aspinall KW, Hendy PG: Clinical evaluation in cats of a new anaesthetic, CT 1341. *J Small Anima Pract* 13:479–486, 1972.
14. Twung-Han L, Shaul MS, Etsten BE: Decreased adrenal venous catecholamine concentrations during methoxyflurane anesthesia. *Anesthesiology* 29:1145–1152, 1968.

15. Hetzel WM: Use of methoxyflurane in veterinary medicine. *Prac Vet* 48:4–15, 1976.
16. Munson ES, Tucker WK: Doses of epinephrine causing arrhythmia during enflurane, methoxyflurane, and halothane anesthesia in dogs. *Canad Anaesth Soc J* 22:496–501, 1975.
17. Sumikawa K, Ishizaka N, Suzaki M: Arrhythmogenic plasma levels of epinephrine during halothane, enflurane, and pentobarbital anesthesiology. 58:322–325, 1983.
18. Tucker WK, Rackstein AD, Munson ES: Comparison of arrhythmic doses of adrenaline, metaraminol, ephedrine and phenylephrine during isoflurane, and halothane anaesthesia in dogs. *Br J Anaesth* 46:392–396, 1974.
19. Peterson ME: Treatment of canine and feline hypoparathyroidism. *J Am Vet Med Assoc* 181:1434–1436, 1982.
20. Peterson ME: Hypoparathyroidism. In Kirk RW (ed): *Current Veterinary Therapy IX*. Philadelphia, WB Saunders, 9:1039–1044, 1986.
21. Babad, AA, Eger EI: The effects of hyperthyroidism and hypothyroidism on halothane and oxygen requirements in dogs. *Anesthesiology* 29:1087–1093, 1968.
22. Murkin JM: Anesthesia and hypothyroidism: a review of thyroxine physiology, pharmacology, and anesthetic implications. *Anesth Analg* 61:371–383, 1982.
23. Weatherill D, Spence AA: Anaesthesia and disorders of the adrenal cortex. *Br J Anaesth* 56:741–749, 1984.
24. Swingle WW, DaVanzo JP, Crossfield HC, Glenister D, Osborn M, Rowen R, Wagle G: Glucocorticoids and maintenance of blood pressure and plasma volume of adrenalectomized dogs subjected to stress. *Proc Soc Exp Biol* 100:617–622, 1959.
25. Feldman EC, Peterson ME: Hypoadrenocorticism. *Vet Clin North Am (Small Anim Prac)* 14:751–766, 1984.
26. Chastain CB, Graham CL, Nichols CE: Adrenocortical suppression in cats given megestrol acetate. *Am J Vet Res* 42:2029–2035, 1981.
27. Peterson ME: Hyperadrenocorticism. *Vet Clin North Am (Small Anim Prac)* 14:731–749, 1984.
28. Kehlet H: A rational approach to dosage and preparation of parenteral glucocorticoid substitution therapy during surgical procedures. *Acta Anaesth Scand* 19:260–264, 1975.
29. Pender JW, Basso LV: Diseases of the endocrine system. In Katz J, Benumof J, Kadis LB (eds): *Anesthesia and Uncommon Diseases: Pathophysiologic and Clinical Correlations*, ed 2. Philadelphia, WB Saunders, 1981, pp 155–220.
30. Wagner RL, White PF: Etomidate inhibits adrenocortical function in surgical patients. *Anesthesiology* 61:647–651, 1984.
31. Twedt DC, Wheeler SL: Pheochromocytoma in the dog. *Vet Clin North Am (Small Anim Prac)* 14:767–782.
32. Pratilas V, Pratila MG, Dimich I: The perioperative management of patients with pheochromocytoma. *Mt Sinai J Med* 46:345–353, 1979.
33. Desmonts JM, Marty J: Anaesthetic management of patients with phaeochromocytoma. *Br J Anaesth* 56:781–789, 1984.
34. Bauer H, Kreuscher H, Menzel H: Antiarrhythmic effects of dehydrobenzperidol in dogs. *Acta Anaethesiol Scand* 151:277–289, 1971.
35. Schaer M: Insulin treatment for the diabetic dog and cat. *Compend Contin Ed* 5:579–588, 1983.
36. Chastain CB: Intensive care of dogs and cats with diabetic ketoacidosis. *J Am Vet Med Assoc* 179:972–978, 1981.
37. Clarke RSJ: The hyperglycaemic response to different types of surgery and anesthesia. *Brit J Anaesth* 42:45–53, 1970.
38. Hsu WH, Hembrough FB: Intravenous glucose tolerance tests in cats: influenced by acetylpromazine, ketamine, morphine, thiopental, and xylazine. *Am J Vet Res* 43:2060–2061, 1982.
39. Hardie EM, Rawlings CA, George JW: Plasma-glucose concentrations in dogs and cats before and after surgery: comparison of healthy animals and animals with sepsis. *Am J Vet Res* 46:1700–1704, 1985.
40. Leifer CE, Peterson ME: Hypoglycemia. *Vet Clin North Am (Small Anim Prac)* 14:873–889, 1984.
41. Leifer CE, Peterson ME, Matus RE: Insulin-secreting tumor: diagnosis and medical and surgical management in 55 dogs. *J Am Vet Med Assoc* 188(1):60–4, 1986.
42. Mehlhaff CJ, Peterson ME, Patnaik AK, Carrillo JM: Insulin producing islet cell neoplasms: Surgical considerations and management in 35 dogs. *J Amer Anim Hosp Assoc* 21:607–612, 1985.
43. Chrisman CL: Postoperative results and complications of insulinomas in dogs. *J Am Anim Hosp Assoc* 16:677–684, 1980.
44. Suffecol SL: Anesthetic management for insulinoma resection. In Brown BR, Blitt CD, Giesecke AH (eds): *Anesthesia and the Patient with Endocrine Disease*. Philadelphia, FA Davis, 1980, pp 11–17.
45. Bourke AM: Anaesthesia for the surgical treatment of insulinomas. *Anaethesiology* 21:239–243, 1966.

PART 8

Anesthetic Considerations of the Gastrointestinal Tract

CYNTHIA M. TRIM, M.R.C.V.S., D.V.A., D.A.C.V.A.

Effects of Anesthetic Agents and Procedures on the Gastrointestinal Tract

GASTROINTESTINAL MOTILITY

Vomition and regurgitation are potential complications of general anesthesia in dogs and cats, and regurgitation is a hazard of anesthesia in ruminants. Aspiration of gastric contents into the lungs will result in pneumonitis and may cause death of the patient. The most commonly used method of decreasing the incidence of gastric reflux is to decrease the volume of the gastrointestinal contents before induction of anesthesia by withholding food and water. Canned meat-based food and dry cereal-based food emptied from the stomach of dogs at the same rate, with a mean half-time for emptying of 2 to 3 hours and complete emptying in 10 hours (1). However, there was a significant variation between dogs in emptying time of food from the stomach. Water emptied completely from the stomach in dogs in a mean time of 54 minutes (2). These experiments justify the current practice of withholding food from dogs and cats before anesthesia for 12 hours and water for 2 hours. Atropine decreases intestinal motility. This may explain the clinical impression that the incidence of vomiting in dogs that have received atropine is decreased after anesthesia. A shorter time of fasting is advisable for animals less than 3 months of age; otherwise they may develop hypoglycemia during or after anesthesia. The rumen of ruminants acts as a reservoir, and a longer withholding time of 36 hours for food and 12 hours for water is recommended.

The influence of anesthetic drugs on gastrointestinal motility is particularly important in horses because of their predisposition to colic. Atropine is not routinely administered for premedication to horses for that reason. In one study, 0.04 mg/kg of atropine decreased intestinal motility for up to 12 hours (3). My preference is to use atropine in horses only for specific treatment to protect against vagal reflex during ocular surgery, to produce bronchodilation in horses with chronic obstructive pulmonary disease, or to treat bradycardia. Food should be withheld for longer than usual after anesthesia from horses that have received atropine to allow time for motility to return.

Recording electrical activity from strain gauges implanted on the intestinal wall has determined that acepromazine decreases electrical activity but increases volume transit (4). Meperidine decreased electrical activity and increased volume transit but was associated with initial forceful contractions that the authors suggested would produce adverse effects on distended or obstructed bowel. Xylazine severely decreased electrical activity for 30 minutes in the colon and cecum (5, 6). Butorphanol and pentazocine inhibited progressive motility in the small intestine (7).

Thiopental or minaxolone injected into dogs caused intense activity in the duodenum and jejunum, but not the stomach or ileum (8). This increase in activity was blocked by premedication with atropine. Ketamine did not alter gastrointestinal activity (8). None of the drugs altered the basal electrical rhythm of the intestine. Halothane anesthesia decreased motility of the stomach, jejunum, and colon of dogs, but contractions returned rapidly after administration was discontinued (9).

Neostigmine is used to reverse nondepolarizing neuromuscular blocking drugs. As an anticholinergic drug it also has vagal effects, and it is usual practice to precede its administration with atropine to prevent bradycardia. Bell and Lewis reported an increased incidence of leakage from anastomoses when neostigmine was used (10). Neostigmine alone increased propulsive activity of the colon in conscious ponies (5) but did not increase activity in the jejunum and delayed gastric emptying time (5, 11). In humans, the administration of atropine or glycopyrrolate before neostigmine did not prevent increased activity of the colon, and there was no difference between the two drugs (12).

SPHINCTER CONTROL

The pressure difference (barrier pressure) across the area between the esophagus and the stomach, which is called the lower esophageal sphincter, plays a large part in preventing gastrointestinal reflux. The barrier pressure has been measured in conscious dogs; decreases in pressure of 73, 61, and 77% were recorded after intravenous injection of atropine (0.03 mg kg^{-1}), acepromazine (0.1 mg kg^{-1}), and xylazine (1.0 mg kg^{-1}), respectively (13). In contrast, intravenous injection of meperidine (5 mg kg^{-1}) produced phasic contractions that were not changed by atropine administration (13). Metoclopramide, which increases gastrointestinal motility, increases barrier pressure, but this effect is abolished by concurrent administration of atropine. Glycopyrrolate produces a decrease similar in barrier pressure to that produced by atropine, at least in humans (14). The threshold of barrier pressure below which regurgitation occurs has not been defined, but it is reasonable to assume that as the pressure decreases, the risk of regurgitation increases.

VOLUME AND COMPOSITION OF SECRETIONS

Anticholinergic drugs, specifically atropine and glycopyrrolate, have been used for premedication to general anesthesia to decrease the volume and acidity of the secretions of the gastrointestinal tract. However, the gastric fluid volume measured after 2 hours of anesthesia in humans anesthetized with 60% nitrous oxide and either fentanyl, enflurane, or halothane was no different when an anticholinergic drug had been included. Atropine and glycopyrrolate decrease the acidity of gastric secretions, and the increase in pH is greater with glycopyrrolate than with atropine. Should pulmonary aspiration occur, the degree of pneumonitis may be less at the higher pH. However, a considerable variation in gastric pH was measured in human patients, and the increase in pH in some patients was not great enough to protect against pulmonary damage (15).

Halothane anesthesia in ponies decreases bile acid excretion and increases bile acid-independent bile flow and conjugated bilirubin excretion (16). These changes may reflect a halothane-induced subclinical hepatopathy because isoflurane under similar experimental conditions only significantly increased biliary bilirubin excretion (17).

INTESTINAL BLOOD FLOW

Intestinal blood flow during anesthesia may have an important influence on the healing of the intestine after surgery. Intestinal blood flow was decreased by 59% in dogs anesthetized with pentobarbital and maintained with halothane (18) and by 53% in dogs anesthetized with methohexital and maintained with 2.0 MAC halothane (19). A 62% decrease in blood flow was measured in ponies anesthetized with 1.0 MAC halothane (20). A smaller decrease was measured during equipotent anesthesia with isoflurane in dogs (36% compared with 53%) (19) and swine (21). In swine it was determined that the percentage of the cardiac output perfusing the gastrointestinal tract was unchanged by anesthesia. The intestinal blood flow was least decreased by halothane and nitrous oxide anesthesia when compared with halothane or enflurane anesthesia because the cardiac output was the least depressed with this drug combination (22). A transient increase in intestinal flow followed by a return to baseline flow was measured in dogs anesthetized with pentobarbital (23). Continuous ketamine infusion in well-oxygenated hypocapnic swine resulted in a decrease in blood flow up to 50% (24).

Anesthetic management will also alter intestinal blood flow. Hypocapnia results in a significant decrease in intestinal blood flow (25), which is an indication that hyperventilation should be avoided. Many clinical patients are hypovolemic or lose blood during surgery. A 10% loss of blood volume over 20 minutes in anesthetized experimental dogs resulted in a significant decrease in colonic blood flow (26). Other important information from this study was that despite the decrease in colon blood flow and cardiac output, arterial pressure was unchanged, and that after the blood was retransfused the colon blood flow did not return to the value obtained before hemorrhage.

INTRALUMINAL PRESSURE

Nitrous oxide inhaled in the anesthetic gases will leave the blood and enter any air space within the body, causing it to expand (27, 28). Thus the administration of nitrous oxide is contraindicated in patients with intestinal distension or pneumothorax. The rate of diffusion of nitrous oxide out of the intestine is slower than its influx, making it impossible to rapidly reverse undesirable distension.

Anesthetic Management for Specific Procedures

ORAL CAVITY AND PHARYNX

A preanesthetic evaluation of the patient should be done before general anesthesia. Patients for elective procedures may have other problems of significance to the anesthetic management, such as old age. Geriatric animals have a reduced requirement for anesthetic drugs; have decreased cardiovascular, pulmonary, hepatic, and renal function; and are more susceptible to hypothermia. Patients with traumatic injuries, such as a fractured jaw, may have had a subdural hemorrhage, and anesthetic drugs or techniques that cause an increase in intracranial pressure should be avoided. These patients may also have pulmonary contusions, blebs, or bullae, predisposing them to pneumothorax, and myocardial contusions, which may result in cardiac dysrhythmias.

Neoplasms in the pharynx may cause airway obstruction during anesthesia or interfere with tracheal intubation. Obstruction should be anticipated; personnel and equipment to facilitate intubation, such as a laryngoscope or endoscope and small size tubes, should be ready. An endotracheal tube that will bend without kinking has a metal spiral embedded in its wall and is available in sizes for dogs. In some animals, placement of a tracheostomy first under local anesthesia may be an appropriate safety precaution.

Any patient having surgery that results in blood loss, loose teeth or debris, or includes water lavage should have an endotracheal tube in place to prevent pulmonary aspiration of foreign material. The tube may simply be pushed to one side to allow access to the surgical site. The endotracheal tube may be removed for assessment of tooth alignment during repair of a fractured jaw, but a better technique in dogs and cats is to provide inhalation anesthesia through an endotracheal tube inserted into the pharynx at the site of placement of a pharyngostomy tube; forceps may have to be introduced through the mouth to direct the endotracheal tube into the larynx. Alternatively, the endotracheal tube may be inserted through a tracheostomy.

The choice of anesthetic drug will depend on the condition of the patient but should be selected to provide a rapid return of pharyngeal and laryngeal reflexes at the end of anesthesia to avoid aspiration or airway obstruction. For old or traumatized dogs, premedication with atropine or glycopyrrolate may be followed by slow intravenous injection of acepromazine or diazepam and oxymorphone, or Innovar-Vet, endotracheal intubation, and maintenance of anesthesia with halothane or isoflurane, with or without nitrous oxide. In healthier animals, the dosage of thiopental in unsedated dogs has been decreased to 11 mg kg^{-1} or less, by administering it with lidocaine in alternate small boluses up to 8 mg kg^{-1} total dose (29). Alternatively, heavy sedation from narcotic drugs has been used to reduce the dosage for induction of anesthesia of thiopental or thiamylal to 2 to 4 mg kg^{-1}. Oxymorphone, 0.11 to 0.22 mg kg^{-1} (30), or Innovar-Vet, 1 ml/30 kg, can be used for this purpose. Methohexital is metabolized at a faster rate than either thiopental or thiamylal and is an excellent drug for induction of anesthesia for oropharyngeal surgery. In cats, chamber induction with halothane is usually followed by a rapid recovery from anesthesia.

A pharyngostomy tube may cause airway obstruction during recovery from anesthesia if it forms a loop in the pharynx. The tube should be observed by direct viewing, not just digital palpation, to pass straight into the esophagus. Before the patient is allowed to recover from anesthesia, blood and fluid should be cleaned from the pharynx, particularly ventral to the epiglottis and around the tube within the larynx. The endotracheal tube should remain in place with the cuff inflated until the patient can swallow. The tube should then be removed with the patient's head lowered below table level and with the cuff should be partially inflated. Corticosteroids should be administered to prevent airway obstruction, and placement of a tracheostomy tube should be considered, when swelling is anticipated after surgery (soft palatectomy or cryosurgery for neoplasia). Because swelling may be initiated by barking or eating or drinking, the patient should be observed for several hours after recovery from anesthesia.

ESOPHAGUS

An animal that has a lacerated esophagus from a dog fight should be examined carefully for tracheal rupture or a penetrating wound of the thorax. Animals with esophageal obstruction that are depressed and dehydrated should receive sufficient intravenous fluid before anesthesia to restore blood volume. Patients with aspiration pneumonia should be supplied with oxygen by face mask or oxygen cage for several minutes before anesthesia and also during induction of anesthesia to avoid hypoxemia. Fluid that has accumulated cranial to the obstruction may be regurgitated during induction of anesthesia. Anesthesia should, therefore, be induced rapidly so that an endotracheal tube may be inserted and the cuff inflated before regurgitation can occur.

A long endotracheal tube of noncollapsing material, which will extend at least to the thoracic inlet, should be used for surgery involving the cervical portion of the esophagus to avoid tracheal collapse during retraction. If an esophageal foreign body is to be removed by esophagoscopy and the obstruction is within the thorax or during dilation of an esophageal stricture, the anesthetist should be prepared for the sudden development of a pneumothorax. Signs may include increased depth of spontaneous breathing, increased resistance to manual inflation of the lungs, progressive expansion of the thorax (tension pneumothorax), and cyanosis. Surgery of the intrathoracic portion of the esophagus involves all the anesthetic considerations of a thoracotomy.

Oxygen supplementation should be provided during recovery from anesthesia until the animal is able to maintain adequate oxygenation on room air.

STOMACH AND INTESTINES

Animals with gastric fluid retention may regurgitate during anesthesia. Premedication with glycopyrrolate 45 minutes before anesthesia should decrease the acidity of gastric fluid so that it may cause less pulmonary damage if aspirated. The patient should be held in a sternal position during induction of anesthesia to decrease the incidence of regurgitation; its head should be held up until the trachea is intubated.

Weight loss is a consistent problem in animals with chronic gastrointestinal disease, and the significance is in the decreased volume for distribution of drugs. Anesthesia from thiobarbiturates will last longer and complete recovery to full function will be slow. The requirement for all anesthetic drugs is often decreased in these patients. Dogs may be intubated with small doses of acepromazine or diazepam and oxymorphone, or Innovar-Vet, and an inhalation agent may be used for maintenance of anesthesia. Nitrous oxide should not be used if the stomach or intestines are gas-filled because the distension will be increased. The addition of a neuromuscular blocking drug to provide muscle relaxation during light anesthesia with neuroleptanalgesia and a low concentration of halothane or isoflurane may provide optimum conditions for severely compromised animals.

Patients that have been vomiting may have a metabolic alkalosis and should receive 0.9% saline for their maintenance fluid. Fluid loss by evaporation from visceral surfaces is considerable, and fluids should be infused at 10 ml kg^{-1} hr^{-1} with continuous reevaluation of the fluid balance. The fluids should be warmed before infusion because heat loss from exposed intestines may cause severe hypothermia. The animal should lie on a hot water circulating pad during surgery, and the intestines should be covered wherever possible.

Hypotension may occur suddenly when catecholamines are released by handling during operation of a carcinoma of the gastrointestinal tract. Anesthetic administration should be discontinued, and the rate of intravenous infusion of fluids should be increased. When a narcotic drug has been used, it should be reversed by intravenous injection of naloxone, 0.02 mg kg^{-1}. Peripheral vasodilation is usually present, and infusion of a vasoconstricting drug may increase the blood pressure. Alternatively, dopamine (Intropin) or dobutamine (Dobutrex), 5 μg kg^{-1} min^{-1} (40 mg in 500 ml lactated Ringer's solution or 0.9% saline; 80 μg/ml), may be useful by increasing cardiac contractility. Similarly, hypotension may develop from release of vasoactive substances after manipulation of ischemic intestine, or an intussusception and flunixin meglumine (Banamine) should be injected in addition to infusion of fluid and dopamine. Dogs treated with flunixin meglumine during experimentally induced sepsis had higher blood pressures, lower packed cell volumes, less metabolic acidosis, and higher survival rates than those that were not treated (31).

A severe decrease in arterial pressure may also occur when intestines are removed from the thoracic cavity during repair of a ruptured diaphragm. Vessels in the trapped intestines may dilate, pooling blood and reducing the volume of blood returning to the heart. In most cases, pressure will be restored by rapid infusion of electrolyte solution (10 ml kg^{-1}). It is important that once the abdominal viscera are removed from the thorax the collapsed lung is not immediately inflated, otherwise pulmonary edema will develop (32). Reinflation should be allowed to progress gradually while the diaphragm is being repaired.

During endoscopy of the colon or rectum, the patient should be closely monitored. Intestinal distension may cause sudden severe bradycardia or may prevent adequate spontaneous ventilation. In addition, prolonged inflation may cause retrograde movement of intestinal fluid and regurgitation into the esophagus or pharynx.

GASTRIC DISTENSION/VOLVULUS

Preanesthetic Preparation

The importance of adequately decompressing the stomach and restoring adequate cardiovascular function before anesthesia in decreasing intra- and post-operative mortality cannot be overemphasized. A large indwelling venous catheter should be inserted and blood should be collected for laboratory analysis. Rapid intravenous infusion of lactated Ringer's solution (up to 90 ml kg^{-1} hr^{-1}) should be given to restore circulating blood volume, and a stomach tube should be passed to relieve intra-abdominal pressure. Gastric distension severely decreases cardiac output and the volume of ventilation so that further depression by anesthetic drugs can kill the patient. The magnitude of the effect has been quantitated experimentally. A 64% decrease in cardiac output was produced when the stomach was inflated to 30 mm Hg pressure (33), and an 89% decrease in cardiac output and 45% decrease in mean arterial pressure was produced by 50 mm Hg pressure distension (34).

Cardiac rhythm disturbances may be present on admission, or they may appear during or after surgery. A survey of 115 dogs with gastric distension/volvulus (GDV) identified 42% developing dysrhythmias, usually between 12 and 36 hours after onset of distension (35). This may be the result of myocardial ischemia because histological changes of myocardial degeneration and necrosis have been seen in clinical and experimental dogs with GDV (35) and a 50% decrease in coronary blood flow has been measured in experimental dogs with gastric distension (34). Acid-base and electrolyte abnormalities and increased circulating vasoactive compounds may contribute to myocardial irritability.

The dysrhythmias are most commonly sinus tachycardia or ventricular premature depolarizations (35, 36) and therefore are potentially life-threatening. Lidocaine (1 to 2 mg/kg) is the initial drug of choice as a bolus injection, followed by an additional dosage up to 8 mg kg^{-1} in 10 minutes if necessary. Blood lidocaine concentration may be maintained by an infusion of lidocaine up to 0.08 mg kg^{-1} min^{-1} (25 ml 2% lidocaine in 475 ml lactated Ringer's solution; 1 mg/ml). Procainamide may be added if lidocaine does not provide sufficient control (37). Procainamide (0.5 mg kg^{-1}) may be injected as an intravenous bolus every 3 to 5 minutes until normal sinus rhythm is established or until 6 mg kg^{-1} is reached. Blood concentration may be maintained by a constant infusion of 0.04 mg kg^{-1} min^{-1} (1 mg/ml solution).

The metabolic status cannot be assessed from the physical status of the patient. A metabolic alkalosis may develop as sequestration of H^+ occurs in the stomach. The decreased cardiac output and inadequate ventilation from gastric distension result in decreased oxygen delivery to the peripheral tissues and lactic acidosis. Either a metabolic alkalosis or a metabolic acidosis may predominate, or they may cancel each other out. The best way to be sure is to measure electrolyte concentrations and arterial pH and PCO_2 or total CO_2 whenever possible. Laboratory measurements on 20 dogs with GDV showed no difference in pH, bicarbonate, anion gap, or electrolytes from values obtained from normal dogs (38). Another survey also showed no significant differences from normal dogs, but when considered individually, over one-half had a metabolic acidosis (39). Hypokalemia was present in about one-third of the dogs. Hypokalemia is important because it predisposes the patient to cardiac dysrhythmias and also results in decreased gastrointestinal motility, which may delay recovery of normal intestinal function after surgery. Intravenous treatment with solutions containing high levels of potassium should not exceed an infusion rate of 0.5 meq K^+ kg^{-1} hr^{-1}.

Anesthetic Management

Anesthetic drugs that sensitize the myocardium to dysrhythmias should be avoided. Xylazine and, to a lesser extent, thiopental and thiamylal decrease the threshold for ventricular dysrhythmias during halothane anesthesia (40–42). The incidence of dysrhythmias occurring during induction of anesthesia with thiopental may be reduced by inducing anesthesia with a combination of lidocaine with thiopental (29), but the lowered threshold caused by barbiturates has been demonstrated to persist for several hours after the anesthetic effects have dissipated (41, 42). Anesthesia may be induced by slow intravenous titration of Innovar-Vet, up to 1 ml 30 kg^{-1}, or diazepam, up to 0.5 mg kg^{-1}, and oxymorphone, up to 0.2 mg kg^{-1}. Intravenous injection of diazepam and ketamine, 2 to 4 mg kg^{-1}, has also been used for induction of anesthesia in these patients. Isoflurane may be a better drug than halothane for maintenance of anesthesia because it causes less sensitization of the myocardium to catecholamines and less depression of cardiac output. Nitrous oxide is contraindicated when the stomach or intestines are distended with gas. Preanesthetic condition varies from relatively healthy to moribund; therefore, sedatives and anesthetic drugs should be administered in small increments to avoid overdosing.

The dog should be preoxygenated, and precautions should be taken against pulmonary aspiration of gastric fluid, as previously described. Controlled ventilation must be instituted immediately after induction of anesthesia. A more rapid rate than usual (15 breaths/min^{-1}) have to be used because the high intra-abdominal pressure will limit the tidal volume. The inspiratory pressure should not be allowed to exceed 40 cm H_2O; otherwise, a further decrease in blood pressure will be observed. The electrocardiogram and arterial blood pressure should be continuously monitored. Hypotension must be treated with increased intravenous fluid infusion and dopamine or dobutamine infusion, up to 5 μg/kg/min.

Intensive monitoring of the patient should be continued into the recovery period, particularly as dysrhythmias may not develop until hours after the surgical operation. Oxygen should be supplied after extubation when the dog is still depressed or until ventilation is judged to be adequate.

PORTACAVAL SHUNT

A dog with portacaval shunt that has hepatic encephalopathy and central nervous system depression will need very little drug for anesthesia. Drug action will be longer because blood by-passing the liver decreases the amount of drug presented to the liver for detoxification. Hypoalbuminemia may increase the activity of anesthetic drugs that are protein bound (barbiturates). The dog may be premedicated with diazepam, or premedication may be omitted and anesthesia may be induced and maintained with isoflurane or halothane. Arterial pressure should be monitored when the shunt is ligated for early recognition of hypotension which may result from decreased blood return to the heart. Absorption of endotoxin may be a problem and administration of flunixin meglumine may be protective.

PERINEUM

Preanesthetic evaluation of a dog with a perineal hernia must include examination to determine whether the urinary bladder is involved and laboratory tests to rule out azotemia. Many of these patients are geriatric, with the corresponding anesthetic considerations, or have cardiac disease that also requires special management.

Positioning during anesthesia must be done with knowledge of the effect of a prone, head down position has on the cardiovascular and respiratory systems. Cardiac output and arterial pressure will decrease when the animal is put into a head down position, and a greater than 30° tilt should be avoided. This position should not be used if the patient has cardiac disease, pulmonary disease, or head trauma. Anesthetized dogs usually hypoventilate when placed in a prone position; controlled ventilation is advisable, particularly if the patient is old, obese, or has cardiac disease. Breathing may be made easier if a sandbag is placed under the animal's pubis so that the abdomen is partially lifted away from the table.

Anesthetic drugs should be chosen according to the status of the patient. Nitrous oxide should not be used initially if loops of intestine are present in the hernia. Epidural analgesia is a useful alternative to general anesthesia for some patients. Lidocaine may not provide sufficient time for surgery but 0.75% bupivacaine (Marcaine) will provide 5 to 6 hours of analgesia in dogs (43). The dosage used is 1 ml/4.5 kg to block forward to the first lumbar vertebra, and 1 ml/3.4 kg to produce analgesia to the fifth thoracic vertebra, with an onset of action of 10 to 20 minutes.

Signs of severe pain may be exhibited by dogs after rectal or perineal surgery and should be anticipated. An analgesic drug, such as meperidine (2 mg kg^{-1}) or butorphanol (0.2 mg kg^{-1}) should be injected intramuscularly at the end of anesthesia before the patient regains consciousness.

Gastrointestinal Surgery in Horses

In a survey of 1301 horses with colic admitted for treatment to 9 University Veterinary Teaching Hospitals, 446 had surgery; 42.8% lived, 22.8 died, and 34.4% were euthanized (N.A. White, personal communication, 1983). No doubt the disease has progressed too far for treatment in many horses, but as our methods of treatment improve, the number of animals surviving must increase. Various clinical and laboratory parameters have been correlated with mortality rate. In 1982, Bristol reported that out of 90 horses treated for colic, no animal with an anion gap exceeding 24 meq/liter survived (44). Today, horses with anion gaps of up to 40 meq/liter are surviving. Low systolic blood pressure on admission to hospital has been correlated with a low survival rate (45, 46). With new vasoactive drugs available and the results of potential research into reperfusion injury, more animals will survive. It is important to begin correction of physiological abnormalities before anesthesia because anesthesia and surgery cause additional adverse hemodynamic changes and jeopardize the patient's chance for survival.

PREANESTHETIC PREPARATION

Hypovolemia and dehydration usually develop in horses with colic, resulting in decreased cardiac output and peripheral perfusion. If anesthesia is induced before circulating blood volume is restored, the patient may die due to an intolerable decrease in cardiac output produced by the anesthetic drugs. In addition, a significant decrease in survival rate after anesthesia was identified in a retrospective survey of 341 operations for colic in horses that had received insufficient fluid to decrease the packed cell volume (PCV) below 45% (47). Clinical signs of a weak peripheral pulse, slow capillary refill time, pale or bluish mucous membranes, together with laboratory measurements of increased PCV and plasma protein (PP) or increased blood urea nitrogen (BUN) are indications for intravenous fluid administration before surgery. The practice of infusing dimethylsulfoxide (DMSO) in an attempt to decrease reperfusion injury of the intestine does not appear to alter the response to anesthetic drugs. Infusion of DMSO (20 mg kg^{-1} to 1 g kg^{-1}) to three healthy anesthetized horses produced no significant change in arterial pressure or cardiac output (D. Allen and C. M. Trim, unpublished observations).

The metabolic status of horses with colic cannot be accurately assessed from the history and physical examination. Each surgical condition does not consistently produce the same metabolic derangement, so that it may range from a mild metabolic alkalosis (base excess of 7 meq/liter) to severe metabolic acidosis (base deficit of 15 meq/liter). Measurement of arterial base deficit from pH and PCO_2 or measurement of total CO_2 should be done if possible. Blood gas and acid-base values for normal horses vary according to their degree of interest in the environment, which alters ventilation, and the nature of their food. Approximate values are pHa, 7.38 to 7.43; $PaCO_2$, 38 to 42 mm Hg; base excess, 0 to 5 meq/liter; arterial bicarbonate, 24.0 to 29 meq/liter; arterial TCO_2, 25.0 to 30.0 meq/liter; and venous TCO_2, 26 to 32 meq/liter. Lactated or acetated Ringer's solutions contain bicarbonate precursor (27 to 50 meq/liter) that is only sufficient to treat a mild metabolic acidosis. A moderate to severe acidosis should be corrected because acidosis decreases myocardial function. The milliequivalent of sodium bicarbonate required can be calculated from the formula:

deficit × kg bodyweight × 0.3 (volume of extracellular fluid); this can be infused intravenously over 45 to 60 minutes. When measurements are not available and acidosis is suspected, sodium bicarbonate (1.5 meq kg^{-1}) should be infused over 30 minutes.

Low serum potassium concentration has been measured in some horses with colic. Hypokalemia may predispose the anesthetized patient to cardiac dysrhythmias and may be a problem after surgery by causing muscle weakness and ileus. For these patients, the potassium concentration of fluids infused before anesthesia should be increased up to 20 meq/liter and the rate of infusion of (K^+) controlled so that it does not exceed 0.5 meq/liter/hr (48). The earliest sign of hyperkalemia in horses during infusion of potassium is diarrhea (48), which may not be observed in horses with obstruction. The electrocardiogram should be monitored for narrow peaked T waves and shortened QT intervals, which would indicate hyperkalemia, but plasma potassium concentration may be excessive before electrocardiogram changes appear.

Low blood calcium concentration of 8 or 9 mg/dl (normal values are 10.2 to 14.3 mg/dl), without clinical signs, may be present in some horses. In addition, a respiratory or metabolic alkalosis will result in a low ionized calcium fraction. Calcium is essential for normal cardiovascular function, and hypocalcemia has been associated with hypotension during anesthesia (49). Intravenous infusion of calcium borogluconate (23%, up to 200 ml/450 kg) over 20 minutes should increase the blood calcium concentration the normal range.

Abdominal distension interferes with breathing and also decreases cardiac output. In the conscious animal, cecal trocharization may be necessary for the animal to survive. Rapid deterioration may occur in these patients after induction of anesthesia when the respiratory and cardiovascular systems are further depressed by anesthetic drugs. The operating room and personnel should be organized so the time from induction of anesthesia to abdominal incision is short, and ventilation should be controlled from the beginning.

Each patient should be auscultated for cardiac dysrhythmias on admission to hospital and immediately before anesthesia. Although not common, ventricular premature depolarization or ventricular tachycardia may be present. Ventricular tachycardia should be treated with lidocaine before induction of anesthesia.

Some horses with colic also have hepatitis (50), which may be made worse by anesthesia. If appropriate to the surgical condition, performing the laparotomy with the animal standing should be considered. Isoflurane is a better choice for general anesthesia in these patients because it is not metabolized and has less effect on the liver.

ANESTHETIC DRUGS

Sedation and analgesia may be necessary before surgery. Acepromazine should be avoided because it produces peripheral vasodilation that is difficult to counteract during anesthesia should cardiovascular deterioration occur. Xylazine (1.1 mg kg^{-1}) and butorphanol (Torbugesic) (0.2 mg kg^{-1}) provided analgesia in healthy ponies and horses during experimental cecal distension (51, 52). In clinical practice, these drugs are often effective in quietening a horse with colic, but are usually used at a lower dosage. Less xylazine is used because xylazine decreases cardiac output, decreases intestinal motility, and increases urine volume and potassium excretion. Less butorphanol is used because the high dose rate results in ataxia and because a lower dose usually provides an adequate effect. Neuroleptanalgesic drug combinations provide adequate sedation while allowing a smaller dose of xylazine to be used. The dosage is xylazine (0.3 to 0.6 mg kg^{-1}) with either butorphanol (0.025 to 0.05 mg kg^{-1}), pentazocine (Talwin-V) (0.3 to 0.5 mg kg^{-1}), oxymorphone (0.01 to 0.022 mg kg^{-1}), or meperidine (0.5 to 1.0 mg kg^{-1}).

Detomidine hydrochloride (Domosedan) is a sedative that is licensed for horses in Europe and is on clinical trial in the United States. Detomidine has cardiovascular effects similar to xylazine but produces a much longer lasting sedation. Anesthetic drugs must be administered cautiously after detomidine has been used because, although the sedative effects may appear to have worn off, the anesthetic requirement for other drugs is still decreased. The horses are much quieter and sleep longer in recovery when detomidine has been used.

The physiological condition of horses with colic requiring anesthesia for surgical operation varies from good to severely abnormal and consequently the anesthetic management must be tailored to the individual patient. Several drug combinations can be used safely provided that the degree to which drug dosages must be decreased is assessed before anesthesia. The author's preference is to use guaifenesin alone to immobilize the severely ill patients for tracheal intubation and guaifenesin and barbiturate (at one-half the usual dose) or guaifenesin and ketamine in the less sick patients (53). Guaifenesin provides control of the animal so that the anesthetic drugs can more easily be titrated to meet the patient's reduced requirement. The horse may be premedicated with a neuroleptanalgesic drug combination or a low dose of xylazine; in some cases, preanesthetic sedation may be omitted. Horses with little physiological change may be anesthetized with drugs normally used in healthy animals. Inhalation anesthesia is generally the best method for maintaining anesthesia for surgery. Halothane is most commonly used, but use of isoflurane for horses with colic is increasing because the cardiovascular system is less depressed and recovery from anesthesia is more rapid and coordinated.

Anesthesia in foals is easily induced and maintained with either halothane or isoflurane without premedication. Alternatively, preanesthetic sedation may include a small dose of xylazine, xylazine and pentazocine or butorphanol, or diazepam and pentazocine or butorphanol. Anesthesia may also be induced in the sedated foal with ketamine titrated to effect.

ANESTHETIC MANAGEMENT

Immediately before induction of anesthesia, accumulated gastric fluid should be removed to reduce the potential for regurgitation during induction of anesthesia, and the stomach tube should be left in place. The mouth should be flushed with water to prevent tracheal contamination with food material with the endotracheal tube. The heart should be reauscultated for dysrhythmias. Preoxygenation is advisable for horses with inadequate cardiopulmonary function and can be provided by insufflating oxygen (15 liters/450 kg) through a tube inserted several inches up the nose for a few minutes before and during induction of anesthesia.

Horses producing a large volume of gastric reflux may regurgitate before intubation is accomplished and may aspirate fluid into the lungs. This may be prevented in some animals by supporting them in a sternal position after induction of anesthesia and intubating the trachea and inflating the cuff before allowing the animal to fall onto its side. The vaporizer dial setting immediately after induction should be lower than usual until the requirement of the individual patient becomes obvious. The strength of the pulse should be assessed when the animal is rolled onto its back because severe hypotension may occur at that time. Most horses will survive if allowed to breathe spontaneously, but hypoventilation in these patients is often severe, and the acidemia usually further decreases the cardiac output. Controlled ventilation is recommended, and a respiratory rate of 10 breaths/min with a tidal volume of 11 ml/kg will maintain a normal arterial carbon dioxide concentration of 40 mm Hg. A larger tidal volume of 15 ml/kg will be necessary to achieve adequate ventilation in foals. If a ventilator is not available, compression of the reservoir bag to 22 cm H_2O will produce adequate volume in a thin or starved animal, but an inspiratory pressure of 30 to 35 cm H_2O is frequently needed for horses with intestinal distension. Pressures greater than 40 cm H_2O will severely decrease the cardiac output. Intravenous fluid administration should continue during anesthesia, at a rate of 10 ml/kg/hr if sufficient fluid to replace blood volume was given before anesthesia, at a faster rate if not. The degree of hemodilution should be followed by measurement of PCV and PP hourly.

Close monitoring of the cardiovascular system is essential. This should include observation of capillary refill time and mucous membrane color and measurement of heart rate and arterial blood pressure. Vigorous treatment is necessary if the mean arterial pressure decreases to 55 mm Hg (systolic pressure of 75 mm Hg), and efforts should be made to maintain the mean pressure above 70 mm Hg (systolic pressure above 90 mm Hg). Treatment includes decreasing anesthetic administration, maintaining arterial oxygenation and normocapnia, and infusing intravenous fluid. Vasoactive drugs such as dopamine or dobutamine (3 to 5 μg/kg/min) may be used to increase cardiac contractility. Infusion of calcium borogluconate may also increase arterial pressure, particularly if peripheral vasodilation is marked. Sudden cardiovascular deterioration can occur when ischemic intestine is handled due to release of vasoactive substances (54). As soon as compromised bowel is observed on opening the abdomen, anesthetic delivery should be decreased or turned off; if not already given, flunixin meglumine (Banamine) should be injected to block some of the effects of endotoxin (55). If hypotension ensues, dopamine or dobutamine should be infused, and sodium bicarbonate (1 meq/kg) should be injected. If only small amounts of endotoxin are released, circulating norepinephrine concentration increases and cardiac output and arterial pressure are initially increased, followed by progressive deterioration and a significant decrease in arterial oxygenation to below 100 mm Hg (56). Dopamine infusion may maintain adequate cardiac output and arterial pressure but will not prevent the decrease in oxygenation or lactic acidosis produced in response to endotoxin (57). Sodium bicarbonate will be needed to treat the metabolic acidosis. Injection of dexamethasone without propylene glycol may be beneficial in patients with endotoxemia. Dexamethasone (1.0 mg kg^{-1}) injected into experimentally studied ponies before the administration of endotoxin prevented prolongation of thrombin time and modified the prolongation of activated partial thromboplastin time (58). Lactate accumulation in these ponies was less than with endotoxin alone, although the decrease in arterial pH was similar. In awake ponies, prednisolone sodium succinate (30 mg kg^{-1}) prevented the severe decrease in arterial PO_2 produced by endotoxin, but lactic acidosis developed more rapidly (59). An additional problem is that the cost of this drug used at the dosages recommended for use in shocked animals is prohibitive.

RECOVERY

The arterial blood pressure should be monitored when the animal is turned onto its side because hypotension may occur at this time. The patient should be allowed to breathe 100% oxygen until the depth of anesthesia has lightened and spontaneous breathing has resumed. During recovery from anesthesia, hypoxemia may be present despite adequate alveolar ventilation and normal arterial carbon dioxide concentration. The inspired air should be enriched with oxygen supplied either by nasal or tracheal tube (15 liters/450 kg) or by ventilation with an air/oxygen mixture using a Bird ventilator or demand valve (Hudson). The nasal cavity should be examined for mucosal edema produced by congestion when the head is positioned lower than the body. If edema is present, the nose should be elevated in recovery; if resistance to breathing is still present at the time of extubation, a smaller endotracheal tube should be inserted through the ventral meatus until the tip lies in the pharynx or trachea. The tube should be left until edema has decreased or until the horse stands up. Additional sedation may be needed to ensure a smooth recovery from anesthesia, and this may be provided by xylazine, (0.2 mg kg^{-1}) or butorphanol (0.02 mg kg^{-1}).

If the stomach tube was removed for recovery, it should be replaced and accumulated gastric fluid should be removed. Monitoring of fluid and metabolic status should be continued.

References

1. Burrows CF, Bright RM, Spencer CP: Influence of dietary composition on gastric emptying and motility in dogs: potential involvement in acute gastric dilatation. *Am J Vet Res* 46:2609–2612, 1985.
2. Leib MC, Wingfield WE, Twedt DC, Williams AR: Gastric emptying of liquids in the dog: serial test meal and modified emptying-time techniques. *Am J Vet Res* 46:1876–1880, 1985.
3. Ducharme NG, Fubini SL: Gastrointestinal complications associated with the use of atropine in horses. *J Am Vet Med Assoc* 182:229–231, 1983.
4. Davies JV, Gerring EL: Effect of spasmolytic analgesic drugs on the motility patterns of the equine small intestine. *Res Vet Sci* 34:334–339, 1983.
5. Adams SB, Lamar CH, Masty J: Motility of the distal portion of the jejunum and pelvic flexure in ponies: Effects of six drugs. *Am J Vet Res* 45:795–799, 1984.
6. Clark ES, Moore JN: The effects of xylazine on cecal arterial blood flow and cecal mechanical activity in conscious horses. *Proceedings of the Fourth Annual Veterinary Medical Forum*, Vol II, 14-5, 1986.
7. Sojka JE, Adams SB, Lamar CH: The effect of two opiate agonist-antagonists on intestinal motility in the pony. Abstract. Second Equine Colic Research Symposium, Athens, Georgia, 1985.
8. Healy TEJ, Foster GE, Evans DF, Syed A: Effect of some i.v. anaesthetic agents on canine gastrointestinal motility. *Br J Anaesth* 53:229–233, 1981.
9. Marshall FTV, Pittinger CB, Long JP: Effects of halothane on gastrointestinal motility. *Anesthesiology* 22:363–366, 1961.
10. Bell CMA, Lewis CB: Effect of neostigmine on integrity of ileorectal anastomoses. *Br Med J* 3:587–588, 1968.
11. Adams SB, MacHarg MA: Neostigmine methylsulfate delays gastric emptying time of particulate markers in horses. *Am J Vet Res* 46:2498–2499, 1985.
12. Child CS: Prevention of neostigmine-induced colonic activity. A comparison of atropine and glycopyrronium. *Anaesthesia* 39:1083–1085, 1984.
13. Strombeck DR, Harrold D: Effects of atropine, acepromazine, meperidine, and xylazine on gastroesophageal sphincter pressure in the dogs. *Am J Vet Res* 46:963–965, 1985.
14. Cotton BR, Smith G: Comparison of the effects of atropine and glycopyrrolate on lower esophageal sphincter pressure. *Br J Anaesth* 53:875–879, 1981.
15. Stoelting RK: Gastric fluid volume and pH after fentanyl, enflurane, or halothane-nitrous oxide anesthesia with or without atropine or glycopyrrolate. *Anesth Analg* 59:287–290, 1980.
16. Engelking LR, Dodman NH, Hartman G, Valdez H, Spivak W: Effects of halothane anesthesia on equine liver function. *Am J Vet Res* 44:607–615, 1984.
17. Engelking LR, Dodman NH, Hartman G, Valdez H: Effects of isoflurane anesthesia on equine liver function. *Am J Vet Res* 45:616–619, 1984.
18. Thulin L, Andreen M, Irestedt L: Effect of controlled halothane anaesthesia on splanchnic blood flow and cardiac output in the dog. *Acta Anaesth Scand* 19:146–153, 1975.
19. Gelman S, Fowler KC, Smith LR: Regional blood flow during isoflurane and halothane anesthesia. *Anesth Analg* 63:557–565, 1984.
20. Manohar M, Goetz TE: Cerebral, renal, adrenal, intestinal, and pancreatic circulation in conscious ponies and during 1.0, 1.5, and 2.0 minimal alveolar concentrations of halothane-O_2 anesthesia. *Am J Res* 46:2492–2497, 1985.
21. Lundeen G, Manohar M, Parks C: Systemic distribution of blood flow in swine while awake and during 1.0 and 1.5 MAC isoflurane with or without 50% nitrous oxide. *Anesth Analg* 62:499–512, 1983.
22. Tranquilli WJ, Manohar M, Parks CM, Thurmon JC, Theodorakis MC, Benson GJ: Systemic and regional blood flow distribution in unanesthetized swine and swine anesthetized with halothane and nitrous oxide, halothane, or enflurane. *Anesthesiology* 56:369–379, 1982.
23. Bond JH, Prentiss RA, Levitt MD: The effect of anesthesia and laparotomy on blood flow to the stomach, small bowel, and colon of the dog. *Surgery* 87:313–318, 1980.
24. Tranquilli WJ, Thurmon JC, Benson GJ: Organ blood flow and distribution of cardiac output in hypocapnic ketamine-anesthetized swine. *Am J Vet Res* 44:1578–1582, 1983.
25. Gilmour DG, Douglas IHS, Aitkenhead AR, Hothersall AP, Horton PW, Ledingham IM: Colon blood flow in the dog: effects of changes in arterial carbon dioxide tension. *Cardiovasc Res* 14:11–20, 1980.
26. Gilmour DG, Aitkenhead AR, Hothersall AP, Ledingham IM: The effect of hypovolemia on colonic blood flow in the dog. *Br J Surg* 67:82–84, 1980.
27. Steffey EP, Johnson BH, Eger EI II, Howland D: Nitrous oxide: Effect on accumulation rate and uptake of bowel gases. *Anesth Analg* 58:405–408, 1979.
28. Moens Y, De Moor A: Diffusion of nitrous oxide into the intestinal lumen of ponies during halothane-nitrous oxide anesthesia. *Am J Vet Res* 42:1751–1753, 1981.
29. Rawlings CA, Kolata RJ: Cardiopulmonary effects of thiopental/lidocaine combination during anesthetic induction in the dog. *Am J Vet Res* 44:144–149, 1983.
30. Hartsfield SM: Gastrointestinal system—Anesthetic considerations. In Slatter DH (ed): *Textbook of Small Animal Surgery*. Philadelphia, WB Saunders Co, 1985, pp 2611–2620.
31. Hardie EM, Rawlings CA, Collins LG: Canine *Escherichia coli* peritonitis: Long-term survival with fluid, gentamicin sulfate, and flunixin meglumine treatment. *J Am Anim Hosp Assoc* 21:691–699, 1985.
32. Ray RJ, Alexander CM, Chen L, Williams J, Marshall BE: Influence of the method of re-expansion of atelectatic lung upon the

development of pulmonary edema in dogs. *Crit Care Med* 12:364–366, 1984.

33. Orten EC, Muir WW: Hemodynamics during experimental gastric dilatation-volvulus in dogs. *Am J Vet Res* 44:1512–1515, 1983.
34. Horne WA, Gilmore DR, Dietze AE, Freden GO, Short CE: Effects of gastric distension-volvulus on coronary blood flow and myocardial oxygen consumption in the dog. *Am J Vet Res* 46:98–104, 1985.
35. Muir WW, Weisbrode SE: Myocardial ischemia in dogs with gastric dilatation-volvulus. *J Am Vet Med Assoc* 181:363–366, 1982.
36. Muir WW, Lipowitz AJ: Cardiac dysrhythmias associated with gastric dilatation-volvulus in the dog. *J Am Vet Med Assoc* 172:683–689, 1978.
37. Muir WW, Bonagura JD: Treatment of cardiac arrhythmias in dogs with gastric distention-volvulus. *J Am Vet Med Assoc* 184:1366–1371, 1984.
38. Wingfield WE, Twedt DC, Moore RW, Leib MS, Wright M: Acid-base and electrolyte values in dogs with acute gastric dilatation-volvulus. *J Am Vet Med Assoc* 180:1070–1072, 1982.
39. Muir WW: Acid-base and electrolyte disturbances in dogs with gastric dilatation-volvulus. *J Am Vet Med Assoc* 181:229–231, 1982.
40. Muir WW, Werner LL, Hamlin RL: Effects of xylazine and acetylpromazine upon induced ventricular fibrillation in dogs anesthetized with thiamylal and halothane. *Am J Vet Res* 36:1299–1303, 1975.
41. Atlee JL, Malkinson CE: Potentiation by thiopental of halothane-epinephrine-induced arrhythmias in dogs. *Anesthesiology* 57:285–288, 1982.
42. Bednarski RM, Majors LJ, Atlee JL: Epinephrine-induced ventricular arrhythmias in dogs anesthetized with halothane: Potentiation by thiamylal and thiopental. *Am J Vet Res* 46:1829–1831, 1985.
43. Heath RB, Broadstone RV, Wright M, Grandy JL: Bupivacaine and mepivacaine lumbosacral epidural analgesia in dogs. *Proc 2nd Intl Cong Vet Anes*, 162–163, 1985.
44. Bristol DG: The anion gap as a prognostic indicator in horses with abdominal pain. *J Am Vet Med Assoc* 181:63–65, 1982.
45. Gay CC, Carter J, McCarthy M, Mason TA, Christie BA, Reynolds WT, Smyth B: The value of arterial blood pressure measurement in assessing the prognosis in equine colic. *Equine Vet J* 9:202–204, 1977.
46. Parry BW, Anderson GA, Gay CC: Prognosis in equine colic: a comparative study of variables used to assess individual cases. *Equine Vet J* 15:211–215, 1983.
47. Pascoe PJ, McDonell WN, Trim CM,Van Gorder J: Mortality rates and associated factors in equine colic operations: a retrospective survey of 341 operations. *Can Vet J* 24:76–85, 1983.
48. Hood DM: Fluid balance in the critically ill horse. *Proc 1st Equine Colic Research Symposium* 285–287, 1982.
49. Drop LJ: Ionized calcium, the heart, and hemodynamic function. *Anesth Analg* 64:432–451, 1985.
50. Moore JN, Traver DS, Coffman JR: Large bowel obstruction and chronic active hepatitis in a horse. *Vet Med/Small Anim Clin* 71:1457–1463, 1976.
51. Kalpravidh M, Lumb WV, Wright M, Heath RB: Effects of butorphanol, flunixin, levorphanol, morphine, and xylazine in ponies. *Am J Vet Res* 45:217–223, 1984.
52. Muir WW, Robertson JT: Visceral analgesia: Effects of xylazine, butorphanol, meperidine, and pentazocine in horses. *Am J Vet Res* 46:2081–2084, 1985.
53. Trim CM: Anesthetic management of the horse with colic. In *Proceedings of the Veterinary Seminar on the Equine Acute Abdomen at the University of Georgia*, Vol 1. Lawrenceville, NJ, Veterinary Learning Systems, 1986, in press.
54. Trim CM: Anesthetic management of the horse with acute intestinal obstruction. *Proc Assoc Vet Anes G Br Ir* 7:28–41, 1977.
55. Moore JN, Garner HE, Shapland JE, Hatfield DG: Prevention of endotoxin-induced arterial hypoxaemia and lactic acidosis with flunixin meglumine in the conscious pony. *Equine Vet J* 13:95–98, 1981.
56. Trim CM, Moore JN, Slade EA, Graham DM, Hardee MM, Hardee GE: Effects of prostacyclin infusion in anesthetized normal and endotoxemic horses. In *Proceedings of the Second Equine Colic Research Symposium at the University of Georgia*, Vol 2. Lawrenceville, NJ, Veterinary Learning Systems, 1986, in press.
57. Trim CM, Moore JN, White NA: Cardiopulmonary effects of dopamine hydrochloride during endotoxemia in anesthetized horses. *Proc Am Coll Vet Anes Scientific Meeting*, 33–34, 1983.
58. Frauenfelder HC, Fessler JF, Moore AB, Bottoms GD, Boon GD: Effects of dexamethasone on endotoxic shock in the anesthetized pony: hematologic, blood gas, and coagulation changes. *Am J Vet Res* 43:405–411, 1982.
59. Moore JN: Effects of prednisolone sodium succinate in endotoxemia in ponies. PhD dissertation, University of Missouri, 1980.

CHAPTER 13

Clinical Anesthesia in Various Animal Species and Conditions

PART 1

Special Considerations for Equine Anesthesia

CHARLES E. SHORT, D.V.M., M.S., D.A.C.V.A.

The horse provides the veterinarian with a variety of unique challenges during anesthesia induction, maintenance, and recovery. In addition to its unique size and speed of motion, one must consider the temperament of the individual horse, the response to preanesthetic medication, the physical aspects of anesthetic induction, cardiopulmonary and other physiological functions during the maintenance of anesthesia, and the potential for stress and injury during the recovery period.

An evaluation of the physical status, clinical and pathological data, and history of the individual horse before the administration of preanesthetics and the induction of anesthesia is desirable. When this is not feasible, it is then necessary to take as many precautions as possible to assure safe and effective anesthesia.

Preanesthetics

ANTICHOLINERGICS

The anticholinergics, such as atropine or glycopyrrolate, are not as routinely utilized as preanesthetics in the horse as in dogs, cats, and human subjects. They are effective in reducing the tendency to bradycardia. This will be of special interest to the veterinarian when xylazine or xylazine-like products are used to control pain or as preanesthetics because these medications are known to produce marked slowing of the heart rate. Anticholinergics are of added benefit in the presence of narcotics, which may slow the heart rate, especially when used in conjunction with anesthetics. Anticholinergics have been shown to be beneficial in the control of reduced heart rates in the presence of higher concentrations of halothane and other potent anesthetic agents.

There are surgical procedures and manipulations that may contribute to slowing of the heart or even cardiac standstill. These procedures include ocular surgery, which can produce ocular-cardiac reflexes resulting in dramatic slowing of the heart; in some cases, cardiac arrest has occurred (1).

The predominant reason for not using anticholinergics is concern over reducing the peristalsis of the intestinal tract, which can result in colicky symptoms. Colic symptoms after high doses of atropine sulfate can be expected, especially if there is food in the intestinal tract. Recent feeding of horses before the administration of anticholinergics can easily lead to reduction in intestinal motility, gas accumulation, intestinal distention, colic symptoms, and even cardiopulmonary distress. The same has been observed in horses under general anesthesia that received no anticholinergics. The withholding of feed for at least 4 to 6 hours prior to the administration of anticholinergics will help to assure that gastrointestinal distress is not as likely to occur following the administration of anticholinergics. Intestinal colic has been observed in animals that have received atropine as an ophthalmic ointment. As a result, selective utilization of anticholinergics in those horses in which protection is required against bradycardia or heart block should be considered. After the intravenous administration of anticholinergics, a period of 45 to 60 minutes of partial to complete relaxation of the intestinal tract may occur. This lasts for potentially longer periods after intramuscular or subcutaneous administration.

The anticholinergic protection to the heart against bradycardia and heart block may last from 30 to 120 minutes depending upon the dosage of anticholinergic and the potential of other medications to produce bradycardia and/or heart block. Dilatation of the pupil after systemic utilization of anticholinergics may last for up to 24 hours. Caution should be used to avoid exposing the horse to bright sunlight or artificial lighting during this period. At least one case of transient blindness has been observed by the author in a horse with atropine-induced dilatation of the pupil.

Sedatives and Tranquilizers

During the last several years, xylazine, a potent sedative, analgetic, and tranquilizer, has been used in many horses as a preanesthetic agent (2–8). It has been shown to possess the characteristics of sedation needed for the control of pain, reduction of excitement, and desirable responses as a preanesthetic, especially before ketamine anesthesia. Its predominant undesirable side effect is reduction of heart rate and/or production of heart block, which is controllable with an anticholinergic. It produces hyperglycemia and hypoinsulemia and is usually associated with an increase in urine volume (6, 7). It has been shown to be one of the most effective preanesthetics for ketamine induction in the horse.

Of the phenothiazine-derivative tranquilizers, acetylpromazine has continued to be one of the more popular tranquilizing agents used by equine practitioners in America. It usually causes smooth production of tranquilization with few undesirable side effects (9, 10). Hypotension may occur; on rare occasions, transient paralysis of the penis may occur in stallions. Transient responses in the hemopoietic system, especially hematocrit and hemoglobin levels, may occur (11). Individual horses may not show full tranquilizing effect of the phenothiazine-derivative tranquilizers, especially if they are administered in less than ideal circumstances where there is excessive noise, handling, or other forms of excitement.

Because of the tendency of some horses to kick when handled after receiving xylazine and the desire to have a combination of medications that offers both tranquilization and analgesia, combinations of acepromazine and xylazine have been used (12–15). The hemodynamic and respiratory effects of this combination have been studied and may be stable if low doses of each agent are used. If the desirable responses of profound tranquilization can be accomplished through the use of partial dosages of phenothiazine-derivative tranquilizers (acetylpromazine) along with the sedative and analgetic effects of xylazine, the individual horse may demonstrate favorable results. This is usually accomplished through the administration of smaller volumes not exceeding 50% of normal recommended dosages of each of the two agents (14). The administration of full recommended doses of both xylazine and acetylpromazine can cause bradycardia or heart block via the effects of xylazine and hypotension because of the alpha-blocking vasodilating effect of acetylpromazine. This results in an animal that has both a slow heart rate and hypotension, producing a form of shock from which the animal may collapse. The incidence of this problem has been limited; however, several cases of transient physiological changes, including reduced intraocular pressure (15), and at least one death from higher doses of this combination have been reported.

Diazepam (0.2 to 0.4 mg/kg i.v.) has been used as a preanesthetic in the horse. It is not as likely to change arterial cardiac output, blood gases, and pH as other agents and produces mild sedation for up to 2 hours (16). Butorphanol (0.11 to 0.22 mg/kg) (17) has been used as an adjunct to xylazine prior to ketamine anesthesia, as has diazepam. Such other analgetics as morphine, meperidine, methadone, fentanyl (20 μg/kg i.v.), and the non-narcotic pentazocine (1 mg/kg) have been used as preanesthetics alone or in combination with the tranquilizers (18–19). The evaluation of azaperone (0.6 to 1.2 mg/kg i.m.) (20) and polamivet (21) has continued the quest to find the ideal preanesthetic to help accomplish the calming effect of the horse. Azaperone may produce excitement, prolapse of the penis, sweating, and trembling. Polamivet (0.06 ml/kg i.v.) have reduced undesirable responses compared to azaperone.

Perphenazine (22) and chloropromazine have been shown to produce undesirable effects on the horse; as a result, their utilization as preanesthetics is discouraged. The use of agents that affect the function of the horse for the specific needs at the time of administration are encouraged. The most predictable remain acetylpromazine for tranquilization and xylazine or detomidine for sedation and analgesia. The concurrent use of two or more agents may result in undesirable responses. Xylazine and acetylpromozine have been administered at partial dosages in combination. Caution is advised to avoid hypotension with excessive medication.

Neuroleptanalgesia

Utilization of xylazine, 1.1 mg/kg i.v., and butorphanol, 0.1 mg/kg i.v., to produce neuroleptanalgesia in the horse has resulted in synergistic analgesic activity. When tranquilizers are used with a narcotic, neuroleptanalgesia should occur. Less depression is anticipated when xylazine is combined with butorphanol (23, 24) than with a number of combinations (24), including xylazine, 0.7 mg/kg, with methadone, 0.1 mg/kg. Xylazine and morphine, although reportedly not producing statistically undesirable cardiopulmonary depression (26), will on occasion give results of hypotension, slow capillary refill time, bradycardia, and evidence of cyanosis. Undesirable heart block may also occur. On many other occasions, excellent analgesia will be observed even to the point of completing short surgical procedures under neuroleptanalgesia alone (24–26). Consequently, xylazine, 0.7 mg/kg i.v., and morphine, 0.12 mg/kg i.v., should be used with caution. It is recommended the veterinarian evaluate cardiopulmonary function by determining heart rates and capillary refill time after the administration of this combination of drugs. An anticholinergic agent may be used for correction of severe bradycardia, and calcium chloride may be used to improve cardiac performance in those individual cases that may require measures to protect the cardiovascular system. Supplemental oxygen in cases of undue respiratory depression will assist in correction of oxygen deficits.

A combination of azaperone, 0.2 to 0.8 mg/kg, and metomidate, 3.5 mg/kg, to produce neuroleptanalgesia has been used in the horse (27, 28). There was an increase in blood lactate concentration and reductions in plasma potassium, calcium, and magnesium with a 20% increase in heart rate and a decrease in arterial blood oxygen.

Etorphine (29) in combination with tranquilizers to produce neuroleptanalgesia in the horse is in use in other countries, especially in England. This combination produces not only analgesia, but immobilization. The degree of relaxation is incomplete, with muscle tremors occurring in as many as 80% of cases. The muscle tremors are sometimes severe enough to cause sweating and hinder surgery. Respiration may be depressed, and there is usually tachycardia and a reduction in the animal's ability to oxygenate, as exemplified by reductions in recorded arterial oxygen levels. It would appear at this time that the predominant utilization of the immobilizing agent etorphine (Immobilon) in the horse is limited to those individuals who are quite difficult to catch or restrain. The utilization of a narcotic antagonist as early as possible to avoid prolonged muscle tremors, changes in body temperature, reductions in arterial oxygen levels and other cardiopulmonary disturbances is recommended (29–34). The veterinarian is cautioned that etorphine is supplied in an extremely potent concentration. Accidental injection of etorphine in man can result in severe depression and/or death.

Induction of Anesthesia

Induction of anesthesia in the horse usually is by one of three methods (35). The first is the utilization of a tranquilizer or some form of premedication followed by intravenous administration of barbiturates, usually with a phenothiazine-derivative tranquilizer, (such as acetylpromazine), followed after the full effects of the tranquilization have been realized with an ultra-short barbiturate. The phenothiazine-derivative tranquilizers may be replaced by xylazine (36) as a preanesthetic followed by thiopenthal or thiamylal for induction of anesthesia. Unless xylazine as a premedication is followed by an anticholinergic, such as atropine, the likelihood of producing severe cardiac depression or heart block during the rapid administration of barbiturate anesthesia is more likely to occur in xylazine-pretreated horses than with the phenothiazine-derivative tranquilizer (36, 37). Oxygen levels will drop rapidly after induction with xylazine and barbiturates.

Physical precautions should be taken prior to rapid administration of barbiturates to avoid the animal crashing to the ground. This includes the utilization of restraint halters, a tail tie, or other mechanical devices to assure that the animal's body can be eased to recumbency rather than suddenly falling with the potential of trauma. Rapid induction is frequently associated with a transient apnea, and the duration of unconsciousness will vary from 5 to 20 minutes (37–38). The utilization of tranquilizers as a preanesthetic agent will help to assure that recovery will not be as excitable as when ultrashort barbiturates are used alone.

A second popular approach to the induction of anesthesia in the horse has been the utilization of guaifenesin as a muscle relaxant in combination with ultrashort barbiturates. This technique usually follows preanesthetic tranquilization. The guaifenesin is used in concentrations of 5 to 15% depending on individual preferences and the availability of the drug (38, 39). To the guaifenesin is added 2 to 3 g of ultrashort-acting barbiturate per 50 g of guaifenesin. The drug combination is usually administered simultaneously. It is given through a large-bore needle or catheter as rapidly as possible by gravity flow until the animal becomes recumbent; this usually does not require more than 2 ml of the mixture per kilogram of body weight. An alternate method is to administer the combination under pressure to obtain a faster administration of the required doses. This can result in as much as a 50% reduction in the dose required for unconsciousness and recumbency.

An alternate method to administer guaifenesin and ultrashort barbiturates after tranquilization is to initially administer guaifenesin as a sole agent until the horse is relaxed and has some difficulty with coordination. At that time, 1 g of ultrashort-acting barbiturate in the average 500-kg horse is administered rapidly to complete the induction of anesthesia (40–45). The induction of anesthesia by guaifenesin and barbiturates is not as likely to produce complete respiratory apnea or excessive cardiac change as barbiturates; however, some degree of respiratory depression and significant decreases in blood pressure, cardiac output, and PaO_2 may occur (40–44). In studies using 32 horses at our laboratories, administering guaifenesin as the sole agent until the animals were recumbent resulted in major respiratory depression in 1 of 32 animals and moderate depression of respiration in 2 others. In its common use in combination with ultrashort-acting barbiturates with careful monitoring and control of rate of flow, safe levels of anesthesia can be achieved after the production of unconsciousness and relaxation. Discontinuing further medication will result in only 10 to 20 minutes of general anesthesia. Prolongation of anesthesia can be accomplished by intubation and administration of inhalant anesthesia or further administration of additional guaifenesin and barbiturate. Continuation of anesthesia with combinations of guaifenesin and barbiturate have been accomplished safely for up to 1 hour or more of continuous anesthesia. As additional drug is administered for the continuation of anesthesia, the maintenance of slight palpebral and corneal reflexes, adequate respiratory volume, and cardiovascular function is essential. The lack of attention to rate of flow of the combination of guaifenesin and barbiturate can result in profound depression. Veterinarians using untrained personnel to assist in administration of these medications are warned to judge levels of anesthetic concentration and the rate of administration of the drug appropriately.

The attempt to maintain levels of anesthesia with guaifenesin alone results in less cardiopulmonary depression in most instances than combinations of guaifenesin and barbiturates. However, when guaifenesin is used alone, consciousness will return before muscle strength and coordination. Pain sensation will return at a faster rate when guaifenesin is used alone rather than in combination with barbiturates. Thus the type of manipulation and surgical procedure being completed with further administration of guaifenesin must be carefully considered. The utilization of extensive amounts of guaifenesin without barbiturates during the later stages of anesthesia to maintain prolonged recumbency to finish mild surgical or manipulative procedures can result in undesirable recovery patterns of the horse. This undesirable recovery pattern is frequently exemplified by extensive efforts of the horse to rise without sufficient muscle coordination to control its body movements. This can result in self-inflicted trauma to the individual equine patient or to the attendees and obviously does not favorably impress the owner of the horse.

The third method of inducing anesthesia has incorporated the utilization of a dissociative anesthetic, ketamine, in combination with preanesthetics (45–50). Neither ketamine nor other dissociative anesthetics should be administered to the horse as a sole agent. The dissociative agents can cause central nervous system (CNS) stimulation in the horse. They do not produce a degree of unconsciousness similar to barbiturates or true anesthesia as with inhalant agents such as halothane, isoflurane, and other fluoronated hydrocarbons. The most commonly used preanesthetic before administration of ketamine is xylazine. Detomidine may be used instead of xylazine. The veterinarian is cautioned to assure that there are full tranquilizing and sedative effects with xylazine prior to the administration of xylazine, 1.1 mg/kg i.v. If the animal has not become sedate, do not administer ketamine. Rather, one should administer either more xylazine to produce this sedation or administer diazepam or other agents to assure needed levels of sedation prior to the administration of the dissociative agent. The administration of ketamine in inadequately sedated horses will result in an animal that does not become unconscious and recumbent or an animal with signs of CNS excitement and muscle tremors. Because xylazine has a tendency to reduce heart rates and ketamine has a tendency to produce CNS stimulation, the combination of the two drugs usually results in a stable cardiovascular system during the first 15 to 18 minutes of the anesthetic procedure after the administration of the ketamine. At that time, one normally observes a rapid recovery from the ketamine anesthesia. In contrast, a slowing of the heart rate may occur at 15 to 18 minutes after ketamine, especially if the animal is being maintained on halothane or other potent inhalant anesthetics.

Xylazine and ketamine anesthesia can be prolonged after the 18- to 20-minute time period using injectables alone by either supplemental administration of partial doses of both xylazine and ketamine, the administration of guaifenesin barbiturate, or connection to an inhalation anesthetic unit. When continuing anesthesia with ketamine and xylazine, increases in muscle fasiculation or muscle rigidity is indicative of excessive response to ketamine with inadequate levels of xylazine. Animals that demonstrate excessive relaxation, reductions in heart rate, or heart block are showing excessive response to xylazine with less than ideal response to xylazine rather than too high concentrations of ketamine (45–53).

The utilization of ketamine and guaifenesin as an induction combination or for maintenance is discouraged. Ketamine alone can produce CNS stimulation even to the extent of seizure. The administration of guaifenesin in sufficient concentrations to avoid these muscle fasiculations and other signs of CNS activity will only reduce the outward CNS symptoms. Outwardly the horse will appear to be well relaxed and unconscious, but considerable undesirable CNS activity is probable.

Cardiac difficulties after ketamine and xylazine induction and halothane maintenance, such as severe bradycardia or cardiac arrest, have occurred. They are rare but extremely rapid in occurrence and extremely difficult to convert. This is probably due to losing the stimulating effect of ketamine, thus allowing the alpha-1 activity of xylazine, with the tendencies for bradycardia combined with the potential for hypotension by halothane to produce major cardiac depression which can result in asystole.

Recoveries from xylazine and ketamine are usually smooth and without excessive complications. Acetylpromazine, methadone, and ketamine have been used with some success in horses (54). Xylazine and ketamine anesthesia is not highly satisfactory in the mule or donkey (54).

There has been interest in finding methods to antagonize the effects of xylazine and ketamine anesthesia (55). Yohimbine and 4-aminopyridine have been used to antagonize this combination. These medications significantly reduce the recovery time in horses with antagonism of xylazine. If xylazine is reversed prior to 20 minutes after the administration of ketamine, CNS stimulation may reoccur.

Saffan has been investigated as a method of inducing anesthesia in the horse (56). Induction was associated with excitement for up to 30 seconds; recovery was associated with marked tactile and audible hyperanesthesia with only slight stimulation necessary to produce twitching and violent kicking movements that might last up to 15 minutes. At best, the agent offers no advantage over other anesthetic agents currently used to induce anesthesia, and the adverse reactions reported indicate its use should be avoided.

Anesthesia can also be induced by inhalation anesthetic methodology. This is usually accomplished in foals and very high risk patients. The procedure is normally accomplished using a face mask or nasal endotracheal tube with relatively high oxygen flows (1 liter/50 kg/min) to assure oxygenation of the patient. Oxygen should be initiated prior to the administration of the inhalant agent to accustom the animal to the movement of air and the presence of the devices. This will reduce the excitement and avoid the potential of hyperventilation and accumulation of excessive concentrations of anesthetic agents in the early phases of induction. Once anesthesia is induced, oral intubation can be accomplished, the tube is connected to the anesthetic equipment, and the procedure continues in a normal manner for maintenance of inhalant anesthesia. Anesthetic concentrations required for induction vary with condition of the animal. Healthy animals require a brief period of 4 to 5% halothane vaporizer settings, whereas toxic ones may be induced with less than 1.5% settings within 3 to 10 minutes, depending on individual responses. Anesthetic concentrations are reduced to 0.25 to 2.0% for maintenance.

In years past, "anesthetic induction" was on many occasions accomplished with the combination of ultrashort barbiturates and succinylcholine, or succinylcholine as a sole agent was used to paralyze the horse into a recumbent position. Utilization of succinylcholine by either method will rapidly produce immobilization of the horse but also eliminates the animal's ability to ventilate adequately. Without preoxygenation and supplemental oxygen at the time that the paralysis occurs, rapid onset of hypoxemia and related cardiac arrhythmias will occur. If the animal has been exposed to organic phosphate insecticides or parasiticides, permanent muscle paralysis can occur due to inadequate levels of pseudocholinesterase to metabolize the succinylcholine molecules. Muscle relaxants can be effectively and beneficially used without interfering with cardiovascular response provided there is proper maintenance of oxygenation through mechanical or manually assisted ventilation. It is recommended, however, that the animals already be on supplemental oxygen at the time the muscle relaxant is administered to avoid undesirable complications. As a result, the utilization of paralytic agents to immobilize a horse or as part of anesthetic induction without supplemental oxygen is strongly discouraged.

Inhalant Anesthetics

Historically, inhalant anesthesia in the horse included the use of diethyl ether or chloroform during the early development of the anesthetic agents. Utilization of these two agents was associated with a variety of complications. One of the obvious reasons for these complications was the lack of uniform administration of anesthetic vapor. The use of a mask containing gauze sponges saturated with diethel ether or chloroform through which the animal breathed atmospheric air not only gave inconsistent concentrations of anesthetic agent, but partially obstructed airway flow, and the air inhaled contained a maximum of 20% oxygen. As a result, any respiratory depression that occurred could result in a related degree of hypoxia. Diethyl ether and chloroform were quite capable of producing cardiac irregularities, severe bradycardia, or cardiac arrest in patients receiving excessive concentrations. The percentage of cases experiencing complications subsided as anesthetic equipment was developed. The rapid development of halothane, isoflurane, and enflurane anesthesia in the horse coincided historically with the development of precision vaporizers and more appropriately designed and manufactured anesthetic units for the administration of anesthetics to large animals.

Inhalant anesthesia in the horse is usually administered after induction of anesthesia with some form of intravenous medication. Intubation normally is accomplished by blind approach. The head and neck are extended or flexed to an angle appropriate relative to the endotracheal tube used. Seldom is it necessary to rotate the tube more than 30° to enter the trachea. The horse is connected to the anesthetic unit. A minimum oxygen flow of 1 liter/100 kg of body weight should be used. Due to the ventilation perfusion characteristics of the horse and the tendency for CO_2 accumulation and reduction in blood pH, closed-system anesthetic technique is not as desirable as semiclosed methods. Unfortunately, even with the present CO_2 absorption systems, there is a tendency with time for CO_2 levels to accumulate unless relatively high flows of oxygen are administered and a semiclosed system is used. Immediately upon intubation and connection to the anesthetic unit, the anesthetic concentrations administered are relatively high, usually in the range of 4 to 5% vaporizer setting. These settings are dramatically reduced during the next 3 to 5 minutes. The concentrations required and the speed with which concentrations may be altered will be dependent on the premedications, the method of induction of anesthesia, and the response of the horse. Arterial blood pressures frequently decrease immediately after induction and usually do not begin to rise until at least 10 minutes after maintenance on halothane after acetylpromazine premedication and induction with guaifenesin and sodium thiamylal (57). The same has been shown with other methods of induction with maintenance on halothane anesthesia (58).

During halothane anesthesia in the horse, cardiac parameters will be decreased proportional to anesthetic concentration. It has been shown that increasing the alveolar halothane concentration results in a progressive decline in systemic arterial pressure and left ventricular work (59). Cardiac output decreased as a result of the decrease in stroke volume. Heart rates, total peripheral resistance, pulmonary artery pressure, hematocrit, plasma protein concentration, arterial oxygen tension, and arterial pH usually remain constant over the same range of anesthetic concentrations (60). Clinical studies, illustrated in Table 13.1, indicate careful attention to anesthetic administration during the first few minutes of the procedure is necessary until cardiovascular parameters stabilized. Blood cell count and biochemical values are altered very little by halothane anesthesia (60). There is minimally depressed renal function during halothane anesthesia, but this usually returns to normal after the first day postanesthesia. The degree of reduction in renal function will be effected by blood pressure and level of hydration.

There will be an increase in blood oxygen levels in horses on halothane anesthesia in most instances (61). This is predominantly due to the supplemental oxygen administered compared to injectable anesthesia. Due to the inability of the CO_2 absorption system to be completely effective in the removal of CO_2 and the ventilation perfusion characteristics of the horse, accumulations of arterial CO_2 are common in the horse. The behavior of blood gases in halothane-anesthetized horses are illustrated in Table 13.2. Mechanical ventilation is often necessary even in healthy horses to assure stable arterial pH and awake level $PaCO_2$.

The uptake of anesthetic in muscle depends significantly on the fat content of the muscle with more absorption of anesthetic agent than those tissues containing more fat (62).

Unpublished and published data (63, 73) on the results of inhalation anesthesia in the horse using halothane have revealed wide acceptance of this drug for equine anesthesia. Although halothane had become one of the most widely used of the inhalant anesthetics in the horse, studies to compare it with enflurane and isoflurane were needed.

Early studies to evaluate enflurane compared to

Table 13.1
Responses of Thoroughbreds to Intermittent Positive Pressure Ventilation versus Spontaneous Respiration

		Beginning of Surgery	+30 Minutes	+60 Minutes
Halothane concentration (%)[c]	A[b]	2.1 ± 0.5[c]	1.9 ± 0.7	1.2 ± 0.5
	B[d]	2.2 ± 0.4	1.6 ± 0.4	1.5 ± 0.4
Systolic blood pressure (mm Hg)	A	89.2 ± 15.8	111.6 ± 15.9	127.2 ± 12.2
	B	115.0 ± 23.2[e]	96.1 ± 17.6[a]	101.3 ± 19.9[f]
Diastolic blood pressure (mm Hg)	A	32.0 ± 4.5	44.8 ± 7.8	52.8 ± 10.9
	B	67.9 ± 21.2[f]	44.9 ± 12.3[a]	58.3 ± 24.6[a]
Heart Rate (bpm)[a]	A	36.0 ± 7.9	35.2 ± 5.4	37.2 ± 3.9
	B	37.3 ± 6.0	33.3 ± 3.7	33.3 ± 3.3
Respiratory rate (breaths/min)	A	10.4 ± 4.6	10.4 ± 4.3	11.2 ± 3.9
	B	7.1 ± 1.5	7.1 ± 1.5	7.1 ± 1.5

[a] Not significantly different for either system.
[b] A, spontaneous respiration.
[c] Mean values ± SD.
[d] B, Intermittent positive pressure ventilation, ventilatory pressure 24.3 cm H_2O, O_2 flow 7.6 liter/min, $V_T = 7$.
[e] Significantly different at $P < 0.1$.
[f] Significantly different at $P < 0.01$.

Table 13.2
Respiratory Responses in Thoroughbreds

	Mechanical Ventilation	Spontaneous Respiration
Guaifenesin/thiamylal induction/halothane maintenance		
Arterial pH	7.393 ± 0.065[a]	7.254 ± 0.050
$PaCO_2$ (torr)	45.3 ± 8.8	69.2 ± 13.9
PaO_2 (torr)	487.1 ± 50.1	375.0 ± 69.2
Bicarbonate	27.3 ± 2.1	29.4 ± 2.7
Total CO_2	28.9 ± 2.5	31.4 ± 3.0
Xylazine/ketamine induction/halothane maintenance		
Arterial pH	7.418 ± 0.033	7.257 ± 0.015
$PaCO_2$ (torr)	42.0 ± 2.9	68.7 ± 2.1
PaO_2 (torr)	374.0 ± 56.8	283.0 ± 191.9
Bicarbonate	27.3 ± 1.3	27.7 ± 1.5
Total CO_2	27.9 ± 1.4	31.7 ± 1.5
Combined responses to A or B induction/halothane maintenance		
Arterial pH	7.402 ± 0.055[b]	7.255 ± 0.039[b]
$PaCO_2$ (torr)	44.1 ± 7.2[b]	69.0 ± 10.5[b]
PaO_2 (torr)	446.0 ± 75.8[b]	340.1 ± 125.5[b]
Bicarbonate	27.3 ± 1.8	29.5 ± 2.2
Total CO_2	28.7 ± 2.1	31.5 ± 2.4

[a] Mean values ± SD.
[b] Highly significant, $P < 0.01$.

halothane in the horse revealed some difficulty in maintaining sufficient anesthesia with enflurane for surgery, with greater respiratory depression than halothane and without significant differences in cardiovascular function (64). Recovery from anesthesia was significantly faster in horses receiving enflurane than halothane, but the pattern was not as desirable. Further study of enflurane in the pony (65) revealed significant depression of blood pressure during enflurane anesthesia and a slower respiratory pattern with enflurane than halothane; however, adequate respiration continued with either agent. In the pony, postanesthetic complications were not observed with either agent. Our own experiences using enflurane anesthesia revealed a slower respiratory rate than with halothane; there was a faster recovery but with more excitement of the patient during the recovery period and more difficulty in maintaining stable surgical plane anesthesia. It did not appear the selection of enflurane was advantageous over the use of halothane anesthesia for routine usage in the horse.

With the development of isoflurane anesthesia, it was of interest to determine the responses of the horse. In early studies I found isoflurane to have the rapid action of enflurane, and a stable plane of anesthesia was observed. There was a tendency for respiratory rates to be slower and for recovery to be fast and without complication. Studies have compared the circulatory and respiratory effects of isoflurane and halothane anesthesia in the horse (66). Isoflurane, similar to halothane, can produce a dose-related depression of cardiovascular function that is less severe during spontaneous ventilation and associated hypercapnia. The two anesthetic agents produce similar circulatory effects during controlled ventilation with constant arterial carbon dioxide tension. Except for a significantly less depressed cardiac output during isoflurane anesthesia, isoflurane was no more depressing to circulatory and respiratory function than halothane. Isoflurane was not associated with undesirable changes in blood cell counts and biochemical values even when prolonged anesthesia was maintained (67). Isoflurane and enflurane have similar physical and chemical characteristics. Induction and maintenance of anesthesia and recovery were smoother with fewer complications with isoflurane than with enflurane (68). There were fewer instances of abnormal muscle twitching with isoflurane than with enflurane. Although either agent can be used, isoflurane is better tolerated by the horse than enflurane.

As a result of clinical experience and research studies indicating that safe anesthesia could be accomplished with halothane, enflurane, or isoflurane in the horse, a comparative study of the potency of these agents was completed (69). Equipotent concentrations in the horse are 1.12% for enflurane, 0.88% for halothane, and 1.31% for isoflurane. The alveolar concentration required to produce at least 60 seconds of apnea was determined as being a minimum alveolar concentration of 2.26, 2.60, and 2.33% for enflurane, halothane, and isoflurane, respectively.

It has always been a goal to reduce the concentration of potent anesthetic agents in the horse and other species to provide anesthesia with less cardiac depression. As a result, nitrous oxide has frequently been considered as an addition to the anesthetic regime. Nitrous oxide in humans does provide this option, especially because humans are sensitive to the analgetic qualities of nitrous oxide. Nitrous oxide in animals does not have as potent an effect as part of the anesthetic regime as in human anesthesia (70). The effect of the addition of nitrous oxide on minimal alveolar concentration of halothane has been studied. Halothane alone in oxygen was found to require 0.93 volume %. Alveolar concentrations of 25 and 50% nitrous oxide reduced the halothane requirements 12 and 25%, respectively. However, in these horses halothane plus 50% nitrous oxide also decreased cardiovascular function. Cardiovascular responses to three concentrations of halothane in oxygen and halothane in 50% nitrous oxide and oxygen were studied (71). Cardiac output was greater during halothane/nitrous oxide anesthesia than with halothane alone. The potency of nitrous oxide was found to be less in the horse than in humans. Studies of blood gas and acid-base responses during anesthesia in the horse with halothane and nitrous oxide combinations show there was depression of arterial pO_2 and an increase in arterial pH when nitrous oxide was added. There are more detrimental effects after 2 hours of anesthesia than during the first 2 hours (72). In prolonged anesthesia with halothane and nitrous oxide, a smaller concentration of halothane was needed to maintain surgical anesthesia, but a greater volume of oxygen was needed to maintain normal function (73).

Studies have been completed to evaluate responses to enflurane plus nitrous oxide (74). The patients were stabilized; oxygen levels were decreased and carbon dioxide was increased. The level of respiratory acidosis did not significantly impair the function of the horse. Anesthesia was induced faster with the enflurane/nitrous oxide combination than with halothane alone, and the nitrous oxide made it easier to control the level of anesthesia with enflurane.

Horses with respiratory depression, pulmonary complications, gas-filled loops of intestine, or pneumothorax should not receive nitrous oxide. This is due to the diffusion of nitrous oxide into those gas-filled areas, further complicating the situation. Secondly, one must decide whether the slight improvement in cardiovascular function with anesthetic nitrous oxide combinations will adequately offset the reduced concentration of oxygen available during ventilation. Oxygen flow must not be reduced during the administration of nitrous oxide; adequate oxygenation must occur.

During recovery from anesthesia, nitrous oxide should be discontinued at least 5 to 10 minutes before discontinuing oxygen. Even maintaining the animals on oxygen for 10 minutes before disconnecting oxygen flow, I have observed two cases of severe diffusion hypoxia after the use of nitrous oxide. Due to the potential complications and the poor analgesic properties of nitrous oxide in animals, it is difficult to justify the use of nitrous oxide for most equine procedures.

Potent inhalant agents can affect hepatic function. Investigations have been conducted to determine if this is significant in the horse (75–79). There is biotransformation of halothane during and after anesthesia in the horse. There is an increase in liver and enzymatic activity. However, there is little evidence of permanent damage to hepatic cells. During halothane anesthesia there is an increase in bilirubin excretion and a decrease in biliary bile acid concentration and reduction of bile acid excretions. Although I have observed increases in serum enzyme levels after halothane anesthesia, I have administered halothane to aged horses on repeated occasions without observing irreversible hepatic damage. When considering halothane anesthesia for a horse, remember that pre-existing hepatic disease or toxicity can predispose to complications. Isoflurane has been shown to have less acute effect on liver function. Enflurane does not appear to adversely affect hepatic function. The recovery of the horse from inhalant anesthesia has been compared for duration and quality of recovery after 2-hour anesthetic periods with equally potent alveolar concentrations of isoflurane, enflurane, halothane, and methoxyflurane (80). Recovery was shortest after isoflurane, followed by enflurane, halothane, and methoxyflurane. The quality of recovery was rated highest with isoflurane, followed by methoxyflurane, halothane, and enflurane. Muscle coordination was excellent after isoflurane recovery. The primary difficulties during halothane recovery are occasional shivering and sometimes delayed coordination upon standing.

Cardiovascular Responses

The effect of halothane anesthesia on arterial blood pressure measurements in the horse were studied (81). Cardiovascular responses in horses are sensitive to halothane anesthesia. The degree of reduction in blood pressures is dose-dependent. The mean awake blood pressure in thoroughbreds has been reported as 111/68 mm Hg systolic/diastolic. During anesthesia, when mean pressures fall below 50 mm Hg, action is usually taken to assure an increase in blood pressure to maintain organ perfusion. Further studies comparing cardiac output of conscious and anesthetized horses reveals the cardiac output can decrease proportionately with the concentration of anesthetic agent (82). This was further determined as the rate of change of left ventricular blood pressure (d.p./d.t.) showing a negative inotropic effect of halothane on the myocardium (83). Acetylpromazine as a premedicant reduces central venous pressure significantly more than xylazine premedication, but after induction of anesthesia and maintenance on halothane for 75 minutes, values for horses in lateral recumbency were significantly higher than those in dorsal recumbency (84). Because it has been recognized both experimentally and clinically that inhalant anesthesia in the horse may be associated with hypotension, efforts have been made to determine the most appropriate ways of maintaining cardiac function. In initial cardiac depression resulting in hypotension, administration of calicum chloride (1 to 5 g) in adult horses for rapid increases in myocardial contraction, improvement in heart rate, and a transient improvement in arterial blood pressure has been successful. Isoproterenol, dopamine, and dobutamine have been evaluated in the experimental laboratory as well as in clinical practice. Isoproterenol infusion will increase heart rate, may increase the sensitivity of the myocardium, and can be utilized by slow infusion to improve cardiovascular performance. Dopamine hydrochloride has been studied experimentally and clinically to improve cardiopulmonary performance during halothane anesthesia at dosage levels of 0.5, 2.5, and 5.0 μg/kg/min. Cardiac output increased significantly at 2.5 and 5.0 μg/kg/min (85). The heart rate, facial artery pressure, and pulmonary artery pressure remained unchanged. Total peripheral resistance was significantly decreased by 30 minutes with 2.5 μg/kg/min at 5.0 μg/kg/min (85). It was shown that dopamine at higher concentrations could cause dysrhythmias in the horse.

When comparing the hemodynamic responses in halothane-anesthetized horses to infusions of dopamine versus dobutamine (86), an increase in systemic arterial blood pressure at lower infusion rates of dobutamine than dopamine is observed. Cardiac output increased in horses receiving 3 μg/kg/minute of dobutamine and 5 and 10 μg/kg/min of dopamine. We have found dobutamine infusions have been very effective in improvement of cardiac output and blood pressure responses. Dopamine is more effective at lower concentrations (5 μg/kg/min) to improve cardiac output, probably through reduction in peripheral resistance. However higher concentrations of dopamine (15 μg/kg/min) in the horse have produced vascular constriction and reduction in renal output.

Pulmonary Function and Ventilation

During halothane anesthesia there is a sharp rise in alveolar arterial oxygen concentration (87). It has been shown that an increase in arterial carbon dioxide levels can occur rapidly in halothane-anesthetized horses (88). Studies to evaluate the retention of carbon dioxide at more frequent or convenient intervals than arterial sampling have used a carbon dioxide analyzer (capnometer) (89). Comparisons of arterial to end-tidal CO_2 tension and alveolar dead space in halothane- and isoflurane-anesthetized ponies have been made (90). The correlation between the end-tidal partial pressure of CO_2 ($PETCO_2$) and the $PaCO_2$ shows that the end-tidal partial pressure of CO_2 is a useful trend indicator for CO_2 during the first hour of halothane anesthesia and 90 minutes of isoflurane anesthesia. It was shown that there was a greater tendency for CO_2 to accumulate during halothane anesthesia than with isoflurane after 1 hour.

There is much concern about the influence of body position and regional blood flow or pulmonary ventilation in the horse (91–96). CO_2 levels will accumulate rapidly in closed systems. Artificial respiration is essential in poor risk animals and in horses with metabolic acidosis (91). Horses have been shown to develop hypoxemia even in lateral recumbency (92). Regional blood flow measured with radioactive labeled microspheres did not show significant differences for the perfusion of the dependent lung versus the standing animal (93). The gradient of pulmonary ventilation in the horse is matched by a similar gradient of perfusion (94). Most horses are predictably improved with controlled positive-pressure ventilation, but regardless of type of ventilation and operating body position, they become hypoxic in the immediate postanesthetic period (96). It has been suggested that the predominant reason for the reduction in lung volume during anesthesia is more relative to posture than to the effects of the anesthetic agents (95). As a result of these concerns, radiographic studies have been done to identify the diaphragmatic activity during anesthesia with a general pattern of diaphragmatic displacement that appeared to be relatively unchanged by increasing the depth of anesthesia (97). It was necessary to use controlled ventilation to alter the pattern of diaphragmatic activity.

There is justifiably some concern about the cardiovascular effect of mechanically controlled ventilation in horses. Most horses will have an increase in oxygen levels and a decrease in CO_2 levels with appropriately controlled mechanical ventilation (Table 13.2).

There are possibilities of ventilation perfusion mismatch that can result in a true shunt (98). Muscle relaxants have been used to ease the control of ventilation in mechanical ventilation. Gallamine triethiodide, 0.3 mg/kg every 30 minutes, has been used to assist in maintaining controlled breathing during halothane anesthesia in horses (99). Ventilators such as the Bird Corporation Ventilator/Respirator Mark VII have a unique feature that is easy to set in a self-triggering mode to correlate assisted breathing with spontaneous efforts. This results in an increase in tidal volume with each breath coordinated at the rate of the animal's own stimulation. There is a demonstrated improvement in lung ventilation utilizing the Bird Mark IX ventilator during general anesthesia (100). The applicability of controlled ventilation during routine anesthesia in the horse has been evaluated (101). Even with controlled ventilation, it appears that nitrous oxide in addition to the anesthetic regime can reduce the level of oxygenation.

It has been my experience that mechanical ventilation can improve the level of oxygen and reduce the level of CO_2 accumulation in a high percentage of horses. There is a tendency for CO_2 to accumulate during anesthesia. This occurs more rapidly in animals in dorsal recumbency than lateral, and faster in lateral recumbency than in the standing individual. It has been easier to control levels of oxygen and CO_2 through early initiation of mechanical respiration versus attempts to correct oxygen and CO_2 disturbances once they have occurred. This is especially true if the accumulation of CO_2 and low levels of oxygen are a result of ventilation profusion mismatch in the lung after which mechanical ventilation with standard available respirators has not been predictably effective in correcting the hypoxia. The respiratory rate used during mechanical ventilation can be a major factor in the influence of oxygen-CO_2 levels versus reductions in cardiac output. Cardiac output does decrease during the pressure cycle of mechanical ventilation. If the period of inspiration and increased pulmonary pressure is high proportional to the pause between breaths (I:E ratio), greater reduction in cardiac output will occur. The same phenomenon can be observed in other species if rapid rates of respiration along with prolonged periods of end expiratory pressure are maintained (PEEP). It is, therefore, important to appropriately set the inspiratory-expiratory ratio and to maintain at least a 1:3 ratio to assure a period of cardiovascular recovery. Respiratory rates in the horse greater than 25% of the cardiac rate are more likely to cause reductions in cardiac output.

Investigations have been made to determine if positive end expiratory pressure can improve oxygenation in horses, as it has been shown to do in certain conditions in human patients. The imposition of positive end inspiratory pressure in spontaneously breathing horses resulted in additional accumulation of CO_2 and a reduction in cardiac output (102). Studies of effects of 0, 5, 10 and 15 cm H_2O pressure maintained in a group of horses revealed that PEEP was contraindicated in lateral recumbent spontaneous-ventilated anesthetized horses. PEEP resulted in alveolar hypoventilation and did not improve pulmonary gas exchange (103). A crucial factor in the ability to administer intermittent positive pressure breathing is the flow rate that can be generated by the delivery apparatus for the horse (104).

Respiration in newborn foals revealed that hemoglobin became saturated at a lower blood O_2 tension in newborn foals than in adults (105). Even when conscious, newborn foals have a mean pulmonary PaO_2 less than that of their dams. As a result, the rapidity with which oxygen deficits may occur in anesthetized foals is of more concern (106).

Hypoxia is difficult to manage during the equine abdominal crisis (107, 108). In addition to the usual responses to anesthesia and position is the potential of distention of the equine gut to interfere with ventilation and profusion. There is electrolyte and fluid imbalance, and the potential need for mechanical ventilation is increased. Early administration of oxygen and the early utilization of mechanical ventilation in these horses may contribute significantly to success.

Neurological Responses

Very little study has been made of specific neurological responses to anesthetics in the horse. Electroencephalographic (EEG) patterns of clinically normal, sedated, and tranquilized newborn foals and adult horses has been made (109). Acetylpromazine was found to have little effect on the EEG recordings, whereas xylazine exerted a substantial effect. Further studies of xylazine and ketamine on the EEG in the horse revealed that xylazine-sedated horses had a demonstrated slowing of the electrical activity of the brain, whereas there was an increase in high voltage activity upon administration of ketamine (110). This could be correlated with the characteristics of the drugs evaluated. Further studies revealed that guaifenesin produced only slight changes of the EEG characteristic of very superficial anesthesia, whereas halothane anesthesia produced significant changes in the EEG pattern characteristic of those produced by general anesthetics (111). In combination with nitrous oxide, halothane produced hypoxia accompanied by EEG patterns characteristic of very deep anesthesia.

Muscle Relaxants

Muscle relaxants in equine anesthesia have predominantly consisted of the administration of guaifenesin-like products for additional muscle relaxation. However, succinylcholine, gallamine, and pancuronium are among those muscle relaxants that have been used in conjunction with anesthesia in the horse (112–117). These are effectively described elsewhere in this text. Of concern during the recovery and immediately postanesthetic period in horses are the problems of postanesthetic myopathy or the development of malignant hyperthermia-like problems. Malignant hyperthermia or a similar phenomenon has been observed after succinylcholine in the horse. Serum enzymes have been shown to increase during the postanesthetic period when myositis has been observed (118–128). Dantrolene sodium has been used as a preventative and therapeutic measure for the control of myositis or malignant hyperthermia-like syndromes in the horse. The principle problem at the present time appears to be the diagnosis of malignant hyperthermia-like symptoms. The utilization of dantrolene in undiagnosed

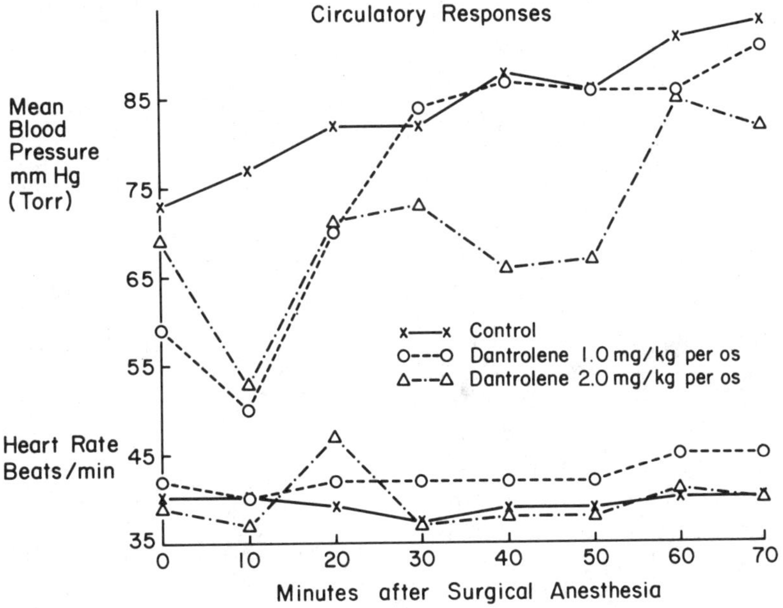

Figure 13.1. Mean arterial pressure and heart rate responses during halothane anesthesia in horses premedicated with dantrolene.

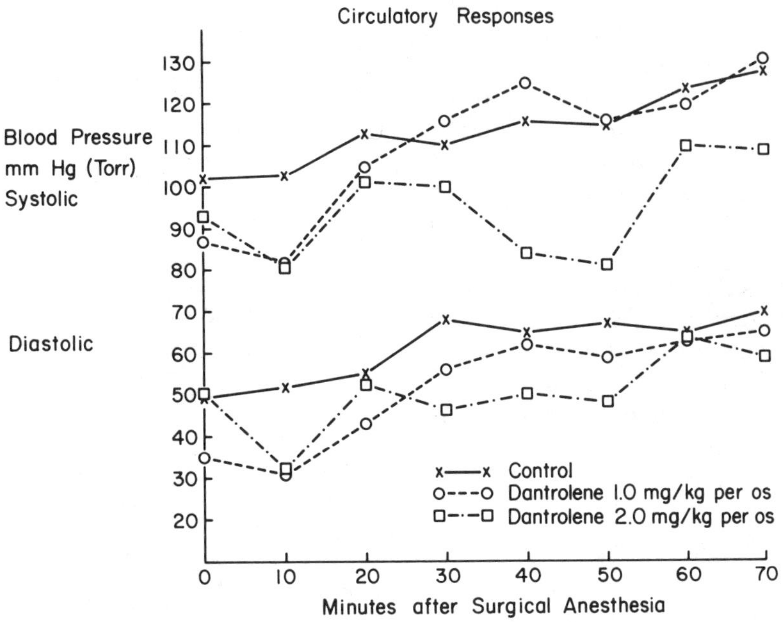

Figure 13.2. Systolic and diastolic blood pressure responses in horses during halothane anesthesia with dantrolene premedication.

Table 13.3
Ventilation Responses

	Arterial pH	$PaCO_2$	PaO_2	Bicarbonate	Total CO_2
		Spontaneous breathing			
1[a]	7.215[b]	77	179	29	32
2[c]	7.220	67	225	26	28
3[d]	7.236	66	241	27	29
		Mechanical respiration			
1[a]	7.467	35	396	25	26
2[c]	7.398	39	409	24	25
3[d]	7.294	57	152	27	28

[a] Group 1 controls—received no dantrolene sodium.
[b] Values are expressed as means.
[c] Group 2 received 1 mg/kg dantrolene sodium as preanesthetic.
[d] Group 3 received 2 mg/kg dantrolene sodium as preanesthetic.

malignant hyperthermia syndrome horses can be associated with hypotension, reduced pO_2, increased pCO_2, and need for mechanical ventilation in horses during halothane anesthesia (Figs. 13.1 and 13.2 and Table 13.3). Further discussion of this syndrome occurs in another chapter of this text.

Although the horse receives many of the same medications as other species, it has many unique characteristics and requirements. The horse has a far greater potential for injury or complications during recovery than many other species. The need for pads, recovery stalls, and grass plots to reduce injuries is evident. Supplemental oxygen can be used during early recovery to avoid hypoxemia, but this can not always be maintained long enough due to movement of the horse; alternatively, availability of O_2 may be limited.

Extubation may be considered early or late during recovery. The advantage of early extubation is reduction of laryngeal spasms and trauma to the larynx and trachea. The disadvantage is maintenance of an open airway if there is an elongated soft palate. Late extubation maintains the airway, but the animal can occlude the airway by bending the tube, may damage the airway, or may have laryngeal spasms upon extubation. The horse should be monitored during and immediately after extubation to assure adequate ventilation.

Horses subjected to prolonged anesthetic procedures may suffer from edema of the upper airway including the nostrils. This may mechanically interfere with the passage of air. The use of a neosynephrine nasal spray to reduce edema has inproved the recovery pattern by improving airway flow of gases.

References

1. Short CE, Rebhun WC: Complications caused by the oculocardiac reflex during anesthesia in a foal. *J Am Vet Med Assoc* 176(7):630–631, 1980.
2. Kerr DD, Jones EQ, Huggins K, Edwards WC: Sedative and other effects of xylazine given intravenously in horses. *Am J Vet Res* 33(3):525–532, 1972.
3. Short CE, Tumbleson ME, Merriam JG: Comparative effects of Bay Va 1470 (Xylazine), promazine and halothane on serum electrolytes in the horse. *VM/SAC* 67(7):747–750, 1972.
4. McCaskin FB, Gobel AA: Evaluation of xylazine as a sedative and preanesthetic agent in horses. *Am J Vet Res* 36(10):1421–9, 1975.
5. Garcia-Villar R, Toutain PL, Alvinerie M, Ruckebusch Y: The pharmacokinetics of xylazine hydrochloride: an interspecific study. *J Vet Pharmacol Ther* 4(2):87–92, 1981.
6. Thurmon JC, Neff-Davis C, Davis LE, Stoker RA, Benson GJ, Lock TF: Xylazine hydrochloride-induced hyperglycemia and hypoinsulinemia in thoroughbred horses. *J Vet Pharmacol Ther* 5(4):241–245, 1982.
7. Thurmon JC, Steffey EP, Zinkl JG, Woliner M, Howland D Jr: Xylazine causes transient dose-related hyperglycemia and increased urine volumes in mares. *Am J Vet Res* 45(2):224–227, 1984.
8. Brouwer, GJ, Hall LW, Kuckel TR: Intravenous anaesthesia in horses after xylazine premedication. *Vet Rec* 107(11):241–245, 1980.
9. Parry BW, Anderson GA: Influence of acepromazine maleate on the equine haematocrit. *J Vet Pharmacol Ther* 6(2):121–126, 1983.
10. Harbison WD, Slocombe RF, Watts SJ, Stewart GA: Thiambutene and acepromazine as analgesic and preanaesthetic agents in horses and sheep. *Austral Vet J* 50(12):543–546, 1974.
11. Skarda R: Effect of propionylpromazine, acepromazine, atropine, thiopental, and halothane on the haematocrit value, erythrocyte count, haemoglobin content and mean corpuscular haemoglobin concentration in the horse. *Schweizer Archiv Tierheilkunde* 115(12):587–596, 1973.
12. Muri WW, Skarda RT, Sheeham W: Hemodynamic and respiratory effects of a xylazine-acetylpromazine drug combination in horses. *Am J Vet Res* 40(11):1518–1522, 1979.
13. Kerr DD, Jones EW, Holbert D, Huggins K: Comparison of the effects of xylazine and acetylpromazine maleate in the horse. *Am J Vet Res* 33(4):777–784, 1972.
14. Chary JF: Sedation of the horse with an acepromazine-xylazine combination. *Pratique Veterinaire Equine* 12(2):97–98.
15. McClure JR Jr, Gelatt KN, Gum GG, Manning JP: The effect of parenteral acepromazine and xylazine on intraocular pressure in the horse. *VM/SAC* 71(12):1727–30, 1976.
16. Muir WW, Sams RA, Huffman RH, Noonan JS: Pharmacodynamic and pharmacokinetic properties of diazepam in horses. *Am J Vet Res* 43(10):1756–1562, 1982.
17. Tranquilli W, Thurmon JC, Turner TA, Benson GJ, Lock TF: Butorphanol tartrate as an adjunct to xylazine-ketamine anesthesia in the horse. *Eq Pract* 5(6):26–29, 1983.
18. Combie J, Dougherty J, Nugent E, Tobin T: The pharmacology of narcotic analgesics in the horse. IV. Dose and time response relationships for behavioral responses to morphine, meperidine, pentozocine, anileridine, methadone, and hydromorphone. *J Eq Med Surg* 3(8):377–385, 1979.
19. Tobin T, Combie J, Miller JR, Crisman MW, Blake JW: Pharmacology of narcotic analgesic in the horse II. Studies on the detection, pharmacokinetics, urinary clearance times and behavioral effects of pentozocine and fentanyl in the horse. *Irish Vet J* 33(10):169–176, 1979.
20. Leglise J de: General anaesthesia. Use of azaperone in the premedication of horses. *Thes Ecole Nationale Veterinaire d'Alfort* 1973.
21. Ehmke J: Stresnil (azaperone) combined with polamivet for sedation and anaesthetic premedication in the horse. *Deutsche Tierarztliche Wochenschrift* 79(21):539–543, 1972.

22. Kovalev MI: Use of etaperazine (per phenazine) in horse, cattle, swine and dog. *Veterinariya USSR* 1:71–72, 1979.
23. Robertson JT, Muir WW: A new analgesic drug combination in the horse. *Am J Vet Res* 44(9):1667–1669, 1983.
24. Nolan AM, Hall LW: Combined use of sedatives and opiates in horses. *Vet Rec* 114(3):63–67, 1984.
25. Kalpravidh M, Lumb WV, Wright M, Heath RB: Effects of butorphanol, flunixin, levorphanol, morphine and xylazine in ponies. *Am J Vet Res* 45(2):217–223, 1984.
26. Muir WW, Skarda RT, Sheehan WC: Hemodynamic and respiratory effects of xylazine-morphine sulfate in horses. *Am J Vet Res* 40(10):1417–1420, 1979.
27. Serrano L, Lees P, Hillidge CJ: Influence of azaperone/metomidate anaesthesia on blood biochemistry in the horse. *British Vet J* 132(4):405–415, 1976.
28. Hillidge CJ, Lees P, Serrano L: Influence of azaperone and metomidate on cardiovascular and respiratory functions in the pony. *British Vet J* 13(1):50–64, 1975.
29. Jenkins JT, Crooks JL, Charlesworth C, Blaine GF: The use of etorphine-acepromazine (analgesic-tranquilizer) mixtures in horses. *Vet Rec* 90(8):207–210, 1972.
30. Dobbs HE, Ling CM: The use of etorphine/acepromazine in the horse and donkey. *Vet Rec* 91(2):40–41, 1972.
31. Hillidge CJ, Lees P: Influence of the neuroleptanalgesic combination of etorphine and acepromazine on the horse: blood gases and acid-base balance. *Equine Vet J* 7(3):148–154, 1975.
32. Lees P, Hillidge CJ: Neuroleptanalgesia and cardiovascular function in the horse. *Equine Vet J* 7(4):184–191, 1975.
33. Lees P, Hillidge CJ: Immobilon: Some comment on its action. *Vet Rec* 99(3):55–56, 1976.
34. Short CE, Brunson DB: General anesthesia in pleasure horses. *Cornell Vet* 68(7):276–283, 1978.
35. Frankland AL, Camburn MA: Induction of anaesthesia using thiopentone sodium in the horse. *Vet Rec* 100(22):472, 1977.
36. Brouwer GJ, Hall LW, Kuchel TR: Intravenous anaesthesia in horses with xylazine premedication. *Vet Rec* 107(11):241–245, 1980.
37. Butera ST, Garner HE, Moore JN, Amed JF: Xylazine/sodium thiopental combination for short-term anesthesia in the horse. *VM/SAC* 75(5):765–768, 770, 1980.
38. Schatzmann U, Tschudi P, Held JP, Muhlebach B: An investigation of the action and haemolytic effect of glyceral guaiacolate in the horse. *Equine Vet J* 10(4):224–228, 1978.
39. Grandy JL, McDonell WN: Evaluation of concentrated solutions of guaifenesin for equine anesthesia. *J Am Vet Med Assoc* 176(7):619–622, 1980.
40. Hubbell JAE, Muir WW, Sams RA: Guaifenesin: cardiopulmonary effects and plasma concentrations in horses. *Am J Vet Res* 4(11):1751–1755, 1980.
41. Schatzmann U, Koehli M, Dudan F, Jones RS: Some cardiopulmonary effects of glyceryl guaiacolate in combination with preanesthetics in the standing horse. *Equine Pract* 6(2):17–21, 1984.
42. Kalhoro AB, Rex MAE: Observations on the use of glyceryl guaiacolate as an adjunct to general anaesthesia in horses. *Australian Vet J* 61(2):49–53, 1984.
43. Anderson IL: An unusual reaction in a horse during anaesthesia. *New Zealand Vet J* 31(5):85, 1983.
44. Browuer GJ: Use of guaiacolyglycerine ether in clinical anaesthesia in the horse. *Equine Vet J* 17(2):133–136, 1985.
45. Muir WW, Skarda RT, Sheehan W: Evaluation of xylazine, guaifenesin, and ketamine hydrochloride for restraint in horses. *Am J Vet Res* 39(8):1274–1278, 1978.
46. Butera TS, Moore JN, Garner HE, Amend JF, Clarke LL, Hatfield DG: Diazepam/xylazine/ketamine combination for short-term anesthesia in the horse. *VM/SAC* 73(4):490, 495–499, 1978.
47. Fisher RJ: A field trial of ketamine anaesthesia in the horse. *Equine Vet J* 16(3):173–179, 1984.
48. Hall LW, Taylor PM: Clinical trial of xylazine with ketamine in equine anaesthesia. *Vet Rec* 108(23):489–493, 1981.
49. Baumgartner M, Keller H: Ketamine hydrochloride anaesthesia in horses. *Deutsche Veterinarmedizinische Gesellschaft*, 177–186, 1982.
50. Komar E: Ketamine anaesthesia of horses. *Medycyna Weterynaryjna* 39(9):528–530, 1983.
51. Tranquilli WJ, Thurmon JC, Neff-Davis CA, Davis LE, Benson GJ, Hoffman W, Lock TF: Hyperglycemia and hypoinsulinemia during xylazine-ketamine anesthesia in thoroughbred horses. *Am J Vet Res* 45(1):11–14, 1984.
52. Muir WW, Skarda RT, Milne DW: Evaluation of xylazine and ketamine hydrochloride for anesthesia in horses. *Am J Vet Res* 38(2):195–201, 1977.
53. Kaka JS, Klavano PA, Hayton WL: Pharmacokinetics of ketamine in the horse. *Am J Vet Res* 40(7):978–981, 1979.
54. Parsons JE, Walmsley JP: Field use of an acetylpromazine/methadone/ketamine combination for anaesthesia in the horse and donkey. *Vet Rec* 111(17):395, 1982.
55. Kitzman JV, Wilson RC, Hatch RC, Booth NH: Antagonism of xylazine and ketamine anesthesia by 4-amino-pyridine and yohimbine in geldings. *Am J Vet Res* 45(5):875–879, 1984.
56. Eales FA: Effects of saffan administered intravenously in the horse. *Vet Rec* 99(14):270–272, 1976.
57. Wright M, McGrath CJ, Raffe M: Indirect blood pressure readings in horses before and after induction of general anesthesia with acetylpromazine, glyceryl guaiacolate and sodium thiamylal. *Vet Anesth* 6(3):41–43, 1979.
58. Neumann H, Wintzer H-J: Systolic blood pressure during halothane anesthesia in the horse. *Berliner Munchener Tierarztliche Wochenschrift* 88(19):365–367, 1975.
59. Steffey EP, Howland D Jr: Cardiovascular effects of halothane in the horse. *Am J Vet Res* 39(4):611–615, 1978.
60. Steffey EP, Farver T, Zinkl J, Wheat JD, Meagher DM, Brown MP: Alterations in horse blood cell count and biochemical values after halothane anesthesia. *Am J Vet Res* 41(6):934–939, 1980.
61. Schulz-Ohrt S: Behavior of blood gases after pre-anaesthetic medication and during halothane-oxygen anaesthesia in the horse. *Inaugural Dissertation, Freie Universitat, Berlin*, 1978.
62. Weaver BM, Webb AI: Tissue composition and halothane solubility in the horse. *Br J Anaesth* 53(5):487–93, 1981.
63. Busetti R, Grudi M, Cassani M, Medri MS, Masetti L: Nine years of inhalation anaesthesia in the horse: retrospective study of 988 cases. *Atti Del congresso Nazionale della Societa Italiana di Ippologia* 6:89–98, 1983.
64. Taylor PM, Hall LW: Clinical anesthesia in the horse: comparison of enflurane and halothane. *Equine Vet J* 17(1):51–57, 1985.
65. Orsini JA, Taylor JI: Enflurane anesthesia in the pony: a comparative study between enflurane and halothane. *Cornell Vet* 70(1):50–66, 1980.
66. Steffey EP, Howland D Jr: Comparison of circulatory and respiratory effects of isoflurane and halothane anesthesia in horses. *Am J Vet Res* 41(5):821–825, 1980.
67. Steffey EP, Zinkl J, Howland D Jr: Minimal changes in blood cell counts and biochemical values associated with prolonged isoflurane anesthesia of horses. *Am J Vet Res* 40(11):1646–1648, 1979.
68. Steffey EP: Enflurane and isoflurane anesthesia: a summary of laboratory and clinical investigations in horses. *J Am Vet Med Assoc* 172(3):367–373, 1978.
69. Steffey EP, Howland D Jr, Giri S, Eger EI: Enflurane, halothane and isoflurane potency in horses. *Am J Vet Res* 38(7):1037–1039, 1977.
70. Steffey EP, Howland D Jr: Potency of halothane-N_2O in the horse. *Am J Vet Res* 39(7):1141–1146, 1978.

71. Steffey EP, Howland D Jr: Alterations in anesthetic requirements (MAC) and cardiovascular responses accompanying the addition of nitrous oxide to halothane-O_2 in horses. *Fed Proceed* 37(3):508, 1978.
72. Herken A: Behavior of blood gases and the acid-base equilibrium during halothane/nitrous oxide anaesthesia in the horse. *Inaugural Dissertation, Tierarztleche Hochscule, Hannover,* 1977.
73. Masetti L, Busetto R: Prolonged anaesthesia in the horse with halothane and nitrous oxide. *Clinica Veterinaria* 101(8):493–498, 1978.
74. Korbner F, Zeller R: Changes in blood gases, acid-base equilibrium and blood pressure during anaesthesia of horses with enflurane and nitrous oxide. *Deutsche Veterinarmedizinische Gesellschaft* 193–201, 1982.
75. DeMoor A, Van Den Hende C, Moens Y, Desmet P: Increased plasma bromide concentration in the horse after halothane anesthesia. *Am J Vet Res* 39(10):1624–1626, 1978.
76. Gopinath G, Ford EJ: The influence of hepatic microsomal amidopyrine demethylase activity on halothane hepatotoxicity in the horse. *J Pathol* 119(2):105–112, 1976.
77. Lees P, Mullen PA, Travernor WD: Influence of anaesthesia with volatile agents on the equine liver. *Br J Anaesth* 45(6):570–578, 1973.
78. Bue M del, Botti P, Ubaldi A, Corbella E: Serum enzyme variations—SGOT, SGPT, gamma-GT, AP, CHE following anaesthesia with halothane in the horse. *Clinica Veterinaria* 102(2):158–165, 1979.
79. Engelking LR, Dodman NH, Hartman G, Valdez H, Spivak W: Effects of halothane anesthesia on equine liver function. *Am J Vet Res* 45(4):607–615, 1984.
80. Aver JA, Garner HE, Amend JF, Hutchenson DP, Salem CA: Recovery from anesthesia in ponies: a comparative study of the effects of isoflurane, enflurane, methoxyflurane and halothane. *Equine Vet J* 10(1):18–23, 1978.
81. Taylor PM: Techniques and clinical application of arterial blood pressure measurements in the horse. *Eq Vet J* 13(4):271–275, 1981.
82. Hillidge CJ, Lees P: Cardiac output in the conscious and anaesthetised horse. *Equine Vet J* 7(1):16–21, 1975.
83. Hillidge CJ, Lees P: The rate of rise of intraventricular pressure as an index of myocardial contractility in conscious and anaesthetised ponies. *Res Vet Sci* 21(2):176–183, 1976.
84. Klein L, Sherman J: Effects of preanesthetic medication, anesthesia, and position of recumbency on central venous pressure in horses. *J Am Vet Med Assoc* 170(2):216–219, 1977.
85. Trim CM, Moore JN, White NA: Cardiopulmonary effects of dopamine hydrochloride in anaesthetised horses. *Equine Vet J* 17(1):41–44, 1985.
86. Swanson CR, Muir WW, Bednarski RM, Skarda RT, Hubbell JA: Hemodynamic responses in halothane anesthetized horses given infusions of dopamine or dobutamine. *Am J Vet Res* 46(2):365–370, 1985.
87. Moor A de: Oxygenation during general anaesthesia, with special reference to halothane anaesthesia in the horse. *Vlaams Dieigeneeskundig Zijdschrift* 43(2):92–111, 1974.
88. Hubbell JA, Muir WW 3d: Rate of rise of arterial carbon dioxide tension in the halothane anesthetized horse. *J Am Vet Med Assoc* 186(4)374–376, 1985.
89. Moens Y, DeMoor A: Use of infra-red carbon dioxide analysis during general anaesthesia in the horse. *Equine Vet J* 13(4):229–234, 1981.
90. Meyer RE, Short CE: Aterial to end-tidal CO_2 tension and alveolar dead space in halothane or isoflurane anesthetized ponies. *Am J Vet Res* 46(3):597–599, 1985.
91. Moors A de, Hende C van den: Inspiratory concentrations of O_2, N_2 and N_2O, arterial oxygenation and acid-base status during closed system halothane anaesthesia in the horse. *Zentralblatt Veterinarmedizin* 19A:1–7, 1972.
92. Moor A de, Desmet P, Verschoot en F: Influence of change body position on arterial oxygenation and acid-base status in the horse in lateral recumbancy, anaesthetized with halothane and efficiency of postanaesthetic oxygen administration. *Zentralblatt Veterinarmedizin* 21A:525–531, 1974.
93. Staddon GE, Weaver BM: Regional pulmonary perfusion in horses: a comparison between anaesthetised and conscious standing animals. *Res Vet Sci* 30(1):44–48, 1981.
94. Amis TC, Pascoe JR, Horn of W: Topographic distribution of pulmonary ventilation and perfusion in the horse. *Am J Vet Res* 45(8):1597–1601, 1984.
95. Sorenson PR, Robinson NE: Postural effects on lung volumes and asymchronous ventilation in anesthetized horses. *J Appl Physiol* 48(1):97–103, 1980.
96. Steffey EP, Wheat JD, Meagher DM, Norrie RD, McKee J, Brown M, Arnold J: Body position and mode of ventilation influences arterial pH, oxygen, and carbon dioxide tensions in halothane anesthetized horses. *Am J Vet Res* 38(3):379–382, 1977.
97. Benson GJ, Manohar M, Kneller SK, Thurmon JC, Steffey EP: Radiographic characterization of diaphragmatic excursion in halothane anesthetized ponies: spontaneous and controlled ventilation systems. *Am J Vet Res* 43(4):617–621, 1982.
98. Weaver BMQ, Walley RV: Ventilation and cardiovascular studies during mechanical control of ventilation in horses. *Equine Vet J* 7(1):9–15, 1975.
99. Capaul EG, Aberti CD, Catalano C, Desmaras E, Mombello R: General anaesthesia with controlled breathing in horses. *Revista Medicina Veterinaria* 53(6):521–525, 1972.
100. Backes G, Skarda R: Improvement of lung ventilation with the respiratory Mark 9 during general anesthesia in the horse. *Schweizer Archiv Zierhdilkunde* 114(1):13–23, 1972.
101. Schatzmann U: Investigation of the applicability of controlled ventilation during routine anesthesia in the horse. *J Eq Med Surg* 2(10):453–458, 1978.
102. Hall LW, Trim CM: Positive end-expiratory pressure in anesthetized spontaneously breathing horses. *Br J Anaesth* 47(8):819–824, 1975.
103. Beadle RE, Robinson NE, Sorenson PR: Cardiopulmonary effects of positive end-expiratory pressure in anesthetized horses. *Am J Vet Res* 36(10):1435–1438, 1975.
104. Steffey EP, Berry JD: Flow rates from an intermittent positive pressure breathing anesthetic delivery apparatus for horses. *Am J Vet Res* 38(5):685–687, 1977.
105. Littlejohn A: Aspects of respiration in anaesthetized newborn foals. *J Reprod Fertil* 23:681–684, 1975.
106. Littlejohn A, Heerden JS van: Respiration in newborn Percheron foals when anaesthetized at a medium altitude of 1300 M. *Br Vet J* 131(1):40–49, 1975.
107. Garner HE, Moore JN, Amed JF, Johnson JH, Tritschler LG, Traver DS, Coffman JR: Post-operative management of hypoxia in the equine abdominal crisis. *Proceedings 23rd Conv AAEP* 177–187, 1978.
108. Short CE, Blais-DiFruscia D, Gleed R, Demson MV, White KK, Hackett RP, Smith DF: Anesthesia and supportive therapy during surgery for equine colic. *VM/SAC* 76(3):419–424, 1981.
109. Mysinger PW, Redding RW, Vaughan JT, Purohit RC, Holladay JA: Electroencephalographic patterns of clinically normal, sedated, and tranquilized foals and adult horses. *Am J Vet Res* 46(1):36–41, 1985.
110. Purohit RC, Mysinger PW, Redding RW: Effects of xylazine and ketamine hydrochloride on the electroencephalogram and the electrocardiogram in the horse. *Am J Vet Res* 42(4):615–619, 1981.
111. Schneider J, Moens V, Moor A de: Electroencephalographic examination of ponies with artificially induced hypoxaemia.

Monatschefte fur Veterinarmedizin 36(15):576–581, 1981.
112. Manley SV, Steffey EP, Howitt Ga, Woliner M: Cardiovascular and neuromuscular effects of pancuronium bromide in the pony. *Am J Vet Res* 44(7):1349–1353, 1983.
113. Hildebrand SV, Howitt, GA: Dosage requirements of pancuronium in halothane anesthetized ponies: a comparison of cumulative and single dose administration. *Am J Vet Res* 45(11):2441–2444, 1984.
114. Klein L, Hopkins J, Beck E, Burton B: Cumulative dose responses to gallamine, pancuronium and neostigmine in halothane anesthetized horses: neuromuscular and cardiovascular effects. *Am J Vet Res* 44(5):786–792, 1983.
115. Hildebrand SV, Howitt GA: Antagonism of pancuronium neuromuscular blockade in halothane anesthetized ponies using neostigmine and edrophonium. *Am J Vet Res* 45(11):2276–2280, 1984.
116. Klein L, Hopkins J, Beck E, Burton B: Mechanical responses to peroneal nerve stimulation in halothane-anesthetized horses in the absence of neuromuscular blockade and during partial nondepolarizing blockade. *Am J Vet Res* 44(5):781–785, 1983.
117. Benson GJ, Hartsfield SM, Smitzer DL, Thurmon JC: Physiologic effects of succinylcholine chloride in mechanically ventilated horses anesthetized with halothane in oxygen. *Am J Vet Res* 40(10):1411–1416, 1979.
118. Manley SV, Kelly AB, Hodgson D: Malignant hyperthermia-like reactions in three anesthetized horses. *J Am Vet Med Assoc* 183(1):85–89, 1983.
119. Hildebrand SV, Howitt GA: Succinylcholine infusion associated with hyperthermia in ponies anesthetized with halothane. *Am J Vet Res* 44(12):2280–2284, 1983.
120. Waldron-Mease E, Klein LV, Rosenberg H, Leitch M: Malignant hyperthermia in a halothane-anesthetized horse. *J Am Vet Med Assoc* 179(9):896–898, 1981.
121. Serteyn D, D'Ieteren G, Spyropoulas E, Klutz JP, Philippart C, Lamy M: Changes in some serum enzymes in equine postanaesthetic myopathy. *Ann Med Veterinaire* 128(4):291–297, 1984.
122. Serteyn D, D'Ieteren G, Philippart C, Lanny M: Post-anaesthetic myopathy of horses: measurement of ions, haematocrit, blood glucose and serum proteins after halothane anaesthesia. *Ann Med Veterinaire* 128(5):385–392, 1984.
123. Johnson BD, Heath RB, Bowman B, Phillips RW, Rich LD, Voss JL: Serum chemistry changes in horses during anesthesia: a pilot study investigating the possible causes of postanesthetic myositis in horses. *J Eq Med Surg* 2(3):109–123, 1978.
124. Klein L: A review of 50 cases of post-operative myopathy in the horse. Intrinsic and management factors affecting risk. *Proc AAEP*:89–94, 1979.
125. Short CE, White KK: Anesthetic/surgical stress-induced myopathy (myositis). Part I. Clinical occurrences. *Proc AAEP*:101–106, 1979.
126. White KK, Short CE: Anesthetic/surgical stress-induced myopathy (myositis). Part II. A post-anesthetic myopathy trial. *Proc AAEP*: 107–114,1979.
127. Lindsay WA, Pascoe PJ, McDonell WN, Burgess ML: Effect of protective padding in fore limb intracompartmental muscle pressures in anesthetized horses. *Am J Vet Res* 46(3):688–91, 1985.
128. Lindsay WA, McDonell W, Bignell W: Equine postanesthetic forelimb lameness: intracompartmental muscle pressure changes and biochemical patterns. *Am J Vet Res* 41(12):1919–1924, 1980.

PART 2

Special Anesthesia Considerations in the Ruminant

CYNTHIA M. TRIM, M.R.C.V.S., D.V.A., D.A.C.V.A.

More manipulative and surgical procedures are performed on ruminants using physical restraint and local analgesia techniques than general anesthesia. Reasons for this are the relative ease with which a ruminant can be restrained by physical means, the high risk of aspiration of regurgitated rumen contents that may occur during general anesthesia, and, in some cases, financial considerations. Nerve block techniques are described in Chapter 8. Intravenous regional analgesia is a form of local anesthesia that is often used in ruminants and will be described here.

Intravenous Regional Analgesia

Analgesia for procedures such as claw amputation or interdigital fibroma removal may be produced by securing a tourniquet around the limb and injecting a local anesthetic drug intravenously distal to the tourniquet (1, 2). The drug is distributed through the limb via the veins and diffuses out into the tissues. Experimental evidence suggests that analgesia is due to blockade of small nerves or nerve endings and not of major nerve trunks, as was previously believed (3). Onset of analgesia is in 5 to 10 minutes and persists until the tourniquet is removed. In some animals, a weak residual effect persists for up to 30 minutes. No significant concentration of lidocaine has been measured in the systemic circulation after the tourniquet is released, provided that sufficient time has elapsed since injection for the drug to be absorbed into the tissues.

The patient is usually restrained on its side manually or with the aid of sedatives. The tourniquet can be placed at any point on the limb (Fig. 13.3). In the adult bovine, the tourniquet is usually placed either above the fetlock or above the hock. In the latter case, padding such as a 4-inch roll of gauze must be inserted between the leg and the tourniquet to fill the gaps and allow even compression. In the small ruminant, the tourniquet is often placed just below or above the elbow or above the hock. Blood will not ooze at the surgical site if the limb is exanguinated first with an Esmarch bandage, but the collapsed veins may make venipuncture difficult. This may be circumvented by preplacing a needle or catheter in the vein. The courses of peripheral veins are illustrated in Figure 13.3. Unlike the dog, the cephalic vein of the sheep and goat runs obliquely across the forearm (Fig. 13.4). Lidocaine without epinephrine should be used. If the needle is directed toward the digits, there will be minimum resistance to injection. Injection of an equal volume of saline after the lidocaine further distributes the anesthetic and has been demonstrated to accelerate the onset of analgesia (4). A small gauge needle should be used, and pressure should be applied to the site of venipuncture after the needle has been removed to prevent hematoma formation, which may be substantial if precautions are not taken. A dosage of 30 ml of 2% lidocaine is adequate for an adult bovine and 3 to 10 ml for a small ruminant, depending on the size of the animal, but not exceeding 4 mg of lidocaine/kg of bodyweight. Complete failure of analgesia is due either to a loose tourniquet or to perivascular injection. Occasionally, sensation persists in the interdigital cleft. Complete analgesia may then be produced by injecting lidocaine subcutaneously on the center midline of both cranial and caudal surfaces of the fetlock.

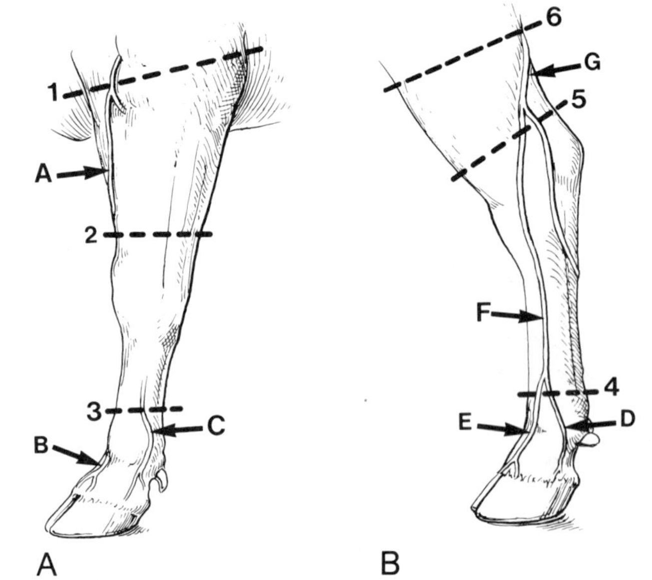

Figure 13.3. Analgesia of a limb can be produced by placing a tourniquet around the limb at one of the points *1* to *6* indicated on the diagram and injecting lidocaine into a peripheral vein, labelled *A* to *G*, distal to it.

Drugs Used for Sedation

Adverse effects may occur in humans who ingest meat or milk containing anesthetic drugs. The total excretion time of some anesthetic drugs is known, and the waiting time before slaughter may appear on the packaging. Many anesthetic drugs used in ruminants are not approved by the Food and Drug Administration (FDA); when these are used, the animal must not be sent for slaughter in the near future. Chloral hydrate,

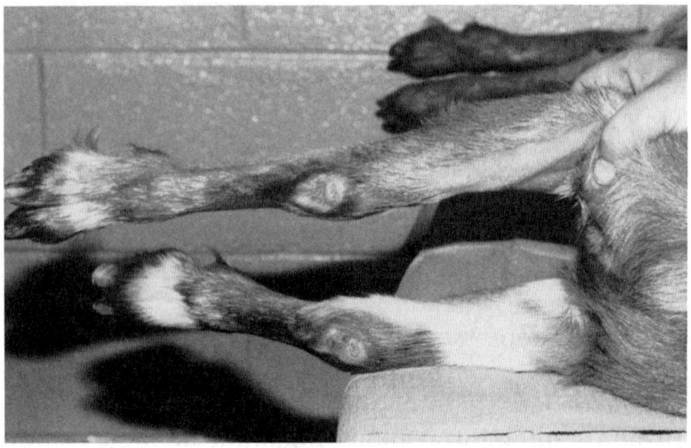

Figure 13.4. The cephalic vein of goats, shown here raised on the right forelimb, runs obliquely from the cranial to the medial surface of the proximal one-third of the radius.

phenothiazines, xylazine, diazepam, and barbiturates pass into the milk, which should be discarded.

CHLORAL HYDRATE

Chloral hydrate is used in adult cattle to produce sedation or basal narcosis. It may be administered orally by stomach tube in a large volume of water or by intravenous injection. Chloral hydrate is also used in combination with magnesium sulfate by intravenous injection. This combination provides better sedation at a lower dose of chloral hydrate. Chloral hydrate will cause tissue necrosis if injected perivascularly. In the blood and liver, chloral hydrate is reduced to its inactive form, trichlorethanol. This metabolite is slow to cross the blood-brain barrier, and consequently several minutes must elapse after intravenous injection before full effect is obtained. A slow infusion of chloral hydrate over several minutes, rather than a bolus injection, is less likely to result in overdose. The usual dose for adult cattle without administration of other drugs is 4 to 7 g/100 kg. The duration of effective sedation from a single administration is 30 to 40 minutes. The low dose or less must be used in depressed or hypovolemic animals. Chloral hydrate decreases cardiac output and arterial blood pressure, and hypotension may occur in the hypovolemic patient. Chloral hydrate has been demonstrated in humans to pass into the milk and into the fetus (5). Metabolites continue to accumulate in the body for at least 2 days. Trichlorethanol is conjugated in the liver with glucuronic acid and excreted in the urine and bile.

Chloral hydrate has also been used in combination with pentobarbital for deep sedation.

PHENOTHIAZINE TRANQUILIZERS

Phenothiazine tranquilizers are used both for tranquilization and for preanesthetic medication. Promazine, acepromazine, triflupromazine, and diethylisobutrazine have all been used in the past, but acepromazine is the most commonly used drug at present. It may be given by intravenous or intramuscular injection at a dosage depending on the physical status of the patient and the required effect. The usual dose for acepromazine is 0.05 to 0.1 mg/kg, with a maximum intravenous dose of 25 mg for preanesthetic medication of adult cattle. Phenothiazine tranquilizers should be avoided in depressed or hypovolemic patients because hypotension may result. Warnings given for triflupromazine are that milk must not be used for food for 10 hours after intravenous injection or for 24 hours after intramuscular injection. Sheep intended for food must not be slaughtered for at least 3 days and cattle for 2 days.

XYLAZINE

Xylazine hydrochloride is licensed for use in cattle in Europe and Canada, but not in the United States. Xylazine has proven to be a very useful sedative in cattle, sheep, and goats, but it has profound effects other than sedation that must be considered before administration to an animal.

Pharmacokinetic studies in horses, cattle, sheep, and dogs have demonstrated remarkably small interspecific differences (6). Rapid distribution of xylazine followed intravenous injection with a half-life of 1.2 minutes in cattle and 1.9 minutes in sheep, compared with 6 minutes in horses. The apparent volume of distribution was large, suggesting that xylazine diffused extensively. After intramuscular injection, absorption was rapid with a half-life of absorption of 5.5 minutes in sheep, although the extent of absorption was only 40% in this species. Plasma concentrations of xylazine were not detected in cattle after intramuscular injection, despite obvious sedation, and it was suggested that the drug effects in this species were due to one or more metabolites. Xylazine is metabolized, and most of the metabolites are excreted in the urine. Very little intact drug was measured in sheep urine collected every 10 minutes after injection (6). In experimental studies of xylazine (0.33 mg/kg by intramuscular injection), residues in milk were decreased to 0.01 ppm by 60 hours after injection, and at 72 hours the total residue measured in tissues was less than 0.1 ppm (J. A. Shmidl, personal communication, 1980).

Not only is there a difference between species in sensitivity to xylazine, in that ruminants only require one-tenth of the dose used for horses or dogs, but there is also an indication that difference in sensitivity exists between breeds of cattle. In an investigation using 34 Holstein and Hereford cattle between 10 and 24 months of age, 84% of Herefords spontaneously lay down after xylazine administration, but only 22% of Holsteins lay down; the rest remained standing (7). A further difference was noted in that the Herefords were down for a mean time of 93 minutes, whereas the Holsteins were down for 52 minutes. There have also been verbal reports that the Brahman is very sensitive to the effects of xylazine.

The dosage for xylazine by intramuscular injection in healthy adult ruminants is between 0.025 and 0.22 mg/kg. This dose range may also be used for intravenous injection, but the lower dosages are less likely to cause complications. Adult cattle will usually remain standing when given the lowest dose intramuscularly (8 to 10 mg total dose). At higher dosages, the animal may assume recumbency. The dosage should be severely decreased for animals which are depressed, and newborn animals should be given only the lowest dose. Xylazine should be administered to small ruminants as a 20 mg/ml solution using a 1 ml syringe and a 25 or 23 gauge needle to allow accurate measurement of drug. Xylazine should be avoided in hypovolemic animals. In contrast, a higher dosage appears to be necessary in wild or excited cattle (8), but this may result in a relative overdosage (Trim, personal observations).

Xylazine impairs thermoregulation in cats for several hours, resulting in hypothermia (9). Small ruminants anesthetized with xylazine and ketamine in an air conditioned surgery room will become hypothermic, and shivering does not begin until long after the animals have recovered from anesthesia. Others have remarked that cattle sedated with xylazine will become hyperthermic if left in the sun (8).

Heavy sedation with xylazine is accompanied by depression of the cough reflex and loss of the swallowing reflex. Swallowing may not return for several hours, even after the animal has regained its feet. Aspiration of ruminal contents is possible if regurgitation occurs. Xylazine has been reported to decrease the respiratory rate in cattle (10) and in calves (11). Several investigations of xylazine have demonstrated mild to severe decreases in arterial PO_2 and decreases and increases in arterial PCO_2 (7, 10–12). The decrease in arterial oxygenation may be gradual and not recognized until the animal collapses or dies. Xylazine decreases gastrointestinal motility, resulting in bloat, which will further impair ventilation. Acute pulmonary edema, manifested as wheezy, labored breathing, has been reported to occur in sheep 15 minutes after injection of xylazine (13). Some of the animals recovered spontaneously, and the symptoms resolved in others given atropine. The complication did not appear to be dose-related and was fatal in some cases. Administration of xylazine to cattle was also accompanied by a progressive increase in pH and base excess over 2 hours (10).

Xylazine causes a decrease in heart rate in cattle (7), calves (11, 14), sheep (15), and goats (Trim, personal observations). The decrease in heart rate can be partly reversed by the administration of atropine. The mean arterial pressure was reported to be increased 5 minutes after xylazine administration and decreased by 15 minutes (11) or decreased at all times of sedation (14). Cardiac output was decreased by 25% in calves receiving an intramuscular injection of 0.22 mg/kg of xylazine, and peripheral vascular resistance was increased (14). Second degree heart block was recorded in 1 out of 5 calves receiving xylazine (14). No atrioventricular heart block was recorded in sheep after xylazine (15).

A 200% increase in plasma glucose and a 400% increase in hepatic glucose production (16–18) with decreased plasma insulin concentration (17, 18) were documented in cattle after xylazine administration. Approximately a 64% increase in blood glucose was recorded in sheep (19, 20).

A 6- to 8-fold increase in urine volume has been measured in cattle, with the greatest increase occurring during the first hour of xylazine sedation and a decreasing effect for 2 to 3 hours (21). Consequently, potential overdistension and rupture of the bladder should be considered before use of xylazine in animals with urethral obstruction.

Administration of xylazine during advanced pregnancy is not advisable. Measurement of intrauterine pressure in cows after an intravenous injection of xylazine or oxytocin has demonstrated similar increases in pressure, and that a greater number of uterine contractions occurred after xylazine (22). In four pregnant cows, a tetanic uterine contraction that increased in pressure with time was produced, and one cow aborted 72 hours later. This cow had developed the highest pressure in response to xylazine and a suggested cause of fetal death was hypoxia from prolonged vasoconstriction of blood vessels in the myometrium and placenta.

Fluid feces have been observed in some cattle 12 to 24 hours after xylazine sedation (8). No treatment appears to be necessary.

There are a variety of antagonists to xylazine sedation. Doxapram (Dopram) will antagonize xylazine and is currently available as a respiratory stimulant. Other more effective drugs or combinations may be commercially available in the future. In cattle, the time of recovery to standing was decreased by intravenous injection of doxapram (1 mg/kg); doxapram and yohimbine (0.125 mg/kg); doxapram and 4-aminopyridine (4-AP; 0.3 mg/kg); or 4-AP and yohimbine, from a mean time of 50 minutes to 17, 4.3, 3.3, and 4.5 minutes, respectively (23). The incidence of relapse was small. The quality of recovery varied and was considered to be relatively smooth after doxapram and 4-AP or 4-AP and yohimbine, but the animals which received doxapram or doxapram and yohimbine made repeated unsuccessful attempts to rise. The combination of doxapram and 4-AP was determined to be the most effective antagonist. Preliminary investigation of idazoxan (0.05 to 0.1 mg/kg), an alpha-2 antagonist, has demonstrated complete reversal of xylazine sedation in calves after intravenous injection (24). Tolazoline, 1.5 mg/kg injected intravenously, also reversed xylazine effects in cattle and sheep (25).

DIAZEPAM

Intravenous injection of diazepam (Valium), 0.04 to 0.5 mg/kg, has been reported to cause sedation in cows (26). It was observed that the cows lay down within 2 minutes of injection of 0.5 mg diazepam/kg, but that intramuscular injection resulted in an unpredictable effect. The high cost of the drug precludes its use in adult cattle at these dosages. In small ruminants, diazepam, 0.2 to 0.5 mg/kg, has been used satisfactorily as premedication to ketamine anesthesia.

NEUROLEPTANALGESIC COMBINATIONS

Some combinations, for example xylazine and butorphanol (Torbugesic), have been used in cattle, but the results have been variable.

General Considerations of Sedation and General Anesthesia

The ruminant is subject to some of the problems encountered with general anesthesia in horses, such as inadequate ventilation and postanesthetic lameness. An additional hazard is regurgitation followed by aspiration of ruminal material into the lungs. The risk is sufficiently high to warrant the use of local analgesia instead of general anesthesia whenever possible. The cost of a general anesthetic technique may also preclude its use in some animals.

REGURGITATION

In the conscious animal, contraction of the reticulum forces ingesta against the cardia. Reflux into the pharynx during rumination is controlled by the pharyngoesophageal sphincter and esophagus, which are innervated by the parasympathetic nervous system. It has been suggested that the incidence of regurgitation may be reduced by atropine, but the effect would be outweighed by the incompetence of the pharyngoesophageal and gastroesophageal sphincters caused by relaxation from anesthetic drugs. Anesthesia induced by either thiopental, pentobarbital, or halothane in nonfasted sheep resulted in a 60 to 80% incidence of reflux (27). Esophageal activity was abolished and the frequency and amplitude of ruminal activity greatly decreased during thiopental and pentobarbital anesthesia. During deep halothane anesthesia, activity in the esophagus and rumen was depressed; in light anesthesia, however, pressure waves were consistently observed in the esophagus. Many of these waves were initiated in the lower part of the thoracic esophagus and progressed toward the rumen. Reflux in light anesthesia appeared to provoke considerable peristaltic esophageal activity. It was also observed that sheep that were anesthetized by either of the barbiturates did not regain the defensive swallowing and esophageal responses to reflux until very late in the recovery phase when animal was able to maintain sternal recumbency.

An important factor contributing to the incidence of regurgitation is the pressure inside the rumen and reticulum. An effective method of decreasing the pressure is to decrease the volume of contents of the gastrointestinal tract and minimize gas production by witholding food and water. This was confirmed in sheep in that the frequency of ruminal reflex was significantly decreased when animals were starved for 24 hours before anesthesia compared with those that were allowed to eat (28). The incidence of regurgitation was less when the table that the animal was lying on was tilted into a head-up position compared with head-down and when the animal was lying on its left side compared with its right. Depriving cattle of feed and water for 48 hours resulted in decreases in rectal temperature, heart rate, and respiratory rate and a 14% increase in packed cell volume (PCV) (29). The animals did not gorge themselves when reintroduced to food, and the PCV had returned to prefasting levels by 8 hours. In sheep, mild metabolic alkalosis was produced by 48 hours of starvation, and intrarumenal bacterial flora were slow to return (30). These effects appear to be minimal compared with the benefit of reducing the incidence of regurgitation during anesthesia.

Other factors that may contribute to increased intrarumenal pressure are the assumption of recumbency during induction of anesthesia, tight belly bands used to secure the animal to a table, rolling the animal from side to side or onto its back, or coughing stimulated during the process of tracheal intubation. Forceful regurgitation sometimes occurs in a lightly anesthetized animal during endotracheal intubation. Retrograde esophageal contractions are easily observed and are a warning of imminent regurgitation. It may be that stimulation of the larynx causes the glottis to close and inspiration at that time results in a large negative intrathoracic pressure. The pressure difference may cause rumenal contents to enter the esophagus and initiate peristaltic contractions that move the material into the pharynx. Clinical impression suggests that, when inducing general anesthesia, this type of regurgitation occurs less often when sufficient drug is administered to abolish jaw and tongue movements. General anesthesia should be avoided in an animal with abomasal torsion because regurgitation usually occurs during induction of anesthesia.

Food and water should be withheld before heavy sedation or general anesthesia to decrease the incidence of regurgitation. The author's preference is to withhold food for 36 hours and water for 8 to 12 hours. Nursing animals are withheld from milk for several hours. Other precautions are to intubate the trachea in all anesthetized animals, to position the head with the mouth lower than the larynx so that saliva and regurgitated fluid can drain, and not moving the animal after induction of anesthesia unless an endotracheal tube has been inserted. Negligence may be successfully claimed if aspiration occurs directly as a result of rolling an animal before intubation (31). Regurgitation occurring when an endotracheal tube is in place should not be a problem provided that the pharyngeal area is elevated to allow free drainage and prevent fluid accumulation in the larynx. Alternatively, a cuffed endotracheal tube may be positioned in the cranial part of the esophagus to ensure any reflux drains. Before extubation, the mouth should be cleared of food material and, preferably, the nose should be flushed with water. The tube should not be removed when chewing movements are first observed; this should be delayed until swallowing occurs and the animal has reasonable control of tongue movement. Extubation with the cuff partially inflated may help to prevent aspiration of fluid collected at the laryngeal entrance.

INADEQUATE VENTILATION

An increase in arterial PCO_2 and decrease in PO_2 commonly occurs during general anesthesia due to the combined effects of central depression of respiration by anesthetic drugs and ventilation-perfusion inequality caused by collapse of the dependent lung. The degree of change depends on drug dosage and drugs used. No significant change from awake values for arterial PO_2, PCO_2, ventilation-perfusion ratio, or intrapulmonary shunt was recorded in sheep lightly anesthetized with pentobarbital (32). Halothane-nitrous oxide anesthesia resulted in decreased arterial PO_2 ventilation-perfusion inequality, and increased shunt from 1.4 to 10.6% (32). Ruminal tympany and advanced pregnancy will also severely decrease ventilation during recumbency and anesthesia. Inflation of the rumen of awake, healthy experimental cows to pressures commonly recorded during bloat has been demonstrated to decrease lung volume and lung compliance and significantly increase arterial PCO_2 and decrease PO_2 (33).

Adequate ventilation should be facilitated by withholding food to decrease pressure on the diaphragm and by keeping drug dosages low to minimize depression of ventilation. A large bore stomach tube introduced through the mouth deep into the esophagus may permit evacuation of rumen fluid and gas.

Inadequate ventilation can be effectively treated by endotracheal intubation and controlled ventilation with oxygen. Arterial oxygenation can usually be maintained in animals with mild to moderate hypoventilation by insufflating oxygen into the nasal cavity, or endotracheal tube, via rubber tubing from an oxygen cylinder and a flowmeter. A flow of oxygen of 15 liter/min is necessary in an adult bovine to produce an improvement in arterial oxygenation. Small ruminants can also be intubated and artificially ventilated with air using a resuscitator (Ambu) bag.

LAMENESS

Myositis or radial nerve damage of the underneath forelimb are possible complications of general anesthesia in the large ruminant (Figure 13.5) (34). Traumatic injury to the hindlimbs may occur if the animal makes an incoordinated movement when standing up after anesthesia.

Myositis or radial nerve damage occurs as a consequence of ischemia, either from low systemic arterial pressure or from local compression of tissues. When the anesthetized animal is lying on its side, the underneath forelimb should be pulled forward to prevent pressure on the radial nerve, and the upper limb should be supported parallel to the ground to prevent its weight compressing the median artery. A large inflated tire inner tube can be strapped to the table or to the cow before induction of anesthesia so that the shoulder is centered over the hold and no pressure is applied to the muscles of the shoulder when the animal is anesthetized. Anesthesia should be managed to prevent hypotension.

Treatment of myositis or radial nerve damage is supportive. The animal's movement should be limited to minimize oxygen demands on the damaged muscle and to avoid further injury due to incoordination. The paralyzed limb should be wrapped to avoid abrasion

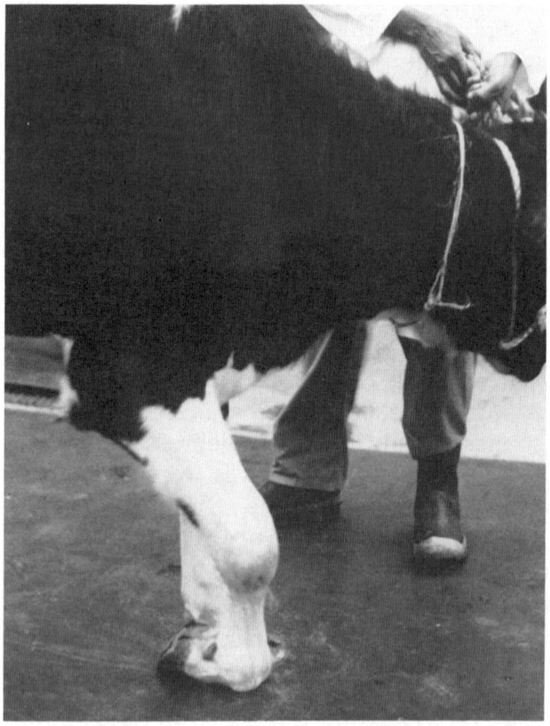

Figure 13.5. This 310-kg Holstein bull had radial nerve paralysis after 1.5 hours of halothane anesthesia for radiography. *Published with permission from Trim CM: Sedation and general anesthesia in ruminants. Calif Vet* 35(4):29–36, 1981.

when it is dragged on the ground, and a support bandage on the sound limb may be advisable. Analgesics should be administered if severe myositis appears to be causing pain. Diuresis by intensive intravenous fluid therapy may be necessary to avoid renal failure in animals with myositis. The lameness usually resolves in a few days.

Anesthetic Drug Combinations for General Anesthesia

A physical examination should be conducted on each animal to be anesthetized and basic hematological and biochemical laboratory tests performed whenever possible to aid in the preanesthetic evaluation. Respiratory or metabolic diseases should be considered when planning anesthetic management. Abnormalities such as hypovolemia or hypocalcemia should be corrected before induction of anesthesia. Food should be withheld for 36 to 48 hours and water for 8 to 12 hours in animals scheduled for elective procedures. Immediately before anesthesia, it is advisable to flush the patient's mouth with water to remove pieces of food that might be inhaled during anesthesia or carried into the trachea during intubation.

Premedication of ruminants with atropine has both advantages and disadvantages. The quantity of saliva produced is decreased, which facilitates the process of tracheal intubation. Atropine will also prevent bradycardia from xylazine or general anesthesia. A disadvantage of atropinization is that saliva production in the ruminant does not completely cease, and the viscid saliva produced may cause respiratory obstruction (35). There is also the clinical impression that the arterial carbon dioxide tensions are higher in atropinized ruminants during anesthesia and that the appetite of animals that have received atropine is slow to return after anesthesia. The author's preference is not to administer atropine routinely but to use it therapeutically at 0.02 mg/kg by intravenous injection when bradycardia develops. Preanesthetic sedation is commonly used before ketamine anesthesia and may be used with other drugs depending on the temperament of the patient.

When a restraining table is available, the cow or bull can be immobilized and rotated onto its side before anesthesia is induced. Alternatively, the animal may be allowed to "free fall" to the ground, but induction of anesthesia is more controlled if the animal is first cast with ropes. Sheep are easily restrained in the sitting position, and goats are usually allowed to stand. Young ruminants and depressed animals may be positioned on the surgery table from the start.

The jugular vein is used for intravenous injection in all species, but the cephalic or recurrent tarsal veins are more accessible in sheep. The vein is more easily located if hair or wool is clipped from the site first. A 14 (A-Cath, Delmed Inc.) or 10 gauge (Medicut, Argyle) 5-inch catheter is suitable for placement in the jugular veins of adult cattle, and 14 gauge 3.5 inch catheters are suitable for calves. Catheters (A-Cath; Sovereign, Sherwood Medical) or wing infusion sets (MediWing, Argyle; Adaptic IV, Jelco; Intrawing, Burron Medical) commonly used in dogs are satisfactory for the small ruminants.

BARBITURATES

The thiobarbiturates thiopental and thiamylal sodium produce satisfactory anesthesia in ruminants. The method of administration of the two agents is similar, although if the same dose rate is used, the duration of anesthesia from thiopental will be shorter than from thiamylal. Thiobarbiturates are usually administered to adult cattle as a bolus intravenous injection at 1 g thiopental/90 kg bodyweight or 1 g thiamylal/140 kg, with an initial maximum dose of 5 and 3.5 g, respectively. Anesthesia should last about 10 minutes. Anesthesia can be prolonged by additional small intravenous doses, according to clinical assessment of the depth of anesthesia, but the use of barbiturates alone to provide anesthesia for more than 20 minutes should be avoided. Less barbiturate should be used if the animal is depressed or debilitated or if preanesthetic sedation is used. Mild sedation will reduce the dose by one-quarter to one-half the dose. The recommended dosage for young calves is 30% less than that used in larger animals. Barbiturates should not be used in animals less than 2 months of age because they tend to be lethargic for several days after anesthesia. Thiopental or thiamylal provides an excellent means of induction of anesthesia in healthy sheep and goats. Although the standard dose to produce anesthesia in healthy animals is 20 mg/kg, the dose rate needed to produce anesthesia in clinical patients varies considerably between individuals and cannot be correlated to weight or age. Without preanesthetic sedation, the range is 7 to 20 mg/kg. To avoid overdosage, an initial bolus of 5 mg/kg should be injected over several seconds. Animals that require the low dose will become partially anesthetized and only a small quantity more needs to be injected to produce surgical anesthesia. Those that require a higher dose will only be sedated, and additional thiobarbiturate should be injected over about 1 minute to produce anesthesia.

Methohexital sodium (Brevital) provides satisfactory anesthesia in cattle, but is not frequently used. In sheep and goats, intravenous injection of methohexital,

4 mg/kg of a 2.5% solution, provides 5 to 7 minutes of anesthesia (36). Recovery may be complicated by violent jerking. Premedication with diazepam or xylazine results in a 50% reduction in methohexital dose and a smooth recovery from anesthesia (36).

Recovery from pentobarbital is too long to be acceptable anesthesia in cattle. In contrast, adult sheep metabolize pentobarbital at a more rapid rate than other species. Slow intravenous injection of pentobarbital, mean dose 24 mg/kg, produces 15 to 30 minutes of surgical anesthesia. A similar dose rate has been used in goats, producing about 20 minutes of anesthesia and recovery in 40 to 60 minutes (37).

GUAIFENESIN

Guaifenesin (glyceryl guaiacolate, Guailaxin) is a centrally acting muscle-relaxing drug that also causes some central nervous system depression (38). It is not licensed for use in ruminants. Although healthy horses immobilized with guaifenesin alone appear to be anxious during induction and recovery, this effect has not been observed in cattle. Guaifenesin can be used alone to provide restraint for procedures such as radiography, but local or general anesthesia must be included if pain is involved. A 5% concentration of guaifenesin has been recommended because bovine red cells are susceptible to hemolysis. An approximate dosage for guaifenesin in cattle is 110 mg/kg infused intravenously, but a lower dose may be adequate in domestic cattle (39); a higher dose, 130 mg/kg, is necessary for buffalo calves (40). Administration of guaifenesin to cattle results in a decrease in tidal volume and an increase in respiratory rate (39). Excessive administration causes hypotension and hypoxemia. Loss of fetal movements has been noted in cows given guaifenesin (39). Guaifenesin is metabolized in the liver, and the metabolites are excreted by the kidney. Guaifenesin can be used in goats, but other agents are used more easily and are less expensive.

A combination of guaifenesin and thiobarbiturate (50 g guaifenesin to 2 g thiobarbiturate) is frequently used, either alone or for induction of anesthesia to inhalation agents. When used in combination, the dosage of each drug is decreased, and the drugs can be titrated to the individual's requirement. Male buffalo calves weighing between 80 and 136 kg were apparently anesthetized by a mean dose of 1.8 ml solution/kg (90 mg guaifenesin and 3.6 mg thiopental/kg) (42). The same average dosage has been used on cattle of beef and dairy breeds and cross-breeds between 200 and 545 kg bodyweight at the University of Georgia. Much less guaifenesin and thiobarbiturate will be needed if the animal has been sedated with xylazine. The anesthetic drug requirement, on a milligram per kilogram basis, decreases in larger animals. In a study of mostly unpremedicated adult bulls and steers, an average dose of 70 to 80 mg of guaifenesin/kg and 2.4 mg of thiobarbiturate/kg was required to produce anesthesia sufficient for tracheal intubation (41). Infusion of guaifenesin and thiopental in cattle results in decreased arterial pressure and increased heart rate (40, 41). Arterial hypoxemia has been recorded immediately after induction of anesthesia, with no change in carbon dioxide concentration (40).

Guaifenesin may also be used with ketamine. The animal may be immobilized by an infusion of guaifenesin and a bolus of ketamine, 1 to 2 mg/kg, injected to facilitate tracheal intubation. Alternatively, 1 g of ketamine may be added to a solution containing 50 g of guaifenesin and the combination infused intravenously until the desired effect is achieved.

KETAMINE

Ketamine is marketed for use in small ruminants in the United Kingdom but is not licensed for this use in the United States. Ketamine may be used to produce anesthesia in adult cattle but is usually administered intravenously because the large volume required for intramuscular use is too expensive. Ketamine may be administered to small ruminants by either intramuscular or intravenous injection, alone or in combination with other drugs. When used alone, ketamine causes muscle rigidity and opisthotonus. Other drugs such as xylazine, acepromazine, diazepam, or guaifenesin are usually included to improve the quality of anesthesia. The dosage of ketamine varies according to the size of the animal. Anesthesia may be produced in large cattle by intravenous injection of xylazine, 0.1 mg/kg, followed immediately or in a few minutes by ketamine, 2 mg/kg (42–44). Swallowing reflexes are depressed; in one study, 5 out of 24 animals regurgitated (44). The duration of anesthesia is short, with the animals regaining their feet in 25 to 40 minutes (44). This anesthetic combination may be used for initial control of the animal to allow restraint with ropes to be applied. Analgesia for surgery should then be provided by local infiltration of lidocaine or nerve block. In animals in the approximate weight range of 150 to 350 kg, xylazine, 0.1 mg/kg, and ketamine, 6 mg/kg, injected intramuscularly will provide similar or slightly longer duration of anesthesia. Anesthesia of 30 to 40 minutes is produced in young calves with xylazine, 0.1 mg/kg, and ketamine, 4.4 to 10 mg/kg, given intramuscularly (33, 45–47). The duration of anesthesia is 50% longer when the drugs are administered simultaneously compared with injection of xylazine 10 minutes before ketamine (45). Intravenous injection of ketamine, 11 mg/kg, produced a moderate decrease in arterial blood pressure, but heart rate and respiratory rate were unchanged (11). Xylazine and ketamine combination produced a significant decrease in mean arterial pressure and arterial PO_2 (47, 48). Heart rate was unchanged when the drugs were administered simultaneously. Respiratory rate increased, and a mild respiratory acidosis was recorded (47, 48). Apnea occasionally occurs in calves that have been given the highest dose of ketamine. Ketamine, 2.2 mg/kg, injected intravenously into buffalo calves after tranquilization with a phenothiazine resulted in 11 minutes of analgesia (49).

Ketamine may be combined with xylazine, acepromazine, or diazepam to provide anesthesia in healthy sheep or goats (50–55). Xylazine, 0.1 mg/kg, and ketamine, 10 mg/kg, may be administered together intramuscularly. The animal will become recumbent in a few minutes. If anesthesia is not complete (chewing movements interfering with tracheal intubation), additional xylazine can be administered up to a total dose of 0.2 mg/kg. Thirty to 40 minutes of anesthesia are produced, and anesthesia can be prolonged by supplemental doses of ketamine or xylazine and ketamine. Supplemental injections of one-third the initial dose of both xylazine and ketamine will produce between 10 and 20 minutes of additional anesthesia. Bradycardia may develop after multiple dosing with xylazine, and treatment with atropine may be necessary. Acepromazine, 0.05 to 0.1 mg/kg, or diazepam, 0.2 to 0.5 mg/kg, can be substituted for the xylazine. When the patient is ill or depressed, it is better to administer the xylazine (or other sedative) first, at a lower dose rate than usually used, in order to evaluate the patient's response. Subsequent dosage of ketamine should be modified to meet the patient's needs. Ketamine may also be administered intravenously at 2 to 6 mg/kg. The lowest dose should be used for depressed animals and may be satisfactory for short procedures in healthy animals. Larger doses of ketamine, 22 to 44 mg/kg, have been used in healthy sheep, and all sheep survived (50, 51). Ketamine, 2 to 3 mg/kg, may be used alone in goats for physical restraint, but muscle tension will be strong. Endotracheal intubation should be possible (56).

STEROID ANESTHETIC DRUGS

The steroid anesthetic agent alphaxalone/alphadolone (CT 1341, Saffan) has been reported to be a useful anesthetic drug in sheep (57, 58), newborn lambs (59), goats (58), and calves (58). It has been used as a sole anesthetic agent and for induction of anesthesia followed by inhalation agents. At least 1.65 mg alphaxalone/alphadolone/kg bodyweight injected intravenously was found to be necessary to produce general anesthesia in adult sheep, and a dose of 3 mg/kg was found to be most useful clinically, producing 5 to 10 minutes of anesthesia (57, 58). It was found that increasing the dose to 6 mg/kg increased anesthesia to 20 minutes, but that respiratory depression was marked. It was suggested that for more than 10 minutes of anesthesia, anesthesia be induced with 3 mg/kg and prolonged by supplemental doses of 1 to 2 mg/kg (58). An alternative regime was induction of anesthesia with 2 mg/kg alphaxalone/alphadolone followed by an infusion of 0.234 mg/kg/min using a 1.6 mg/ml solution (57). In each case, intubation of the trachea was recommended. Injection of alphaxalone/alphadolone, 4.4 mg/kg, intravenously over 10 seconds into adult experimental sheep produced anesthesia for approximately 15 minutes (57). The palpebral reflex was abolished, mydriasis was present, and jaw relaxation was good. Heart rate and the arterial PO_2 were decreased by 20%. Rapid injection of 2.2 mg/kg produced a severe transient (3 minutes) decrease in mean arterial pressure to 55% of the preinjection value. Experimental data indicate that the cardiovascular depression is due to direct myocardial depression and not mediated through the CNS (57). The animals recovered rapidly from anesthesia without residual depression, but were sensitive to auditory and tactile stimuli during the recovery.

Lambs aged between 1 and 11 days (mean, 5 days) appeared to be less sensitive to alphaxalone/alphadolone than adult sheep (59). An intravenous dose of 6 mg/kg was needed to produce anesthesia for 9 minutes in the lambs. A single intramuscular injection of 9 mg/kg produced inconsistent results, but when it was divided in half and injected at two sites, it produced 10 minutes of anesthesia. At these dosages, significant decreases in heart rate and respiratory rate were recorded, but the mucous membranes remained pink and the capillary refill time was unchanged. Shivering was observed in all the lambs at some stage of anesthesia. Recovery was smooth, and no hyperesthesia was observed.

Alphaxalone/alphadolone has been reported to be a safe method of producing anesthesia for disbudding goats when injected intravenously at 6 mg/kg, 1 to 2 ml, depending on the size of the goat (60, 61). The kids were able to stand in 15 to 30 minutes.

Minaxolone differs from alphaxalone in that it is water-soluble. Pharmacological studies in sheep have determined the therapeutic ratio (fatal blood concentration to anesthetic concentration) to be three to four when no respiratory support is provided (62). When artificial ventilation was instituted, the therapeutic ratio increased to 30. The degree of respiratory depression accompanying minaxolone anesthesia may limit its use in the ruminant under field conditions, but further investigations should be performed.

INHALATION AGENTS

Halothane is the most commonly used inhalation agent in ruminants. Methoxyflurane is used in small ruminants, but an adequate depth of anesthesia can be difficult to achieve in adult cattle. Nitrous oxide may be used, but it causes progressive distension of the gastrointestinal tract. Isoflurane appears to have the same advantages in ruminants that have been observed in horses. The minimum alveolar concentration (MAC) of halothane in 3- to 8-week old calves was 0.76% (63). There appeared to be an age-related increase in MAC in that calves of less than 5 weeks had a mean MAC of 0.69%, whereas calves older than 5 weeks had a MAC of 0.83%. Addition of 50% nitrous oxide decreased MAC by about 27% (63). The MAC values for halothane, methoxyflurane, and isoflurane in adult ewes were 0.97%, 0.26%, and 1.58%, respectively (64). Pregnancy decreased these values by 25%, 32%, and 40%, respectively.

Inhalation anesthesia in adult cattle is usually preceded by tracheal intubation performed during heavy xylazine sedation (65) or anesthesia produced by injectable drugs. Induction of anesthesia with an inhalation agent by facemask administration is easily accomplished in young animals. Healthy adult sheep and goats may resent application of the mask and prior sedation or induction or anesthesia with injectable drugs may be necessary to avoid excitement. The inhalation agent should be administered through a large animal circuit to adult cattle; through a human adult circuit to sheep, goats, and calves of less than 140 kg bodyweight; and through a nonrebreathing system to lambs and kids. Initial oxygen flow for a cow or bull should be 6 to 8 liters/min, and the halothane vaporizer should be set to deliver 3.5%. The high oxygen flow should be maintained for about 10 minutes to flush expired nitrogen from the circuit and to supply sufficient halothane. The oxygen flow should then be decreased to 3 liters/min and the vaporizer setting progressively decreased according to the clinical assessment of the depth of anesthesia. A lower flow of 0.5 to 2 liters/min and a vaporizer setting of 2% or less should be satisfactory for small ruminants.

Halothane anesthesia in Holstein cows previously sedated with xylazine resulted in significant decreases in cardiac output, heart rate, and arterial pressure (66). In bulls and steers, anesthesia with guaifenesin and thiobarbiturate maintained with halothane resulted in a significant decrease in cardiac output, no change in heart rate, and systemic arterial hypertension (41). Hypertension was also recorded in cows and bulls anesthetized with a combination of xylazine, guaifenesin, thiopental, halothane, and 50% nitrous oxide (67). An increase in halothane administration from 1.0 to 2.0 MAC in calves during controlled ventilation resulted in significant decreases in cardiac output and arterial pressure (63). A nonsignificant decrease in arterial pressure from the awake value was measured in pregnant ewes during a light plane of halothane or isoflurane anesthesia (68, 69). Deep levels of halothane and isoflurane anesthesia produced greater decreases in maternal cardiac output and arterial pressure, and the fetuses became hypoxemic and acidotic (68). At 1.0 and 1.5 MAC methoxyflurane anesthesia in pregnant ewes, arterial pressure and cardiac output were slight to moderately decreased (70). Cardiac output was decreased by 34% and arterial pressure by 37% from awake values during 2.0 MAC anesthesia.

Anesthetic Management

INTUBATION OF THE TRACHEA

Intubation of the trachea of a ruminant is usually accomplished by one of 3 methods: introduction of a hand into the animals' mouth in order to palpate the opening to the larynx and guide the endotracheal tube into it, directly viewing the introduction of a tube into the larynx using a laryngoscope, or "blind" introduction of the tube through the pharynx. Large ruminants are most easily intubated by direct palpation of the larynx. With a mouth speculum or wedge firmly in place to prevent the jaws closing, the tube is inserted into the mouth by hand (Fig. 13.6). The arm should be dorsal to the tube and the fingers should extend beyond the end of the tube by a few inches so that the epiglottis can be palpated and depressed. Using the opposite hand, the tube should then be advanced until the tip lies on the epiglottis. The hand inside the mouth should then be advanced further and two fingers used to separate the arytenoid cartilages (Fig. 13.6). The tube can then be pushed into the larynx and down the trachea. In medium-sized animals, the hand may have to be introduced at right angles to the horizontal surface of the teeth in order to be able to pass beyond the last molars. When the mouth is not large enough to accomodate the forearm and endotracheal tube, an alternative method is to introduce a stomach tube or 6-foot rod into the trachea and then use it as a guide to feed the endotracheal tube into the trachea. This may be facilitated by a spiral movement of the endotracheal tube as it is advanced over the stomach tube. Direct viewing of the laryngeal entrance is difficult because the jaws do not open wide, the pharynx is narrow, and the view may be obstructed by the laryngoscope blade. In addition, the dorsum of the tongue is prominent and tends to deflect the endotracheal tube off midline and into the esophagus. In the adult bovine, a long laryngoscope blade (Rowson) or a bovine laryngoscope or vaginal speculum with light source (Jorgensen Laboratories Inc., Loveland, CO.) may be used to introduce a metal rod into the trachea. The laryngoscope should then be removed and the endotracheal tube fed over the rod into the trachea. In small ruminants the same technique may be used, or the endotra-

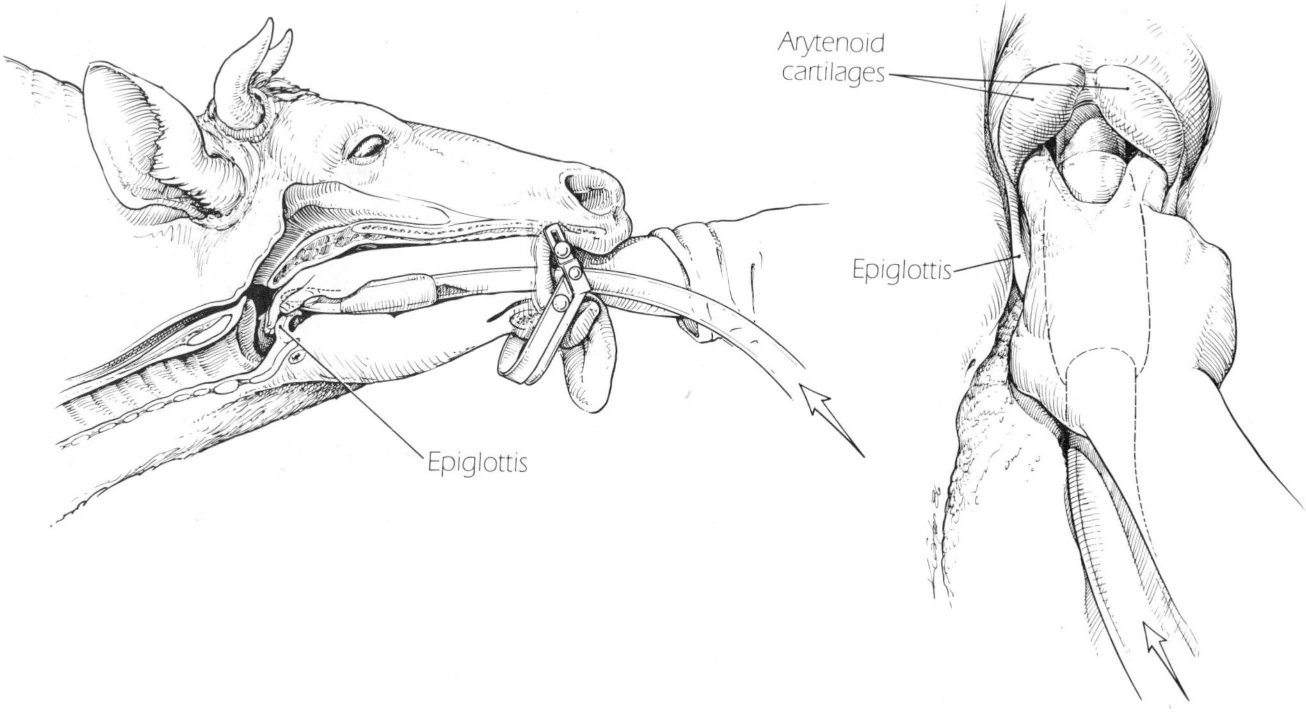

Figure 13.6. The trachea of adult cattle may be intubated by direct palpation of the laryngeal entrance. With a mouth speculum firmly in place, a hand should be inserted into the pharynx. First the epiglottis should be depressed and the tip of the tube advanced onto it. Then the arytenoid cartilages should be spread with two fingers so that the endotracheal tube may be pushed into the trachea.

cheal tube may be introduced directly utilizing a laryngoscope or a penlite laryngoscope inserted inside the tube. The procedure may be facilitated by stiffening the tube with a metal stilette and rotating the tube 90 to 180° as it is advanced through the larynx. Whenever intubation is to be performed, it is essential to have the head and neck fully extended (Fig. 13.7) to ensure that the oral cavity and trachea are in a straight line. The third technique of intubation is blind intubation; it can be used on both large and small ruminants. The tube should be introduced into the mouth with one hand while the other hand is used to hold the larynx. With the curvature of the tube in line with the curvature of the head and neck, the tube is fed into the larynx. Some rotation of the tube may be necessary to advance the tip past the epiglottis.

Large ruminants must not be rolled before the trachea is intubated. The position of the small ruminant (prone, on its side or back) for tracheal intubation is often dependent on personal preference. Regurgitation may be less likely if the animal is in a sternal position, but when the animal is on its side, saliva will drain out of the mouth and not obscure the view of the larynx. It is advisable to have two endotracheal tubes available so that if the animal begins to regurgitate before the trachea is intubated, one tube can be inserted into the esophagus to channel material out of the pharynx and the second can be introduced into trachea. Some people recommend leaving a tube in the esophagus so that any material that is regurgitated does not collect in the pharynx. A tube introduced down the esophagus into the rumen may be effective in

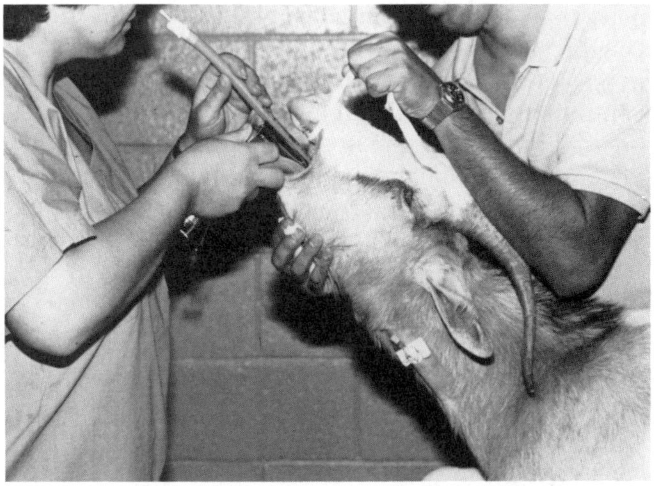

Figure 13.7. Intubation of a small ruminant by direct viewing of the larynx with a laryngoscope is most easily accomplished when the oropharynx and trachea are positioned in a straight line. Inserting a stilette into the endotracheal tube to stiffen it may assist correct placement of the tube.

preventing gas accumulation, but it frequently becomes occluded by ingesta. The head should be positioned with the nose lower than the pharynx to allow fluid to drain (Fig. 13.8).

MONITORING

Signs referable to depth of anesthesia vary according to the drugs used. The position of the eye in the orbit, correlated with the strength of the palpebral reflex, provides useful information. During the transition from light to medium depth anesthesia with the barbiturates, guaifenesin and thiobarbiturate, or inhalant agents, the eye rolls ventrally (Fig. 13.9) (occasionally, rostroventrally or caudodorsally) and the palpebral reflex decreases from brisk to weak. As a deeper plane of anesthesia is induced, the eye moves into a central position in the orbit and the palpebral reflex is abolished. Thus if the eye is eccentrically placed in the orbit, excessive CNS depression is not present. Ketamine maintains extraocular muscle tone so that the eye remains in a central position. The palpebral reflex also remains strong. The eye will begin to rotate ventrally as the influence of ketamine decreases.

Respiratory rates during anesthesia should be between 20 and 35 breaths/min. Although inadequate ventilation can occur at any respiratory rate, severe hypercarbia is most likely with rates less than 20 and more than 40 breaths/min and will occur if the animal is lying on its back. Adult cattle almost invariably hypoventilate during halothane anesthesia. Controlled ventilation with a tidal volume of 5 to 6 liters and 10 breaths/min will result in normal arterial carbon dioxide tensions. In small ruminants, a tidal volume of 12 ml/kg or peak inspiratory pressure of 25 cm H_2O and a frequency of 10 to 12/min should provide adequate ventilation. Alternatively, a peak inspiratory pressure of 30 cm H_2O at 6 breaths/min can be used. The animal should be "sighed" periodically by inflating the lungs to 35 cm H_2O pressure. In research conditions in which maintenance of high arterial oxygen tensions is essential, this may be achieved in small ruminants by ventilating with a tidal volume exceeding 20 ml/kg, adding deadspace or carbon dioxide to maintain normal PCO_2, and imposing 5 to 10 cm H_2O positive end expiratory pressure (71).

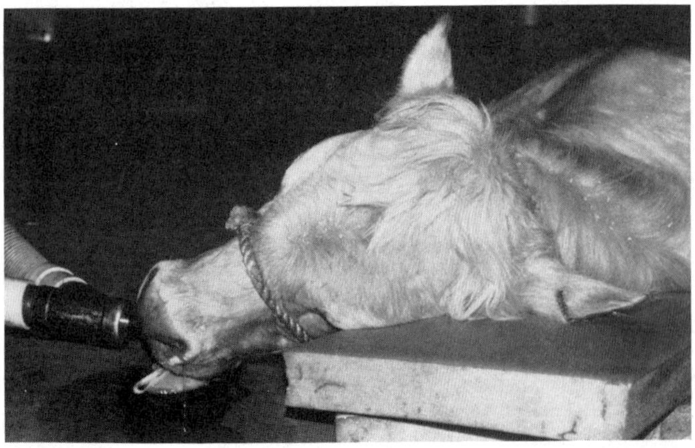

Figure 13.8. The head of the anesthetized ruminant should be positioned to place the nose lower than the pharynx to encourage drainage of saliva and any regurgitated ruminal fluid. Foam pads were placed under the head of this anesthetized bull, and the pool of saliva accumulating on the floor confirms that they were effective.

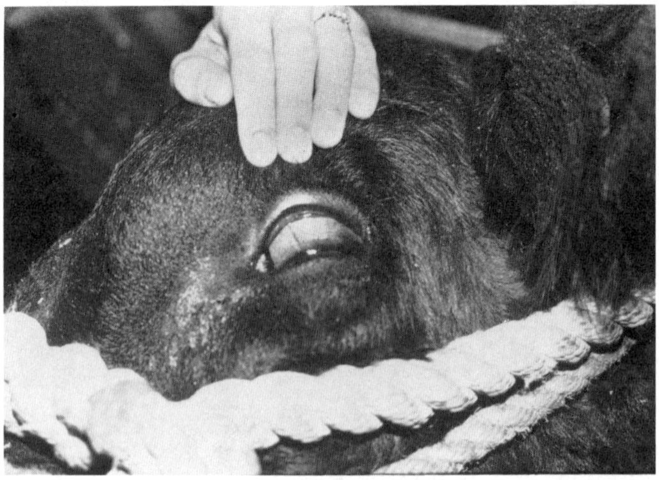

Figure 13.9. During halothane anesthesia, the eye rotates ventrally during a light plane of anesthesia and then returns to the central position as anesthesia deepens. This animal had a weak palpebral reflex and constricted pupils, and the eye was beginning to rotate back centrally. These signs were interpreted as a medium plane of anesthesia. The animal did not move in response to surgery.

Heart rates in conscious cattle are between 60 and 70 beats/min; in sheep and goats, heart rates are 70 to 90 beats/min with increases up to 140 beats/min if the animal is excited. The heart rate tends to be higher in the spontaneously breathing ruminant anesthetized with thiobarbiturate or an inhalation agent due to sympathetic stimulation from hypercarbia. The animal should be checked to see if it is breathing adequately if the heart rate exceeds 100 beats/min. In addition, the process of tracheal intubation causes a transient (10-minute) increase in heart rate. Xylazine and ketamine anesthesia frequently results in heart rates between 50 and 60 beats/min.

A wide range of arterial pressure has been reported in nonanesthetized cattle. Systolic and diastolic pressures varied between 118/62 and 275/195 mm Hg, depending on whether the cows were quiet or stimulated (72). During anesthesia, arterial pressure should not be allowed to decrease much below resting awake value. The peripheral pulse can be palpated on the dorsal surface of the ear (median auricular artery) (Fig. 13.10), on the caudomedial surface of the forelimb at or just above the carpus (radial artery), and above the

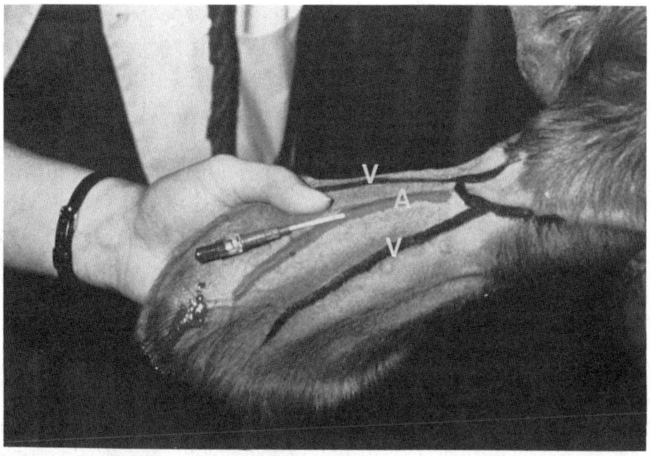

Figure 13.10. The median auricular artery (*A*) and adjacent veins (*V*) have been identified by ink marks on the dorsal surface of this cow's ear. An 18-gauge catheter has been inserted into the artery. The artery may be used for palpation of the pulse, measurement of arterial pressure, and collection of arterial blood for pH and blood gas analysis. The veins may be used for injection of fluids or nonirritating drugs.

fetlock (metacarpal arteries). The femoral artery can be palpated in small ruminants. Arterial pressure can be measured indirectly by placing a cuff and probe on the tails of cattle or limbs of sheep and goats or by directly inserting a needle or catheter into one of the arteries on the ear.

Balanced electrolyte solution, 10 ml/kg/hr, should be infused intravenously for all major or prolonged surgeries. The healthy ruminant has a mild metabolic alkalosis, but saline infusion should be substituted for balanced electrolyte solution when the animal has a severe metabolic alkalosis. Cardiovascular function may also be improved by the infusion of dopamine hydrochloride (Intropin), 3 to 5 μg/kg/min.

Small ruminants may become cold during anesthesia if precautions are not taken. These animals appear to have difficulty after anesthesia in restoring body temperature without external application of heat if it has decreased below 36° C (97°F), especially if they have received xylazine.

NEUROMUSCULAR BLOCKING DRUGS

These agents are not routinely used in ruminants in veterinary practice. Facilities for controlled ventilation and intensive monitoring of the patient must be available if neuromuscular blockade is induced during anesthesia. Pancuronium, 0.07 mg/kg, or alcuronium, 0.08 mg/kg, have been used successfully during anesthesia of adult cattle (66, 72). In calves, the dose of pancuronium to produce 90% to 99% reduction of twitch tension of hindlimb muscles was 0.043 mg/kg; this is less than in other species (73). Twitch height recovered to 50% of baseline values in a mean time of 26 minutes. Pancuronium, 0.027 mg/kg, restored paralysis for 20 minutes, with full recovery in 37 minutes. Similar to ponies but in contrast to other species, the facial muscles were more resistant to paralysis than limb muscles and could not be used to reliably monitor the degree of paralysis.

RECOVERY

The animal should be supported in sternal position as soon as possible to allow the release of gas trapped in the rumen. The nasal cavity may be flushed with water if regurgitation has occurred. The trachea should not be extubated before the animal is sternal and swallowing, which may be some time after chewing movements first began. The tube should be removed with the cuff partially inflated. Additional sedation for recovery is not usually needed in the ruminant. Analgesics, such as an intramuscular injection of meperidine, 3 mg/kg, may be administered in recovery after orthopedic surgery.

Electroimmobilization

A commercial instrument is available that produces generalized rigidity of voluntary muscles when an electrical current is passed through the animal from electrodes placed at the head and tail. The animal is thus unable to stand or move. This technique provides convenience and safety for the veterinarian and removes the danger of an accident during surgery due to sudden movement of the patient. However, it is probable that the technique is inhumane when surgery is performed without the addition of local analgesia. Evidence also indicates that the procedure is unpleasant for the animal. Measurement of blood cortisol concentrations as an indicator of stress in cattle during dehorning did not indicate a significant difference between cattle that had been immobilized and those that had received local analgesia (75). Subjective observations were that flinching around the head and neck occurred when the horns were severed from the immobilized cattle, an effect which was not observed in cattle with a cornual nerve block. Aversion to electroimmobilization has been identified in cattle and sheep. Holstein cows trained to lead through stocks developed a reluctance to enter the stocks after a treatment with the electroimmobilizer (76), and a similar effect was noted in sheep that had been electroimmobilized for shearing compared with sheep that had been physically restrained (77). Other results from the latter investigation were that the degree of aversion was not related to the duration of immobilization but was greater when a high current was used. It seems clear that whereas it may be necessary to use this technique in certain conditions, care must be taken to provide adequate analgesia for surgery using lidocaine or other drugs.

Bovine Sedatives under Development

A new sedative, R51163, is under development by Janssen Pharmaceutica, Beerse, Belgium. The cardiovascular, respiratory, and gastrointestinal effects of R51163 have been compared to xylazine in cattle by Degryse and Ooms (78).

Xylazine (Rompun) is an alpha$_2$-adrenoceptor agonist widely used in veterinary medicine as a sedative with analgesic and muscle relaxant properties on both domestic and wild animals. R51163 is a newly synthetized purine alkyl piperidine that produced reliable sedation in cattle after i.v. and i.m. injection at doses of 0.05 and 0.1 to 0.15 mg/kg, respectively. The subjects were adult healthy cattle of either sex and different breeds. The compounds studied were R51163 and xylazine. R51163 was dissolved at a concentration of 10 mg/ml in 20% propylene glycol with 3 equivalents of lactic acid and was injected i.v. at a dose of 0.05 mg/kg. Xylazine was used as the commercially available preparation (Rompun, Bayer; 20 mg/ml) and was injected at 0.04 mg/kg i.v. in the cardiovascular experiment and at 0.05 mg/kg i.v. in the gastrointestinal experiment (78).

CARDIOVASCULAR AND RESPIRATORY RESPONSES

Compared to the control value, R51163 increased heart rate. In contrast, xylazine produced a reliable and pronounced decrease in heart rate. Both R51163 and xylazine significantly depressed respiratory rate throughout the 10- to 16-minute period after injection. R51163 significantly decreased both systolic and diastolic blood pressure at 50 and 60 minutes after injection. Xylazine also decreased blood pressure, but at no time interval did this decrease reach statistical significance.

Venous blood gas analysis revealed an increase in oxygen saturation and pO_2 at 30, 50, and 60 minutes after injection of R51163. After injection of xylazine, pCO_2, base excess, and HCO_3 were increased throughout the 60-minute experimental session. Arterial blood gas analysis revealed a short-lived decrease in pH and pO_2 after R51163 and xylazine, whereas pCO_2 values showed only insignificant increases (78).

GASTROINTESTINAL RESPONSES

Xylazine caused a profound depression of rumen motility; it completely blocked rumination for at least 2 hours and reduced antegrade and retrograde contractions by 92 and 64%, respectively, during the first hour after injection. In contrast, R51163 did not inhibit rumination and decreased antegrade and retrograde contractions by no more than 21 and 55%, respectively, in the first hour. Although not presently approved for clinical usage, R51163 may be a sedative with desirable features that the veterinarian may consider in the future.

References

1. Weaver AD: Intravenous local anesthesia of the lower limb in cattle. *J Am Vet Med Assoc* 160:55–57, 1972.
2. Prentice DE, Wyn-Jones G, Jones RS, Jagger DW: Intravenous regional anesthesia of the bovine foot. *Vet Rec* 94:293–295, 1974.
3. Lillie PE, Glynn CJ, Fenwick DG: Site of action of intravenous regional anesthesia. *Anesthesiology* 61:507–510, 1984.
4. Tyagi RPS, Kumar R, Manohar M: Studies on intravenous retrograde regional anesthesia for the forelimbs of ruminants. *Aust Vet J* 49:321–324, 1973.
5. Harvey SC: Hypnotics and sedatives. In Gilman AG, Goodman LS, Gilman A (eds): *The Pharmacological Basis of Therapeutics*, ed 6. New York: McMillan Publishing Co, 1980, p 361.
6. Garcia-Villar R, Toutain PL, Alvinerie M, Ruckebusch Y: The pharmacokinetics of xylazine hydrochloride: an interspecific study. *J Vet Pharmacol Therap* 4:87–92, 1981.
7. Raptopoulos D, Weaver BMQ: Observations following intravenous xylazine administration in steers. *Vet Rec* 114:567–569, 1984.
8. Hopkins TJ: The clinical pharmacology of xylazine in cattle. *Aust Vet J* 48:109–112, 1972.
9. Ponder SW, Clark WG: Prolonged depression of thermoregulation after xylazine administration to cats. *J Vet Pharmacol Therap* 3:203–207, 1980.
10. DeMoor A, Desmet P: Effect of Rompun on acid-base-equilibrium and arterial O_2 pressure in cattle. *Vet Med Rev* 2:163–169, 1971.
11. Aouad JI, Wright EM, Shaner TW: Anesthesia evaluation of ketamine and xylazine in calves. *Bovine Practice* 2:22–31, 1981.
12. Mitchell B, Williams JT: Blood gas changes in sheep associated with feeding. *Proc Assoc Vet Anaesth G Br Ir* 6:37–47, 1976–1977.
13. Uggla A, Lindquist Å: Acute pulmonary oedema as an adverse reaction to the use of xylazine in sheep. *Vet Rec* 113:42, 1983.
14. Campbell KB, Klavano PA, Richardson P, Alexander JE: Hemodynamic effects of xylazine in the calf. *Am J Vet Res* 40:1777–1780, 1979.
15. Freire ACT, Gontijo RM, Pessoa JM, Souza R: Effect of xylazine on the electrocardiogram of the sheep. *Brit Vet J* 137:590–595, 1981.
16. Symonds HW: The effect of xylazine upon hepatic glucose production and blood flow rate in the lactating dairy cow. *Vet Rec* 99:234–236, 1976.
17. Symonds HW, Mallison CB: The effect of xylazine and xylazine followed by insulin on blood glucose and insulin in the dairy cow. *Vet Rec* 102:27–29, 1978.
18. Eichner RD, Prior RL, Kvasnicka WG: Xylazine-induced hyperglycemia in beef cattle. *Am J Vet Res* 40:127–129, 1979.
19. Brockman RP: Effect of xylazine on plasma glucose, glucagon and insulin concentrations in sheep. *Res Vet Sci* 30:383–384, 1981.
20. Muggaberg J. Brockman RP: Effect of adrenergic drugs on glucose and plasma glucagon and insulin responses to xylazine in sheep. *Res Vet Sci* 33:118–120, 1982.
21. Thurmon JC, Nelson DR, Hartsfield SM, Rumore CA: Effects of xylazine hydrochloride on urine in cattle. *Aust Vet J* 54:178–180, 1978.
22. LeBlanc MM, Hubbell JAE, Smith HC: The effect of xylazine

hydrochloride on intrauterine pressure in the cow and the mare. *Proc Ann Meeting Soc Theriogenol* 211–220, 1984.
23. Zahner JM, Hatch RC, Wilson RC, Booth NH, Kitzman JV, Brown J: Antagonism of xylazine sedation in steers by doxapram and 4-aminopyridine. *Am J Vet Res* 45:2546–2551, 1984.
24. Doherty T: Idazoxan: a novel xylazine antagonist. *Vet Rec* 117:135, 1985.
25. Roming LGP: Tolazolin als xylazin-antagonist beim rind. *Dtsch Tierärztl Wschr* 91:154–157, 1984.
26. Rehm WF, Schatzman U: Benzodiazepines as sedatives for large animals. *J Assoc Vet Anaesth G Br Ir* 12:93–106, 1984.
27. Hossain MDA, Camburn MA: The influence of different anaesthetic agents on the reflux of rumen contents and oesophageal and rumen function in anaesthetised sheep. *J Assoc Vet Anaesth G Br Ir* 12:107–114, 1984.
28. Hossain MA, Camburn MA; Reflux, regurgitation and oesophageal activity in anaesthetised sheep. *J Assoc Vet Anaesth G Br Ir* 11:190–199, 1983.
29. Rumsey TS, Bond J: Cardiorespiratory patterns, rectal temperature, serum electrolytes and packed cell volume in beef cattle deprived of feed and water. *J Anim Sci* 42:1227–1238, 1976.
30. Mitchell B, Williams JT: Blood gas changes in sheep associated with feeding. *Proc Assoc Vet Anaesth G Br Ir* 6:37–47, 1976–1977.
31. Porter ARW: The legal aspects of death in a bull. *Proc Assoc Vet Anaesth G Br Ir* 5:58–62, 1974–1975.
32. Dueck R, Rathburn M, Greenburg AG: Lung volume and VA/Q distribution response to intravenous *versus* inhalation anesthesia in sheep. *Anesthesiology* 61:55–65, 1984.
33. Musewe VO, Gillespie JR, Berry JD: Influence of ruminal insufflation on pulmonary function and diaphragmatic electromyography in cattle. *Am J Vet Res* 40:26–31, 1979.
34. Trim CM: Sedation and general anesthesia in ruminants. *California Vet* 35:29–36, 1981.
35. Hall LW, Clarke KC: *Veterinary Anaesthesia*, ed 8. London, Balliere-Tindall, 1983, p 68.
36. Hall LW, Clarke KC: *Veterinary Anaesthesia*, ed 8. London, Balliere-Tindall, 1983, p 282.
37. Booth NH: Intravenous and other perenteral anesthetics. In Booth NH, McDonald LE (eds): *Veterinary Pharmacology and Therapeutics*, ed 5. Ames, Iowa State University Press, 1982, p 203.
38. Van Dieten, JSMM: The use of muscle relaxants in large animals—An European view. *Proc Assoc Vet Anaesth G Br Ir* 10(suppl):189–197, 1982.
39. Funk KA: Glyceryl guaiacolate: a centrally acting muscle relaxant. *Equine Vet J* 2:173–178, 1970.
40. Agrawal KBP, Prasad B, Sobti VK: Clinical observations with glyceryl guaiacolate and its combination with thiopental sodium or chloral hydrate in buffalo calves (Bos bubalis). *Indian Vet J* 60:536–539, 1983.
41. Semrad SD, Trim CM, Hardee GE: Hypertension in bulls and steers anesthetized with guaifenesin-thiobarbiturate-halothane combination. *Am J Vet Res* 47: July, 1986.
42. Agrawal KBP, Prasad B, Sobti VK: Physiological and biochemical effects of glyceryl guaiacolate-thiopentone sodium anaesthesia in buffalo calves. *Res Vet Sci* 35:53–57, 1983.
43. Fuentes VO, Tellez E: Mid-line caesarian section in a cow using ketamine anesthesia. *Vet Rec* 99:338, 1976.
44. Tadmor A, Marcus S, Eting E: The use of ketamine hydrochloride for endotracheal intubation in cattle. *Aust Vet J* 55:537–538, 1979.
45. Mbiuki SM: Xylazine and ketamine anesthesia in cattle. *Vet Med Sm Anim Clin* 77:251–253, 1982.
46. Waterman AE: Preliminary observations on the use of a combination of xylazine and ketamine hydrochloride in calves. *Vet Rec* 109:464–467, 1981.
47. Waterman AE: Effect of a combination of ketamine and xylazine on respiratory gas tensions and acid-base status in calves. *Vet Rec* 113:517, 1983.
48. Rings DM, Muir WW: Cardiopulmonary effects of intramuscular xylazine-ketamine in calves. *Can J Comp Med* 46:386–389, 1982.
49. Pathak SC, Nigam JM, Peshin PK, Singh AP: Anesthetic and hemodynamic effects of ketamine hydrochloride in buffalo calves (Bubalus bubalis). *Am J Vet Res* 43:875–878, 1982.
50. Nowrouzian I, Schels HF, Ghodsian I, Karimi H: Evaluation of the anaesthetic properties of ketamine and a ketamine/xylazine/atropine combination in sheep. *Vet Rec* 108:354–356, 1981.
51. Thurmon JC, Kumar A, Link RP: Evaluation of ketamine hydrochloride as an anesthetic in sheep. *J Am Vet Med Assoc* 162:293–297, 1973.
52. Byagagaire SD, Mbiuki SM: Duration of analgesia in sheep under xylazine/ketamine anesthesia. *Vet Rec* 114:15–16, 1984.
53. Kumar A, Thurmon JC, Hardenbrook HJ: Clinical studies of ketamine HCl and xylazine HCl in domestic goats. *Vet Med Sm Anim Clin* 71:1707–1713, 1976.
54. Kumar A, Thurmon JC, Nelson DR, Link RD: Effects of ketamine hydrochloride on maternal and fetal arterial blood pressure and acid-base status in goats. *Vet Anesth* 5(2):28–33, 1978.
55. Kumar A, Thurmon JC, Nelson DR, Benson GJ, Tranquilli WJ: Response of goats to ketamine hydrochloride with and without premedication of atropine, acetylpromazine, diazepam, or xylazine. *Vet Med Sm Anim Clin* 78:955–960, 1983.
56. Tadmor A, Zukerman I: The use of ketamine hydrochloride for endotracheal intubation in goats. *Aust Vet J* 57:303–304, 1981.
57. Waterman AE: Evaluation of the actions and use of alphaxalone/alphadolone (CT 1341) in sheep. *Res Vet Sci* 30:114–119, 1981.
58. Camburn MA: Use of alphaxalone-alphadolone in ruminants. *Vet Rec* 111:166–167, 1982.
59. Eales FA, Small J: Alphaxalone/alphadolone anaesthesia in the lamb. *Vet Rec* 110:273–275, 1982.
60. McKeating FJ, Pilsworth RC: "Disbudding" of kids. *Vet Rec* 115:419, 1984.
61. Williams BM: Disbudding kids. *Vet Rec* 116:480, 1985.
62. Mather LE, Gourlay GK, Parkins KS, Roberts JG: Pharmacodynamics of minaxolone, a new steroidal anesthetic. *J Pharmacol Exp Ther* 217:481–488, 1981.
63. Steffey EP, Howland D: Halothane anesthesia in calves. *Am J Vet Res* 40:372–376, 1979.
64. Palahniuk RJ, Shnider SM, Eger EI II: Pregnancy decreases the requirement for inhaled anesthetic agents. *Anesthesiology* 41:82–83, 1974.
65. Adetunji A, Pascoe PJ, McDonell WN, Horney FD: Retrospective evaluation of xylazine/halothane anesthesia in 125 cattle. *Can Vet J* 25:342–346, 1984.
66. Warren RG, McDonell W, Adetunji A, Horne JA: Cardiopulmonary effects of xylazine/halothane anesthesia in mature cows. *Proc Am Coll Vet Anesth Ann Meeting* Atlanta, 1983.
67. Schatzmann U, Held JP, Rohr W: Experiences with inhalation anesthesia, peripheral relaxation and controlled ventilation in the bovine. *Assoc Vet Anaesth G Br Ir* 8:108–119, 1978–1979.
68. Palahnuik RJ, Shnider SM: Maternal and fetal cardiovascular and acid-base changes during halothane and isoflurane anesthesia in the pregnant ewe. *Anesthesiology* 41:462–472, 1974.
69. Biehl DR, Tweed WA, Cote J, Wade JG, Sitar D: Effect of halothane on cardiac output and regional flow in the fetal lamb in utero. *Anesth Analg* 62:489–492, 1983.
70. Smith JB, Manning FA, Palahniuk RJ: Maternal and foetal effects of methoxyflurane anaesthesia in the pregnant ewe. *Canad Anaesth Soc J* 22:449–459, 1975.
71. Gardaz JP, Perez-Chada D, Sykes MK: Oxygenation during mechanical ventilation in goats. *Anesthesiology* 56:491–492, 1982.
72. Doyle JT, Patterson JL, Warren JV: Observations on the circulation of domestic cattle. *Circ Res* 8:4–15, 1960.
73. Watney GCG: Effects of posture and intraruminal pressure on the bronchial calibre of cattle during xylazine/halothane anesthesia. *Res Vet Sci* 40:166–172, 1986.
74. Hildebrand SV, Howitt GA: Neuromuscular and cardiovascular

effects of pancuronium bromide in calves anesthetized with halothane. *Am J Vet Res* 45:1549–1552, 1984.
75. Carter PD, Johnston NE, Corner LA, Jarrett RG: Observations on the effect of electro-immobilization on the dehorning of cattle. *Aust Vet J* 60:17–19, 1983.
76. Pascoe PJ, McDonell WN: Aversive conditioning used to test the humaneness of a commercial electroimmobilization unit in cattle. *Proc Am Coll Vet Anes Ann Sci Meet* 3, 1984.
77. Rushen J: Observations on the aversion of sheep to electro-immobilization and physical restraint. *Aust Vet J* 63:63–64, 1986.
78. Degryse A-D, Ooms LAA: Comparative studies on cardiovascular, respiratory, and gastrointestinal effects of the sedatives R51163 and xylazine in cattle. *Drug Development Res* 8:433–441, 1986.

PART 3

Anesthetic Considerations in the Canine and Feline

CHARLES E. SHORT, D.V.M., M.S., D.A.C.V.A.

Anesthetic management in dogs and cats involves an understanding of the individual patient and breed responses and the proper selection of medications and equipment. The discussion of specific medications and their dosages will be limited because they are discussed in detail in the first section of this text, and specific disease conditions will not be discussed in this chapter because they too are covered elsewhere. Small animal anesthesia may include a wide range of techniques.

Preanesthetics

The most common preanesthetics used in canine and feline anesthesia are the anticholinergics. Although atropine sulfate is most commonly used, glycopyrrolate has been shown to be a safer agent. Atropine may contribute to sinus tachycardia or ventricular arrhythmia. In contrast to the routine use of anticholinergics, present practice indicates that selective use of these agents in dogs and cats is appropriate.

Anticholinergics are indicated when there is preexisting bradycardia or as preventive medication when the anesthetics to be used cause excessive salivation or slowing of the heart or heart block. The anticholinergics are especially indicated when xylazine usage is planned in dogs and cats or narcotics or neuroleptanalgesia including Innovar is used in dogs. The anticholinergic will prevent the resulting bradycardia commonly associated with these agents. Innovar in dogs or ketamine in cats may produce excessive salivation. Because diethyl ether is seldom used, ketamine is the most commonly used agent that may cause salivation sufficient to need anticholinergic control.

Many drugs are available for use as tranquilizers. The most commonly used in the dog is acetylpromazine. When used as a preanesthetic, acetylpromazine should be administered at low dosage rates, usually between 0.05 and 0.1 mg/kg. Acetylpromazine dramatically reduces the dosage of barbiturate required to produce unconsciousness. Less than 10 mg/kg of ultrashort-acting barbiturate as a total dosage is needed in most cases. Acetylpromazine is an effective preanesthetic for either ketamine or barbiturate induction in cats.

Xylazine is frequently used as a sedative/tranquilizer. It produces profound sedation with a period of transient analgesia. Unfortunately, bradycardia or heart block can occur unless an anticholinergic is used. Xylazine greatly reduces dosage of barbiturates. Rapid administration of high concentrations of barbiturates can result in cardiac arrest that frequently does not respond well to cardiopulmonary resuscitation efforts.

Xylazine (1.1 mg/kg i.v.) in combination with atropine (0.04 mg/kg) and ketamine (11 mg/kg) i.v. has been administered in dogs (1). The combination causes hypoventilation, increased $PaCO_2$, and up to a 30%

decrease in cardiac index. Arterial blood pressure, left atrial pressure, and peripheral resistance usually increase. This effect lasts for approximately 30 minutes. Without the atropine, slowing of heart rate due to the effect of xylazine is frequently observed. At this dosage level of ketamine, without adequate tranquilization muscle rigor or even seizure-like activity may occur in the dog.

A similar dosage has been more frequently administered by intramuscular injection. There is less incidence of cardiopulmonary depression or change. Dogs may exhibit also muscle fasciculations or seizure-like activity after this technique. The frequency of occurrence is not as great, but duration is longer. Most dogs receiving xylazine-ketamine combinations have safe anesthesia; death has occurred in only a low percentage of dogs.

Diazepam (0.37 mg/kg i.v.) has been administered to cats in conjunction with ketamine anesthesia (2). This produced no significant respiratory depression. It has also been administered intramuscularly for similar purposes. Diazepam has been used as a premedication in dogs as well. Diazepam does not produce the significant level of depression of the cardiopulmonary system of more potent tranquilizers and sedatives, but the animals are also more active. Diazepam is a more likely choice if the animal has a history of seizures or if ketamine is to be used for induction.

Narcotics are commonly used for preanesthetics in dogs; their use is less frequent in cats. They can greatly reduce the anesthetic concentrations needed for surgical anesthesia. Neuroleptanalgesia may be useful to produce a gradual, progressive induction. In high risk patients, neuroleptanalgesia should be combined with supplemental oxygen to avoid hypoxemia. The use of Innovar or other neuroleptanalgesia combinations by intramuscular injection is especially helpful to control vicious dogs. Ketamine and tranquilizer combinations are used for a similar purpose in cats.

Induction of Anesthesia

The induction methodology must be compatible with the method of anesthetic maintenance. Induction can be accomplished quickly using ultrashort barbiturates or dissociative anesthetics and more deliberately with narcotic combinations or mask or chamber inhalant techniques.

Ultrashort barbiturates with or without tranquilizers produce rapid induction of anesthesia. Careful attention is needed to avoid extravascular injection of drug, which may cause major tissue irritation including tissue sloughs. The insertion of intravenous catheters before induction aids in avoiding this complication. If this is to be done, it is more important to administer preanesthetic medications to avoid stimulation of the dog or cat during placement of catheters. In contrast, small gauge needles are helpful to avoid pain and physical activity during induction. The author frequently uses 25 gauge needles in cats and 1% ultrashort barbiturates for control of injection. In dogs, less than 3% concentration is frequently used to avoid tissue irritation if administered extravascularly, especially in small subjects. If the volume injected is large, tissue irritation may still occur. Concentrations greater than 2.5% can be conveniently used in larger dogs.

Cardiac arrhythmias can occur with a wide range of concentrations. A blind study completed at our hospital showed a similar incidence of arrhythmias after 2.5 or 5% solutions of sodium thiamylal for induction. The incidence of ventricular arrhythmias during and after induction is predominately related to dosage and speed of injection of the barbiturate. Rapid injections are more likely to produce transient apnea and cardiac arrhythmias. Administration of oxygen corrects over 90% of ventricular arrhythmias associated with induction regardless of concentration used.

Intravenous lidocaine has been shown to control most induction-related arrhythmias. The use of thiopental/lidocaine combinations has been reported to reduce the incidence of arrhythmias. Cardiopulmonary stability was demonstrated (3). The effectiveness of lidocaine to control arrhythmias has been demonstrated; however, it is frequently unnecessary. The ventricular arrhythmias associated with ultrashort barbiturate inductions are quite responsive to oxygenation. The rapid onset of anesthesia produces mild to severe transient apnea. Preoxygenation before induction prevents arrhythmias, whereas adding oxygen immediately after induction corrects arrhythmias. The presence of arrhythmias is frequently indicative of inadequate oxygenation. The cause of the problem should be corrected; it is not enough only to control the symptoms.

Intubation and oxygenation should be considered if maintenance with barbiturates is considered and there is respiratory depression. Immediately after induction, animals are intubated and placed on oxygen if inhalants are to be used. Intubation can be greatly facilitated by adequate anesthesia, appropriate size endotracheal tubes, and an laryngoscope. Cetacaine should not be used to aid intubation because it may cause respiratory complications.

Neuroleptanalgesia may be considered part of induction. In most instances, supplemental oxygen is added in high risk cases. Concurrent use of N_2O will reduce the time required for induction because the combination of narcotics and N_2O can produce adequate analgesia. N_2O alone does not provide adequate surgical anesthesia unless there is considerable central nervous system (CNS) depression from other causes.

Neuroleptanalgesia induction commonly precedes balanced anesthesia.

Ketamine and a tranquilizer or Telazol may be the initial medication used for induction, Ketamine has been used extensively in cats and has growing popularity in dogs. Xylazine and ketamine usage in dogs is normally safe but has occasionally resulted in adverse responses of bradycardia, tachycardia, seizures, or cardiopulmonary distress. Either diazepam, acetylpromazine, or xylazine may be used with ketamine in cats.

The greatest use of saffan for anesthetic inductions has been in the British Isles. Most procedures using saffan in cats have been safe and successful. Complications that have been associated with saffan usage in cats includes hyperemia or edema of the pinnae or forepaws (4). Less common but more disturbing is the occurrence of laryngeal spasm or edema, which may lead to cynosis and hypoxemia. Saffan appears to be losing popularity as an anesthetic, and it is not likely to be available in the United States.

Mask and chamber inductions are usually safe for the patient. The inhalant agent used will usually be the same as the primary agent used for maintenance. Methoxyflurane inductions are the slowest of the available agents. N_2O can accelerate induction. Mask and chamber induction should be reserved for high risk or unique circumstances because of the occupational hazards of waste gases created. Of the two approaches, mask induction is the safest to both patient and personnel. Chamber induction results in extremely high atmospheric concentrations with rapid increases as soon as the chamber is opened. The animals' skin and hair absorbs much inhalant anesthetic, and the vapor is present for prolonged periods of time. It exceeds levels recommended by the National Institute of Occupational Safety and Health. The technique has its primary advantages with difficult to manage small dogs and cats that may be injured during restraint or other induction techniques. Mask induction is a safe approach in depressed patients. The time required is shortened, and the level of CNS depression can be accurately controlled.

Anesthetic Maintenance

Barbiturates may be used by supplemental injections of 10 to 50% of the initial dosage to maintain anesthesia. The principal complication is prolonged recovery when multiple doses are used. The dosage administered should be given slowly and to effect. Repeat dissociative anesthesia can be used providing adequate fluid intake and renal function are maintained. Usually no more than 50% additional drug is used. Balanced anesthesia of narcotic-tranquilizer plus muscle relaxants and N_2O can be used. The concentration of N_2O is held constant with supplemental doses of narcotics and muscle relaxants. The muscle relaxant dosage should be reduced to 50% of the preceeding level with each injection. Well-trained personnel should be available to use monitoring equipment, and respiratory support capability is essential. Monitoring should continue even after reversal of narcotics and muscle relaxants because muscle relaxation or narcosis may reoccur.

Inhalant anesthetics are frequently used for maintenance of anesthesia in both dogs and cats and are the easiest to maintain stable levels of anesthesia. The most common agents used are halothane and methoxyflurane. Enflurane has been used in a considerable number of dogs, especially in the presence of renal or hepatic dysfunction. High concentrations can result in muscle rigidity or seizures, but concentrations over 3.5% are seldom needed. Isoflurane produces excellent anesthesia in both dogs and cats. Even in the presence of hepatic and renal dysfunction or cardiac irregularities, isoflurane provides stable anesthesia with few complications.

The techniques for administration of anesthetics to dogs and cats obviously varies with size, age, health status, and the requirements of the surgical or diagnostic procedure. Congenital or inherited diseases and conditions influence anesthetic management when they are present.

Low oxygen flow versus high oxygen flow techniques are common contrasting techniques. A low flow technique has been more frequently used with methoxyflurane. A total flow rate of 15 ml/min/kg using 1:1 nitrous oxide and oxygen and methoxyflurane used in a study in dogs revealed elevated end-tidal oxygen levels of 230 mm Hg and low carbon dioxide during a 4-hour procedure. Lower flows than 15 ml/min/kg resulted in less than 200 mm Hg oxygen tension and collapse of the rebreathing bag (5). Nonrebreathing systems require higher oxygen flows to eliminate carbon dioxide buildups.

Oxygen levels administered, cardiopulmonary function, and depth of anesthesia contribute to the level of myocardial oxygen supply. During prolonged anesthesia, metabolic oxygen requirements of the heart increase (6). This can create an unfavorable effect on the myocardial oxygen supply-demand relationship and is a partial explanation of the undesirable responses observed in animals during prolonged anesthesia with low oxygen flow. The methods used for ventilation influence the carbon dioxide level. It has been shown that ventilatory support of the anesthetized patient markedly improves blood gas and acid-base status compared with that of unsupported, spontaneously breathing dogs (7).

Anesthesia produces a significant reduction in lung compliance and an increase in chest wall compliance in dogs. There is a significant reduction (16.9%)

in the functional reserve capacity (FRC) of anesthesia induced dogs in the supine position (8). Positions on the table including dorsal recumbency may worsen these responses. Care should be taken to ensure that the extremities are not adversely positioned so as to reduce the animals' ability to breath. Dogs and cats are affected by disease conditions, concentrations of anesthetic, and choice of anesthetic agents. Isoflurane is less likely to produce cardiac arrhythmias in dogs and cats (9) than halothane. This is especially true in animals with myocardial sensitivity due to disease or trauma.

Intestinal motility may be present in dogs receiving thiopentone or ketamine (10). Inhalant anesthesia appears to be more effective in reducing intestinal motility. In contrast, ketamine and acepromazine anesthesia in cats may greatly reduce intestinal motility.

Nitrous oxide increases the rate of increase of bowel gases during anesthesia (11). Studies have demonstrated breathing of oxygen without nitrous oxide may reduce the accumulation rate of bowel gases and provide less interference in intestinal surgery. Anesthesia in the presence of cardiovascular stabilization does not cause a redistribution of blood flow away from the mucosal layers of the intestinal tract (12). During gastrointestinal surgical procedures, maintenance of levels of anesthesia that do not adversely influence systemic circulation assures needed function.

This does not prevent changes in other abdominal organ functions. Halothane may reduce renal output due to reductions in blood pressure and flow to the kidney. Renal output returns during arousal. Even N_2O and fentanyl in artificially ventilated dogs will reduce renal function (13). If animals receiving ketamine or other medications requiring renal clearance also receive potent inhalant anesthetics that reduce renal function, prolonged recoveries may occur due to slower excretion of the injectable agent.

Efforts to reduce recovery times after ketamine anesthesia have been effective if improvement in renal function has been achieved. Yohimbine (0.1 mg/kg i.v.) will reduce the recovery time in xylazine-ketamine anesthesia (14). The mode of action should be the reversal of the xylazine, an alpha-adrenoreceptor medication for which yohimbine is a selective antagonist. There is some evidence that yohimbine may have an effect on reversal of ketamine, but efforts to reproduce the results have not been predictably successful.

Hypothermia is a greater problem in dogs and cats than in large animals. Heated and humidified air has been used effectively during inhalant anesthesia in dogs (15) and cats (16) to prevent hypothermia. Circulating warm water blankets are effective in preventing or treating hypothermia (17). Electric heating pads should not be used for anesthetized dogs and cats because their continued contact can result in burns.

The cost of administering anesthesia is highly variable. The cost of pentobarbital is extremely low compared to many other techniques. The combination of acetylpromazine-thiamylal-halothane is one of the most inexpensive methods to provide inhalant anesthesia in dogs. Isoflurane adds to cost (18). It is cheaper to induce with barbiturates than by mask or chamber induction. The financial outlay must be balanced with the safe and effective administration of newer or physiologically safer agents. Anesthesia for elective surgery in healthy dogs and cats can be completed with cost-effective agents. In the high risk patient, it becomes more critical to consider the safety of anesthesia rather than inexpensive techniques.

Congenital Problems in Canine Breeds

An extensive list of congenital conditions has been observed or diagnosed in the purebred breeds (19); awareness of these is of value in anticipating and avoiding potential anesthetic problems. These problems do not occur frequently but can significantly influence anesthetic management if present. Reported congenital abnormalities that do not influence anesthetic management have not been included.

Specific problems in the affenpinscher that may influence anesthetic management include an occasional patent ductus arteriosis in the young dog or mitral valve insufficiency in animals over 8 years of age. The Afghan is sensitive to anesthetic agents, and low doses of anesthetic agents are recommended. The Afghan is sensitive to anesthetics for the same reason as all sight hounds are sensitive, which is because it has little body fat for anesthetic redistribution; neither does it retain body temperature or other physiological functions well during recumbency. The airedale accepts pain and distress without outward signs of distress in many instances. As a result, the airedale can be in relatively severe pain without appearing uncomfortable, which may influence the dosage of an analgetic agent required. The akita may have nervous disorders that can develop into tremors. It has been shown to be very sensitive to anesthetics, possibly relative to thyroid imbalance, which is common in the breed. Lower dosage levels may be adequate. During recovery, causes of postanesthetic tremors may be difficult to determine accurately. The Alaskan malamute occasionally has been shown to have hemopoetic anemia, which can influence the uptake of oxygen during anesthesia. Techniques using inhalant anesthesia with oxygen should be considered. The malamute may also have renal cortical hypoplasia, which is characterized by polydypsia and polyuria. Care should be taken if methoxyflurane is administered for prolonged periods. The heavy hair coat may contribute to elevated body temperatures during summer. Increased body temperature of this type could be confused with malignant hyperthermia. The American foxhound has few problems that influence anesthesia. More prominent among the inherited characteristics are potential thrombocytopathy, a blood disease that manifests itself as moderate to severe bleeding. Maintenance of adequate blood pressure or prevention of shock is of concern. The American staffordshire terrier has an extremely high pain threshold when excited and heavy dense muscle masses that can influence anesthetic management. Anesthetic dosages to overcome the excitement may be high, resulting in prolonged recoveries. The dense muscle mass can contribute to postanesthetic myopathy. The redistribution of anesthetic agents can be influenced by the muscle mass ratio to other body tissues.

The basenji may have inherited characteristics of anemia. It may also have renal tubular dysfunction with a history of polydypsia and polyuria with persistent weight loss. Care should be taken if methoxyflurane is used to avoid prolonged anesthesia. A higher level of allergic responses to substances occur in the basenji than in many other breeds. The breed may have asthma-like symptoms (see Chapter 23). If allergic responses to narcotics, barbiturates, or muscle relaxants occur, prompt treatment is necessary. The animals may have pyruvate kinase deficiency, sleep a great deal, and tire easily. Seriously affected dogs may become unconscious. They sometimes have pale mucous membranes and tachycardia. Anesthetics must be administered with care, and blood transfusions prior to or during anesthesia may be necessary.

The bassett hound has been known to be subject to a platelet disorder that can result in moderate to severe bleeding. The beagle is considered by many to be almost totally safe for anesthesia because it has been used in laboratory procedures so often. However, it too may have pyruvate kinase deficiency and urinary problems. This is of special concern if agents that can contribute to renal dysfunction are used. Epilepsy has also been reported in the beagle, which again may influence the selection of anesthetic agent or tranquilizer used for premedication. Enflurane may contribute to the problem even though experimentally it is not well defined. The bearded collie predominately has an inherited characteristic of idiopathic epilepsy. Animals showing seizure-like activity can be difficult to manage during anesthesia. Acetylpromazine, which may lower seizure threshold, should be avoided. Barbiturate induction is usually indicated. The Bedlington terrier may have renal cortical hypoplasia. Other Bedingtons have been diagnosed as having chronic progressive hepatitis. This hepatic dysfunction should be considered in the selection of anesthetic agents that undergo biotransformation by the liver. At the present time, isoflurane or enflurane are safer agents to use in these cases than halothane or methoxyflurane. The Belgian sheepdog has been shown to have epilepsy. This breed has been reported to have sensitivity to tranquilizers and anesthetics, including acepromazine. Although we might assume this has been relative to size-dose relationship, caution is justified. The Belgian tervuren may have a lack of sufficient thyroid hormone; anesthesia considerations as described under endocrine dysfunction are appropriate. Epilepsy has also been shown in Belgian tervurens. Diazepam or xylazine may be needed as a preanesthetic.

The Burmese mountain dog occasionally has cerebral degeneration of a genetic basis. This can lower the concentration of anesthetic required to produce unconsciousness. The predominant inherited characteristic of the bichon frise that may influence anesthetic management is epilepsy, which occurs more in this breed than in larger breeds of dogs. The black and tan coonhound is considered by some to be easily controlled and easily anesthetized; however, it is susceptible to polyneuritis, the so-called coonhound paralysis. Because this is a muscular-skeletal disorder, careful examination of the animal before anesthesia and certainly before the administration of muscle relaxants should be made to avoid anesthetic complications. Diagnosis of this condition before anesthesia can avoid embarrassing complications. Black and tan coonhounds may also have hemophilia B as a sex-linked hereditary trait characterized by prolonged bleeding. The bloodhound is relatively free from congenital abnormalities that influence anesthesia; the primary consideration is that they require a smaller dose of sedating drug in relation to their size than many smaller breeds. The border collie does not appear to have special anesthetic considerations, but the border terrier may present with congenital ventricular septal defects.

The borzoi, also known as the Russian wolfhound, responds to anesthetics, especially barbiturates, in an unpredictable fashion. Extremely long sleeping times or violent recoveries may occur, especially when anesthesia is administered without preanesthetics. The large size of the borzoi can make the dose unit body weight determination extremely critical. Most of the prolonged recoveries are probably due to relative overdosage of barbiturates. Volatile anesthetics are more predictable and easier to control than tranquilizers and barbiturates and should be considered when possible. The Boston terrier may have respiratory difficulties, but they are not as likely to be as significant as in the English bull dog. The Boston terrier may have hydrocephalis or heart defects, especially patent ductus arteriosis, which influences cardiovascular responses during anesthesia. The patency of the upper airway should be verified before administering anesthetics. There are sufficient anatomical problems of the airway in the Boston terrier to consider intubation during injectable anesthesia whenever possible. The bouvier de Flanders occasionally may have excessive soft palate that may contribute to laryngeal spasm during induction of or recovery from anesthesia. Occasional cardiac defects may be noticed; these should be evaluated during the preanesthetic examination.

The boxer has a variety of abnormalities that can influence anesthetic management. Gastric torsion frequently occurs. Individuals within the breed have been diagnosed as having subaortic stenosis, pulmonary stenosis, atrial septal defects, multiple cardiac defects, blood deficiency problems, and sinus arrhythmias. The boxer has been diagnosed in some instances as having excessive vagal tone, which can contribute to vagal/vagal syncope. The need for anticholinergics in this breed is greater than others. Refer to the section on cardiovascular considerations during anesthesia elsewhere in this text.

Gastric torsion may occur in the briard, and it has also been diagnosed in some instances as being hypothyroid. Brittanys may have hemophilia with prolonged bleeding. The English bull dog is a classic respiratory problem during anesthesia because of its upper airway structure. As with other brachycephalic breeds, stenotic nares are a frequent occurrence. The elongated soft palate can certainly contribute to respiratory failure during anesthesia. The breed may also have hypoplasia of the trachea. The size of endotracheal tube that can be used is smaller than in other breeds. Preoxygenation before induction is desirable but not always practical. It should not be used if excessive physical restraint is necessary. The principal consideration in the bull mastiff is to appropriately titrate dosage, as in other large breeds. Utilization of injectables on a milligram per unit body weight base can result in anesthetic overdose.

Cairn terriers may suffer from globoid cell leukodystrophy. This is a disease that produces demyelinating nervous disease symptoms characterized primarily by the destruction of the myelin sheaths. Less coordination is present because locomotion is affected, and motor deficits may progress to paralysis. An awareness of the symptoms of this problem in the cairn terrier can avoid the complications associated with utilization of muscle relaxants during these conditions. Care must also be used if reflexes of the extremities are used as the primary means of determining depth of anesthesia.

Circulatory defects have been reported in Chihuahuas and include pulmonic stenosis and mitral valve defects. Chihuahuas are a highly nervous breed; this may in some instances contribute to overdose of anesthetics. The collapsed trachea may be an inherited characteristic of the Chihuahua; it often results in respiratory difficulties during anesthesia. The Chihuahua is a classic example of the breed requiring attention to airway and delivery system management. The tidal volume is quite small, and nonrebreathing systems are desirable.

The desired head structure of the chow is brachycephalic. As a result, anesthesia must be approached with the same extreme care as with other brachycephalics, although it is usually not as troublesome as with the bulldog. The chow is often sensitive to narcotics, including morphine and meperidine, and may show laryngeal spasm during the administration of intravenous barbiturates. The aggressive nature of the chow sometimes contributes to overdose of an anesthetic agent due to concern about controlling these animals. In the event of an overdose of anesthetic in the chow, difficulty in determining levels of oxygenation are further complicated by the blue or black color of the tongue.

The cocker spaniel may have a sex-linked recessive trait for hemophilia and as a result have anemia problems. Renal cortical hypoplasia has been reported in a few with proteinuria that persists and increases in intensity. Cardiac abnormalities have been documented in the breed as well. Because of the unpredictable temperament of the cocker, unusually excessive levels of tranquilization have been used to assure a calm and easily managed patient. This sometimes results in excess hypotension or other undesirable responses to the tranquilizer. Owners should be warned that the animal may have a period of personality change after anesthesia. This breed is not always predictable without tranquilizers. The owners should be warned to handle the dog with caution until recovery is total. The collie can have hemophilia as well, and epilepsy has been reported in some collies. However, the principal anesthetic problem in the collie is frequently that of anesthetic overdose. This is partially because of the extensive haircoat. Collies are frequently much ligher in weight than they appear to be, so careful physical examinations is necessary. The curly coated retriever may suffer from Cushing's syndrome or low thyroid function or have an inability to metabolize calcium. This can result in variations in anesthetic management and control in cardiovascular function, especially heart rate, contractile force, and blood pressure.

It is not unusual for the dachshund to develop diabetes mellitus. When presented with a dachshund with this condition, refer to the anesthetic and endocrine disorder discussion elsewhere in this text. The Dalmatian may have urinary calculi. As a result, renal dysfunction is a condition that often occurs and can influence not only the choice of anesthetic but the dosage, especially in cases of uremia. All anesthetics that must be excreted via the urine must be considered with caution. The Doberman pincher frequently has cervical vertebral instability often referred to as wobbler's syndrome. This can result in incoordination or complete paralysis and can be especially troublesome in recovery from anesthesia. Anesthetics for radiological examinations should be used with caution to avoid further deterioration of the condition. Bundle of His degeneration has been reported as a cause of sudden death in Dobermans. If this happens to occur during anesthesia, it is difficult to explain. Congenital renal hypoplasia has been reported in Dobermans as well; this can influence renal function and elimination of anesthetics.

The English setter tends to be a long sleeper with acepromazine and other phenathiazine derivative tranquilizers and narcotics. English springer spaniels may suffer from blood deficiencies. The English toy spaniel is prone to diabetes mellitus, and there have been instances of congestive heart defects.

Pulmonic stenosis has been reported in fox terriers, as has persistent aortic arch. If these conditions are evident, appropriate management of the cardiovascular system must be taken into account. The principal problem associated with anesthesia in the German shepherd has been the temperament and size of the animal. Relatively common complications of anesthesia in the German shepherd have been the administration of high levels of preanesthetics such as acetylpromazine, xylazine, or neuroleptanalgesia for control of the animal without sufficient reduction in the dosage of inducing agents, resulting in overdepression.

The German short haired pointer may show signs of subaortic stenosis or blood disorders, particularly of the platelets. This can influence the overall management. Cerebellar hypoplasia has been reported in the golden retriever. The Gordon setter may have thyroid imbalance or cerebellar corticoabiotrophy, which contributes to ataxia and can influence recovery from anesthetics. Great Danes are prone to gastric torsion or dilatation, which can result in an emergency anesthetic situation. Great Danes often have low tolerance to tranquilizers, and the dose of injectable anesthetics required for induction is frequently much lower than expected. Great Danes may also have wobbler's syndrome, so recovery can be difficult. Other neurological problems, including progressive ataxia, spinal cord degeneration, and necrotizing myelopathy, have been recorded, as well as cerebral hypoplasia. These factors influence the coordination of Great Danes in recovering from anesthesia and influence dose requirements to induce or maintain anesthesia.

Great Pyrenees frequently require less than calculated inducing doses of anesthetics, and they may also have cardiovascular problems that should be identified. The greyhound is highly susceptible to injectable barbiturates. Methohexital is preferred over either sodium thiamylal or thiopenthal for induction of anesthesia. Maintenance of anesthesia with inhalants is preferred over injectables to assure faster recovery and stability of the vital functions.

The ibizan hound is in a similar category to the greyhound with the same considerations for anesthesia. The Irish setter is frequently not mentally or emotionally mature until about 3 years of age; as a result, utilization of tranquilizers to calm the animals prior to induction of anesthesia is more important than in many other breeds. The Irish terrier has a tendency to develop cystine stones. An awareness of this condition can avoid undue anesthetic complications. The Irish wolfhound does not require the same proportional dose of ultrashort barbiturates for induction at per unit of body weight as does smaller breeds. As a result, care must be taken during injectable barbiturate anesthesia to avoid excessive drug administration. They usually require much less than 50% of the calculated dose per unit of body weight. The Italian Greyhound should be considered as similar to the American Greyhound for anesthetic dose determinations because they are so sensitive to barbiturate anesthesia. Gas anesthesia is recommended.

Epilepsy is common in the keeshond. Renal corticohypoplasia has been seen with signs of polydypsia, vomiting, polyuria, convulsions, anemia, and weakness, which will certainly influence the dose of anesthetic required and the importance of fluid and electrolyte balance. Efforts to correct these imbalances may be necessary before anesthesia. There are reports that the komondorok may not tolerate sodium penobarbital well. Low doses of ultrashort barbiturates followed by volatile anesthesia would be better tolerated. The Labrador retriever may have hemophilia and muscle disorders. The muscle disorders are characterized by deficiency of Type two muscle fibers.

Pulmonic stenosis has been found in miniature schnauzers. They may have von Willebrand's disease and can suffer from mild to severe bleeding. The Newfoundland may present with acute gastric dilatation. Newfoundlands require lower doses of tranquilizers and anesthetics than smaller breeds. The Norwegian elkhound may require lower doses of tranquilizers. They may also suffer from renal cortical hypoplasia.

The old English sheepdog may suffer from wobbler's syndrome and have recovery problems. They frequently require greatly reduced doses of tranquilizers or anesthetics.

Otter hounds may have canine thrombocytopathy. As a result, blood clotting may be affected due to blood platelet defects. They should be screened for this condition. The Pekingese has upper airway and stenotic nares characteristic of brachycephalic breeds that can influence ability to breathe. The soft palate is often elongated, contributing further to airway difficulties. The Pekingese combines the bradycephalic problems of the pug or English bulldog with the size requirements for anesthetic equipment presented by the Chihuahua. The Pembroke Welsh corgi is prone to bladder stones and urinary tract difficulties. Use of methoxyflurane or other agents that affect renal functions should be considered with caution.

Patent ductus arteriosus may be a problem in the Pomeranian. During barbiturate induction, dilution of ultrashort barbiturates (0.5 to 1.0% solution) makes control of dosage easier. The Pomeranian may also have a collapsed trachea or hypoglycemia. Its management is similar to that of the Chihuahua. Epilepsy, patent ductus arteriosus, or diabetes may be observed in the poodle. Poodles presented for cataract surgery with diabetes have a high incidence of coexisting problems.

The pug has respiratory difficulty without anesthesia. It must be considered during anesthesia, and intubation is frequently essential. Rapid intubation is needed, and much caution should be used during extubation. Rhodesian ridgebacks may require lower dosage per unit weight than small dogs. The same can be said for the rottweiler and the St. Bernard. In addition, the St. Bernard may have diabetes mellitus. They are prone to gastric torsion, hemophilia, and epilepsy.

The saluki's response to barbiturates is unpredictable. Tranquilizers and barbiturates should be given with caution, and inhalants should be used when possible. The samoyed is predisposed to Hemophilia A, pulmonic stenosis, and diabetes. The Scottish deerhound is prone to gastric torsion. Scottish terriers may show thyroid or urinary problems.

The shar pei should be anesthetized with extreme caution and after careful physical examination. They are prone to rapid CNS depression and cardiopulmonary collapse and are high anesthetic risks. Careful induction is necessary, and inhalant anesthetic management is desirable.

Shetland sheepdogs may have hemophilia. The shih tzu has a problem with renal cortica hypoplasia and potential uremia. The Siberian husky may exhibit ventricular septal defects and Hemophilia A. The silky terrier may have tracheal collapse, hydrocephalus or congenital cardiovascular abnormalities, and diabetes mellitus as factors contributing to anesthetic complications.

Tibetan terriers may require lower anesthetic concentrations than other breeds. The Welsh springer spaniel sometimes has epileptic seizures. West Highland white terriers can have globoid cell leukodystrophy (canine Krabbe-type) of myelin degeneration. The whippet is sensitive to anesthetics, especially tranquilizers and barbiturates. The Yorkshire terrier may show hypoglycemia. There is a high frequency of congenital hydrocephalus.

Conclusion

Although many congenital conditions in purebred dogs have been discussed, this list does not assure that other problems may not be encountered. It can aid the veterinarian in the evaluation of patients and selection of agents and dosages so as to avoid complications when congenital abnormalities that can influence anesthetic management exist. Most animals presented for anesthesia do not suffer from congenital abnormalities.

There are many techniques of administering anesthesia in dogs and cats. Their size encourages the adaptation of drug combinations and methods used in human anesthesia. There is a physical convenience not enjoyed during anesthesia in horses and cattle, especially during induction and recovery. Maintenance of body temperature and the control of cardiac arrhythmias are two especially important areas of concern in dogs and cats.

References

1. Kolata RJ, Rawlings CA: Cardiopulmonary effects of intravenous xylazine, ketamine, and atropine in the dog. *Am J Vet Res* 43(12):2196–2198, 1982.
2. Lee MJ, Clemont JG: Respiratory depression produced by diazepam in cats: effect of anaesthesia. *Arch Int Pharmacodyn Ther* 248(2):289–293, 1980.
3. Rawlings CA, Kolata RJ: Cardiopulmonary effects of thiopental/lidocaine combination during anesthetic induction in the dog. *Am J Vet Res* 44(1):144–149, 1983.
4. Dodman NH: Complications of saffan anaesthesia in cats. *Vet Rec* 107(2):481–483, 1980.
5. Haskins SC, Knapp RG: Effect of low carrier gas flows (50% oxygen/50% nitrous oxide) on inspired oxygen tension in anesthetized dogs. *J Am Vet Med Assoc* 180(7):735–738, 1982.
6. Ritter JW, Shigezowa GY, Roe SD Sr, Sullivan SF: Increasing myocardial oxygen demand during prolonged halothane anesthesia in dogs. *Anesth Analg* 62(9):788–792, 1983.
7. Hightower CE, Kiopes AL, Butler HC, Fedde MR: End-tidal partial pressure of CO_2 as an estimate of arterial partial pressure of CO_2 during various ventilatory regimes in halothane-anesthetized dogs. *Am J Vet Res* 41(4):610–612, 1980.
8. Southorn P, Rehder K, Hyatt RE: Halothane anesthesia and respiratory mechanics in dogs lying supine. *J Appl Physiol* 49(2):300–305, 1980.
9. Hubbell JA, Muir WW 3rd, Bednarski RM, Bednarski LS: Change of inhalation anesthetic agents for management of ventricular premature depolarization in anesthetized cats and dogs. *J Am Vet Med Assoc* 185(6):643–646, 1984.
10. Healy TE, Foster GE, Evan DF, Syed A: Effect of some IV anaesthetic agents on canine gastrointestinal motility. *Br J Anaesth* 53(3):229–233, 1981.
11. Steffey EP, Johnson BH, Eger EI II, Howland D Jr: Nitrous oxide: effect on accumulation rate and uptake of bowel gases. *Anesth Analg* 58(5):405–408, 1979.
12. Bond JH, Prentiss RA, Levitt MD: The effect of anesthesia and laporotomy in blood flow to the stomach, small bowel and colon of the dog. *Surgery* 87(3):313–318, 1980.
13. Hunter JM, Jones RS, Utting JE: Effect of anaesthesia with nitrous oxide in oxygen and fentanyl on renal function in the artifically ventilated dog. *Br J Anaesth* 52(3):343–348, 1980.
14. Hsu WH, Lu ZX: Effect of yohimbine on xylazine-ketamine anesthesia in cats. *J Am Vet Med Assoc* 185(8):886–888, 1984.
15. Raffe MR, Martin FB: Effect of inspired air, heat and humidification on anesthesia-induced hypothermia in dogs. *Am J Vet Res* 44(3):455–458, 1983.
16. Haskins SC, Patz JD: Effect of inspired-air warming and humidification in the prevention of hypothermia during general anes-

thesia in cats. *Am J Vet Res* 41(10):1669–1673, 1980.
17. Haskins SC: Hypothermia and its prevention during general anesthesia in cats. *Am J Vet Res* 42(5):856–861, 1981.
18. Bednarski RM, Bednaski LS, Muir WW 3rd: Cost comparison of anesthetic regimes in the dog and cat. *J Am Vet Med Assoc* 185(8):869–872, 1984.
19. Clark RD, Stainer JR: *Medical and Genetic Aspects of Purebred Dogs*. Edwardsville, KA, Vet Med Publishing Co, 1985, pp 1–474.

PART 4

Special Anesthesia Considerations of Swine

JOHN C. THURMON, D.V.M., M.S., D.A.C.V.A., and
G. JOHN BENSON, D.V.M., M.S., D.A.C.V.A.

Introduction

Three important points must be taken into account when considering anesthesia of swine. First, a mature pig is difficult to restrain for intravenous injection. Adding to the difficulty is the sparsity of peripheral veins suitable for catheterization and injection of large volumes of fluids. Finally, the economic value of the average pig will not permit the extensive use of expensive drugs and equipment.

Swine have become important research animals because their cardiovascular system and other anatomical features, such as skin and gastrointestinal tract, are similar to those of humans. They are the animals of choice for studying the well-known familial human condition malignant hyperthermia. Although this chapter is written primarily for the veterinary student, practitioner, and academic clinician, some of the techniques will be useful to the researcher working with swine. Recommendations for drug dose, rate, and route of drug administration are for the average healthy pig. Individuals may vary greatly in their response to a given drug or combination of drugs administered under nearly identical circumstances. Although such variability suggests the need for further investigation of these agents, it also highlights the importance of a thorough understanding of the physiological and pharmacological responses peculiar to swine. From this standpoint, the veterinarian must exercise his or her sound professional judgment when administering potentially lethal agents such as anesthetics. Judicious administration of anesthetic and anesthetic-related agents with close monitoring of response is essential for safe anesthesia.

In swine, anesthesia may be safely induced with injectable or inhalation agents. The shape of the pig's nose is well suited to a nose cone for administration of an inhalation anesthetic. Further, anesthetic equipment used in humans or small animals such as dogs and cats is ideal in size for swine. However, cost effectiveness must be considered. When an injectable agent must be given by the intravenous route, restraint and immobilization of the pig's head is essential. Placement of an intravenous catheter will prevent perivascular injection (Fig. 13.11). Cannulation of a central dorsal ear vein in mature swine with light skin and large ears is relatively simple (Figs. 13.12 to 13.17). This is far from the case in dark-skinned pigs with small ears. Intravenous injection of 1 to 2 ml of 2% lidocaine with a 23 to 25 gauge needle into the vein prior to attempting catheter placement will dilate the vein, aiding catheterization. The practice of using ear notches in pigs for identification often disrupts continuity of peripheral ear veins, destroying their suitability for drug administration.

It is possible to percutaneously cannulate the anterior vena cava, as is illustrated in Figure 13.18. Direct injection after needle placement into this large vessel is discouraged because pigs often struggle during the

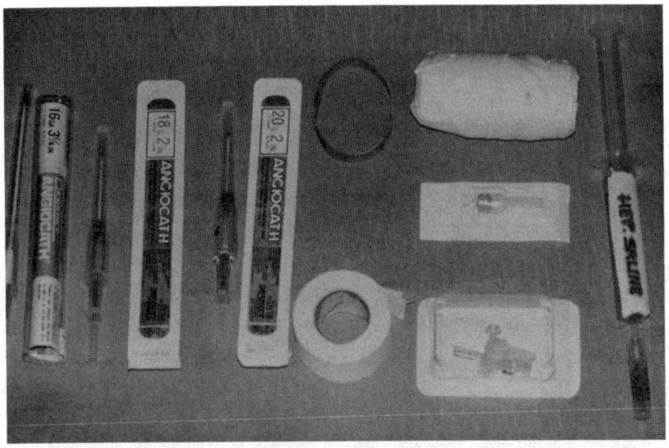

Figure 13.11. Supplies used to catheterize an auricular vein. A 16-gauge catheter is preferred in mature swine. A rubberband placed around the ear at its base will promote venous engorgement. Dilation may be further enhanced by injecting 1 to 2 ml of 2% lidocaine directly into the vein using a 23- to 25-gauge needle. A gauze roll placed inside the ear will provide stability when taping the catheter in place.

injection procedure, increasing the likelihood of perivascular injection, which may result in pleuritis and/or mediastinitis. When injecting into an auricular vessel without a catheter, it is advisable to use a short length of fine gauge tubing between the needle or catheter and syringe (Fig. 13.19). This technique will prevent the pig from dislodging the intravascular needle if it struggles or shakes its head during injection.

Some drugs, such as ketamine or atropine, may induce a satisfactory response when given by the intramuscular route. However, it must not be forgotten that most pigs have a thick subcutaneous layer of fat that must be penetrated before an intramuscular injection can be made. A 3.5- to 4-cm needle will be required in most healthy mature pigs, whereas a 2- to 2.5-cm needle will be satisfactory in piglets.

Preparation for Anesthesia

When possible, food should be withheld for 12 hours and water for 4 to 6 hours before general anesthesia. Although the incidence of vomiting is relatively low in pigs, it does occur; thus withholding food and water before general anesthesia is prudent. When food and water are to be withheld from one pig in a group, it is less stressful to the isolated pig if it is allowed to have sight and nose contact with its pen mates. When the gastrointestinal tract is full of fresh food, administration of an anticholinergic (e.g., atropine or glycopyrrolate) will accentuate development of gastrointestinal tympany. Accumulation of bowel gas will increase intra-abdominal pressure, pressing the diaphragm forward into the thoracic cavity and decreasing functional residual lung capacity and alveolar ventilation. This undesirable effect is accentuated by deep surgical anesthesia and by manually restraining pigs by their hind limbs with the head and thorax in a downward position. After surgery, the pig should only be placed with other pigs when it has fully recovered from anesthesia. Pigs have been known to mutilate their anesthetized penmates. Sows presented for Caesarean section may be toxic and hypotensive. Administration of fluids and other therapy is advisable before induction of anesthesia.

Restraint

Manual restraint of baby pigs is easily accomplished by placing one hand over the back and the other under the sternum. If handled gently, squealing will be minimal. Pigs will not tolerate rough handling, especially during hot weather. They can easily become stressed and die from heat exhaustion. In mature swine, a rope or cable snare with the loop placed around the upper jaw and behind the canine teeth is the most common form of mechanical restraint. Other devices include a head catch similar to that used for cattle but designed specifically for swine. For some time, we have used a webbing-topped mobile table to restrain swine for transport to and from the laboratory and for induction of anesthesia (Fig. 13.20). This device was constructed in our workshop of galvanized steel pipe and nylon webbing. When the pig is placed on the conveyance, its feet are allowed to slide through the webbing. The two front and two rear feet are secured with tape encircling the pig's legs just above the fetlocks. The pig may struggle and squeal at first but will quickly quiet down once the taping process is completed. As a matter of fact, once the conveyance is moving, the pig actually appears to enjoy the ride to the surgical suite. We have found the webbed conveyance to be ideal for restraint of pigs during induction of anesthesia by either inhalation or intravenous injection technique. In addition, epidural or subarachnoid injection can be easily accomplished by pulling the rear feet forward, causing the back to arch at the lumbosacral joint. For minor surgical procedures, this webbed table may serve quite well as a surgical table (Fig. 13.20).

Tracheal Intubation

Because the dose of an anesthetic (i.e., barbiturate) required to induce surgical anesthesia is extremely close to that which will cause respiratory arrest, tracheal intubation is essential for safe management of

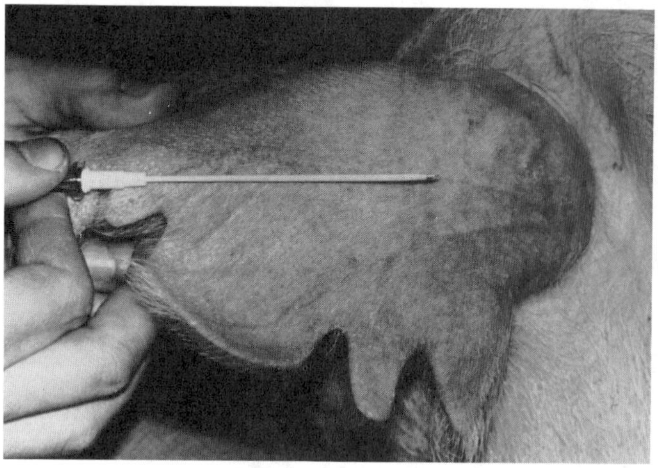

Figure 13.12

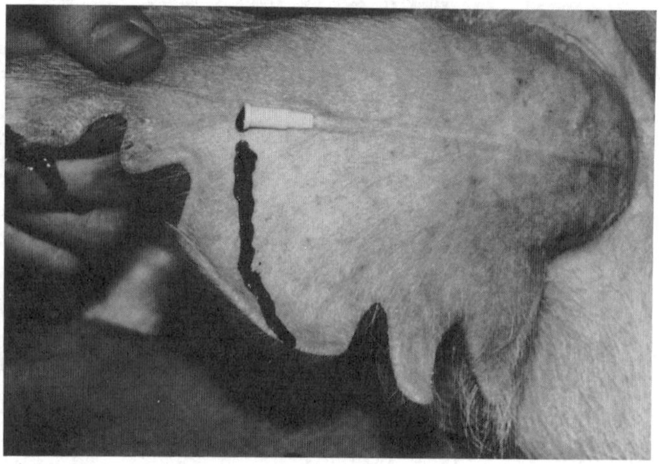

Figure 13.15

Figures 13.12 to 13.17. Placement of a 16-gauge catheter in a central ear vein. The catheter is secured in place by taping around a gauze roll placed inside the pig's ear.

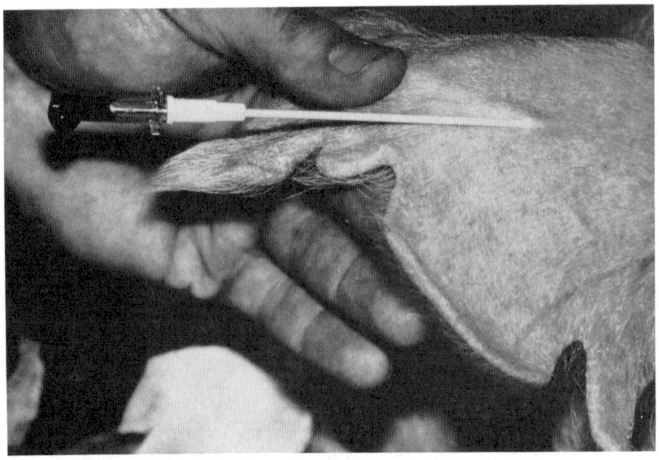

Figure 13.13

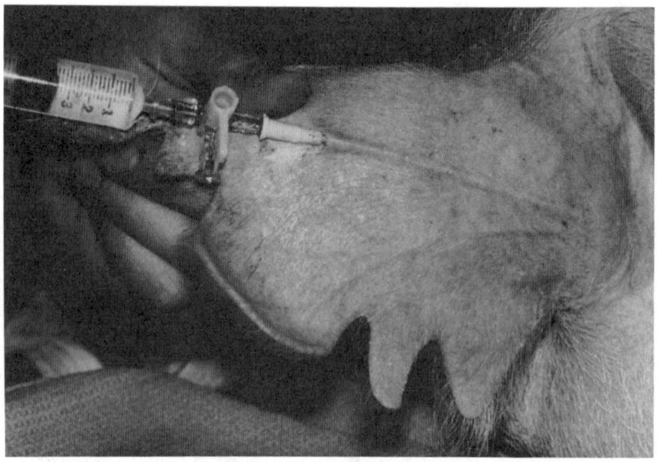

Figure 13.16

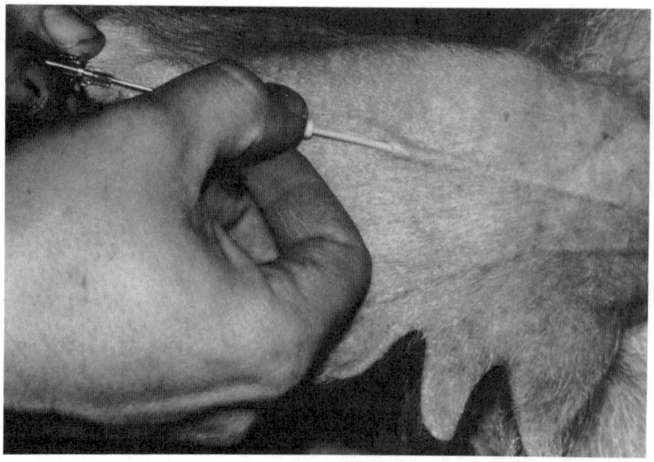

Figure 13.14

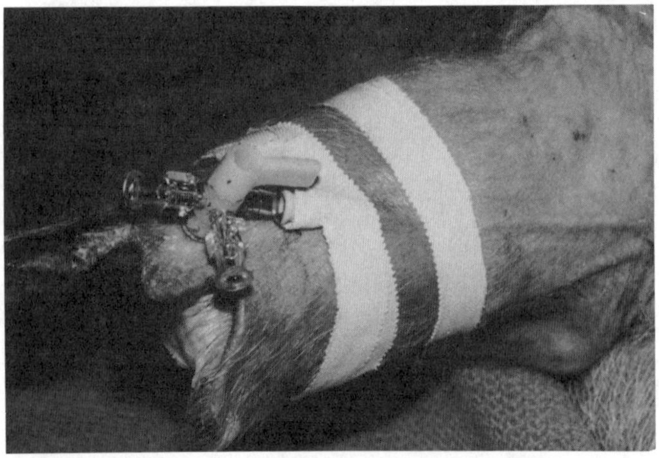

Figure 13.17

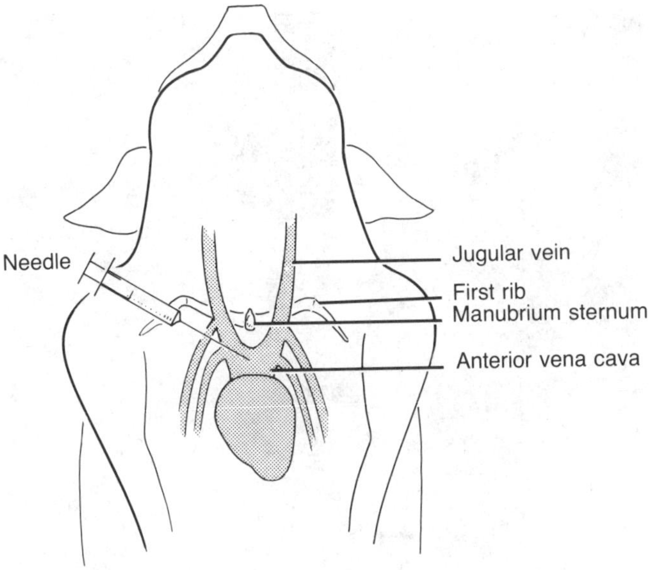

Figure 13.18. Percutaneous puncture of the anterior vena cava (courtesy CRC Press) (3).

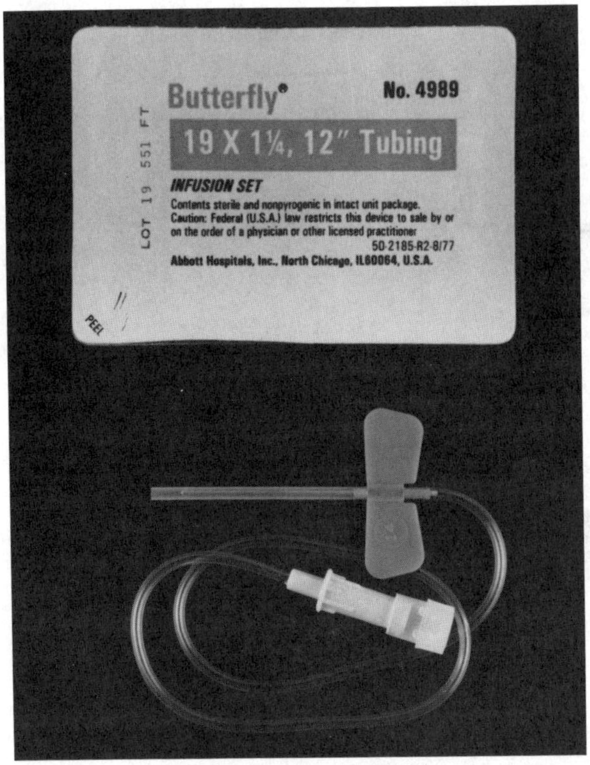

Figure 13.19. A "butterfly" system will help prevent dislodging of needle if the pig shakes its head during the injection process.

general anesthesia. The shape of the pig's head is well suited to the use of a nose cone for induction of anesthesia with an inhalation agent. Inhalation anesthesia may also be administered using nasal tubes and a Carlen's adapter. Neither method ensures a patent airway nor prevents aspiration of secretions or vomitus. The use of either technique can be disastrous when mechanical ventilation is required to manage apnea because gases will be forced into the stomach, causing gastric tympany. Gastric dilatation will increase intra-abdominal pressure, which may severely limit alveolar ventilation in spite of mechanical support. Thus, tracheal intubation, although essential, adds a measure of difficulty to maintenance of safe anesthesia in swine.

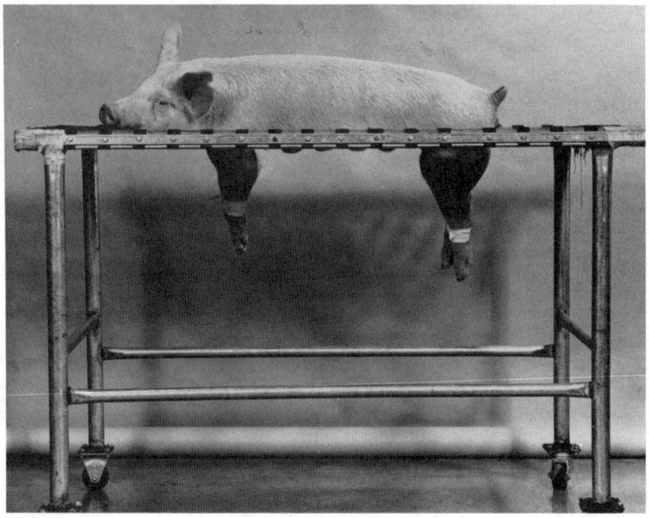

Figure 13.20. A webb-topped mobile table for transporting and restraining swine for induction of anesthesia (courtesy CRC Press) (3).

The pig's mouth cannot be opened wide. In addition, the pig has a small larynx that slopes downward, creating a very sharp angle to the tracheal opening. These anatomical features are responsible for the difficulty often encountered when attempting intubation. Repeated attempts to intubate often elicit laryngeal spasms. The incidence is highest and spasms are more severe in piglets less than 2 months of age (1), but is a common occurrence in all lightly anesthetized swine. Rough treatment of the extremely delicate laryngeal mucosa during intubation may be accompanied by laryngeal edema and spasms that become apparent during the recovery period. Once the endotracheal tube is removed, such responses may be life-threatening because it is nearly impossible to intubate a struggling hypoxic pig. Often the only practical solution to the problem is a tracheostomy. For this reason, it is extremely important to observe the pig closely during recovery, especially after extubation, to ensure a patient airway and adequate ventilation. Attempting to mechanically ventilate the pig with a nose cone will most often compound the problem by creating gastric tympany, further hindering alveolar ventilation. The problems of laryngeal edema and laryngeal spasms are easily prevented by inducing surgical anesthesia before attempting to intubate and using sound, gentle, atraumatic technique. In lightly anesthetized swine, laryngeal spasms may be prevented by spraying the larynx with 2 to 4% lidocaine solution before attempting to intubate. Succinylcholine (1 to 2 mg/kg i.v.) may be given to prevent or treat laryngeal spasms. Administration of succinylcholine should be followed immediately by tracheal intubation and mechanical support of ventilation, which should be continued (6 to 8 breaths/min) until spontaneous breathing resumes. One should be aware that succinylcholine can trigger malignant hyperthermia in susceptible swine. Thus the pig should be monitored for the classic symptoms of the syndrome after the use of succinylcholine.

Intubation Technique

Anesthesia may be achieved by intravenous injection (e.g., thiopental sodium 10 to 12 mg/kg i.v.) or with an inhalation agent via nose cone (e.g., halothane in oxygen). A guide to the selection of appropiate size endotracheal tubes is shown in Table 13.4. After a light surgical plane of anesthesia has been achieved, the mouth is opened and the tongue is withdrawn. A laryngoscope is used to expose the epiglottis and visualize the laryngeal opening for spraying with 2 to 4% lidocaine. If anesthesia is being induced with an inhalation agent, the nose cone is replaced after spraying the larynx, and induction is continued for 3 to 4 minutes while the lidocaine takes effect. With the pig in sternal recumbency, short lengths of cotton rope are placed around the upper jaw behind the canine teeth and around the lower jaw behind the canine teeth to open the pig's mouth wide. The head and neck are extended, the tongue is drawn forward, and a laryngoscope (Fig. 13.21) is used to provide an unobstructed view of the laryngeal opening. A plastic or metal stylet may be passed into the trachea, serving as a guide over which the endotracheal tube can be passed (Fig. 13.22). The stylet should be at least three times the length of the endotracheal tube and should be held stationary while the tube is placed. Otherwise, the stylet could be advanced along with the endotracheal tube, resulting in injury to bronchial and peribronchial tissues. The authors have witnessed the occurrence of tension pneumothorax in a goat when the stylet was improperly used. When the endotracheal tube is placed without the aid of a stylet, its natural curvature is positioned ventrally. When the tip of the tube has reached mid-

Table 13.4
Endotracheal Tube Sizes for Swine

Piglets	3 to 4 mm
10 to 15 kg	4 to 6 mm
20 to 50 kg	6 to 9 mm
100 kg and larger	10 to 16 mm

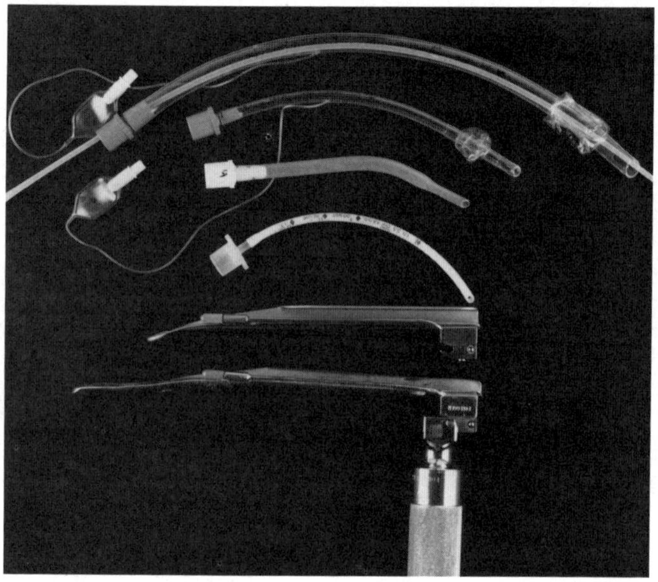

Figure 13.21. Cuffed and uncuffed (Cole's tube) endotracheal tubes used in swine. A plastic stylet for aiding passage of the tube through the larynx is shown in the uppermost tube. A laryngoscope with a standard blade (*top*) and a blade to which an extension has been added are shown below.

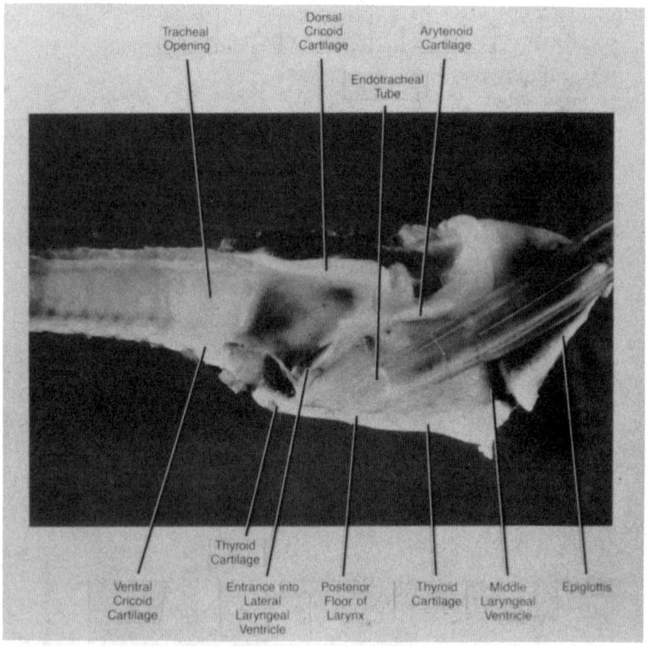

Figure 13.22. Sagittal section of pig larynx illustrating the sharp angle through which an endotracheal tube must pass before entering the trachea (courtesy CRC Press) (3).

point of the larynx, it is rotated 180° on its long axis, directing the tube through the cricoid ring into the tracheal opening. If the tube is not rotated while passing through the larynx, its tip will become entrapped in the posterior floor of the larynx, anterior to the cricoid ring, preventing its passage into the trachea (Fig. 13.22). When the endotracheal tube has been properly positioned, the cuff is inflated to provide an airtight seal with the tracheal wall and connected to the anesthetic machine. Apnea is simply dealt with by squeezing the rebreathing bag 4 to 8 times per minute until spontaneous breathing resumes. Apnea in a pig maintained with injectable agents is easily managed with an Ambu bag.

During recovery, the pig should be monitored rather closely. Signs of respiratory or circulatory embarrassment should be dealt with promptly. Extubation should not be attempted until strong signs of recovery are apparent (i.e., chewing, swallowing, shivering, coughing, and ability to maintain sternal recumbency). Clinical signs of laryngeal edema, laryngeal spasm, and hypoxia are major problems that are often only identified after tracheal extubation. When major surgery has been performed, postoperative pain may be accompanied by hypoventilation, hypercapnea, and hypoxemia. In such instances, administration of oxygen by nasal tube or nose cone will effectively correct hypoxemia but may have only a limited effect on hypercapnia and associated respiratory acidosis. An analgesic that does not depress respiration may be used effectively to overcome the latter problem. Morphine, although promoting analgesia, may cause further respiratory depression and in some instances central nervous excitation. Because of the varied response of swine to morphine and other opiate agonists, one of the following agonist-antagonists may be more appropriate for swine when treating postoperative pain (3): pentazocine (0.4 to 5 mg/kg i.m.), butorphanol (0.1 to 0.3 mg/kg i.m.), nalbuphine (0.15 to 0.2 mg/kg i.m.), and buprenorphine (0.004 to 0.008 mg/kg i.m.).

Preanesthetic Medication

ANTICHOLINERGIC AGENTS

Induction with an inhalation agent (e.g., halothane in oxygen) or ketamine may be associated with profuse salivation and airway obstruction. Attempts to intubate the pig's trachea during a light plane of anesthesia can elicit a vagovagal response resulting in bradycardia. Such responses may be prevented by preanesthetic administration of an anticholinergic. Atropine (0.06 to 0.08 mg/kg i.m.) is often chosen for this purpose, but its administration is followed by tachycardia. In pigs in which tachycardia is undesirable, glycopyrrolate (0.01 mg/kg i.m. or i.v.) may be more suitable than atropine). In addition, glycopyrrolate tends to increase gastric pH, rendering gastric secretion less irritating to airway tissues should they be aspirated prior to tracheal intubation. For these reasons, glycopyrrolate would appear to be a desirable anticholinergic in swine.

SEDATIVES AND TRANQUILIZERS

Because mature pigs are more difficult to restrain than most other domestic animals and are usually highly vocal, it is often desirable to administer a tranquilizer or sedative by intramuscular injection before applying restraint required for induction of anesthesia. In order to ensure prompt onset of action and full response to a tranquilizer, pigs should be handled as gently as possible during the injection procedure. It should be left undisturbed until the desired clinical response is achieved. Repeated stimulation in order to assess the pig's reaction, prior to full onset of tranquilization, will often result in less than a desirable response. A number of agents have been used for this purpose. Either of the short-acting barbiturates pentobarbital or secobarbital (6 to 12 mg/kg i.m. of a 3% solution) will induce sedation and decrease vocalization during the induction procedure. However, a sedative dose of barbiturate will not provide any degree of analgesia; in fact, pigs appear to become hyperalgesic. Administering xylazine (1 to 2 mg/kg i.m.) will tend to offset the hyperalgesic effect of barbiturates. Other classes of agents used to induce sedation and/or tranquilization include phenothiazines, butyrophenones, benzodiazepines, and opiates.

PHENOTHIAZINE TRANQUILIZERS

The phenothiazine derivatives exert their effects centrally and peripherally. Their principal central site of action is the basal ganglia, where they interfere with the neurotransmitter dopamine (4). Administration of a phenothiazine results in a dose-related state of hypotension. This hypotensive state is caused by depression of central activity, direct myocardial depression, and a dilation of blood vessels resulting from specific peripheral alpha-adrenergic receptor blockade. The use of these agents should be avoided in ill or debilitated swine because of their tendency to aggravate hypovolemia, anemia, hypothermia, shock, and hepatic dysfunction. Their use in high dosages as adjuncts to epidural or spinal analgesia is discouraged unless a large gauge vascular catheter is in place so that fluid loading can be initiated promptly when required. Hypotension associated with tranquilizer administration is best treated by fluid loading with balanced electrolyte solution (e.g., 20 to 40 ml/kg). Specific peripheral alpha-adrenergic agonists (i.e., methoxamine (3 to 5 mg i.v. or 10 to 20 mg i.m.) or phenylephrine (0.8 mg i.v. or 5 mg s.c. or i.m.) have been used as effective adjuncts in cases not responding to fluid therapy alone. Although ephedrine (0.15 to 0.2 mg/kg i.v.) acts centrally and has minimal arterial vasoconstrictor properties, it increases venous tone and promotes venous return (preload), resulting in increased cardiac output. Thus, it may be the catecholamine of choice for treating hypotension induced by alpha-adrenergic blockade. The phenothiazine most commonly used in clinical practice is acetylpromazine administered by the intramuscular route; onset of action is rather slow, requiring 20 to 30 minutes for peak effect. Acetylpromazine induces very little analgesia; thus intravenous puncture may be accompanied by vigorous head and ear movement when swine are not restrained with a nose loop or head catch.

Some accepted clinical doses of phenothiazine tranquilizers are: acetylpromazine (Acepromazine) (0.03 to 0.22 mg/kg i.m.), chlorpromazine (Thorazine) (0.55 to 3.3 mg/kg i.v. or 2.0 to 4.0 mg/kg i.m.), promazine (Sparine) (0.44 to 1.0 mg/kg i.v. or i.m.), triflupromazine (Vetame) (0.88 mg/kg i.v. or 1.3 mg/kg i.m.), and propiopromazine (Tranvet) (0.55 to 1.0 mg/kg i.v. or i.m.).

THIOXANTHENE DERIVATIVES

Chlorprothixene (Taractan) is a relatively potent tranquilizer possessing chemical and pharmacological properties similar to those of the piperazine phenothiazines. Taractan is a satisfactory tranquilizer for swine when administered by the i.v. route at a dose of 0.3 to 1.0 mg/kg (5) or 3.3 mg/kg i.m. (6). It is reportedly an effective drug for treating postpartum hysteria in sows. Jones reports that sows "savaging" their piglets would allow the neonates to be returned to the pen where they could play and crawl around the mother's mouth with impunity 10 min after she was injected with 0.4 to 0.5 mg/kg i.v. of Taractan (6).

BUTYROPHENONE TRANQUILIZERS

This group of tranquilizers is frequently referred to as "neuroleptics." When combined with an opiate, the term "neuroleptanalgesic" is used to describe this drug combination. Drugs of this group induce physiological responses similar to those induced by phenothiazine administration. Degree of cardiopulmonary depression is dose-dependent and appears, in part, to be related to depression of the central actions of dopamine and norepinephrine (4). These agents are also peripheral alpha-adrenergic receptor blockers. Thus, high doses can induce severe hypotension, predisposing to hypothermia.

The *only* tranquilizer approved for use in swine is azaperone (Stresnil). This agent is approved for prevention of aggression among newly mixed pigs. It has also been used for treatment of postpartum hysteria and as an immobilizing agent of large swine prior to induction of anesthesia. As with other tranquilizers, when swine are subjected to rough handling, kept in noisy surroundings, or otherwise frequently stimulated prior to full onset of azaperone's action, swine may become agitated instead of tranquilized. Signs of agitation are often preceded by sneezing and incoordinated movement. Thus, swine should be left undisturbed for 20 to 30 minutes before attempting diagnostic or other manipulative procedures. The response to azaperone is dose-dependent. The following doses have been found satisfactory: for light sedation, 1 mg/kg i.m.; to decrease aggressiveness, 2.5 mg/kg i.m.; and for deep sedation and immobilization, 5 to 8 mg/kg i.m. The initial dose of azaperone should always be given intramuscularly; when given intravenously, "violent excitement" may occur (7). Azaperone does not induce significant analgesia. Painful manipulations can cause swine to awaken suddenly in an agitated state. A similar response is likely to occur when painful procedures are attempted without local or general anesthesia or during recovery, particularly when ketamine has been given intramuscularly to provide the analgesia absent with azaperone immobilization. However, ketamine and azaperone appear to be a workable combination of drugs if used judiciously.

In European countries, a frequently used injectable immobilizing combination is azaperone and metomidate (Hypnodil). The latter is a hypnotic agent that induces only minimal analgesia. Thus, this drug combination is often followed by general anesthesia (e.g., halothane in oxygen) or by local or regional analgesia (8). Otherwise, painful manipulations may result in abrupt, violent arousal. When the azaperone-metomidate combination is employed, azaperone is given at a dose of 2 mg/kg i.m. followed in 20 to 30 minutes with an initial dose of 3 to 4 mg/kg of metomidate i.v. To prolong restraint beyond 10 to 20 minutes, repeated administration of metomidate is required. Intraperitoneal administration of metomidate (10 mg/kg) after azaperone (2 mg/kg) has been advocated (9–11). However, the intrapertoneal route is followed by a rather long recovery (approximately 3 hours) and "peritonitis and the formation of adhesions" (7). Thus, its use by this route cannot be recommended.

Lenperone (Elanone-V) and droperidol (Inapsine) are two other butyrophenones that have been advocated for use in swine. Lenperone is administered at a rate of 0.4 to 1.6 mg/kg i.m. (12). Responses are similar to those of pigs receiving azaperone. Droperidol has been used to delay the onset of malignant hyperthermia in susceptible swine in doses of 0.02 to 2 mg/kg i.m. A dose of 0.18 mg/kg was effective for this purpose (13). Most commonly, droperidol is combined with fentanyl (Innovar-Vet) and used as a neuroleptanalgesic. Innovar-Vet is an expensive but satisfactory preanesthetic medication in swine if preceded by an anticholinergic (14), such as glycopyrrolate or atropine, to prevent fentanyl-induced bradycardia. The dose of Innovar-Vet is 1 ml/15 kg i.m. given 20 to 30 minutes before attempting i.v. catheter placement and induction of anesthesia (14). Another neuroleptanalgesic combination we have found useful in swine is lenperone (1 mg/kg i.m.) and butorphanol (Torbugesic) (0.3 mg/kg i.m.). The addition of ketamine (11 mg/kg i.m.) results in sufficient analgesia for hernia repair.

BENZODIAZEPINE

Of the benzodiazepine sedative hypnotics, only diazepam (Valium) has been used to any extent in swine. When used at the most frequently recommended dose, diazepam (1 to 2 mg/kg) has only a minimal effect upon cardiopulmonary function and thus has a high therapeutic index. Further evidence of diazepam's high therapeutic index is supported by the large dose (8.5 mg/kg) used to produce "excellent" sedation in swine. At this dose, pentobarbital requirements for general anesthesia were decreased by approximately 50% (5). Diazepam is an effective central muscle relaxant with long duration of action. Its sedative hypnotic effect is ideally suited for control of seizures, convulsions, and hyperexcitation that may be associated with dissociative anesthesia (e.g., ketamine). Because diazepam is relatively expensive, its use in pigs is limited.

THIAZINE DERIVATIVES

Xylazine (Rompun) possesses sedative, analgesic, and muscle-relaxing properties. Its potency is dose- and species-dependent. In swine, only marginal sedation occurs at a dose 10 times that inducing deep sedation, analgesia, and immobilization in cattle. However, xylazine's sedative, analgesic, and muscle-relaxing effects appear to be greater than additive when given in conjunction with an anesthetic agent (e.g., ketamine or a barbiturate). When used as a preanesthetic (1 to 2 mg/kg i.m.), the pig may vomit. We have also observed vomiting during the recovery period. At a dose of 1 to 2 mg/kg i.m., sedation is minimal, but a decreased response to injection or catheter placement suggests that a dose-dependent level of analgesia is present. Xylazine induces salivation and bradycardia; thus, it appears prudent to administer an anticholinergic. The use of xylazine in pigs is generally limited to its combination with anesthetic agents such as ketamine or barbiturates. Techniques that include xylazine will be discussed later.

Injectable Anesthetics

The injectable agents will be discussed under the headings of barbiturates, nonbarbiturates, and combinations of injectable anesthetics. The barbiturates consist of a very large number of compounds, but only pentobarbital (Nembutal), thiopental (Pentothal), thiamylal (Biotal), and methohexital (Brevital) are used to any extent in swine. Unfortunately, barbiturates are poor analgesics. In fact, sedative doses render swine hyperalgesic. Herein lies a major problem encountered with barbiturate anesthesia. When swine are given a barbiturate, the dose required to induce surgical anesthesia is very near the apneic dose. Thus, frequent repeated administration of small doses are required to maintain surgical anesthesia but may induce apnea. This practice leads to saturation of body tissue stores (e.g., muscle), which is accompanied by a prolonged recovery period. Even though barbiturates have been used extensively in all domestic species, fully establishing their safety and reliability under many circumstances, their major undesirable properties (e.g., poor muscle relaxation, severe respiratory depression, and poor analgesia) prevent them from fulfilling the criteria of the ideal injectable anesthetic agent for swine.

PENTOBARBITAL

Pentobarbital may be administered intramuscularly (4 to 6 mg/kg of a 3% solution) for sedation or controlling seizures or hyperexcitation. The later may be encountered during recovery of mature swine receiving intramuscular ketamine. The intramuscular route is not recommended for induction of surgical anesthesia because of the exceedingly large dose required. The intraperitoneal route may be used in individuals not having accessible veins for intravenous injection. By the intraperitoneal route, needle placement in the peritoneal cavity must be ensured by aspiration. With the pig held by its rear limbs so that the viscera gravitate toward the diaphragm, the needle is placed just off the midline and anterior to the pubic symphysis. For this purpose, a needle with a rounded tip (e.g., metal teat tube) will aid in ensuring that pentobarbital is not injected directly into visceral tissues. The dose ranges from 25 to 30 mg/kg. While the response to intraperitoneal pentobarbital is less predictable than when given intravenously, the maximum depth of anesthesia is attained in 20 to 30 minutes (7). Variation in response to intraperitoneal pentobarbital ranges from moderage sedation requiring local analgesia before surgery can be performed to deep surgical anesthesia with respiratory depression that may require mechanical ventilation. In the latter, provided apnea is effectively controlled, large doses of pentobarbital are well tolerated by healthy swine even though recovery may be quite prolonged.

Pentobarbital has been injected directly into the testicles of large boars to induce anesthesia for surgical castration. Anesthesia develops in 10 to 15 minutes after administration of 40 to 50 mg/kg. Castration should be performed as soon as anesthesia is present so that excess pentobarbital will be removed with the testicle, thus decreasing recovery time. Testicular tissue of these boars should be kept out of reach of other animals; otherwise its consumption could result in fatal toxicity. Intravenous pentobarbital (8 to 10 mg/kg) will induce a brief period of surgical anesthesia sufficient for castration of large boars. Experience with intratesticular injection of ketamine and xylazine (4 to 8 mg/kg and 2 to 3 mg/kg, respectively) has shown it to be effective. In our hands, this drug combination is superior for castration of large boars and has more or less replaced the use of pentobarbital.

Pentobarbital given intravenously for induction and maintenance of surgical anesthesia in swine is given at a dose of 30 mg/kg in pigs up to 50 kg. In mature swine, the dose is decreased by 10 to 20%. The injection should be made slowly with titration of the dose until the desired plane of anesthesia is achieved. Rapid administration, whether for initial induction or for supplementation of maintenance anesthesia, can easily result in apnea requiring respiratory support if death is to be prevented. Thus, tracheal intubation and maintenance of a patent airway is essential. Surgical anesthesia is of short duration (30 to 40 minutes). To prolong anesthesia, frequent supplemental doses must be given. This practice is often complicated by a prolonged period of immobilization and respiratory depression, with full recovery requiring as much as 6 to 8 hours, even though analgesia and muscle relaxation are insufficient for surgical manipulation. Surgery under such circumstances requires regional or locally induced analgesia (e.g., lidocaine infiltration of the surgical site).

METHOHEXITAL

Methohexital (2.5 to 5% solution) has been used satisfactorily for minor surgical procedures such as castration and detusking and to induce anesthesia followed by maintenance with an inhalation agent. Swine recovering from methohexital anesthesia may reveal signs of excitement characterized by vigorous head shaking. These signs are not observed when surgical anesthesia is maintained for a period of time with an inhalation agent following methohexital induction. For induction of a brief period of anesthesia, methohexital may be given intravenously at a dose of 8 to 12 mg/kg. Premedication with azaperone (1 to 2 mg/kg i.m.) will decrease the dose of methohexital and also enable safe prolongation of anesthesia with small incremental doses of methohexital without prolonging recovery (7).

THIOBARBITURATES (THIOPENTAL AND THIAMYLAL)

Because thiamylal's potency is between 1.25 and 1.5 times that of thiopental, it is more widely used in veterinary anesthesia. The thiobarbiturates are most often mixed as a 5% solution for adults or a 2.5% solution for young pigs. A 10% solution can be used, but it causes phlebitis, which may result in ear tissue necrosis. When pigs are premedicated with azaperone (1 to 2 mg/kg) and left undisturbed for 20 minutes, the dose of thiobarbiturate required to induce and maintain anesthesia is reduced considerably. It appears that azaperone antagonizes the respiratory depressing effect of the thiobarbiturates (7). It is quite possible that this impression is a direct result of the smaller dose of thiobarbiturate required to induce and maintain anesthesia in swine receiving a butyrophenone tranquilizer. In anesthetic doses, thiobarbiturates profoundly depress respiration. Rapid intravenous injection is frequently followed by 15 to 30 seconds of apnea. A slow rate of injection will prevent this problem. The excitatory response often encountered in the dog with slow intravenous injection is seldom observed in swine. The margin of safety of the thiobarbiturates is quite broad provided respiratory support is effectively used. Apnea occurring intraoperatively as a result of repeated administration of a barbiturate is more serious than the transient apnea frequently encountered upon induction. Thus, anesthesia of swine other than for a brief period of time for minor surgery should always be accompanied by tracheal intubation. Respiratory arrest in swine receiving thiobarbiturates should be of less concern if an endotracheal tube is in place and an Ambu bag or some other respiratory support device is immediately at hand to support ventilation. Cardiac dysrhythmias taking the form of bigeminal rhythm often occur after intravenous injection of thiamylal. This abnormal cardiac rhythm generally goes unnoticed unless the electrocardiogram (ECG) is monitored closely. Bigeminal rhythm in healthy swine receiving intravenous thiamylal appears to be of little importance.

The thiobarbiturates should be administered by the intravenous route. An auricular vein is most often chosen for this purpose. Originally, one-half of the calculated dose is injected rapidly. If apnea occurs, injection is discontinued until spontaneous breathing resumes, at which point injection is continued at a slow rate, titrating the injection to the desired state and plane of anesthesia. Incremental doses may be given to prolong surgical anesthesia. It must be understood that this practice will drastically increase the total recovery time and that apnea occurring during supplemental dosing is much more serious than that occurring after injection of the initial induction dose. It is imperative that apnea occurring during supplemental dosing be treated with mechanical ventilation if a catastrophic outcome is to be avoided.

We have found thiopental (10 to 20 mg/kg i.v.) or thiamylal (6 to 18 mg/kg i.v.) adequate for induction of anesthesia in swine. Preanesthetic medication with a tranquilizer (e.g., azaperone) or sedative (e.g., xylazine) will decrease the dose accordingly.

Combination of Injectable Agents

A thiobarbiturate may be combined with guaifenesin for induction and maintenance of short-term general anesthesia of swine. Guaifenesin is a central-acting muscle relaxant. It blocks transmission of nerve impulses at the internuncial neuron of the spinal cord (15), resulting in paralysis of the extremities. Diaphragmatic function is minimally affected; thus spontaneous respiration continues after its administration. Guaifenesin is mixed as a 5% solution in 5% dextrose in water. To this solution is added 2 mg/ml of thiamylal or 3 mg/ml of thiopental (GT). The solution is administered rapidly via a catheter placed in an auricular vein. When a small diameter catheter of perhaps 18 to 20 gauge is used, gravitational flow of GT will be slow and insufficient for induction of anesthesia in large swine. This problem may be overcome by pressurizing the bottle with air injected through the vent port. The dose required for induction of anesthesia is 1.0 ml/kg. Anesthesia may be maintained by continuing to drip GT to effect. The total dose should not exceed 4 ml/kg over a period of 1 hour.

A combination of agents that we have found effective for induction and maintenance of surgical anesthesia in swine is guaifenesin, ketamine, and xylazine (GKX) (16). We refer to this drug combination as "Triple 500" because the combination is prepared by adding 500 mg ketamine and 500 mg xylazine to 500 ml of 5% guaifenesin (prepared in 5% dextrose). In swine receiving atropine or glycopyrrolate, the induction dose is 1 ml/kg. If a preanesthetic (i.e., tranquilizer or sedative) is given, the induction dose may be reduced by as much as one-half. Surgical anesthesia may be safely extended by administering the mixture as a continuous i.v. infusion at a rate of 2.2 ml/kg/hr or to effect. The infusion rate is calculated as follows using a standard disposable i.v. administration set with a transparent drip chamber (Venoset-Abbott) for a 100-kg pig. Initially, the pig receives 100 ml (100 kg × 1 ml/kg), the loading or induction dose. Infusion is continued at a rate of 55 drops/min (15 drops/ml × 2.2 ml × 100 kg/60 min). Muscle relaxing and analgesic qualities are excellent. In contrast to thiobarbiturates alone and GT, apnea with GKX is encountered only with gross overdose. Studies in our laboratory and clinic confirm that respiration is only minimally affected by administration of a maintenance dose of GKX. In these studies, $PaCO_2$ values remained near 40 torr throughout 2 hours of surgical anesthesia, maintained with a continuous drip of GKX (16). Recovery is not accompanied by excitement and is quite rapid when compared to that of barbiturates. Recovery rate may be enhanced by reversal of the sedative effects of xylazine with yohimbine (0.125 mg/kg i.v.) and/or doxapram (0.5 to 1.0 mg/kg i.v.). Tolazoline (1 to 2 mg/kg i.v.) is also an effective reversal agent for xylazine sedation. The major drawback to use of GKX is the requirement for intravenous administration, which may be a problem in dark-skinned swine and in those in which veins have been disrupted by previous intravenous injection or by ear notching for purposes of animal identification.

KETAMINE

Since the first reports in the veterinary literature of the use of ketamine in swine (17, 18), it has become a major component of most anesthetic regimens used in this species. The unconscious state induced by ketamine has been described as "dissociative" or "cataleptoid" anesthesia. In swine, this state is not accompanied by visceral or somatic analgesia sufficient for major surgical intervention and thus it is generally supplemented with a sedative analgesic (xylazine), local analgesic (lidocaine), anesthetic (barbiturate), or tranquilizer (azaperone). Muscle tone is not obtunded as with other anesthetic agents (e.g., halothane), and tendinous reflexes are often exaggerated, resulting in frequent involuntary movement of extremities. Respiration is moderately depressed and characterized by an apneustic pattern, which promotes mild hypercapnia and hypoxemia. Oral and upper airway protective reflexes remain intact in proportion to the dose of ketamine. Other agents used to supplement ketamine may further obtund protective reflexes; thus tracheal intubation is advisable in order to fully ensure airway protection from aspiration of vomitus and oral secretions and provide a means for managing apnea.

In adult swine receiving ketamine by the intramuscular route, excitement during recovery is rather common. The response is accentuated if the animal is handled roughly during the induction procedure or disturbed during the recovery period. During recovery, sows receiving ketamine should be left undisturbed in a darkened warm area. If under such circumstances excitement does occur, it may be treated effectively with pentobarbital (2 to 6 mg/kg i.v. or 6 to 8 mg/kg i.m.). Diazepam (0.25 to 0.5 mg/kg i.v.) may be used in place of a barbiturate but is no more effective and much more expensive. Gentle handling and appropriate preanesthetic medication is generally all that is required to prevent excitement during the recovery period.

Administering ketamine rapidly by the intravenous route may cause apnea much like that encountered with barbiturates. Apnea induced by supplemental doses is much more life-threatening than that occurring at induction and thus requires immediate respiratory support if a catastrophy is to be avoided. Because ketamine tends to relax bronchial smooth muscle and dilate the bronchi, its choice in animals suffering from bronchial constrictive disease may promote better alveolar ventilation. This may be of significance in pigs reared in total confinement.

The cardiovascular effects of ketamine are a result of central sympathetic nervous stimulation and direct myocardial depression (19). Overall response is dose-related, with small doses causing central nervous system stimulation and larger doses resulting in myocardial depression (20). Clinically, cardiovascular response to ketamine is characterized by tachycardia, increased cardiac output, increased arterial blood pressure, and increased myocardial oxygen consumption when a moderate dose is given in unpremedicated swine (21). Ketamine possesses direct myocardial antidysrhythmic properties. However, its central actions can increase circulating catecholamines (20). Thus, the incidence of dysrhythmias may be increased by ketamine in patients receiving agents that sensitize the myocardium to circulating catecholamines. Unquestionably, ketamine is a useful and reliable anesthetic agent for swine when judiciously combined with supplemental agents. The large number of favorable reports in the veterinary literature fully supports this conclusion (2, 14, 16–18, 22, 23).

Administration of Ketamine

In swine, ketamine has become a major component of most injectable anesthetic regimens. Ketamine may be administered by either the intramuscular or intravenous route. Mature swine may react violently when ketamine is given by the intramuscular route if they have not received preanesthetic medication, for instance, with xylazine, diazepam, or azaperone (24). The most popular adjunct to ketamine anesthesia is xylazine, even though it does not induce pronounced sedation in swine when given i.m. at a dose of 1 to 2 mg/kg. Satisfactory anesthesia of short duration may be achieved with atropine (0.044 mg/kg i.m.) followed by xylazine (2.2 mg/kg i.m.) and ketamine (12 to 30 mg/kg i.m.). A mixture of ketamine and xylazine (0.5 to 1 ml of 100 mg/ml xylazine and 1 ml of 100 mg/ml ketamine) may be combined in the same syringe and given i.v. to safely prolong anesthesia. This mixture should be injected slowly if apnea is to be avoided.

A combination of xylazine (2 mg/kg i.v.), oxymorphone (0.075 mg/kg i.v.), and ketamine (2 mg/kg i.v.) mixed in the same syringe has been used to induce anesthesia in swine ranging from 40 to 100 kg in body weight. Narcosis, muscle relaxation, and analgesia were reported to be good. Cardiovascular and respiratory function were reasonably stable. Recovery was not accompanied by the delerium or aberrant behavior often occurring when ketamine is given as the sole anesthetic. By doubling the intravenous dose, a satisfactory response may be achieved by the intramuscular route (25).

Diazepam (1 to 2 mg/kg i.m.) may be used to supplement ketamine anesthesia. It will promote muscle relaxation through its central actions and ensure a smooth recovery. However, diazepam is not as strong as analgesic as xylazine, and it is much more expensive. Innovar-Vet (1 ml/15 kg i.m.) in pigs up to 45 kg pretreated with atropine (0.044 mg/kg i.m.) may be followed by ketamine (12 to 16 mg/kg i.m.) for 30 to 40 minutes of anesthesia satisfactory for hernia repair. Ketamine (2 to 3 mg/kg i.v. or 6 to 8 mg/kg i.m.) may be given as required to extend anesthesia (14). Cost, as with most injectable anesthetic regimens in swine, is a major drawback to this drug combination.

Acetylpromazine (0.4 mg/kg i.m.) followed in 30 minutes by ketamine (15 mg/kg i.m.) has been used to immobilize swine for 1 to 1.5 hours (22). Analgesia is poor, thus requiring local or regional analgesia for surgery of more than a minor nature. Azaperone (2 to 8 mg/kg i.m.) followed in 20 to 30 minutes by ketamine (10 to 20 mg/kg i.m.) will immobilize swine. Analgesia is sufficient for surgical manipulation. Swine should not be handled roughly during the administration process; otherwise an unfavorable response to this drug combination may result. Recently, in our hospital, we have combined ketamine (11 mg/kg i.m.), xylazine (2 mg/kg i.m.), and butorphanol (0.22 mg/kg i.m.) for anesthesia in pigs (5 to 20 kg) for umbilical hernia repair. Butorphanol appears to enhance analgesia without causing noticeable respiratory depression. A laboratory study is underway to further validate the safety and efficacy of this drug combination.

Steroidal Anesthetics

Saffan is a combination of alphaxolone (9 mg/ml) and alphadolone (3 mg/ml) with a total concentration of 12 mg/ml of steroids. These agents are poorly water-soluble. To overcome this problem, the steroids are prepared in a polyoxyethylated castor oil compound (cremophore EL). Because of the rather high incidence of hypersensitive reactions, which appear to be related to the solubilizing agent, approval of saffan for the veterinary market in the United States has been delayed. Saffan is approved for use in Canada and European countries, and it is from there that most reports on veterinary use have come. Clinical experience and reports from the veterinary literature suggest that saffan induces excellent muscle relaxation and profound analgesia, making it a useful drug in swine. Saffan may be given by either the intramuscular or intravenous route. Because of its low concentration (12 mg/ml), the intravenous route is preferred in order to decrease injection volume and cost. Induction is rapid following i.v. injection (4 to 6 mg/kg) and of short duration (10 to 15 minutes). Onset of anesthesia after intramuscular injection is slower but of longer duration and requires twice the intravenous dose. Anesthesia may be safely prolonged by intravenous supplementation (1 to 2 mg/kg). Recovery is smooth and rapid even after repeated intravenous injections with animals being able to stand approximately 30 minutes after the last injection (26). When swine are premediated with azaperone (4 mg/kg i.m.), the induction dose of saffan may be decreased by approximately 50% (7). In neonatal pigs, deep sedation, analgesia, and muscle relaxation may be induced with saffan (2 to 3 mg/kg i.m.) allowing placement of an i.v. catheter that will permit induction of anesthesia (saffan, 2 to 3 mg/kg i.v.). Anesthesia has been safely maintained for up to 2 hours in neonatal pigs with intravenous incremental injections (27).

Inhalation Anesthesia

Administration of inhalation anesthetics to swine requires an understanding of the physical and pharmacological characteristics of the inhalation agents and the machinery required for their administration (Chapter 14). Fortunately, the anatomical features of the pig's head make it well suited for the use of a nose cone for induction of anesthesia with an inhalation agent. Machines designed for use in small companion animals, such as dogs and cats, and humans are ideally suited for use in swine. Characteristics and operation of these machines are described in detail in Chapter 14. Nose cones are commerically available for small swine but not large mature animals. This problem is easily overcome by fashioning a nose cone from a plastic bottle such as a large soda pop bottle. After the bottom of the bottle has been cut away, the edges should be padded with rubber or plastic foam so that an airtight seal can be maintained between the edges of the nose cone and the pig's snout; otherwise, inhalation will entrain atmospheric air around the edges of the nose cone, diluting the inspired anesthetic concentration and prolonging induction. With a properly fitted nose cone, anesthesia may be induced and maintained with any of the volatile inhalation agents, such as halothane, isoflurane, or enflurane. These volatile agents may be supplemented with nitrous oxide (N_2O) for its additive effect. Nitrous oxide may be used to hasten induction by utilizing the "second gas effect." The "second gas effect" is employed by allowing the pig to breath an inhalation agent (e.g., halothane) in oxygen until signs of onset of anesthesia are apparent (e.g., gradually increasing halothane concentration up to 3 to 5% in 4 liters of oxygen over a period of 3 to 4 minutes), at which time oxygen flow is decreased to 2 liters and N_2O flow is quickly increased from no flow to 4 liters/minute. Induction of anesthesia with this technique is achieved quickly with only minimal struggling. Induction of surgical anesthesia is followed by tracheal intubation (endotracheal tube sizes are given in Table 1) and maintenance of surgical anesthesia with halothane (2% in oxygen) or a combination of halothane (1.5 to 2% in oxygen) and N_2O (50 to 70%). For an average-size pig of 45 to 90 kg, settings on the anesthetic machine for maintenance of surgical anesthesia might be oxygen flow, 1.5 to 2 liters/min, and N_2O, 1.5 to 3 liters/min with a halothane vaporizer setting of 1.5 to 2%, depending on the depth of anesthesia required. When N_2O is not employed, reasonable machine settings for maintenance of surgical anesthesia are oxygen flow, 1 to 3 liters/min with a halothane vaporizer setting of 2 to 2.5%. In the final stages of surgery, halothane concentration may be decreased to 1 to 1.5%. When N_2O has been used as part of the maintenance regimen, it should be discontinued and the pig allowed to breath oxygen alone for at least 5 minutes before disconnecting the endotracheal tube from the anesthetic machine. This measure will prevent the development of "diffusion hypoxia" as N_2O rapidly diffuses from the blood into the alveoli.

In the author's experience, isoflurane, like halothane, is a highly desirable anesthetic in swine. Its major drawback, as in other species, is cost. Due to the low economic value of the individual market pig, inhalation anesthetics in general are not cost-effective in swine. However, in valuable breeding stock, inhalation anesthetic techniques can be used effectively and economically. Inhalation techniques (i.e., halothane or halothane and N_2O) are commmonly employed for a Caesarean delivery of specific pathogen-free pigs.

Specific Anesthetic Agents

NITROUS OXIDE

Nitrous oxide, as mentioned earlier, can be used effectively when employing the "second gas effect" for purposes of induction. Otherwise, it is not a potent anesthetic in swine. Because the anesthetic effect of two or more inhalation agents is additive (28), N_2O is often combined with the more potent agents (e.g., halothane, isoflurane, or enflurane). The minimum alveolar concentration (MAC) for N_2O in swine has recently been determined by using an extrapolation technique based upon the fact that the accumulative effects among inhalation agents are additive (29, 30). Results of these studies show that N_2O MAC of swine (195% to 277%) is considerably greater than that of humans (100 to 105%) (31). Unless hyperbaric conditions are employed, anesthesia of swine with N_2O alone cannot be achieved. If the MAC value for N_2O of people is used for swine, then swine will be less deeply anesthetized. Thus, the practice of using a narcotic dose of N_2O and a potent muscle relaxant such as pancuronium, as has been reported in some cardiovascular studies, cannot be recommended as an anesthetic regimen in swine because of the low potency of N_2O in this species. Because the N_2O MAC for swine is approximately twice that of humans N_2O should only be used in combination with a potent analgesic to ensure the absence of pain during surgery.

HALOTHANE

Halothane is a potent anesthetic that has been studied extensively in swine. In this species, halothane produces dose-dependent depression of cardiovascular function characterized by decreased cardiac output, stroke volume, arterial blood pressure, rate pressure product, and ventricular work. The decrease in cardiac output is a reflection of left ventricular myocardial depression in as much as heart rate is altered only slightly at clinically useful concentrations (i.e., 1 to 1.5 MAC) (32, 33). Halothane does not alter heart rate in response to decreased arterial blood pressure. This suggests that it depresses baroreceptor-mediated reflexes (34). However, a recent study has shown that halothane induces bradycardia in neonatal pigs (35). Whether or not bradycardia in these piglets is a reflection of the relationship of age to the effects of halothane is unknown at this time. However, it is possible that baroreceptors become more responsive as pigs age (36).

ISOFLURANE

Isoflurane is less potent (MAC 1.58; average of MAC values reported for swine, which range from 1.45 to 1.75; variation in MAC values may be related to breed, age, circadian rhythm, body temperature, type of stimulus, and other factors) than halothane (MAC (0.91). Because of its low blood-gas solubility, however, anesthesia may be rapidly induced via nose cone (4 to 5% in oxygen). The addition of N_2O (60 to 70%) employing the "second gas effect," as discussed with halothane, will increase the speed of induction. Because of isoflurane's low solubility, as compared to halothane or methoxyflurane, the depth of anesthesia can be rapidly altered to meet existing surgical requirements. Recovery is rapid and free from excitement. With light surgical levels of anesthesia, cardiovascular function is well maintained (37). As the depth of anesthesia is increased, dose-dependent decrease in cardiopulmonary function occurs (38), but seizure activity as may occur with enflurane is absent (37). However, results of most studies in swine and other species indicate that isoflurane is less depressing to cardiovascular function than is halothane at comparable depths of anesthesia (37). Blood flow to most body tissues is well maintained in swine with isoflurane (38). Isoflurane, as other halogenated ethers, does not predispose the myocardium to epinephrine-induced dysrhythmias to the same degree as does halothane. It has been suggested that intraoperative dysrhythmias occurring with halothane (i.e., in dogs and cats) may be ameliorated by switching to isoflurane (39).

ENFLURANE

Enflurane is an ether derivative similar to isoflurane but more soluble and less potent (MAC 2.2 in the dog). In our laboratory, we have observed that high inspired concentrations of enflurane are often characterized by seizure activity in swine. Cardiovascular function is depressed to a greater degree with enflurane than with either halothane or isoflurane. When anesthesia in young swine was maintained with 4% inspired influrane, mean arterial blood pressure, cardiac output, stroke volume, left ventricular work, systemic vascular resistance, and rate pressure product were all decreased significantly (40).

Methoxyflurane

Methoxyflurane is a halogenated ether, as is isoflurane and enflurane. It is high soluble in blood and body tissues. This physical characteristic causes a prolonged induction time unless it is used with N_2O employing the "second gas effect" (41). Methoxyflurane depresses cardiovascular function in a dose-dependent manner that is characterized by decreased cardiac output, stroke volume, stroke work, mean arterial blood pressure, and systemic vascular resistance (42, 43). An increase in heart rate is thought to be in response to hypotension and an intact baroreceptor reflex mechanism (43).

Even though inhalation anesthesia, for example with halothane, isoflurane, enflurane, or methoxyflurane), is accompanied by a dose-dependent decrease in cardiovascular function, it offers a stable, readily controllable form of anesthesia. The main disadvantage of inhalation anesthesia centers around cost of the agents and equipment required for administration. Although compatible with the inhalation agents, peripheral-acting muscle relaxants are used infrequently in swine under clinical conditions. A full discussion of these agents is presented in Chapter 9.

Malignant Hyperthermia

Malignant hyperthermia (MH) is a genetically linked condition of swine (44) and humans that is encountered infrequently in other mammalian species. Although MH has been diagnosed in all breeds of swine, it occurs most commonly in Pietrain, Landrace, Spotted Swine, Poland China, and swine of Large White breeding. The incidence in the Duroc breed appears to be relatively low. Swine possessing the MH trait will often experience sudden onset of the condition when subjected to the stress of restraint and handling, vigorous exercise, high environmental temperature, transportation, or combining with unfamiliar swine. Chemical restraint can also initiate the occurrence of MH. In highly susceptible individuals, breathing halothane in oxygen will quickly trigger the onset of MH. Less susceptible pigs not reacting to halothane alone will often develop MH following succinylcholine administration. Anesthesia induced and maintained with thiopental and N_2O in oxygen may not induce MH in swine with low susceptibility. The addition of halothane and/or succinylcholine in such swine can quickly trigger onset of the condition.

Clinically, MH is characterized by rapid onset of muscle rigidity, tachycardia, tachpnea, and hyperthermia; rectal temperature may reach 108°F or more. Dyspnea follows, progressing to apnea, cardiac dysrhythmias, bradycardia, and death. In light-skinned pigs, erythematous splotches will develop, particularly on the ventral-most portion of the abdomen. Death is a result of severe acidosis, hyperkalemia, hyperchatecholemia, and finally, circulatory failure.

In our hospital and laboratory, we have observed the onset of MH in a matter of minutes in pigs breathing halothane in oxygen via nose cone. At the other extreme, susceptible pigs receiving intravenous thiopental and administered halothane in oxygen after tracheal intubation did not develop clinical signs of MH for some 20 to 30 minutes after receiving halothane. The delayed response in the latter pigs may have been due to the protective effects of thiopental (45) or the lack of stress accompanying restraint of pigs required for nose cone induction with halothane. Recently, it has been shown that treatment of MH-susceptible swine with acetylpromazine prior to anesthesia with halothane in oxygen will effectively delay onset of the condition (46). When MH has reached a stage of development characterized by muscle rigidity, dyspnea, and appearance of cardiac dysrhythmias, most swine will die in spite of attempts to reverse the condition. When MH is recognized early in its course of development, quickly removing the pig from halothane and instituting supportive measures (i.e., body cooling by emersing the pig in ice water, intravenous sodium bicarbonate, ventilation with oxygen free from all traces of halothane, and so on) may be helpful in arresting further development of the condition. Only dantrolene (5 to 10 mg/kg i.v.) has been shown to be effective in treating and preventing MH in susceptible swine (47). More recently, a smaller dose of dantrolene (2 to 3 mg/kg i.v.) has been shown to effectively reverse malignant hyperthermia of swine (48).

References

1. Lee JC, Stoll BJ, Downing SE: Properties of the laryngeal chemoreflex in neonatal piglets. *Am J Physiol* 233:R30–R36, 1977.
2. Riebold TW, Thurmon JC: Anesthesia in swine. In Tumbleson, ME (ed): *Swine in Biomedical Research* 1986 (in press).
3. Thurmon JC, Tranquilli WJ: Anesthesia for cardiovascular research. In Stanton HC, Mersmann JH (eds): *Swine in Cardiovascular Research*. Boca Raton, FL, CRC Press Inc, 1986, in press.
4. Booth NH: Psychotropic agents. In Booth NH, McDonald LE (eds): *Veterinary Pharmacology and Therapeutics*, ed 5. Ames, The Iowa State University Press, 1982, p 321.
5. Ragan HA, Gillis MF: Restraint, venipuncture, endotracheal intubation, and anesthesia of miniature swine. *Lab Anim Sci* 23:409–419, 1975.
6. Jones RS: A review of tranquilization and sedation in large animals. *Vet Rec* 90:613–617, 1972.
7. Hall LW, Clark KW: *Veterinary Anesthesia*, ed 8. London, Bailliere Tindall, 1983, p 287.
8. Anderson IL: Anesthesia of swine. *N Z Vet J* 25:319–321, 1977.
9. Ravaud M: Une nouvelle methode d'anesthesia dela truie lors de cesariennes realisees pour obtenirdes animaux. *SPF Recl Med Vet EC Alfort* 148:1245–1249, 1972.
10. Callear JFF, Van Gestel JFE: An analysis of the results of field experiments in pigs in the U.K. and Eire with the combination anesthetic azaperone and metomidate. *Vet Rec* 92:284–287, 1973.
11. Porter DB, Slasser CA: Azaperone: a review of a new neuroleptic agent for swine. *Vet Med* 80:88–92, 1985.
12. Short CE: Preanesthetic medication in ruminants and swine. In Thurmon JC (ed): *Veterinary Clinics of North America, Food Animal Anesthesia*. Philadelphia, WB Saunders 1986, in press.
13. McGrath CJ, Rempel WE, Addis PB, Crinn AJ: Acepromazine and droperidol inhibition of halothane-induced malignant hyperthermia (porcine stress syndrome) in swine. *Am J Vet Res* 42:195–198, 1981.
14. Benson GJ, Thurmon JC: Anesthesia of swine under field conditions. *J Am Vet Med Assoc* 174:594–596, 1979.
15. Westhues M, Fritsch R: *Animal Anesthesia, General Anesthesia*. London, Oliver and Boyd, 1965, vol 2, p 184.
16. Thurmon JC, Tranquilli WJ, Benson GJ: Glyceryl guaiacolate, ketamine, and xylazine: balanced anesthesia by intravenous infusion in swine. *Vet Surg* (abstract) 14:17, 1985.
17. Thurmon JC, Nelson DR, Christie GJ: Ketamine anesthesia in swine. *J Am Vet Assoc* 162:293–297, 1972.
18. Roberts FW: Anesthesia in pigs, intramuscular ketamine as an induction agent. *Anesthesia* 26:445–449, 1971.
19. Dowdy EA, Kaya K: Studies of the mechanism of cardiovascular response to CI-581. *Anesthesiology* 29:931–935, 1968.
20. Roberts JG: Intravenous anesthetic agents. In Prys-Roberts C (ed), *The Circulation in Anesthesia, Applied Physiology, and Pharmacology*. Oxford, Blackwell Scientific Publications, p 459, 1980.
21. Tranquilli WJ, Thurmon JC, Benson GJ: Organ blood flow and distribution of cardiac output in hypocapnic ketamine-anesthetized swine. *Am J Vet Res* 46:1578–1582, 1983.
22. Gray KN, Roulston GL, Flow BL, Jardine JH, Huchton JI: Repeated immobilization of miniature swine with an acepromazine-ketamine combination. *Southwest Veterinarian* 31:27–30, 1978.
23. Trim CM, Gilroy BA: Cardiopulmonary effects of a xylazine and ketamine combination in pigs. *Res Vet Sci* 38:30–34, 1985.
24. Thurmon JC: Injectable anesthetic agents and techniques in ruminants and swine. In *Veterinary Clinics of North America Food Animal Anesthesia*. Philadelphia, WB Saunders 1986, in press.
25. Breese C, Dodman NH: Xylazine-ketamine-oxymorphone: an injectable anesthetic combination in swine. *J Am Vet Med Assoc* 184:182–183, 1984.
26. Cox JE, Done SH, Lee SP, Walton JR: Preliminary studies of the actions of alphaxolone and alphadalone in the pig. *Vet Rec* 97:497–498, 1975.
27. Green CJ, Halsey MJ, Precious S, Wardley-Smith B: Alphaxolone-alphadalone anesthesia in laboratory animals. *Lab Anim* 12:85–89, 1978.
28. DiFazio CA, Brown RE, Ball CG, Heckel CG, Kennedy SS: Addi-

tive effects of anesthetics and theories of anesthesia. *Anesthesiology* 36:57–63, 1976.
29. Weiskopf RB, Bogetz MS: Minimum alveolar concentrations (MAC) of halothane and nitrous oxide in swine. *Anest Analg* 63:529–532, 1984.
30. Tranquilli WJ, Thurmon JC, Benson GJ: Anesthetic potency of nitrous oxide in young swine (*sus scrofa*). *Am J Vet Res* 46:58–60, 1985.
31. Quasha AL, Eger EI II: MAC. In Miller RD (ed): *Anesthesia*, New York, Churchill Livingston, 1981, p 257.
32. Brower R, Merin RG: Left ventricular function and compliance in swine during halothane anesthesia. *Anesthesiology* 50:409–415, 1979.
33. Merin RG, Verdow PD, deJong JW: Dose-dependent depression of cardiac function and metabolism of halothane in swine (*sus scrofa*). *Anesthesiology* 46:417–423, 1977.
34. Duke PC, Fownes D, Wade JG: Halothane depresses baroreflex control of heart rate in man. *Anesthesiology* 46:184–187, 1977.
35. Boudreaux JP, Schieber RA, Cook DR: Hemodynamic effects of halothane in the newborn piglet. *Anesth Analg* 63:731–737, 1984.
36. Gootman PM, Gootman N, Buckley BJ: Maturation of central autonomic control of the circulation. *Fed Proc* 42:1648–1655, 1983.
37. Eger EI II: *Isoflurane: A Compendium and Reference*. Madison, WI, Ohio Medical Products (Anaquest), 1985.
38. Lundeen G, Manohar M, Parks C: Systemic distribution of blood flow in swine while awake and during 1.0 and 1.5 MAC isoflurane anesthesia with and without 50% nitrous oxide. *Anesth Analg* 62:499–512, 1983.
39. Hubble JAE, Muir WW, Bednarski RM, et al: Change of inhalation anesthetic agents for management of ventricular premature depolarization in anesthetized cats and dogs. *J Am Vet Assoc* 185:643–646, 1984.
40. Tranquilli WJ, Manohar M, Parks CM, Thurmon JC, Theodorakis MC, Benson GJ: Systemic and regional blood flow in unanesthetized swine and swine anesthetized with halothane + nitrous oxide, halothane, or enflurane. *Anesthesiology* 56:369–379, 1982.
41. Benson GJ, Hartsfield SM, Thurmon JC: A method of anesthetizing pigs using small animal inhalation anesthetic equipment. *Pract Vet* 49:20–25, 1977.
42. Sawyer DC, Lumb WV, Stone HL: Cardiovascular effects of halothane, methoxyflurane, pentobarbital, and thiamylal. *J Appl Physio* 30:36–43, 1971.
43. Hickey RF, Eger EI II: Circulatory effects of inhaled anesthetics. In Prys-Roberts C (ed): *The Circulation in Anesthesia: Applied Physiology and Pharmacology*. Oxford, Blackwell Scientific Publications, 1980, p 441.
44. Campion DR, Topel DG: A review of the role of swine skeletal muscle in malignant hyperthermia. *J Anim Sci* 41:779–786, 1975.
45. Harrison GG, Saunders SJ, Biebuyck JF, Hickman R, Dent DM, Weaver V, Terblanche J: Anesthetic-induced malignant hyperpyrexia and a method of its prediction. *Brti J Anesth* 41:844, 1969.
46. McGrath CJ, Rampel WE, Addis PB, Crimi AJ: Acepromazine and droperidol inhibition of halothane-induced malignant hyperthermia (porcine stress syndrome) in swine. *Am J Vet Res* 42:195–198, 1981.
47. Gronert GA, Milde JH, Theye RA: Dantrolene in porcine malignant hyperthermia. *Anesthesiology* 44:488–495, 1976.
48. Alitalo I, Schulman A: Halothane induced pòrcine malignant hyperthermia reversed by dantrolene. *Nord Vet-Med* 35:239–242, 1983.

PART 5

Avian and Wildlife Anesthesia

Avian Anesthesia

KATHLEEN A. LINN. D.V.M., and ROBIN D. GLEED, B.V.Sc., M.R.C.V.S., D.V.A., D.A.C.V.A.

Introduction

Because of the obvious differences between birds and mammals, as well as lack of familiarity with the multitude of avian species, many veterinarians are reluctant to anesthetize birds. However, with the increasing popularity of pet birds and rising interest in wild bird medicine, more veterinarians will need this skill. It is the purpose of this section to review some of the principles that must be understood to anesthetize birds safely.

Local Anesthesia

Local anesthesia is seldom used on birds for a number of reasons. First, cutaneous sensation in birds is limited compared with that of mammals, and thus minor procedures such as the suturing of skin lacerations seem to cause them little pain (1). Secondly, although local anesthesia may deaden any pain the patient is perceiving, it does little to protect it from stress. More than one pet budgerigar has been known to die during handling. With wild birds who have had little contact with humans, the effects of manipulation can be equally as devasting. It is often safer to avoid the stress factor as much as possible by rendering the bird in hand unconscious. Finally, the small size of many avian patients makes overdosage of local anesthesia agents a real danger. A volume of 2% lidocaine as small as 0.5 ml administered to a budgerigar well exceeds the 50% lethal dose (LD_{50}) reported for dogs on a milligram per kilogram basis (2). Dosages of 2% lidocaine reported to be reasonably safe for birds are in the range of 20 mg/kg or less (1). Birds do seem to tolerate small amounts of topical anesthetics, such as proparicaine eye drops and lidocaine ointment (1).

Injectable General Anesthetics

Injectable anesthetics require little equipment and are convenient for many of the short procedures common to birds, such as radiography, wound repair, and laparoscopy. A few problems attend the use of agents given by this route, however. The weight of the bird must be known so that drug dosage can be accurately calculated. Determining an appropriate dosage may be difficult when the patient is a small bird with a large tumor, which is a rather common occurrence in budgerigars (3). Most importantly, once the drug has been injected, it is difficult to control the depth and duration of anesthesia. Thus, injectable agents are less desirable for long procedures or critically ill patients.

BARBITURATES

Many of the barbiturates have been tried in birds with varying degrees of success. Ultrashort-acting barbiturates have been used in some of the larger raptors and were found to provide about 10 minutes of useful anesthesia (1, 4). The approximate dose of sodium thiamylal is 0.2 ml/kg i.v. of a 2.5% solution given slowly (1).

Pentobarbital is one of the more versatile of the barbiturates. It has been used in a wide number of species and can be given by intramuscular, intravenous, and even oral routes (4, 5). Duration of the anesthesia induced by any of these routes is about 30 minutes in most species (4), but recovery is generally prolonged and may take up to 12 hours (3). The recommended i.m. dosage is 50 mg/kg (1).

A combination of pentobarbital, chloral hydrate, and magnesium sulfate has been used in a large number of species with relative success (1, 6). The i.v. dosage is 1.0 to 1.5 ml/kg; the i.m. dosage is 2.5 ml/kg (2.0 ml/kg in obese or debilitated birds) (1). Induction by the more commonly used intramuscular route takes from 10 to 35 minutes, and duration of action is from 25 to 90 minutes (7). Muscle necrosis may occur when the drug is given intramuscularly (1).

In general, although barbiturates can be used successfully, their relatively narrow margin of safety and prolonged recovery period make them less desirable than some of the other agents available.

METOMIDATE

Metomidate is not available in the United States, but has been used for avian anesthesia, especially on raptors, in other countries. Its duration of action is usually 10 to 40 minutes (4). The dosage may be repeated to prolong its effect (8). The drug is administered i.m., and dosages vary from 3 to 20 mg/kg (4), with the lower dose providing immobilization (9) and the higher doses provide light anesthesia for minor procedures (8). Metomidate is a poor analgesic, and deeper planes of anesthesia are not possible (10), rendering it appropriate for major surgical procedures. A major drawback to the use of metomidate is the long recovery period most birds experience. This ranges from less than 6 to more than 40 hours, depending on the species of bird and dose received (11). In addition, it produces copious salivation that is nonresponsive to atropine (11). This could be dangerous in small birds whose airways are easily obstructed.

CT 1341 (SAFFAN)

CT 1341 (Saffan, made by Glaxco Laboratories Ltd) is a steroid anesthetic that, like metomidate, is not available in America. Given by the i.v. route at a dose of about 10 mg/kg, it rapidly produces a surgical plane of anesthesia (9) lasting from 5 to 15 minutes (3, 12, 13). This dosage can be repeated if necessary (14). Saffan has been given by the i.m. route, but the volumes required are so large as to be prohibitive in many birds, and the plane of anesthesia produced is so light as to be appropriate for restraint only (9). The chief advantage to the use of Saffan is the relatively rapid recovery birds make from this drug. In all species, recovery takes less than 30 minutes (10, 14), and most are standing and feeding within 15 minutes (9). However, episodes of sinus arrest, cardiac arrhythmias, and apnea and occasional deaths have been reported in birds receiving the recommended intravenous dose of this drug (12–14). Red-tailed hawks appear to be especially sensitive to Saffan, and a dosage of 5 mg/kg is recommended for them (12). All birds appear to develop a transient bradycardia on induction that rapidly gives way to a tachycardia (13, 14). In general, Saffan appears to be a useful injectable anesthetic agent, but careful monitoring of cardiac and respiratory function must accompany its administration.

KETAMINE

Of the injectable anesthetics available in this country, ketamine is the most widely used. Given intramuscularly, it takes from 3 to 5 minutes to produce anesthesia of approximately 10 to 30 minutes duration. Its recovery period is longer than that associated with Saffan; birds take from 30 minutes to 5 hours to stand after administration of ketamine (1). Dosage varies from species to species, but in general it is inversely proportional to body weight on a per kilogram basis. The most widely cited intramuscular dosage scheme is that proposed by Boener and Wright (Table 13.5) (15). Large raptors seem to do best when given between 25 and 50 mg/kg (1). Our experience indicates 30 to 40 mg/kg i.m. has worked well to anesthetize raptors for radiography and laparoscopy.

Ketamine can be given intravenously to larger birds; this rapidly induces anesthesia that lasts from 15 minutes to several hours (16, 17). It may be combined with intravenous diazepam to smooth induction and recovery and enhance muscle relaxation. The usual dosage of ketamine is 30 to 40 mg/kg and of diazepam is 1.0 to 1.5 mg/kg (17). As with the intramuscular route, there is substantial variation in the amount of anesthetic required by different species. Owls appear to be especially sensitive. It has been suggested that the optimal dosage for strigiforms is 25 mg/kg, with the exception of the barred owl, which needs only a dosage of 10 mg/kg (17). It is important to inject the drug slowly and to give the drug in divided doses separated by a few minutes if the total amount given is more than 50 mg because too much ketamine given too quickly can result in apnea and even cardiac arrest (17).

Ketamine dosage by either route can be repeated if necessary (1, 17). The duration of anesthesia as well as the recovery time is dose-dependent; birds given heavier doses take longer to wake up (15, 18). Depth of anesthesia is also dependent on dose. However, analgesia appears to be incomplete even at the highest dosages (1, 11, 16).

When ketamine is administered properly it has little effect on respiration, but heart rate does tend to decrease (3, 17). There are several problems with the use of ketamine. The questionable degree of analgesia obtained has already been mentioned. Also, the recovery period can be rather long on occasion. Excessive salivation has been reported (17), although this does not seem to occur as consistently as it does with metomidate. Most workers have found muscle relaxation to be poor under ketamine, with tremors and wing flapping quite common. Recovery can also be quite violent (1, 15, 16). This can be a real problem during orthopedic procedures. The addition of intravenous diazepam to the anesthetic protocol appears to alleviate this problem somewhat (19). Xylazine (up to 5 mg/kg i.m.) has been administered to large birds as a premedication to ketamine (10 to 20 mg/kg i.m.), thus increasing the muscle relaxation and analgesia produced by the ketamine (1). However, this combination may produce profound cardiovascular and central nervous system depression. Finally, although ketamine is generally considered a safe anesthetic agent for birds, its therapeutic index (at least in chickens) is only 4.85 (16), making accurate dosage critical. It is possible to overdose birds if they have a higher than average amount of body fat (19).

Table 13.5
Intramuscular Dosages of Ketamine by Body Weight (Boener & Wright 15)[a]

Body Weight (g)	Intramuscular Dosage (mg/g)	Intramuscular Dosage (mg/kg)
100	0.1–0.2	100–200
250–500	0.05–0.1	50–100
500–3000	0.02–0.1	20–100
3000	0.02–0.05	20–50

[a] In using this table it is helpful to remember that the average budgerigar weighs 30 g, the average pigeon weighs 300 g, and great horned owls tend to weigh about 1 kg.

Inhalation Anesthesia

Inhalation anesthesia is the method of choice for lengthy or involved procedures because it can be maintained for as long as necessary and the depth of anesthesia can be controlled. Because recovery from some of the inhalation anesthetic agents is quite rapid, this is also a desirable method for anesthetizing patients for short procedures.

Avian anatomy differs considerably from that of mammals, and this has some important implications for how birds should be given inhaled anesthetics. The avian respiratory system is composed of a group of cranial and caudal air sacs connected to each other via large mesobronchi and to the lungs through ventrobronchi and dorsobronchi (Figure 13.23). Gas exchange in the lungs occurs in tubular parabronchi rather than in dead-ended alveoli such as mammals have. During

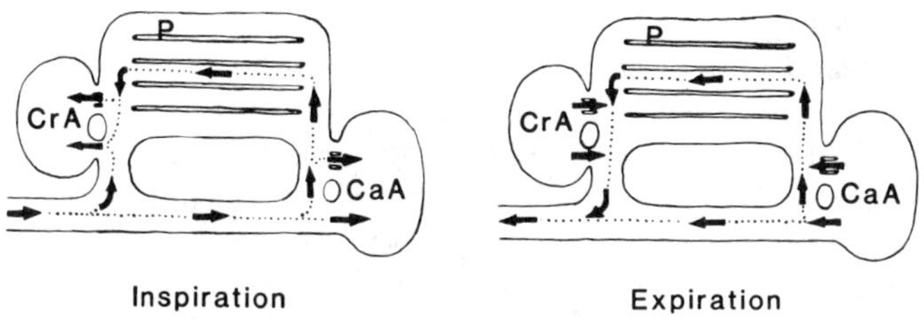

Figure 13.23. Schematic representative of the avian respiratory system. Note the unidirectional flow in the parabronchi (P) during both inspiration and expiration. CrA, cranial air sac group; CaA, caudal air sac group.

respiration, air flows into and out of the air sacs, which serve largely as reservoirs, but parabronchial airflow remains unidirectional throughout inspiration and expiration (20). Compared to that of mammals, the avian lung has a much higher surface to volume ratio and a thinner blood-air barrier, making it more efficient at gas exchange (21). This may account for the more rapid induction times seen in avian anesthesia as well as the sudden and dramatic changes in anesthetic concentration or respiratory rate (10, 22). Birds have about the same total volume of gas in their respiratory systems (proportional to body size) as mammals (21), largely because of the presence of their air sacs. This means that birds have far less functional residual capacity in their parabronchi than mammals do in their alveoli. Blood oxygenation can only occur if a constant flow of gas is maintained in the parabronchi. Apnea, therefore, results in death much more quickly in birds than in mammals. Some researchers feel that the large amount of gas stored in the air sacs makes birds relatively inefficient at eliminating inhaled anesthetics (7). They suggest that oxygen should be continued after anesthetics are turned off while the birds are clearing their air sacs of residual anesthetic gases.

Because birds lack diaphragms, air is pumped through their respiratory systems by a bellows-like contraction and expansion of their ribcage and sternum. Anything which prevents them from moving their chests will prevent them from breathing. Great care must be taken while restraining birds not to restrict their breathing movements. During surgery the anesthetist must be vigilant enough to prevent weight on the bird's sternum, whether from draping, instruments, or the surgeon's heavy hands, from causing apnea. On small birds, artificial respiration can be accomplished by mimicking pumping action with intermittent pressure on the sternum (3). Larger birds can be given positive pressure ventilation in the same way as mammals.

The depth and frequency of avian respiration is controlled by many of the same mechanisms that influence mammalian breathing. However, birds are especially sensitive to carbon dioxide concentrations in inspired air. They possess carbon dioxide-sensitive pulmonary receptors that play a role in regulating respiratory frequency (23). Respiration is vastly reduced in the absence of carbon dioxide. When pure oxygen is instilled into the air sacs, birds may become apneic (2). Systems that allow some carbon dioxide to be rebreathed may be desirable for avian anesthesia.

Two rather different methods exist for delivering anesthetic gases to birds. A nonrebreathing system utilizing an Ayre's T-piece or a Bain apparatus works well for birds, which generally lack the tidal volume and force to overcome the resistance inherent in a circle system. Gas can be administered either by face mask or (better) through an endotracheal tube. The recommended gas flow for a bird on a nonrebreathing system is at least 660 ml/kg min. Generally flow rates of 1 to 3 liters/minute are used (7, 10).

Another gas delivery system makes use of the constant undirectional flow through the parabronchi described earlier. By this method gas that has been bubbled through warm water to moisturize it is instilled into an air sac through a needle, catheter, or teat cannula so that it passes from the air sac through the parabronchi and out through the trachea (21). Usually either the interclavicular (22, 24) or abdominal (22) air sac is used for this instillation. Because most of the air flowing through the parabronchi during expiration comes from the caudal air sac group (20), the abdominal air sac seems the most logical choice for cannulation. However, because there is little communication between the caudal air sacs and lungs from one side of the bird to the other, perhaps a cannula placed in each of the abdominal air sacs would be best. Birds anesthetized by this method are apneic despite adequate oxygenation because the instilled gas contains no carbon dioxide (23). This removes the most important parameter usually monitored for depth of anesthesia, respiratory rate, making careful observation of heart rate and reflexes critical. However, this method ensures adequate ventilation of patients and carries with it the added bonus of supplying moisturized air to the respiratory membranes. Dead space and stored anesthetic gas problems are eliminated (23), making more rapid control of anesthetic depth possible. Gas is generally delivered at a rate of about 1 liter/kg/min (3). This method is not recommended for birds weighing less than 50 g (22), probably because such birds would require such a small total gas flow that there would be inconsistent vaporization of anesthetic and inaccurate measurement of the amount of gas being instilled into the air sacs. Because aspiration can still occur, birds are usually intubated during air sac instillation (23).

Induction can be accomplished by any of a number of methods. Ketamine can be given intravenously or intramuscularly to anesthetize the patient enough to perform intubation. Alternatively, inhalation anesthesia may be used. Birds that are easily restrained can be mask-induced. A cat face mask works well for caged birds (1, 14, 25), whereas smaller specimens can be subdued by use of a face mask fashioned from a syringe case (25). A tank induction chamber may also be used. One may even anesthetize a bird in its own cage by enclosing the cage in a plastic bag containing oxygen and anesthetic gases administered through an opening in the bag (26). A clear plastic bag is preferred to enable one to monitor the degree of relaxation and response to anesthetics. The bird is adequately induced when it is no longer flapping its wings and its neck is fairly limp, but is breathing well and has its palpebral, corneal, and pedal reflexes intact (1).

Intubation can be accomplished in any bird weighing 100 g or more (22). An illustration of the glottis to facilitate intubation is shown in Figure 13.24. For most birds, small uncuffed Cole tubes work well. Cuffed tubes may be used in larger birds, but care must be taken not to overinflate the cuff, because avian tracheas have circumferential rings and are therefore unable to expand (1, 10, 16). To minimize dead space, any tube used should be cut so that it does not protrude beyond the end of the beak (7). Birds are easily intubated because the glottis is large and visible at the base of the tongue. Because endotracheal tubes are generally not passed deep into the trachea, it is important to secure them by taping them to the lower beak (7). If this is not done, the tube can become easily dislodged during surgery or at least be moved around enough to provide a substantial chemical tracheitis. Because in most birds the trachea and endotracheal tubes have a small lumen, it is easy for them to become occluded, sometimes with disasterous results. Signs of airway obstruction include increased respiratory effort, squeaking noises, and eventually apnea. Birds may appear to be at lighter planes of anesthesia than they were previously (22). If there is any doubt, the tube should be removed and checked for patency. Atropine at a dose of 0.04 to 0.1 mg/kg has been suggested to decrease secretions. However, this seems to cause what secretions are present to become more viscid and therefore more likely to cause obstruction. Some of the secretion promoted by ketamine and metomidate is reported to be unresponsive to atropine administration (11, 19). The following agents have been used successfully for inhalant anesthesia of birds.

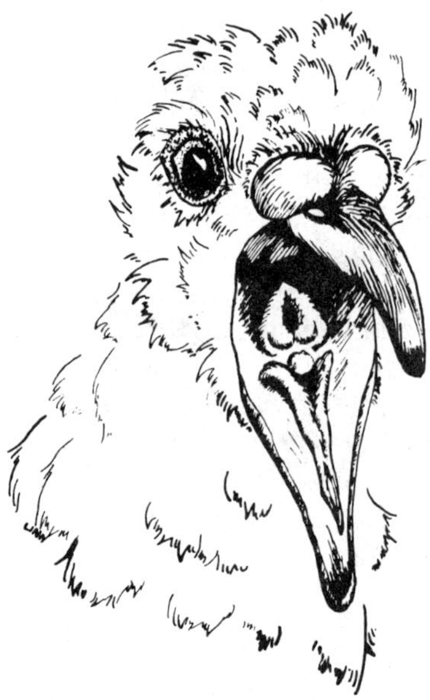

Figure 13.24. In most species of birds the glottis is easily visible at the base of the tongue. This facilitates tracheal intubation.

ETHER

Ether is administered most frequently by open-drop face mask technique. Induction and recovery are very rapid; both occur within minutes (27). Unfortunately, ether is very explosive, rendering electrocautery (among other things) dangerous. It is also very difficult to control depth of anesthesia with ether, especially when an open-drop method is used (25). Because of these problems, ether has largely been replaced as an anesthetic by new volatile agents.

NITROUS OXIDE

When used alone, nitrous oxide is incapable of producing anesthesia in birds. Even a 90% concentration fails to anesthetize chickens (11). It has been used in combination with halothane and methoxyflurane to speed induction (whether or not this actually occurs is unclear) (7, 28, 29) and to decrease the concentration of other anesthetic agents necessary to induce and maintain anesthesia. Usually the concentration of halothane or methoxyflurane can be reduced one-quarter to one-third when nitrous oxide is added to the gas mixture (7, 10). The phenomenon of diffusion hypoxia is assumed to occur if ample oxygen is not given at the anesthetic period (especially considering the gas storage that occurs in the air sacs), but this has never been reported.

METHOXYFLURANE

Methoxyflurane can be administered by open drop technique or through a standard anesthetic apparatus with a vaporizer. It is thought to produce a more stable plane of anesthesia than halothane does (22, 24), but induction and recovery take longer when methoxyflurane is used. Generally, an initial 3% concentration is used to induce anesthesia (1). This takes from 4 to 15 minutes in most birds (7). Anesthesia can usually be maintained at 0.5 to 1.5% vaporizer concentrations (7). Recovery can be prolonged. Larger birds often take from 45 minutes to 1 hour to stand after surgery completed with methoxyflurane (4, 22).

HALOTHANE

Halothane must be administered through an anesthetic system using a calibrated vaporizer. Concentrations delivered to the bird using open-drop technique can be lethally high (27). Induction usually takes from 2 to 4 minutes (7) and requires anesthetic-vaporizer concentrations of approximately 2% for small birds and 2.5 to 3% for larger ones (1, 27). Concentrations required for maintenance vary between 0.5 and 1.5% (1, 10). Recovery usually takes from 3 to 5 minutes (1, 10). Bradycardia, hypotension, and hypothermia can occur with halothane, as with other anesthetics (1, 10). This is reported to resolve rapidly once the anesthetic is turned off. Nevertheless, it may be of considerable concern during a surgical procedure.

ISOFLURANE

Isoflurane is a relatively new agent in avian anesthesia, but it has been studied by Harrison (30) and is used extensively in the Avian Clinic at the New York State College of Veterinary Medicine. Between September 1983 and May 1984, 17 birds (including English sparrows, pigeons, red-tailed hawks, great horned owls, a peregrine falcon, a mynah bird, and a crow) were anesthetized with isoflurane for orthopedic procedures. The crow became apneic and subsequently died about an hour after anesthesia was induced due to an endotracheal tube occluded with mucus. The other birds were maintained at a satisfactory level of anesthesia and recovered uneventfully. Induction with isoflurane is rapid; usually 1 to 2 minutes at a concentration of 3% renders a bird ready for intubation. A vaporizer concentration of 1.5% is effective for maintenance of analgesia. Harrison reported maintenance concentrations of around 3% (30). Recovery from isoflurane anesthesia is almost immediate. Most birds are standing within 5 minutes. We have noticed a decrease in the heart rate of birds undergoing isoflurane anesthesia, but this is not as marked as that which has been reported for halothane. Usually heart rate only decreases 20 to 40 beats/min in hawk-sized birds. The birds do become hypothermic during anesthesia.

Monitoring of Anesthetized Birds

The most reliable indication of the depth of anesthesia and the well-being of the patient is respiratory rate and character. Respiration becomes slower and more shallow as the plane of anesthesia deepens (7). Because apnea rapidly results in death, immediate measures must be taken to lighten anesthesia and provide ventilation should the bird stop breathing spontaneously. Average respiratory rates vary inversely with size. Most raptors breath 10 to 16 times/min under halothane anesthesia; smaller birds breath more rapidly (7).

Heart rate should also be monitored. This can be done by listening through a stethoscope (external or esophageal); because this is frequently difficult on a draped bird during surgery, it is useful to monitor the electrocardiogram. Leads can be placed on the bird's back and sternum or in more conventional positions at the base of the wings and legs (1, 7). Heart rate tends to vary with size, as with respiration. Large raptors given halothane usually have heart rates between 80 and 140, whereas in smaller birds the heart rate may be greater than 400 beats/min (1). It may be reassuring to know that the RS complex in Lead II is normally negative in birds (1).

Special reflexes are useful for monitoring the depth of anesthesia. The palpebral reflex is present only in very light planes, as is reflexive movement in response to stimulation. The corneal reflex (manifested by the movement of the third eyelid across the eye in response to corneal stimulation) and the pedal reflex (withdrawal of the foot in response to toe stimulation) remain longer and are generally slow but just present at a surgical plane of anesthesia (1, 7). The pedal reflex may be less reliable in raptors than in other species (10).

Special Problems with Avian Patients

Most problems encountered in avian anesthesia are related to the small size of most birds. For one thing, it is very difficult to monitor a very small patient swathed in layers of surgical draping. The use of clear plastic drapes helps to alleviate this problem by allowing respiration to be seen rather than guessed at (7). Secondly, the loss of even a little blood can be life-threatening in smaller birds. The loss of just 1 ml of blood from a budgerigar, for example, represents a reduction of that bird's blood volume by one-third. Fluids can be given subcutaneously or intravenously, depending on the size of the patient. Intravenous fluids may be placed in the brachial vein near the elbow. Alternatively, the right jugular vein or medial metatarsal vein may be used. If a transfusion is deemed necessary, it is best to take blood from a conspecific with the patient. However, it has been reported that pigeon blood may be a "universal donor." As it is very easy to overhydrate very small creatures, careful monitoring is needed on the amount of fluids a bird is actually receiving. Birds with fractures may need fluids, special anesthetic considerations, and postoperative care (31).

The most commonly encountered problem is that of hypothermia. Being small, birds have a high surface-to-volume ratio that predisposes them to heat loss when they are not moving. Normal body temperature is usually between 105 and 112°F (18, 27), but it may drop up to 18° during halothane anesthesia (10). This is especially important in birds because hypothermia markedly decreases their respiratory rate (4, 21). All birds undergoing anesthesia should be kept on heating pads throughout surgery and the recovery period. Small birds may be kept warm by placing them on warm bags of intravenous fluid or even surgical gloves filled with warm water and knotted. Alcohol scrubs prior to surgery should be avoided. Hypothermia can be compounded by hypoglycemia, which is common in debilitated birds. It is important not to fast birds (except for those at least 1 kg in weight) before surgery because fasting for even a few hours may produce hypoglycemia (1). If a candidate for surgery is found to be hypoglycemic, administration of 5% dextrose solution i.v. or s.c. will help it maintain its body temperature (1).

Large birds are capable of causing injury to personnel. Care and caution should be taken during the preanesthetic period to properly handle the bird both for its safety, and to avoid personal injury. Large birds, especially the ostrich, may attack the eyes and can deliver a damaging blow with the head.

Anesthetic management in the bird is indeed an interesting challenge.

Anesthetics and Wild or Exotic Mammals

WILLIAM J. BOEVER, D.V.M.

Introduction

Various nondomestic animals in need of chemical restraint are occasionally presented to the veterinary practitioner. In general, inhalation anesthetics can be used on most species with excellent results. Intramuscular agents and their dosages are discussed because it would be difficult to administer inhalation agents to many animals without some form of injectable induction of anesthesia. Intramuscular agents are administered either by dart gun, blowdart, pole syringe, or hand syringe. General guidelines are presented because it would be difficult to list all available dosages for individual needs. Additional information concerning the chemical immobilization of nondomestic animals, including general principles and individual dosages, can be obtained by consulting Reference 32.

PRIMATES

Ketamine HCl intramuscularly is the most commonly used agent for immobilizing primates. As a general guideline, 8 to 10 mg/kg of body weight i.m. will provide good restraint for minor procedures, and 15 to 30 mg/kg of body weight will produce surgical anesthesia.

Small primates and prosimians	20 to 30 mg/kg ketamine HCl i.m.
Medium-sized primates	10 to 20 mg/kg ketamine HCl i.m.
Great apes	6 to 10 mg/kg ketamine HCl i.m.

The initial restraint dosage of ketamine may be followed by maintenance with inhalant anesthetics when complete anesthesia is desired.

RODENTS

Most small rodents are easily immobilized in an inhalation chamber. If the intramuscular route is necessary, ketamine HCl can be used at a dosage of 4.4 mg/100 g i.m. in the small species and 11 mg/kg in larger species for short-term immobilization. The addition of xylazine, promazine, or acepromazine will result in longer immobilization with more complete relaxation.

RABBITS

Rabbits can be immobilized utilizing inhalation anesthesia or they can be immobilized with a combination of 35 to 50 mg/kg ketamine HCl and 5 mg/kg xylazine i.m.

INSECTIVORES

Tenrecs, hedgehogs, shrews, and moles are easily immobilized with inhalation anesthesia administered in a Bell jar or chamber. If injectable anesthetics are needed, ketamine HCl, 1 to 2 mg/100 g i.m. along with 0.2 mg of xylazine/100 g of body weight i.m. produces an effective anesthetic regime.

FELINES

Exotic felids responds in a similar manner to domestic cats to anesthetic once immobilization has been accomplished. Ketamine HCl at 10 to 20 mg/kg i.m. and xylazine 2 mg/kg i.m. will produce immobilization for 15 to 20 minutes. Additional maintenance dosages can be given, or inhalation and anesthetics can be used to maintain anesthesia for longer periods of time.

Small cats	20 to 35 mg/kg ketamine HCl i.m.
Medium sized cats	10 to 20 mg/kg ketamine HCl i.m.
Large cats	5 to 10 mg/kg ketamine HCl i.m.

CANIDS

Wild exotic canids are treated like domestic dogs. Ketamine HCl 10 mg/kg i.m., along with xylazine at 2 mg/kg i.m., will provide 15 to 20 minutes of anesthesia. Supplemental doses may be given, or anesthesia can be maintained with inhalation anesthetics.

RACOONS AND OTTERS

Immobilization can be accomplished with 15 mg/kg ketamine HCl i.m. and 2 mg/kg xylazine i.m.

BEARS

Ketamine HCl administered at 4 to 10 mg/kg i.m. in conjunction with 2 mg/kg xylazine i.m. may be used to immobilize most bears. Smaller bears may require a higher dosage rate.

Small bears	8 to 10 mg/kg ketamine HCl i.m.
Larger bears	4 to 8 mg/kg ketamine HCl i.m.

MARINE MAMMALS

Inhalation anesthesia is preferred for both pinnipeds and cetacians. Physical restraint is necessary until the animal is induced via mask and intubated for maintenance.

ELEPHANTS, RHINOCEROS, TAPIRS, AND ZEBRAS

Etorphine HCl (M99) i.m. is still the drug of choice for the elephant, rhinoceroses, tapir, and zebra. This drug has a specific antagonist, diprenorphine HCl (M50-50), which is given intravenously at two times the etorphine HCl dose to reverse the effects of etorphine when the procedure is complete.

Elephants	4 to 8 mg total dose of M99 i.m.
Rhinoceros	2 to 4 mg total dose of M99 i.m.
Tapirs	1 to 3 mg total dose of M99 i.m.
Zebra	2 to 5 mg total dose of M99 i.m.

Xylazine may be used in combination with etorphine HCl (M99) to effect a smooth immobilization. Xylazine alone may be used in elephants at 0.08 to 0.15 mg/kg i.m.

RUMINANTS

Etorphine HCl (M99) i.m. continues to be the drug of choice for most exotic ruminants. The drug has a specific antagonist, diprenorphine HCl (M50-50), which is given i.v. at two times the etorphine HCl dose when the procedure is completed.

Xylazine can be used in combination with etorphine HCl at 0.2 to 0.5 mg/kg i.m. The average total dose of etorphine HCl for ruminants weighing less than 50 kg is 0.5 to 2.0 mg; for those weighing between 50 and 125 kg, the dose is 1.5 to 3.0 mg; and for those weighing more than 125 kg, the dose is 3.0 to 5.0 mg. The effective dose of etorphine HCl for immobilizing exotic ruminants is species-dependent rather than weight-dependent.

Camels	2 to 4 mg etorphine HCl i.m.
Llama	1 to 3 mg etorphine HCl i.m.
Muntjac deer	1 to 3 mg etorphine HCl i.m.
White-tailed deer	3 to 6 mg etorphine HCl i.m.
American elk	3 to 6 mg etorphine HCl i.m.
Giraffe	3 to 8 mg etorphine HCl i.m.
Greater kudu	4 to 7 mg etorphine HCl i.m.
Eland	5 to 10 mg etorphine HCl i.m.
Bison	6 to 10 mg etorphine HCl i.m.
Addax	5 to 8 mg etorphine HCl i.m.
Gazelle	2 to 3 mg etorphine HCl i.m.
Big horn sheep	2 to 4 mg etorphine HCl i.m.

References

1. Altman RB: Avian anesthesia. *Comp Cont Ed* 2(1):39–43, 1980.
2. Booth NH: Local anesthetics. In Booth NA, McDonald LE (eds): *Veterinary Pharmacology and Therapeutics*, ed 5. Ames, The Iowa State University Press, 1982, pp 357–363.
3. Sanford J: Avian anesthesia. In Soma, LR (ed): *Textbook of Veterinary Anesthesia*. Baltimore, Williams & Wilkins, 1971, pp 359–368.
4. Fedde MR: Drugs used for avian anesthesia: a review. *Poult Sci* 57:1376–1399, 1982.
5. Spellerberg IF: Capturing and immobilizing McCormick Skuas. *J Am Vet Med Assoc* 155(7):1040–1043, 1969.
6. Grandal CP: Satisfactory general anesthesia in birds. *J Am Vet Med Assoc* 128:332–334, 1956.
7. Hartsfield SM: A review of avian anesthesia. *Southwestern Vet* 35(2):117–125, 1982.
8. Cooper JE: Metomidate anesthesia of some birds of prey for laparotomy and sexing. *Vet Rec* 94:437–440, 1984.
9. Cooper JE, Frank L: Use of the steroid anesthetic CT 1341 in birds. *Vet Rec* 92:474–479, 1973.
10. Haigh JC: Anesthesia of raptorial birds. In *Recent Advances in the Study of Raptor Diseases. Proceedings of the International Symposium on Diseases of Birds of Prey*. London, Chiron Publications, 1981, pp 61–66.
11. Houston DC, Cooper JE: Use of the drug metomidate to facilitate the handling of vultures. *International Zoo Yearbook*. 1973, pp 269–273.
12. Cooper JE: Unexpected reactions to the use of CT 1341 by red tailed hawks. *Vet Rec* 97:352, 1975.
13. Cribb PH, Haigh JC: Anesthetic for avian species. *Vet Rec* 100:472–473, 1977.
14. Harcourt-Brown NH: Avian anesthesia in general practice. *J Avian Pract* 19:573–582, 1978.
15. Boener WJ, Wright W: Use of ketamine for the restraint and anesthesia of birds. *VM/SAC* 70:86–88, 1975.
16. McGrath CJ, Lee JC, Campbell VL: Dose-responsive anesthetic effects of ketamine in the chicken. *Am J Vet Res* 45(3):531–534, 1984.
17. Salerno A, Van Tienhoven A: The effect of ketamine on heart rate, respiration rate and EEG of white leghorn hens. *Comp Biochem Physiol* 556:69–76, 1975.
18. Petrak ML: *Diseases of Cage and Aviary Birds*, ed 2. Philadelphia, Lea & Febiger, 1984.

19. Redig PT, Duke GE: Intravenously administered ketamine HCl and diazepam for anesthesia of raptors. *J Am Vet Med Assoc* 169(9):886–888, 1976.
20. Scheid P, Slama H, Piiper J: Mechanisms of undirectional flow in parabronchi of avian lungs: measurements in duck lung preparations. *Respir Physiol* 14:83–95, 1972.
21. Burger RE, Lorenz FW: Artificial respiration in birds by undirectional air flow. *Poult Sci* 39:236–238, 1960.
22. Klide AM: Avian anesthesia. In *Veterinary Clinics of North America*. Philadelphia, WB Saunders, 1973, pp 175–186.
23. Boeverot D: Control of breathing in birds compared with mammals. *Physiol Rev* 58(3):604–655, 1978.
24. Whittow GC, Ossorio N: A new technique for anesthetizing birds. *Lab Anim Care* 20:651–656, 1970.
25. Dolphin RE, Olsen DE: Anesthesia in the companion bird. *VM/SAC* 72(2):1761–1765, 1977.
26. Mandelker L: Anesthesia for parakeets and other birds. *J Am Vet Med Assoc* 157(2):1081, 1970.
27. Arnall L: Anesthesia and surgery on captive and aviary birds. *Vet Rec* 73:139–142, 1961.
28. Frost RDI: Anesthesia of birds of prey (Letter). *Vet Rec* 108:195–196, 1981.
29. Wingfield WE, DeYoung DW: Anesthetic and surgical management of eagles with orthopedic difficulties. *VM/SAC* 67:991–993, 1972.
30. Harrison GJ: Avian medical and surgical seminar. Avian Society of the Southern California V.M.A., Pico Rivera, CA, 1984.
31. Elkins AD, Herron MR: Management of avian fractures I. anesthetic and intraoperative considerations. *VM/SAC* 77(4):587–591, 1982.
32. Wallach JD, Boever WJ: Diseases of Exotic Animals. Philadelphia, WB Saunders Co, 1983.

PART 6

Anesthesia for Neonatal and Geriatric Patients

ROBERT E. MEYER, D.V.M., D.A.C.V.A.

Introduction

At first glance, there would appear to be little common ground between neonatal and geriatric animals with respect to anesthesia. The newly born and the nearly dead represent the widest extremes of the life experience. What the very young and the very old patient have in common is that both are undergoing physiological changes—maturation in the very young and degeneration in the very old—that significantly modify their response to anesthesia. Clinicians are most comfortable anesthetizing animals in their early adult and middle years, largely because physiological responses to anesthesia and anesthetic drug pharmacology are best described for these patients. Much of human neonatal and pediatric physiology and pharmacology is based on experimental animal work, but few, if any, comprehensive reviews are available to tie this body of knowledge together as it specifically relates to anesthesia of the domestic species. Studies on geriatric domestic animal physiology and pharmacology are even fewer. However, many of the changes described for neonatal and geriatric humans have been assumed to be similar for the domestic animal species. This chapter serves a two-fold purpose: to review the ways in which the maturation process in the neonate and the degeneration process in the older animal can affect anesthetic management and 2 to discuss anesthetic management of these patients.

Rates of maturation and degeneration are species-dependent, and increasing physiological age may not parallel increasing chronological age for all species and breeds. Definitions of the neonatal and the geriatric periods are required for the purpose of discussion within this chapter. The neonatal period has been defined for the canine and feline species as the first 2 weeks and the pediatric period as the first 12 weeks of postnatal life (1). The same time periods will be applied to the other domestic animal species. The transition from middle to old age can not be arbitrarily defined but depends largely on the anticipated life expectancy of the species or breed in question. The last 20 to 25% of the anticipated natural life span has been suggested as the geriatric phase of life for dogs (2); this appears to be a reasonable estimate for the other domestic animal species as well.

Pharmacological and Physiological Considerations

Whether an anesthetic drug has the desired effect in young or aged animals depends on the interrelationship between pharmacokinetic processes and physiological functions. The pharmacokinetic processes of uptake (absorption), distribution, metabolism, and elimination affect drug concentrations in plasma as well as at receptor sites. Substantial differences in these processes exist in both neonates and geriatric patients compared with the average adult, and most adverse reactions to drugs exhibited by animals in either age group given average adult dosage levels can be attributed to differences in distribution and elimination (3). Physiological function can be thought of as describing a parabolic arc, with the peak region of function during the adult years and decreased function during the leading and trailing neonatal and geriatric phases. The reasons for decreased function during the neonatal and geriatric phases are not necessarily the same.

UPTAKE (ABSORPTION)

Anesthetic drugs are commonly administered to neonatal and geriatric patients by intravenous, intramuscular, and inhalant routes, but rarely by mouth. Uptake of drugs after intramuscular injection is not consistent in neonates. Absorption will depend on regional blood flow at the injection site and coexisting disease states (4). The effects of drugs administered by this route will also depend on the apparent volume of distribution (V_d), as discussed in the section on distribution.

There are a number of physical changes associated with aging that are expected to alter parenteral drug absorption. Among these changes are generalized wasting of the skin, loss of elastic tissue and collagen, and loss of subcutaneous tissue. Bruising and hematoma formation often occurs after injection, and the venipuncture process can be more difficult. However, there has been little evidence to suggest that these factors are of any major significance in the uptake of parenterally administered drugs in the older patient compared with the younger adult (5). On the other hand, there have been few systematic studies of drug uptake in the elderly (6).

Uptake of inhalant anesthetics is more rapid in the newborn and pediatric patient, and marked fluctuations in the level of anesthesia may occur with changes in ventilation. Alveolar surface area is one-third and oxygen consumption is two to three times that of the adult, so that respiratory rate and resting alveolar ventilation are increased to the same extent. The ratio of alveolar ventilation to functional residual capacity (FRC) is 5 to 1 in human infants and 1.5 to 1 in adults. The advantage of a large minute ventilation to FRC ratio is that induction and recovery from inhalant anesthetics will be more rapid. The disadvantage of a low FRC is that the FRC acts like an oxygen reservoir for the body; the elevated oxygen requirement of the neonate is not matched by the reserve in the FRC, and hypoxia will occur more quickly. The responses of neonates to increased $PaCO_2$ and low PaO_2 are depressed compared with adults. Newborns may respond to hypoxia with depressed ventilation. The neonate has a high percentage of fetal hemoglobin (70 to 80%), which has a higher affinity for oxygen than adult hemoglobin and carries a greater percentage of oxygen at a low partial pressure. Hemoglobin levels are highest in the newborn (17 g%) and drop to near 10 g% by 2 weeks of age (1). This "anemia of infancy" is associated with increased 2,3-diphosphoglycerate (2,3-DPG), a metabolic product that alters the ability of oxygenated hemoglobin to give up oxygen and accept H^+ ions. The increased 2,3-DPG compensates for the defect in oxygen delivery to the cells by reducing oxygen affinity for hemoglobin.

Uptake of inhalant anesthetics in the geriatric patient would be expected to be abnormal for several reasons, including decreased pulmonary function and the presence of degenerative cardiovascular disease. The incidence of heart disease in older dogs has been reported as 25% between 9 and 12 years of age and 33% in dogs 13 years and older and has been associated with chronic valvular disease (7). In humans, the cardiac index decreases approximately 1% per year after age 30 (8). Lung elasticity has been shown to decrease in aged beagle dogs (9), and this has been associated with increased closing volume of the small airways (2, 10). As closing volume increases, greater portions of tidal ventilation occur at lung volumes below closing volume, causing air trapping, worsened ventilation/perfusion (V/Q) mismatch, and decreased resting PaO_2. Diffusion capacity and pulmonary capillary blood volume have also been shown to decrease in aged dogs (11). With slower circulation in the geriatric patient, a faster onset of action of inhalational agents would be expected because of a faster increase in alveolar concentrations. This does not appear to occur in the older patient, however, because of the decreased effectiveness of ventilation. The overall net effect of the decreased cardiac performance and decreased ventilation is either a normal or decreased rate of rise of alveolar anesthetic levels. Conversely, recovery will tend to be prolonged for the same reasons.

DISTRIBUTION

Newborn and geriatric patients demonstrate increased sensitivity to central nervous system (CNS) depressant drugs. Two possible explanations for increased responsiveness to anesthetic drugs in the newborn and geriatric patient are an increase in target cell or organ sensitivity, resulting in an increased response for a given drug concentration, and that the amount of drug within the body is modified through altered redistribution and changes in organ size and weight in these patients.

Neonates initially show increased sensitivity to CNS depressant drugs, followed by decreased sensitivity as measured by the minimum alveolar concentration (MAC) of inhalant anesthetics required to abolish response to painful stimuli. Lerman et al. (12) determined the anesthetic requirements for halothane in neonates and in pediatric humans 1 to 6 months of age. They reported a MAC for halothane of 0.87% in neonates and a MAC for halothane of 1.2% in 1- to 6-month-old infants. They postulated three reasons for the low MAC in neonates: elevated progesterone levels, immature CNS, and a combination of high circulating beta endorphines and an immature CNS. Progesterone is thought to be the cause of the 30% decrease in MAC observed in pregnant human patients; it crosses the placenta, and levels are measurable in the human neonate during the first 10 days of life. The immature neonatal CNS may result in a lower appreciation of pain or conversely a higher threshold to elicit the pain response. Neonates have higher beta endorphin levels than adults; although endorphins do not normally cross the adult blood-brain barrier, the immature blood-brain barrier may allow passage, resulting in a lower MAC value.

The blood-brain barrier restricts the diffusion of drugs and endogenous substances into the CNS. It has been shown in lambs that the immature blood-brain barrier is more permeable in the neonate because of open tubulocisternal endoplasmic reticulum components of the cerebral endothelial and choroid plexus epithelial cells rather than incomplete tight junctions between the cells (13). The permeability of the blood-brain barrier to drug penetration decreases as the animal advances into the older neonate and pediatric stages. Penetration of intravenous anesthetics that have their desired effects in the brain may be much more rapid in neonates than in the older pediatric patient (3).

Marked fluctuations in the level of anesthesia in neonates may also occur with changes in cardiac output. The relatively greater distribution of cardiac output to such vessel-rich tissues as the brain has been speculated to lead to more rapid and profound CNS effects of both intravenous and inhalant agents in the neonate. Maintenance of heart rate is important in neonates because cardiac output is rate-dependent. The neonatal heart has immature innervation and is less able to increase the force of contractility. Vasomotor control is poor. Inhalant anesthetics cause dose-dependent vasodilation and decreased myocardial contractility. Studies comparing compensatory responses to halothane-induced hypotension in newborn and adult rabbits have shown depressed baroreceptor activity in the neonate, resulting in decreased heart rate (14), and therefore decreased cardiac output. Atropine is recommended to maintain heart rate in children and young animals (15), but may have little or no effect in neonatal puppies less than 14 days old because of immature vagal innervation (16).

Geriatric patients demonstrate reduced anesthetic requirements. The MAC for halothane in oxygen has been shown in humans to decrease from 1.2% in pediatric patients (12) to 0.64% in the eighth decade of life (17, 18). The elderly human demonstrates an increased response to thiopental, requiring only 70% of the dose needed for younger patients; $T_{1/2}$ is increased, V_d is increased, and rate of clearance is 50% less compared with the younger human (19). Decreased local anesthetic requirement per epidural segment has also been demonstrated in the geriatric human (20). Cerebral oxygen consumption decreases with age (21), and cerebral blood flow declines 0.5% per year beyond age 30 in humans, while cardiac output falls 1% per year. A higher overall percentage of cardiac output, and thus anesthetic agent, will be delivered to the brain of geriatric patients. Circulation time is prolonged with advancing age, and the subsequent delay in anesthetic effect may predispose the geriatric group to overdose unless injection rate is reduced. Changes in anatomical structure may also contribute to the decreased anesthetic requirement. The blood-brain barrier is altered in older rats, allowing more drug to enter the brain (22). In humans, the brain decreases 20% in weight from the second to eighth decades of life. Accumulation of lipofucsin pigments, loss of neurons from the cerebral cortex, changes in metabolism of catecholamines and neurotransmitters, and endocrine changes have been associated with the increased CNS response to drugs in the geriatric patient.

The apparent volume of distribution, defined as the ratio of blood concentration to the total amount of drug in the body (V_d), is influenced by many factors, including the actual volume of tissue compartments, blood flow per unit mass of tissue, the binding of drugs to serum proteins, and the binding of drugs in tissue. Distribution volumes normalized for body weight tend to be larger in neonates than in adults, and the relative mass of tissues tends to change throughout maturation (23). Total body water of the neonate accounts for a greater percentage of body weight (70 to 75% compared with 50 to 60% in the adult). The extracellular fluid volume is nearly doubled in the neonate and decreases with increasing age. Drugs that are normally confined to the extracellular space will have a larger distribution volume in the neonate than in the adult. Atropine, succinylcholine, and meperidine appear to be less potent in the neonate because of the larger fraction of total body water for a given body weight, resulting in a larger V_d (3).

Body composition changes with increasing age, with fat replacing metabolically active tissue. In humans, body fat increases by 18 to 36% in males and 33 to 48% in females during the period from 15 to 60 years of age (6). As a result, lean body mass decreases in proportion to total body weight. Lipid-soluble drugs would be expected to show increased V_d (especially in females), whereas water-soluble drugs should demonstrate higher plasma concentrations due to decreased V_d. This is precisely what has been demonstrated for thiopental (19) and diazepam (24) in the older human patient. Total body water decreases 10 to 15% in humans from 20 to 80 years of age (25); intracellular water decreases from 42% at age 25 to 33% at age 75, while extracellular water remains constant at 20% and constitutes a greater portion of the total body water (5).

Adipose tissue content, in contrast, is very low in the neonate (2 to 3%) and increases with age. Although neonates are relatively lacking in adipose tissue, lipid-soluble drugs have a larger V_d in the neonate than in the adult. Increased blood flow to lipid-rich organs such as the brain and liver has been speculated to be the cause of the increased V_d observed with the local anesthetics lidocaine and mepivacaine (26, 27).

The exaggerated effects of intravenous anesthetics in both neonatal and geriatric patients can be explained through the combination of decreased plasma protein binding, increased V_d, increased blood-brain barrier permeability, and decreased metabolism. Drugs bind less extensively to serum proteins of neonates than to the serum proteins in older pediatric patients or adults. This appears to be true for acidic drugs that bind primarily to albumin as well as basic drugs that are bound more avidly to globulins. The lower concentration of plasma albumin in the neonate of most species contributes to the lower plasma drug concentration and provides a relatively larger fraction of the unbound active drug for extravascular distribution (28). Because only the unbound drug fraction is available for diffusion to sites of activity and biotransformation, changes in unbound drug concentration will increase the net effect of highly protein-bound anesthetic drugs. The presence of competing ligands, such as bilirubin in hemolytic disease of the newborn foal, will decrease basic drug binding to globulins.

Total protein concentrations remain constant into the geriatric phase; however, albumin concentrations have been reported to fall in the elderly human by 0.4 to 0.6 g/dl, whereas globulin levels tend to rise (5). Decreases in albumin levels accompany inflammatory disease, burns, pressure sores, and severe infection and would be expected to increase the unbound fraction of acidic drugs such as thiopental. Hospitalized geriatric animals are frequently receiving several drugs concurrently; competition for similar binding sites may cause increased displacement of drugs from binding sites. Recent studies have also shown decreased binding of meperidine, diazepam, and pentazocine to red blood cells with increasing age in humans (29, 30). Increased globulin levels tend to increase the amount of binding of basic drugs, such as lidocaine, propranolol, and quinidine, while reducing the amount of free, active drug in plasma. The unbound fraction of diazepam has been shown to be correlated with increasing age in humans, but only in females (29); this may be related to increased V_d for lipid-soluble drugs and the greater female fat stores associated with aging.

METABOLISM

The liver is the major site of drug metabolism. Hepatic drug metabolism can activate a drug, terminate its pharmacological action, and in some cases generate a more polar ionized metabolite to allow for increased renal excretion. The ability of the neonatal liver and the geriatric liver to metabolize drugs is generally depressed compared with the adult. Not all metabolic pathways are equally affected. The rate of development of different metabolic pathways with respect to age is not well described and may vary with the species of animal (31). There appears to be a great deal of variation in geriatric decline of hepatic drug metabolism, such that prediction of how an animal will react to a particular drug based strictly on age is difficult.

Hepatic microsomal oxidation, often followed by glucuronide conjugation, is the principal metabolic pathway for a large number of lipid-soluble drugs, including thiopental. The drug-metabolizing activities of the cytochrome P450-dependent mixed function oxidase system and the glucuronide conjugation reaction are decreased in neonates. Development of the microsomal-mediated pathways is rapid during the first 3 to 4 weeks after birth and approaches adult activity at 6 to 12 weeks (3). Thiopental undergoes desulfuration by an additional oxidative step to pentobarbital. Pentobarbital hydroxylase activity is not detectable at birth in beagle dogs, rises from Day 1 to Day 9, undergoes partial decrease to Day 25, and subsequently increases to adult levels by Day 135 after birth (32). Hydroxylation of diazepam and mepivacaine is reduced more than is demethylation in newborns (33). Drugs that are metabolized by these pathways will have prolonged $T_{1/2}$ in neonates.

Age, by itself, does not appear to impair the usual metabolic indicators of hepatic function in the domestic animals; bilirubin clearance does not change with age, and significant changes in serum glutamic oxaloacetic transaminase (SGOT) serum glutamic pyruvic transaminase (SGPT), and alkaline phosphatase are not seen. Plasma sulfobromophthalein sodium (BSP) levels have been shown to increase with increasing age due to reduced hepatic retention (34). Decreased hepatic function in the geriatric patient can be attributed, in part, to decreased hepatic blood flow and decreased drug binding with albumin. In humans, cardiac output decreases 30 to 45% by age 65, and hepatic blood flow decreases 12 to 40%. Anesthesia will tend to reduce hepatic blood flow; in the presence of hypotension, hepatic blood flow may be decreased an average of 40 to 81%.

Half-lives for drugs in geriatric patients, like hepatic metabolism, are highly variable. The half-life of a drug ($T_{1/2}$) is determined by the ratio between its V_d and its clearance. Changes in metabolism are reflected more accurately by changes in clearance, which means an increase in duration of action of many drugs. The classic example is that of diazepam, in which $T_{1/2}$ increases proportionately with increasing V_d (and age) and not as a function of decreased metabolism (35). Although plasma drug concentrations may be similar to those seen in the younger adult population, drug concentrations at the receptor sites may be quite different in the older patient due to changes in clearance, $T_{1/2}$, and V_d. Specific values for the anesthetic drugs are lacking in the domestic animals.

ELIMINATION

The kidney is the major route of elimination of most drugs, either as the unchanged drug or as the metabolic byproduct. The renal mechanisms for handling drugs include: (*a*) glomerular filtration of unbound molecules in the plasma, (*b*) carrier-mediated excretion of certain polar organic molecules by the proximal tubule, and (*c*) pH-dependent passive reabsorption of the nonionized lipid-soluble portion of drugs that are weak organic acids or bases. Both neonates and geriatric patients exhibit decreased renal function, but for different reasons.

The mechanisms of renal excretion are not completely developed in the neonates of most species. Glomerular filtration rate and renal plasma blood flow are reduced in the human infant and in neonatal pigs, dogs, rats, and rabbits. On the other hand, glomerular function and active tubule secretion are much better developed at 1 to 2 days of age in calves, lambs, and kids. The situation in the neonatal foal has not been reported (3). Response to diuretics may be limited in neonates because of the low glomerular filtration and immature tubule function. Active proximal tubule secretion is linked with increase of renal tubule mass, and attainment of function tends to have a slower onset than glomerular filtration. Functionally, the neonate is less able to conserve fluids, is less able to tolerate fluid overload, and will tend to lose Na^+ during the first days after birth. Overall renal function matures within the first 1 to 2 weeks after birth in ruminants (36) and pigs (3); in other species, this may take up to 4 weeks. The urine pH is acidic in neonates, which will delay excretion of weak organic acids. Because of the decreased hepatic microsomal oxidation in the neonatal liver, more lipid-soluble drug may reach the distal tubule and be available for reabsorption.

Information on geriatric renal function in domestic animals is lacking. Some general comments can be made based on the canine and human literature. Aged dogs demonstrate reduced renal weight, which represents a decrease in the size and number of nephrons, and the space between tubules is widened by increased interstitium connective tissue (37). Glomerular filtration rate decreases with increasing age. With increasing age, the renal tubules gradually lose the ability to reabsorb water, resulting in a decreased mean maximum urine-specific gravity. The ability to conserve Na^+ and reabsorb phosphate is also reduced. Distal tubule function becomes impaired and results in decreased acid excretion when faced with an acid load. Chronic nephritis, pyelonephritis, and glomerulonephritis accounted for 5% of canine mortality in a postmortem survey, with renal disease the second most common cause of death after cancer (38). Acid-base metabolism and electrolyte balance will thus be impaired. As hepatic function decreases, more lipid-soluble drugs will be filtered by the glomerulus and be available for tubule reabsorption. Agents that rely entirely (i.e., ketamine in cats and gallamine) or partially (i.e., pancuronium) on renal clearance will demonstrate prolonged $T_{1/2}$ in the older patient with renal dysfunction.

Anesthetic Recommendations

One can conclude from the information presented in the previous discussion that neonatal and geriatric patients share increased overall sensitivity to anesthetic agents for similar yet different reasons. The choice of an appropriate anesthetic protocol must be considered in light of the pharmacokinetic and physiological changes expected for each age group and the physical and pathological signs presented by the individual patient. Age alone should not be the primary determinant as to how a particular patient will be anesthetized, but it should be taken into account along with presenting signs, coexisting disease, type and length of procedure, available facilities, and the skill and experience of all involved personnel.

As a general rule, the best plans are the simplest plans. Minimizing the number of anesthetic agents helps keep things straightforward by decreasing potential drug interactions and reducing dependence on the processes of uptake, distribution, metabolism, and elimination. Through knowledge of the drug class, mode of action, and method of termination of action, the clinician can choose anesthetic agents that will cause the least homeostatic disruption and not depend on immature or poorly functioning organ systems for termination of action or elimination. With fewer drugs, there is also less clinician confusion as to level of anesthesia.

Inhalant anesthesia with an agent of low solubility, such as isoflurane or halothane, is safe and particularly well suited for both neonatal and geriatric patients. The chief advantages of inhalants are their rapid uptake and elimination via the lungs, which provides a high degree of control, and their administration in higher than normal oxygen levels. Both large animal and small animal neonates can be masked down. The method requires practice for proficiency. The mask is placed near or over the animal's nose, and oxygen is initially administered to accustom the patient to the mask. The inhalant is added to the oxygen flow (0.25%/30 seconds) so that the patient is gradually introduced to the agent; breath holding and struggling are reduced. The animal will begin to relax before entering the excitement phase. At this point, the vaporizer setting is increased. In order to pass through the excitement phase as quickly as possible, nitrous oxide is added in a 2:1 or 3:1 mixture with oxygen to invoke the second gas and the concentration effects. The nitrous oxide may be discontinued after endotracheal intubation, and the animal can be maintained for the procedure on the inhalant agent. Small animal neonates can also be placed in an aquarium-type induction chamber for anesthetic induction. Inhalant inductions may also be conducted in neonatal large animals by passing a lubricated nasal catheter into the pharynx after desensitization of the nose with a local anesthetic; the catheter can be connnected to the outlet of a precision calibrated vaporizer. Webb (39) has described a similar technique for passing a cuffed endotracheal tube into the trachea through the nasal passages of awake foals before induction of anesthesia. Guaifenesen, a centrally acting neuromuscular relaxant with minimal cardiovascular effects, may be titrated to effect (25 to 50 mg/kg i.v.) to facilitate endotracheal intubation of foals before maintenance with inhalant anesthetics.

Debilitated, depressed, or especially calm geriatric small animal patients can also be safely masked with low solubility inhalant anesthetics. A poorly performed mask induction, however, may be more detrimental to the older patient than a well-chosen injectable anesthetic induction. Catecholamines and myocardial oxygen demand will be increased, and the overall increase in cardiac output and muscle blood flow will tend to delay the rate of rise of alveolar concentration of anesthetic. Injectable anesthetics for geriatric patients should be chosen for homeostatic neutrality and lack of dependence on metabolism for return to consciousness and function. Low intramuscular doses of narcotics are preferred for sedation over phenothiazine or butyrophenone tranquilizers because narcotics have minimal effects on peripheral vascular control and cardiovascular performance aside from bradycardia. Should bradycardia occur before or after induction, either atropine or glycopyrrolate can be administered intravenously. A major advantage of narcotics in the geriatric patient is that systemic effects can be reversed by means of specific narcotic antagonists. Should an adverse reaction to the narcotic occur, such as severe ventilatory depression, airway obstruction, or prolonged recovery, a specific antagonist can be administered. Oxygen should be administered by mask after administration of narcotics; this will not prevent the dose-related increase in CO_2 associated with narcotics but will help prevent hypoxia by increasing the available oxygen through nitrogen washout of the FRC of the lung. Induction of anesthesia can be safely performed by using intravenous agents that do not cause excessive cardiovascular depression or require extensive metabolism or clearance for termination of anesthetic action. Agents in this category include: hypnotic doses of thiobarbiturates (4 to 6 mg/kg i.v., administered to effect), diazepam (0.2 mg/kg i.v.; 5 mg maximum) combined with the hypnotic agent etomidate (1.5 to 3.0 mg/kg i.v.), and administration of additional sedative-narcotic combinations (neuroleptanesthesia; i.e., diazepam, 0.2 mg/kg i.v., and oxymorphone, 0.05 to 0.1 mg/kg i.v.). Rather than use excessive amounts of injectable or inhalant anesthetics to allow endotracheal intubation and abolish nociceptor-induced reflex movement, a muscle relaxant can be added to each of the above protocols. Atracurium (Tracrium, Burroughs Wellcome) is a competitive neuromuscular relaxant that spontaneously breaks down at body temperature and pH into inactive metabolites through metabolism-independent Hoffmann elimination; neuromuscular blockade will not be prolonged in the face of renal or hepatic failure. The recommended dose of 0.4 mg/kg i.v. will provide between 20 and 40 minutes of relaxation in dogs (40). Epidural anesthesia can be utilized in debilitated older patients; however, the dose is reduced compared with younger patients. Should sedation and restraint be needed or if the procedure becomes more involved than originally planned, a general anesthetic may provide better conditions for both the patient and the surgeon. Intravenous regional anesthesia (Bier block) combined with neuroleptanesthesia provides an excellent means to work on the distal limb of the older patient.

The otherwise healthy older patient that does not require preanesthetic sedation can be anesthetized with a combination of diazepam (0.2 mg/kg i.v., 5 mg maximum) followed by thiobarbiturate (8 to 12 mg/kg, to effect); this combination allows quick return of protective reflexes and function. The combination of diazepam (0.5 mg/kg) and ketamine (10 mg/kg) is used by many clinicians in older dogs. This combination has minimal effects on canine cardiovascular and pulmonary function; however, it provides poor muscle relaxation, and vomition at induction has been reported (41). Maintenance is with a low-solubility inhalant agent. Xylazine should be avoided in the older patient; it greatly potentiates any subsequent anesthetic agents, can cause atrioventricular blockade, and sensitizes the myocardium to catecholamines (42).

Temperature regulation, fluid and electrolyte replacement, and blood glucose requirements should be aggressively managed in both neonatal and geriatric patients. Hypothermia will occur during general anesthesia for several reasons, including depression of the thermoregulatory centers, reduced or absent skeletal muscle activity, and direct radiative and conductive heat loss to the environment. Anesthesia depth will be increased and recovery prolonged because of reduced metabolism and clearance of agents. Heat can be provided through circulating water blankets or frequently changed water balloons. These measures will also tend to insulate the patient from the table. Clipping should be minimized, surgical scrub materials should be warmed, and the surgical site should be scrubbed without completely soaking the patient. Lactated Ringer's solution with dextrose is recommended for neonates during anesthesia at 4 ml/kg/hour through a pediatric minidrip (1); geriatric patients can be given 10 ml/kg/hour of lactated Ringer's solution unless anuric or in heart failure, in which case central venous pressure and urine output are used to determine administration rate and reduced Na^+-containing fluids are substituted. Serial blood glucose levels can be obtained easily by needle hub blood aspiration with capillary tubes using a commercially available test strip (Dextrosrix, Ames; Chemstrip, Boerringer Mannheim Diagnostics); in neonates, a marginal ear vessel can be pricked and the drop of blood aspirated with the capillary tube.

The preceding chapter has attempted to present the pharmacological and physiological changes expected in neonatal and geriatric patients as they concern the anesthetic process. These changes provide the base on which concurrent disease processes will be superimposed. Rather than provide an extensive list of empirical do's and don't's for all possible combinations of disease and age, it is hoped this discussion will aid in the making of rational decisions for the anesthetic management of these patients. The key lies in the recognition of the unique pharmacological differences between these patients and the more familiar adult animal in the prime of life.

References

1. Robinson EP: Anesthesia of pediatric patients. *Comp Cont Ed Pract Vet* 5:1004–1011, 1983.
2. Dodman NH, Seeler DC, Court MH: Aging changes in the geriatric dog and their impact on anesthesia. *Comp Cont Ed Pract Vet* 6:1106–1113, 1984.
3. Baggot JD, Short CR: Drug disposition in the neonatal animal, with particular reference to the foal. *Equine Vet J* 16:364–367, 1984.
4. Green TP, Mirkin BL: Clinical pharmacokinetics: pediatric considerations. In Benet LZ, Massoud N, Gambertoglio JG (eds): *Pharmacokinetic Basis for Drug Treatment.* New York, Raven Press, 1984, pp 269–282.
5. Massoud N: Pharmacokinetic considerations in geriatric patients. In Benet LZ, Massoud N, Gambertoglio JG (eds): *Pharmacokinetic Basis for Drug Treatment.* New York, Raven Press, 1984, pp 283–310.
6. Crooks J, O'Malley K, Stevenson IH: Pharmacokinetics in the elderly. *Clin Pharmacokinet* 1:280–296, 1976.
7. MacDougall DF, Barker J: An approach to canine geriatrics. *Br Vet J* 140:115–123, 1984.
8. Evans TI: The physiological basis of geriatric general anesthesia. *Anesth Intensive Care* 1:319–322, 1973.
9. Robinson NE, Gillespie JR: Lung volumes in aging beagle dogs. *J Appl Physiol* 35:317–321, 1973.
10. Evans T: Anesthesia for the geriatric patient. *Vet Clin North Am: Small Animal Practice.* 11:653–667, 1981.
11. Robinson NE, Gillespie JR: Pulmonary diffusing capacity and capillary blood volume in aging dogs. *J Appl Physiol* 38:647–650, 1975.
12. Lerman J, Robinson S, Willis MM, Gregory GA. Anesthetic requirement for halothane in young children 0–1 month and 1–6 months of age. *Anesthesiology* 59:421–424, 1983.
13. Saunders NR: The blood-brain barrier in the foetal and newborn lamb. *Ann Rech Vet* 8:384–395, 1977.
14. Wear R, Robinson S, Gregory GA: The effect of halothane on the baroresponse of adult and baby rabbits. *Anesthesiology* 56:188–191, 1982.
15. Short CE: Pediatric animal anesthesia. In Short CE (ed): *Clinical Veterinary Anesthesia.* St. Louis, CV Mosby Co, 1974, pp 145–151.
16. Fox MW: *Canine Pediatrics.* Springfield, IL, Charles C Thomas, 1966.
17. Gregory GA, Eger EI, Munson ES: The relationship between age and halothane requirement in man. *Anesthesiology* 30:488–491, 1969.
18. Nicodemus HF, Nassairi-Rahimi C, Bachman LB: Median effective dose (ED_{50}) of halothane in adults and children. *Anesthesiology* 31:344–348, 1969.
19. Christensen JH, Andreasen F, Jansen JA: Influence of age and sex on the pharmacokinetics of thiopentane. *Br J Anaesth* 53:1189–1195, 1981.
20. Bromage PR: Aging and epidural dose requirements. *Br J Anaesth* 41:1016–1021, 1969.

21. Ellison N: Problems in geriatric anesthesia. *Surg Clin North Am* 55:929–945, 1975.
22. Witts DJ, Bowkay AA, Garland M: Studies in the elderly: pharmacokinetic aspects. *Age Aging* 8:271–281, 1979.
23. Rane A, Wilson JT: Clinical pharmacokinetics in infants and children. *Clin Pharmacokinet* 1:2–24, 1976.
24. Wilkinson GR: Effects of aging and liver disease on disposition of lorazepam. *Clin Pharmacol Ther* 24:411–419, 1978.
25. Vestal RE: Drug use in the elderly. A review of problems and special considerations. *Drugs* 16:358–382, 1978.
26. Mihaly GW, Moore RG, Thomas J: The pharmacokinetics and metabolism of the anilide local anesthetics in neonates. *Eur J Clin Pharmacol* 13:143–152, 1978.
27. Moore RG, Thomas J, Triggs EJ: The pharmacokinetics and metabolism of the anilide local anesthetics in neonates. III. Mepivacaine. *Eur J Clin Pharmacol* 13:203–213, 1978.
28. Short CR, Sexton RL, McFarland K: The binding of ^{14}C-salicylic acid and ^{14}C-pentobarbital to plasma proteins of several species during the perinatal period. *Biol Neonate* 26:58–65, 1975.
29. Greenblatt DJ, Allen MD, Hartmatz JS, Shader RI: Diazepam disposition determinants. *Clin Pharmacol Ther* 27:301–311, 1980.
30. Hayes MJ, Langman MJS, Short AH: Changes in drug metabolism with increasing age: phenytoin clearance and protein binding. *Br J Clin Pharmacol* 2:73–79, 1975.
31. Short CR: Drug elimination in the newborn animal. *Proc Symp Vet Pharmacol Ther* 2:81–99, 1980.
32. Peters EL, Farber TM, Heider A, Ritter DL: The development of drug-metabolizing enzymes in the young dog. *Fed Proc* 30:560, 1971.
33. Wood AJJ: Drug disposition and pharmacokinetics. In Wood M, Wood AJJ (eds): *Drugs and Anesthesia: Pharmacology for Anesthesiologists.* Baltimore, Williams & Wilkins, 1982, pp 3–59.
34. Thompson E, Williams R: Effect of age on liver function with particular reference to bromsulphalein excretion. *Gut* 6:266–269, 1965.
35. Klotz U, Avant GR, Hayumpa A: The effects of age and liver disease on the disposition and elimination of diazepam in adult man. *J Clin Invest* 55:347–359, 1975.
36. Friis C: Postnatal development of renal function in goats. In Ruckebusch Y, Toutain P-L, Koritz GD (eds): *Veterinary Pharmacology and Toxicology.* Lancaster, MTP Press, 1983, pp 57–62.
37. Kaufman GM: Renal function in the geriatric dog. *Comp Cont Ed Pract Vet* 6:1087–1095, 1984.
38. Bronson RT: Variation in age of death of dogs of different sexes and breeds. *Am J Vet Res* 43:2057–2059, 1982.
39. Webb AI: Nasal intubation in the foal. *J Am Vet Med Assoc* 185:48–51, 1984.
40. Jones RS, Hunter JM, Utting JE: Neuromuscular blocking action of atracurium in the dog and its reversal by neostigmine. *Res Vet Sci* 34:173–176, 1983.
41. Haskins SC, Farver TB, Patz JD: Cardiovascular changes in dogs given diazepam and diazepam-ketamine. *Am J Vet Res* 47:795–798, 1986.
42. Muir WW, Werner LL, Hamlin RL: Effects of xylazine and acetylpromazine upon induced ventricular fibrillation in dogs anesthetized with thiamylal and halothane. *Am J Vet Res* 36:1299–1303, 1975.

PART 7

Special Anesthetic Considerations for Caesarean Section

G. JOHN BENSON, D.V.M., M.S., D.A.C.V.A., and JOHN C. THURMON, D.V.M., M.S., D.A.C.V.A.

Introduction

The ideal anesthetic protocol for Caesarean section should provide adequate analgesia, muscle relaxation, and sedation or narcosis for optimal operating conditions and safety to the mother without unduly depressing or compromising the fetus. Drugs that induce analgesia, sedation and narcosis, such as anesthetics, analgesics, tranquilizers, and sedatives, must of necessity cross the blood-brain barrier. Because the physicochemical properties that allow drugs to cross the blood-brain barrier also allow their placental transfer, it is not possible to anesthetize the mother selectively while sparing the fetus. Fetal depression and hence decreased viability is directly proportional to the degree of maternal depression. Caesarean section is often an emergency procedure. Frequently, the physical condition of the mother and fetus is less than optimal because veterinary assistance has been delayed. Thus, the veterinarian is faced with the dilemma of having to anesthetize the mother, who may already be compromised, without adversely affecting the fetus.

No anesthetic or anesthetic protocol is ideal for all parturients. The choice of anesthetic protocol is based upon safety to the mother and fetus, patient comfort, convenience to the surgeon to allow rapid completion of the procedure, and familiarity with the anesthetic technique. Further, the choice of anesthetic protocol must be based upon knowledge of the physiological alterations induced by pregnancy and labor, the pharmacology of the agents when administered in the perinatal period and their direct and indirect effects on the fetus and neonate, the benefits and risks of the techniques chosen, and the significance of obstetric complications in anesthetic management. Regardless of the technique used, agents should be chosen and administered to minimize fetal depression. Minimizing time from induction to delivery, and especially that between isolation of the uterus and fetal removal, will decrease fetal exposure to anesthetic drugs and the period of maternal cardiopulmonary depression induced by anesthetic agent and recumbency.

Table 13.6
Physiological Alterations Induced by Pregnancy

Variable	
Heart rate	Increased
Cardiac output	Increased
Blood volume	Increased
Plasma volume	Increased
Packed cell volume, hemoglobin, and plasma protein concentration	Decreased
Arterial blood pressure	Unchanged
Central venous pressure	Unchanged; increases during labor
Minute volume of ventilation	Increased
Oxygen consumption	Increased
Arterial blood gases and pH	pH and oxygen tension unchanged; carbon dioxide tension decreased
Total lung capacity and vital capacity	Unchanged
Functional residual capacity	Unchanged
Gastric emptying time and intragastrical pressure	Increased
Gastric motility and pH of gastric secretions	Decreased
Gastric C1 and enzyme concentration	Increased
SGOT, LDH, and BSP retention time	Increased
Plasma cholinesterase concentration	Decreased
Renal plasma flow and glomerular filtration rate	Increased
BUN and creatinine	Decreased
Na^+ and water balance	Unchanged

Physiological Alterations Induced by Pregnancy

Metabolic demands of gestation and parturition are met by altered physiologic function (Table 13.6). Most of the data describing these physiological alterations has been obtained from women and ewes. Although little similar work has been done in other species, the changes should be comparable, even if not of equal magnitude. Birth weight expressed as percent of maternal weight for people, sheep, dogs, and cats is 5.7%, 11.4%, 16.1%, and 13.2%, respectively (1). This suggests that the physiological burden and therefore physiological alterations may be greater in animals than in women.

CARDIOVASCULAR ALTERATIONS

Pregnancy induces alterations in normal cardiovascular variables which affect the response to anesthetic agents and adjuncts. Because of increased heart rate and stroke volume, cardiac output increases during pregnancy to 30 to 50% above normal near term (2, 3). During labor and immediately postpartum, cardiac output increases an additional 10 to 25% as a result of blood being extruded from the contracting uterus (4). Cardiac output during labor is also influenced by the parturient's body position, pain, and apprehension (5). During pregnancy, blood volume increases by approximately 40%; plasma volume increases more than red cell mass, resulting in decreased hemoglobin concentration and packed cell volume (5). Systolic and diastolic blood pressure remains unchanged during pregnancy as a result of decreased peripheral vascular resistance. During labor, systolic pressure increases 10 to 30 mm Hg. While central venous pressure does not change during pregnancy because of increased venous capacity, it increases slightly (4 to 6 cm H_2O) during labor and has been reported to increase by 50 cm H_2O during painful fetal extraction (6). Dorsal recumbency can result in compression of the posterior vena cava and aorta by the enlarged uterus and its contents. This can cause decreased venous return and cardiac output with resultant decreased uterine and renal blood flow. Therefore, time spent restrained or positioned in dorsal recumbency should be kept to a minimum (7, 8).

Clinical Implications

Because cardiac work is increased during pregnancy and at parturition, cardiac reserve is decreased. Pulmonary congestion and heart failure may occur in patients with previously well-compensated heart disease. In such patients, additional stress induced by pain and anxiety should be relieved. However, care must be taken to avoid excessive cardiac depression and decompensation induced by excessive doses of analgesics, sedatives, or anesthetics. The use of ecbolic agents during or after parturition can adversely affect cardiovascular function. Oxytocin in large or repeated doses induces peripheral vasodilation and hypotension, which can adversely affect both mother and fetus through decreased tissue perfusion. Ergot derivatives induce vasoconstriction and hypertension. Severe hypertension and cardiac failure may occur if they are given after delivery when cardiac output is highest (9). Because venous engorgement decreases the size of the epidural space, the dose of local anesthetic agent required for epidural analgesia should be reduced by approximately one-third (5).

PULMONARY ALTERATIONS

During pregnancy, increased serum concentration of progesterone increases the sensitivity of the respiratory center to arterial carbon dioxide tension ($PaCO_2$). As a result of increased minute volume of ventilation, $PaCO_2$ decreases and is near 30 torr at parturition. This respiratory alkalosis does not affect arterial pH because of long-term renal compensation. Oxygen consumption increases 20% due to the developing fetus, placenta, uterine muscle, and mammary tissue, but arterial oxygen tension remains unchanged. Ventilation may be further increased during labor by pain, apprehension, and anxiety (5).

Pregnancy also affects the mechanics of ventilation. Airway conductance is increased and total pulmonary resistance is decreased as a result of hormone-induced relaxation of bronchial smooth muscle. Lung compliance is unaffected. Functional residual capacity (FRC) is decreased by anterior displacement of the diaphragm and abdominal organs by the gravid uterus. In addition, FRC decreases further during labor due to increased pulmonary blood volume subsequent to intermittent uterine contraction. Due to the decrease in FRC, airway closure at end exhalation develops in approximately one-third of parturients during tidal ventilation (5). Total lung capacity and vital capacity are unaltered.

Clinical Implications

Because FRC is decreased, hypoventilation induces hypoxemia and hypercapnia more readily in pregnant than nonpregnant patients. Hypoxemia is exacerbated by increased oxygen consumption during labor. Thus, induction of anesthesia must be smooth and rapid. Excitation and struggling associated with excessive restraint and poor technique must be avoided. Intubation should be accomplished quickly and ventilation supported to ensure adequate oxygenation. Adequacy of ventilation may be assessed by observing rate of respiration, excursion of the chest wall and/or reservoir bag, and color of mucous membranes. Close monitoring is essential.

Induction of anesthesia with inhalation agents is more rapid in pregnant than nonpregnant patients. The rate of equilibration between inspired and alveolar anesthetic partial pressure is increased by the increased alveolar ventilation and decreased FRC. In addition, pregnancy decreases anesthetic requirements. MAC (minimum alveolar anesthetic concentration that prevents purposeful movement in response to a noxious stimulus in 50% of patients) values are reduced by 25% for halothane, 32% for methoxyflurane, and 40% for isoflurane in pregnant compared to nonpregnant animals. Thus, anesthetic induction may be extremely rapid requiring as little as one-fourth to one-fifth the time required for nonpregnant patients (10). Therefore, care must be taken to prevent overanesthetization of pregnant patients.

GASTROINTESTINAL FUNCTION ALTERATIONS

Physical displacement of the stomach by the gravid uterus, decreased gastric motility, and increased serum progesterone delay gastric emptying. Acid, chloride, and enzyme concentrations in gastric secretions are increased. Lower esophageal sphincter tone is decreased, and intragastric pressure is increased. Pain and anxiety during labor (5) decrease gastric motility further.

Clinical Implications

As a result of altered gastric function, the risk of regurgitation (both active and passive) and aspiration is greater in the parturient. Frequently, patients presented for Caesarean section have been fed or the time of the last feeding is unknown. In all cases, parturients should be regarded as having a full stomach. Tracheal intubation should be performed rapidly upon induction of general anesthesia to gain control of the airway and prevent aspiration of foreign material. Incidence of vomiting is increased by opiates, xylazine, hypotension, hypoxia, and toxic reactions to local anesthetics. Smooth induction of general anesthesia and prevention of hypotension during epidural anesthesia will decrease the incidence of vomiting. Because silent regurgitation can occur when intragastric pressure is high, a cuffed endotracheal tube is desirable. Passive regurgitation can be induced by positive pressure ventilation with a face mask or succinylcholine-induced fasciculations. Atropine given intravenously may increase gastroesophageal sphincter tone, thereby helping to prevent regurgitation (6).

HEPATIC AND RENAL FUNCTION ALTERATIONS

Pregnancy induces minor alterations in hepatic function. Plasma protein concentration decreases slightly, but total plasma protein is increased due to the increase in blood volume. Bilirubin concentration is unaltered. Serum enzyme concentrations serum glutamic oxaloacetic transaminase (SGOT) and lactic dehydrogenase (LDH) are slightly increased, and sulfobromophthalein sodium (BSP) retention is increased. Plasma cholinesterase concentration decreases. In spite of these alterations, overall liver function is generally well maintained and adequate (5).

Renal plasma flow and glomerular filtration rate are increased by approximately 60% in pregnant patients. As a result, blood urea nitrogen and creatinine concentrations are lower than in nonpregnant patients (6). Sodium and water balance are unaffected.

Clinical Implications

Decreased plasma cholinesterase may result in prolonged action of succinylcholine in the pregnant patient, particularly if they have been exposed recently to organophosphate parasiticides (e.g. anthelmintics, flea collars, or dips). Normal or slightly elevated blood urea nitrogen or creatinine levels may indicate renal pathology or compromise in parturient patients. It would appear wise in such patients to avoid drugs with known nephrotoxic potential, such as tetracyclines, aminoglycoside antibiotics, and methoxyflurane.

UTERINE BLOOD FLOW ALTERATIONS

Fetal and maternal homeostasis and neonatal survival are dependent upon maintenance of the uteroplacental circulation. Uterine blood flow is directly proportional to perfusion pressure and inversely proportional to uterine vascular resistance. Obstetrical anesthesia may decrease uterine blood flow and thereby contribute directly to reduced fetal viability. In addition, uterine vascular resistance is indirectly increased by uterine contractions and hypertonia (oxytocic response). Arterial hypotension is induced by hypovolemia or sympathetic blockade. Vasoconstriction is induced by endogenous sympathetic discharge or by exogenous sympathomimetics having alpha-1 adrenergic effects, such as epinephrine, norepinephrine, methoxamine, phenylephrine, or metaraminol (5, 11, 12).

Clinical Implications

Hypotension induced by anesthetic agents or adjuncts and increased uterine tone induced by ecbolics should be avoided when possible. Either condition alone or in combination will decrease uteroplacental circulation with adverse fetal effects.

SUMMARY

Because cardiac reserve diminishes during pregnancy, cardiac decompensation or failure can occur. Likewise, pregnant patients are prone to hypoventilation, hypoxia, and hypercarbia due to altered pulmonary function. Inhalation anesthetic dose is decreased, thus increasing the likelihood of overdose and excessive depression with these agents. Finally, vomition or regurgitation and aspiration can occur if induction and intubation are not performed expediently. Thus because of the physiological alterations induced by pregnancy, parturient patients are at greater anesthetic risk. Physiologic changes associated with pregnancy and labor are further summarized in Table 13.6.

Perinatal Pharmacology

Alterations in physiological function induced by pregnancy will variably effect the uptake, distribution, and final disposition of anesthetic agents and adjuncts. The concentration of free drug in maternal plasma, which is the portion of the administered dose exerting maternal and fetal effects, is dependent upon several complex processes that occur simultaneously. These include uptake from the site of administration, protein binding, distribution to maternal tissues, biotransformation by maternal liver, excretion, placental transfer, and fetal distribution and metabolism. Because quantitative studies of drug disposition in pregnant patients are sparse, the effects of pregnancy upon drug disposition are largely unknown (13). The effects of pregnancy on drug biotransformation and excretion are variable and not fully understood. Inhalation anesthetic dose (MAC) is reduced due to an unknown mechanism. Hepatic biotransformation of barbiturates appears to be decreased in pregnancy (13). As a result of decreased plasma cholinesterase concentrations, succinylcholine and procaine metabolism is decreased, although usually not significantly (13). The increase in renal blood flow and glomerular filtration should favor renal excretion of drugs.

The placenta was once regarded as a relative barrier to passage of drugs from mother to fetus. It is now recognized as being quite permeable to anesthetics and anesthetic adjuncts. Any drug administered to the mother will cross the placenta at a rate unique to each drug and induce its effect upon the fetus. These effects will be proportionate to those observed in the mother. Factors that determine placental transfer of drugs and their distribution into and ultimate removal from fetal tissues include: physiochemical properties of the compound; the anatomical features of the maternal circulation, placenta, and fetus; and the hemodynamic and pharmacokinetic events that occur within them (13).

Medications administered at parturition affect the fetus either directly as a result of placental transfer or indirectly through their effects on the mother. Placental transfer of drugs can occur by several mechanisms: simple diffusion, facilitated diffusion via carrier systems, active transport, and pinocytosis. Of these, by far the most important is simple diffusion. The amount of drug crossing the placenta and entering the fetal circulation is described by the Fick equation:

$$Q/t = K \frac{A(Cm - C_f)}{D}$$

where:

Q/t = amount of diffused substance per unit time,
K = diffusion constant of a given substance,
A = surface area available for diffusion,
D = thickness of the membrane (placenta),
Cm = concentration of the substance in the maternal blood perfusing the placenta (uterine artery concentration), and
Cf = concentration of drug in fetal blood perfusing the placenta (umbilical artery concentration).

Surface area and thickness of the placenta are determined by the type of placenta present in a given species. The common domestic farm animals have thick epitheliochorial placentas with relatively small areas for diffusion, due to their cotyledonary or patchy diffuse distribution. The dog and cat have thinner endotheliochorial placentas with somewhat larger zonary areas of implantation. Women and rodents have the thinnest type of placenta, which is the hemochorial (14, 15). Thus, the placental diffusion barrier, although not of great significance, is greatest in ruminants, pigs, and horses, intermediate in the dog and cat, and least in rodents and women.

The diffusion constant (K) is unique to each drug and affected by the conditions present in the dam at the time of its administration. The diffusion constant is determined by molecular weight, degree to which the drug is bound to maternal plasma proteins, lipid solubility, and degree of ionization. Drugs with low molecular weight (MW < 500), a low degree of protein binding, high lipid solubility, and poor ionization have high K values and diffuse rapidly across the placenta. Those with high molecular weights (MW > 1000) that are highly protein bound, have low lipid solubility, and are highly ionized cross the placenta slowly. Most anesthetics and anesthetic adjuncts have high K values due to their low molecular weight, high lipid solubility, low degree of ionization, and low degree of protein binding. The muscle relaxant drugs are an exception. These agents are highly ionized and of low lipid solubility. Thus, their K value is low and, although they can be recovered from fetal blood, they are generally regarded as having minimal placental transfer and negligible direct fetal affects (13, 16). The degree to which a drug is ionized in the body is determined by its pKa and the pH of the patient's body fluids. The pKa is the pH at which the ionized and nonionized forms of the drug exist in equal proportions and is unique to each drug. Drugs that are weak acids will be less highly ionized as pH decreases (16). For example, thiopental is a weak acid with a pKa of 7.6. Thus, when administered to a patient with pH of 7.4, 61% of the drug is nonionized and active. In acidemic patients with pH's less than 7.4, a greater proportion of the administered dose will be nonionized. Therefore, acidemia decreases the required anesthetic dosage of thiopental and other barbiturates. In addition, as the degree of ionization decreases, so does the fraction of the dose that is protein bound and thus not available to exert its effect. Weakly basic drugs such as opiates and local anesthetics are more highly ionized at pH's below their pKa (17). In addition to the effect upon degree of ionization and thus the fraction of the dose in active form, distribution of drug between mother and fetus is influenced by their blood pH and drug pKa. Normally, the fetal pH is 0.1 units less than that of the mother. Thus, weakly basic drugs such as opiates and local anesthetics will be found in higher concentration in fetal tissues and plasma than in those of the mother due to "ion trapping." The nonionized form can cross the placenta but, due to the maternal-fetal pH difference, ionization occurs in the fetus. This decreases the concentration of fetal nonionized drug maintaining the maternal-fetal concentration gradient and more nonionized drug can cross the placenta to the fetus (18).

Maternal blood concentration of drug is dependent upon total dose, site and route of administration, rate of distribution and uptake of the drug by maternal tissues, and maternal metabolism and excretion. Thus, drugs with rapidly declining plasma concentration after administration of a fixed dose (e.g., thiopental or succinylcholine) result in a short period of exposure of the fetus and placenta to high maternal blood drug concentration. This can be contrasted to the sustained maternal blood levels of drugs administered by continuous infusion and inhalation anesthetics which result in continuous placental transfer of drug to the fetus (13, 18).

Fetal drug concentration is the result of passive

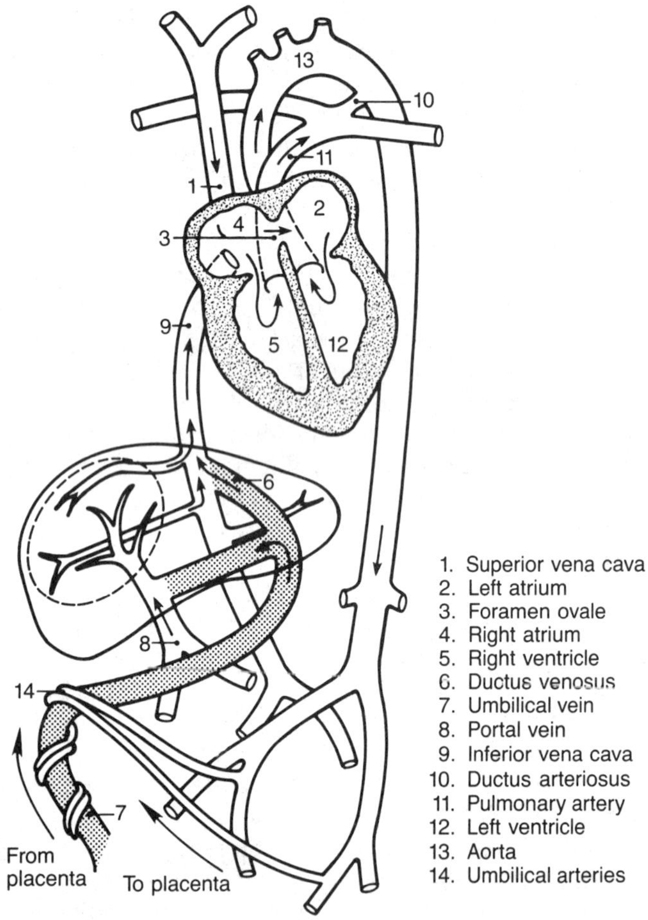

Figure 13.25. Major vasculature of the fetus. *Arrows* indicate direction of blood flow. Umbilical venous blood (*stippled*) perfuses the liver via the portal vein or enters the inferior vena cava via the ductus venosus. Right to left shunting of blood occurs through the foramen ovale and the ductus arteriosus, which close after birth.

diffusion across the placenta and is altered by fetal redistribution, metabolism, and protein binding. The concentration of drug in the umbilical vein is not that which is available to the fetal target organs (brain, heart, and other vital organs). As much as 85% of umbilical venous blood initially passes through the fetal liver, where drug may be sequestered or metabolized. In addition, umbilical venous blood containing drug enters the inferior vena cava via the ductus venosus and mixes with drug-free blood returning from the lower extremities and pelvic viscera (Fig. 13.25). In this way the fetal circulation buffers vital fetal tissues from sudden high drug concentrations. Binding of drug to fetal proteins may limit the amount of available drug and thus reduce toxicity (13, 16). Fetal metabolism of drugs is not as efficient as in the adult because the fetal liver microsomal enzyme system is not as active as in later life. Drug concentrations and effects can be considerably greater and of longer duration than in the mother. Finally, fetal drug toxicity can be enhanced by fetal or maternal metabolism to more toxic metabolites and by drug interaction (18).

CLINICAL IMPLICATIONS

Anesthetic and anesthetic adjunct drugs should be carefully chosen and properly administered to avoid undue maternal and fetal depression and to maximize neonatal vigor and viability. No agent should be used unless distinctly indicated.

Some drugs that induce sedation and/or tranquilization include the barbiturates, phenothiazines, butyrophenones, benzodiazepines, and xylazine. All of these agents rapidly cross the placenta, resulting in neonatal depression. Barbiturates cause neonatal respiratory depression, sleepiness, and decreased activity. Suckling activity is decreased and has been reported to be depressed for 4 days in the human neonate (18).

Phenothiazine and butyrophenone tranquilizers are frequently used as preanesthetic agents and are often used in conjunction with opiates. Phenothiazines potentiate opiate-induced depression but add little to analgesia. They induce hypotension via alpha-adrenergic blockade, as well as central nervous depression. This results in respiratory depression and decreased ability to regulate body temperature. Their duration of action is long, lasting up to 8 hours (6, 18). The use of tranquilizer-sedative drugs should be restricted to the markedly apprehensive or excited parturient and then only in doses sufficient to induce a calming effect without undue generalized depression. There is little indication for the routine use of these agents in the parturient patient (18).

Diazepam (Valium), when used to induce maternal sedation, can induce neonatal lethargy, hypotonus, and hypothermia (13). These effects are avoided by administering less than 0.14 mg/kg i.v. (18).

Xylazine (Rompun) is a potent sedative-hypnotic with significant analgesic properties. However, this agent rapidly crosses the placenta and induces both maternal and fetal respiratory and circulatory depression. When used in conjunction with ketamine, there are significant and potentially life-threatening cardiopulmonary changes resulting in decreased tissue perfusion in healthy dogs (19). Thus, use of xylazine or xylazine-ketamine combinations probably should be avoided in patients presented for Caesarean section. Similar effects have recently been reported for ketamine-acepromazine in the cat (20).

Opiates rapidly cross the placenta and can cause neonatal respiratory and neurobehavioral depression that may last up to 24 hours (18, 21, 22). In addition, fetal elimination may require 2 to 6 days. It appears that depression is proportional to degree of analgesia; equal analgesic doses of opiates induce equal degrees of depression. Thus, the choice of an opiate is based upon the duration of action desired. The most commonly used opiates are fentanyl, meperidine, and oxymorphone, in order of increasing duration of action (18). Recently, agents having opiate agonist and antagonist activity have been used to induce analgesia. These agents are nalbuphine and butorphanol. They reportedly induce less respiratory depression than pure opiate agonists. In addition, a narcotics license is not required for use of these agents. One of the advantages of opiate agonists is that direct antagonists are available to reverse their action. Of the antagonist agents, naloxone (0.04 mg/kg) appears to be one of the most effective. It is a pure antagonist without opiate agonist action. Because nalorphine and levellorphan possess opiate activity of their own, they can increase depression induced by other nonopiate agents (e.g., barbiturates, phenothiazines, and inhalation agents).

Because all opiate antagonists rapidly cross the placenta, maternal administration before delivery has been advocated to reverse opiate-induced neonatal depression. This technique deprives the mother of analgesia at the time when it is needed most. Therefore, these agents should be administered directly to the neonate.

Finally, because naloxone has a shorter duration of action than most opiate agonists, renarcotization may occur when naloxone is metabolized and excreted. Thus, both mother and neonates should be carefully monitored after opiate reversal with naloxone for recurring signs of narcosis (18). Should this occur, additional naloxone should be given.

The most commonly used intravenous induction agents are the ultrashort-acting barbiturates thiopental, thiamylal, or methohexital. When administered in low doses (less than 4 mg/kg) to women, fetal depression is minimal (18). Ketamine can be given intravenously to induce anesthesia for intubation rather than a barbiturate. In women, doses of less than 1 mg/kg induced minimal neonatal depression (18, 23). Because effective induction doses for these agents are higher in dogs and cats than humans, some neonatal depression is more likely to be associated with their use.

Some other injectible short-acting nonbarbiturate anesthetics are currently in use in the United Kingdom and Europe. These agents are not approved for use in the United States at this time but may become available in the future. Saffan is a combination of two progesterone-like steroids (Alphaxalone, 9 mg/ml, and Alphadolone, 3 mg/ml). This agent can be administered intravenously or intramuscularly to cats. Anesthetic induction is smooth and rapid. Cardiovascular depression is proportionate to dosage and similar to that of equivalent doses of thiopental or methohexital. Saffan induces less respiratory depression than barbiturates. Saffan is compatible with the commonly used preanesthetics, muscle relaxants, and inhalation anesthetics (23). Due to its short duration of action, the agent is best suited for induction of anesthesia for Caesarean section. Saffan has been shown to cross the placenta. Its use in the dog is limited because the solubilizing agent causes severe histamine release. However, it has been used to induce anesthesia in dogs pretreated with antihistamines (24).

Etomidate is a short-acting nonbarbiturate hypnotic. In dosages suitable for anesthetic induction, etomidate induced rapid safe anesthesia with no significant cardiovascular effects in dogs. On the basis of its cardiopulmonary effects, etomidate has been judged to be superior to thiamylal for anesthetic induction in the dog. In women, induction and recovery occur more rapidly with etomidate than with thiopental (25). Fetal tissue perfusion is enhanced, as shown by more rapid initiation of neonatal spontaneous breathing and greater fetal vitality at delivery than with thiopental (26).

Skeletal muscle relaxants cross the placenta to a very limited degree and induce little effect on the neonate when used in reasonable clinical doses (16); thus these agents are very useful in balanced anesthesia techniques for Caesarean section (23, 24). The most commonly used agents are succinylcholine and pancuronium. Succinylcholine, due to its rapid onset and short duration of action, is especially useful when combined with an ultrashort-acting barbiturate for induction or where muscle relaxation of short duration is desired. Pancuronium can be used to induce muscle relaxation of longer duration (45 minutes). Gallamine may also be used; however, because this drug appears to cross the placenta more readily than the other muscle relaxants and because it offers no distinct advantages, its use in obstetrics has diminished (18).

Atracurium and vecuronium are nondepolarizing muscle relaxants. Because both these agents are rapidly metabolized in the liver and atracurium is metabolized by Hoffman elimination, they have a short duration of action similar to that of succinylcholine. These agents have fewer cardiovascular side effects than the other muscle relaxants. However, due to economic considerations, their use in veterinary medicine is limited at this time.

Inhalation anesthetics readily cross the placenta with rapid fetal and maternal equilibration. Thus, the degree of neonatal depression is proportional to the depth of anesthesia induced in the mother. Deep levels of maternal anesthesia cause maternal hypotension, decreased uterine blood flow, and fetal acidosis. The less soluble agents halothane, isoflurane, and enflurane are preferable to highly soluble agents such as methoxyflurane because induction and recovery of mother and neonate are more rapid. Nitrous oxide can be used to potentiate the more potent volatile agents, thus decreasing the total amount of volatile agent administered. If nitrous oxide is administered at 60%, fetal depression is minimal and neonatal diffusion hypoxia does not occur upon delivery (18, 24, 25).

Administration of oxygen to the mother is not associated with a significant decrease in uterine blood flow or fetal acidosis (18). Fetal red blood cells are low as compared to the adult in 2,3-diphosphoglycerate (2,3-DPG) concentration. This anion competes with oxygen for the binding site on the hemoglobin molecule. Thus fetal hemoglobin can carry more oxygen at low oxygen tensions than adult hemoglobin. Physiologically, this is important in that it ensures a higher level of hemoglobin saturation at the normally low oxygen partial pressures (PO_2 of umbilical vein equals 30 torr) (26), to which the fetus is exposed. Maternal oxygen administration can result in a significant increase in fetal oxygen content. Therefore, oxygen administration is indicated regardless of the anesthetic protocol. Inspired oxygen concentrations of 50% or more during general anesthesia result in more vigorous neonates because of improved oxygenation (18).

The total effect of carbon dioxide on the fetus is not clear, but passive hyperventilation of the dam results in hypocapnia with decreased uterine artery blood flow. This decreased placental perfusion causes fetal hypoxia, hypercapnia, and acidosis. Maternal active hyperventilation may have the same effect. With adequate arterial oxygenation, a modest increase in $PaCO_2$ is well tolerated by the fetus (18).

Local anesthetic agents are frequently used in combination with other agents or as the sole anesthetic agent for regional techniques. Esters of para-aminobenzoic acid, such as procaine or tetracaine, are metabolized by maternal and fetal pseudocholinesterase. Thus, there is little accumulation of these agents in the fetus. Amide derivatives (e.g., lidocaine, mepivicaine, bupivicaine, and etidocaine) are metabolized by hepatic microsomal enzymes. After absorption from the site of injection, blood levels decrease slowly but can reach significant levels in the fetus. Neonatal blood concentrations in excess of 3 μg/ml of lidocaine or mepivicaine cause neonatal depression at delivery. These concentrations rarely occur after epidural administration but can occur with excessive volumes of drug used for local infiltration (18). Use of these agents can indirectly affect the fetus. Sympathetic blockade resulting in maternal hypotension and decreased uteroplacental perfusion may occur after epidural injection. This can be controlled by judicious administration of intravenous fluids to offset increased capacity of the vascular tree (25). In addition to intravenous fluids, vasopressors can be used to treat maternal hypotension resulting from sympathetic blockade. Because ephedrine acts centrally and has minimal arterial vasoconstrictor properties while increasing venous tone and thereby preload, it is used to treat maternal hypotension, thus restoring uterine blood flow. Mephentermine acts in a similar manner. Other agents with alpha-adrenergic activity increase maternal blood pressure by increasing systemic vascular resistance. This results in decreased uterine blood flow, and fetal deterioration often occurs. In addition, these agents stimulate hypertonic uterine contractions, further decreasing uteroplacental perfusion (18, 25).

Anticholinergic agents, such as atropine or glycopyrrolate, should be administered to most parturient patients (23, 27) to decrease salivation and inhibit excessive vagal tone that may occur when traction is applied to the uterus. Many parturients have recently eaten, increasing the likelihood of regurgitation, which is enhanced by hypoxia or hypotension. The influence of anticholinergics upon vomition is controversial (6, 28). In women, atropine has not been shown to decrease the incidence of vomition at parturition (29). Glycopyrrolate increases gastric pH, thus decreasing severity of Mendelson's syndrome should regurgitation and aspiration of vomitus occur (30). Additionally, because glycopyrrolate does not readily cross the placenta, it does not effect the fetus to the same extent as atropine. Therefore, it may be a more appropriate anticholinergic (31).

Anesthetic Techniques for Caesarean Section

Satisfactory anesthesia for Caesarean section can be induced by a number of methods. Caesarean section can be accomplished either by regional or general anesthesia. Advantages of general anesthesia include speed and ease of induction, reliability, reproducibility, and controllability. General anesthesia provides optimum operating conditions with a relaxed immobile patient. Tracheal intubation ensures control of the maternal airway, thereby preventing aspiration of vomitus or regurgitated rumen contents. In addition, it provides a route for maternal oxygen administration, thereby improving fetal oxygenation. When general anesthesia is properly administered, maternal cardiopulmonary function is well maintained (23, 25). In addition, most veterinarians are more confident of their ability to induce general anesthesia safely than to induce regional anesthesia successfully. General anesthesia is not without disadvantages, however, because it induces greater neonatal depression than regional anesthesia. If the anesthetic plane is too light, maternal catecholamine release can result in hypertension and decreased uteroplacental perfusion, leading to both maternal and fetal stress and deterioration of cardiopulmonary function (11, 12, 21). Aspiration and problems of airway management with general anesthesia are more likely to occur when the trachea is not properly intubated. Aspiration and inability to successfully intubate the trachea are the leading causes of maternal mortality associated with Caesarean section in women (23, 25). Fortunately, dogs, cats, and horses are relatively easy to intubate because of their anatomical features. However, ruminants and swine are relatively difficult to intubate, and this presents problems for most veterinarians on the farm. General anesthesia is essential in mares and may be more appropriate than regional anesthesia in selected clinical situations in other species. These include maternal hypovolemia, prolonged dystocia in which the mother is exhausted and the fetus is severely stressed, maternal heart disease or failure, morbid obesity, cases in which the mother is so aggressive or fractious as to preclude regional anesthesia, brachycephalic dogs with upper airway obstruction, and instances in which the veterinarian is inexperienced in regional anesthetic techniques.

Many different techniques for induction of general anesthesia for Caesarean section have been shown to be satisfactory (24, 27, 32). The following can be used as guidelines to establish a protocol to meet the individual patient's requirements.

SMALL ANIMALS

Premedicate with atropine (0.04 mg/kg) or glycopyrrolate (0.011 mg/kg) i.m. or i.v. 10 to 20 minutes before induction. Avoid tranquilizers, sedatives, hypnotics, and opiates unless indicated by an overly apprehensive, aggressive, or fractious patient. If possible, preoxygenate for 3 to 5 minutes by mask.

Induction should be smooth, rapid, and efficient. The transition from the awake to the anesthetized state should be as physiological as possible. Intubation should be performed rapidly upon induction to gain contrtol of the airway, ensure adequate oxygenation, and prevent aspiration. Spraying the larynx with lidocaine will aid in prevention of laryngospasm, and coughing and ease intubation. Drugs used for induction include thiamylal Na (6 to 8 mg/kg i.v.), thiopental Na (8 to 10 mg/kg i.v.), methohexital Na (5 mg/kg i.v.), droperidol-fentanyl (Innovar-Vet; not suitable for use in cats) (1 ml/20 to 30 kg i.v.), diazepam (0.2 to 0.5 mg/kg i.v.) and ketamine HCl (not approved for use in dogs) (2 to 4 mg/kg i.v.), and acepromazine-oxymorphone (not suitable for use in cats) (0.1 mg/kg to a maximum of 4 mg acepromazine i.m. or i.v. and 0.11 mg/kg oxymorphone i.v.). Succinylcholine (0.3 mg/kg i.v.) can be administered to ease intubation with any of the above induction agents. When this drug is used, intubation must be rapid and ventilation must be controlled until spontaneous breathing resumes.

After intubation, oxygen should be administered. If available, nitrous oxide can be administered in a 50-50 mixture of nitrous oxide and oxygen.

Halothane, methoxyflurane, isoflurane, or enflurane can be administered to induce additional analgesia and narcosis as needed; vaporizer concentration should be low before delivery (0.5 to 1%, 0.5% to 0.75%, 0.7 to 1.39, and 0.8 to 1.7%, respectively), after which the concentration can be increased as needed for surgical closure. In addition, muscle relaxants may be given to induce relaxation at light planes of anesthesia, thus avoiding excessive anesthetic-induced fetal depression. These agents include: succinylcholine (0.2 to 0.4 mg/kg for 15 minutes), gallamine (0.4 mg/kg for 20 to 40 minutes), and pancuronium (0.06 to 0.14 mg/kg for 30 to 60 minutes). Muscle relaxation induced by gallamine or pancuronium may be reversed with neostigmine (0.06 to 0.2 mg/kg) or edrophonium (0.1 to 0.2 mg/kg). Either of these agents should be preceded by atropine (0.04 mg/kg) to prevent bradycardia.

LARGE ANIMALS

Premedicate with atropine or glycopyrrolate i.m. or i.v. 10 to 20 minutes before induction. Avoid tranquilizers, sedatives, and hypnotics unless indicated by an overly apprehensive, aggressive, or fractious patient.

Induction should be smooth, rapid, and efficient. The transition from the awake to the anesthetized state should be as physiological as possible. Intubation should be performed rapidly upon induction to gain control of the airway, ensure adequate oxygenation, and prevent aspiration. In swine, spraying the larynx with lidocaine will aid in prevention of laryngospasm and bronchospasm and ease intubation. Induction techniques include the following.

Horse

Induction is with an ultrashort-acting barbiturate in 5% guaifenesin or 1.1 mg/kg of xylazine i.v. followed in 5 minutes by 2.2 mg/kg of ketamine i.v. Anesthesia is maintained with halothane or isoflurane in oxygen.

Cattle

Induction is with an ultrashort-acting barbiturate in 5% guaifensin or 50 mg of xylazine and 500 mg of ketamine in 500 ml of 5% guaifenesin to effect.

Sheep and Goats

Induction is with an ultrashort-acting barbiturate in 5% guaifenasin or 50 mg of xylazine and 500 mg of ketamine in 500 ml of guaifenesin to effect, or 0.22 mg/kg of xylazine i.m. followed in 5 minutes by 11 mg/kg of ketamine i.m., or mask induction with a volatile inhalation anesthetic.

Swine

Induction is with an ultrashort-acting barbiturate, 500 mg of xylazine and 500 mg of ketamine in 500 ml of guaifenesin to effect i.v., or mask induction with volatile inhalation agents.

General anesthesia may be maintained in ruminants and swine with inhalation agents or by continuous infusion of the induction agents to effect. After completion of surgery, the mother is allowed to recover in a quiet area and extubated. Because vomiting and aspiration can occur on recovery as well as induction, extubation should be delayed until the mother can maintain sternal recumbency and defend her airway.

Regional anesthesia for Caesarean section is a well-established technique (24, 27, 33). Local infiltration or field block may be used, but it has several disadvantages when compared to the epidural technique. Infiltration requires larger amounts of anesthetic agent, which are absorbed and depress the fetus. Muscle relaxation and analgesia are not as profound or as uniform as with epidural techniques. Therefore, field block is often supplemented with heavy sedation or tranquilization, contributing to profound maternal and fetal depression. For these reasons, this type of approach should be abandoned for either general anesthesia or epidural anesthesia.

Because the spinal cord terminates at the level of the sixth lumbar vertebra in the dog and cat, subarachnoid (true spinal) injection of the anesthetic agent is not common when made at the lumbosacral junction. Because the spinal cord terminates at the midsacrum in swine and ruminants, subarachnoid injection can occur at the lumbosacral junction. Spinal anesthesia (epidural or subarachnoid) has the advantages of simplicity of technique, minimal exposure of the fetus to drugs, less intraoperative bleeding, and, because the mother remains awake, minimal risk of aspiration. In addition, muscle relaxation and analgesia are optimal. Disadvantages include hypotension secondary to sympathetic blockade. Nausea and vomiting can occur during the procedure as a result of hypotension and visceral manipulation. Because the dam remains conscious, movement of the forelimbs and head often occurs (33). This precludes the use of spinal technique in highly excited or fractious patients and in mares because they become hysterical when they are unable to stand. Finally, the successful induction of epidural anesthesia requires that the veterinarian be well acquainted with the technique. However, the skill required is well within the reach of anyone wishing to utilize this approach and can be readily acquired with minimal practice of the techniques, which are fully described in Chapter 8. The hypotension induced by epidural anesthesia can be readily offset by concurrent fluid and catecholamine administration. Lactated Ringer's solution, normal saline, or half-strength saline mixed with equal volumes of 5% dextrose solution can be administered at approximately 20 ml/kg over 15 to 20 minutes to maintain arterial blood pressure. When hypotension is severe, ephedrine may be administered (0.15 mg/kg i.v.). As with general anesthesia, anticholinergic agents are indicated to prevent bradycardia.

Spinal anesthesia will induce recumbency, which may not be desirable in large ruminants because of adverse effects on cardiopulmonary function. If the veterinarian prefers, standing Caesarean section in cattle may be performed using either a proximal or distal paralumbar block (see Chapter 8). In cows that are in poor condition, exhausted, or in shock, the distal technique is preferred because it does not induce a scoliosis-like position and the cow is more likely to remain standing throughout the procedure. These techniques may also be used in sheep and goats; however, most veterinarians find it convenient to place small ruminants in lateral recumbency for Caesarean section. Therefore, spinal techniques are preferable to regional techniques in sheep and goats.

Spinal techniques work well in sows. The technique is well established and not difficult to perform. When utilizing this technique, it is sometimes necessary to restrain the sow's head and forelimbs. If this is done, usually by placing a rope around the upper jaw, it is important that the head not be placed in extension. If pigs are sedated and restrained in lateral recumbency with the head extended, the soft palate may occlude the airway and the patient may suffocate. The authors have observed this occurrence in sows and gilts undergoing Caesarean section with spinal anesthesia without additional sedative or tranquilizers. Because Caesarean section in swine is often viewed as a last-ditch effort by producers, it is often delayed until the sow's condition has deteriorated severely. Often, the sow has been traumatized by repeated efforts to manually extract the piglets and has received large repeated doses of oxytocin. Thus a high percent of sows presented for Caesarean section are hypovolemic and hypotensive. In the authors' experience, success or failure is often predicated on restoring effective circulating blood volume before anesthesia and surgery. Fluids can be readily administered to sows via indwelling catheters placed percutaneously into the ear veins. Prior to anesthetic administration, 1 to 3 liters of lactated Ringer's solution or other balanced electrolyte solution can be given rapidly. This will restore circulating volume and offset hypotension induced by spinal techniques. Fluid administration can be continued throughout surgery to maintain a patent vein for administration of other supportive therapy as indicated.

As with general anesthesia, anticholinergic agents should be used to prevent vagal bradycardia.

Care of the Newborn

After delivery, the head should be cleared of membranes and the oropharynx should be cleared of fluid. The umbilical vessels should be milked toward the fetus to empty them of blood, clamped approximately 2 to 5 cm from the body wall, and severed from the placenta. The neonate can then be gently rubbed with a towel to dry it and stimulate breathing. It may also be helpful to gently swing the neonate in a head-down position to help clear the respiratory tree of fluid. The head and neck should be supported to avoid a whiplash action and prevent injury.

When general anesthesia is used in ruminants or horses, an alternate method of managing the neonate may be used to good advantage. After uterine incision, the fetal head is delivered through the incision, the oropharynx is cleared of fluid, and the trachea is intubated with a cuffed tube. The fetus can then be delivered and the umbilicus severed. Because the uteroplacental and umbilical circulation is preserved until the airway is secured, hypoxia is prevented. Once the fetus is delivered, ventilation can be supported if necessary via an Ambu bag.

Doxapram can be used to stimulate breathing in the neonate. In the pup, the dosage is 1 to 5 mg (approximately 1 to 5 drops from a 20 to 22 gauge needle). In the kitten, the dosage is 1 to 2 mg (1 to 2 drops) administered topically to the oral mucosa or injected intramuscularly or subcutaneously (34). Newborns are susceptible to chilling and should be kept warm (35). After completion of surgery and recovery from anesthesia, the young can be introduced to their mother. If regional anesthesia was used, they can be placed with their mother as soon as the surgery is complete.

Conclusion

Successful induction of anesthesia for Caesarean section is both challenging and rewarding. With proper attention to the physiological alterations induced by pregnancy and consideration of perinatal pharmacology, the properly performed technique can provide safe, effective anesthesia for mother and offspring.

References

1. Dawes GS: *Foetal and Neonatal Physiology*. Chicago, Year Book Medical Publishers Inc, 1968, p 15.
2. Kerr MG: Cardiovascular dynamics in pregnancy and labor. *Br Med Bull* 24:19, 1968.
3. Ueland K, Parer JT: Effects of estrogens on the cardiovascular system of the ewe. *Am J Obstet Gynecol* 96:400, 1966.
4. Ueland K, Hansen JM: Maternal cardiovascular dynamics. II: Posture and uterine contractions. *Am J Obstet Gynecol* 103:1–7, 1969.
5. Shnider SM: The physiology of pregnancy. *Annual Refresher Course Lectures*. Park Ridge, IL, American Society of Anesthesiologists, 1978, pp 1251–1258.
6. James FM III: Physiologic Changes during Pregnancy. *Annual Refresher Course Lectures*. Park Ridge, IL, American Society of Anesthesiologists, 1980, pp 1251–1255.
7. Marx GF: Physiology of pregnancy—High risk implications. *Annual Refresher Course Lectures*. Park Ridge, IL, American Society of Anesthesiologists, 1979, pp 1251–1254.
8. Kerr MG, Scott DB: Inferior vena caval occlusion in late pregnancy. In G Marx (ed): *Clinical Anesthesia*. Philadelphia, FA Davis, 1973, vol 10–2, p 38.
9. Lipton B, Hershey SG, Baez S: Compatibility of oxytocics with anesthetic agents. *JAMA* 179:410–416, 1962.
10. Palahniuk RJ, Shnider SM, Eger EI III, Lopez-Manzanara P: Pregnancy decreases the requirements of inhaled anesthetic agents. *Anesthesiology* 41:82–83, 1974.
11. Wright RG, Shnider SM, Levinson G, et al: The effect of maternal stress on plasma catecholamines and uterine blood flow in the pregnant ewe. Abstract, Annual Meeting of the Society of Obstetric Anesthesia and Perinatology, 1978, p 17.
12. Morishema HO, Yeh M-N, James LS: The effects of maternal pain and hyperexcitability upon the fetus—Possible benefits of maternal sedation. Abstract, Scientific Session of American Society of Anesthesiologists Annual Meeting, 1977.
13. Alper MH: Perinatal pharmacology. *Annual Refresher Course Lectures*. Park Ridge, IL, American Society of Anesthesiologists, 1979, pp 1261–1267.
14. Ramsey EM: *The Placenta of Laboratory Animals and Man*. New York, Holt, Rinehart and Winston, 1975, pp 73, 142, 154, 160.
15. Nalbandov AV: *Reproductive Physiology*. San Francisco, WH Freeman, 1958, p 196.
16. Finster M: Perinatal pharmacology. *Annual Refresher Course Lectures*. Park Ridge, IL, American Society of Anesthesiologists, 1980, pp 1261–1264.
17. Collins VJ: *Principles of Anesthesiology*, ed 2. Philadelphia, Lea & Febiger, 1976, p 199.
18. Gutsche B: Perinatal pharmacology. *Annual Refresher Course Lectures*. Park Ridge, IL, American Society of Anesthesiologists, 1978, pp 1291–1299.
19. McDonnell W, Van Gorder J: Cardiopulmonary effects of xylazine/ketamine in dogs. Abstract, Annual Scientific Meeting, American College of Veterinary Anesthesiologists, 1982.
20. Becker M, Beglinger R: Effects of ketamine and its combination with acepromazine on the cardiovascular system of the cat. Abstract, 1st International Congress of Veterinary Anesthesia, 1982.
21. Palahniuk RJ: Obstetric anesthesia in the healthy parturient. *Annual Refresher Course Lectures*. Park Ridge, IL, American Society of Anesthesiologists, 1979, pp 1271–1274.
22. Hodgkinson R, Bhatt M, Wang CN: Double-blind comparison of the neurobehavior of neonates following the administration of different doses of meperidine to the mother. *Can Anaesth Soc J* 25:405, 1978.
23. Hall LW: Althesin in the large animal. *Postgrad Med J* 48 (Supplement 2):55–58, 1972.
24. Corbet HR: The use of saffan in the dog. *Aust Vet Pract* 7(3–4):184–188, 1977.
25. Nagel ML, Muir WW, Nguyen K: Comparison of the cardiopulmonary effects of etomidate and thiamylal in dogs. *Am J Vet Res* 40, 2:193–196, 1979.

26. Downing JW, Buley RJR, Brock-Utne JG, Houlton PC: Etomidate for induction of anaesthesia at caesarian section: comparison with thiopentone. *Br J Anaesth* 51:135–140, 1979.
27. Gibbs CP: Anesthesia for cesarian section: general. *Annual Refresher Course Lectures.* Park Ridge, IL, American Society of Anesthesiologists, 1981, pp 2181–2185.
28. Datta S, Alper MH: Anesthesia for cesarean section. *Anesthesiology* 53:142–160, 1980.
29. Goodger WJ, Levy W: Anesthetic management of the cesarean section. In CE Short (ed): *Veterinary Clinics of North America,* vol 3, No 1. Philadelphia, WB Saunders, 1973, p 85.
30. Guyton AC: *Textbook of Medical Physiology,* ed 4. Philadelphia, WB Saunders, 1971, p 978.
31. Sawyer DC: The anesthetic period. In *Predictable Problems in the Practice of Small Animal Anesthesia.* Philadelphia, WB Saunders, 1982, p 194.
32. Ratra CK, Badola RP, Bhargava KP: A study of factors concerned in emesis during spinal anaesthesia. *Br J Anaesth* 44:1208–1211, 1972.
33. Dow TGB, Brock-Utne JG, Rubin J, et al: The effect of atropine on the lower esophageal sphincter during pregnancy. *Obstet Gynecol* 51:426–430, 1978.
34. Baraka A, Saab M, Salem MR, et al: Control of gastric acidity by glycopyrrolate premedication in the parturient. *Anesth Analg* (Cleve) 56:642, 1977.
35. Proakis AG, Harris GB: Comparative penetration of glycopyrrolate and atropine across the blood-brain and placental barriers in anesthetized dogs. *Anesthesiology* 486:339–344, 1978.
36. Soma LR: Anesthetic management. In *Textbook of Veterinary Anesthesia.* Baltimore, Williams & Wilkins, 1971, pp 303–309.
37. Klide AM: Epidural analgesia. In LR Soma (ed): *Textbook of Veterinary Anesthesia.* Baltimore, Williams & Wilkins, 1971, pp 450–467.
38. Reports on File. Pharmacology Department, AH Robins Company, Richmond, Virginia.
39. Mosier JE: Incubators and puppy survival. In *Nutrition and Management of Dogs and Cats.* St. Louis, Ralston Purina Company, 1981, p M10.

PART 8

Anesthetic Considerations in the Conditioned Animal

CHARLES E. SHORT, D.V.M., M.S., D.A.C.V.A.

Introduction

In both animal and human medicine, most consideration for anesthetic regimes has been given to the sick or injured patient with special concerns described when extensive pathophysiology exists. As evidenced in other chapters in this text, extensive information is available when considering anesthesia in patients with diseases of the heart, lungs, or other internal organs and in various species. Surprisingly, the literature is almost devoid of information on anesthesia in the conditioned animal or the human athlete. This is in spite of the tremendous upsurge in emphasis on human physical fitness and athletic competition and our enjoyment of animals, especially horses, in various performance activities. This has encouraged physical development, conditioning, breeding programs, nutrition, and other efforts to achieve peak performance. However, we associate athletes, animal or human, with such high levels of athletic performance that we seldom consider that they may require diagnostic or surgical procedures. Anesthetic management considerations for these patients are thus regarded as insignificant except in those cases in which complications occur. When anesthetic complications occur to a well-known athlete, the public is appalled, especially if the end result is death.

The need for anesthesia for diagnostic or surgical procedures in the athlete may occur during training, during high levels of performance, or after competition during the time that the physiological function of the athlete may be influenced by the training or competitive activity. Most of the competitive activities in nonequine animals concern greyhound racing. Equine performance includes a variety of events, varying from short races to extensive endurance rides of up to 100 miles. The differences in physical requirements of the

Thoroughbred, Standardbred, Quarterhorse, and other breeds for racing, dressage events, steeplechase, polo, and horse show events should be appreciated. Likewise, a difference in the mental attitude, physical capabilities, and stress of competition should be appreciated in comparing the Tennessee Walking Horse, the American Saddlebred, the Arabian, and other breeds.

Animal athletes respond to training for special events in many ways similar to the human athlete. There certainly is an expected difference in performance capability comparing long-distance runners to sprinters or ice-hockey players to football players. Figure 13.26 illustrates the conditioning and mental attitude of these competitive animal athletes.

Most athletic injuries in animals are contact injuries or injuries to the extremities occurring during competition. Anesthesia for orthopedic surgery or repair of soft tissue lesions occurring during training or athletic competition or after competition requires varying dosages of medication. Anesthesia for the repair of simple lesions varies greatly from general anesthesia with requirements for the completion of involved orthopedic procedures. In many instances, the most complicated part of the procedure may be postoperative recovery after the animal has responded well to the anesthetic regime during maintenance of oxygenation, fluid therapy, and other supportive measures. With these complexities of management of the athlete, it is only fitting to consider the physiology of exercise and how it may relate to selection of medications and anesthetic techniques for this group of animals. An extensive review of the literature reveals the responses to exercise discussed in this chapter.

Responses in Man That May Relate to Conditioned Animals

Reactivity of airways to short-term exercise was tested in 15 healthy subjects and repeated on 8 of the group using Stead-Wells and wedge spirometers and

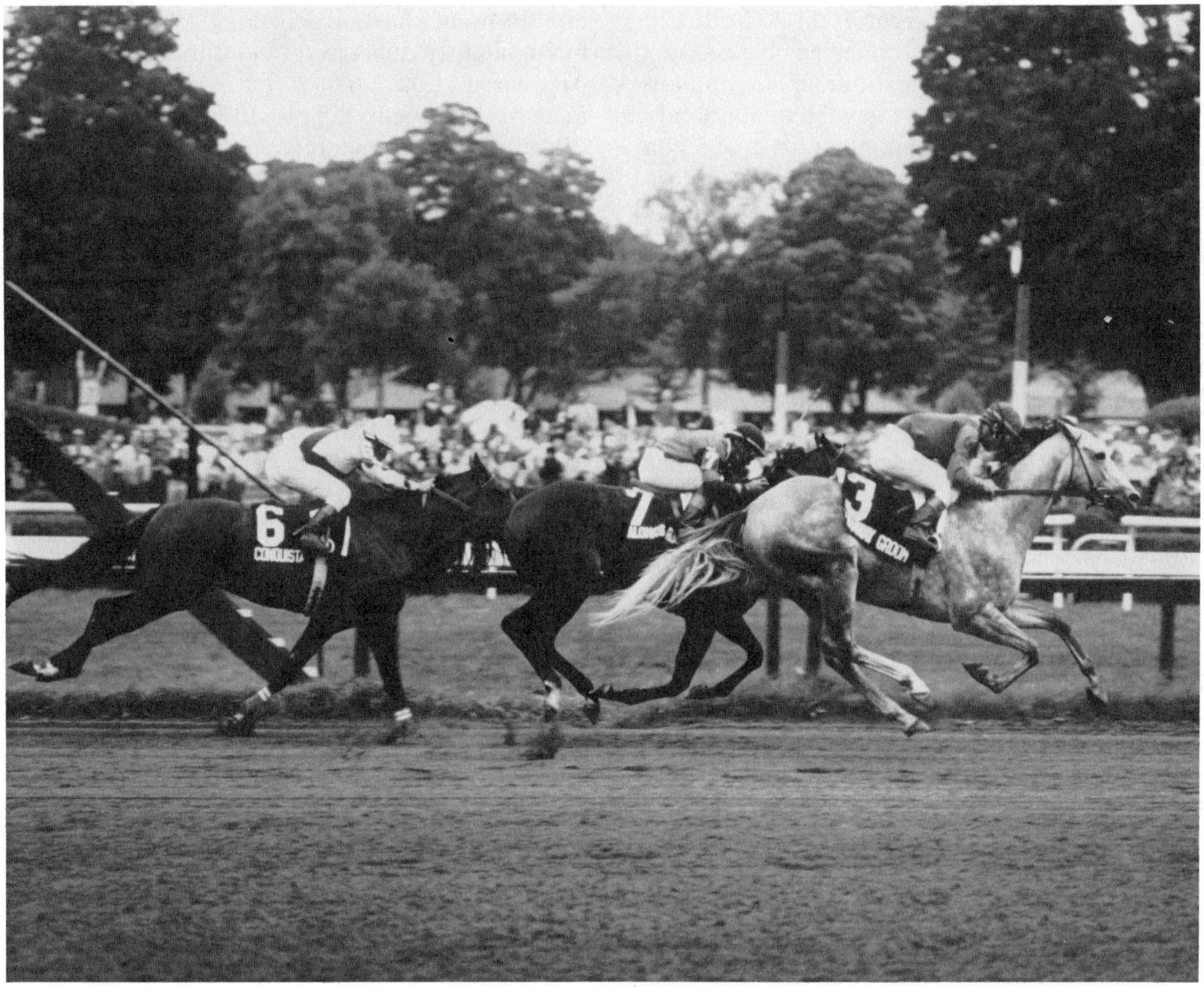

Figure 13.26. The competitive responses of conditioned Thoroughbreds in action. Photo of the Travers Stakes, Saratoga Race Track, 1983. Conquistador Cielo (6), Aloma's Ruler (7), and Runaway Groom (3). Photo courtesy of Mr. and Mrs. Albert P. Coppola.

body plethysmograph. The pulmonary function tests were performed at rest and shortly after exercise, and the data were studied by means of a randomized block analysis of variance. It was demonstrated that overall postexercise pulmonary functions were not statistically different from the pre-exercise baseline in humans (1). This does not explain the pulmonary hemorrhage often seen in race horses.

Cardiovascular and respiratory parameters were measured during and after release of pressure in thigh cuffs that occluded circulation to the legs of four human subjects exercising on a bicycle ergometer. The subjects exercised at 200 kg/min while thigh cuffs were inflated for 4 minutes and then released. Responses from six to eight identical experiments were ensemble-averaged so the precise timing of delays could be obtained. At 5 to 10 seconds after cuff release, end-tidal CO_2 increased, marking arrival of the trapped blood at the lungs. At 10 to 18 seconds after this increase in end-tidal CO_2, ventilation, respiratory rate, and tidal volume increased. This delay in ventilation must have resulted in an increase in arterial PCO_2 and suggests that arterial chemoreceptors mediated the responses and that no venous chemoreceptors or CO_2 flux or disequilibrium receptors in the lung need be postulated (2). Although this study was completed in humans, evidence is presented that gives partial explanation for the CO_2 responses seen during anesthesia in the conditioned animal if reduced perfusion of the extremities develops. Hypercarbia may be observed in conditioned animals even with excellent cardiopulmonary capability. Racehorses show increases in CO_2 in many cases.

The cardiorespiratory demands involved in playing ice hockey were reviewed in terms of their relation to short races. Heart rate (HR) monitoring by radiotelemetry during actual game performance has indicated near-maximal cardiorespiratory efforts for the 2.5- to 3-minute on-ice shifts. Analyses of the temporal characteristics of the game and thus the intermittent exercise (IE) schedules involved were also utilized to elucidate the cardiorespiratory demands of the sport. Compared to continuous exercise at the same average power output, IE performance represents a greater demand on both the central circulation and oxidative metabolism in the muscle cell. In IE with time and intensity components typical of those found in ice hockey as compared to continuous exercise, laboratory data showed a higher cardiac output and yet a widened arteriovenous oxygen difference in the active muscles compensating for a lower muscle blood flow. Further, it is suggested that there is reduced efficiency of the thermoregulatory system in IE, placing added demand on the cardiorespiratory system. The analysis suggests that training programs to increase aerobic power would be beneficial for ice hockey players (3). This indicates that the conditioned athlete needing anesthesia for a surgical procedure would have peak cardiopulmonary function. Conditioning for short bursts of high intensity physical activity (during which an injury requiring surgery may occur) would not cause cardiopulmonary compromise.

Adaptive cardiac responses to isotonic training were studied with echocardiographic measurement of cardiac dimensions and function in 20 endurance runners whose maximal aerobic capacity on the treadmill was 4.88 ± 0.13 (mean standard error of mean) liters of oxygen/minute. This may relate well to responses in horses during endurance rides. They were compared with 26 young sedentary control subjects whose capacity was 3.34 ± 0.11 liters of oxygen/minute ($P < 0.001$). A modest degree of right and left ventricular chamber enlargement and left ventricular hypertrophy was observed in endurance runners (left ventricular mass index, 140 ± 6 G/M2 compared with 107 ± 4 G/M2 in sedentary control subjects ($P < 0.001$). Resting heart rate was slower in endurance runners (51 ± 2 versus 62 ± 2 beats/minute, $P < 0.001$). Resting left ventricular function as evaluated with ejection fraction and maximal posterior wall shortening velocity and mean circumferential shortening velocity (VCF) was comparable or slightly depressed in endurance runners (0.98 ± 0.03 versus 1.02 ± 0.05 circumferences/second, difference not significant). This study suggests that isotonic training results in adaptive changes in ventricular volume and mass, slower heart rates that may be associated with more efficient pumping function (that is, increasing stroke volume), and insignificant alterations in resting ejection phase indexes of left ventricular function (4).

A battery of noninvasive graphic techniques was used, including echocardiogram (ECG), apexcardiogram, carotid pulse, electrocardiogram, vectorcardiogram (VCG), phonocardiogram, systolic time intervals, and treadmill stress testing, in 12 professional marathon runners, mean age 33.8 ± 11.1. A group of 20 nonathletes matched for age, height, sex, and weight served as a control group. Left ventricular (LV) end-diastolic dimension in marathon runners averaged 5.53 ± 0.5 cm compared to 4.81 ± 0.04 cm in nonathletes ($P < 0.001$). LV end-diastolic volume was 172.69 ± 43.3 ml compared to 113.57 ± 30.41 ml in nonathletes ($P < 0.001$). Stroke volume was 122.27 ± 32.8 ml compared to 78.42 ± 20.44 ml in nonathletes ($P < 0.001$). The thickness of the posterior LV wall was 1.0 ± 0.2 cm compared to 0.7 ± 0.1 cm in nonathletes ($P < 0.001$), and LV mass was significantly increased, 212.43 ± 55.8 G compared to 123.48 ± 24.54 G in nonathletes ($P < 0.01$). Left atrium and aortic root were also relatively larger in athletes ($P < 0.01$). Right ventricular end-diastolic dimension was enlarged in marathon runners (2.02 ± 0.65 cm). The carotid tracing had a bisferious pulse in 5 marathon runners. These abnormalities were related to the overload type of heart as proven by echocardiogram. Early repolarization syndrome (abnormal RS-T segment elevation) and notched T waves in the ECG had a counterpart of a semilunar configuration in the VCG. Three athletes met ECG criteria and one met VCG criteria of left ventricular hypertrophy (LVH). The treadmill exercise ECG was negative in ECG was negative in all 12 athletes. Biventricular enlargement and increased left ventricular mass are present in the marathon runner's heart. Myocardial contractility at rest was, however, not statistically different from nonathletes (5). One would expect similar responses in endurance horses.

Relationships between physical activity and plasma lipids and between cardiorespiratory (CR) fitness and plasma lipids were investigated in 152 young adults. There were no significant correlations in either females or males between the physical activity indicators and any of the plasma lipids investigated. Plasma triglycerides were negatively correlated with CR fitness in the males. It was suggested that the two fitness components, aerobic capacity and percent fat, may be related to certain plasma lipid differences in males and females (6).

Three groups of five women aged 18 to 25 years participated in a 12-week training program. Cardiovascular responses up to 85% maximum oxygen consumption ($\dot{V}O_2$ maximum) to interval (ITG) and continuous (CTG) training were studied in two groups, before training and after 4, 8, and 12 weeks of training four times per week. A control group was assessed before and after 6 and 12 weeks. Both exercise groups demonstrated significant increases in arterial-venous oxygen difference (CAO2-CVO2) after 8 weeks with only slight further increases after 12 weeks (CTG was 8.9% and ITG was 20.0% at 85% of maximum oxygen consumption ($\dot{V}O_{2max}$). No significant changes were noted in either group in stroke volume (SV) or in their cardiac output (QC). These results indicated that, in response to high intensity training, females may demonstrate the same cardiovascular adaptations to training that have been observed for males (7). Little sex difference in response to anesthetics should be seen if both are equally conditioned.

Ten female hockey players were studied to determine if prolonged dynamic conditioning results in an increased left ventricular internal dimension at end diastole (LVIDD) and if this increase correlates with maximal oxygen consumption ($\dot{V}O_{2max}$). At peak season, echocardiograms were obtained and $\dot{V}O_{2max}$ determined during maximal treadmill exercise. $\dot{V}O_{2max}$, LVIDD index (LVIDD/body surface area (BSA)), and ventricular septal and posterior wall thickness were compared to age-matched nonathletic women. Mean LVIDD index was significantly greater in athletes than in controls: 29.3 ± 0.99 mm/m^2 vs. 26.3 ± 0.6, $P <$ 0.005. Echocardiographic wall measurements did not differ significantly in the two groups. Mean $\dot{V}O_{2max}$ for the athletes was significantly greater than controls: 51.7 ± 4.0 ml O_2·kg·min vs. 41.2 ± 2.1, ($P < 0.001$). $\dot{V}O_{2max}$ correlated significantly with the LVIDD index ($R = 0.92$; $P < 0.001$). Female athletes show an increased LVIDD in response to dynamic conditioning similar to that seen in male athletes. The proficiency of athletic performance as measured by $\dot{V}O_{2max}$ may be related to the heart's ability to increase LVIDD because there is a high correlation between $\dot{V}O_{2max}$ and LVIDD index (8).

To study the factors limiting the O_2 supply in heavy exercise, O_2 uptake at exhaustion was determined by the progressive loading method with a bicycle ergometer in 33 well-trained male runners and 34 sedentary male adults. Pulmonary ventilation, oxygen removal, respiratory rate, tidal volume, pulmonary diffusing capacity, alveolar-capillary oxygen difference, cardiac output, arterial-venous oxygen difference, stroke volume, and heart rate was measured. It was found that pulmonary diffusing capacity, cardiac output, and stroke volume were correlated with the difference in O_2 uptake at exhaustion between athletes and nonathletes (9). One may thus conclude that the physiological responses to exercise in males and females are similar.

Training reduced heart rate and increased maximum duration and estimated oxygen consumption of treadmill exercise. Compared to pretraining, the echogram in the post-training period revealed an increased LV end-diastolic dimension (EDD), a decreased end-systolic dimension (ESD), and thus an increased stroke volume (EDD3-ESD3) and shortening fraction (EDD-ESD)/EDD). Cardiac output (CO) and peripheral vascular resistance (BP/CO × 80) were identical preconditioning and postconditioning. Importantly, an increase in mean fiber shortening velocity was observed post-training as were increases in LV wall thickness, ECG voltage of S in lead V1 + R in lead V5, and LV mass. Thus endurance training was accompanied by increases in both LV dimension and mass as well as LV shortening fraction and contraction velocity as observed by echocardiogram (10).

LV dimensions and wall stress were measured echocardiographically before and immediately after exercise in 14 athletes and 7 control subjects. The findings suggest that afterload is an important determinant of cardiac performance and wall hypertrophy in athletes. In spite of major changes in heart rate and blood pressure, left ventricular wall stress remains unchanged after submaximal exercise in trained and untrained hearts. It would appear that the changes in heart size during exercise are to a large extent limited in untrained ventricles, as smaller LV dimensions are required to "normalize" wall stress. This results in a lower stroke volume for a given stroke dimensional change. Consequently, cardiac output is a function of heart rate rather than stroke volume in untrained subjects. The effect of increased muscle mass in athletes is to permit larger LV dimensions for a given afterload; thus stroke volume can be augmented. The study suggests that afterload is more important than preload in the development of LV hypertrophy (11). This should be considered in the evaluation of responses of the conditioned patient during anesthesia.

Responses in Conditioned Dogs

Myocardial contractility and the enzymatic (ATPase) activity of cardiac contractile proteins were examined after exercise training using the chronically instrumented, unanesthetized dog as an experimental model. Before training, heart rate and the maximum rate of left ventricular pressure development (max dP/dT) were measured at rest and during submaximal exercise. Animals were then subjected to an 8- to 10-week treadmill running program. Training was verified by the establishment of a 10 to 20 beat/minute reduction in heart rate during submaximal exercise. After training, max dP/dT was within normal limits at rest but significantly elevated during submaximal exercise. When max dP/dT was plotted as a function of heart rate, either with the animal standing quietly on the treadmill or during submaximal exercise, a marked elevation in max dP/dT at any given heart rate was observed after training. Myofibrillar protein yield and ATPase activity values were nearly identical in left ventricles from exercise-trained and sedentary control dogs. Although exercise training by treadmill running improved contractile function in the unanesthetized dog myocardium, this response does not appear to involve alterations in myofibrillar ATPase activity (11).

Myocardial O_2 extraction rate was studied during exercise-induced augmentation of cardiac work in dogs (12). The O_2 extraction rate at rest was 75% of arterial content. Progressive levels of exercise increased the animals' O_2 consumption from 7 ml/min/kg up to 91 ml/min/kg. Cardiac output rose from 108 ml/min/kg at rest to 484 ml/min/kg at the highest exercise level. The increase in myocardial O_2 consumption from 9 ml/min/100 g at rest up to 57 ml/min/100 g at the highest exercise level was met by an increase in coronary flow from 59 to 256 ml/min/100 g and a rise of myocardial arterial oxygen concentration from 15 to 22 vol %. Thus the latter contributed 40% to the augmented myocardial O_2 requirements. Coronary venous O_2 saturation decreased to 9% saturation during highest levels of exercise. This low value was not the result of a limited coronary dilatory capacity, inadequate state of exercise training, or a relative underperfusion of the inner layers of the left ventricle. Thus, augmentation of myocardial O_2 extraction rate seems to be a mechanism of physiological relevance during exercise-induced elevation of myocardial O_2 requirements in dogs and may be explained by capillary recruitment in the myocardium (13). Animals undergoing anesthesia for injuries soon after extensive exericse should have procedures with supplemental oxygen to protect against further myocardial oxygen needs.

Exercise in Chronic Obstructive Pulmonary Disease

The effect of physical training on cardiopulmonary function in 21 patients with chronic obstructive pulmonary disease (COPD) was compared to the results of similar observations in 8 untrained patients. The training consisted of daily walking on a treadmill at increasing speeds and grades and other graded physical exercises. Evaluation of pulmonary function, including spirometric studies, lung volumes, and arterial blood gas levels, showed no significant change after training. Hemodynamic functions, including heart rate, cardiac index, stroke index, pulmonary vascular resistance, and arteriovenous oxygen content difference, were similarly unchanged at comparable submaximal loads. Pulmonary arterial wedge pressure increased after training in the treated group at rest and during exercise, but this may be related to changes in respiratory mechanics. Consumption of oxygen and minute ventilation decreased in the treated group during treadmill exercise, suggesting improved neuromuscular coordination and efficiency of walking on the treadmill. Total work performed on the treadmill increased significantly in the trained group. Improvement in the capacity for exercise after physical training for 4 weeks was not associated with improvement in cardiopulmonary function at submaximal exercise (14).

Cardiac syncopes appeared in four heavily trained male patients without a history of cerebral or heart disease. Three were young athletes participating in competitive sport; one had trained intensively for years after poliomyelitis complicated by paraplegia. On admission, all patients had sinus bradycardia; one had second degree atrioventricular (AV) block at rest, and one had transient sinoatrial (SA) block. His bundle studies demonstrated prolonged recovery time of the SA node (SAN) in two, prolonged atrio-His interval in three, and appearance of second degree AV block at abnormally low pacing rates in two. Refractory periods of the AV node (AVN), determined in three subjects, tended to reach the upper limit of the normal range. The dysfunction of SAN and AVN was temporarily abolished in all patients by 1 mg of atropine i.v., the dysfunction disappeared during exercise by the three young athletes as well. The patient with paraplegia and one of the young athletes who had second degree AV block at rest were given atropine, 0.5 mg 6 times a day, and all three active sportsmen reduced training activity considerably. After 6 to 12 months, all patients were re-examined. None had cerebral symptoms or other complaints. They were in regular sinus rhythm and in excellent physical condition (15). An awareness of potential cardiac syncopes in highly conditioned subjects may avoid potential complications during anesthesia.

Effect of Ambient Temperature

Three relatively fit subjects performed duplicate 20- to 25-minute cycle ergometer exercise bouts at moderate and heavy intensities (40% and 70% $\dot{V}O_{2max}$) in ambient temperatures of 20, 26, and 36° C. They approached a steady state in internal body temperature in all but the heavy exercise in the heat, where body temperature rose consistently, averaging 38.84° C at the termination of exercise. Cardiac output (Q), estimated by a rebreathing technique, was proportional to VO2 and independent of the body temperatures, except during the lower exercise intensity in the heart, where Q averaged 1.3 liter/min higher throughout. In any environment, forearm blood flow was linearly related to body temperature above the temperature threshold for vasodilation, but during heavy exercise in the heat this relationship was severely attenuated above a body temperature around 38.0° C. Plasma volume decreases during exercise were primarily a function of the intensity of exercise. During heavy exercise in the heat, the relative vasoconstriction contributes to the maintenance of an adequate stroke volume preventing a fall in cardiac output. In this case, circulatory regulation has precedence over temperature regulation (16). Conditioned animals with high-level or long-term performance during high ambient temperatures should be suspected of undergoing more stress than at lower temperatures.

Responses in the Conditioned Horse

The well-conditioned horse has increased capability for maximum performance. Competition requires excellent physical response and supportive physiological function. Figure 13.27 illustrates a highly competitive performer. If anesthesia is required for a horse of this type, the conditioning program, time since racing, mental attitude, and value of the horse both as an athletic competitor and later as a breeding animal should be considered.

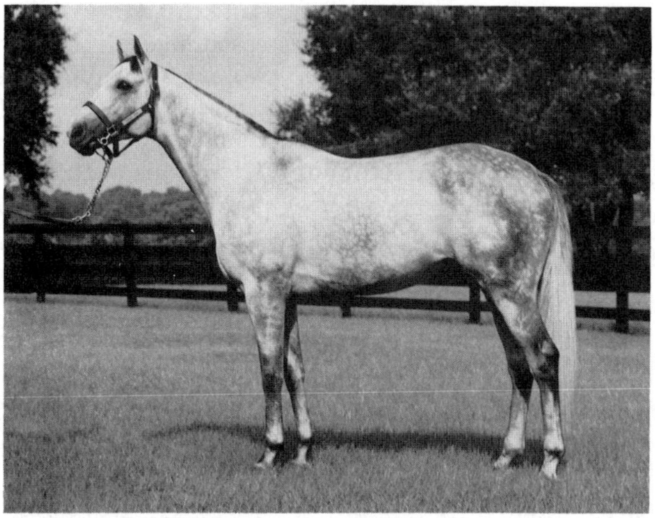

Figure 13.27. Runaway Groom, winner of the Travers Stakes (N.Y.), the Breeder's Stakes, (Can.), and the Prince of Wales Stakes (Can.). An example of the well-conditioned horse for which special consideration should be given if anesthesia is required. Photo courtesy of Mr. and Mrs. Albert P. Coppola.

Respiratory function may be related to the type of event and the breed of horse. The horse has a large capacity for transfer of O_2 and CO_2 across the pulmonary capillary membrane. The racing horse has the capability for substantial increases in cardiac output (17). This capacity of respiration and cardiac output may well influence the uptake of inhalant anesthetic agents.

The horse's oxygen consumption and pulmonary ventilation are almost linearly related to velocity. At a gallop of 550 m/min and a heart rate of 182 ± 12 bpm, mean oxygen uptake in four horses was 60 ± 5 liter/min. The galloping horse respires more frequently and with lower tidal volume. The minute volume may increase from 157 ± 63 liter/min at rest to 1337 ± 165 liter/min at a fast gallop (18). Care should be taken to assure adequate oxygen delivery in anesthetized horses.

In ponies at rest or exercised at 3 or 6 mph, cardiac output (Qc), blood pressure, and arterial O_2 content (CaO_2) were measured. A rapid, work load-dependent increase in CaO_2 and Qc was observed in exercising ponies in the first minute of work. The subsequent overshoot in Qc may be related to a hematological response. The possibility of reflex mechanisms adjusting Qc to maintain nearly constant O_2 delivery during exercise is suggested (19).

Blood-gas tensions and acid-base status were examined in 8 healthy grade ponies at rest (heart rate 55 ± 3 bpm) and during moderate (fast trot, heart rate 155 ± 3 bpm) and severe (gallop, heart rate 218 ± 7 bpm) exercise performed on a treadmill. Arterial oxygen tension and hemoglobin-oxygen saturation of exercising ponies did not change from the resting values.

Arterial oxygen content increased greatly during exercise as a consequence of increased hemoglobin concentration. The total oxygen content, as well as the saturation of hemoglobin with oxygen in the mixed venous blood, decreased at each intensity of exercise. Arterial carbon dioxide tension decreased with moderate (16%) and severe (29%) exercise, indicating hyperventilation. In galloping ponies during steady-state severe exercise, pronounced metabolic acidosis developed, as indicated by a sharp increase in the arterial concentration of lactic acid, accompanied by a decrease in arterial pH and bicarbonate concentration (20).

When related to the cardiac ventilatory and hematological changes for normal and carotid body-denervated ponies, it was demonstrated that VO2 kinetics during exercise is affected relatively more by the cardiac and hematological response, whereas VCO2 kinetics is affected relatively more by alveolar ventilation kinetics (21).

Hemoglobin concentration, partial pressures of oxygen and carbon dioxide, oxygen content, and pH were determined in the arterial and mixed venous blood of five normal and three abnormal horses with COPD at three stages of an exercise distance of 1200 m. Arterial and mixed venous samples were collected simultaneously by means of an automatic technique during the walk, trot, and gallop at 0–100 m, at 500–600 m, and at 1100–1200 m. The standard bicarbonate and the lactic and pyruvic acid concentrations were also determined in arterial and mixed venous blood. Highly significant changes in the mean value of the partial pressure of oxygen in mixed venous blood (PvO2), O_2 content, and DELTA arterial-venous oxygen (a-v O_2) content occurred during exercise in COPD subjects, and significant changes in PvO2 and DELTA a-v O_2 content occurred during exercise in normal subjects. It is concluded that COPD subjects compensated for respiratory dysfunction during exercise by extracting more oxygen from the blood than did normal horses. There was a highly significant correlation between the changes in standard bicarbonate and the changes in lactic acid concentration during exercise in both normal and COPD subjects. This led to the conclusion that lactic acid production was primarily, but not completely, responsible for the metabolic acidosis of exercise in horses (22). Anesthetic administration in these horses should consider level of respiratory function and contributing metabolic acidosis.

The anatomy and physiology of the pharynx was investigated in an attempt to elucidate the causes of exercise-induced upper airway obstruction in horses, particularly suffocative attacks suffered by racehorses (choking down syndrome). Obstruction of the nasopharyngeal airway occurs when the soft palate and larynx become separated. This may result from the soft palate being sucked, pushed, or lifted dorsally away from the larynx or by the larynx being pushed, pulled, or lifted away from the soft palate. Dislocation may be brought about during exercise by retraction of the tongue, open mouth swallowing, head flexion, fatigue, or nervous excitement under stress. Laryngopalatal dislocation may be affected by conditions such as hypoplasia and hyperplasia of the soft palate, stenosis of the posterior nares, adenoiditis, chronic pharyngitis, and pharyngeal hemiplegia (23). Horses receiving anesthetics with these airway problems would have more adequate function during gas anesthesia and O_2 administration. Intubation is sometimes difficult, and a smaller diameter endotracheal tube may be required. Supplemental O_2 during recovery is beneficial.

Some confusion exists in the interpretation of laryngoscopic findings in horses. In an attempt to clarify the significance of asynchronous abduction, an endoscopic survey of horses in training was made. Over a 5-year period, 537 horses were examined. Of these, 168 were examined on more than two occasions; 156 horses were recorded as being unchanged in degree of asynchronous abduction observed. In the 12 horses in which changes were observed, asynchrony at no time progressed to hemiplegia. It is suggested that asynchronous laryngeal abduction is normal in the horse (24). Hemiplegia may result in more difficult placement of an endotracheal tube during induction or recovery complications to airway flow.

Six different groups of horses were examined to determine the frequency of exercise-induced pulmonary hemorrhage (EIPH) after competitive exercise. The prevalence of EIPH was 65.6 to 75.4% in Thoroughbred flat dirt racing, 67.7% in steeplechase racing, 14.3% in flat turf racing, 66.7% in timber racing, 38.3 to 65.6% in flat training gallop, 40% in cross-country event, and 0% in 100-mile endurance races. The average speeds were 240 m/min during endurance rides with no bleeding to 1050 m/min during flat dirt track racing, where 75.4% showed bleeding. The frequency of hemorrhage is greater in older competitive animals (25).

During the course of a Hong Kong Thoroughbred racing season, 485 individual horses were examined with a flexible endoscope after racing in order to detect the presence or absence of blood in the proximal trachea. Of these, 29 had bled from their nostrils. The blood at the nostrils and proximal trachea comes from the lungs and is known as EIPH. Of the runners, 46.8% had EIPH, but in those examined more than three times, an incidence of 82% was recorded. Postmortem examinations carried out on 117 horses that had been trained in Hong Kong showed that 82% had signs of previous hemorrhage in the posterior lobes of the lungs. Histological examination revealed that 96% of horses had evidence of old alveolar hemorrhage and bronchiolitis.

The endoscopic examination did not assist in predicting whether an animal would bleed from the nostrils at its next start or in assessing the degree of lung hemorrhage, but results did reveal that EIPH had an effect on performance and increased with age (26).

In 10 Thoroughbred racehorses that developed epistaxis during a race, the mean pulmonary arterial diastolic pressure (PADP) was significantly higher and the mean pulmonary arterial oxygen tension (PaO2) was significantly lower than the corresponding mean values of a sample of 14 clinically normal Thoroughbreds in training. It is concluded that in horses with epistaxis during a race, pulmonary dysfunction may persist for up to two months after the episode and that the results indicate a need for pulmonary function studies before anesthesia in order to resolve problems concerning EIPH (27).

EIPH is a condition of uncertain etiology. It seems to be caused by mechanical stress in the dorsal region of the lung (28).

In the horse with a history of postexercise epistaxis, blood may be present in the airway or lungs. The presence of blood indicates that some trauma to the pulmonary tissues has occurred and pulmonary dysfunction may be observed. This may influence the uptake of inhalant agents or alter ventilation.

Determination of the effect of furosemide on possible changes in pulmonary blood pressure, renal function, or electrolyte balance is necessary. The concurrent usage of furosemide and withdrawal of food and water before anesthesia can result in dehydration and an increased need for fluid administration. In the horse with pulmonary hemorrhage and loss of body fluids, rapid administration of fluids during anesthesia, especially if in dorsal recumbency, can result in pulmonary edema.

The hemorrhage appears to occur predominately in the posterior lobes of the lung. Furosemide frequently has been used to alter hemostasis in Thoroughbred horses exhibiting postexercise epistaxis. Furosemide has been shown to reduce right atrial and pulmonary artery pressure without change in cardiac output. Furosemide was shown to increase the trend in platelet aggregation to reverse the bleeding trend (29).

Arterial, capillary, and mixed venous blood samples were taken immediately on capture and at specified intervals thereafter from wild zebra subjected to forced exercise under simulated capture conditions. All animals exhibited a profound acidemia down to pH 6.5. The pH levels were not rectified during the ensuing 30 minutes and tended to fall further in spite of hyperpnoea and hypocapnea. The results indicate that at least the acute phase of overstraining disease is commensurate with a metabolic acidosis. The postmortem findings are consistent with those of other workers describing deaths from capture myopathy. The fall in pH that results after a short chase of only a few kilometers proved lethal in untreated animals, whereas those in which the acidemia was rectified by infusion survived. Treatment in six cases consisted of an infusion of 1000 meq sodium bicarbonate in 1 liter of Normosol solution. This treatment reduced the acidemia, improved the general condition, restored the heart and respiratory rates to more normal levels, and resulted in a pronounced clinical improvement. Animals treated in this way survived, whereas untreated animals died within 12 hours. The indications are that this form of therapy may be usefully employed for animals captured after a short chase at the animal's maximum speed in which there is clinical evidence of a persistent acidemia (30). The responses in the zebra are severe compared to conditioned horses, but this illustrates the ultimate potential of severe exercise stress.

The effects of prolonged strenuous exercise on arterial and venous oxygen tension, carbon dioxide tension, pH, bicarbonate, standard bicarbonate, base excess, hemoglobin, packed cell volume, and total plasma protein were studied in 36 horses during a 100-km endurance ride. There were significant changes when preride values were compared with both mid-ride and end of ride values. The prominent changes were the development of dehydration and a metabolic alkalosis. At the mid-ride sampling time, those horses with higher heart rates had a greater degree of metabolic alkalosis than those with lower heart rates. The first four horses in the race completed the ride with speeds of 322 to 330 m/min and exhibited a metabolic acidosis (31).

CARDIOVASCULAR CONSIDERATIONS

Resting heart rates in conditioned animals are usually slow, but rates above 200 bpm frequently occur during heavy exercise or racing. In the 450- to 550-kg horse with a heart rate of 32 to 45 bpm, cardiac output is 30 to 45 liter/min with a stroke volume of 600 to 1000 ml/beat. At trotting speeds with a heart rate of 137 bpm, cardiac output increased to 134 liter/min. During work, there is an increase in mean carotid artery pressure, cardiac output, stroke volume, heart rate, oxygen consumption, and lactic acid production (32).

The anticipatory response to exercise may be evidenced by an increasing heart rate. The conditioned horse requiring anesthesia during the racing season may show this increase in heart rate and related increases in cardiovascular function as it is lead from the stall unless adequately sedated. In addition to cardiac stimulation, CNS hyperactivity may be observed. These observations may encourage a higher dosage of tranquilizers, sedatives, or induction agents. The use of anticholinergics is seldom considered, either because of higher heart rates or concern for reduction in intestinal activity. As a result, soon after induction, significant drops in cardiovascular function during the peak levels of anesthetic concentration may be evident.

Studies have shown that coronary vasodilator reserve exists even with maximum exercise. Further exertion is not limited because of coronary circulation (33).

Anesthesia in the conditioned animal is not expected to be influenced by pre-existing cardiac arrhythmias from myocardial ischemia. An index to the effects of conditioning in the equine is illustrated in Table 13.7. Although these values were determined in ponies, there is relative value to other breeds when considering the influence of exercise on anesthetic consideration (34).

In healthy adult ponies, moderate exercise (heart rate, 154 ± 3 bpm) increased the cardiac output, mean aortic pressure, right ventricular systolic and end-diastolic pressure (EDP), LV EDP, LV max dP/dt, and transmural myocardial blood flow (MBF). Severe exercise (32 km/h, heart rate 225 ± 7 bpm) resulted in further increases in all these values. With adenosine infusion during severe exercise, transmural MBF was able to increase further. There remained a significant transmural coronary vasodilator reserve (CVR) during severe exercise. In a study of blood flow to the brain, kidneys, diaphragm, and skeletal muscles, response to severe exercise in the pony seemed to be similar to that in human beings. In ponies in which tachycardia was produced by ventricular pacing, CVR in the deeper layers of the LV was exhausted at a heart rate of 250 bpm (35).

Table 13.7
Cardiodynamic Effects of Exercise in Ponies

Expressed as Mean Values	Control (at Rest)	Maximal Exercise
Heart rate (bpm)	56	225
Cardiac output (ml/min/kg)	139	649
Stroke volume (ml/beat/kg)	2.5	2.9
Aortic systolic pressure (mm Hg)	155	218
Mean aortic pressure (mm Hg)	120	160
Aortic diastolic pressure (mm Hg)	103	131
Left ventricular (LV) end-diastolic pressure (mm Hg)	11	36
Peripheral vascular resistance (mm Hg/ml/min/kg)	0.88	0.23
LV min dP/dt (mm Hg/sec)	1,336	8,099
LV max dP/dt (mm Hg/sec)	3,238	12,079
Rate-pressure product (mm Hg × bpm)	8,680	49,050
Left ventricular work (kg/mm/min/kg)	226	1,432
Right ventricular (RV) systolic pressure (mm Hg)	39	101
RV end-diastolic pressure (mm Hg)	11	22
RV systolic work (kg/mm/min/kg)	75	919
RV myocardial blood flow (ml 4 min/g)	0.46	4.80
RV coronary vascular resistance (mm Hg/ml/min/g)	267	30
LV myocardial blood flow (ml/min/g)	0.89	5.34
LV coronary vascular resistance (mm Hg/ml/min/g)	130	27

A microprocessor and a semiorthogonal lead system were used to record vector-cardiograms from 217 Standardbred horses. The recordings were subjected to temporospatial analysis by computer, and manual measurements of QRS duration were also made. Computer-measured and manually determined QRS durations were compared, and the former were also compared with special features of the QRS loop; with age, sex, and body parameters; and with performance.

The results provided some support for the use of the average of three limb leads in the determination of heart score and give an insight into the probable physiological basis of its relationship with performance. However, the significant influence of many confounding variables, the primary influence of the pattern of depolarization in the ventricular septum, the lack of any relationship with performance for geldings, and the weakness of the relationship for mares and stallions indicate that the heart score concept has very limited value in performance prediction (36).

ECGs were recorded from 153 racehorses and 10 Olympic 3-day event horses. The horses were then grouped into those presented for routine examination, those in which there was a complaint of poor performance, those going to the Montreal Olympics, and those with upper respiratory tract abnormalities. When the ECGs of the four groups were compared on the basis of detection of abnormality, it was found that 93% of the poor performance group showed abnormalities of various types. The routine examination group showed 21% with abnormal ECGs, and over one-half of these had raced unsuccessfully. In particular, this applied to those horses with T wave abnormalities in four or more leads and to those with intra-atrial block. There were significant T wave changes in 50% of the Olympic horses; 43.7% of horses with laryngeal hemiplegia showed abnormality. It is concluded that T wave changes are important ECG findings (37).

ECGs, full blood counts, and a range of plasma biochemical measurements were recorded in 131 horses with a history of poor racing performance. A comparison group of 129 horses (routine group) presented for musculoskeletal problems or heart score determination also had ECGs recorded. The incidence of various ECG abnormalities in the two groups of horses were compared by chi square analysis; the age of the horses, P wave duration, P-R interval, mean QRS interval (Leads I, II, and III), Q-T interval, and electrical axis were compared in the two groups using an unpaired Student's t test.

The hematological and plasma biochemical values for horses in the poor performance group were all within the normal ranges for their laboratory. The poor performance group of horses had significantly higher incidences of second-degree atrioventricular block and T wave abnormalities in three or more leads and than horses in the routine group. Other abnormalities in the poor performance group included intra-atrial block, intraventricular block, and atrial fibrillation. These ECG abnormalities were not found in the routine group. There were no significant differences in the age of the horses nor in any of the various ECG intervals when the two groups of horses were compared (38).

Of primary interest to anesthesiology is the determination that slow heart rates are not related to heart block but rather are a result of conditioning. ECG analysis is helpful in this determination. Exercise-related heart block may be seen. Medications should be chosen that do not contribute to further slowing of the heart.

ECG recordings made on 40 foals during training between 13 and 15 and 17 and 20 months of age (with 40 untrained foals serving as controls) failed to reveal any effect of training on the angle of the electrical cardiac axis, although it did increase the magnitude of the ventricular vector as a result of ventricular hypertrophy (39).

Values were obtained by telemetry from three horses fitted with carotid loops several months previously, both when standing under the rider and during exercise. During steady gallop at a mean speed of 548 ± 90 m/min, heart rate rose from the standing value of 38 ± 5 bpm to 184 ± 23, systolic pressure from 83 ± 10 to 116 ± 12, mean pressure from 97 ± 12 to 160 ± 20, and pulse pressure from 32 ± 9 mm Hg to 89 ± 19. When the speed of the horses was increased progressively from walk through trot to gallop, both the mean arterial blood pressure and the pulse pressure rose in proportion to the speed (40).

Studies on the ventilation, cardiac output, heart rate, and blood pressure in ponies exercised at 1.8, 3, or 6 mph suggest that mean right ventricular pressure, pulmonary CO_2 flow, $PaCO_2$, and mixed venous PCO_2 do not provide the primary stimuli for exercise hyperpnoea in ponies (41).

Six male Thoroughbred and Anglo-Arab horses were used to measure the blood lactate concentration and heart rate after galloping 200 m, 1000 m, and 1600 m and after exhaustion running. Both speed and duration of exercise affected heart rate. Maximum heart rate may not be reached at top speed running for 2 minutes; up to 5 minutes at nearly the fastest speed may be needed. Maximum blood lactate developed after 1 to 2 minutes of exercise at greatest speed and did not correspond to the appearance of highest heart rate. There was no correlation between maximum heart rate and performance measured in work tests (42).

AV dissociation and synchronous diaphragmatic flutter (SDF) were seen in a horse after prolonged strenuous exercise. The horse had hypokalemic, hypocalcemic, hypochloremic alkalosis from the loss of electrolytes during exercise. The low levels of potassium or calcium or their combination were thought to have produced the condition in which the phrenic nerve responded to the sinoatrial depolarization, producing SDF, and in which a quiescent pacemaker in the ventricle functioned independently, producing the AV dissociation. Intravenous and oral electrolytes seemed adequate for restoration of normal electrolyte balance (43).

The cardiorespiratory and metabolic responses to various levels of tethered swimming were evaluated in five sedentary horses. Cardiac output (Q) and heart rate (HR) correlated highly with work effort (WE) expressed as kg pulled/kg body weight × 100. While swimming, stroke volume (SV) was reduced at the lowest workloads, but increased with increased WE so that at the highest workloads it had returned to the on-land resting SV. Pressures in the pulmonic as well as on both sides of the systemic circulation were considerably elevated by this form of exercise, although only mean carotid artery pressure correlated with WE. During tethered swimming, plasma lactic acid rose exponentially from 1 to 10 mm/liter with increasing HR over the range 150 to 200 bpm. Oxygen consumption ($\dot{V}O_2$) increased linearly from 25 to 112 ml/kg/min over the WE range of 3.0 to 7.8 kg/pulled/kg body weight × 100. The aerobic capacity of the horse would appear to be twice that of humans. The greater increase in $\dot{V}O_2$ in the exercising horse cannot be explained solely on the basis of increases in Q. Therefore, alterations in hematocrit, hemoglobin, and oxygen extraction appear to play a more important role in the horse during exercise than they do in humans (44).

Blood flow to the brain, heart, kidneys, diaphragm, and skeletal muscles was studied at rest and during graded treadmill exercise using radionuclide-labeled microspheres (15 microμ diameter) in 11 healthy adult ponies. Exercise brought about pronounced increases in cardiac output, mean aortic pressure, left ventricular end-diastolic pressure, and right ventricular systolic and end-diastolic pressures. Blood flow to the brain stem and cerebral hemispheres was unchanged during both moderate exercise (heart rate 154 ± 3 beats/min) and severe exercise (heart rate 225 ± 7 beats/min). Despite pronounced hypocapnia during severe exercise, cerebellar blood flow increased by 32%. Myocardial blood flow increased transmurally with both levels of exercise, although it remained proportional to total ventricular perfusion. During severe exercise, renal blood flow decreased to 19% of its control value. Blood flow to the diaphragm exceeded that to the skeletal muscles during both intensities of exercise. Blood flow to the exercising muscles of the brachium and thigh increased 31 to 38 times during moderate exercise and 70 to 76 times during severe exercise. It is concluded that the cardiovascular responses to strenuous exercise in the pony included an increase in blood flow to the cerebellum, myocardium, diaphragm, and exercising skeletal muscles, while blood flow was diverted away from the kidneys (45).

Data on resting HRs, pre-exercise HRs, the anticipatory rises before exercise, the influence of speed of work, and recovery HRs have been determined. A linear relationship between HR and working speed within the range of 400 to 800 m/min was observed. When the speed of work was between 400 and 800 m/min, horses with resting ECG classed as abnormal had significantly higher heart rates than those regarded as normal (46).

MUSCLE RESPONSES

Biopsy samples from the gluteus medius muscle of 68 clinically healthy horses and 59 horses with the tying-up syndrome were examined under electron and light microscopy, histochemically, and biochemically. In adult healthy horses, the following three types of muscle fiber were identified: those displaying high ATPase staining intensity with low oxidative activity (FT), 22%; those displaying high ATPase staining intensity with high oxidative activity (FTH), 54%; and those with low ATPase staining intensity (ST), 24%. The size of all the fibers increased with age and training. The muscle glycogen concentration was 95 mM in foals and 126 mM glucose units × kg in adults; FTH and ST fibers had low glycogen concentration. Maximal or near-maximal trotting for 700 to 1000 m was necessary for achieving not only high HRs but also a high demand on the anaerobic energy release. FTH and ST fibers were active at all intensities and were most involved during work at slower trotting speeds; at high speeds, FT fibers were most active. Biopsy samples taken from horses within 4 hours of onset of acute tying-up revealed low glycogen, ATP, and creatine phosphokinase and high lactate concentrations. Light microscopy showed focal localization of the hyaline degeneration type of muscle change. Electron microscopy revealed myofibrillar degeneration and necrosis with invasion of inflammatory cells. These changes were more pronounced 18 to 24 hours after the onset of acute symptoms. No apparent etiology of the disease could be established, but it is suggested that the disease be named "equine rhabdomyolysis" (47).

Morphometric methods allow a quantitative description of the ultrastructural composition of tissue sections. They are therefore useful tools in analyzing structure-function correlations in skeletal muscle tissue. Histochemical methods permit the separation of muscle fiber populations into subgroups with distinct physiological and biochemical characteristics, although it has proved rather difficult to extract quantitative information from conventionally processed histochemical preparations. A serial-sectioning technique to analyze muscle fibers by both histochemical and morphometric methods has been used. The aim of the study was to estimate the volume density of mitochondria in the individual fiber types of equine semitendinosus muscle. The highest mean volume density of mitochondria ws found in Type IIA fibers (6.7%). Type IIA was followed by Type IIC (6.5%), Type I (5.6%), Type IIB ox (oxidative-glycolytic; 3.25%), and Type IIB gly (glycolytic; 0.7%). The study also demonstrated a considerable variability of mitochondrial content and fiber size within all fiber types of equine semitendinosus muscle (48).

Muscle biopsies were obtained from both the left and right gluteal and semitendinosus muscles of 10 Standardbred colts 6 to 8 months of age. All 10 colts were raised by the same farm during the following year, 5 of them (T group) were subjected to regular controlled exercise 4 to 5 days/week, while the only physical activity of the other 5 foals (C group) consisted of that usually occurring in a group of yearlings. Muscle biopsies were again obtained from all 10 yearlings at 4 and 10 months after the first biopsies had been taken. No difference in either fiber composition (Type I, IIA, or IIB) or oxidative and glycolytic enzyme activities was found when the two groups were compared at the time when the biopsies were taken. However, large variations in muscle characteristics existed among the yearlings. The Type I/Type II ratio did not change with age, but Type IIA/Type IIB ratio increased in both groups. Fiber areas increased by 30 to 70% in all fiber types. The oxidative enzyme citrate synthase showed a significant increase with age only in the T group, while 3-OH-acyl CoA dehydrogenase (HAD) was unchanged in both groups. The glycolytic enzymes triose phosphate dehydrogenase and lactate dehydrogenase were significantly decreased (20 to 40%) in both groups. No significant training effect was detected in this study; the yearlings in the T group that were physically activated demonstrated an almost similar adaptation in muscle to the yearlings in the C group. This does not exclude the possibility of other training regimes influencing muscle characteristics. Furthermore, the potential for adaptation in skeletal muscle may depend on hereditary factors because large variations in muscle characteristics existed among the foals even before training (49).

Biopsies of the middle gluteal muscle were obtained from 14 Thoroughbred yearlings before the start of training. The horses were then trained and raced through their 2-year-old season, and biopsies were again taken during the last week of the season.

The muscle samples were analyzed for fiber composition, fiber areas, and enzyme activities. By the end of the racing season, the proportion of Type IIA fibers had increased from 31 to 38%, while the proportion of IIB fibers had decreased from 56 to 49%. There was no significant change in fiber areas.

Increased oxidative capacity of the muscle was demonstrated by about a two-fold increase in citrate synthase (28 to 60 μM/g/min) and HAD (14 to 23 μM/g/min). The glycolytic enzyme lactate dehydrogenase was unchanged, whereas, triosephosphate dehydrogenase decreased in activity. There was a large individual variation among horses in the proportion of fiber types and enzyme activities in muscle (50).

Fiber type composition and enzyme activity data from the gluteus medius muscle of foals at 2 to 4 weeks and 8 months of age demonstrated a significant reduction in fast twitch highly oxidative fibers from 37.1 to 25.6% and an increase in fast twitch fibers of intermediate oxidative capacity from 20.5 to 27.6% of the population. Slow twitch fibers (14.7 and 16.0%) and fast twitch low oxidative fibers (29.4 and 30.8%) did not change over the period.

A significant increase in phosphofructokinase and decrease in succinate dehydrogenase activities over this same period suggested that the foals enhanced the anaerobic, rather than the aerobic, component of muscle metabolism during the first 8 months of life. Fiber cross-sectional areas at 2 to 4 weeks of age were substantially smaller than those in older foals and adult horses (51).

The skeletal muscle metabolism of 18 Standardbred and North-Swedish trotting horses with a wide range of cardiocirculatory capacities was studied in relation to muscle fiber composition during a standardized near-maximum exercise test. Although the same amount of work was performed by all horses, the amount of triglycerides and glycogen used and lactate accumulated differed widely. Both blood and muscle lactate accumulation was positively related to the amount of glycogen used. These factors were in turn positively associated with the percentage of Type IIB fibers and consequently negatively associated with the percentage of Type IIA fibers. The percentage of Type IIB fibers was negatively correlated with the activities of the oxidative enzymes citrate synthase and HAD and positively associated with the lactate dehydrogenase activity. The results indicate that horses with a high proportion of Type IIB fibers had a lower muscle oxidative capacity and were, therefore, more dependent upon glycolysis with subsequent lactate accumulation for energy production, than horses that had a high proportion of Type IIA fibers. The different metabolic properties of the muscle fiber type indicate that the pattern of muscle fiber recruitment could have a significant effect on intramuscular substrate utilization (52).

The middle gluteal muscle of 5 2-year-old untrained trotters was investigated by repeated needle biopsy over a training period of 6 months. A second group of 5 3-year-old untrained horses was included to examine the effect of growth. After the training period, there were increases in the relative distribution of slow twitch (ST) fibers from 18 to 25% and fast twitch (FTa) fibers from 36 to 45% and a decrease in FTb fibers from 46 to 30%. A proportionally equal reduction (about 18%) in the cross-sectional area of all fiber types was observed after the first 2 months of training, succeeded by an increase to about pretraining levels at the end of the period. The number of capillaries per fiber was increased from 1.7 to 2.4. Proliferation of capillaries occurred around fibers of all types. The metabolic adaptations showed on increases of 50% in the activities of HAD and citrate synthase (31%). Growth had no effect on the relative fiber type distribution nor the capillary per fiber ration, but as the mean fiber area increased 36% (primarily because of increases in FT fibers), the number of capillaries/mm^2 was lower in the older untrained horses (350 capillaries/mm^2) compared with the younger untrained ones (460 capillaries/mm^2). Increase with growth was found in the activity of phosphorylase and HAD and a decrease was seen in the activity of hexokinase. It is concluded that training induced alterations that improved the aerobic capacity of the muscle (53).

Enzyme levels were assayed before, during, and after long-distance exercise (approximately 22,000 m at trot and slow canter) performed for 5 consecutive days by one 9-year-old and two 5-year-old healthy horses. Exercise was adjusted to maintain heart rate at about 170 bpm. Creatine kinase activity (A) increased during exercise, and thereafter remained high or increased further. Aspartate amino-transferase activity (B) and fructosediphosphate aldolase activity (C) increased gradually during exercise and were maximal about 1 hour after exercise ended, before gradually decreasing or remaining unchanged. Magnitude of response was low for B, slightly higher for C, and highest for A. Enzyme levels were influenced by the previous day's exercise, but whereas A changed in phase with fluctuating intensity of exercise, B and C increased steadily over the exercise period. When training ceased, A increased for 1 day and then fell, whereas B and C generally decreased (although B remained high for 1 week in one horse). Red cell count was low 5 hours after exercise. In two horses, erythrocyte sedimentation rate (ESR) decreased during the first half of exercise and then increased; in one horse it increased throughout the exercise period. Packed cell volume (PCV) reached a peak at the middle or end of exercise, then fell abruptly. There was an approximately inverse relationship between PCV and ESR. Body weight decreased gradually throughout and was still depressed after 7 days' rest. Creatine kinase is a good indicator of severity of exercise and degree of training, and aspartate amino-transferase indicates fatigue (54). This should be considered when laboratory values can be determined prior to anesthesia.

Blood lactate concentrations were determined in 16 horses (3 Thoroughbreds, 7 Standardbreds, and 6 polo ponies) before and 5 minutes after galloping over distances of 200, 300, and 400 m at maximum speed. The highest net lactate concentration of 14 to 15 mM/liter was attained by the polo ponies and the highest speed by the Thoroughbreds. The maximum rate of lactate production was about 35 mM/liter/min for the polo ponies and 20 to 25 mM/liter/min for the Standardbreds and Thoroughbreds. Values were similar to those measured in human athletes after exhaustive work. The increase in lactate production related to increasing speed (55). Depending on the relation between performance and anesthesia, high lactate concentrations may still be present.

Effects of training at an increasing exercise rate on heart rate, output, stroke volume, and venous lactic acid were determined using a standardized exercise test on previously trained, sedentary, healthy adult Standardbred horses. Heart rate, cardiac output, and stroke volume did not significantly decrease with training. Venous lactic acid was the only measured value that changed significantly during training. It appeared that training increased the uptake, but not the delivery of oxygen, to the muscles of these horses (56).

Arterial blood samples were collected from six human student volunteers, mean 21.5 years old and 70.4 kg in weight, during an initial resting phase of 75 minutes, an exercise period of 20 minutes pedaling a bicycle ergometer in the supine position at a work load that increased the heart rate to nearly 140 bpm at an ambient temperature of 23° C, and a recovery period of 125 minutes. The study was repeated at 40°C. HR and rectal temperature were significantly greater during exercise and recovery in the hot environment than in the cool. The mean increases in lactate, pyruvate and glycerol were significantly greater and the mean decrease of glucose was smaller in hot conditions, whereas the mean decreases in free fatty acids and 3-hydroxybutyrate did not differ significantly. Compared to their corresponding mean resting values, the mean changes in all six blood values were significantly greater during recovery in the hot environment than in the cool (57).

Eight Thoroughbred horses of varying ages were investigated by needle biopsy sampling of the middle gluteal muscle. Fiber types, mean fiber areas, capillary/fiber ratios, and the number of capillaries/mm^2 are given for all horses. The foals had a lower proportion of IIA fibers and a higher proportion of IIB fibers than the rest of the horses. The capillary density was also lower in the foals. As these horses had smaller mean fiber areas, this was predominantly caused by lower capillary/fiber ratios. The effect of maturation was investigated by resampling the foals 7 months later. On both occasions these biopsies were further analyzed for properties of the individual fiber types. Although proliferation of capillaries was observed around fibers of all types, this did not affect the capillary densities, which remained unaltered (58). Thus the perfusion of muscle during anesthesia is not influenced by the number of capillaries per mm^2 in the conditioned horse.

Heat acclimatization was induced in a group of healthy young men by walking on a treadmill (5.6 km/hour at 49 and 27°C, 90 min/day for 7 days) and was confirmed by significantly reduced final rectal temperatures and heart rates on the 7th day of exercise in the heat. A second group of men, paired for maximum oxygen consumption and bodyweight, remained sedentary in the same environmental conditions. Although the mild exercise combined with the severe heat induced significant hyperkalemia on the first and final days, there was an attenuated response with significantly reduced plasma K^+ after 45 minutes on the 7th day compared with first-day values.

No significant inter- or intragroup differences in plasma Na^+ values were found, although the Na^+ content of 24-hour urine samples showed that men exercising in the heat retained an increase ability to conserve Na^+, whereas sedentary subjects consistently showed increased excretion of Na^+. It is concluded that even the mild exercise affected hyperkalemia at each sampling time, but the degree of hyperkalemia was attenuated after acclimatization. Although Na^+ was conserved in the exercising men, no such adaptive process occurred in sedentary subjects (59).

The effects of trotting at 3.3 to 12.5 m/sec for 400 to 2000 m, continuous trotting for 1 to 2 hours, and racing were studied in clinically healthy Standardbred horses aged 4 to 8 years in good training condition. Temperature and heart rate were measured and blood and muscle biopsy samples were taken in the 5-minute rest intervals between work bouts and at the end of each exercise. Mean muscle temperature, which was 37°C at rest, increased to 41°C after the highest trotting speed and racing. The heart rate increased from 40 to 140 bpm in most of the tests, but rose to 240 bpm in racing and at close to maximal trotting speed maintained for at least 700 m.

Muscle and blood lactate values increased and glycogen levels decreased rapidly near maximal speed, although critically low levels were never reached. Further evidence of increased glycolysis during racing was the 8- to 10-fold increase in glucose-6-phosphate levels found in muscle immediately after a race. It is concluded that a number of short training bouts would be preferable to a single long exercise period, and that six 100-m trots at close to maximal speeds produced stresses similar to those of racing (60).

Biopsy samples were collected from the left middle gluteal muscle of horses participating in three competitive endurance rides. Six horses were sampled the day before and 30 minutes after completion of 40 km (Ride 1), nine horses were sampled the day before and 30 minutes after 110 km (Ride 2), and eight horses were sampled 30 minutes after completing 160 km (Ride 3). In addition, muscle samples were collected 24 and 48 hours after Ride 2 and 20 hours after Ride 3.

Serial muscle sections were studied histochemically for myosin adenosine triphosphatase activity after acid preincubation and for glycogen content using the periodic-acid Schiff (PAS) reaction. When the rides were compared, there was progressive recruitment from I to IIB fibers, according to the distance completed. This appeared to be independent of the speed of exercise, as horses in all rides were exercised at similar intensities. Elite horses in Ride 3 had higher percentages of Type I and Type IIA fibers and lower percentages of Type IIB fibers than the horses in the two other rides, which were considered to be only average competitors. There was, however, considerable variation in muscle fiber types when the nine horses in Ride 2 were sampled repeatedly in the same muscle. This would appear to limit any possible predictive value of muscle biopsy (61). Endurance horses presented for anesthesia soon after competition may be expected to have greater muscle glycogen depletion than noncompeting horses.

In order to fully appreciate the physiological effects of alterations in fluid and electrolyte balance during exercise, it is necessary to first consider the fluid compartments from which these losses occur. The total body water (TBW) of normal 450- to 500-kg horses is approximately 300 liters.

Approximately one-third of this fluid (100 liters) is distributed to the extracellular fluid (ECF) compartment. We can reasonably assume that 90% or more of the weight loss during exercise is due to water loss. A heavily sweating endurance horse with a weight loss of 40 kg has probably lost 36 to 40 liters of body water. If the initial serum Na concentration was 140 mM/liter and did not change after exercise, the exchangeable cation loss (i.e., Na + K) would be 140 mM/liter × 36 to 40 liters, or 5000 to 5600 mM. It would be valuable to have an estimate of the Na and K loss. One way to make this estimate is simply to multiply this figure by the relative amount of Na and K lost in sweat and urine.

If Na accounts for 70% of the cation loss, the calculated Na loss would be around 3500 to 4000 mM, while the K loss would be 1500 to 1600 mM. This large loss of Na-containing fluid would result in a decrease in ECF volume of 25 to 28 liters. If the decrease in plasma volume was proportional, plasma volume would also be reduced by 25 to 28% or by about 6 to 7 liters in a 500-kg horse with a resting plasma volume of 24 liters. If the same horse with exactly the same electrolyte deficits had consumed sufficient water to reduce its net water loss to 20 liters, the serum Na concentration would have decreased from 140 to around 130 mM/liter.

Provision of electrolyte supplementation for heavily sweating endurance horses may be beneficial in certain circumstances. Well-conditioned endurance horses performing in cool climates may not require such supplements because they seldom develop major imbalances. In hot and humid environments, sweat losses may be massive. In these situations replenishment of the accumulated water deficit is of overriding importance. Electrolyte supplementation designed to replenish sweat losses should contain Na and Cl in roughly equal proportions; the K content should be one-third to one-half that of Na. Ca and Mg may be added in relatively small amounts. The amount of such supplements required depend upon the individual and environmental conditions. Electrolyte supplementation for endurance horses performing normally should not be overzealous (62).

The effects of exercise on blood coagulation, platelet function, and fibrinolysis were studied in five fit Thoroughbred horses that were galloped at maximal speed for 1200 m. Blood samples were collected 4 hours before exercise (resting sample), after saddling the horse and walking him to the track (track sample), and 5 minutes after exercise (postexercise sample). Activated partial thromboplastin times, one-stage prothrombin times, and thrombin times did not significantly differ in any of the samples, nor were fibrinogen/fibrin degradation products detected at any stage. The slopes of the ADP-induced platelet aggregation curves were reduced, but not significantly, when results from track samples were compared with resting sample findings. Exercise induced a significant reduction in the slopes of all ADP-induced aggregation curves. It was hypothesized that this response was an indirect effect of increased plasma catecholamine levels, possibly mediated via the release of increased amounts of prostacyclin from vascular endothelium (63).

The packed cell volume, red blood cell count, plasma protein concentration, and plasma lactate levels all increased with exercise and peaked postexercise.

Fifteen biochemical tests were performed on plasma samples from Thoroughbred horses in training.

Of the 128 horses initially bled, only 63 were bled on a sufficient number of occasions during the 2-month conditioning period and the first 2 months of racing to be acceptable for statistical analysis. This analysis showed that stage of training had a significant effect on the majority of plasma constituents tested, although trends were apparent for only a few: increases in creatinine and bilirubin and decreases in urea, phosphorus, and lactate dehydrogenase during the training period. Sex-related influences and age did not have such a general effect. It was found that total protein, lactate dehydrogenase, and aspartate aminotransferase differed between the sexes and that inorganic phosphorus, alkaline phosphatase, and lactate dehydrogenase tended to decrease with age, whereas bilirubin and total protein tended to increase with age (64).

Four diets supplying the same energy and with 4, 8, 12, and 16% dietary fat (as soya bean oil) were given to four horses at four intervals according to a Latin square design. After 3 weeks of conditioning, dietary effects were evaluated by trotting all horses at 3.2 m/s for 6 hours. Pre- and post-trotting responses were estimated in muscle and liver glycogen, serum long-chain fatty acids, serum electrolytes, serum enzymes, serum cholesterol, plasma glucose, packed cell volume, and hemoglobin. Dietary fat was highly correlated with exercise-induced plasma glucose changes and with cholesterol concentrations. Regardless of the diet, linoleate concentration was about eight times higher than that of the other fatty acids, and it increased slightly as dietary fat increased. Stearate concentration also increased with increasing dietary fat, but palmitic and oleic acid decreased. Increases in fat intake also resulted in slight increases in liver glycogen at the resting level. Conditioning resulted in a significant decrease in exercise-induced fluctuations of serum enzymes and electrolytes but significantly increased plasma long-chain fatty acid concentrations. Resting muscle glycogen increased by 37% as a result of conditioning, but there was no effect on liver glycogen at rest or after exercise (65). Conditioning should not reduce the capability of the liver for hepatic biotransformation of anesthetic agents.

Venous blood samples and middle gluteal muscle biopsy samples were obtained from 21 horses taking part in 50- or 100-km endurance rides. Group A consisted of 7 horses competing over 100 km (4 horses completed the ride); Group B consisted of the 6 horses that were among the 10 best over 50 km, while the other 8 horses of Group C completed 50 km at a slower speed. Blood lactate, glycerol, and creatine kinase increased in all groups, but aspartate aminotransferase levels were higher only in Group A. No change was found in blood glucose in Groups B and C, although horses in Group A had lower levels after the ride. Neither fiber composition, fiber areas, nor enzyme activities differed between the groups. Intramuscular glycogen content was similar before the ride in all groups. After the ride, glycogen had decreased only one-half as much in Group C as compared to Groups A and B. Group C had a higher intramuscular triglyceride content at rest than Group B. The greatest decrease in triglyceride content after the ride was found in Group C. In Groups A and B, many Type I, IIA, and IIB fibers were glycogen depleted after the ride, whereas in Group C mainly Type I and some Type IIA fibers were depleted. The results of this study show that intramuscular carbohydrate and lipid stores are both important fuel during endurance rides (66). Glycogen depletion should be considered in the performance under anesthesia and in recovery.

Four Thoroughbreds performed four gallops (g1–g4) with intervals of 5 minutes over a distance of 620 m on a circular track. Biopsy samples taken under local anesthesia before g1, immediately after each gallop, and during 30 minutes of recovery were examined for muscle metabolites. In three horses, mean gallop times increased from 46.7 sec for g1 to 60.0 sec for g4, whereas, in the fourth horse, g1 was approximately 10% slower than the other horses; subsequent gallops were marginally faster. In all four horses there was a decrease in ATP, especially in the three fatigued animals, with no resynthesis occurring within 30 minutes. No changes occurred in ADP or AMP concentrations, while a stoichiometric increase in inosine monophosphate (IMP) in relation to the ATP decreases was found. The decrease in ATP appeared to be related to the anaerobic stress of the exercise, as shown by a progressive increase in muscle lactate and decrease in blood pH. In the three fatigued horses, little or no decrease in muscle lactate concentrations had occurred after 30 minutes. Exercise resulted in extremely large increases in hexose monophosphate (up to 34 mM/kg dry muscle) and glycerol 1-phosphate (up to 19 mM/kg dry muscle), reflecting the high proportion of fast twitch fibers in this breed (67).

Before and after they were given 100 g (C^{13}) glucose, seven male students 21 to 25 years old walked on a 10% uphill treadmill for 2 or 4 hours at between 4 and 5 km/hour to induce a metabolism close to one-half that of maximum oxygen consumption. After intake of C^{13} glucose, expired CO_2 became enriched with C^{13} in as little as 15 minutes and reached a maximum within 1 to 2 hours when utilization of exogenous glucose was between 500 and 650 mg/min, which represented as much as 55% of the carbohydrate metabolism and 24% of the total energy expenditure (68).

Muscle biopsies were collected from the left middle gluteal muscle of 12 horses the day before and within 30 minutes of completion of an 800-m barrier trial. A further 6 horses were sampled the day before and within 30 minutes of completion of a 1200-m barrier trial. Serial muscle sections were examined histochemically for myosin adenosine triphosphatase activity after acid preincubation to demonstrate Type I, IIA, and IIB fibers. The glycogen content in the individual fibers was assessed using PAS reaction. Total glycogen in muscle was measured fluorimetrically after hydrolysis to glucose. Significant decreases in total muscle glycogen of 167.1 ± 22.2 and 158.1 ± 23.2 mM glucose units/kg occurred from pre- to post-trial samples for horses in both 800- and 1200-m trials, respectively. There were no significant differences between the decreases in total muscle glycogen from horses in either 800-m or 1200-m trials. In both 800-m and 1200-m trials, there was a significant decrease in the percentage of IIA and IIB fibers classified as having high PAS staining intensity and a significant increase in the percentage of fibers classified as having medium staining intensity when samples taken after the trial were compared to those taken before the trial (69).

In Standardbred trotters, glycogen depletion was slight (0.3 mM/kg/min) at slow trotting speed (0.3 km/min) but rose to nearly 14 mM/kg/min at maximal trotting speed (+0.75 km/min) for six trials at 400 m. At slow speeds, predominantly the slow twitch fibers became depleted; once that had occurred, the fast twitch, high oxidative fibers also became subject to depletion. During maximal speed, after six trials at 400 m, the fast twitch, low oxidative fibers became strikingly depleted as well. There is thus a preferential fiber recruitment with increase in speed and duration of exercise. Lactate accumulation in the blood did not increase strikingly until speeds exceeded 10 m/sec. Repeated 700- to 1000-m exercise sessions at maximum to near-maximum speed, respectively, appears to be appropriate for training of fast twitch fibers, as well as for achieving a high heart rate and a high demand on anaerobic energy release (70). The effects of glycogen depletion on anesthetic management are less likely to be important in the horse running short races than the endurance horse.

The effect of physical training on the in vitro activities of enzymes that provide quantitative information on the maximum capacities of anaerobic and aerobic metabolism was investigated. Surprisingly, training had no effect on the activities of 6-phosphofructokinase or creatine kinase, suggesting that there was no effect on the capacity of anaerobic metabolism in this muscle. However, the activities of hexokinase and citrate synthase were increased, indicating that training increased the capacity of aerobic metabolism (71).

Experiments were conducted on six geldings subjected to an effort test (gallop of 2400 m on a steep course) before and after 4 months of training. Physical exericse caused an increase of 2,3-DPG and ATP levels in whole blood and a decrease in glucose concentration. In erythrocytes taken from horses after physical exercise, a fall of glucose utilization was observed during incubation in plasma, whereas the same erythrocytes incubated in Krebs-Henseleit buffer did not show this effect. Possibly, in horses during physical exercise, some substances were synthesized or activated in plasma that inhibit glycolysis in erythrocytes, because the pH value of blood was not affected. After 4 months of training, a decrease of 2,3-DPG concentration in erythrocytes was observed. These erythrocytes also utilize glucose more rapidly than the erythrocytes of untrained horses, and this occurs both before and after exercise (72).

Muscle biopsy samples were collected from the left middle gluteal muscle of six Thoroughbreds the day before and within 30 minutes of completing the second day (speed and endurance test) of a 3-day event. A decrease in total muscle glycogen of 306 ± 34.6 mM glucose units/kg occurred in samples collected after exercise (73).

Standard metabolic rate (SMR) and energy use of two newly weaned ponies were determined by indirect calorimetry in a metabolism chamber. Ponies weighing 55 and 68 kg had calculated SMRs of 60 and 71 kcal/hour compared to measured values of 63 and 72 kcal/hour, respectively. Chamber values for oxygen consumption ranged from 11 to 33 liters/hour, and RQ values were within an acceptable range from 0.77 to 1.77 O_2. Oxygen consumption values obtained on exercising animals with a specially designed face mask ranged from 51 liters/min before exercise to 401 liters/min after a 30-minute trot, with RQ range from 0.55 to 1.56. Resting heart rate tended to decrease and recovery rate to increase through training. Muscle lactic acid concentration increased from approximately 5 μg of muscle at rest to 9, 11, and 17 μg for 30 minutes and 1 and 1.25 hour bouts of walking, respectively. Lactic acid concentration after 15- and 30-minute bouts of trotting decreased to 0.3 and 0.5 μg (74).

To study changes in glucose metabolism with training, the glucose tolerance test was carried out in four female Thoroughbreds who had all recorded more than one win during their racing life. The clearance rate of exogenous glucose from plasma is much slower in the horse than in any other monogastric animal. A delay in immunoreactive insulin (IRI) secretion was observed in horses with a complete resting condition 4 months after they left the racecourse that were stabled during this period. In these horses, 6 weeks after training, the IRI secretion was stimulated and the clearance rate became more than three times as high as that before the training (as high as, or higher than that in any other monogastric animal). It is concluded that glucose metabolism in the racehorse is influenced largely by exercise and that the main reason for the change is not an increase in IRI sensitivity, but a greater and more rapid secretion of insulin from the pancreas (75).

Four horses were trained twice daily, 6 days/week, for 7 weeks. Exercise consisted of 1 minute walking (110 m/min) followed by trotting (200 m/min) for 5 minutes increasing by 1 minute each week to 12 minutes after 7 weeks. Biopsy samples of the middle gluteal muscle, collected before training and at 1, 3, 5, and 7 weeks, were examined for fiber types, oxidative capacity, capillary numbers, citrate synthase, HAD, lactate dehydrogenase, and total glycogen. Over the 7 weeks, fiber types and capillary numbers were unchanged; Type IIB fiber oxidative capacity, citrate synthase, and HAD increased, and lactate dehydrogenase decreased. Glycogen utilization fell progressively by 35% from levels measured before training began (76). The addition of glucose to fluid administration during anesthesia may be indicated.

In the horse, the dominant glucocorticoid is cortisol. An elevated blood cortisol level occurs during or immediately after exercise in most species, including the horse. This increase is greater under heavy work loads or in stressful situations. Adrenaline stimulates a large number of mechanisms required for vigorous exercise. It promotes the conversion of muscle glycogen to glucose phosphate, activates tissue lipases, inhibits insulin release, stimulates the heart, increases cardiac output and promotes redistribution of blood flow to muscles from organs not involved in exercise, facilitates neuromuscular transmission in skeletal muscle, stimulates contractile processes in fast twitch fibers, relaxes bronchioles, and stimulates respiration. Most of the effects of adrenaline are due to increased cyclic adenosine monophosphate production after binding to beta-receptors. Noradrenaline, which combines weakly with beta-receptors, has many of the above effects, but because it also binds more firmly to alpha-receptors, a few responses differ. Unlike thyroid and steroid hormones, catecholamines exert their effects within minutes. It is not surprising that they play the major hormonal role in acute exercise.

During exercise, an increase in plasma noradrenaline that is almost linearly proportional to exercise intensity occurs. A nine-fold increase in plasma noradrenaline occurs in the horse after brief maximal exercise and a 50% increase occurs after an endurance ride. By contrast, there is little increase in plasma adrenaline with light work loads, whereas during heavy exercise, especially if it is accompanied by emotional stress, a marked increase occurs. Unlike adrenocortical hormones, catecholamines increase less in trained subjects, although basal levels are unchanged.

The interaction of adrenaline with many other hormones can be important in exercise. For example, thyroid hormones both enhance the sensitivity to excitement as a stimulus for adrenaline release and increase the peripheral effects of adrenaline. In prolonged exercise, mobilization of the fuel for muscular work becomes important. Glucagon acts on the liver, causing glycogenolysis and gluconeogenesis. The primary signal for glucagon release is hypoglycemia, and the glucagon rise after an endurance ride is consistent with the hypoglycemia induced by prolonged exercise (77). These increased levels of adrenaline and noradrenaline may explain some of the dose-dependent responses to anesthetics.

In a study in Thoroughbred racehorses, blood samples were collected within 10 minutes after races over distances of 1000 to 2402 m. After racing, marked increases in hematocrit and circulating concentrations of glucose, glycerol, lactate, pyruvate, uric acid, and cortisol occurred. A moderate increase in total plasma protein, sodium, and phosphate with no change or a slight elevation in potassium and no change in chloride and urea concentrations were observed. The large increase in blood lactate concentration resulted in changes in the acid-base status of the horses, with a venous pH as low as 6.900 being recorded in some horses. A consistent and generally small increase in both creatine kinase and aspartate aminotransferase activities occurred. There appeared to be no relationship between distance raced and degree of change seen (78). The results recorded from the races at Newmarket, England are shown in Table 13.8.

Carotid artery blood samples were sequentially collected for acid-base and blood gas measurements from five fit Thoroughbred horses during maximal exercise. Each horse galloped 1.6 km, and samples were collected via a catheter when the horse was at rest, after 0.8 km and 1.6 km of galloping, immediately upon stopping, and 5 minutes after exercise. The arterial oxygen tension (PaO_2) and pH decreased progressively during exercise in all horses, and four of them developed an obvious hypercapnea. Each animal became progressively more acidemic in the time it took to pull it up and in the succeeding 5 minutes. The horses developed a respiratory alkalosis, however, and the PaO_2 returned to a level higher than that measured at rest. It was concluded that this phenomenon possibly limits performance in racing horses. The reasons for the development of hypoxemia and hypercapnea are not clear, although there are several possible causes, including the existence of marked ventilation-perfusion inequalities due to arteriovenous shunting, an increase in the blood-alveolar diffusion distance, and alveolar hypoventilation. Further work is needed to assess the possible role of each of these factors in affecting performance during maximal exercise (79). It should be noted that the figures in Table 13.9 evaluating arterial blood values show more definite effects of ventilation capability than venous blood in the study illustrated in Table 13.8. The trend to acidosis is simi-

Table 13.8
Postrace Blood Chemistries in Thoroughbreds

	Prerace Resting	1201 m	1401 m	1602 m	2002 m	2402 m
Plasma cortisol (mM/liter)	79 ± 39	265 ± 84[a]	367 ± 24[a]	267 ± 24[a]	350 ± 82[a]	443 ± 155[a]
Creatine kinase (IU/liter)	132 ± 15	207 ± 86[a]	160 ± 66[a]	181 ± 58	176 ± 47[a]	181 ± 36[a]
Aspartate aminotransferase (IU/liter)	342 ± 128	424 ± 120[a]	388 ± 67	372 ± 30	337 ± 78	372 ± 23
Hematocrit (l/liter)	0.42 ± 0.05	0.59 ± 0.03[a]	0.59 ± 0.04[a]	0.63 ± 0.04[a]	0.64 ± 0.02[a]	0.62 ± 0.05[a]
Total plasma protein (g/liter)	62.3 ± 3.7	71.6 ± 4.1[a]	75.5 ± 3.2[a]	80.7 ± 5.7	78.5 ± 5.8[a]	77 ± 5.8[a]
Sodium (mM/liter)	136 ± 3.8	147 ± 3.5[a]	144 ± 3.5[a]	149 ± 1.0	141 ± 2.9	147 ± 2.8
Potassium (mM/liter)	3.6 ± 0.5	4.0 ± 0.4	4.1 ± 0.4[a]	4.5 ± 0.4	3.6 ± 0.2	4.3 ± 0.8
Phosphate (mM/liter)	1.23 ± 0.12	1.64 ± 0.18[a]	1.44 ± 0.15[a]	1.38 ± 0.06	1.45 ± 0.12	1.45 ± 0.06
Glucose (mM/liter)	5.6 ± 0.5	9.3 ± 0.7[a]	9.2 ± 1.4[a]	10.1 ± 3.4[a]	8.9 ± 0.8[a]	9.4 ± 0.6[a]
Glycerol (mol/liter)	20 ± 6	760 ± 256[a]	763 ± 323[a]	750 ± 353[a]	993 ± 486[a]	697 ± 248[a]
Lactate (mm/liter)	0.3 ± 0.1	26.6 ± 4.3[a]	25.5 ± 2.7[a]	29.6 ± 2.1[a]	25.0 ± 3.4[a]	27.3 ± 2.4[a]
Pyruvate (mol/liter)	40 ± 10	330 ± 60[a]	300 ± 50[a]	—	320 ± 30[a]	320 ± 80[a]
Urea (mM/liter)	4.8 ± 1.0	5.1 ± 0.8	5.2 ± 1.4	5.7 ± 0.8	6.5 ± 0.9	5.8 ± 0.9
Uric acid (mol/liter)	—	90 ± 30	100 ± 30	100 ± 52	90 ± 10	88 ± 72
pH	7.403 ± 0.031	7.013 ± 0.065	6.968 ± 0.010	6.990 ± 0.038	6.984 ± 0.036	6.998 ± 0.010
pCO_2 (mm Hg)	48.7 ± 4.0	26.4 ± 3.9[a]	25.5 ± 1.0[a]	22.0 ± 1.4[a]	25.1 ± 2.5[a]	24.3 ± 0.6[a]
pO_2 (mm Hg)	40.4 ± 5.9	60.6 ± 7.7[a]	65.8 ± 2.5[a]	69.2 ± 1.9[a]	66.6 ± 4.3[a]	64.3 ± 14.8[a]
HCO_3 (mm/liter)	30.0 ± 2.4	6.7 ± 1.6[a]	5.8 ± 0.3[a]	5.5 ± 0.7[a]	6.0 ± 0.9[a]	5.9 ± 0.2[a]
Base excess (mm/liter)	5.1 ± 2.4	−24.1 ± 3.0[a]	−26.2 ± 0.5[a]	−25.1 ± 1.3[a]	−25.5 ± 1.8[a]	−25.1 ± 0.5[a]
Speed (m/sec)		15.8	15.8	15.8	15.5	15.4

[a] Significant change during racing.

Table 13.9
Arterial Acid-Base and Blood Gas Responses in Thoroughbreds Performing a Maximal Exercise Test[a]

	At rest	After 0.8 km	After 1.6 km	On stopping	5 minutes post exercise
pH	7.398 ± 0.01	7.207 ± 0.05	7.120 ± 0.02	7.069 ± 0.03	7.032 ± 0.03
PaO_2 (mm Hg)	96.2 ± 6.0	64.7 ± 2.5	61.5 ± 2.1	78.6 ± 8.4	106.3 ± 1.3
$PaCO_2$ (mm Hg)	44.5 ± 1.6	49.8 ± 2.2	50.8 ± 4.3	40.4 ± 5.4	27.1 ± 1.0
HCO_3 (mM/l)	26.6 ± 1.1	19.5 ± 2.9	15.4 ± 0.9	10.6 ± 0.9	6.6 ± 0.8
BE	1.8 ± 0.9	−9.7 ± 4.1	−15.4 ± 1.1	−20.9 ± 1.6	−25.7 ± 2.4
O_2 Sat (%)	96.2 ± 0.5	82.5 ± 2.8	77.4 ± 1.6	82.7 ± 4.4	91.32 ± 0.5

[a] Data are expressed as the mean ± SEM. HCO_3, bicarbonate; TCO_2, total carbon dioxide; BE, base excess; O_2 Sat, oxygen saturation.

lar. The arterial samples show the reduction in oxygen saturation of hemoglobin. Perhaps this explains the tolerance of some horses to low pH values during anesthesia.

Sixteen plasma biochemical variables and blood lactate were measured in Thoroughbred racehorses before exercise and during the first hour after exercise. When horses were exercised at a canter, changes occurred in a number of blood constituents. With the exception of creatinine, phosphorus, and potassium, all variables returned to their pre-exercise values within 1 hour. Phosphorus and potassium, however, were below their pre-exercise value after 1 hour. Exercise at a gallop resulted in changes in blood lactate and in all plasma constituents assayed, except chloride and conjugated bilirubin. Of the constituents altered, only sodium, potassium, cholesterol, and alkaline phosphatase returned to their respective pre-exercise values after 1 hour. At this time, bicarbonate, phosphorus, and total bilirubin were below their resting values, whereas glucose, urea, creatinine, urate, calcium, lactate dehydrogenase, creatine kinase, and blood lactate were above their pre-exercie values (80).

Various hematological analyses were performed on daily preride and postride blood samples collected from 20 randomly sampled horses participating in the South African National Endurance Ride of 1981. The ride is an annual 3-day event during which distances of 80 km, 80 km, and 50 km are covered over the 3 days, respectively. The values of the majority of parameters increased during the ride on each of the 3 days and returned to approximately preride values overnight. The blood glucose decreased during the ride and also returned to preride values overnight. An exception was the plasma urea concentration, which showed a cumulative increase during the 3 days. Only minor changes occurred in the concentrations of the plasma cations.

The horses were ridden faster on the first day of the ride, and the alterations in the blood constituents were more marked on this day than on the 2 subsequent days. The greater alterations in the concentration of blood constituents observed in less fit horses ridden at average speeds exceeding 19 km/hour suggest that they were more stressed than the fit or more slowly ridden horses (81).

Plasma creatine kinase in an 80-km endurance ride increased from 72 μ/liter pre-race to 389 after the 80-km ride. Plasma cortisol increased from 309 to 671 nmol/liter. Blood glucose levels were relatively stable (82).

Plasma activities of creatine kinase (CK) and aspartate aminotransferase (AST) were measured in 70 horses before and after competitive endurance rides. Both preride levels and the magnitude of the increases during the competitions were extremely variable and were not related to subjective assessments of degree of fatigue. The same enzymes were measured in four horses that took part in a controlled (16 to 18 km/hour) 80-km ride on two occasions each. Measurements in these horses were continued for 6 months after the rides. Again, neither preride enzyme activities nor the magnitude of the increases during the rides were related to observed degree of fatigue. Two horses showed elevated and fluctuating enzyme levels during the following months, although no clinical muscle problems were seen. It is suggested that elevated plasma CK and AST activities in endurance horses may be a common occurrence and that they should not be interpreted as an adverse indication unless clinical evidence of muscle damage is also present (83).

Is the adaptation to physical training effective when superimposed on the metabolic demands of growth in yearling Standardbreds? Several cardiorespiratory and metabolic variables were studied in a group of 10 colts during a 1-year observation period. The variables studied were: the red-cell volume (CV) calculated from the Evans blue dilution space and the postexercise hematocrit; the oxygen uptake at a heart rate of 200 bpm was extrapolated from a stepwise treadmill exercise test; the pulse/work relationship (V_{200}) expressed as the extrapolated treadmill velocity at a 10% slope performed with a heart rate of 200 bpm in a standard exercise tolerance test; the postexercise blood lactate level (LAO′); the extrapolated blood lactate level at a heart rate of 200 bpm (LA_{200}); and the extrapolated treadmill velocity performed with a blood lactate of 4 mM/liter (V_{LA4}). The horses were examined before the start of the program and in the middle and at the end of the observation period.

The results indicated that physical activation in the yearling induces a transition of energy metabolism during exercise from anaerobic to aerobic predominance mainly by adaptation of functional capacities such as peripheral oxygen utilization and mitochondrial enzyme activities rather than by increasing cardiorespiratory dimensions. This adaptation is not sufficient, however, to prevent a relative decrease of the oxygen uptake capacity due to the rapid growth during this period of life (84).

Five Standardbred trotters were first submitted to an incremental work test at intervals during a 5-week graded treadmill training program and then to 5 weeks of detraining. There was no significant change related to training or detraining in mean values of arterial or mixed venous blood gas tensions, pH, cardiac output, or oxygen uptake, at rest or at 8.5 m/sec. (the comparative reference speed) during the work tests. During each work test, all these variables changed significantly from resting values. Arterial PCO_2 rose from 6.26 ± 0.54 kPa at rest to 7.60 ± 0.76 kPa at 8.5 m/sec.,whereas arterial PO_2 dropped from 14.06 ± 1.15 kPa to 8.30 ± 2.06 kPa. Mixed venous PCO_2 rose from 7.14 ± 0.46 kPa at rest to 14.17 ± 1.13 kPa at 8.5 m/sec. whereas mixed venous PO_2 dropped from 5.48 ± 0.59 to 2.06 ± 0.31 kPa. Arterial pH dropped from 7.390 ± 0.036 at rest to 7.255 ± 0.058 at 8.5 m/sec. whereas mixed venous pH dropped from 7.358 ± 0.034 to 7.139 ± 0.060. There was an immediate and significant change toward resting values in all variables upon cessation of work, except in mixed venous PCO_2, which was unchanged at 15 seconds and then declined exponentially until 90 seconds after exercise. There was a 37.6-fold increase in oxygen uptake to which increased cardiac output (8.3 times) contributed approximately two-thirds and muscular oxygen extraction contributed approximately one-third. Stroke volume increased only 1.5 times. There was no difference in mean arterial and mixed venous lactate concentrations. Mixed venous lactate concentration at rest did not change with training or detraining, whereas that at 8.5 meters/sec. declined significantly from 9.58 ± 2.16 mM/liter before training to 5.66 ± 1.31 mM/liter after training. There was no further change with detraining (85).

ENDURANCE RIDES

Observations were made on the day before the ride, at stops every 3 hours, and at the end. Packed cell volume increased by 20% after 30 miles and remained high. Total plasma protein was increased by 7% at the first stop, returned to preride levels by 83 miles, and was only increased by 2% at the end. Blood glucose decreased by 22.5%, and free fatty acids increased five-fold. There was little change in blood lactates.

Creatinine phosphokinase increased four-fold. Mean chloride and calcium levels were reduced by 8 to 10% and phosphorous and potassium by 45 and 14%, respectively (86). Muscle damage does occur during long endurance rides. This affects the level of relaxation during anesthesia, but more critically may affect the recovery after anesthesia.

As part of a study of the metabolic effects of long distance riding, the results of biochemical analyses of blood samples taken from horses before, immediately after, and 1 hour after an 80 km ride were reported. The results show that the horses were moderately dehydrated; they were working aerobically using fats as metabolic substrates, and blood glucose was reduced. There was no evidence of postexercise ketosis, and circulating alanine levels fell. Metabolic hormone levels were related to the availability of substrates for gluconeogenesis. There was evidence of reduced kidney and liver function that showed little sign of recovery in the first hour after the ride (87).

Blood samples were taken before and immediately after 80-km and 40-km rides held on consecutive days. Samples were analyzed for hematocrit, blood glucose and lactate, plasma sodium, potassium, calcium, albumin, free fatty acids (FFA), glycerol, bicarbonate, insulin, cortisol, glucagon, urea, creatinine, uric acid, bilirubin, and aklakine phosphatase. Unusually hot weather probably contributed to hemoconcentration with a significant increase in hematocrit and plasma albumin values.

A fall in blood glucose and a rise in FFA and glycerol were consistent with long distance riding and were associated with a reduction in plasma insulin and a rise in cortisol and glucagon. The results suggested that the horses were working aerobically, and the small increase in blood lactate was likely to be a result of reduced tissue perfusion. Plasma urea, cretinine, and bilirubin increased during the 80-km ride and were still high the next morning. Blood samples were taken from two horses that became exhausted and were forced to retire; the results from these animals indicated a slow rate of recovery. It is suggested that hemoconcentration with reduced tissue perfusion might contribute to exhaustion during long distance exercise and that the speed of recovery might be improved by the intravenous administration of balanced electrolyte solutions (88). This is an important consideration when anesthesia is required before total recovery from the ride.

The reliability of heart rate (HR) and respiratory rate (RR) recovery as an assessment of fitness was examined after endurance exercise under different conditions of environmental temperature, distance, and speed. Blood samples were collected 30 minutes after a 100-km endurance ride and 30 minutes after a 160-km endurance ride to determine whether significant correlations existed for HR and RR with various plasma biochemical parameters. In horses competing in a 100-km ride, significant correlations were found for HR with total protein (TP), albumin, cholesterol, creatinine, bilirubin, creatine kinase (CK), alkaline phosphatase (AP), and lactate dehydrogenase (LD). Significant correlations were found for RR with TP, albumin, creatinine, bilirubin, CK, and LD. After the 160-km ride, significant correlations were found for HR and CK, LD, alpha-hydroxybutyrate dehydrogenase (HBD), AP, albumin and cholesterol. The only significant correlation found for RR was with creatinine. It was concluded that measurement of HR recovery provided a good objective assessment of the degree of fatigue suffered by a horse during endurance exercise (89).

Venous blood samples were collected before and immediately after an 80-km ride and a 42-km race. They were analyzed for blood glucose and lactate and for plasma nonesterified fatty acids, insulin, pancreatic glucagon, pancreatic polypeptide, gastrin, gastric inhibitory peptide, somatostatin, and vasoactive intestinal polypeptide concentrations. The 80-km ride was associated with marked hypoglycemia and a slight lactic acidemia together with an increase in plasma glucagon, somatostatin, pancreatic polypeptide, and vasoactive intestinal polypeptide values. The 42-km race produced hyperglycemia and marked lactic acidemia together with an increase in plasma glucagon, somatostatin, and vasoactive intestinal polypeptide. The increase in these peptides is not related to alterations in blood glucose or the relative contributions of aerobic and anaerobic muscle metabolism (90). This influences the responses to anesthetics.

Blood samples were collected from 13 horses before, during, and at the end of the ride, as well as 1 hour and 16 hours after the completion of the ride. Decreases were observed in serum concentrations of chloride, potassium, and calcium. An increase in the serum concentration of phosphorous was also observed. The mean concentrations of chloride and calcium remained reduced in the 16-hour postride sample. A small but significant increase in sodium and a decrease in glucose concentrations were observed in the midride sample. Although midride samples did not show a significant change in blood pyruvate concentration, a significant increase was observed at the end of the ride. Hematocrit and the total protein concentration increased. The horses showed increases in concentrations of free fatty acids, serum enzymes, and lactate during the ride. The elevated values of creatine kinase and lactate dehydrogenase decreased, although the aspartate aminotransferase values remained increased long after completion of the ride. The lactate and free fatty acids, which rose significantly during the ride, decreased to approximately preride values by 16 hours after the ride. It is concluded that the changes in serum electrolytes, enzymes, and blood metabolites reflect sweating, muscle damage, and increased dependence on anaerobic glycolysis and lipid mobilization (91).

This indicates anesthesia for surgical correction of injuries within the 16-hour postride period should include fluid administration to correct electrolyte imbalances.

Blood samples were collected from 16 Thoroughbred horses before, during, and after the second day of a 3-day event. Plasma osmolality and concentrations of sodium, potassium, chloride, urea, creatinine, glucose, bilirubin, iron, total protein, albumin, alkaline phosphatase, aspartate aminotransferase, alanine aminotransferase, creatine kinase, calcium, inorganic phosphate, uric acid, cholesterol, triglycerides, and nonesterified fatty acids were measured. Significant differences from starting values were found in all components, with the greatest changes being found after the cross-country phase. Most values showed significant rises after exercise, with the exception of calcium and chloride, which decreased. It was deduced from the changes in biochemistry that dehydration, reduced glomerular filtration rate, increased glycogenolysis, and increased lipid metabolism were a result of this form of competitive exercise (92). During anesthesia, reduced cardiac function may be observed due to lower calcium levels.

Four Thoroughbred horses were ridden for a distance of up to 80 km on two occasions at a speed of 16 to 18 km/hour. Blood, sweat, urine, and muscle samples were collected at various times before, during, and after the ride. Mean body weight loss was 7%. Increases occurred in hematocrit values and plasma proteins during the ride; plasma chloride fell. Hypoglycemia was evident at the end of the ride, and large increases were noted in free fatty acids and glycerol. Activities of all enzymes, particularly creatine kinase, increased during the ride, but the magnitude of the increases was not related to the observed degree of fatigue. A neutrophilia occurred during the ride and was still evident 48 hours later. Rate of urine formation and urea, sodium, and potassium excretion were not significantly different from the resting state, but the chloride excretion rate decreased by 64%. Sweat concentrations of all electrolytes were hypertonic to plasma, and total electrolyte losses during the ride were 6.03 mol sodium, 1.90 mol potassium, and 6.34 mol chloride. Muscle glycogen decreased progressively throughout the ride with complete depletion being seen after the ride on five occasions. Depletion occurred initially in the Type I and IIA fibers, with the IIB fibers only being recruited in the latter stages. The pattern for repletion in the fibers was the reverse of depletion, with only some of the fibers being repleted after 24 hours. The measurements that appeared to correlate best with the observed degree of fatigue were depletion of muscle glycogen stores and elevation of plasma uric acid (93).

Total and individual nonesterified fatty acids, pyruvate, lactate, alpha ketoglutarate, acetoacetate, beta hydroxybutyrate, glucose, and insulin were measured in horses during an 80-km endurance ride and during 4 days of food deprivation. In the latter group venous, blood-gas and acid-base parameters and plasma cortisol concentrations were also measured. During exercise and food deprivation, the nonesterified fatty acids became considerably elevated; the predominant ones were oleic (35%), palmitic (24%), linoleic (19%), and linolenic (10%). By 1 hour after feeding, total nonesterified fatty acids fell to approximately 20% of 12-hour fasting concentrations. This was associated with a fourfold rise in insulin. Small but significant increases occurred in lactate, acetoacetate, and beta hydroxybutyrate after the 80-km endurance ride. It was concluded that a ketone pathway is relatively unimportant in the horse, probably due to the ability of the liver to maintain glycogenolysis (94). Xylazine must be used with caution even though it may be effectve. Xylazine produces a drop in insulin levels and hyperglycemia, the opposite of exercise.

EXERCISE AND DISEASE

Five normal horses and four COPD subjects were exercised at the walk, trot, and gallop speeds of 1.5, 4, and 7.7 meters/sec, respectively. Arterial and mixed venous blood samples were collected anaerobically and simultaneously by means of an automatic technique at 0 to 100 m, at 500 to 600 m, and at 1100 to 1200 m over a work distance of 1200 m. Blood gas and acid-base values and lactate and pyruvate concentrations were determined. HRs were measured by telemetry. Highly significant changes in mean $P\bar{v}O_2$, O_2 content, $\Delta a\text{-}\bar{v}O_2$ content, and $PaCO_2$ occurred during exercise in COPD subjects. In the normal subjects, significant changes occurred in mean $P\bar{v}O_2$ and $\Delta a\text{-}\bar{v}O_2$ content. The increase in HR was greater in COPD subjects than in normal subjects during the trot. It was concluded that the horses with COPD compensted for lung dysfunction by extracting more oxygen from blood than normal horses and increasing the HR. In all subjects, the $PaCO_2$ decreased within 12 seconds of the start of the gallop to a level that remained constant for the duration of the exercise period. HR and hemoglobin mobilization, on the other hand, only approached maximum values at the 600-m mark (95).

During anesthesia, horses with COPD will have greater need for supplemental oxygen to maintain high blood oxygen levels. Inhalant anesthetic uptake and elimination may be altered due to changes in respiratory function.

HRs were measured in healthy horses (17) and in horses with chronic emphysema (7), extreme chronic bronchitis (5), moderate chronic bronchitis (15), slight chronic bronchitis (4), heart valve disease (3), and atrial fibrillation (2) during a defined course of exercise.

Horses had to cover a course at a walk, trot, canter, and fast gallop (400 m/minute) without a pause. ECG was recorded on to a cassette recorder worn by the rider. The recovery rate of pulse and respiration of the horses with lung diseases after a 20-minute trot on the lunge was also recorded. The changes in HR were correlated with the clinical signs exhibited by the horses. In the horses with lung disease, there was a close correlation between the stage of the disease and the HR during the exercise test. In 3 animals with heart valve disease, there was no apparent difference in HR compared with healthy horses, but the HR of horses with atrial fibrillation showed a significant increase.

The recovery rate of pulse and respiration after a 20-minute trot did not show any correlation with the stage of disease or the results of gradually stepping up the exercise in horses with lung disease (96). All these conditions would increase the risk of anesthesia.

It was noteworthy to review the literature on influence of exercise in patients with diabetes because exercise influences insulin levels. Two hundred human patients with overt diabetes mellitus who were over age 30 were investigated for the presence of ischemic heart disease. Thirty patients had abnormalities in the resting ECG indicative of myocardial infarction, ischemic ST-T depression, or left bundle branch block. When 170 patients were subjected to Master's two-step exercise test, another 29 were found to have postexercise ST-T segment depression. The frequency of ischemic heart disease as judged by ECG was 29.5% in these patients. There was a significant correlation between associated systemic hypertension and presence of ischemic heart disease (97).

A total of 76 male diabetics and 46 male controls were studied with exercise tests in similar conditions. During exercise, systolic blood pressure was significantly higher in the diabetic than in the control at all rates. In 36 diabetics with normal postexercise ECG, cholesterol, triglycerides, and systolic and diastolic blood pressure were significantly lower than in diabetics with pathological postexercise ECG depressions. There were 12 diabetics with clinical or ECG myocardial infarction and 1 control subject with ECG sign of myocardial infarction (98).

A total of 29 adult iron deficient anemic subjects with Hb from 4.0 to 12.0 g/100 ml blood were divided into Fe treatment and placebo groups. Hematological, cardiorespiratory, and performance data were collected before, during, and after treatment and compared with data from a control group of subjects. Hb for the treated group improved from 7.7 to 12.4 g for the women and from 7.1 to 14.0 g for the women and men. The placebo group showed hardly any change over the 80-day period (8.1 to 8.4 g for women and 7.7 to 7.4 g for men). Peak exercise HRs (5 minute 40-cm step test) were significantly reduced after treatment from 155 to 113 for the treated men and 152 to 123 for the women compared with the placebo group, which showed no change. In response to the exercise test, no difference in oxygen consumption was found between the Fe treatment and placebo group, although 15% more O_2 was delivered per pulse in the treated group. Blood lactates were significantly higher in the placebo than the treated group both at rest (1.18 versus 0.64 mM/liter) and 1 minute after exercise (5.30 versus 2.68 mM/liter). The results support the concept that performance requiring high oxygen delivery is significantly affected by Hb (99). The same would be true during anesthesia.

Cardioversion through varying quinidine sulphate treatments was achieved in three riding horses with auricular fibrillation. The horses were subjected to continual telemetric ECG registration before and after reversion in a uniform exercise-tolerance test. A comparison of the HR curves showed a strong decline of the heart beat frequency during the exercise phase after synchronization. The decrease in heart rate during exercise was greater than 30% in all 3 cases. Therefore, antiarrhythmic treatment is recommended for horses with auricular fibrillation and without concurrent heart disease (100). Treatment of this nature should be known before anesthesia is induced.

EFFECTS OF MEDICATION

Various cardiorespiratory parameters of five horses were studied before, during, and at various times after submaximal exercise in the swimming pool. The response to intravenous administration of furosemide was also evaluated. It was concluded that the cardiovascular system of these horses responded to swimming in a manner qualitatively similar to running forms of exercise. The respiratory response to exercise differed qualitatively and quantitatively between swimming and running. The effects of furosemide on right atrial and pulmonary arterial pressure in horses after swimming were similar to those in resting horses (101).

Plasma concentrations of phenylbutazone (PBZ) and its metabolites were measured in horses after dosing schedules that simulated conditions under the "no treatment for 24 hours before racing" rule. In 16 Thoroughbreds or Standardbreds at pasture given PBZ at 4.4 mg/kg/day i.v. for 4 days, mean plasma PBZ increased from 0.77 μg/ml on Day 2 to 2.5 μg/ml on Day 5 (24 hours after the last dose). In a second trial, this group was given PBZ at 8.8 mg/kg/day orally for 3 days and 4.4 mg/kg i.v. on Day 4. Mean plasma PBZ was 3.4 μ/ml on Day 2 and 3.5 μg/ml on Day 5. In a third trial, 62 Thoroughbreds in training were dosed as in the second trial. Mean plasma PBZ increased to

5.3 μg/ml on Day 5 (102). PBZ influences the protein binding of barbiturates used in anesthesia.

The effects of prolonged exercise on plasma concentrations of corticosteroids, insulin, glucose, lactate, and beta-hydroxybutyrate were studied in a group of horses competing in a 160-km endurance ride. Of the 53 horses included in the study at the outset, 23 completed the course. Plasma corticosteroids increased and glucose and insulin decreased during exercise. Little change occurred in plasma lactate or beta-hydroxybutyrate. No consistent significant differences were found between individuals that completed and those that did not complete the course (103).

In another study, nine horses were treated with amphetamine alone, with atropine alone, and with amphetamine and atropine in combination. Cardiac effects of these drugs studied by ECG during resting and exercising states and immediately after exercise differed significantly for each treatment; the most rapid decrease in heart rate was found after the amphetamine treatment. Amphetamine caused second-degree atrioventricular (AV) block in each horse during the postexercise period. Amphetamine also caused ectopic beats either during or immediately after exercise in six horses. Second-degree AV block was not found when atropine was used alone or when it was used in combination with amphetamine. Fewer ectopic beats were found when atropine was used with amphetamine. Heart rate responses indicated that the direct effect of amphetamine was greater than the reflex effect at rest and during exercise. Second-degree AV block during the postexercise period was attributed to vagotonia due to baroreceptor stimulation. Release of adrenaline by amphetamine probably caused many of the ectopic beats by increasing automaticity of subordinate pacemakers (104).

Exercise initiates cardiovascular and respiratory responses and also results in a series of biochemical changes. In the evaluation of the effects of drugs on speed and performance, horses were subjected to a number of standardized exercise tests in which an assessment of cardiac and respiratory changes was also made. Physiological changes associated with racing and severe exercise have three components; preliminary excitement, a major phase during the actual exertion, and a recovery phase of cardiac and respiratory deceleration. Stimulants of the CNS were generally effective in increasing speed in at least some of the tests; a short 200-m gallop appeared to be the most sensitive indicator of the effect of this class of drug. With the exception of methylamphetamine, which increased the changes in pre-exercise excitement, increased effects on HR and respiratory rate during exercise and a prolongation of the recovery phase depended upon the increases in running speed caused by the administration of the drug. Increases after exercise were recorded in blood glucose, lactate, pyruvate, FFA, and glycerol. Serum concentrations of creatine kinase, aldolase, and lactic dehydrogenase were also increased. Similar increases can be demonstraed after the injection of adrenaline, but the results do not suggest that the biochemical changes of exercise are entirely due to the release of this agent (105).

A galloping test simulating racing conditions was established. A marked increase in the HR and respiratory rate was observed when the horses walked onto the race track prior to exercise. The mean HR/min at different times was: before exercise, 40; at 1 minute after exercise, 121; at 10 minutes, 100; at 30 minutes, 75; and at 60 minutes, 45. Changes in respiratory rate paralleled changes in heart rate. Cardiac arrhythmia observed at 1 minute disappeared by 3 minutes after exercise. The effect of i.v. administration of amphetamine sulphate, 0.2 mg/kg, promazine hydrochloride, 0.5 mg/kg, and thiamine hydrochloride, 5 mg/kg, 30 to 60 minutes before the exercise test was determined. Promazine depressed the respiratory rate, increased heart rate at 1 minute (which decreased below control levels at 30 and 60 minutes), and decreased speed by 15%. Amphetamine caused an increase in respiratory rate before the test but had no consistent effect on respiration after exercise. One minute after the exercise, there was a marked depression of the heart rate and a nonphasic cardiac arrhythmia, which disappeared at 3 to 5 minutes. Thiamine did not affect cardiac or respiratory rates before or after the test. The last two drugs had no effect on speed (106).

Six mature Standardbred horses during an 8-week period of training over a distance of 16,000 m increased speed from 604 to 690 m/min. Every second week, each horse was given one of our drugs i.v. an averge of 17 minutes before a submaximal exercise test (ST) of 1810 m at 557 m/min. The sequence of drug administration was by a modified latin square design. Control data were obtained on alternate weeks. The drugs and dosages were: methylprednisolone sulphate, 0.44 mg/kg; promazine hydrochloride, 0.544 mg/kg; amphetamine sulphate, 0.55 mg/kg; or furosemide, 1.1 mg/kg. From the observable response of the horses, it could not be accurately determined which drug had been given. Amphetamine and promazine caused an increase in heart rate at 1810 m of ST (telemetry), and amphetamine and furosemide caused the heart rate immediately after ST to be higher than the control data. Amphetamine caused venous lactate to be higher than the control values during the 60 minutes after ST (107).

Studies in Standardbreds reveal stimulation from narcotics. Horses trotted faster after increasing doses of fentanyl for 0.5, 2, 4, and 8 mg/500 kg body weight. Etorphine at as little as 0.00002 mg/kg resulted in locomotor stimulation. In addition, methadone, 0.05

mg/kg; morphine, 0.05 mg/kg; and meperidine, 1.0 mg/kg, resulted in locomotor stimulation (108). This gives some explanation of the stimulating effect of narcotic analgesics administered to injured racehorses at the track to control pain.

Physiological data were recorded from mature Standardbred horses on 2 consecutive days weekly (1 day drug, 1 day placebo) for 8 weeks during and after a submaximal exercise test (st). The horses were in an 8-week training program during which they progressed from a speed of 604 to 690 m/min over a distance of 1600 m. In these blind trials, 0.55 mg/kg of amphetamine sulphate, 0.55 mg/kg of methylphenidate, or a placebo were administered intravenously an average of 17 (15 to 20) minutes before ST.

Both drugs made the horses eager to go fast and pull on the reins. In addition, methylphenidate made the horses hyperresponsive to auditory and visual stimuli; they tended to make fast movements sideways on and off the track.

Both drugs caused venous lactate, HR, respiratory rate and rectal temperature to increase after exercise. Cardiac output also tended to be greater than in the controls, being significantly higher 10 minutes after exercise following methylphenidate administration (109).

To evaluate the effects of theophylline and some nonsteroidal anti-inflammatory drugs (NSAID), namely flunixin, meclofenamic acid, and nefopam, on circulatory and metabolic parameters related to exercise tolerance, each of five experimental horses performed a standard exercise tolerance test on a high-speed treadmill 4 hours after administration of each drug.

Theophylline caused a significant decrease of the extrapolated treadmill velocity with a heart rate of 200 (speed of 200 meters/sec). (V_{200}, m/s). Among the NSAIDs, only flunixin had a significant effect on the heart rate response to exercise. The accumulation of lactate in the blood after exercise was significantly lower after administration of all three NSAIDs. The same tendency was noted for the extrapolated blood lactate level at an exercise heart rate of 200 (LA_{200},mM/liter), but was significant only after administration of meclofenamic acid. The "anaerobic threshold" (i.e. the extrapolated treadmill velocity performed with a blood lactate level of 4 mM/liter) was significantly higher after meclofenamic acid administration (110). The presence of medications that either depress or stimulate the horse may greatly affect dosage requirements of anesthetics and response to anesthetic management.

Blood samples were collected from 11 horses presented for prolonged surgery before, after, and at 30-minute intervals during anesthesia lasting up to 4 hours. Anesthesia was induced with atropine (20 mg i.m.), promazine (250 mg i.v.), and pentothal (2 g i.v.) and maintained with halothane (2%), oxygen (6 liters/min), and nitrous oxide (2 liters/min). Horses were restrained in lateral recumbency on a large table padded with a water-filled mattress. Leg restraints were removed as soon as surgical anesthesia was attained. Another group of 4 horses fed a diet supplemented with rolled oats (2 kg/dat) for 2 weeks and confined before anesthesia were challenged with hypoxia, acidosis, and poor padding during deeper anesthesia. Blood samples were collected as before. The blood samples were subjected to a wide battery of clinical tests. One of the horses developed myositis. In both groups there was a steady increase in inorganic phosphate and a steady decline in serum calcium, causing a marked change in the Ca:P ratio. Although Ca decreased enough to produce tetany, this did not occur. The stressed group also showed marked increases in blood glucose and potassium and, in the 2 animals tested, a decrease in chloride. A proposed mechanism for postoperative myositis is that anesthesia and prolonged recumbency cause a state of regional hypoperfusion and partial uncoupling of oxidative phosphorylation in which creatine phosphate becomes the principle energy source for skeletal muscle. The products of the altered metabolism reduce the activity of myophosphorylase, which produces a local tetany similar to that described for McArdle's disease (111).

In an evaluation of isoflurane, halothane, enflurance, and methoxyflurane, the EEG changed with the deepening of anesthesia from high frequency/low amplitude to low frequency/high amplitude. With administration of either isoflurane or enflurane, additional changes during deep anesthesia included burst suppression, spike, and isoelectric periods (112).

The maximal alveolar concentration (MAC) for halothane was determined in the presence of varying concentrations of N_2O in 11 young, healthy, normothermic horses. Ventilation was mechanically controlled, and CO_2 tension averaged 38 mm Hg. Alveolar N_2O concentrations of 25 and 50% reduced the halothane-0_2 MAC of these horses from 0.93 ± 0.04 volume % to 0.82 ± 0.5 and 0.70 ± 0.05%, respectively. Cardiovascular (CV) responses to three concentrations of halothane-oxygen and halothane-50% N_2O-O_2 were studied in 8 of these horses. Except for a greater cardiac output and left ventricular work with N_2O at MAC multiples of 1.0 and 1.5, there was no significant difference in the CV changes produced by the two forms of anesthesia. The potency of N_2O at concentrations that permit adequate oxygenation was less in the horse than in humans (113).

Enflurane and isoflurane, which are chemically similar to methoxyflurane but have physical properties and clinical characteristics more closely resembling those of halothane, successfully induced general anesthesia. Induction and emergence from anesthesia were generally rapid and smooth, and postanesthetic complications were not seen. Reductions of cardiovascular function and abnormal muscle twitching appeared less during isoflurane anesthesia. From these initial observations in healthy horses, it appears that both enflurane and isoflurane may be used as inhalant anesthetics for the horse; however, isoflurane is probably better tolerated by the horse over a wider range of anesthetic doses (114).

The cardiopulmonary effects of positive end-expiratory pressures (PEEP) of 0, 5, 10, and 15 cm of H_2O were determined in anesthetized, spontaneously breathing horses. Cardiac output, alveolar-arterial oxygen tension difference, alveolar ventilation, dead space/tidal volume ratio, and carbon dioxide elimination were not significantly altered by the procedure. As PEEP was increased, alveolar and arterial oxygen tensions, respiratory exchange ratio, and pH decreased, whereas arterial carbon dioxide tension and oxygen consumption increased. These results indicate PEEP is contraindicated in laterally recumbent spontaneously ventilating anesthetized horses breathing air, because it causes alveolar hypoventilation and does not improve pulmonary gas exchange (115).

Heart rate responses to elevation or decrease in systemic arterial pressure produced by phenylephrine or nitroglycerine were studied in healthy, awake horses during a control period, after beta-adrenergic blockade produced with propranolol, after vagal efferent blockade produced with atropine, and after blockade of both beta-adrenergic and vagal efferent activities. Cardiac slowing in response to increase in systemic arterial pressure results from increase in vagal efferent activity. Cardiac acceleration in response to decrease in systemic arterial pressure results from decrease in vagal efferent activity. Cardiac acceleration (in excess of that produced by atropine) during maximal excretion results from increase in sympathetic efferent activity (116).

Controlled ventilation/peripheral relaxation was applied to 85 adult horses given a halothane, nitrous oxide, and oxygen mixture. The respiratory minute volumes and the administration of nitrous oxide were adjusted to maintain arterial PCO_2 and PO_2 within normal limits. The respiratory minute volumes/kilogram of body weight were compared with those of a group of 81 anesthetized horses breathing spontaneously. The addition of nitrous oxide was found to be restricted by a progressive fall in arterial partial oxygen pressure. According to the results, the described technique proved to be effective in maintaining external respiration of horses for several hours (117).

Effects of body position and type of ventilation were determined on arterial blood gases and pH during and immediately after clinical halothane anesthesia in 36 young, physically conditioned horses. Horses in dorsal recumbency had a lower oxygen tension than did similarly breathing horses in a lateral position. Predictably, controlled positive-pressure ventilation improved arterial oxygenation and permitted maintenance of a normal carbon dioxide tension. Most horses, regardless of type of ventilation and operative body positioning, were hypoxemic in the immediate postanesthetic period (118).

Both propranolol (0.2 mg/kg) and metoprolol (0.2 mg/kg) reduced the elevation in HR seen immediately after exercise and reduced performance because it took longer to perform each gallop. Rises in plasma glucose, glycerol, and lactate and the fall in blood pH seen after exercise were attenuated by both drugs. However, a greater increase in plasma FFAs occurred. Exercise increased plasma noradrenaline by 9 to 12 times. Neither drug had any effect on resting levels of noradrenaline, but after metoprolol, the levels during exercise were increased (119).

A long-lasting increase of the plasma bromide concentration was found in 25 horses after clinical halothane anesthesia. In 18 horses, peak values were reached between 48 and 72 hours after anesthesia. Eighteen days after horses had been anesthetized, the plasma bromide concentration was still high. There was little correlation between the total dose of halothane and the plasma bromide concentration. In one horse anesthetized with halothane 4 days after initial halothane anesthesia, the plasma bromide concentration increased to high concentrations (120).

Clinical Anesthetic Management of the Animal Athlete

CANINE ATHLETES

Even before considering the changes due to conditioning and racing, the racing greyhound requires selection of anesthetic agents and dosages for a breed of canine with an extremely lean body mass that influences the uptake distribution and elimination of anesthetic agents. Without the fat component, a greater proportion of circulating anesthetic agent remains in the highly perfused tissues during anesthesia. There is a greater tendency for the animal to develop hypothermia if in contact with cold metal surfaces or in rooms with lower ambient temperatures. The hypothermia may prolong the speed of recovery because hypothermia can slow the elimination of muscle relaxants and anesthetic agents. The thoracic structure of the greyhound also may contribute to some cardiopulmonary dysfunction during prolonged procedures in lateral recumbency.

If barbiturate inductions are anticipated, methohexatol with a faster redistribution and elimination is desirable. If it is unavailable, lower doses of thiobarbiturates are indicated. High concentrations of barbiturates that may result in prolonged recovery should be avoided. Mask inductions as well as maintenance of anesthesia with potent inhalants, including methoxyflurane, halothane, or isoflurane, may be used. The utilization of enflurane may be contraindicated in some racing greyhounds because there appears to be a higher incidence of CNS seizure activity in some racing greyhounds after peak performance than in either nonracing greyounds or in some other breeds. The utilization of diazepam to control extrasensitivity of the CNS as either a preanesthetic or in conjunction with other medication to control CNS activity post-anesthetically may be indicated. Evaluation of fluid and electrolyte imbalance and correction with appropriate fluid therapy is beneficial in the control of CNS disturbances.

There is extensive muscle activity and muscle fiber development in the racing greyhound. There are stresses on bones and joints at a fast gallop to a much greater extent than those at a walk. The range of movement is also greater. With extensive exercise of the muscles during peak performance, use of energy sources occur relative to the rate of running. At the fastest speeds, energy is derived from local concentrations of high-energy phosphate bonds. Adenosine triphosphate (ATP) is broken down to adenosine diphosphate (ADP); the ADP is immediately reconverted to ATP by reaction with creatine phosphate (CP). This CP supply may change in a matter of 5 to 10 seconds. Contracting muscle uses ATP; the energy for the conversion of ADP to ATP comes from the breakdown of glycogen. The breakdown of glycogen generates pyruvate, which is converted to lactic acid. As a result, animals with extensive breakdown of ATP during exaggerated muscle activity will show increasing levels of creatine phosphate and lactic acid. If there has been insufficient time for the recovery of muscle fibers for the elimination of excessive lactic acid during racing before anesthesia is performed, additional recovery problems may be encountered.

Many greyhounds participating in racing perform in high ambient temperatures, such as in races in Florida and Nevada. Ambient temperatures during summer months are high enough to increase body temperatures. As assessment of body temperature before anesthesia should be made to avoid confusion of higher body temperatures during anesthesia with the potential onset of malignant hyperthermia. In contrast, in racing greyhounds in the Northeast, especially during the winter months, low body fat content may result in hypothermia. This too can result in a reduction of metabolism during anesthetic procedures.

Anesthetic regimes should be designed to provide low concentrations of medications when possible. The selection of agents that are fast acting with few complications in the recovery periods produced by prolonged anesthesia is desirable. It is more appropriate to consider a rapid and complete arousal from anesthesia even when postoperative analgetics are required than to produce a more prolonged anesthetic recumbent state, which may contribute to further deterioration of stressed muscle or compensated cardiopulmonary function. One should remember, especially during procedures required after racing, that the greyhound has run at speeds from 15 to 60 km/hour. The lower running speeds of 15 to 25 km/hour can be supported almost completely by the use of oxygen, but at the higher running speeds, anaerobic metabolism of glycogen will become a more crucial factor in the development of total energy.

ANESTHETIC CONSIDERATION IN THE CONDITIONED HORSE

Endurance Horse

Anesthetic considerations of the endurance horse fall into the category of those changes that take place at slower speeds but with more prolonged exercise. These animals are more likely to have extreme fatigue. They may suffer from marked changes in ambient temperature. The necessity of providing fluid replacement for dehydration, electrolyte balance, and general support will be evident. Without fluid replacement, caution should be exercised when considering acetylpromazine or other phenothiazine-derivative tranquilizers that may result in hypotension due to alpha-blocking effect. With electrolyte disturbances, caution prior to the administration of xylazine is indicated. Supplementing with fluids and achieving electrolyte balance will add greatly to the safety of utilization of either of these medications. A clear definition of whether xylazine, which produces an increase in blood glucose and a drop in insulin levels, is contraindicated or desirable has not been established because in extremely fatigued individuals blood glucose may be low and insulin levels elevated. It would be helpful to have laboratory results indicating the levels of glucose and insulin. Unfortunately, there is frequently the need to use xylazine as a sedative analgetic for the repair of minor wounds and lacerations occurring during endurance rides. Careful assessment after the administration of preanesthetics, tranquilizers, or sedatives to determine HRs and relative pulse pressure responses is indicated.

The horse undergoing extensive exercise during training or in competition with adjustments of body fluids and electrolytes can usually be more safely induced for anesthesia techniques that provide gradual induction in contrast to crash inductions. Although injectable anesthetic techniques may be used, the addition of inhalant anesthesia is desirable because it provides supplemental oxygenation. This is beneficial to body tissues during metabolic acidosis. The increased oxygenation will provide respiratory compensation for the metabolic acidosis.

Determination of level of anesthesia may be critical in the animal suffering from physical exhaustion. It is not unusual for the horse to require less than anticipated concentrations of anesthesia to maintain surgical planes. Without attention to this detail, excessive depression of the cardiopulmonary system may occur. Many of these animals may have an elevated heart rate at the time they are presented. This may be especially noticed in the Arabian, which has a tendency to experience partial recovery from the rigors of exercise and may become excitable in the new environment of the veterinary hospital.

Recovery is more complex because the muscle damage that has occurred during extensive exercise produced fatigue. This along with the depression by anesthetics and a potential further relaxation with products such as guaifenesin may result in incoordination or weak recovery patterns. When available, supplemental oxygen and fluid therapy during recovery are beneficial. In many circumstances, however, they are unavailable because of the location in which the procedures must be accomplished.

Anesthetic Considerations in Show Horses

The principal difference in anesthetic considerations in show horses compared to exhaustive endurance riding is more psychological than physical. Conditioning is beneficial. The show horse has a higher food intake to maintain body size and appearance versus lean body mass for ultimate physical performance. The walking horse show, as an example, is not as exhaustive as a 100-mile endurance ride. The Tennessee walking horse is prone to highly excitable states geared for peak performance. CNS alertness requires careful handling to avoid further excitement and the dumping of circulating catecholamines. Adequate time after the administration of tranquilizers or sedatives should be allowed before induction of anesthesia to reduce the complications of induction and the potential cardiovascular changes that may take place during anesthetic management. Care should be taken during the administration of halothane, especially if xylazine has been used as a premedication without the concurrent use of anticholinergics, to avoid sudden depression of heart rate. In rare instances, utilization of xylazine as premedication followed by either ketamine or barbiturate induction and halothane maintenance can result in sudden cardiac complication. This, in the author's experience, has been more likely to occur in the conditioned animal with a greater level of circulating catecholamines or one which has recently worked in a high-performance sporting event.

The circulating catecholamine level may sensitize the myocardium to halothane. The combination of xylazine and halothane is more likele to cause a reduction in HR than many other combinations. Acepromazine followed by barbiturate-guaifenesin induction and isoflurane maintenance of anesthesia should result in fewer cardiac irregularities. Supplemental injections of xylazine to provide additional analgesia should either be avoided or given with extreme caution because it can produce dramatic slowing of the heart or heart block, especially during halothane anesthesia.

Recovery of the walking horse or the American saddlebred after show ring performance when anesthesia and surgery are necessry can be anticipated to be less stressful than in endurance horses because of the reduced amount of muscle trauma which occurs as a result of performance.

Anesthetic Considerations in Quarterhorses and Other Breeds in Rodeo Events

This group of horses requires consideration because of exercise, CNS excitement in the competition arena, and the performance of these events in various ambient conditions. Many of these horses compete in regions of the country where temperatures are adequately high to produce dehydration and elevated body temperature responses to competition. This increase in body temperature results in greater depletion of the muscle fibers because of increased metabolism. One must give similar considerations in rodeo horses to endurance horses relative to fluid electrolyte management but also consider excitement of the nervous system. The secretion of catecholamines in the rodeo may cause responses to medications similar to show horses.

Anesthetic Considerations for the Standardbred and Thoroughbred

There are two principal differences in the anesthetic considerations for the Standardbred and the Thoroughbred. First of all is the difference in the mental attitude of the two breeds. Standardbred competition requires the horse to be semicontrolled to maintain either the trot or pace gait during competition. As a result, the Standardbred during preanesthesia, induction of anesthesia, and recovery usually has less excitement or added stress from a mental attitude of competitiveness than has been observed in the Thoroughbred. The speed the animal develops around the track is slower for the Standardbred than the Thoroughbred. As a result, those conditions that affect anesthesia will be more exaggerated in the Thoroughbred. An example of this difference is shown in the extent of respiratory function indicated in the studies included in this chapter. The incidence of exercise-induced pulmonary hemorrhage is greater in Thoroughbreds than Standardbreds. As a result, maintaining respiratory function may be influenced by the number of times that horses have had pulmonary hemorrhage after training and racing. The extent of this hemorrhage can influence both respiratory function and the uptake of inhalant anesthetics. In instances in which active hemorrhage is still present, the utilization of intermittent positive pressure ventilation, although beneficial for additional oxygen to the horse, may be associated with some further damage to the anatomical structures of the respiratory system if pressures are not well controlled.

After repeated instances of pulmonary hemorrhage, damage to the lungs may further compromise ventilatory exchange in dorsal recumbency. Rapid administration of fluids can result in pulmonary edema. Judicious care for respiratory function and the balance of fluids and electrolytes with appropriate monitoring to avoid an increase in pulmonary water can be beneficial.

The HRs and cardiodynamics of the Standardbred and Thoroughbred are normally excellent. Depending on the time of preanesthetic evaluation, the Thoroughbred or Standardbred at rest may show pronounced bradycardia as a result of conditioning or an increase in HR because of excitement. If adequate care to avoid stimulation of the horse at the time of the examination is not exercised, erroneous preanesthetic data may be determined. The HRs during peak performance in these horses well exceeds 200 bpm and slow heart rates in the resting state may show signs of bradycardia, sinus arrhythmia, or heart block. A diagnosis of sinus bradycardia may justify an ECG to determine whether bradycardia exists because of conditioning or heart block or other undesirable cardiac arrhythmias are present. Anticholenergics may be needed to avoid severe bradycardia if cardiac depressing medications will be part of anesthetic management.

There is anticipation by the racehorse when it is led from the stall or paddock for anesthesia. A more desirable effect can be accomplished if after the administration of tranquilizers and sedatives the animal is kept in a quiet area away from the stimulation of crowds or other activities until the animal becomes tranquil or sedate. This will result in a lower dosage of medication required to produce anesthesia. Without this quietness and calmness in handling horses, especially in some Thoroughbreds, utilization of xylazine plus ketamine has resulted in ultimate failure to produce anesthesia at all. In other instances, high levels of excitement have been observed. Xylazine has been inadequate to overcome the CNS stimulation of competition in some horses. In the horse without sufficient sedation from the xylazine, ketamine has resulted in further stimulation of the CNS, rather than a production of smooth analgesia in anesthesia.

The utilization of acepromazine followed by guaifenesin and barbiturates for producing anesthesia has been more predictable in this group of horses. Anesthetic maintenance with inhalant anesthetics is very helpful. Halothane has been more commonly used, but exceptionally high concentrations of halothane have been required in some instances in which horses come from the track for anesthesia. In a few instances, horses required an abnormally high halothane vaporizer setting of 3 to 4% for as long as 30 to 40 minutes after the induction of anesthesia. This is an extremely high setting; it is of concern, but it is occasionally necessary to keep the animal relaxed enough to stay on the table. Unfortunately, lower concentrations in some instances do not result in adequate surgical plane anesthesia. At the same time, sudden depression of the cardiovascular system affecting both HRs and severe drops in blood pressure may result. Obviously, at concentrations well above 2 MAC, sudden drops in cardiovascular function can be highly detrimental to the patient.

An explanation of the reason for such high levels of anesthesia in the horses from the track may be the high levels of circulating catecholamines. During this period of stimulation of the heart and CNS alertness, exceptionally high levels of anesthetics are required to produce similar planes of surgical anesthesia. The myocardium is more sensitive. In at least two horses in this situation, excessive sweating occurred during the 30 to 40 minutes requiring high concentrations of anesthetics. Very careful attention must be given any time excessive concentrations of anesthetics are required to produce minimum surgical plane anesthesia in racing horses. Supplemental doses of xylazine during halothane should be avoided. The counteraction of stimulation of the circulating catecholamines during these procedures may be sudden. Horses suffering from extreme fatigue may require very low anesthetic concentrations.

The availability and potential utilization of medications such as isoproterenol, dopamine, or dobutamine to help support the heart in severe failure should be available. Under these circumstances at high concentrations of halothane, one anticipates a greater likelihood of ventricular arrhythmia than with isoflurane. The availability of lidocaine to control ventricular arrhythmias and the utilization of ECG monitoring to determine potential arrhythmias is indicated. Unfortunately, the occurrence of single ectopic beats or other minor arrhythmias may be followed suddenly by more severe arrhythmias. The time between insignificant arrhythmias and life-threatening arrhythmias may be especially short. Fortunately, after induction, especially if muscle relaxants such as guaifenesin are used during induction, these excessively high concentrations of halothane or isoflurane are not required for anesthesia in the majority of racing Standardbreds and Thoroughbreds.

The monitoring of the patient is very crucial. Ideally, one is able to achieve adequate surgical plane anesthesia and sufficient relief of pain from the surgical stimulus.

Recovery in the racehorse is not without a percentage of complications. Many of the complications that are observed relate to the types of procedures that have been corrected during the anesthetic regime. The recovery of the racehorse with a leg in a cast does not simplify the procedure. The extent of muscle damage that has occurred during conditioning or racing may further exacerbate the complications of muscle functions at the time. Careful consideration of the calcium levels as they may affect muscle responses is indicated. In some horses, calcium levels will be low, and supplemental calcium can be beneficial for a better recovery. The recovery can be further complicated by the degree of excitement that the racehorse undergoes because of its own efforts to move quickly. Highly padded stalls are desirable for recovery.

Anesthetic Management in Horses Participating in Equestrian Events or Polo

The anesthetic considerations in these horses are a combination of the factors discussed previously. These must be highly conditioned animals. Their performance is relative to not only speed of activity, but also extensive efforts in competition exist with some reduction in body fluid levels. There is a potential for muscle fatigue and high levels of circulating catecholamines because of the excitement of competition. It should be noted that a number of these horses have quite a large body size and are at the same time expected to perform at high speeds. Not only must the temperament of the Thoroughbred in flat track racing be considered, the stress of performance by horses with a large body mass will frequently be encountered in horses participating in equestrian events. Polo horses, although not as large, are subjected to the stresses of many quick turns and more prolonged exercise than in short races.

One can conclude that anesthesia in the conditioned animal, especially in the conditioned horse with its body size and speed, is a challenge to the veterinarian's knowledge of anesthesiology as well as understanding of the fundamentals of exercise physiology. This is further complicated by administration of anesthesia to an animal considered to be at a high level of physiological function. Ordinarily the risk of anesthesia in this group of animals is almost nonexistent in the opinion of many lay people. In reality, the risk of anesthesia in the conditioned horse may be even greater than the very sick. It is difficult for the owner of a well-conditioned performance horse to understand the complications that may develop during or after anesthesia. It is not only for the safety and well being of the patient that an understanding of the risks and considerations of anesthetizing conditioned animals in important. Persons involved in the care of the conditioned animal should be so advised.

References

1. Chen WY: Reactivity of normal airways to short-term exercise. *Eur J Appl Physiol* 38(4):277–280, 1978.
2. Hildebrandt JR, Winn RK, Hildebrandt J: Cardiorespiratory responses to sudden release of circulatory occlusion during exercise. *Respir Physiol* 38(1):83–92, 1979.
3. Paterson DH: Respiratory and cardiovascular aspects of intermittent exercise with regard to ice hockey. *Can J Appl Sport Sci* 4(1):22–28, 1979.
4. Gilbert CA, Nutter DO, Felner JM, Perkins JV, Heymsfield SB, Schlant RC: Echocardiographic study of cardiac dimensions and function in the endurance-trained athlete. *Am J Cardio* 40(4):528–533, 1977.
5. Zoneraich S, Rhee JJ, Zoneraich O, Jordan D, Appel J: Assessment of cardiac function in marathon runners by graphic noninvasive techniques. *Ann NY Acad Sci* 301:900–917, 1977.
6. Schwane JA, Cundiff DE: Relationships among cardiorespiratory fitness, regular physical activity, and plasma lipids in young adults. *Metabolism* 28(7):771–778, 1979.
7. Cunningham DA, McCrimmon D, Vlach LF: Cardiovascular response to interval and continuous training in women. *Eur J Appl Physiol* 41(3):187–197, 1979.
8. Zeldis SM, Morganroth J, Rubler S: Cardiac hypertrophy in response to dynamic conditioning in female athletes. *J Appl Physiol* 44(6):849–852, 1978.
9. Yamaji K, Miyashita M: Differences in cardio-respiratory responses to exhaustive exercise between athletes and non-athletes. *Eur J Appl Physiol* 38(4):233–238, 1978.
10. Demaria AN, Neumann A, Lee G, Fowler W, Mason DT: Alterations in ventricular mass and performance induced by exercise training in man evaluated by echocardiography. *Circulation* 57(2):237–244, 1978.
11. Cahill NS, O'Brien M, Rodahl A, Allen JF, Knight D, Dolphin C: A pilot study on left ventricular dimensions and wall stress before and after submaximal exercise. *Br J Sports Med* 13(3):122–129, 1979.
12. Dowell RT, Stone HL, Sordahl LA, Asimakis GK: Contractile function and myofibrillar atpase activity in the exercise-trained dog heart. *J Appl Physiol* 43(6):977–982, 1977.
13. Von Restorff W, Holtz J, Bassenge E: Exercise induced augmentation of myocardial oxygen extraction in spite of normal coronary dilatory capacity in dogs. *Pfluegers Arch* 372(2):181–185, 1977.
14. Chester EH, Belman MJ, Bahler RC, Baum GL, Schey G, Buch P: Multidisciplinary treatment of chronic pulmonary insufficiency. 3. The effect of physical training on cardiopulmonary performance in patients with chronic obstructive pulmonary disease. *Chest* 72(6):695–702, 1977.
15. Rasmussen V, Hauns S, Skagen K: Cerebral attacks due to excessive vagal tone in heavily trained persons. A clinical and electrophysiologic study. *Acta Med Scand* 204(5):401–5, 1978.
16. Nadel ER, Cafarelli E, Roberts MF, Wenger CB: Circulatory regulation during exercise in different ambient temperatures. *J Appl Physiol* 46(3):430–437, 1979.
17. Gillespie JR, Pascoe JR: Respiratory function in the exercising horse: a review. In Snow DH, Persson SGB, Rose RJ (eds): *Equine*

Exercise Physiology: Proceedings of the First International Conference. Cambridge, Granta Editions, 1983, pp 1–6.
18. Hornicke H, Meixner R, Pollmann U: Respiration in exercising horses. In Snow DH, Persson SGB, Rose RJ (eds): *Equine Exercise Physiology: Proceedings of the First International Conference*. Cambridge, Granta Editions, 1983, pp 7–16.
19. Pan LG, Forster HV, Bisgard GE, Dorsey SM, Busch MA: O_2 transport in ponies during treadmill exercise. *J Appl Physiol: Respir, Environ, and Exercise Physiol* 57(3):744–752, 1984.
20. Parks CM, Manohar M: Blood-gas tensions and acid-base status in ponies during treadmill exercise. *Am J Vet Res* 45(1):1–19, 1984.
21. Forster HV, Pan LG, Bisgard GE, Dorsey SM, Britton MS: Temporal pattern of pulmonary gas exchange during exercise in ponies. *J Appl Phys: Respir, Environ and Exercise Physiol* 57(3):760–767, 1984.
22. Littlejohn A, Bowles F: Studies on the physiopathology of chronic obstructive pulmonary disease in the horse. V. Blood gas and acid-base values during exercise. *Onderstepoort J Vet Res* 48(4):239–249, 1981.
23. Cook WR: Some observations on form and function of the equine upper airway in health and disease. I. The pharynx. II. Larynx. *Proc Amer Assoc Equine Pract* 27:355–391, 393–451, 1982.
24. Baker GJ: Laryngeal asynchrony in the horse: definition and significance. In Snow DH, Persson SGB, Rose RJ (eds): *Equine Exercise Physiology: Proceedings of the First International Conference*. Cambridge, Granta Editions, 1983, pp 46–50.
25. Sweeney CR, Soma LR: Exercise-induced pulmonary haemorrhage in horses after different competitive exercises. In Snow DH, Persson SGB, Rose RJ (eds): *Equine Exercise Physiology: Proceedings of the First International Conference*. Cambridge, Granta Editions, 1983, pp 51–56.
26. Mason DK, Collins EA, Watkins KL: Exercise-induced pulmonary haemorrhage in horses. In Snow DH, Persson SGB, Rose RJ (eds): *Equine Exercise Physiology: Proceedings of the First International Conference*. Cambridge, Granta Editions, 1983, pp 57–63.
27. Littlejohn A, Howell W, Killeen V: Pulmonary arterial haemodynamics and blood gas values of Thoroughbred racehorses with a history of epistaxis during a race. *Vet Res Communications* 8(1):41–45, 1984.
28. Clarke AF: Review of exercise induced pulmonary haemorrhage and its possible relationship with mechanical stress. *Equine Vet J* 17(3):166–172, 1985.
29. Bayly WM, Meyers KM, Keck MT, Huston LJ, Grant BD: Effects of furosemide on exercise-induced alterations in haemostasis in Thoroughbred horses exhibiting postexercise epistaxis. In Snow DH, Persson SGB, Rose RJ (eds): *Equine Exercise Physiology: Proceedings of the First International Conference*. Cambridge, Granta Editions, 1983, pp 64–70.
30. Harthoorn AM, Young E: A relationship between acid-base balance and capture myopathy in zebra (Equus burchelli) and an apparent therapy. *Vet Rec* 95(15):337–342, 1974.
31. Rose RJ, Ilkiw JE, Martin ICA: Blood-gas, acid-base and haematological values in horses during an endurance ride. *Equine Vet J* 11(1):56–59, 1979.
32. Fregin GF, Thomas DP: Cardiovascular response to exercise in the horse: a review. In Snow DH, Persson SGB, Rose RJ (eds): *Equine Exercise Physiology: Proceedings of the First International Conference*. Cambridge, Granta Editions, 1983, pp 76–90.
33. Manohar M, Parks C: Transmural coronary vasodilator reserve in ponies at rest and during maximal exercise. In Snow DH, Persson SGB, Rose RJ (eds): *Equine Exercise Physiology: Proceedings of the First International Conference*. Cambridge, Granta Editions, 1983, pp 91–104.
34. Parks CM, Manohar M: Transmural distribution of myocardial blood flow during graded treadmill exercise in ponies. In Snow DH, Persson SGB, Rose RJ (eds): *Equine Exercise Physiology: Proceedings of the First International Conference*. Cambridge, Granta Editions, 1983, pp 105–120.
35. Parks CM: Exercise in ponies: a study of myocardial blood flow, coronary vasodilator reserve, regional distribution of cardiac output and effects of heart rate on coronary flow. *Dissertation Abstracts International B* 43(9):802–822, 1983.
36. Physick-Sheard PW, Hendren CM: Heart score: physiological basis and confounding variables. In Snow DH, Persson SGB, Rose RJ (eds): *Equine Exercise Physiology: Proceedings of the First International Conference*. Cambridge, Granta Editions, 1983, pp 121–134.
37. Rose RJ, David PE: The use of electrocardiography in the diagnosis of poor racing performance in the horse. *Australian Vet J* 54(2):51–56, 1978.
38. Stewart JH, Rose RJ, Davis PE, Hoffman K: A comparison of electrocardiographic findings in racehorses presented either for routine examination or poor racing performance. In Snow DH, Persson SGB, Rose RJ (eds): *Equine Exercise Physiology: Proceedings of the First International Conference*. Cambridge, Granta Editions, 1983, pp 135–143.
39. Hanak J: Effect of training Thoroughbred foals on the angle of their electrical cardiac axis and magnitude of the ventricular vector. *Acta Veterinaria Brno* 51(1/4):69–73, 1982.
40. Hornicke H, Engelhardt WV, Ehrlein H-J: Effect of exercise on systemic blood pressure and heart rate in horses. *Pfluegers Archiv* 372(1):95–99, 1977.
41. Pan LG, Forster HV, Bisgard GE, Dorsey SM, Busch MA: Cardiodynamic variables and ventilation during treadmill exercise in ponies. *J Appl Physiology: Resp, Environ Exercise Physiol* 57(3):753–759, 1984.
42. Kubo K, Takagi S, Murakami M, Kai M: Heart rate and blood lactate concentration of horses during maximal work. *Bull Equine Res Inst* Tokyo, Japan 21:39–45, 1984.
43. White NA II, White SL: Atrioventricular dissociation with synchronous diaphragmatic flutter in a horse. *VM/SAC* 70(8):967–971, 974, 1975.
44. Thomas DP, Fregin GF, Gerber NH, Ailes NB; Cardiovascular, respiratory and metabolic adjustments to tethered swimming in the horse. *Fed Proc* 38(3):945, 1979.
45. Parks CM, Manohar M: Distribution of blood flow during moderate and strenuous exercise in ponies (Equus caballus). *Amer J Vet Res* 44(10):1855–1861, 1983.
46. Hall MC, Steel JD, Stewart GA: Cardiac monitoring during exercise tests in the horse. 2. Heart rate responses to exercise. *Australian Vet J* 52(1):1–5, 1976.
47. Lindholm A: Muscle morphology and metabolism in standardbred horses at rest and during exercise. *Akademisk Avhandling*, Kungl. Veterinarhogskolan, Stockholm, Sweden, 1974, p 29.
48. Hoppeler H, Claassen H, Howald H, Straub R: Correlated histochemistry and morphometry in equine skeletal muscle. In Snow DH, Persson SGB, Rose RJ (eds): *Equine Exercise Physiology: Proceedings of the First International Conference*. Cambridge, Granta Editions, 1983, pp 184–192.
49. Essen-Gustavsson B, Lindholm A, McMiken D, Persson SGB, Thornton J: Skeletal muscle characteristics of young Standardbreds in relation to growth and early training. In Snow DH, Persson SGB, Rose RJ (eds): *Equine Exercise Physiology: Proceedings of the First International Conference*. Cambridge, Granta Editions, 1983, pp 200–210.
50. Lindholm A, Essen-Gustavsson B, McMiken D, Persson SGB, Thornton JR: Muscle histochemistry and biochemistry of Thoroughbred horses during growth and training. In Snow DH, Persson SGB, Rose RJ (eds): *Equine Exercise Physiology: Proceedings of the First International Conference*. Cambridge, Granta Editions, 1983, pp 211–217.
51. Thornton JR, Taylor AW: Skeletal muscle characteristics of foals at two to four weeks and eight months of age. In Snow

DH, Persson SGB, Rose RJ (eds): *Equine Exercise Physiology: Proceedings of the First International Conference.* Cambridge, Granta Editions, 1983, pp 218–224.
52. Valberg S, Essen-Gustavsson B, Lindholm A, Persson S: Energy metabolism in relation to skeletal muscle fibre properties during treadmill exercise. *Equine Vet J* 17(6):439–444, 1985.
53. Henckel P: Training and growth induced changes in the middle gluteal muscle of young Standardbred trotters. *Equine Vet J* 15(2):134–140, 1983.
54. Murakami M, Takagi S: Effects of continuous long distance running exercise on plasma enzyme levels in horses. *Exper Rep Equine Health Lab* 11:106–119, 1974.
55. Saibene F, Cortili G, Gavazzi P, Sala A, Faina M, Sardella F: Maximal anaerobic (lactic) capacity and power of the horse. *Equine Vet J* 17(2):130–132, 1985.
56. Milne DW, Gabel AA, Muir WW, Skarda RT: Effects of training on heart rate, cardiac output, and lactic acid in Standardbred horses, using a standardized exercise test. *J Equine Med and Surg* 1(4):131–135, 1977.
57. Irondelle M, Freund H: Carbohydrate and fat metabolism of unacclimatized men during and after submaximal exercise in cool and hot environments. *Europ J Applied Physiol* 37(1):27–38, 1977.
58. Henckel P: A histochemical assessment of the capillary blood supply of the middle gluteal muscle of Thoroughbred horses. A preliminary report. In Snow DH, Persson SGB, Rose RJ (eds): *Equine Exercise Physiology: Proceedings of the First International Conference.* Cambridge, Granta Editions, 1983, pp 225–228.
59. Francesconi R, Maher J, Bynum G, Mason J: Recurrent heat exposure: effects on levels of plasma and urinary sodium and potassium in resting and exercising men. *Aviat Space Environ Med* 48(5):399–404, 1977.
60. Lindholm A, Saltin B: The physiological and biochemical response of Standardbred horses to exercise of varying speed and duration. *Acta Veterinaria Scandinavica* 15(3):310–324, 1974.
61. Hodgson DR, Rose RJ, Allen JR: Muscle glycogen depletion and repletion patterns in horses performing various distances of endurance exercise. In Snow DH, Persson, SGB, Rose RJ (eds): *Equine Exercise Physiology: Proceedings of the First International Conference.* Cambridge, Granta Editions, 1983, pp 229–236.
62. Carlson GP: Thermoregulation and fluid balance in the exercising horse. In Snow DH, Persson SGB, Rose RJ (eds): *Equine Exercise Physiology: Proceedings of the First International Conference.* Cambridge, Granta Editions, 1983, pp 291–309.
63. Bayly WM, Meyers KM, Keck MT, Huston LJ, Grant BD: Exercise-induced alterations in haemostasis in Thoroughbred horse. In Snow DH, Persson SGB, Rose RJ (eds): *Equine Exercise Physiology: Proceedings of the First International Conference.* Cambridge, Granta Editions, 1983, pp 336–343.
64. Judson GJ, Mooney GJ, Thornbury RS: Plasma biochemical values in Thoroughbred horses in training. In Snow DH, Persson SGB, Rose RJ (eds): *Equine Exercise Physiology: Proceedings of the First International Conference.* Cambridge, Granta Editions, 1983, pp354–361.
65. Hambleton PL, Slade LM, Hamar DW, Kienholz EW, Lewis LD: Dietary fat and exercise conditioning effect on metabolic parameters in the horse. *J Anim Sci* 51(6):1330–1339, 1980.
66. Essen-Gustavsson B, Karlstrom K, Lindholm A: Fibre types, enzyme activities and substrate utilisation in skeletal muscles of horses competing in endurance rides. *Equine Vet J* 16(3):197–202, 1984.
67. Harris RC, Snow DH: ATP depletion following intermittent maximal exercise in the horse. *J Physiol* 353:58, 1984.
68. Pirnay F, Lacroix M, Mosora F, Luyckx A, Lefebvre P: Glucose oxidation during prolonged exercise evaluated with naturally labeled (13C) glucose. *J Appl Physiol* 43(2):258–261, 1977.
69. Hodgson DR, Rose RJ, Allen JR, Dimauro J: Glycogen depletion patterns in horses performing maximal exercise. *Res Vet Sci* 36(2):169–173, 1984.
70. Lindholm A: Glycogen depletion pattern and the biochemical response to varying exercise intensities in Standardbred Trotters. *J S Afr Vet Assoc* 45(4):341–342, 1974.
71. Cutmore CMM, Snow DH, Newsholme EA: Activities of key enzymes of aerobic and anaerobic metabolism in middle gluteal muscle from trained and untrained horses. *Equine Vet J* 17(5):354–356, 1985.
72. Debski B: The effect of training and physical exercise on the energetic metabolism of equine erythrocytes. *Zentralbl Veterinaermed (A)* 32(3):190–195, 1985.
73. Hodgson DR, Rose RJ, Allen JR, Dimauro J: Glycogen depletion patterns in horses competing in day 2 of a three day event. *Cornell Vet* 75(2):366–374, 1985.
74. Burke DJ, Albert WW: Methods for measuring physical condition and energy expenditure in horses. *J Anim Sci* 46(6):1666–1672, 1978.
75. Takagi S: Effect of training on glucose utilization in the racehorse. *Bull Equine Res Inst*, Tokyo, Japan, 20:71–76, 1983.
76. Hodgson DR, Rose RJ, Dimauro J, Allen JR: Effects of submaximal treadmill training programme on histochemical properties, enzyme activities and glycogen utilization of skeletal muscle in the horse. *Equine Vet J* 17(4):300–305, 1985.
77. Irvine CHG: The role of hormones in exercise physiology. In Snow DH, Persson SGB, Rose RJ (eds): *Equine Exercise Physiology: Proceedings of the First International Conference.* Cambridge, Granta Editions, 1983, pp 377–388.
78. Snow DH, Mason DK, Ricketts SW, Douglas TA: Post-race blood biochemistry in Thoroughbreds. In Snow DH, Persson SGB, Rose RJ (eds): *Equine Exercise Physiology: Proceedings of the First International Conference.* Cambridge, Granta Editions, 1983, pp 389–399.
79. Bayly WM, Grant BD, Breeze RG, Kramer JW: The effects of maximal exercise on acid-base balance and arterial blood gas tension in Thoroughbred horses. In Snow DH, Persson SGB, Rose RJ (eds): *Equine Exercise Physiology: Proceedings of the First International Conference.* Cambridge, Granta Editions, 1983, pp 400–407.
80. Judson GJ, Frauenfelder HC, Mooney GJ: Biochemical changes in Thoroughbred racehorses following submaximal and maximal exercise. In Snow DH, Persson SGB, Rose RJ (eds): *Equine Exercise Physiology: Proceedings of the First International Conference.* Cambridge, Granta Editions, 1983, pp 408–415.
81. Grosskopf JFW, van Rensburg JJ, Bertschinger HJ: Haematology and blood biochemistry of horses during a 210 km endurance ride. In Snow DH, Persson SGB, Rose RJ (eds): *Equine Exercise Physiology: Proceedings of the First International Conference.* Cambridge, Granta Editions, 1983, pp 416–424.
82. Grosskopf JFW, van Rensburg JJ: Some observations on the haematology and blood biochemistry of horses competing in 80 km endurance rides. In Snow DH, Persson SGB, Rose RJ (eds): *Equine Exercise Physiology: Proceedings of the First International Conference.* Cambridge, Granta Editions, 1983, pp 425–431.
83. Kerr MG, Snow DH: Plasma enzyme activities in endurance horses. In Snow DH, Persson SGB, Rose RJ (eds): *Equine Exercise Physiology: Proceedings of the First International Conference.* Cambridge, Granta Editions, 1983, pp 432–440.
84. Persson SGB, Essen-Gustavsson B, Lindholm A, McMiken D, Thornton JR: Cardiorespiratory and metabolic effects of training of Standardbred yearlings. In Snow DH, Persson SGB, Rose RJ (eds): *Equine Exercise Physiology: Proceedings of the First International Conference.* Cambridge, Granta Editions, 1983, pp 458–469.
85. Thornton J, Essen-Gustavsson B, Lindholm A, McMiken D, Persson S: Effects of training and detraining an oxygen uptake,

cardiac output, blood gas tensions, pH and lactate concentrations during and after exercise in the horse. In Snow DH, Persson SGB, Rose RJ (eds): *Equine Exercise Physiology: Proceedings of the First International Conference.* Cambridge, Granta Editions, 1983, pp 470–486.
86. Fregin GF: General discussion of physiologic observations recorded on 117 horses during 100-mile endurance rides. *Proc. Annual Convention Amer Assoc Equine Pract* 25:315–321, 1980.
87. Lucke JN, Hall GM: Long distance exercise in the horse: Golden Horseshoe Ride 1978. *Vet Rec* 106(18/19/20):405–407, 1980.
88. Lucke JN, Hall GM: Further studies on the metabolic effects of long distance riding: Golden Horseshoe Ride 1979. *Equine Vet J* 12(4):189–192, 1980.
89. Rose RJ: An evaluation of heart rate and respiratory rate recovery for assessment of fitness during endurance rides. In Snow DH, Persson SGB, Rose RJ (eds): *Equine Exercise Physiology: Proceedings of the First International Conference.* Cambridge, Granta Editions, 1983, pp 505–509.
90. Hall GM, Adrian TE, Bloom SR, Lucke JN: Changes in circulating gut hormones in the horse during long distance exercise. *Equine Vet J* 14(3):209–212, 1982.
91. Deldar A, Fregin FG, Bloom JC, Davanipour Z: Changes in selected biochemical constituents of blood collected from horses participating in a 50-mile endurance ride. *Amer J Vet Res* 43(12):2239–2243, 1982.
92. Rose RJ, Ilkiw JE, Arnold KS, Backhouse JW, Sampson D: Plasma biochemistry in the horse during 3-day event competition. *Aust Equine Vet J* 12(3):132–136, 1980.
93. Snow DH, Kerr MG, Nimmo MA, Abbott EM: Alterations in blood, sweat, urine and muscle composition during prolonged exercise in the horse. *Vet Rec* 110(16):377–384, 1982.
94. Rose RJ, Sampson D: Changes in certain metabolic parameters in horses associated with food deprivation and endurance exercise. *Aust Res Vet Sci* 32(2):198–202, 1982.
95. Littlejohn A, Bowles F, Aschenborn G: Cardiorespiratory adaptations to exercise in riding horses with chronic lung disease. In Snow DH, Persson SGB, Rose RJ (eds): *Equine Exercise Physiology: Proceedings of the First International Conference.* Cambridge, Granta Editions, 1983, pp 33–45.
96. Maier-Bock H, Ehrlein H-J: Heart rate during a defined exercise test in horses with heart and lung diseases. *Equine Vet J* 10(4):235–242, 1978.
97. Caplash VK, Khattri HN, Bidwai PS, Rastogi GK: Frequency of ischaemic heart disease in patients with overt diabetes mellitus. *J Assoc Physicians India* 23(6):373–376, 1975.
98. Persson G: Exercise tests in male diabetics. A nine years' follow-up study with special reference to ECG changes and cardiovascular morbidity. *Acta Med Scand* Suppl. 605:7–23, 1977.
99. Gardner GW, Edgerton VR, Barbard RJ, Bernauer EM: Cardiorespiratory, hematological and physical performance responses of anemic subjects to iron treatment. *Amer J Clin Nutr* 28(9):982–988, 1975.
100. Deegen E, Buntenkotter S: Behaviour of the heart rate of horses with auricular fibrillation during exercise and after treatment. *Equine Vet J* 8(1):26–29, 1976.
101. Milne DW, Muir WW, Skarda RT, Fregin GF, Nicholl JK: The hemodynamic response of the horse to swimming with and without furosemide. *J Equine Med Surg* 1(10):331–335, 1977.
102. Chay S, Woods WE, Nugent TE, Weckman T, Houston T, Sprinkle F, Blake JW, Tobin T, Soma LR, Yocum J, Smith JD: Population distribution of phenylbutazone and oxyphenbutazone after oral and i.v. dosing in horses. *J Vet Pharmacol and Therap* 7(4):265–276, 1984.
103. Dybdal NO, Gribble D, Madigan JE, Stabenfeldt GH: Alterations in plasma corticosteroids, insulin and selected metabolites in horses used in endurance rides. *Equine Vet J* 12(3):137–140, 1980.
104. Smetzer DL, Senta T, Hensel JD: Cardiovascular effects of amphetamine in the horse. *Can J Comp Med* 36(3):185–194, 1972.
105. Sanford J, Aitken MM: Effects of some drugs on the physiological changes during exercise in the horse. *Equine Vet J* 7(4):198–202, 1975.
106. Stewart GA: Drugs, performance and response to exercise in the racehorse. 1. Physiological observations on the cardiac and respiratory responses. 2. Observations on amphetamine, promazine and thiamine. *Aust Vet J* 48(10):537–543, 544–547, 1972.
107. Gabel AA, Milne DW, Ray RS, Noonan J, Muir WW, Skarda RT, Weingold MF: A study of the effects of methylprednisolone, promazine, amphetamine and furosemide on physiological parameters in Standardbred horses performing a submaximal exercise test. In Snow DH, Persson SGB, Rose RJ (eds): *Equine Exercise Physiology: Proceedings of the First International Conference.* Cambridge, Granta Editions, 1983, pp 531–537.
108. Tobin T, Kamerling S, Nugent TE: Drugs and equine performance: a review. In Snow DH, Persson SGB, Rose RJ (eds): *Equine Exercise Physiology: Proceedings of the First International Conference.* Cambridge, Granta Editions, 1983, pp 510–520.
109. Gabel AA, Milne DW, Ray RS, Sams R, Muir WW, Skarda RT, Weingold MF: A double blind study of the effects of amphetamine and methylphenidate on physiological parameters in Standardbred horses performing submaximal exercise tests. In Snow DH, Persson SGB, Rose RJ (eds): *Equine Exercise Physiology: Proceedings of the First International Conference.* Cambridge, Granta Editions, 1983, pp 521–530.
110. Kallings P, Persson S: Effects of theophylline and non-steroidal anti-inflammatory drugs on pulse and blood lactate responses in exercise in the horse: a preliminary report. In Snow DH, Persson SGB, Rose RJ (eds): *Equine Exercise Physiology: Proceedings of the First International Conference.* Cambridge, Granta Editions, 1983, pp 538–542.
111. Johnson BD, Heath RB, Bowman B, Phillips RW, Rich LD, Voss JL: Serum chemistry changes in horses during anesthesia: a pilot study investigating the possible causes of postanesthetic myositis in horses. *J Equine Med Surg* 2(3):109–123, 1978.
112. Auer JA,, Amend JF, Garner HE, Hutcheson DP, Salem CA: Electroencephalographic responses during volatile anesthesia in domestic ponies: a comparative study of isoflurane, enflurane, methoxyflurane, and halothane. *J Equine Med Surg* 3(3):130–134, 1979.
113. Steffey EP, Howland D JR: Alterations in anesthetic requirements (MAC) and cardiovascular responses accompanying the addition of nitrous oxide to halothane-O_2 in horses. *Fed Proc* 37(3):508, 1978.
114. Steffey EP: Enflurane and isoflurane anesthesia: a summary of laboratory and clinical investigations in horses. *J Am Vet Med Assoc* 172(3):367–373, 1978.
115. Beadle RE, Robinson NE, Sorenson PR: Cardiopulmonary effects of positive end-expiratory pressure in anesthetized horses. *Am J Vet Res* 36(10):1435–1438, 1975.
116. Hamlin RL, Klepinger WL, Gilpin KW, Smith CR: Autonomic control of heart rate in the horse. *Am J Physiol* 222(4):976–978, 1972.
117. Schatzmann U: Investigations of the applicability of controlled ventilation during routine anesthesia in the horse. *J Equine Med Surg* 2(10):453–458, 1978.
118. Steffey EP, Wheat JD, Meagher DM, Norrie RD, McKee J, Brown M, Arnold J: Body position and mode of ventilation influences arterial pH, oxygen, and carbon dioxide tensions in halothane-anesthetized horses. *Am J Vet Res* 38(3):379–382, 1977.
119. Snow DH, Summers RJ, Guy PS: The actions of the beta-adrenoceptor blocking agents propranolol and metoprolol in the maximally exercised horse. *Res Vet Sci* 27(1):22–29, 1979.
120. De Moor A, Van den Hende C, Moens Y, Desmet P: Increased plasma bromide concentration in the horse after halothane anesthesia. *Am J Vet Res* 39(10):1624–1626, 1978

PART 9

Special Considerations for Anesthesia and Analgesia in Research Animals

RALPH C. HARVEY, D.V.M., M.S., and JAMES WALBERG, D.V.M.

Sedation, tranquilization, pharmacological restraint, or general anesthesia is frequently required in research animals. Many procedures that can be accomplished in other animals without the aid of anesthesia or chemical restraint are otherwise either very difficult or impossible in research animals.

The techniques and drugs used for anesthesia of research animals frequently represent relatively minor variations on those used in the more conventional veterinary species. Although significant differences must be recognized, the principles of good anesthetic care are equally important. The anesthetic plan should be individualized for the procedure and animals to be used. Preanesthetic evaluation should include recognition of unusual or unexpected diseases and dysfunctional conditions. Depressant anesthetic drugs should be titrated to effect, and the airway should be protected when possible. Monitoring of physiological status and postoperative recovery indicates the level of support necessary to maintain cardiopulmonary performance and body temperature. Postoperative analgesics should be considered for all research animals and administered appropriately when their use is indicated.

General Considerations

A thorough preanesthetic physical examination is frequently impractical, difficult, or impossible to perform in research animals (1–3). The temperament of the animal or the numbers of animals involved may prevent as complete an examination as would be indicated for the clinical patient. A hands-off examination in the animal's usual environment is less influenced by stress and excitement than is possible following removal to the laboratory or surgical area. As with exotic animals, observant caretakers and animal health technicians can recognize subtle evidence of disease or dysfunction that may markedly influence responses to anesthetics. Caretakers and technicians familiar with individual animals of the larger species, such as dogs, cats, and primates, that are used over a period of time or in chronic studies can provide valuable insight concerning their temperament, acceptance of handling, and individual need for tranquilization and restraint.

The complexity of anesthetic techniques should be minimized when designing research protocols. This will prevent the anesthetic management from encumbering the investigation and will make completion of assigned tasks on a repeated basis as practical and easy as possible for the personnel involved. The complexity of the technique used will vary greatly with the nature of the research protocol, the species used, and the physiological stress resulting from the intended procedures.

Inadequate ventilation represents the most common adverse complication and life-threatening problem in research animal anesthesia. Most anesthetic techniques are based on injectable agents, and it is unusual that airway protection or assisted ventilation is provided. Frequently, neither supplementary oxygen nor the means for its delivery to the animal are available. The provision of a gas anesthesia machine and associated equipment may represent a significant investment with infrequent utilization to justify the expense of laboratory space devoted to it. If central surgical facilities are used, it is much more likely that this equipment will be available.

Airway protection by placement of an endotracheal tube is both practical and easy in many research animals. Depending upon the species used and the research procedure, it may be absolutely required. In the smaller laboratory animals, such as most rodents, endotracheal intubation becomes increasingly difficult. Although possible, cannulation of the trachea is usually impractical as well as unnecessary in these animals. If required, a mouth speculum can be fashioned from a bent paper clip and an endotracheal tube fashioned from various small tubing. Endotracheal intubation may be facilitated by viewing the larynx through an operative otoscope or by tracheostomy. The provision of supplementary oxygen futhermore enhances patient safety and increases the likelihood for successful outcome regardless of the anesthetic techniques utilized.

Anesthetics Commonly Used in Research Animals

Several anesthetic drugs have been used almost exclusively in research animals. Others are used more commonly in research than in clinical situations. Consideration of the properties and effects of these anesthetics indicates why they are useful in research protocols and facilitates the choice of such anesthetics for specific purposes (1–3).

Many anesthetics cause marked alterations in the autonomic nervous system and cardiopulmonary physiology. This may represent a great problem in certain research in that effects being evaluated may be substantially altered or overshadowed by the influence of the anesthetics. To devise a strategy whereby confounding effects are avoided, chronic instrumentation of the animals or other modifications of the protocol may be necessary. Chronic instrumentation, however, may cause stress and inherent influences. These may be less obvious, but just as significant, as those due to anesthetic drugs. Instrumentation also frequently requires some physical or pharmacological restraint, again with inherent physiological effects.

Hence, the suitability of a research model for the intended purpose may depend on the selection of an anesthetic protocol with minimal or no influence on certain physiological parameters. To minimize influences of anesthetics, agents that characteristically maintain autonomic nervous system stability or preserve spontaneous ventilation and hemodynamic function may be utilized.

CHLORAL HYDRATE

Chloral hydrate acts predominantly as a cerebellar depressant with minimal effect on the brainstem at low hypnotic doses (200 to 300 mg/kg i.p. in rodents). Analgesia is poor, particularly at low doses of chloral hydrate. At higher doses, there is substantial respiratory depression and hypotension. Bradycardia, with occasional heart block, may be severe due to parasympathetic stimulation. Dilute solutions (5% or less) may be given by oral or intravenous routes. Perivascular irritation with necrosis follows accidental extravascular injections. Intraperitoneal injection has been used in rodents, but tissue irritation leads to chemical peritonitis. Adynamic ileus has been a frequently reported complication of intraperitoneal injection of chloral hydrate in rats. Cardiac instability with potential for fibrillation and sudden death is also a problem at higher doses in rats. Chloral hydrate is a poor general anesthetic. However, it may be suitable, at low doses, as a hypnotic agent to produce sleep for prolonged periods. The resulting hypnosis may be augmented by the use of other anesthetics, notably magnesium sulfate and pentobarbital. Other uses for chloral hydrate are inappropriate and have been replaced by newer techniques.

CHLORALOSE

The α-isomer of chloralose is prepared by heating equal quantities of anhydrous chloral and glucose or may be purchased as a crystalline powder. Fresh 1% solutions were prepared with water or saline immediately before use. To avoid precipitation upon cooling, a mixture of 10% polyethylene glycol in water may be used.

Intravenous injection of α-chloralose (80 to 100 mg/kg in rabbits, dogs, and cats) will induce unconsciousness. The resulting narcosis is frequently accompanied by central nervous system (CNS) stimulation as indicated by muscle twitching and increased electroencephalogram (EEG) spike activity. Maximal effect occurs at least 15 minutes after i.v. injection. It is common, therefore, to induce anesthesia with another agent such as an ultrashort-acting barbiturate prior to administration of α-chloralose.

The autonomic nervous system is thought to be unaffected by α-choralose. Blood pressure is maintained or slightly elevated, but heart rate may be greatly elevated. Little respiratory depression occurs at usual doses, although mechanical ventilation should be provided at higher dose levels. Prolonged anesthesia (10 hours) with maintenance of autonomic nervous system stability is achieved with α-chloralose in research animals.

Recovery from chloralose anesthesia is unacceptably prolonged and stormy. Attempts have been made to reduce struggling during recovery by the addition of other anesthetics. In general, however, chloralose is not a suitable anesthetic when recovery is anticipated. It should be reversed for nonsurvival experiments in which prolonged light anesthesia with minimal autonomic disturbance is needed. Chloralose is unacceptable for clinical anesthesia.

URETHANE

Urethane, ethyl carbamate or the ethyl ester of carbaminic acid, is another anesthetic with properties similar to chloralose. Urethane produces prolonged basal narcosis in dogs and cats after i.v. injection at 0.5 to 1.0 g/kg. CNS stimulation does not accompany urethane narcosis, and the drug has been used along with chloralose to suppress muscle twitching. Cardiopulmonary effects are very minimal, except in rabbits. Urethane has been used primarily in cardiopulmonary, physiological, and pharmacodynamic studies. As with chloralose, it is unsuitable when recovery from anesthesia is anticipated.

Unfortunately, urethane has been shown to be mutagenic and carcinogenic, with a high incidence of lung tumors occurring in various animal species regardless of the route of administration. There are substantial risks to personnel as a result of exposure to urethane in the course of laboratory use. Because of these risks and the availability of alternative anesthetics, the use of urethane is not recommended.

PENTOBARBITAL

Sodium pentobarbital has been used extensively in research animal anesthesia in a great variety of species. The advent of modern inhalant anesthetics and ketamine has largely supplanted its use in clinical veterinary anesthesia. In research laboratories, where a gas anesthesia machine may not be available, pentobarbital may remain the agent of choice for many procedures.

Pentobarbital alone does not provide very substantial analgesia, except at higher doses that cause significant respiratory depression. Induction and particularly the recovery from pentobarbital anesthesia can be rather rough. The use of preanesthetic medications and mechanical support of ventilation with either oxygen or air can contribute substantially to achieving a desirable anesthetic state and a successful outcome in many situations.

MUSCLE RELAXANTS

In an attempt to minimize or avoid the side effects of general anesthetics, neuromuscular blocking agents have been used in research protocols. Muscle relaxants, in careful combination with anesthetics, narcotics, tranquilizers, or other CNS depressants, can contribute substantially to a desirable and safe anesthetic protocol. It is essential, however, that adequate analgesia and loss of consciousness be provided by other drugs whenever muscle relaxants are used.

The use of different drugs for the different components of the state of balanced general anesthesia (loss of consciousness, analgesia, and muscle relaxation) can result in a lack of overlap in these components. The greatest potential for this may occur when drugs with differing durations of action are used. An awake but paralyzed condition may result when shorter acting general anesthetics for the induction of anesthesia are combined with longer acting muscle relaxants. This condition is inhumane and must be avoided. Any technique that provides inadequate unconsciousness or inadequate analgesia furthermore distorts the physiological stability of the experimental animal and probably compromises the validity of any results obtained.

ETHER AND CHLOROFORM

The first anesthetics used commonly in veterinary medicine were diethyl ether and chloroform. They both produce generally controllable levels of anesthesia in response to inhaled vapor concentration. There is insufficient justification, however, for the current use of either agent as an anesthetic in any but the most unusual circumstances.

Chloroform has potent cardiovascular, hepatic, and renal toxicities that may lead to death several days after apparent recovery from anesthesia. Trace concentrations in laboratory air may contribute to reproductive disorders in rodent colonies and hepatotoxicity in laboratory personnel.

Diethyl ether has been used successfully in millions of cases, but it has also become outmoded with the introduction of other anesthetics. Respiratory tract irritation, nausea, and delirium are common side effects of ether anesthesia, although organ toxicity is minimal. The highly flammable nature of ether is well known. Explosive peroxides form when ether is exposed to oxygen or air. Improper use and particularly storage of ether has resulted in numerous operating room and laboratory fires and explosions. Considering the numerous alternatives available, these risks are too great to allow for the continued use of ether as an anesthetic.

CARBON DIOXIDE

Brief exposure to a high concentration of carbon dioxide (CO_2), generally 40 to 60%, will result in general anesthesia in a wide variety of animals. The CO_2 may be produced from the solid form or Dry Ice or delivered from a cylinder of compressed gas. When produced from the solid in a container, it is of course necessary to prevent contact with the animal by use of a wire screen or perforated platform well above the Dry Ice. It is important to avoid hypoxia when either the solid or compressed gas form is used. Safety of the technique is greatly improved by the provision of supplementary oxygen.

Induction of anesthesia is generally very smooth and requires only a few seconds. CO_2 anesthesia is generally reserved for very brief procedures in rodents requiring less than 1 minute of anesthesia, such as cardiac puncture. The vasoconstriction produced by CO_2 anesthesia facilitates cardiac puncture and increases the yield obtained in exsanguinations. Recovery is also free of excitement and is generally complete within 1 to 2 minutes. The ease, reliability, economy, and lack of drug residues in tissue or blood samples makes CO_2 anesthesia an attractive option for very brief procedures in rodents. The same advantages lead to the frequent use of CO_2 for humane euthanasia.

Anesthetic Techniques for Research Animals

Techniques for administration of anesthetics are somewhat more varied for research animals than are those used in most clinical veterinary anesthesia. The wider variety of species encountered leads to a greater diversity of appropriate methods employed.

INJECTION OF ANESTHETICS

Intraperitoneal injections of anesthetics and medications is usually reserved for rodents. This route is, however, occasionally used in larger animals, particularly swine. Injection is usually made just lateral to the umbilicus with the rodent held in dorsal or slightly head-down position in an attempt to avoid penetration of the viscera. Even with the best technique, variable effects result from intraperitoneal injections of anesthetics. Usually an increased dose is required relative to that needed with other routes of injection. There is a risk of peritonitis with intraperitoneal injections of anesthetics. Chemical peritonitis may result from the drug itself, whereas septic peritonitis may result from bowel perforation and laceration. Inadvertent injection into abdominal organs may lead to organ toxicity or necrosis. As a result, the validity of the research model may be compromised.

Intravenous injection may be the most desirable but least practical route of administration of injectable anesthetics. In many cases, tranquilization or sedation will be required for venipuncture, and surgical cutdown may be necessary in some species. Sites and techniques for intravenous injection vary considerably with species.

ORAL ADMINISTRATION OF ANESTHETICS

Rodents are often well suited to oral administration of medications, including some anesthetics such as chloral hydrate, by stomach tube or gavage. The technique and proper equipment will vary somewhat with each species. Care must be used to avoid oral, pharyngeal, or esophageal trauma and to protect against aspiration of the drug.

HYPOTHERMIC ANESTHESIA

Hypothermic anesthesia may be successfully used in young rodent pups (1 to 2 days old) for brief minor procedures such as thymectomy. It is important that the animal's body surface is dry and protected from direct contact with very cold surfaces. The technique is not appropriate for older animals.

INHALANT ANESTHESIA

Inhalation of volatile anesthetics provides for the easiest adjustment of depth of anesthesia with changing requirements. This provides considerable safety and speed of recovery from anesthesia.

Commercially available anesthesia machines, patient circuits, and endotracheal tubes are designed for humans or occasionally for the domestic animals usually seen in clinical veterinary medicine, rather than for the usual laboratory animals. As a result, certain adaptations of existing equipment can improve the suitability of anesthetic equipment for use with research animals.

Flow meters and precision vaporizers may be quite suitable for the full range of uses, although gas flow rates may be greatly in excess of those needed to meet physiological requirements of smaller laboratory animals. This may represent an unnecessary use of compressed oxygen, nitrous oxide, and the volatile anesthesics in order to operate the flowmeters and vaporizers in an accurate range. Excess anesthetic gases should be discharged to the scavenger system when possible.

Nonrebreathing patient circuits with minimal mechanical dead space should be used in the smaller animals. If face masks are used, they should be as small as possible to fit the animal with minimum dead space in order to reduce rebreathing and hypercapnea.

Endotracheal tubes for smaller laboratory animals, when needed, may be fashioned from polyethylene tubing of appropriate size if the commercially available endotracheal tubes are too large.

Induction of anesthesia in research animals by inhalation of volatile anesthetics is often most easily performed by introduction of anesthetic gases into a chamber containing the animal. A bell jar or modified aquarium-type container with an airtight lid is usually appropriate. Various transparent, airtight enclosures will suffice and may be selected to correspond to the size of animal to be used.

A gauze or cotton pledget containing a small amount of a liquid volatile anesthetic may be placed in a closed container with the animal as an alternative to use of an anesthesia machine. A screen or platform support should prevent contact of the animal with the liquid anesthetic. This technique has been used for years with chloroform and ether. As discussed previously, both of these anesthetics have substantial disadvantages and should now be replaced with other volatile anesthetics. Methoxyflurane can be used in the same manner as liquid ether or chloroform, with reduced risk of toxicities and without risk of explosion. Inhalant inductions are somewhat prolonged with methoxyflurane, and the delirium characteristics of Stage II of anesthesia may be a problem.

Following induction of anesthesia in the chamber, a face mask or nose cone with methoxyflurane-impregnated gauze can be placed on the muzzle for maintenance of anesthesia by the "open drop" method. Halothane should not be used as a liquid either in a closed chamber or by the open drop method. Lethal concentrations can be readily achieved with halothane or any of the other modern inhalant anesthetics except for methoxyflurane. Open drop administration of methoxyflurane anesthesia also requires considerable care to avoid overdosage. It is also more difficult to provide supplemental oxygen, and there is no practical means of eliminating waste anesthetic gas pollution of the laboratory. The advantage of this technique is that it requires no anesthesia machine and can thereby provide substantial cost savings.

RECOVERY FROM ANESTHESIA

Supervised recovery from anesthesia is often overlooked in laboratory animals but is nevertheless important. Procedures involving anesthesia should be scheduled to allow time for supervised recovery. A warm, darkened, quiet, clean, and comfortable place where the animal can be observed frequently is necessary. Care should be taken to ensure that the animal cannot aspirate food or water or injure itself when trying to stand. Unconscious animals should not be placed with cage mates where they can be attacked. Judicious use of parenteral fluids and postoperative analgesics can help make recovery smooth and rapid.

Anesthesia of Common Research Animal Species

RABBITS

The rabbit is frequently considered to be perhaps the most difficult research animal to anesthetize safely. Inadequate anesthetic techniques for demanding surgical procedures in an animal predisposed to anesthetic problems has lead to this impression. Recognition of factors increasing the risks of general anesthesia in rabbits and adoption of appropriate agents and techniques improves the likelihood of success.

Rabbits are easily frightened, and catecholamine release may be easily triggered. Struggling may result in self-inflicted fractures or other serious injury. They have a relatively large abdominal cavity and a relatively small thorax. The ratio of tidal volume to body weight is exceptionally small in rabbits. There is a high incidence of underlying respiratory disease in clinically normal research rabbits. Endotracheal intubation is difficult, and airway obstruction is a common anesthetic problem.

The digestive tract of the rabbit is voluminous, and its contents may contribute significantly to total body weight. When placed in dorsal recumbency, the abdominal viscera may interfere with diaphragmatic movement and venous return to the heart. Fasting for 12 hours prior to anesthesia is recommended to reduce both the amount of injesta present and the production of digestive gases in the cecum.

There is considerable variation between rabbit breeds and even among animals within a breed with regard to the susceptibility to injectable anesthetic agents. This may be particularly true for the barbiturate anesthetics. There is a narrow margin of safety between the anesthetic dose and the lethal dose of pentobarbital in rabbits. The dose that provides a surgical level of anesthesia will frequently be sufficient to result in respiratory arrest.

In spite of these limitations, pentobarbital anesthesia remains a frequent choice for rabbits. The results frequently contribute to the reputation of rabbits as difficult anesthetic challenges. Careful and quiet technique with appropriate finesse to avoid undue distress will greatly improve the safety of pentobarbital anesthesia in rabbits. Preparation should be made for respiratory support in the event that it becomes necessary. A dilute solution of pentobarbital (average 30 mg/kg) is administered by intravenous injection. A slow injection is of considerable importance in life-threatening respiratory depression.

Pentobarbital is a poor analgesic in rabbits. Only a light surgical plan of anesthesia should be expected with this agent at safe dosage levels. Anesthesia usually will persist for less than 20 minutes, although recovery times vary widely. Repeated injection of pentobarbital in rabbits is associated with an unacceptably high mortality. The limitations and dangers of pentobarbital anesthesia for rabbits have stimulated investigation of numerous alternatives.

The ultrashort-acting barbiturates are useful in rabbits although, as with pentobarbital, there is great variability in dose requirement. As a rough approximation, 30 to 40 mg/kg of thiamylal, 35 to 45 mg/kg of thiopental, or 10 mg/kg of methohexital are usually required for induction of anesthesia. Thiamylal has been advocated as the most adaptable anesthetic for surgical procedures in the albino rabbit. It is usually not associated with respiratory arrest unless administered too rapidly. A single induction dose of thiamylal provides 5 to 10 minutes of anesthesia in rabbits. Induction of anesthesia with an ultrashort-acting barbiturate allows for placement of an endotracheal tube.

Innovar-Vet (Pitman-Moore Co., Washington Crossing, N.J.) (fentanyl 0.4 mg/ml, and droperidol, 20 mg/ml) at 0.2 ml/kg i.m. provides good analgesia and relaxation in rabbits for brief anesthesia (4). It is perhaps most valuable for short periods of restraint, comparable to that provided by ketamine, but with analgesia and muscle relaxation for minor surgical procedures. Cardiac puncture and tatooing are greatly facilitated by the administration of small doses (0.1 ml/kg s.c. or i.m.) of Innovar-Vet. Atropine should be given either prior to or mixed with Innovar-Vet to prevent severe bradycardia. Respiratory depression is commonly encountered, and cyanosis may occur. Rabbits will frequently respond to auditory stimuli while under the influence of Innovar-Vet. Smooth recovery usually occurs within 60 minutes (frequently less), although some sedation may persist for several hours.

Other combinations of narcotics and tranquilizers have been evaluated in rabbits with a primary objective being the avoidance of the respiratory depression that is common with Innovar-Vet. Hyponorm (Janssen Pharmaceutica, Beerse, Belgium), a commercial combination of fentanyl and fluanisone available in the United Kingdom, has been used along with diazepam in rabbits with very favorable results.

High dosages of ketamine (44 mg/kg i.m.) provide good restraint but very little analgesia in rabbits. Muscle rigidity rather than relaxation occurs. Some seizure activity may also occur when ketamine is administered without sedatives. Relaxation and analgesia can be provided by the addition of xylazine (5 mg/kg i.m.) or acetylpromazine (1 mg/kg i.m.) with the ketamine dose reduced to 35 mg/kg. Surgical anesthesia with a duration of approximately 45 minutes results. Diazepam (2 to 10 mg/kg i.m.) with ketamine will provide muscle relaxation and protect against seizure activity. The large dose of diazepam may result in the administration of a substantial amount of the vehicle propylene glycol. This is not without risk, and the potential for cardiovascular shock should be recognized. The combination of ketamine and xylazine is most popular, although respiratory depression is common at doses required for surgical anesthesia. Atropine is recommended to improve ventilation and prevent xylazine-associated bradycardia.

From one-third to one-half of all rabbits have a high level of atropinase activity. Preanesthetic medication with atropine can be effective in rabbits if higher dosages (0.05 to 0.1 mg/kg i.m.) or s.c. at more frequent intervals are administered than in other animals. Anticholinergic medication is not required in all anesthetic techniques. It is recommended prior to barbiturate or ketamine anesthesia to reduce oral and respiratory secretions and with the administration of xylazine and some narcotics, such as fentanyl or oxymorphone, which may otherwise cause substantial bradycardia. The reduction of secretions and reduced airway resistance is crucial to success if ether anesthesia is used. Airway obstruction or increased resistance to ventilation is a very common cause of anesthetic complications in rabbits. Antichlolingeric therapy can be valuable in avoiding this problem.

Respiratory pattern and rate provide the best index to plane of anesthesia in the rabbit. Respirations should be deep, regular, and at a rate of greater than 15/minute. If serious respiratory depression occurs, ventilation should be supported via a snug-fitting mask or an endotracheal tube. Transient ventilatory stimulation can often be provided by the application of light pressure to the lateral thorax, thereby stimulating pressure receptors. In the absence of appropriate support equipment, limited ventilatory assistance may be provided by rocking the animal in such a fashion that inertia of the abdominal viscera causes movement of the diaphragm. Respiratory arrest subsequent to pentobarbital anesthesia in rabbits can be much more refractory to treatment than in other animals. The respiratory stimulant doxapram hydrochloride (2 to 4 mg/kg i.v.) may be of value for treating respiratory depression in rabbits.

Several techniques have been devised to simplify the difficult task of endotracheal intubation in rabbits. The large tongue, skin folds in the diastema, limited range of mandibular opening, and prominent incisors obstruct the placement of an endotracheal tube. Aided by use of a small-blade laryngoscope, visual placement of a small endotracheal tube (2.5 to 3.5 mm Cole tube) becomes routine for some individuals. Blind intubation is possible with the larynx grasped through the skin and tube placement guided by feel. Significant trauma is inevitable, and some blood and laryngeal swelling must be expected.

Other techniques may be less traumatic. The laryngeal opening may be visualized through an operative otoscope cone, and a guide tube (e.g., canine urinary catheter or small polyethylene tubing) may be placed into the trachea. After removal of the otoscope cone, an endotracheal tube may be advanced over the guide tube, which is then removed. This technique is shown in Figure 13.28. A similar guide tube may be placed through the skin overlying the trachea and retrograde out the mouth by use of a long, through-the-needle intravencus catheter. This catheter is then held under tension at both ends and used as a guide

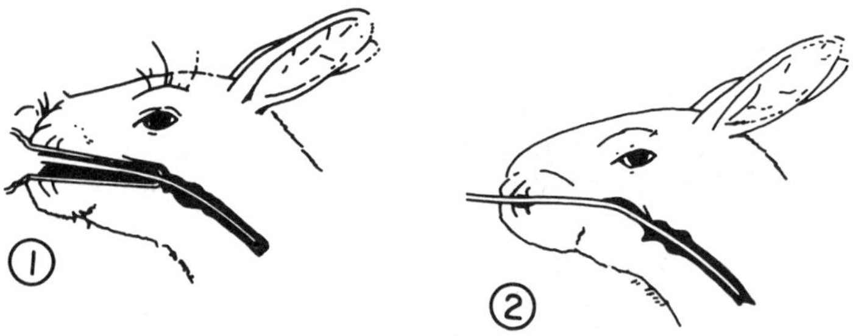

Figure 13.28. Use of otoscope and catheter guide for endotracheal intubation of rabbits. Used by permission. Gilroy BA: Endotracheal intubation of rabbits and rodents. *J Am Vet Med Assoc* 179:1295, 1981.

over which an endotracheal tube is advanced. Each method has been recommended as providing for rapid and easy placement of an endotracheal tube with relatively little trauma. With practice, any of these or other methods may be mastered and become the technique of choice. Nasal intubation may be used as well with 2.5- to 3.0-mm tubing.

Endotracheal intubation is not required in every rabbit anesthesia. Any of the techniques suggested requires practice to insure success without undue delay and injury. The placement of an endotracheal tube, however, makes prolonged anesthesia with inhalant or injectable agents safer, provides for assisted or controlled ventilation, and greatly increases survival in many situations.

RODENT ANESTHESIA

The requirements for surgical anesthesia in rodents are most often met by pentobarbital as the sole agent. In most laboratory rodents, intraperitoneal injection is most practical. Because intravenous injection is relatively easy in some laboratory rodents, such as the rat, this route may be preferred. Although the techniques are more difficult, skilled individuals may easily make intravenous injections in various rodent species using the ear veins or tarsal veins (guinea pig), the penile vein (hamster, guinea pig), or the tail vein (mouse).

Pentobarbital may also be administered orally by gavage tube in rodents. The anesthetic dosage is slightly higher by this route, and the time to effect is slightly longer. Intramuscular injection of barbiturates should generally be avoided due to significant tissue damage. This problem is much more severe with the ultrashort-acting thiobarbiturates thiamylal and thiopental than with the short-acting oxybarbiturate pentobarbital.

Alternative techniques are readily available for situations requiring either a more rapid return to full consciousness than occurs with barbiturates or for avoidance of the enzymatic (hepatic) effects of barbiturate administration.

Mice

Anesthesia for brief procedures may be induced in mice using either carbon dioxide or one of the volatile inhalant anesthetics in a chamber. Induction and recovery are usually quite rapid. Inhalant anesthesia may be prolonged by use of various masks or cones fashioned to the appropriate size. As described above, oxygen or a mixture of oxygen and nitrous oxide is preferred to air as the carrier gas.

Several strains of mice are particularly susceptible to hepatic and renal toxicity of anesthetic gases. Chloroform is quite toxic to some male mice in particular, and deaths attributed to chloroform may occur as long as months after exposure.

In spite of this concern, the inhalant anesthetics are usually quite suitable for mice. The results of different comparisons have ranked either methoxyflurane or halothane as the superior agent. Methoxyflurane offers the advantage of suitability for safe use without an anesthesia machine and vaporizer. Halothane offers the advantage of potentially less toxicity.

Intravenous injections in the ventrolateral tail veins of mice are facilitated by heat-induced vasodilatation and may become easy with practice. Barbiturate anesthesia in the mouse is much safer by intravenous injection than by intraperitoneal injection. A widely variable response to anesthetic doses and a narrow therapeutic index lead to considerable anesthetic mortality with intraperitoneal barbiturates in mice.

Small mammals, such as mice, are more subject to hypothermia than are many other species. The mouse should, therefore, be protected from excessive heat loss during anesthesia. As in other cases, this may be done by covering the animal with thin plastic wrap or metal foil when possible. Procedures can be conducted on warmed surfaces or heat provided from radiant sources. It is also necessary to avoid hyperthermia and injuries due to external heating.

Rats

The long-standing popularity of the rat as a research animal has led to a wealth of options available for anesthetic management. A collection of anesthetic agents that produce relatively minor physiological alterations have been widely used in rat protocols. In situations in which physiological stability is of primary importance and neither survival nor long-term toxicity is of concern, anesthetics such as α-chloralose, chloral hydrate, urethane, chlorobutanol, and paraldehyde have been used. As discussed earlier, newer anesthetic agents and techniques should generally take the place of these approaches.

Ketamine (20 to 60 mg/kg i.m.) may be used as a resistant agent for rats prior to the administration of injectable or inhalant anesthetics. Restraint may be provided for placement of an intravenous catheter or endotracheal tube and subsequent general anesthesia. An anticholinergic may be administered with ketamine to reduce secretions and thereby help maintain a clear airway. Ketamine alone will not produce good general anesthesia. When administered at 80 to 90 mg/kg i.m. along with xylazine (2 to 10 i.m.), phenothiazines, pentobarbital, or other anesthetics, a surgical plane of anesthesia results.

Physical restraint by wrapping the rat in a towel or by placement in a commercially available rat restrainer may be used prior to intravenous injection. For intravenous catheterization, ketamine restraint may be more desirable. The tail is clipped or shaved, and a vasodilator such as xylene or warm water may be applied to the ventral surface of the tail. Placement of an intravenous catheter facilitates repeated injection for prolonged anesthesia or other purposes. Other sites for intravenous injections in rats include the femoral, saphenous, and sublingual veins.

Pentobarbital by intravenous (30 to 40 mg/kg) or intraperitoneal (35 to 50 mg/kg) routes can be injected as either a 3 or 6% solution and provides a dose-dependent depth of anesthesia for up to 1 hour. There may be pronounced variation in dosage requirement with specific strain, age, sex, and environmental factors in rats. Albino strains are reported to have a lower 50% lethal dose (LD_{50}) for pentobarbital than are pigmented strains, although no difference was detected in a study of pentobarbital LD_{50} in albino and pigmented rats of the same strain. Female rats may have a longer duration of anesthesia than males due to slower metabolism of pentobarbital. Rats housed on wood chip bedding may require higher doses of barbiturates due to hepatic enzyme induction. Similarly, animals chronically exposed to increased ammonia gas resulting from soiled bedding may require increased amounts of anesthetic.

The ultrashort-acting thiobarbiturates are not frequently used in rats. Dose-related respiratory depression may be a significant problem. The recommended route is by intravenous injection and at a dose of 20 mg/kg for either thiamylal or thiopental.

For prolonged light anesthesia with minimal physiological effect, α-chlorolase may be administered by intravenous or intraperitoneal injection. Intraperitoneal administration is associated with a significant incidence of postanesthetic adynamic ileus, presumably resulting from a chemical peritonitis.

As for other animal species, the inhalant anesthetics provide for relatively easy adjustment of anesthetic plane in rats and can add safety, particularly for prolonged or otherwise demanding procedures. A wide variety of anesthetic induction chambers, face masks, and nose cones have been devised for rat anesthesia using volatile agents. Several of these may be quickly and inexpensively prepared using commonly available supplies. A Simplex (Cutter Laboratories, Emeryville, CA.) fluid administration set may be used as a nose cone for the administration of anesthetic gases to rats. A face mask for use without an anesthesia machine (open drop method) may be prepared from a syringe barrel as shown in Figure 13.29. The vapor pressure and potency of methoxyflurane makes it particularly well suited for this approach. Methoxyflurane can readily replace most uses of ether anesthesia in the rat by these techniques. Inorganic fluoride, a metabolite product of methoxyflurane, is much more nephrotoxic in Fisher 344 rats than in some other strains. A dose-related diabetes insipidus-like syndrome has been noted after methoxyflurane anesthesia in this strain.

Hamsters

Hamsters are often difficult to handle. A tendency to bite handlers and resist physical restraint makes it necessary to provide pharmacological restraint and sedation in situations that could be otherwise managed in most rodents. The short tails of hamsters precludes intravenous injections by the tail vein, which is so useful in many other rodents.

Pentobarbital (35 mg/kg) is administered by intraperitoneal injection just lateral to the umbilicus.

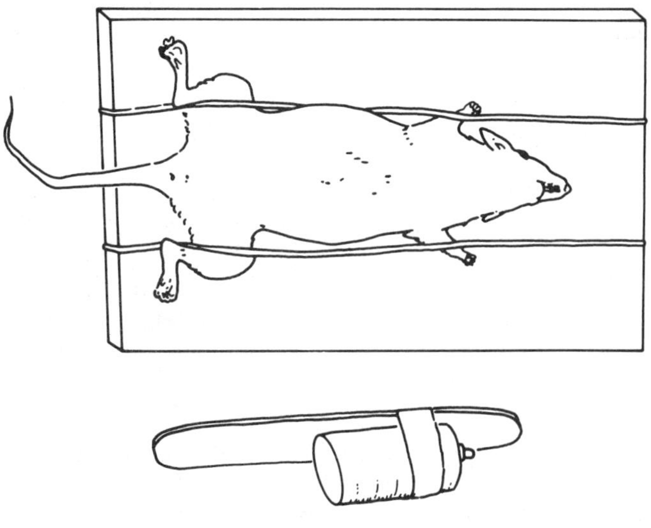

Figure 13.29. Practical low-budget rodent anesthesia/surgery table. Materials: one small cardboard box, two rubber bands, tongue depressor, one 30-ml or 50-ml syringe barrel cut in half, one roll of surgical tape. Method: Tape syringe barrel to tongue depressor and place cotton or gauze in end of syringe barrel. Squirt a few drops of methoxyflurane on cotton. With tranquilized rat in dorsal recumbency, place legs under rubber bands. Slip tongue depressor under the neck of the rat and slide it down until the syringe barrel fits loosely around the rat's face. Adjust depth of anesthesia by moving syringe barrel toward or away from the rat. Used by permission. Kintner B: Rock-bottom low-budget rodent anesthesia/surgery table. *Synapse* 15:28, 1982.

Methohexital (30 mg/kg) and diazepam (5 mg/kg) have been injected together, producing anesthesia rapidly; this lasts for 20 to 25 minutes and can be prolonged by small supplemental doses. The physical compatibility of these two solutions when mixed in the syringe is questionable, and separate injection may be considered advisable.

Ketamine (40 to 150 mg/kg i.m. or 100 to 200 mg/kg i.p.) provides restraint but poor analgesia and muscle relaxation. The addition of xylazine (up to 10 mg/kg i.m. or i.p.) or diazepam (5 mg/kg i.p.) will improve relaxation and provide dose-related analgesia. Innovar-Vet has been recommended for hamsters at a dose of 0.1 ml of a 1:10 dilution. Its use, however, may result in undesirable CNS stimulation. Previous administration of atropine is necessary to prevent serious bradycardia. The use of atropine in hamsters has been associated with cecal atony. Anticholinergics may be necessary if anesthetic agents that are most likely to cause excesive secretions (ketamine) or severe bradycardia (narcotics) are avoided.

Guinea Pigs

Unique aspects of anesthesia of the guinea pig or cavy require special consideration. The relatively docile demeanor of the species facilitates gentle restraint and physical examination, particularly in animals accustomed to frequent handling. Guinea pigs are easily frightened, however. Research animals less frequently handled may easily panic and will usually squeal and wiggle when restrained. Stress should be minimized because it predisposes guinea pigs to pneumonia and other diseases.

The cecum of the guinea pig occupies a considerable volume of its abdominal cavity. The cecal contents constitute a considerable proportion of total body weight independent of the circulating blood volume available for distribution of anesthetic agents. The determination of drug dosages for injectable anesthetics should be adjusted to an estimate of true body weight reduced by some factor to correct for the cecal contents. The cecum also frequently contains a gas cap just as in ruminants and other species in which cecal fermentation plays a prominent role in digestion. This gas-filled cavity can be important with regard to the use of nitrous oxide. Fasting is recommended for 12 hours before anesthesia in the guinea pig. Partial emptying of the intestinal tract may reduce body weight, of which 20 to 40% normally represents ingesta.

Pentobarbital (28 mg/kg i.p.) provides adequate anesthesia for most purposes, although the very narrow therapeutic index and poor analgesia provided by the barbiturate anesthesia for this species. Innovar-Vet (0.66 to 0.88 mg/kg i.m.) with an anticholinergic provides very favorable anesthesia for nonsurvival procedures in guinea pigs. Tissue necrosis and self-mutilation is frequently associated with the use of Innovar-Vet in guinea pigs, and its use cannot, therefore, be recommended for survival procedures in this species.

Surgical anesthesia may be provided for about 1 hour in guinea pigs by i.m. injection of approximately 35 mg/kg of ketamine and 0.2 mg/kg of xylazine. This technique results in a fairly rapid return (4 to 5 hours) to normal hemodynamic values as shown in chronically instrumented animals. This dosage level for xylazine is lower than that frequently recommended and contributes to improved hemodynamic stability and increased safety. A combination of ketamine (35 mg/kg) and xylazine (5 mg/kg) is generally recommended for surgical anesthesia with good muscle relaxation in guinea pigs. Ketamine (44 mg/kg i.m.) as the sole anesthetic produces a quite, immobile status but inadequate analgesia for surgical procedures. Inhalant anesthetics may be added after ketamine restraint.

Inhalant agents may be used in a chamber for induction of anesthesia or applied by mask as an adjunct to chemical restraint, sedation, or other anesthetics. With appropriate recognition of risk factors, the inhalant anesthetics may be used successfully in guinea pigs. Copious bronchial secretions may be produced in guinea pigs after exposure to inhalant anesthetics. The problem is most significant with diethyl ether, a notorious respiratory tract irritant. The tendency toward bronchial secretion is very greatly reduced by utilization of newer inhalant anesthetics, including methoxyflurane, halothane, enflurane, and isoflurane. Any potential problem can be further minimized by preanesthetic medication with atropine (0.05 mg/kg s.c.). Periodic suctioning of the trachea may be used to remove secretions when necessary. Endotracheal intubation in guinea pigs is difficult, but it may be achieved by use of the techniques described for rabbits.

Nitrous oxide may be a valuable adjunct to inhalant induction of anesthesia in guinea pigs but should not be used for prolonged anesthesia. Diffusion of nitrous oxide into the gas-filled cecum and subsequent distention can seriously compromise diaphragmatic movement and ventilation. Carbon dioxide can be used to provide brief anesthesia with remarkable safety if adequate oxygen is provided.

A peculiarity frequently exhibited by the guinea pig as it passes into a surgical plane of anesthesia, particularly with inhalant anesthetics, is a writhing or squirming motion. This movement usually begins with one rear leg and progresses to involvement of the entire body. This should not be taken as a sign of inadequate anesthesia. The administration of additional anesthetics at this time can lead to dangerously excessive dosages. This transient movement may interfere with surgical procedures, and it may be advisable to await this sign of transition prior to surgery.

RUMINANT ANESTHESIA

Small ruminants, particularly sheep and young calves, are being used with increasing frequency in biomedical research. Anesthetic techniques for these animals in research settings are much like those for clinical practice, although there may be increased demands with prolonged anesthesia for more elaborate physiological monitoring and support. Procedures involving extensive instrumentation require specialized management unique to each situation.

SWINE ANESTHESIA

The advent of swine breeds with greatly reduced adult body size has increased the practicality of using pigs as research animals. Information provided elsewhere concerning swine anesthesia in clinical practice, including precautions regarding malignant hyperthermia, will be appropriate for many research applications. As in any species, however, there may be additional requirements for prolonged or invasive procedures.

A combination of xylazine (2 mg/kg), ketamine (2 mg/kg), and oxymorphone (0.075 mg/kg) may be mixed together and given by intravenous injection for light surgical anesthesia in swine. Well-balanced muscle relaxation and analgesia is produced for 20 to 30 minutes.

Preanesthetic medication by intramuscular injection of either Innovar-Vet (1 ml/15 kg) with atropine (0.04 mg/kg) or azaperone (2 to 4 mg/kg) provides moderate tranquilization. Induction of a light plane of anesthesia results from the subsequent injection of ketamine (10 mg/kg i.m.), which is sufficient for basic noninvasive instrumentation and many other minor procedures. Deeper anesthesia is produced by intravenous administration of incremental doses of ketamine (2 mg/kg) or by careful administration of an ultrashort-acting thiobarbiturate.

A very suitable alternative for swine is the administration of inhalant anesthetics in oxygen or oxygen and nitrous oxide by means of a face mask after sedation with injectable agents.

Airway management is more difficult in swine than in any comparably sized animal frequently encountered. An adequate depth of anesthesia is required to achieve relaxation of the massive masseter muscles and will help to avoid laryngospasm, which is common in swine. At a sufficient depth of anesthesia, the larynx is sprayed with liodcaine and an endotracheal tube is placed. A long-bladed laryngoscope and a malleable

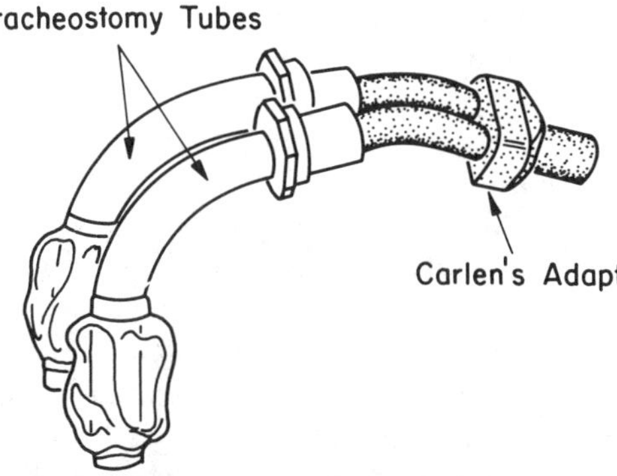

Figure 13.30. Tracheostomy tubes and Carlen's adapter or Y-piece for nasal intubation of swine. Reprinted by permission from Riebold TW, Goble DO, Geiser DR: *Large Animal Anesthesia: Principles and Techniques*. Ames, Iowa, Iowa State University Press, 1982, p 86.

stylet for the endotracheal tube aid successful placement. The laryngeal opening is more ventral and caudal than might be expected. The laryngeal ventricles and other anatomical obstacles impede endotracheal intubation of swine. Slight rotation of the endotracheal tube as the tip is advanced over and beyond the laryngeal opening may be a useful technique.

Use of a tight-fitting face mask and bilateral nasal intubation using two human tracheostomy tubes joined with a Carlen's adapter (shown in Fig. 13.30) are alternatives to endotracheal intubation. These provide for administration of volatile anesthetics and oxygen but may not suffice for controlled ventilation nor protect against aspiration because the trachea is not sealed.

PRIMATE ANESTHESIA

The nonhuman primates frequently must be restrained for even routine physical examination. Physical methods suffice for some species and situations, but more often chemical restraint is required. Chemical restraint is mandatory in the larger, more aggressive, and potentially more dangerous primates, such as baboons, macques, and the great apes.

Ketamine at various dosages (5 to 25 mg/kg i.m.) is the drug of choice for chemical restraint. Ketamine is often administered to primates in a squeeze cage or temporary restraint device. A cataleptic state is produced in primates by ketamine, and variable analgesia occurs. Muscle relaxation remains poor unless a supplementary agent has been given. Diazepam (0.5 mg/kg i.m.) improves relaxation and provides for a smoother, somewhat more prolonged anesthesia and recovery.

Anesthesia may be prolonged or otherwise augmented after ketamine restraint by the administration of other injectable or inhalant agents. A combination of a reduced dose of ketamine with xylazine (0.6 to 2 mg/kg i.m.) produces a greater relaxation and analgesia and faster recovery than higher doses of ketamine alone. There is dose-related respiratory depression and a possibility for bradycardia with xylazine either when given alone or in combination with other agents. Intravenous ketamine, at doses considerably lower than for intramuscular administration, supplements and prolongs the cataleptic state or dissociative anesthesia. With multiple administrations, tolerance to ketamine (increased dose requirement) occurs in some primate species, notably macaques and baboons.

A restraint dose of ketamine followed by pentobarbital (20 to 30 mg/kg i.v.) provides anesthesia for up to 1 hour with the anesthesia and recovery generally smooth and excitement-free. The ultrashort-acting barbiturates may be injected intravenously to facilitate intubation after ketamine restraint and thus prepare the animal for inhalant anesthesia.

Innovar-Vet produces good analgesia and restraint for brief procedures in primates. The characteristic dose-related respiratory depression makes this technique somewhat more dangerous than ketamine for chemical restraint. There is greatly superior analgesia, however, and partial reversal with narcotic antagonists is possible. The dosage of Innovar-Vet required for restraint or minor surgical procedures varies greatly (0.05 to 1.0 ml/kg i.m.) in different primate species. The effects in chimpanzees are reported to be unreliable.

Inhalant anesthesia in nonhuman primates parallels its use in humans. Nitrous oxide may more effectively supplement volatile anesthetics in primates than in other mammals. When injectable anesthetics are contraindicated, inhalant induction of anesthesia may be achieved using chambers for small primates or occasionally by application of a mask in the larger primates. Induction of anesthesia with a mask requires that the nonhuman primate be physically restrained and well trained to accept the restraint. The application of a small amount of fruit-scented extract to the interior of the mask or breathing circuit will greatly improve acceptance of the mask in nonhuman primates, as in children. With recognition of the usual advantages and disadvantages of each agent, any of the modern inhalant anesthetics may be used in primates.

Anticholinergics may be needed to prevent vagal responses associated with endotracheal intubation and to reduce salivary secretions. Atropine (0.04 mg/kg i.m. or s.c.) is often used in combination with ketamine, Innovar-Vet, and the inhalant anesthetics in primates.

Tranquilization or sedation of nonhuman primates, as opposed to more substantial pharmacological restraint, is unacceptable in most situations considering the potential consequences of early arousal from an apparently sedated condition.

Analgesic Therapy for Research Animals

Every effort should be made to avoid or prevent distress and discomfort in research animals. The relief of pain in research animals has fortunately received increasing attention in recent years (5). Several comprehensive reviews have addressed both the recognition and allevation of animal pain (6).

The perception of pain is subjective, and the recognition of pain in animals requires consideration of subtle behavioral changes (7, 8). These may vary greatly in different species. Because evidence of distress may invite aggression from predators or even from animals of the same species, animals are usually less likely to display evidence of pain and suffering than are humans. Pain alters the behavioral patterns of affected animals, frequently leading to decreased activity and food intake and altered interaction with other animals.

Untreated pain in research animals is not only inhumane, but also adversely influences the validity of many research models. Physiological effects may include those attributed to increased stress and may be related to increased catecholamine release. The treatment of pain in research models of human conditions more closely approximates the medical condition in that human patients usually receive necessary analgesics. The routine use of postoperative analgesics will often enhance smooth recovery from anesthesia.

Considerable attention is being devoted to the development of analgesic therapies for research animals. Buprenorphine and other mixed-acting narcotic agonist-antagonist drugs with long duration of analgesia offer great potential for this application as dosages and treatment intervals are further defined (9).

The recommendations in Table 13.10 for analgesic therapy in research animals may serve as a guide for postoperative analgesia. Individual requirements and responses will vary with the animal and peculiarities of each situation (10, 11). In general, if there is a reasonable possibility that pain may result from a procedure or a condition, analgesic therapy should be considered. The duration as well as magnitude of analgesia required should be considered in the choice of analgesics. If pain cannot be relieved by administration of analgesics or prevented by alterations in experimental protocol, the program should be re-evaluated.

Reversal of narcotic effects can be provided by administration of the narcotic antagonist naloxone (0.04 mg/kg i.v., i.m., or s.c.) in any species. Renarcotization can occur especially when long-acting opioids are used. Additional naloxone may thefore be required in some situations. Tolerance and addiction to narcotic analgesics may occur in some rodents.

Table 13.10
Recommended Analgesic Drugs and Dosages for Research Animals

Species	Drug	Dosage	Route	Duration
Dogs	Oxymorphone	0.2 mg/kg[a]	i.v., i.m., s.c.	4–6 hr
	Morphine	0.5 to 1.0 mg/kg	i.m., s.c.	4 hr
	Meperidine	2 to 6 mg/kg	i.m.	1 hr
	Pentazocine	1.5 to 3.0 mg/kg	i.m.	4–6 hr
	Butorphanol	0.2 to 0.5 mg/kg[a]	s.c.	3–4 hr
	Buprenorphine	0.01 to 0.02 mg/kg	i.m., s.c.	8–12 hr
	Aspirin	10 mg/kg	p.o.	8–12 hr
	Phenylbutazone	9 mg/kg	p.o.	8 hr
Cats	Oxymorphone	0.2 mg/kg	i.v., i.m., s.c.	4–6 hr
	Morphine	0.05 to 0.1 mg/kg	i.m., s.c.	4 hr
	Pentazocine	1.5 to 3.0 mg/kg	i.m.	4 hr
	Aspirin	10 mg/kg	p.o.	48–72 hr
Primates	Morphine	1 to 2 mg/kg	i.m., s.c.	4 hr
	Meperidine	2 to 4 mg/kg	i.m.	3–4 hr
	Pentazocine	2 to 5 mg/kg	i.m., s.c.	4 hr
	Buprenorphine	0.01 mg/kg	i.v., i.m.	8–12 hr
	Aspirin	10 to 20 mg/kg	p.o.	6 hr
Rats	Morphine	2 to 5 mg/kg	s.c.	4–6 hr
	Meperidine	20 mg/kg	i.m.	2 hr
	Pentazocine	10 mg/kg	s.c.	4 hr
	Butorphanol	20 mg/kg	s.c.	
	Buprenorphine	0.02 to 0.8 mg/kg	s.c., i.p.	6–8 hr
	Aspirin	100 mg/kg	p.o.	
Mice	Morphine	2 to 8 mg/kg	s.c.	2–4 hr
	Meperidine	20 mg/kg	i.m.	2–3 hr
	Pentazocine	10 mg/kg	s.c.	3–4 hr
	Butorphanol	5 to 10 mg/kg	p.o.	6 hr
		0.1 mg/kg	s.c.	6 hr
	Buprenorphine	2.5 mg/kg	i.p.	6–8 hr
	Aspirin	120 to 300 mg/kg	p.o.	
Rabbits	Morphine	5 mg/kg	i.m., s.c.	2 hr
	Meperidine	10 mg/kg	i.m.	2 hr
	Pentazocine	10 to 20 mg/kg	i.m., s.c.	4 hr
	Buprenorphine	0.02 to 0.05 mg/kg	i.v., s.c.	8–12 hr

[a] Total dose not to exceed 4.0 mg.

Conclusion

Proper selection of anesthetics for research animals requires an understanding of the related pharmacology as well as a familarity with the animal species and the requirements of the research project. In general, anesthetic techniques should be relatively simple and inexpensive and offer a high probability of success with minimal alteration of normal physiology.

The suitability of anesthetics for use in research protocols should be evaluated with regard to any physiological abnormalities that may be integral to the research model. Customary side effects and subclinical toxicities of anesthetic drugs can be of increased importance, particularly when prolonged procedures or physiologically altered animals are required.

Increased concern for the provision of adequate and humane anesthesia and analgesia for research animals is reflected in additional attention to these needs. The well-being and comfort of the animals should always be a primary consideration in the development of research protocols.

References

1. Clifford DH: Preanesthesia, anesthesia, analgesia, and euthanasia. In Fox JG, Cohen BJ, Loew FM (eds): *Laboratory Animal Medicine*. Orlando, Academic Press, 1984, pp 527–562.
2. Hughes HC: Anesthesia of laboratory animals. *Lab Anim* 10(5):40–56, 1981.
3. Soma LR: Anesthesia and analgesic considerations in the experimental animal. *Ann NY Acad Sci* 406:32–47, 1983.
4. Flecknell PA, Mitchell MJM, Shurey C, Simpkins: Neuroleptanalgesia in the rabbit. *Lab Anim* (London) 17:104–109, 1983.

5. Kitchell, RL, Erickson HH, Carstens E, Davis LE (eds): *Animal Pain: Perception and Alleviation*. Bethesda, American Physiological Society, 1983.
6. Flecknell PA: The relief of pain in laboratory animals. *Lab Anim* (London) 18:147–160, 1984.
7. Morton DB, Griffiths PHM: Guidelines on the recognition of pain, distress and discomfort in experimental animals and an hypothesis for assessment. *Vet Rec* 116:431–436, 1985.
8. Wright EM, Marcella KL, Woodson JF: Animal pain: evaluation and control. *Lab Anim* 14(4):20–36, 1985.
9. Heel RC, Brogden RN, Speight M, Avery GS: Butorphanol: a review of its pharmacological properties and therapeutic efficiency. *Drugs* 16:473–505, 1978.
10. Heidrich JE: Use of analgesics after surgery in animals. *J Am Vet Med Assoc* 187:513–514, 1985.
11. Taylor PM, Houlton JEF: Post-operative analgesia in the dog: a comparison of morphine, buprenorphine and pentazocine. *J Small Anim Pract* 25:437–451, 1984.

SECTION 3

Related Clinical Topics

CHAPTER 14

Machines and Breathing Systems for Administration of Inhalation Anesthetics

SANDEE M. HARTSFIELD, D.V.M., M.S., D.A.C.V.A.

Introduction

The halogenated hydrocarbon liqud anesthetics have revolutionized veterinary anesthesia over the last two decades. They have allowed the attainment of readily reversible general anesthesia and are primarily responsible for facilitation of sophisticated, prolonged surgical procedures in both small and large animals. Because of their high potency and volatility, they must be delivered with accuracy and consistency. For precise, safe administration, an anesthetic machine and a breathing system are required. Although numerous machines and systems are available commercially, all machines have the same basic components (Figs. 14.1 and 14.2) and the breathing systems function to accomplish the same goals (1). The primary purpose of a machine and a breathing system are delivery of oxygen, delivery of exact amounts of inhalation anesthetics, removal of carbon dioxide from exhaled gases, and provision for positive pressure ventilation. In 1979, the American National Standards Institute published standards for basic performance and safety for anesthetic machines (2); these have been discussed by Dorsch and Dorsch (3).

The fundamental components of an anesthetic machine are sources of compressed medical gases, specifically oxygen and possibly nitrous oxide; a regulator and a flowmeter for each gas; and a vaporizer for each volatile liquid anesthetic. The anesthetic machine prepares a precise mixture of gases that can be varied by the machine operator, and this mixture is then piped to the breathing system (e.g., circle system) for administration to the patient (3).

Compressed Gases

Small compressed gas cylinders attach directly to an anesthetic machine to supply oxygen and nitrous oxide. Alternatively, medical gases can enter the machine through its pipeline inlets (Fig. 14.3) and are supplied for a central hospital pipeline system. Central sources of nitrous oxide originate from banks of large cylinders; oxygen is available from large cylinder banks, liquid oxygen bulk tanks, or possibly from oxygen-concentrating systems. The latter has yet to be proved reliable and safe (4). Bulk sources of gases are usually more economical (5). Gases are piped to various locations through copper alloy tubes that terminate at wall, floor, or ceiling station outlets. A noninterchangble fitting, present at the station outlet, accepts only its corresponding component, which attaches to an anesthetic machine through a flexible hose. The diameter-indexed safety system (DISS), incorporating threaded connections and a set of concentric bores, prevents inadvertent interchange of medical gases at the station

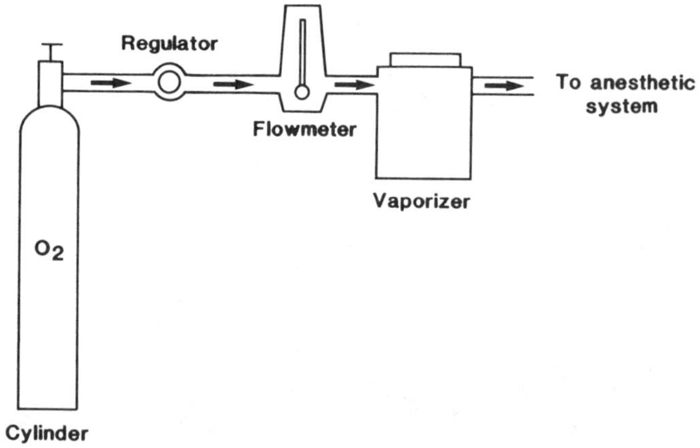

Figure 14.1. Diagram illustrating the four basic components (compressed oxygen source, regulator, flowmeter, and vaporizer) essential to the operation of an anesthetic machine. When attached to a breathing system, the anesthetic machine can deliver a precise mixture of gases to the patient. (Biomedical Learning Resources Center, College of Veterinary Medicine, Texas A & M University, College Station, Texas).

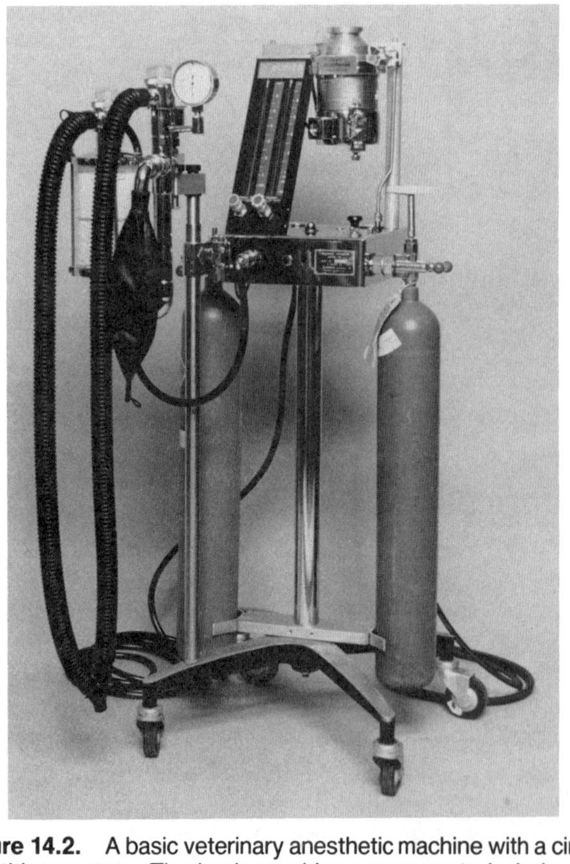

Figure 14.2. A basic veterinary anesthetic machine with a circle breathing system. The basic machine components include gas cylinders, regulators, flowmeters, and a vaporizer located out of the system (Dupaco, San Marcos, California).

outlet. Alternatively, to allow faster attachments, quick connections without threads have been developed for the same purpose. Anesthetic machines equipped to attached to station outlets usually have the capacity

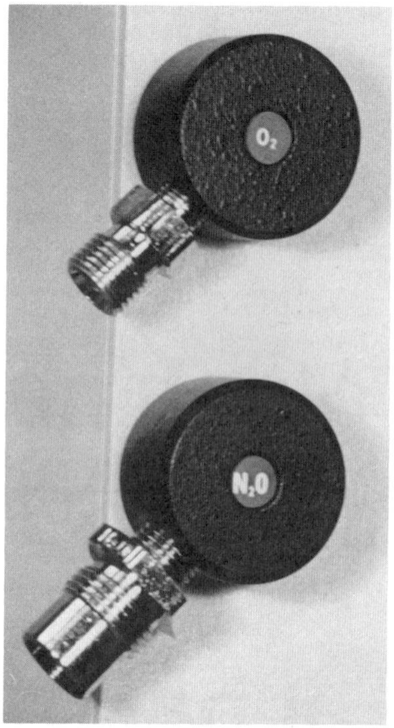

Figure 14.3. Pipeline inlets for oxygen and nitrous oxide on an anesthetic machine. The diameter-indexed safety system prevents inadvertent interchange of medical gases. Note the differences in thread size and bore of the connections (North American Drager, Telford, Pennsylvania).

for small cylinders of oxygen and nitrous oxide as emergency sources. Such cylinders attach to the machines at the hanger yokes.

Steel or steel alloy cylinders for medical gases are strictly controlled and tested during construction and use. A cylinder usually has a service pressure (maximum pressure to which that cylinder can be filled at 70°F) between 1800 and 2400 psig (a psig equals a pound per square inch above atmospheric pressure). Cylinder sizes are indicated alphabetically, with A being the smallest. Sizes E and H are very commonly used for medical O_2 and N_2O. These cylinders have permanent markings stamped near the top of the cylinder, including such information as the type of steel, the service pressure, the serial number, the manufacturer, and testing dates (3, 6). Also, a label on the cylinder wall (Fig. 14.4) gives the name of the gas, its color code (green for O_2 and blue for N_2O in the United States), warnings about principal hazards associated with the cylinder and its contents, and the manufacturer or distributor of the cylinder. Commonly, a cylinder tag is attached to the cylinder valve; it is color-coded, and the printed name of the gas appears on it. Tags have sequential perforated tabs designated as "full," "in use," and "empty" to help track the cylinder contents.

Gases pass to and from the cylinder through a

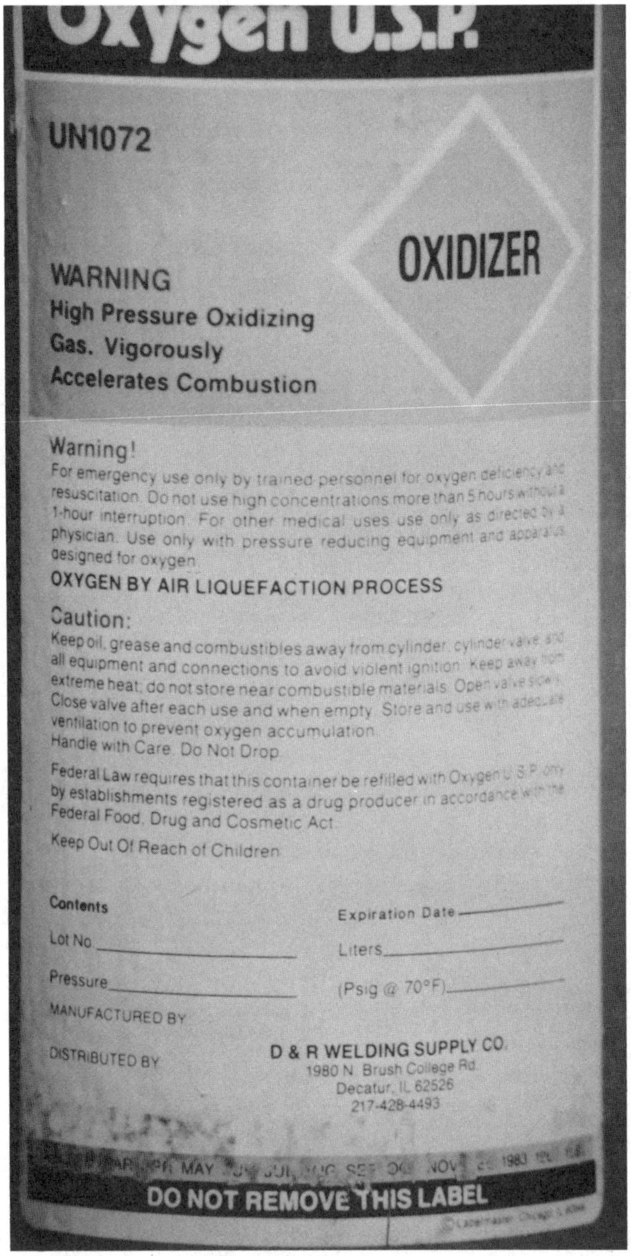

Figure 14.4. A cylinder label for medical oxygen with warnings about principle hazards associated with the cylinder and its contents (Biomedical Learning Resources Center).

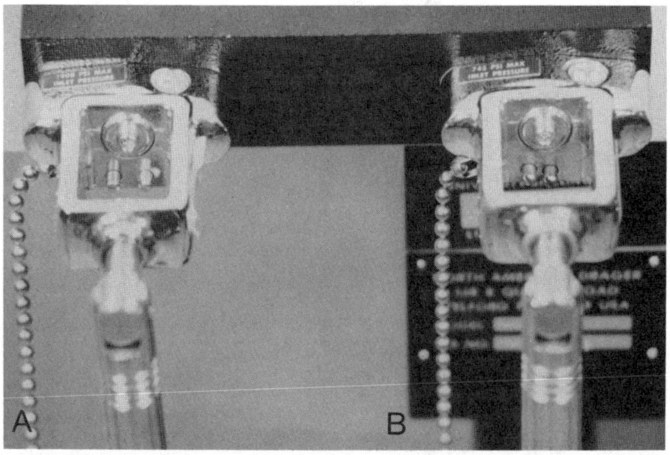

Figure 14.5. Hanger yokes for attachment to valve bodies of O_2 (*A*) and N_2O (*B*) cylinders. The spacing of the nipple and pins with each hanger yoke is integral to the pin index safety system to prevent inadvertent interchange of medical gas cylinders on an anesthetic machine (North American Drager, Telford, Pennsylvania).

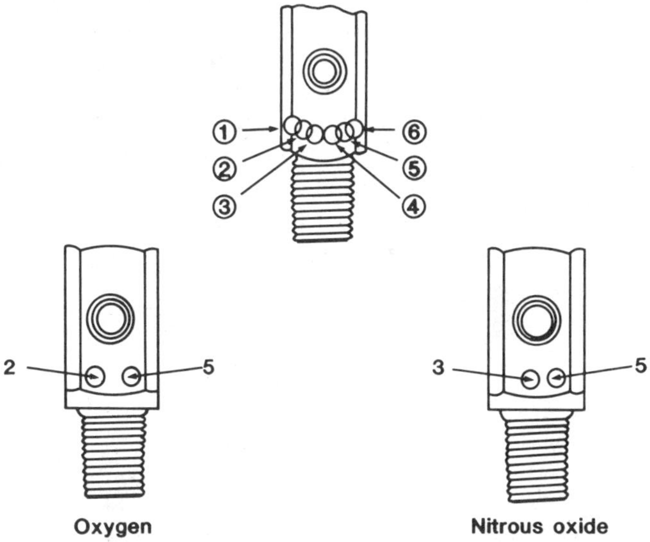

Figure 14.6. Diagram illustrating the spacing between the valve outlet and the pin holes in the valve bodies for oxygen and nitrous oxide cylinders. These correspond to the nipple and pins of hanger yokes on anesthetic machines and function to prevent inadvertent interchange of medical gases (pin-indexed safety system) (Biomedical Learning Resources Center).

valve that is usually made of brass and has a stem for controlling gas flow and a safety relief device to prevent bursting of the cylinder. For example, one device called a fusible plug has a relatively low melting point to allow escape of gases if an elevated temperature develops. Small cylinder valves use the pin index safety system to assure correct attachment to the hanger yokes of anesthetic machines (Fig. 14.5) (3, 6). The two holes and the valve port of the valve are spaced to fit the two pins and the nipple of the hanger yoke. Spacing of the pins varies with each medical gas (Fig. 14.6). Large cyclinder valves have varying diameters and thread types to prevent improper connections.

Numerous safety precautions should be followed when using gas cylinders (3). These include avoiding storage near flammable materials, securing cylinders properly at all times even during transport, not using a cylinder with any defects, and never trying to stop a leak of high pressure gases with one's hand. Before use, full cylinders should be pointed away from the operator, opened briefly to clear the valve port, and then closed before connection to a regulator. After attachment to a regulator or an anesthetic machine, the cylinder valve should be opened slowly to pressurize the regulator. Then, the valve stem should be fully opened during use (3, 6).

When full, O_2 cylinders have service pressures near 2200 psig. At 70°F, an E cylinder at 2200 psig contains about 700 liters of O_2 and an H cylinder contains about 7000 liters of O_2. Oxygen cylinders contain only gaseous O_2, and the pressure is proportional to the remaining contents. An N_2O cylinder, when full, has a pressure near 750 psig under normal environmental conditions. In a full cylinder, N_2O is in both liquid and gas phases because ambient temperature is less than its critical temperature. Therefore, the vapor pressure of the liquid N_2O varies with temperature and determines the cylinder pressure. In a full cylinder, 95% of the volume is liquid (3). A full E cylinder of N_2O contains about 1600 liters, whereas H cylinder contains about 16,000 liters. Vaporization of liquid N_2O results in cylinder cooling, and frosting of the cylinder or its valve may occur. Cylinder contents are not directly proportional to the cylinder pressure, but when the pressure begins to drop after all liquid has been vaporized, about 75% of the N_2O has been used (1). The remaining N_2O and its time of use, depending on flow, have been discussed (7).

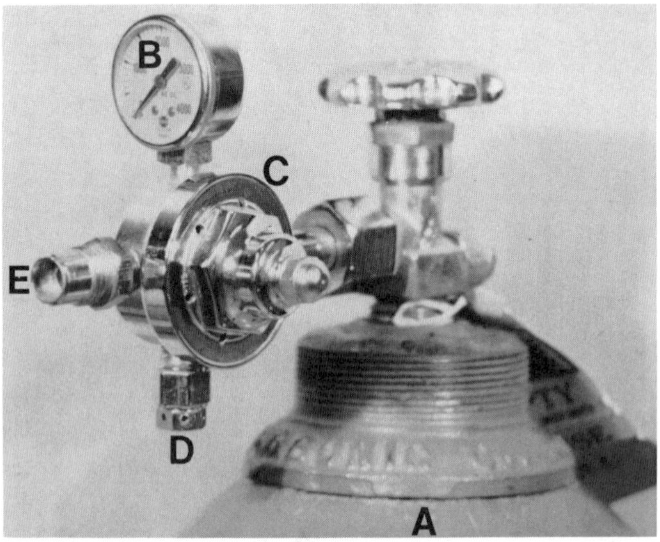

Figure 14.7. A regulator attached to the valve body of a large oxygen cylinder (*A*). A pressure gauge (*B*) is situated atop the regulator (*C*) to indicate the pressure within the cylinder when the cylinder valve is opened. A safety relief mechanism (*D*) is also present. Gases pass from *E* to the flowmeter (Biomedical Learning Resources Center).

Pressure Gauges

A pressure gauge is provided for each compressed gas on an anesthetic machine, and one is attached to each regulator to indicate the gas pressure in large cylinders (Fig. 14.7). Gauges are identified by the chemical symbol or the name of the gas for which they are designed, and gauges are usually color-coded. Pressure is measured, in most instances, as weight per unit of area, and they are often of the Bourdon tube type. The full scale reading of the gauge should be at least one-third greater than the maximum cylinder pressure, and on a given anesthetic machine, all gauges should displace a similar arc from the lowest to the highest reading. The pressure gauge gives the pressure of gas on the high pressure side (cylinder side) of the regulator (3, 6).

Regulators

Pressure regulators, sometimes called pressure-reducing valves (8), are connected to gas cylinders to reduce and control pressure (Fig. 14.7) (3, 6). This allows maintenance of constant flow as cylinder pressure changes (3). A regulator is a valve, often controlled by a diaphragm, to reduce a high pressure to be a present constant lower pressure. In simplest form, a regulator has a high pressure chamber separated by a valve port from a low pressure chamber. Movement of a flexible diaphragm opens or closes the valve, thereby regulating a variable annular gap and the pressure in the low pressure chamber. Increasing pressure on the low side tends to close the valve. The amount of pressure required to close the valve depends on a spring mechanism opposite the diaphragm. Variations in regulator mechanisms exist (6), but their function is the same. Regulators provide a safe operating pressure for the anesthetic machine, the anesthetist, and the patient; prevent flowmeter fluctuations as cylinders empty because a constant pressure is provided; and decrease the sensitivity of the flowmeter to slight movements of the control knob (3, 8). Present standards provide for regulators on anesthetic machines to be set at slightly less than 50 psig, whereas most pipeline systems are set at 50 psig. This allows preferential use of pipeline gases rather than cylinder gases if a cylinder inadvertently remains on after machine attachment to the pipeline gas source (3). Older anesthetic machines may have regulators set at 50 psig, and open cylinders may flow instead of pipeline gases. Regulators are designed for safety relief at two to four times the pressure in the low pressure chamber, with the diaphragm being the relief mechanism in some cases (6). This protects personnel and patients from excess pressures. Components of the anesthetic unit (such as flowmeters attached to an anesthetic machine) are not designed for accurate operation or safety at high pressures.

Flowmeters

A medical gas passes through a flowmeter after leaving the regulator. Flowmeters measure the amount of gases supplied to a breathing system and/or passing through a vaporizer. Flowmeter function depends on the principle that rate of flow through a restriction depends on the pressure difference on the two sides of the restriction. Gases enter the flowmeter at the bottom, pass around a movable indicator, and exit at the top. The glass tube of a flowmeter tapers, being larger at the top (6, 8). As the indicator or float of the flowmeter rises in the tube, more gas flows around it (variable orifice) (Fig. 14.8) (8). A scale behind the tube indicates the rate of gas flow (Fig. 14.9). Flowmeters are calibrated at 760 mm Hg and 20°C, and accuracy may change under variable atmospheric conditions (3, 6). The lowest reading on a flowmeter scale is the first accurate setting, and extrapolation below that mark can be inaccurate (3). Some flowmeters have double tapers (8), a slight taper on the bottom of the tube for accuracy at low flows (ml/min) and a greater taper at the top to allow use of higher flows (liter/min) (Fig. 14.8). The indicator or float of a flowmeter is read at the top (Fig. 14.10) except for the ball type (Fig. 14.9), which is read in the center (3). Newer anesthetic machines are designed to have the O_2 flow control knob as large or larger than other flow control knobs, and

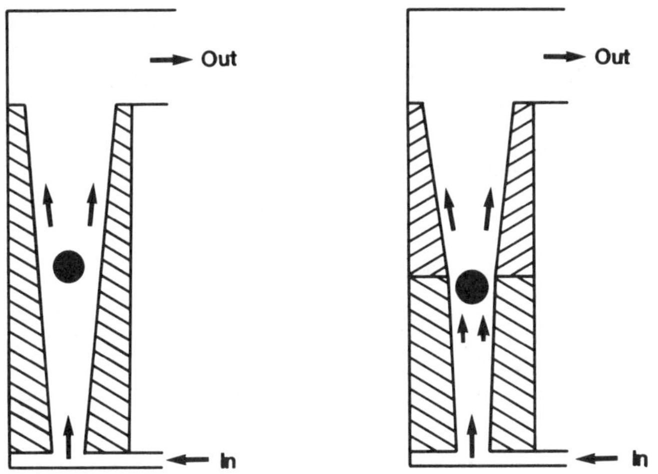

Single taper flowmeter   Double taper flowmeter

Figure 14.8. Diagram illustrating gas flow from bottom to top through flowmeters with single and double tapers. As the indicator (*black dot*) rises, flow increases because orifice size increases. The double taper tube allows increased accuracy at the lower end of the tube while retaining ability to meter high flows at the top (Biomedical Learning Resources Center).

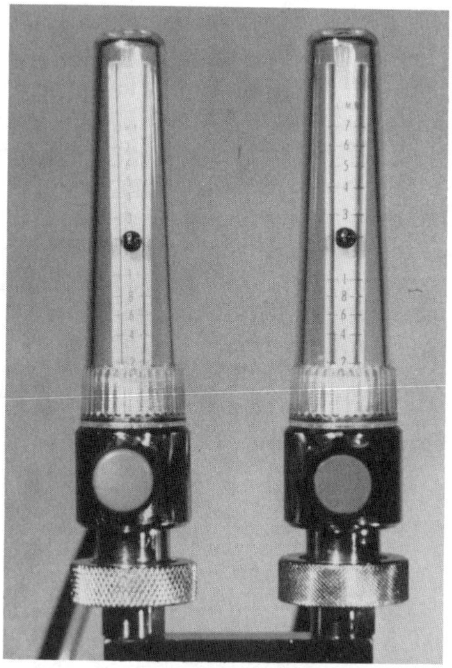

Figure 14.9. Oxygen and nitrous oxide flowmeters with ball-type indicators. The indicator is read in the center; both flowmeters indicate 2 liters/min. Flow of gases is from the bottom of the inside tube to the top. Note the fluted control knob for oxygen, (North American Drager, Telford, Pennsylvania).

the O_2 control knob is fluted (Fig. 14.9) (3). Both allow the operator to feel which gas is being adjusted; they may be said to be touch-coded (9). The knob is labeled with the gas symbol and is color-coded. Good flow controls have fine threads for accuracy and stops to prevent over-tightening, which can damage flow control valves. Newer anesthetic machines, based on current standards, should have only one flowmeter for each medical gas, and the delivery of O_2 should be downstream from all other gases (10). The O_2 flowmeter should be positioned to the right in a flowmeter grouping (3). Flowmeter parts are not interchangable; flowmeters should be off when not in use. Sudden pressure should not be applied to a flowmeter in the on position (e.g., opening a cylinder valve), and flowmeters should be used in the position for which they were originally designed (e.g., vertical or slanted) (3). Flowmeters assure an adequate total volume and an appropriate concentration of each medical gas. Flows should be set to meet or exceed the patient's oxygen consumption demands and to provide an adequate inspired concentration of O_2 (generally greater than 30% in inspired gases).

Flush Valves

The O_2 cylinder or the pipeline O_2 source also supplies gas to the flush valve, a component on most anesthetic machines. The flush valve delivers O_2 to the common gas outlet of an anesthetic machine at a flowrate between 35 and 75 liters/min (3). The flush valve, often set to deliver 50 liters/min of oxygen (1), will quickly fill the breathing system with oxygen that does not pass through the vaporizer. Older machines and "homemade" machines may flush through the vaporizer. As a general rule, small volume pediatric breathing systems should not be filled using the flush valve because of the danger of overpressurizing the patient's respiratory system.

Vaporizers

Except for N_2O and some of the rarely used agents, inhalation anesthetics are delivered by vaporizers. A vaporizer is an instrument designed to facilitate the change of a liquid anesthetic into its vapor and to add a controlled amount of this vapor to the flow of gases to the patient (3). Because the saturated vapor pressures of most volatile liquid anesthetics are above the partial pressures required to produce clinical anesthesia, vaporizers must be accurate. Oxygen, alone or in combination with N_2O, that passes through a vaporizer to obtain anesthetic vapors is called carrier gas. In general, the design of a vaporizer must allow appropriate dilution of saturated anesethetic vapor to produce a clinically safe concentration; that is, the vaporizer must regulate the output of anesthetic vapor.

Understanding the physics of vaporization is necessary to appreciate vaporizer function (1). The molecules in a liquid anesthetic must overcome forces keeping them in the liquid phase. Therefore, heat must be supplied. the heat of vaporization (the number of calories required to convert 1 g of liquid into vapor), used during the vaporization process, causes a temperature decrease in the liquid anesthetic. More heat is required as the liquid cools. The vapor pressure of the liquid is the partial pressure of the gas above a liquid at equilibrium and varies with the temperature. Because the vapor pressure determines the maximum concentration of anesthetic vapor, uncontrolled cooling of the liquid will limit vaporizer output. The specific heats of liquid anesthetics and vapor components are important. Agents with low specific heat require less heat to be added to maintain a stable temperature. A vaporizer made of a substance with a high specific heat (the quantity of heat required to raise the temperature of 1 g of substance 1°C) maintains a more stable temperature during anesthetic vaporization. In addition, a vaporizer constructed of material with high thermal conductivity (a measure of heat flow through a substance) allows rapid transfer of heat from ambient air into the

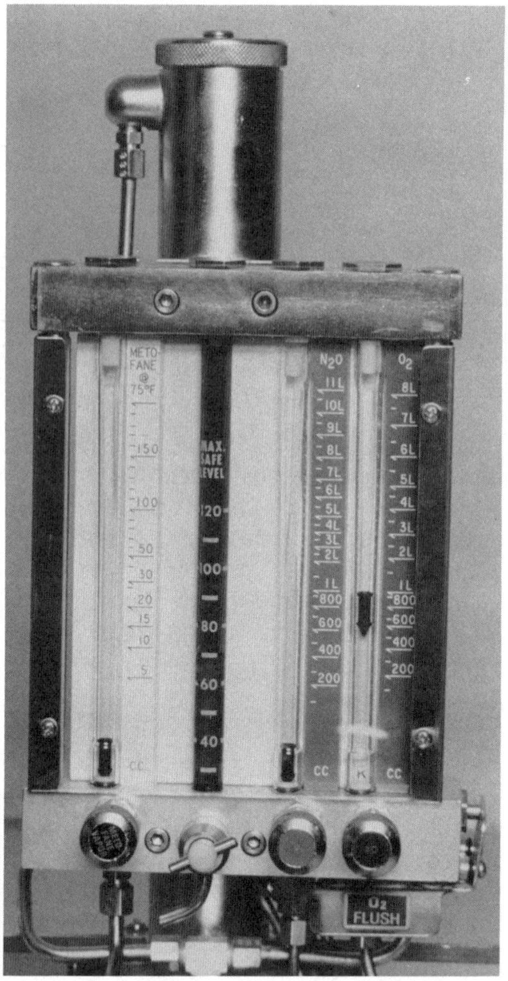

Figure 14.10. Flowmeters for O_2 and N_2O with floats or indicators that are read at the top. The O_2 flowmeter on the right is flowing at 1 liter/min (Ohio Medical Products, Madison, Wisconsin).

vaporizer (3). Most calibrated vaporizers are graduated to express output of anesthetic gas in volumes percent (Fig. 14.11), which compares the number of units of anesthetic vapor to a total volume of 100 units. This relative value will change with barometric pressure (3). Thus, one should be cognizant of the partial pressures of gases delivered from a vaporizer in comparison to barometric pressure if conditions are not standard, as with high altitude.

Certain vaporizers allow compensation for temperature variations, changes in rate of flow of carrier gases, and changes in pressure. Temperature variations can be countered in different ways. Copper or bronze, metals with high specific-heat high thermal conductivity, are used because of rapid conduction of heat into the vaporizer for a more constant temperature. Other mechanisms, such as bimetallic strip values, are used to compensate for temperature changes by altering carrier gas flow (1). In some older vaporizers, manual

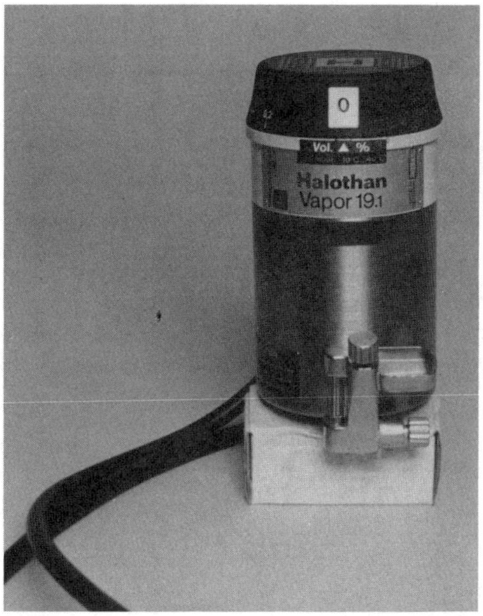

Figure 14.11. A Vapor 19.1 vaporizer showing calibration of output in volumes %. The white button marked "0" is a mechanism for locking the control and must be depressed to activate the control dial (North American Drager, Telford, Pennsylvania).

adjustments in carrier gas flow are required when vaporizer temperature varies. Differences in carrier gas flows through uncompensated vaporizers will also alter vapor output. Newer vaporizers are flow-compensated to produce accurate anesthesic concentrations over a range of 300 ml/min to 10 liters/min. Present machine standards require vaporizers to accept flows of 15 liters/min (3). Older vaporizers may require manual adjustments of flow through the vaporization chamber when total flow changes. Finally, pressure can be transmitted to vaporizers during positive pressure ventilation and during activation of the anesthetic machine's flush valve; under these circumstances, vaporizer output may increase when compared to free flow of gases (3). Newer vaporizers use several different methods to prevent this "pumping effect." These include use of a small vaporization chamber, a long spiral tube at the entrance to the chamber, a pressure check valve just downstream from the vaporizer, and a relief valve at the vaporizer outlet (3).

Other features incorporated into newer vaporizers include keyed filler systems to prevent use of the wrong liquid anesthetic, filler ports situated to prevent overfilling, and sight glasses to allow visualization of the liquid anesthetic. Both help to prevent liquid anesthetic from entering the fresh gas line of the vaporizer. More recent designs prevent liquid from entering the vaporizer's fresh gas line even during tipping or inversion. It is quite common to put two or more vaporizers in series on one anesthetic machine; simultaneous use of two agents and cross contamination can occur. To prevent this, interlock devices and selector valves have been developed (3).

Classification of vaporizers is a complex task, and numerous attempts have been made (3); some use only one characteristic of vaporizers, such as the method of vaporization (5). A useful, although imperfect, scheme is given in Table 14.1. However, it seems reasonable to consider each vaporizer individually, evaluating each characteristic of a vaporizer on its own merits (Table 14.2). Vaporizers have been categorized by five major characteristics: the method of output regulation, the method of vaporization, the location, the mechanism of temperature compensation and agent specificity (3). Regulation of output (control of the percentage concentration of anesthetic agent) can be accomplished by a variable bypass or a measured flow mechanism. Variable bypass vaporizers receive all of the fresh gas flow into the body of the vaporizer, and part of this flow is diverted through and part bypasses the vaporization chamber. The gases rejoin before exiting the vaporizer, delivering an operator-set anesthetic concentration. On the other hand, measured flow vaporizers allow all gases (usually a small flow) entering the vaporizer to go through the vaporization chamber. This fully saturated gas from the vaporization chamber is then diluted by a second source of gas that never enters the vaporizer. Both of these gas flows are determined by the operator.

The second important vaporizer characteristic is the method of vaporization, either flow-over or bubble-through. The flow-over method moves carrier gas over the surface of the liquid anesthetic, and wicks are used to increase the surface area for vaporization. The bubble-through method disperses carrier gas under the surface of the liquid anesthetic, usually through a diffuser. Efficiency of vaporization increases with smaller bubbles, deeper bubble dispersion, and slower carrier gas flow.

Table 14.1
A Useful System for Classification of Vaporizers Commonly Used in Veterinary Anesthesia with Examples (Not All-Inclusive)

- Nonprecision vaporizers
  - Ohio #8
  - Other glass vaporizers with wicks
- Precision vaporizers
  - Automatic vaporizers
    - "Tecs" (Fluotec III, Fortec, etc.)
    - "Matics" (Flumatic, Pentomatic, etc.)
    - Vapor 19.1
    - Other fully compensated vaporizers
  - Semiautomatic vaporizers (vapor)
  - Saturation vaporizers
    - Copper kettle
    - Verni-trol

Table 14.2
Characteristics of Several Vaporizers for Inhalation Anesthetics

Vaporizer	Output Regulation	Method of Vaporization	Location	Temperature Compensation (Range °C)[a]	Agent Specificity	Flow Compensation	Primary Construction Material	Backpressure Compensation Method
Ohio #8	Variable bypass	Flow-over with wick	In the system	None	Multiple	None	Glass	None
"Tec"	Variable bypass	Flow-over with wick	Out of the system	Bimetallic strip valve (20–36°C)	Specific	Resistance mechanism	Copper helix between wicks	Small vaporization chamber
"Matics"	Variable bypass	Flow-over with wick	Out of the system	Plastic thermal mechanism (15–30°C)	Specific	Resistance mechanism	Metal	Small vaporization chamber
Vapor 19.1	Variable bypass	Flow-over with wick	Out of the system	Silicone cone (10–40°C)	Specific	Resistance mechanism	Metal	Spiral inlet tube
Vapor	Variable bypass	Flow-over with wick	Out of the system	Manual	Specific	Resistance mechanism	Copper	Spiral inlet tube
Copper kettle	Measured flow	Bubble-through	Out of the system	Copper construction and manual	Multiple	Manual	Copper	Check valve
Verni-trol	Measured flow	Bubble-through	Out of the system	Bronze construction and manual	Multiple	Manual	Silicon bronze	Check valve

[a] Range of temperature compensation for newer halothane vaporizers.

The third category for vaporizer classification is very important; this is the vaporizer location in relation to the breathing system, either out of the system (Fig. 14.2) or in the system (Fig. 14.12). Out of the system precision vaporizers are required for administration of highly potent, highly volatile agents, such as halothane and isoflurane. It is the configuration used on most newer anesthetic equipment, but in the system configurations are still available. The locations for vaporizers in reltion to the components of anesthetic machines and circle breathing systems are diagrammed in Figures 14.13 and 14.14.

A fourth category, temperature compensation, can be accomplished by supplied heat or variation in flow. Heat may be supplied by constructing the vaporizer with a metal such as copper with a high specific heat and high thermal conductivity (heat sink). In the past, heat has been supplied by electric heaters and warm water jackets. In other vaporizers, thermostatic mechanisms (bimetallic strip valve) or manual adjustments alter flow through the vaporization chamber to maintain output as the liquid anesthetic cools during the vaporization process.

Finally, vaporizers can be either drug-specific or all purpose (used with any volatile liquid anesthetic). The general trend is toward agent-specific vaporizers with temperature, flow, and back-pressure compensation.

Vaporizers should be carefully maintained. They should not be overfilled or tipped when filled. Many vaporizers are not designed to be transported and should be empty if moved. Servicing as recommended by the manufacturer is appropriate, and this includes cleaning, recalibration, and replacement of worn parts. Halothane and methoxyflurane contain preservatives (thymol and butylated hydroxytoluene, respectively) that do not vaporize, but collect in vaporization chambers and can affect anesthetic output. Vaporizers should be drained periodically to eliminate these preservatives (11). Occasionally, flushing a vaporizer with

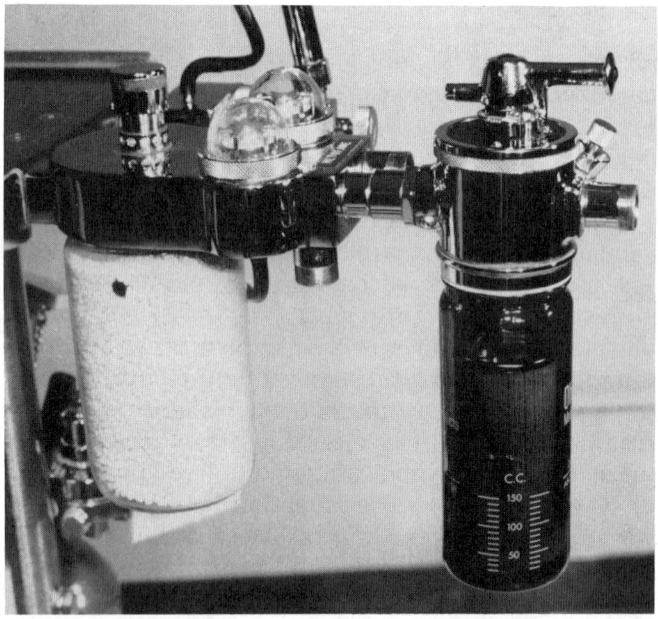

Figure 14.12. An Ohio #8 vaporizer for use with methoxyflurane. The wick present in the brown glass jar improves saturation of carrier gases by increasing surface area for vaporization. The control lever, present at the top of the vaporizer, allows variation of the amount of carrier gas routed to the vaporization chamber (Ohio Medical Products, Madison, Wisconsin).

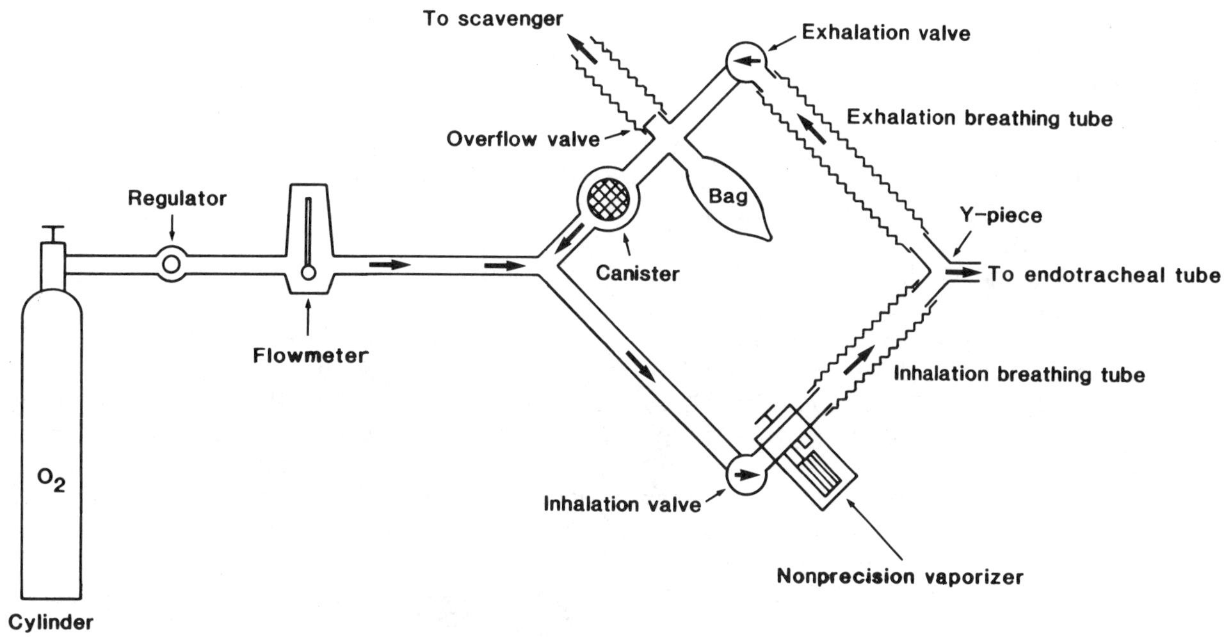

Figure 14.13. Diagram of the relationship of an in the system nonprecision vaporizer to the various components of an anesthetic machine and a circle breathing system (Biomedical Learning Resources Center).

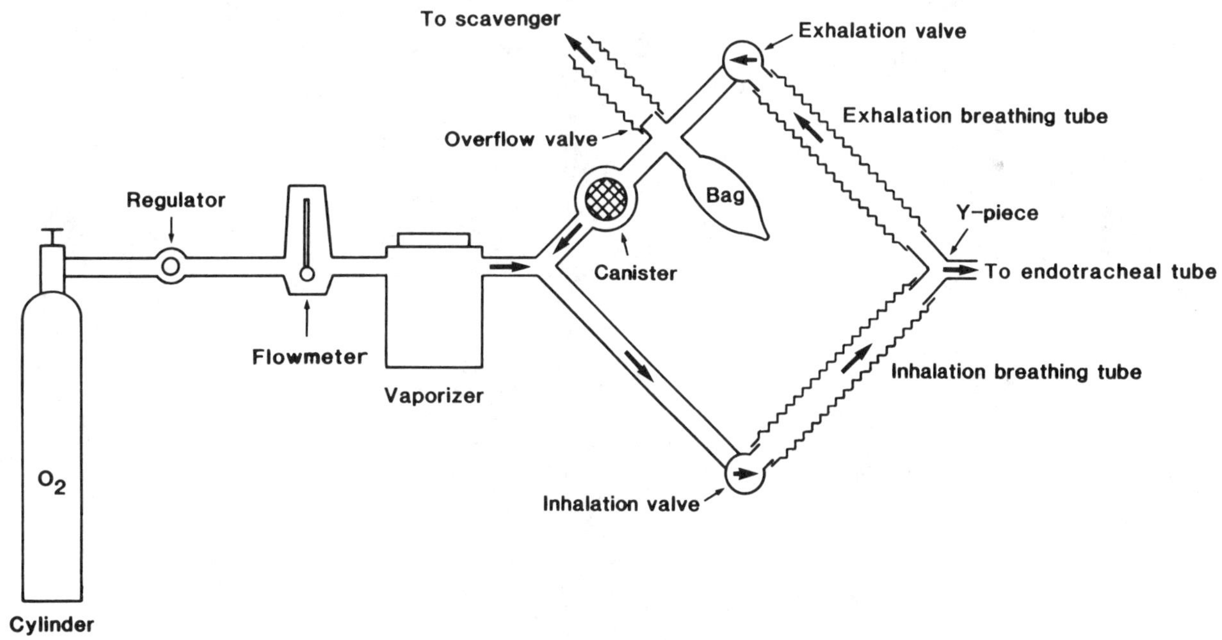

Figure 14.14. Diagram of the relationship of an out of the system precision vaporizer to the various components of an anesthetic machine and a circle breathing system (Biomedical Learning Resources Center).

ether has been recommended to clean the wicks and eliminate the preservative from within the vaporizer (12).

In veterinary anesthesia, several vaporizers are used commonly, and a few of their characteristics deserve mention. Nonprecision vaporizers used in the system include the Ohio #8 (Ohio Medical Products, Madison, Wisconsin) (Fig. 14.12) and others (12). Such vaporizers should be used only for drugs that are low in potency (ether) or low in vapor pressure (methoxyflurane) and never for highly potent, highly volatile agents (halothane and isoflurane) (12). With nonprecision, in the system vaporizers, the inspired anesthetic concentration varies with the patient's respiratory minute volume, use of intermittent positive pressure ventilation, carrier gas flow rate, and changes in vaporizer temperature. At a given setting, increased spontaneous ventilation, intermittent positive pressure ventilation, and lower fresh gas flow increase the inspired anesthetic concentration. On the Ohio #8, the control lever is adjusted from 0, corresponding to no gas flow through the vaporization chamber, to 10, complete gas flow through the vaporization chamber. The precise concentration of anesthetic delivered by these vaporizers cannot be predicted because of the many factors affecting vaporizer output (13).

Precision vaporizers should be used for volative liquid anesthetics when possible. Several types are available and are in common use. "Automatic" vaporizers include the Tecs (Fraser Harlake, Inc., Orchard Park, New York), Vapor 19.1 (North American Drager, Telford, Pennsylvania), and Matics (Foregger, Air Products, Allentown, Pennsylvania), as well as other units. The new models are temperature, flow, and back-pressure compensated. They use temperature-sensitive devices to regulate flow through the vaporization chamber, and wicks are used to increase efficiency of vaporization (Fig. 14.15). The control dial setting for concentration and the vaporizer output are linear over a wide range of flow rates and temperatures. Older Tec vaporizers are not necessarily linear at all carrier gas flows. Consequently, the older Fluotec II was supplied with a calibration chart. In addition, older models may not be back-pressure compensated. Presently available automatic vaporizers are very reliable instruments, but they should be used only with the drug for which they were intended because they are agent-specific vaporizers. Dangerous concentrations of halothane and isoflurane may be delivered if they are delivered with methoxyflurane vaporizers. However, because of their comparable vapor pressures, halothane and isoflurane may be interchanged in their respective agent-specific vaporizers (5) with only minor variations in output from the setting on the concentration control dial (14).

The Vapor vaporizer (North American Drager), sometimes called semiautomatic, is a very accurate instrument. It is constructed of a large mass of copper as a heat sink to prevent excessive cooling during vaporization (11). The concentration dial must be manually adjusted to the temperature of the vaporizer and liquid between 16 and 28°C (Fig 14.16) (12). The unit is flow-compensated over a wide range and has a back-pressure compensation mechanism involving a long coiled tube at the inlet to the vaporization chamber (3).

Saturation vaporizers, including Copper Kettles (Foregger) and Verni-Trols (Ohio Medical Products) (5) are also precision units. These units are no longer being manufactured, but they are often available as used equipment and are functional. However, manual adjustments in flowrates are required to account for variations in both flow and temperature. These calculations (explained below) can be done by application of gas law principles, but a calculator or slide rule (Fig.

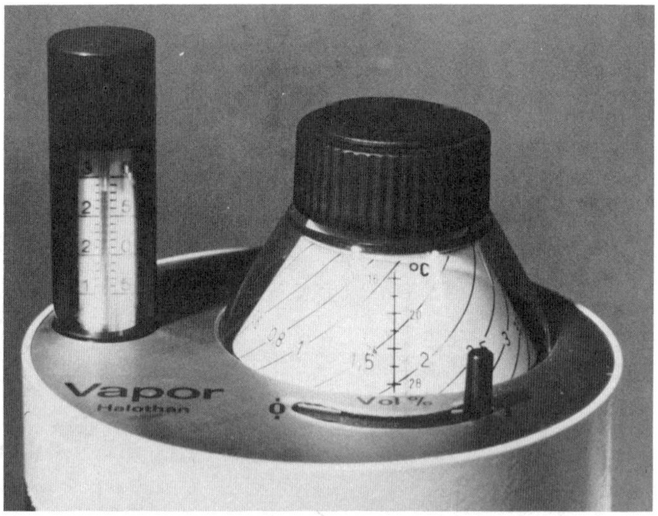

Figure 14.16. Controls on Vapor vaporizer showing the thermometer (*left*) for determining vaporizer temperature and the control dial (*right*) used to adjust the desired concentration line to the appropriate temperature (North American Drager, Telford, Pennsylvania).

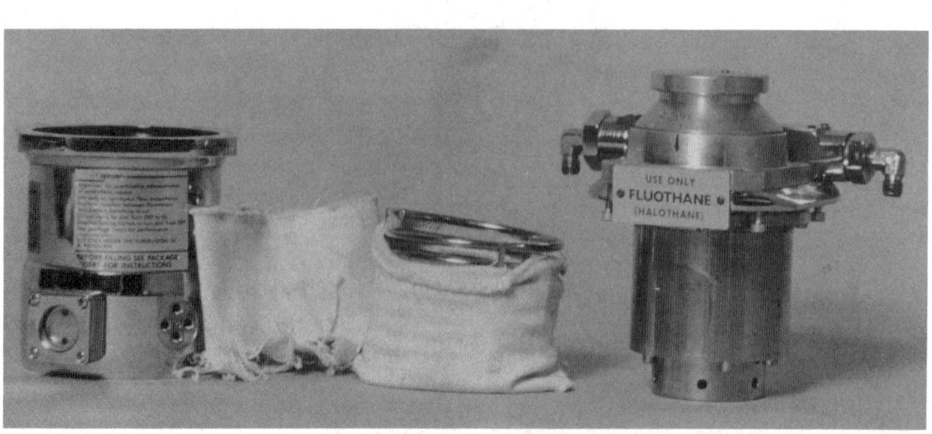

Figure 14.15. A partially disassembled Fluotec III showing the wicks used to increase the surface area for vaporization (Fraser Harlake, Orchard Park, New York).

14.17) is provided for that purpose with each vaporizer. Anesthetic machines with saturation vaporizers have two oxygen flowmeters (Fig. 14.18). One flowmeter routes all its oxygen through the vaporization chamber to be saturated with anesthetic, while the other by-

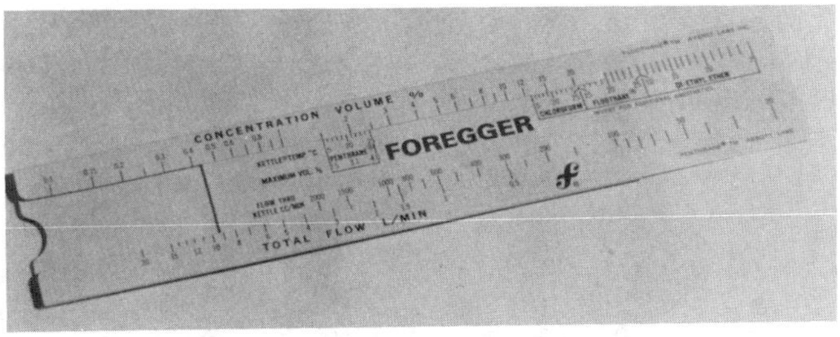

Figure 14.17. A slide rule for calculation of oxygen flows for an anesthetic machine with a Copper Kettle vaporizer. The rule can be used for several different anesthetics used at various flowrates over a range of temperatures (Foregger, Air Products, Allentown, Pennsylvania).

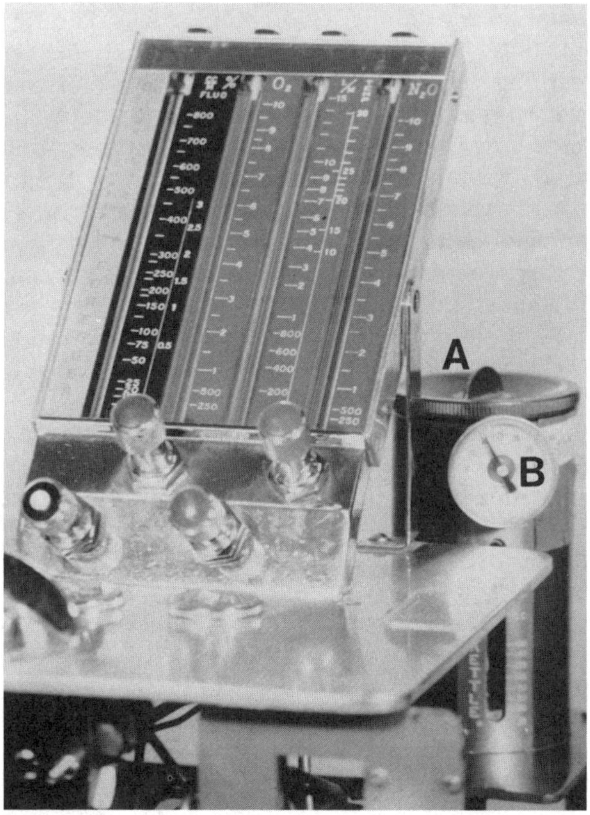

Figure 14.18. An illustration of a saturation vaporizer (Copper Kettle, Foregger, Air Products, Allentown, Pennsylvania) and its required flowmeters. The flow of oxygen through the vaporizer is metered by the flowmeter on the left (black control knob and scale). Bypass oxygen to meet patient and system needs is controlled by the two center flowmeters. Nitrous oxide is delivered by the two center flowmeters. Nitrous oxide is delivered via the flowmeter on the right. The vaporization chamber (*A*) of the vaporizer has a thermometer (*B*) for use in adjustment of flow according to temperature (Biomedical Learning Resources Center).

passes the vaporizer and supplies the oxygen needs of the patient. Both sources of gas combine in a mixing valve to achieve the proper anesthetic concentration before entering the breathing system. Saturation vaporizers are multipurpose and can be used with any volatile liquid anesthetic. They are constructed of copper or silicon bronze for thermostability; back-pressure compensation mechanisms are present on more recent models and can be fitted on older models.

An explanation of calculations for saturation vaporizers is in order. Saturation vaporizers produce an anesthetic concentration equal to the specific anesthetic's saturated vapor pressure, which depends on the temperature of the liquid anesthetic. Thus, if halothane's vapor pressure is 243 mm Hg at 20°C, 32% halothane will exit the vaporization chamber. This concentration must be diluted by gases that bypass the vaporizer to achieve a safe, appropriate concentration in the breathing system (5, 13). Appropriate calculations are needed to determine the required flowrates into the vaporizer and through bypass flowmeters. If a 100-pound patient is to be maintained with a total oxygen flow of 1.5 liters/min and a halothane concentration of 1.5%, then 22.5 ml/min of halothane vapor must reach the breathing system (1.5% · 1.5 liters = 22.5 ml) with 1477.5 ml/min of oxygen. Therefore, 47.8 ml of oxygen must enter the saturation vaporizer each minute to produce an output of 22.5 ml/min of halothane (22.5 ml = 32% · X, thus X = 70.3 ml and 70.3 ml − 22.5 ml = 47.8 ml). The bypass oxygen flow must equal (1500 ml/min − 70.3 ml/min) 1429.7 ml/min. In all calculations, the total gas flow to the patient must be considered, including O_2, N_2O, and vaporizer flows, in determination of anesthetic requirements. For example, if 50% N_2O was used in the example given above, total flow would equal 3 liters/min, and flow through the vaporizer must be doubled. Using similar computations for methoxyflurane at 20°C (vapor pressure = 23 mm Hg), a maximum vaporizer output of 3% can be predicted. Thus, with 1.5 liters of total fresh gas flow to the breathing system and a required maintenance concentration of 1%, 15 ml/min of methoxyflurane must be delivered to the breathing system. To deliver 15 ml/min of flow (15 ml = 3% X, thus X = 500 ml and 500 ml − 15 ml = 485 ml). Thus, 485 ml/min of O_2 must be delivered to the vaporization chamber to result in a total output of 500 ml/min including methoxyflurane. The bypass flow must then be equal to 1000 ml/min in order to achieve a total flow of 1.5 liters/min to the breathing system. Such calculations are eliminated by use of a slide rule, which accounts for vapor pressure, temperature, and total flowrate to give a value for flowrate into the saturation vaporizer. All of the vaporizers discussed can be used with safety if the limitations of each unit are recognized, if the proper drugs are used, and if proper care is exercised during use, storage, and movement.

Anesthetic Breathing Systems

Anesthetic breathing systems consist of components necessary to deliver anesthetic gases and O_2, remove CO_2, and usually allow application of intermittent positive pressure ventilation (IPPV). In a respiratory cycle, gas flow occurs during inhalation and exhalation. Gas flow can be very high during these short periods, and if the dimensions of the system are too small for the size of the patient, breathing systems can add significant resistance to respiration. Although numerous factors affect resistance, a major one is the diameter of the breathing tubes. Simply doubling the radius of the system decreases the resistance 16 times, whereas halving the length of the system only halves the resistance (12). Also, points in a system where gas flow must change directions or move through restrictions create turbulent flow and increase resistance. Therefore, within practical limits, the system should be of minimal length and maximal diameter with few bends or restrictions to gas flow (3). Generally, the smallest diameter in the entire breathing apparatus is the endotracheal tube or its adapter, which emphasizes the need for using the largest endotracheal tube that can be positioned safely.

Classification of anesthetic systems has been approached in many ways; one text lists classifications from eight different authors (3). All methods seem cumbersome and, in some instances, have created confusion rather than understanding. Therefore, references to anesthetic systems in the scientific literature should name and, if necessary, fully describe the specific system, state all gas flowrates, and relate the body weight or oxygen consumption of the patient (15). Even the terms "rebreathing" or "nonbreathing," "adult" or "pediatric," and "closed," "semiclosed," "semiopen," or "open" are not exclusive. Their meanings vary with fresh gas flowrates, system volumes and diameters, and the patients for which they are used. Therefore, this discussion will include references to specific systems, relating guidelines for the use of each in various veterinary patients. The above terms will be used only as common usage dictates.

Elimination of carbon dioxide, mechanisms for maintaining proper direction of gas flow, the method for providing artificial ventilation, fresh gas flow requirements, and the size of patients appropriate for a particular system are important for each system. Each system has appropriate applications and can be used efficiently in certain patients.

Circle Systems

Circle systems, commonly classified as rebreathing systems, are regularly used in veterinary patients. There are pediatric, standard adult (small animal), and large animal circles. Pediatric circles are appropriate for patients weighing less than 6.8 kg (15 lb), standard adult circles for patients between 6.8 kg and 135 kg (300 lb), and large animal circles for larger patients. These divisions are somewhat arbitrary, and slight variations in application can be made if good judgement is exercised regarding flowrates, duration of anesthesia, type of ventilation, and size of the CO_2 absorbent canister.

Circle systems are called circles because gases move in one direction through the system and back to the patient after chemical removal of carbon dioxide. A complete circle can be traced as exhaled gases move from the patient into the Y-piece through the exhalation breathing tube, the exhalation one-way valve, the CO_2 absorbent canister, the inhalation one-way valve, and the inhalation breathing tube to return to Y-piece and the patient (Figs. 14.13 and 14.14). Sizes of some of these components are listed in Table 14.13. The Y-piece, constructed of metal or plastic, is a connector that joins to the endotracheal tube adapter and to the inhalation and exhalation breathing tubes. The Y-piece contributes to the system's mechanical deadspace. Breathing tubes, usually made of rubber or plastic, serve as flexible, low resistance conduits between the Y-piece and the one-way valves. Corrugations are present to prevent kinking and obstructions. Breathing tubes contribute to the length and volume of the system, thus being sources of resistance and causes for increased patient inspiratory effort, but they do not contribute to mechanical deadspace if the one-way valves function properly. The one-way or unidirectional valves (Fig. 14.19) are paired and keep gases moving in only one direction within the system, away from the patient on the exhalation side and toward the patient on the inhalation side. Gases enter a one-way valve from below the disc valve, raise the disc, and pass under the clear plastic dome to reach either the canister (exhalation valve) or the inhalation breathing tube (inhalation valve). Such valves are usually attached to the canister, but in some older systems one-way valves have been located within the Y-piece. The Y-piece location is more likely to be associated with valve sticking, increased resistance, or incompetence. Valves are a source of resistance and should be inspected and cleaned regularly to assure proper function. The CO_2 absorbent canister is located between the one-way valves and is on the side of the circle opposite the patient. It holds the chemical required for absorption of CO_2 from exhaled gases. The most economical use of absorbent is in canisters divided in half to allow one portion of the absorbent to be completely used before it is discarded (3). The plastic canister should contain an airspace between chemical granules equal to or greater than the maximum tidal volume of the patient. The height:width ratio should be 1:1 (12).

Table 14.3
Approximate Sizes of Various Components of Circle Systems[a]

Circle System Component	Pediatric Circle	Adult Circle	Large Animal Circle
Y-piece endotracheal tube connector (i.d.)	15 mm	15 mm	2.5–5 cm (1–2 inches)
Y-piece endotracheal tube connector (o.d.)	Approximately 16 mm	22 mm	5.4 cm (2⅛ inches)
Y-piece breathing tube connectors (i.d.)	15 mm	15–22 mm	4.8–5 cm (1⅞–2 inches)
Y-piece breathing tube connectors (o.d.)	Approximately 16 mm	22 mm	5.4 cm (2⅛ inches)
Breathing tubes (i.d.)	15 mm	22 mm	Approximately 5 cm (Approximately 2 inches)
One-way valves—breathing tube connectors (o.d.)	Approximately 15 mm	22 mm	Approximately 5.4 cm (Approximately 2⅛ inches)
Reservoir bag mount	15 mm	22 mm	Approximately 5.4 cm (Approximately 2⅛ inches)
Reservoir bag, usual sizes	0.5–1 liter	1–5 liters	15–30 liters

[a] Slight variations in sizes will be noted with differences in manufacturer and materials used.

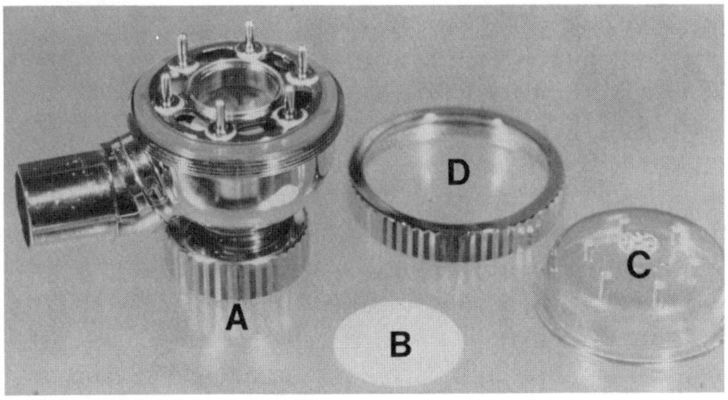

Figure 14.19. A one-way or unidirectional dome valve showing the annular seat between the pin-shaped disc guides on the main body (*A*) of the valve, the white disc valve (*B*), and the clear plastic dome (*C*) next to the threaded ring (*D*) for securing the dome (North American Drager, Telford, Pennsylvania).

Exhaled gases may enter the canister from the top or bottom, depending on the manufacturer, and a canister may have baffles or annular rings to move gases toward the center of the canister to minimize the "wall effect" (lower resistance near the canister wall that may lead to channeling of gases and inefficient absorption of CO_2). In the case of a canister with an annular ring, an entrance diameter smaller than the total diameter of the canister, gases disperse more equally through the absorbent to reduce the wall effect. The most efficient canisters do not have an internal tube for gas return because this enhances the wall effect and channeling.

Other components of a circle system include a fresh gas inlet, an overflow valve, and a reservoir bag. The fresh gas inlet is the point at which gases from the common gas outlet of the anesthetic machine enter the circle system, usually connected through a small diameter rubber hose. The fresh gas inlet is attached to the canister near the inhalation one-way valve or may directly enter the inhalation one-way valve. Such positioning on the inhalation side controls dilution of fresh gases, prevents flushing of chemical dust from the canister toward the patient, and reduces elimination of fresh gases through the overflow valve. The overflow or "pop-off" valve is designed to prevent excessive buildup of pressure within the circle system, and it allows rapid elimination of the system's contents in emergency situations when 100% O_2 is indicated. An overflow valve should be adjusted to allow escape of gases at pressures of 1 to 2 cm H_2O except when the intent of the operator is to use positive pressure ventilation. Gases from the overflow valve should be evacuated from the immediate working area through a scavenging system (Fig. 14.20). Several types of overflow valves are available, but those that are spring-loaded or function with a variable orifice due to movable plates are commonly used. The overflow valve can be located in various places, but it is most convenient and conservative with CO_2 absorbent if located between the exhalation valve and the canister. This location also limits elimination of fresh gases during exhalation, and they are used to meet the peak inspiratory flowrate demands of the patient; these demands are normally in excess of the fresh gas inflow. The bag serves as a means for application of intermittent positive pressure ventilation, and bag excursions during spontaneous breathing allow monitoring or respiratory rate and rough estimations of tidal volume. The usual recommendation for a reservoir bag size is six times tidal volume. A 20-liter bag has been recommended for the average adult horse (12). The appropriate bag size should be chosen because an excessively large bag is more difficult to use for ventilation and is a less

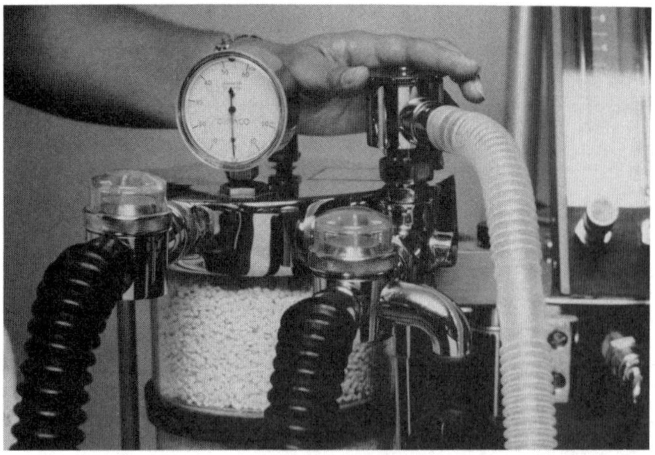

Figure 14.20. An overflow valve being adjusted after it was closed during assisted patient ventilation. Gases enter the valve from the bottom and are discharged through the white plastic scavenger tubing to be eliminated from the operating room (Dupaco, San Marcos, California).

effective monitor; a bag that is too small is less distensible, may be an inadequate reservoir, and may lead to pressure elevation during exhalation. An excessively large bag also lengthens the time for changes in anesthetic concentration from an out-of-system vaporizer to create similar concentrations in the system. Finally, a manometer, usually attached to the canister, but occasionally on the inhalation side of the circle (Fig. 14.21), is a useful addition to a circle system to evaluate pressure, especially during intermittent positive pressure ventilation and sighing of the patient.

Chemical CO_2 elimination is an integral part of a circle system's function. Depending on fresh gas flowrate, all or part of the exhaled CO_2 may be eliminated by chemical absorption. If the flowrate approaches the O_2 consumption of the patient, essentially all of the exhaled CO_2 will be chemically neutralized. Advantages of chemical absorption of CO_2 relate to the lower fresh gas flows that can be used. Less anesthetic gases are required, and cost is reduced. There is less chance for operating room pollution because less gas moves through the overflow valve. Finally, less heat and moisture from exhaled gases are lost through the overflow.

Soda lime and barium hydroxide lime are the two CO_2 absorbents commonly used, and the primary component by weight of each is calcium hydroxide. Small amounts of sodium and potassium hydroxide in soda lime activate the reaction, and silica is added to give hardness to the granules, thereby decreasing formation of alkaline dust that can be damaging to the patient if inhaled. Barium hydroxide lime granules, inherently hard due to bound water molecules, do not require silica (1). A specific water content of 14 to 19% is required in soda lime for optimal performance. However, humidity in exhaled gases does not affect the reaction (3). Water formed during granule reactions with CO_2 can be useful in humidifying dry gases from the fresh gas inlet before they are inhaled. A summarization of the chemical reactions of these absorbents is given in Table 14.4. On the basis of the reactions, unused absorbent granules (soft $Ca(OH)_2$) and used granules (hard $CaCO_3$) can be differentiated. Heat can be detected in an active canister due to the exothermic reaction, especially in large animals. Finally pH indicators added to the absorbents show color changes as reactions proceed. This color change will disappear during storage of the canister but will quickly reappear it if is used again. The amount of CO_2 absorption is about 26 liters/100 g, but it may be less efficient depending on canister design and packing. Absorbent granule size is 4 to 8 mesh and represents a compromise between absorptive activity and air flow resistance (1). Proper packing of a canister with granules is important to prevent preferential passage of gases over a single pathway in the canister. Gentle shaking of the canister upon filling it with an absorbent will avoid loose packing and reduce channeling. Packing too tightly may increase resistance to ventilation.

Fresh gas flowrates into a circle system vary with personal preference. Classically, circle systems have been called "closed" or "semiclosed." Although confusing, these terms are so ingrained in the literature that they deserve some consideration. These terms relate to flowrate specifically compared to the system and the patient's uptake of gases (oxygen and anesthetic gases), and they do not lend information about the patency of the circle's overflow valve, although some gases must be eliminated periodically with semiclosed circle flowrates.

Anesthesia with a closed circle system is "a form of low flow anesthesia in which the fresh gas inflow equals the uptake of anesthetic gases and oxygen by the patient and the system (3). In practice, one must observe the system and adjust flowrates to meet patient needs when using a closed system. Roughly, approximation of a patient's O_2 consumption gives a guideline for fresh gas flowrate (e.g., 11 ml/kg/min in a dog or 2.2 ml/kg/min in a horse). However, minimum flowrates for vaporizers must be taken into account. With such low flow systems, continuous O_2 monitoring is absolutely essential if N_2O is added to inspired gases. With closed systems, denitrogenation or emptying the

Table 14.4
Chemical Reactions of Absorbents with Carbon Dioxide

1. $CO_2 + H_2O \rightarrow H_2CO_3$
2. Barium hydroxide lime intermediate reaction (rapid):
   $H_2CO_3 + Ba(OH_2) \rightarrow BaCO_3 + 2\ H_2O + HEAT$
   Soda lime intermediate reaction (rapid):
   $H_2CO_3 + NaOH \rightarrow Na_2CO_3 + 2\ H_2O + HEAT$
3. $H_2CO_3 + Ca(OH)_2 \rightarrow CaCO_3 + 2\ H_2O + HEAT$

reservoir bag through the overflow and refilling the system with fresh gas should be done two to four times during the first 15 minutes of anesthesia and each 30 minutes thereafter to prevent nitrogen from the patient's exhaled gases from diluting O_2 in the system (5, 17). Such a system is totally dependent on chemical CO_2 absorption and requires longer to alter inspired anesthetic concentration when using out-of-system vaporizers. Closed circle systems are more economical, retain more heat and humidity, and are less likely to produce operating room pollution than are other systems. The economic aspects of low flow techniques for veterinary patients have been discussed recently (18, 19).

When used with higher flowrates (greater than the patient and system's metabolism and absorption of O_2 and anesthetic), a circle is defined as "semiclosed." Therefore, excess gases must be eliminated, usually through the overflow valve. Personal preference dictates the choice of flowrate, but a common guideline is the patient's O_2 consumption times three. For example, if O_2 consumption in a dog is approximately 11 ml/kg/min, fresh gas flow would be 33 ml/kg/min. Use of N_2O would require additional gas flow. If 50% N_2O is desired, O_2 flow would equal 33 ml/kg/min and N_2O flow would equal 33 ml/kg/min, with a total fresh gas flow of 66 ml/kg/min. With a semiclosed circle, nitrogen accumulation within the system leading to dilution of O_2 is not significant because gases are regularly eliminated through the overflow and are replaced through the fresh gas inflow. N_2O can be used safely without continuous in-line oxygen monitoring, the inspired anesthetic concentrations can be altered rather quickly, and dependency on chemical CO_2 absorption is not absolute because CO_2 is partially eliminated through the overflow valve. Scavenging of these higher flow gases is very important. Retention of heat and humidity within the system is less, and the system is less economical.

When using a circle system, a nonprecision, low resistance vaporizer may be located in the system (Fig. 14.13) or a precision, high resistance unit may be located out of the system (Fig. 14.14). Precision vaporizers are much more desirable, as explained previously. With an out of the system vaporizer, the concentration dial setting gives a slightly high estimate of the inspired anesthetic concentration (some anesthetic is absorbed by the rubber and plastic components of the circle); therefore, the anesthetic's minimum alveolar concentration value can be used as a guide to anesthetic requirements of the patient. Increasing the fresh gas flow will increase inspired concentration of anesthetic, and assisted or controlled ventilation can be used without affecting vaporizer output, assuming that the precision vaporizer is back-pressure compensated. With such a vaporizer arrangement, low flowrate can be used with greater safety than with in the system vaporizers (13). However, anesthetic concentrations will rise in any closed system as the patient's tissues decrease anesthetic uptake with time.

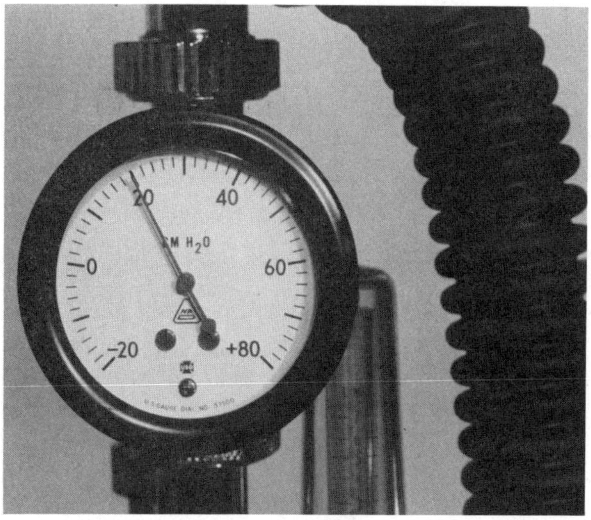

Figure 14.21. A manometer of a circle breathing system during application of intermittent positive pressure breathing. An inspiratory pressure of 20 cm H_2O has been attained (North American Drazer, Telford, Pennsylvania).

With in the system vaporizers, especially with low fresh gas flowrates, increases in spontaneous or manual ventilation may drastically increase anesthetic concentration in the circle. Lower fresh gas flows tend to result in higher anesthetic levels in the system. Thus, economy is achieved at the risk of potentially dangerous anesthetic concentrations (13). Use of low flow technique with an in the system vaporizer requires intensive patient and system monitoring for acceptable safety.

To-and-Fro Breathing Systems

A to-and-fro breathing system (Fig. 14.22) involves a CO_2 absorbent canister placed between an endotracheal tube adapter and a reservoir bag. An overflow valve and a fresh gas inlet are present between the canister and the endotracheal tube adapter. A to-and-fro system can be used for patients of various sizes if appropriately sized canisters are available (13). Such a system designed especially for large animals has been described (12). In a to-and-fro system, gases pass back and forth through the absorbent canister during inhalation and exhalation. This double passage of gases allows very efficient CO_2 removal. Flowrates should be similar to those used for circle systems. If low flowrates are used (approximately equal to the patient's oxygen consumption), the removal of CO_2 is totally by chemical means. If higher flowrates are used (approx-

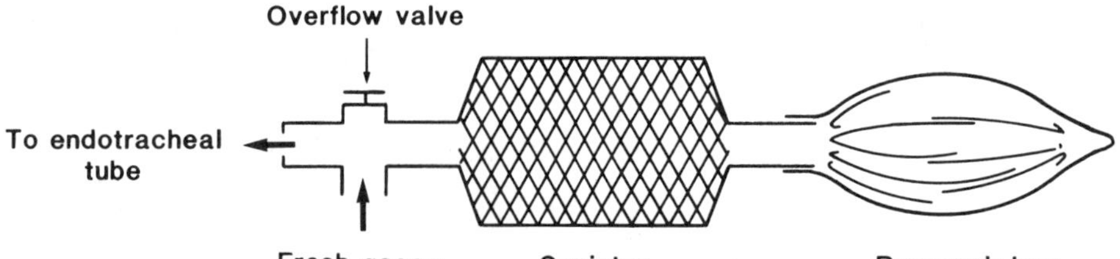

Figure 14.22. Diagram of a to-and-fro breathing system illustrating its usual component parts (Biomedical Learning Resources Center).

imately three times oxygen consumption), some CO_2 will escape through the overflow valve. Low resistance to ventilation and simplicity are the primary advantages of the system. Portability is an advantage for use of the system in the field or stall (12). Disadvantages of the system include heat accumulation due to the proximity of the endotracheal tube to the exothermic soda lime-CO_2 reaction, potential for inhalation of absorbent dust, channeling of gases through the canister leading to inefficient CO_2 absorption, an increase in canister deadspace as absorbent is used, and the inconvenience of placing a canister in close proximity to the patient's head. As with circle rebreathing systems, denitrogenation of the system should be considered, especially if low fresh gas flowrates are used.

Mapleson Systems and Systems with Nonrebreathing Valves

The Mapleson system and systems with nonrebreathing valves are primarily used for pediatric patients in human anesthesia, and they are usually preferred for smaller veterinary patients weighing less than 6.8 kg (20), with a few exceptions to be noted below. For convenience, these systems have been called "nonrebreathing systems" as a group, but this is technically incorrect. The degree of rebreathing of exhaled gases is dependent on the fresh gas flowrate and on the proper function of valves in some systems. Only the commonly used or representative types of these systems will be discussed.

In one study comparing cardiopulmonary variables in cats maintained with halothane using a pediatric circle, an adult circle, and an Ayre's T-piece system, no statistically significant differences were noted. However, respiratory rate in the adult circle group remained above the rates of the other groups, possibly indicating increased respiratory effort to maintain $PaCO_2$ (21). In comparison to adult circle systems, the Mapleson and nonrebreathing valve systems offer some advantages (3). In general, they are simple and easy to use, are easily cleaned and sterilized, are light and compact, can be positioned for convenience, have minimal moving parts, are relatively inexpensive, impart less resistance to respiration, do not require CO_2 absorbents, have minimal deadspace, and allow the concentration of anesthetic in the inspired mixture to remain closer to that coming from the vaporizer. Disadvantages of these systems include the large gas flow requirement (decreased economy), potential for valve malfunction in systems with valves, need for both hands to assist or control ventilation, requirement in valved systems for frequent adjustments in fresh gas flow, and significant heat and humidity loss with the high gas flows.

A Magill system (Fig. 14.23) is classified as Mapleson A and is characterized by an overflow valve near the patient and a corrugated tube separating the valve from a reservoir bag. Fresh gas inflow is into the reservoir bag. Continuous fresh gas inflow washes CO_2-rich gases from the system through the overflow valve, a very efficient system during spontaneous ventilation. Use of the system with assisted or controlled ventilation usually results in some rebreathing of expired gases. Fresh gas inflow should be approximately equal to the patient's minute volume (22), with flows less than 0.7 of minute volume leading to some rebreathing (3). If N_2O is used, it should be calculated as a part of the fresh gas inflow into the system. The volume of the corruguated tubing between the patient and the reservoir bag should be equal to the patient's tidal volume. Because of the location of the overflow valve, the system is more cumbersome than some of the other pediatric systems when applying IPPV.

A Bain coaxial system (Figs. 14.24 and 14.25) is classified as a modified Mapleson D system and is designed as a tube within a tube (23). The internal tube (0.7 mm inner diameter (i.d.)) carries fresh gases to the patient, opening near the endotracheal tube adapter (Fig. 14.26), which reduces dead space. The external tube (22 mm i.d.) carries gases away from the patient. The overflow port and reservoir bag are located away from the patient. The patient end of the system will accept an endotracheal adapter (15 mm i.d.) or a mask (22 mm outer diameter (o.d.)). In a Bain system, fresh gas inflow less than two to three times the minute volume will result in some rebreathing of CO_2. During spontaneous ventilation, one source recommends use

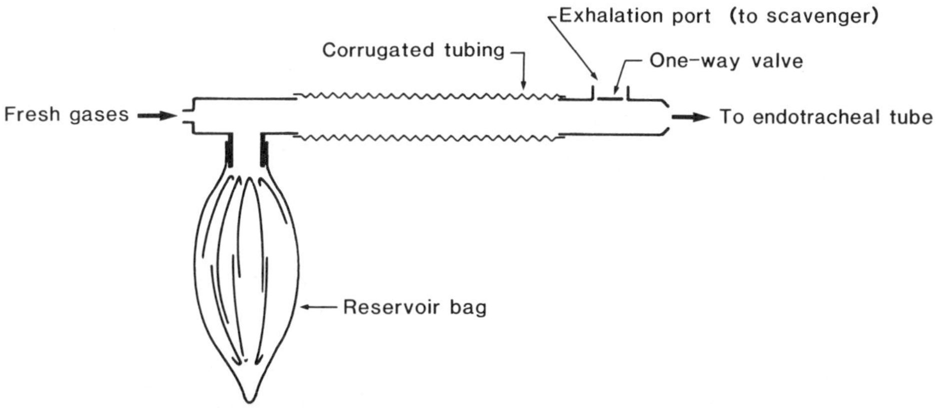

Figure 14.23. A diagram of a Magill system with the basic components illustrated (Biomedical Learning Resources Center).

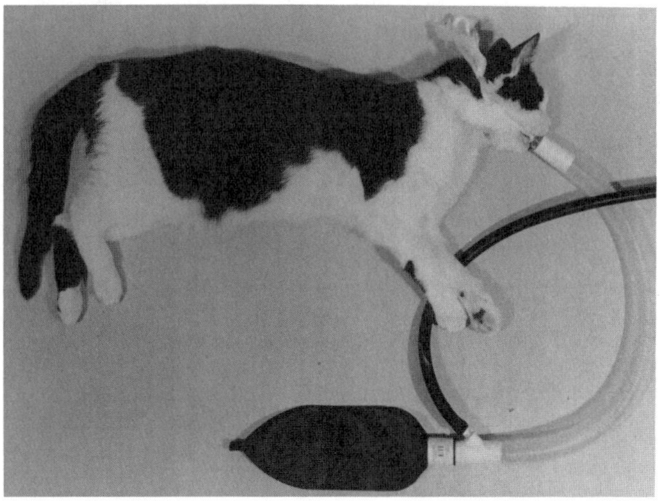

Figure 14.24. A Bain coaxial system being used for maintenance of halothane anesthesia in a cat. The fresh gas inflow enters the system near the reservoir bag, being conducted to the patient end of the system through a tube running inside the corrugated outer tube. Exhaled gases move from the animal through the corrugated tubing to the reservoir bag and out the open end of the bag. These excess gases should be scavenged appropriately (Biomedical Learning Resources Center).

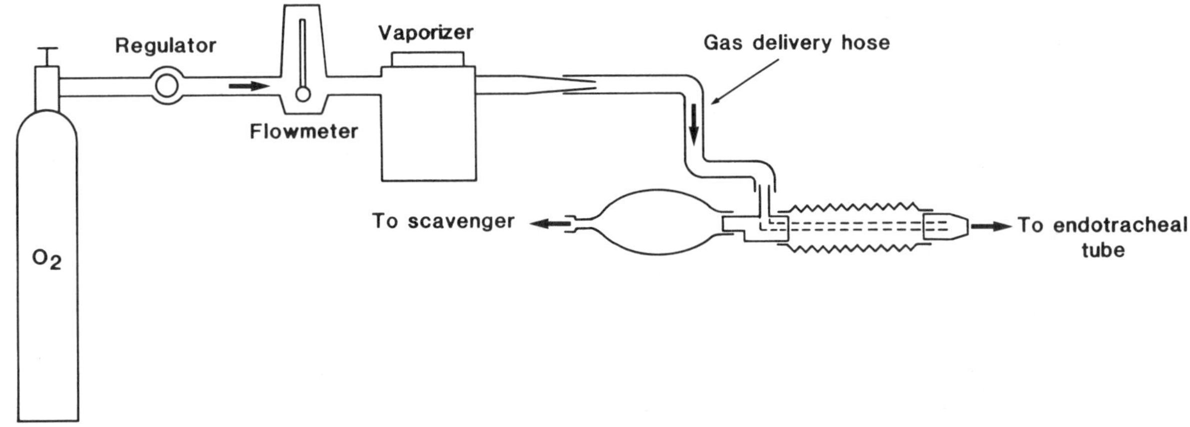

Figure 14.25. Diagram of a Bain coaxial system's attachment to an anesthetic machine. Like other nonrebreathing systems, the Bain unit connects immediately downstream from the vaporizer (Biomedical Learning Resources Center).

of a Bain system at 200 to 300 ml/kg/min (1). For veterinary patients, flowrates of 100 to 130 ml/kg/min have been recommended, with a minimal flow of 500 ml/min and the suggestion for use of higher flows (two to three times minute volume) in obviously hypoventilating patients (24). With controlled ventilation, 100 ml/kg/min is an adequate flowrate for fresh gases. During spontaneous ventilation, a Mapleson D system has been shown to function identically to a Mapleson F system (3). The tube within a tube design is supposed to be effective in reducing heat and water loss from this system (3). This author generally uses the Bain system like a Mapleson F system. Bain systems can be used in patients larger than 6.8 kg, with one study reporting clinical use in dogs weighing up to 35.5 kg (24).

Ayre's T-piece (Figs. 14.27 and 14.28) and Norman mask elbow (Figs. 14.27 and 14.29) systems are Mapleson F systems if they are equipped with an expiratory limb and a reservoir bag (3). They are E systems if no reservoir bag is present. An Ayre's T-piece is a T-shaped tube with an internal diameter of 1 cm. Fresh

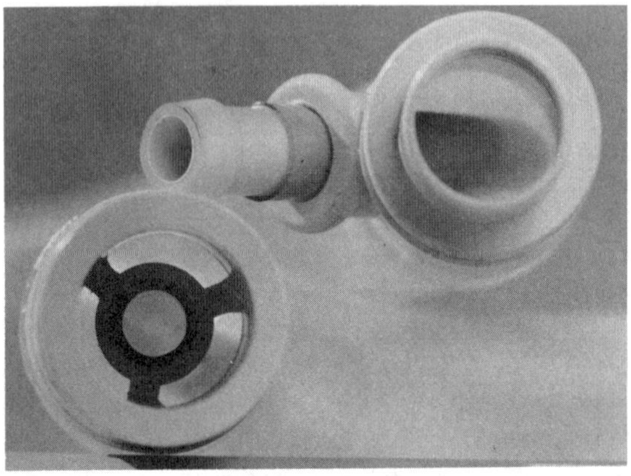

Figure 14.26. The two ends of a Bain coaxial system showing the location for the reservoir bag attachment (*top right*) and for patient/endotracheal tube attachment (*bottom left*). Fresh gases enter at the reservoir end (Y-connection) and move through the small inner tube to the patient end of the system (triangular supports) (Biomedical Learning Resources Center).

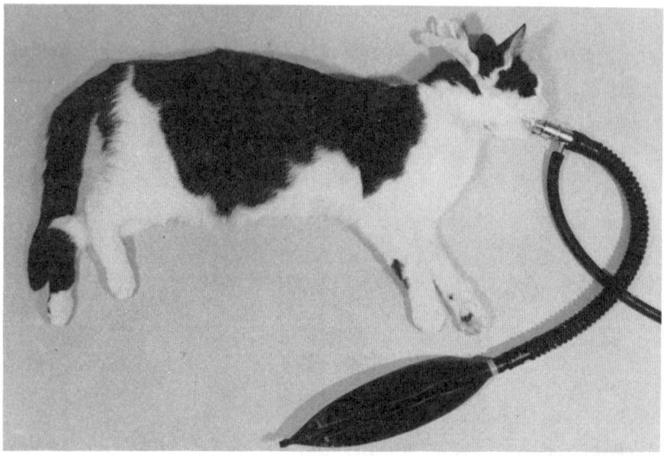

Figure 14.28. An Ayre's T-piece system being used for maintenance of halothane anesthesia in a cat. The fresh gas inflow enters the system perpendicular to the flow of gases during inhalation and exhalation. Exhaled gas flows from the patient through the corrugated tubing to the reservoir bag and out the open end of the bag. These excess gases should be appropriately scavenged (Biomedical Learning Resources Center).

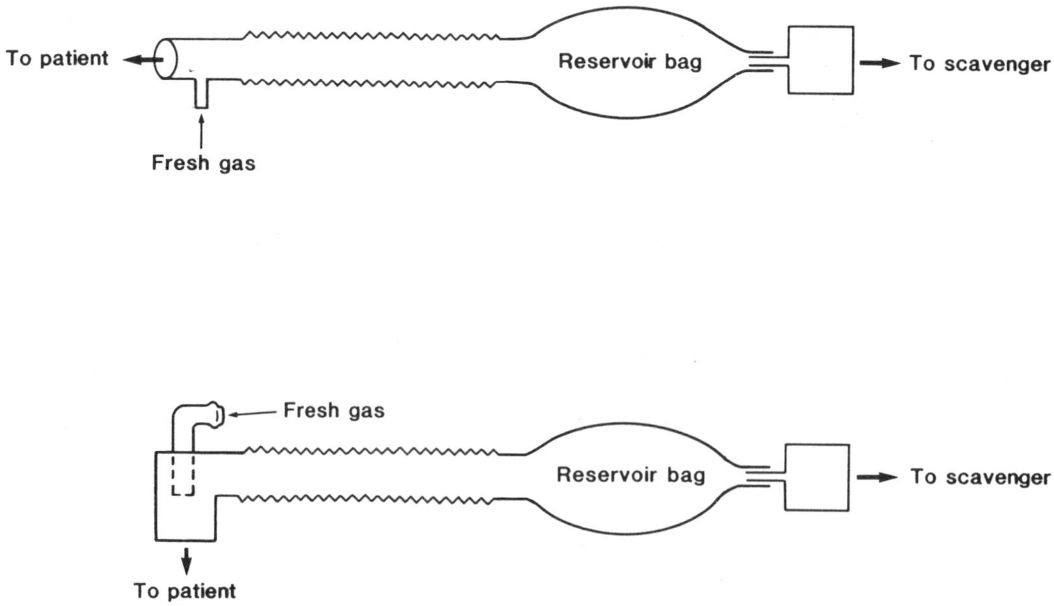

Figure 14.27. Diagrams of an Ayre's T-piece system (*top*) and a Norman mask elbow system (*bottom*) illustrating sites for endotracheal tube and patient attachment, fresh gas sources, reservoir bag locations, and points for exit of exhaled gases to a scavenger system. Note the difference in the entry of fresh gas flow into each system (Biomedical Learning Resources Center).

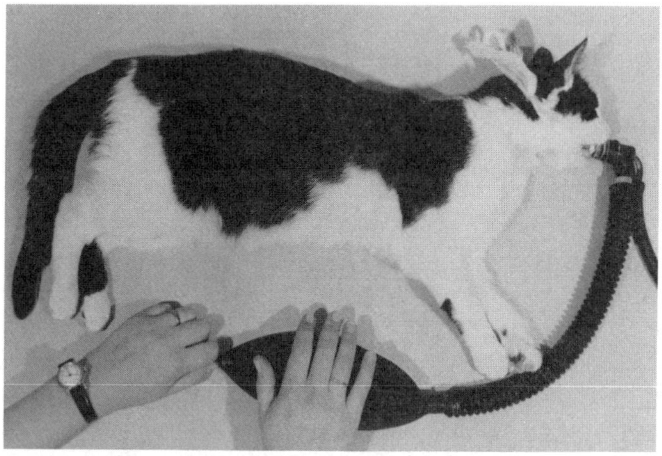

Figure 14.29. A Norman mask elbow system being used for maintenance of halothane anesthesia in a cat. Fresh gas inflow enters the system from the small tube (*right*) and flows parallel to inhalation through the corrugated tube to the reservoir bag and out the open end of the reservoir bag. As shown, IPPV can be applied by occluding the open end of the bag, allowing the bag to fill slightly, and compressing the bag until an adequate tidal volume is produced (Biomedical Learning Resources Center).

gas enters the tube from the side, perpendicular to the direction of gas flow during inhalation and exhalation (Fig. 14.27). One end of the tube attaches to an endotracheal tube adapter, and a Mapleson F system, the other end is attached to an expiratory arm which is connected to a reservoir bag. The reservoir bag is vented for escape of excess gases. Technically, an Ayre's T-piece with expiratory tube and reservoir is a Ree's modification of an Ayre's T-piece or a Jackson-Ree's system (3). During spontaneous ventilation, fresh gas flows toward the patient during inspiration and toward the reservoir during exhalation and prior to the next inspiration. Gas flow direction is determined by the path of least resistance. Inspiratory flow demands in excess of the fresh gas flow presumably are met by moving gases to the patient from the expiratory tube and the reservoir. During exhalation and before inspiration, the high gas flow clears exhaled gases from the expiratory tube. Such a system should have an internal diameter of at least 1 cm to minimize resistance. Generally, two to three times the patient's minute ventilation is recommended to prevent CO_2 rebreathing, and this author uses 440 to 660 ml/kg/min of total fresh gas flow for small dogs and cats. If N_2O is used, the desired concentration is calculated using N_2O as a portion of the total fresh gas flow.

Norman mask elbow systems are similar to Ayre's T-piece systems in design. However, the direction of gas flow into the system is parallel to inhalation-exhalation gas flow (Fig. 14.27). The orifice for fresh gas flow is located in the center of the endotracheal tube end of the system. It reduces dead space slightly more than the Ayre's T-piece system. Also, the endotracheal adapter end of the elbow will accept a mask (22 mm o.d.). Both systems should be used with similar flowrates, exhalation tube volumes, and reservoirs. Controlled ventilation can be used with either system by closing the overflow port and compressing the reservoir bag. To prevent rebreathing during controlled ventilation using a reservoir bag, the expiratory tube should have a greater volume than the patient's tidal volume.

Different guidelines for flow, ventilation, and system volumes may be appropriate if other T-piece modifications are used. For example, the original Ayre's T-piece without an expiratory tube required four to five times the minute volume to prevent a significant amount of inhalation of room air. Also, without a reservoir bag and with an exhalation tube volume of about one-third of the patient's tidal volume, rebreathing of exhaled gases is unlikely at fresh gas flowrates of 1.5 to 2 times minute volume. The Ayre's T-piece and Norman elbow systems described are not used for larger patients because the high flowrates required create excessive resistance to ventilation. However, larger diameter systems have been adapted for use in adults (3).

A Stephens-Slater system (Figs. 14.30 and 14.31) is

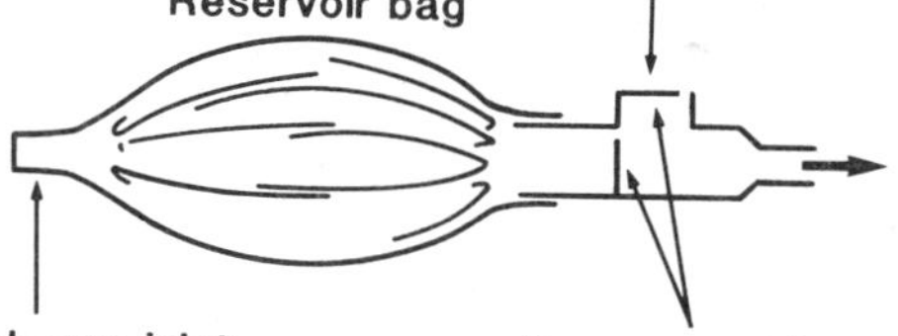

Figure 14.30. Diagram of a Stephens-Slater system illustrating various components in the valved nonrebreathing system (Biomedical Learning Resources Center).

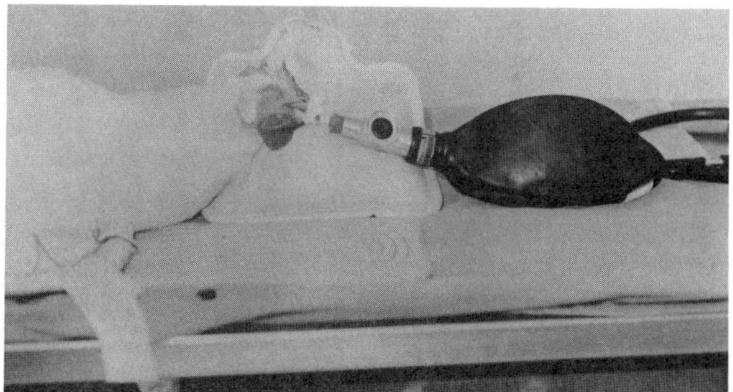

Figure 14.31. A Stephens-Slater system being used for maintenance of halothane anesthesia in a chicken. Fresh gas inflow enters the system through the end of the reservoir bag and passes through the inhalation one-way valve (not seen) and into the patient's respiratory system. Exhaled gases flow from the patient through the black rubber valve in the center of the metal Stephens-Slater body (Biomedical Learning Resources Center).

a nonrebreathing unit employing two one-way valves, one allowing inhalation from a reservoir bag and a second allowing exhalation into the atmosphere or into a scavenger system. The valves usually have rubber or plastic flaps, and the main body of the unit is metal. A raised drapery guard protects the exhalation valve from inadvertent occlusion. Because the valves are small and lightweight, they offer little resistance to ventilation, and the size and design of the system limits dead space. Fresh gases enter the system through the reservoir bag and move toward the patient. The total flow of fresh gases is generally equal to the patient's respiratory minute volume (3, 13) or approximately 220 ml/kg/min as a guideline. If N_2O is used, it is calculated as a part of this total fresh gas flow. This system is more cumbersome than others such as the Bain, and it must be monitored regularly to avoid excessive or inadequate filling of the reservoir bag. Collapse of the reservoir may result in inadequate tidal volume, reduced oxygenation, or inadequate supply of anesthetic. Positive pressure ventilation is applied by manually closing the exhalation valve and compressing the reservoir. Other nonrebreathing valves such as the Digby-Leigh, Ambu, and Fink work similarly.

The Mapleson and nonrebreathing valve systems must receive O_2 and anesthetic gases from an anesthetic machine by their attachment at the common gas outlet (Fig. 14.25). These systems perform the same functions as a circle system, and attachments of the pediatric systems to machines have been described (25).

Masks and Closed Containers

Closed containers (Fig. 14.32) are commonly used for inhalation inductions in small veterinary patients (5, 25). The primary advantage is the lack of need for patient restraint; it is thus particularly useful in cats and laboratory species. Closed containers also can be used for birds, puppies, and small dogs. In aggressive patients, the chamber can be placed over the patient in its cage. Most containers are constructed of glass or clear plastic that allows close observation of the patient during induction. This is particularly important because airway obstruction is possible. To prevent injury should excitement occur, the chamber should be no larger than necessary, but the animal should be able to lie in lateral recumbency without having to flex the neck and possibly impair ventilation (Fig. 14.32). Excess chamber volume will slow the rise in anesthetic concentration and the onset of induction. As soon as the patient is induced and manageable, the induction should be completed by mask, and endotracheal intubation should be accomplished.

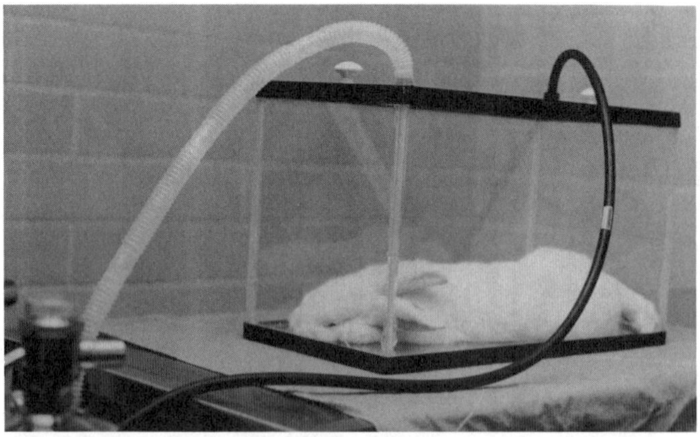

Figure 14.32. A closed container being used for induction of halothane anesthesia in a rabbit. A high fresh gas inflow (5 liters/min) enters the container through the black rubber hose. A low pressure scavenger system (white corrugated tubing) takes excessive gases from the container. This rabbit is ready to be removed from the container for completion of the induction by masking (Biomedical Learning Resources Center).

For chamber inductions, 5 liters/minute are used for total fresh gas inflow. Patients are usually preoxygenated for about 5 minutes; then induction is begun. An inhalation anesthetic, such as halothane, is administered in O_2 or in O_2 plus N_2O. During induction of an adult cat, the halothane concentration is elevated at 0.5% increments approximately every 10 seconds until 4% is reached. Similarly, isoflurane at approximately 5% or methoxyflurane at 3% can be used. Unless N_2O is contraindicated, it can effectively speed induction in concentrations of 60 to 70%. For smaller chambers, total flow requirements are reduced (25). Some rebreathing must occur, but use of high flowrates should minimize effects on $PaCO_2$.

Use of chamber inductions generally causes considerable pollution of room air with anesthetic gases unless one works under a vented hood. Low pressure scavenging systems are useful and decrease loss of gas into ambient air (Fig. 14.32). However, when the patient is removed from the container, some pollution will occur.

Mask inductions can be done using concentrations and flowrates similar to those for closed containers; masks are used to complete inductions started in closed containers. A mask induction is best performed in patients premedicated with a tranquilizer or other depressant medication, although they can be done smoothly in many unpremedicated patients (Fig. 14.33). A mask should be used with an anesthetic system appropriate for the patient so that a reservoir is present to meet the patient's inspiratory flowrate demands if those demands happen to exceed the fresh gas flowrate (Fig. 14.33). In addition, excess flow at times other than inspiration can be scavenged from an overflow valve on a system, because most veterinary

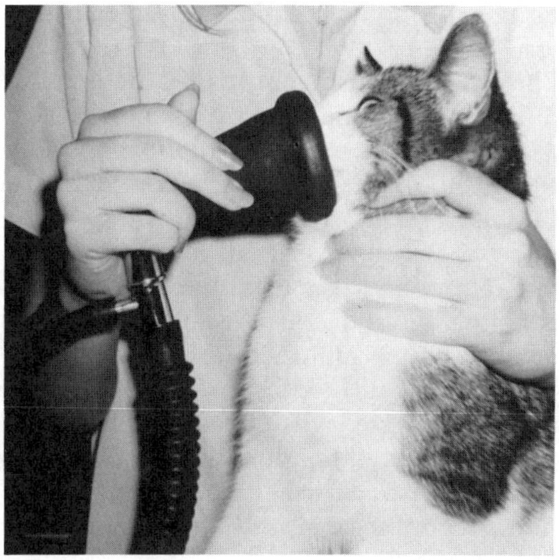

Figure 14.33. A mask induction using halothane and O_2 for a cooperative, unpremedicated cat. The mask has been adapted to an Ayre's T-piece system to provide a reservoir should inspiratory demands exceed the fresh gas inflow and to allow a mechanism for scavenging of excess gases (Biomedical Learning Resources Center).

masks do not provide a scavenging mechanism. Use of high flows (e.g., 5 liters/min) helps in dilution and elimination of CO_2, supplies inhalation anesthetic in adequate quantity so that induction rate can be rapid, and helps to prevent inhalation of room air around masks.

Masks should fit snugly over the muzzle to minimize dead space, and an appropriate size for the patient should be chosen. The author prefers conical rubber masks, but plastic, clear masks are useful and allow visualization of the nares and mouth during their use. During masking or use of closed containers, patient ventilation must be assured at all times.

Scavenging Systems

In recent years, a correlation between exposure to trace anesthetic levels and occupational disease has emerged. Although a cause-effect relationship is yet to be proved in most instances, it seems justified to take appropriate steps to eliminate overflow gases from the environment of veterinary hospitals (26, 27). Persons working in areas of possible contamination need to be aware of the potential risk, and it seems prudent to discourage pregnant women from working in areas where chronic exposure to low levels of anesthetic gases is likely. Persons maintaining and using anesthetic equipment should eliminate leaks from equipment in low, intermediate, and high pressure areas of all anesthetic machines. Care should be exercised when filling anesthetic vaporizers, and keyed filling mechanisms should be considered. Periodic monitoring of anesthetic levels in operating rooms is done in human hospitals and probably should be done in veterinary hospitals.

The major area of anesthetic contamination is overflow gases from anesthetic systems. To prevent this, a scavenger system composed of a gas-capturing assembly, an interface (if high negative pressure scavenging is used), and a disposal system is required. Gas-capturing methods for a circle system and a closed container are shown in Figures 14.20 and 14.32. These are attached by plastic corrugated tubing to a low-pressure evacuation system. A high-pressure evacuation system (Fig. 14.34) required an interface to allow a reservoir bag for gases should the overflow volume exceed the evacuation capacity. It has positive and negative relief valves, also. These mechanisms prevent transfer of pressure back to the system and the patient, and the negative pressure relief valve allows entrapment of room air in the event of excessive vacuum (to avoid taking excessive gases from the patient and sys-

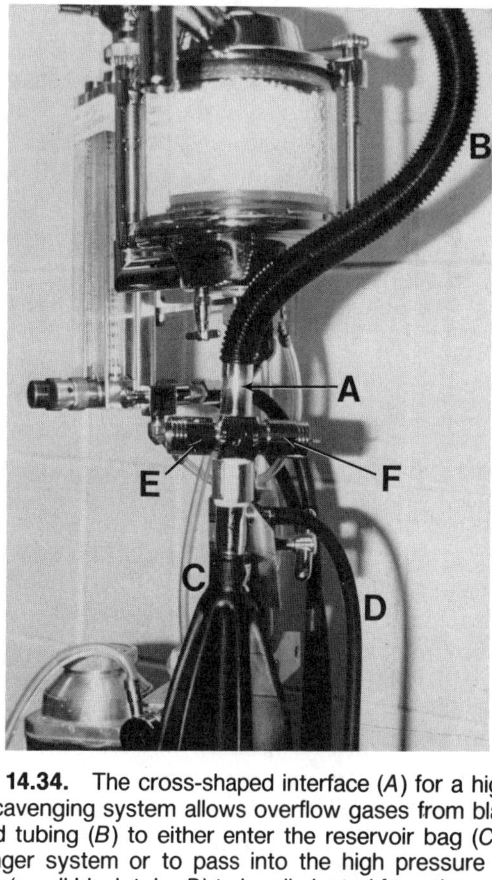

Figure 14.34. The cross-shaped interface (*A*) for a high pressure scavenging system allows overflow gases from black corrugated tubing (*B*) to either enter the reservoir bag (*C*) of the scavenger system or to pass into the high pressure vacuum system (small black tube *D*) to be eliminated from the room. The left side of the interface is a positive pressure relief valve (*E*) to prevent excessive pressure buildup in the scavenger system. The right side of the interface (*F*) is a negative pressure relief valve to allow entrapment of room air if the vacuum becomes excessive (Biomedical Learning Resources Center).

tem). The disposal system can be a nonrecirculating air-conditioning system (return air vent), a hole through an outside wall, a low- or high-pressure central vacuum, or an activated charcoal absorber. The latter must be changed regularly and does not absorb N_2O. With any disposal system, the ultimate elimination of the gas must be at a point that prevents recirculation of gases to any area of the hospital. The key to low contamination is prevention of leakage by good equipment maintenance and good scavenging techniques. There is further discussion of control of anesthetic waste gases in Chapter 24.

Troubleshooting Anesthetic Machines and Breathing Systems

Anesthetic machines and breathing systems may malfunction for many different reasons. It is not the purpose of this section to prepare an exhaustive list for evaluation of equipment. However, certain common problems will be addressed.

In preparation for use of anesthetic equipment, the integrity of the machine and system should be evaluated. Circle systems should be examined for leaks by occluding the Y-piece, closing the overflow valve, filling the system with oxygen, and determining if 30 to 40 cm H_2O pressure can be maintained. If not, the leaking area must be located and corrected. Common locations for leaks include seals around the absorbent canister and deteriorating rubber goods such as reservoir bag and hoses. The water drain in the canister may be open and allow escape of gases. Other connections at various points in the circle should be evaluated as well. Nonrebreathing systems should be filled with oxygen before use, the overflow port and the endotracheal tube connector should be occluded, and 30 to 40 cm H_2O pressure should be applied to assure the system's integrity. Leaks should be prevented to avoid contaminating room air with inhalation anesthetics and to assure IPPV capability when it is needed.

Nondisposable rubber parts on anesthetic systems should be checked regularly for wear and replaced if deteriorated. The various valves of breathing systems should be evaluated for proper function on a regular basis. Inhalation and exhalation valves should be clean and should operate with minimal resistance. Open overflow valves should allow gases to pass at pressures less than 1 to 2 cm H_2O. Circle systems should be free of soda lime dust or particles, and moisture should be wiped from the various components (e.g., one-way valve discs and domes) of the system. The Y-piece of the circle and the connector for attachment of the endotracheal tube in nonrebreathing systems should be clean, free of mucus and moisture, and capable of making tight-fitting connections to endotracheal tube adapters.

In preparation for machine use, the levels of oxygen, nitrous oxide and volative liquid anesthetics should be checked to assure adequate amounts for the expected duration of anesthesia. Also, the freshness of soda lime must be assured in rebreathing systems.

Vaporizer function certainly affects anesthetic machine operation, and it is ideal to evaluate the output of anesthetic vapor with a calibrated instrument (e.g., infrared anesthetic agent monitor) at regular intervals. Methoxyflurane and halothane contain preservatives that do not vaporize, will collect on vaporizer parts (particularly the wick), and may affect anesthetic output. Draining these vaporizers periodically will help to prevent this complication, and the regular servicing of vaporizers as recommended by manufacturers will alleviate this problem. Others have recommended introduction of ether into the vaporizer to remove preservatives, followed by draining of the unit and flowing oxygen through it prior to refilling it with anesthetic. Certain nonprecision vaporizers (Figs. 14.12) have parts that malfunction after extensive use. In some cases, the valves that control carrier gas flow into the vaporization chamber fail to seal properly, and the unit vaporizes anesthetic even in the off position. These valves should be visually inspected from below with the glass jar and wick removed from the vaporizer. Any adjustments or repair should be by qualified service personnel. Except for the most recent types of precision vaporizers, tipping or inversion may affect output, and calibration should be rechecked after such an incident. Finally, leaks involving the vaporizer may occur at the inlet, the outlet, or the filler port, and these should be corrected when discovered.

Flowmeter function should be evaluated periodically. Accuracy is more likely to be a problem at low flows. Estimations of flowrate can be made by flowing gases into a rebreathing bag of known volume over a set period of time. For example, a flowmeter set at 2 liters/min should fill a 2-liter bag in 1 minute. Periodic servicing by qualified personnel is the best way to assure flowmeter function. If a leak occurs in the oxygen flowmeter (e.g., due to a chipped or cracked tube), inadequate amounts of oxygen may be delivered to the patient. If N_2O is being used concurrently, the F_IO_2 (fraction of inspired O_2) may be reduced to dangerous, even fatal, levels. Because of this possibility, continuous monitoring of oxygen levels is practiced more commonly.

Failure of fresh gas to be delivered to the breathing system and to the patient can occur for various reasons. This may then lead to hypoventilation by the patient (3). A leak at the flush valve has been the cause of inadequate delivery of fresh gases and anesthetic vapor (25). Mechanical obstructions can occur within the piping of the anesthetic machine or the breathing system. In addition, the hose that connects the machine's common gas outlet to the breathing system can become kinked or disconnected and prevent fresh gas delivery (3).

Problems with overflow valves on circle systems that lead to sticking or only partial opening can cause pressure build-up within the system that can be transferred to the patient. Similarly, occluded exhalation tubes of nonrebreathing systems can cause pressure increases. If no reservoir bag is present, the pressure can elevate very rapidly. If undiscovered, the consequences of high pressure may include impaired venous return and cardiac output as well as ruptured alveoli and pneumothorax. Scavenger system obstructions can produce similar effects.

Leaks may occur at various locations in the high-pressure (cylinders, regulators, and flush valves) and intermediate-pressure (downstream from the regulator to the flowmeters) areas. These may be detected with "soapy" bubbles applied at various connections; such leaks also may be audible. Leaks at the hanger yoke where a washer is used as a seal next to the cylinder valve port are common and may only require a new washer or tightening of the cylinder within the hanger yoke. Consequences of such leaks include room air contamination with N_2O and inadequate delivery of gases to the system.

Although no list of potential problems can be exhaustive, the above discussion has enumerated several possible locations for machine malfunction. The primary concern is that the machine operator should check the equipment prior to use. Particularly, connections should be secure, gas and anesthetic levels should be assured, the flow of gases should be traced from source to patient, and system function should be evaluated. In general, an anesthetic machine and breathing system must allow free, unrestricted gas flow and application of effective IPPV when the operator occludes the overflow value. Ultimately, the anesthesiologist must monitor both the equipment and the patient to assure safety.

Endotracheal Tubes

The endotracheal tube provides the connecting link between the patient's airway and the anesthetic equipment. In most cases, oral endotracheal tubes are used in animal patients. Exceptions include the use of nasal tubes or tracheostomy tubes (Fig. 14.35). Tubes may be constructed of plastic, real rubber, latex, or silicone. Both disposable and reusable tubes are available in the sizes normally used for small companion animals and the smaller food animal patient. Most large animal tubes are reusable. Endotracheal tube sizes are 2.5 to 14 mm i.d. for small animals and 16 to 40 mm i.d. for large animals. Tracheostomy tube sizes are 6.0 to 30.0 mm i.d. for both small and large animals.

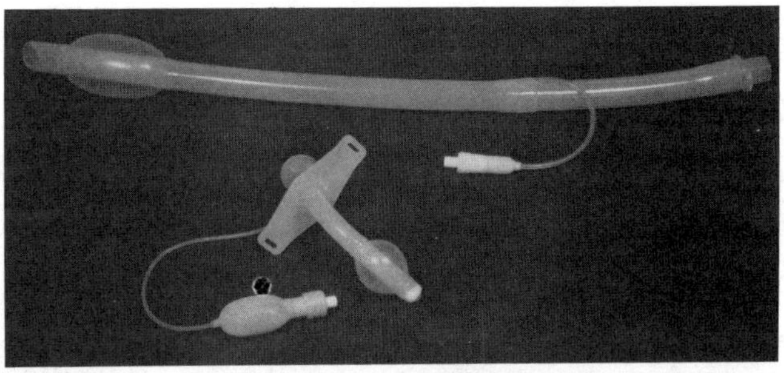

Figure 14.35. Illustration of silicone endotracheal and tracheostomy tubes. Photo courtesy Bivona Surgical Instrument, Inc., Gary, Indiana.

The most common styles of endotracheal tubes are the Cole (noncuffed pediatric) and the Murphy or Magill style, either cuffed or uncuffed. The Murphy style tubes are quite similar to the Magill tubes except there is an opening (eye) opposite the bevel of the tube to assure safe air flow. This opening is commonly referred to as a "Murphy eye." Endotracheal tubes may contain wire reinforcement that is very helpful in avoiding kinking or twisting, especially in small patients or cases in which positioning the hose to the side of the patient is beneficial (Figure 14.36).

The placement of endotracheal tubes into the trachea is significantly enhanced by adequate anesthetic depth and muscle relaxation of the upper airway and oral area. The use of force during intubation should be avoided. Excessive trauma to the larynx can produce laryngeal edema, laryngeal spasm, or excessive stimulation of the vagus resulting in potential bradycardia.

The use of local anesthesia to the laryngeal area may be helpful. Small amounts should be used, and cetacaine should be avoided because it may produce irritation, postanesthetic tracheitis, or other complications.

Endotracheal tubes are commonly placed in the horse by blind approach, whereas a laryngoscope is quite helpful in dogs, cats, calves, sheep, goats, and pigs. The laryngoscope with Miller style blades is quite beneficial in veterinary anesthesia. The large 205-mm Miller blade is very helpful in sheep, wine, goats, and large dogs; the infant size works well for small dogs and cats. The infant McIntosch blade adapts well to cats.

Care should be used to avoid Excess inflation of the cuff to avoid damage to the trachea. Sufficient concern has been shown so that soft cuffs have been developed or noncuffed tubes used. Noncuffed tubes may allow escape of gases or are more likely to allow aspiration of secretions from the oral cavity.

After usage, airway tubes should be cleaned by

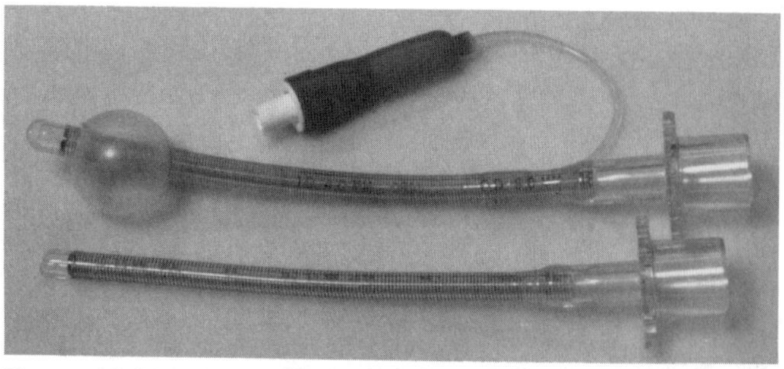

Figure 14.36. Illustration of silicone cuffed wire-reinforced endotracheal tube. Photo courtesy Bivona Surgical Instrument, Inc., Gary, Indiana.

gently scrubbing with a good surgical soap followed by a thorough water rinse. The integrity of the cuff should be determined after each use. The use of chemical sterilizing agents is beneficial if ethyloxide is not available or if the possibility of infection exists. Care should be taken to rinse away all chemical agents before usage. They are not recommended for tubes with foam inserts in the cuff.

Ethylene oxide should be used only according to the recommendations of the manufacturer of the sterilizing equipment. Human exposure should be avoided. Minimum aeration times are 48 hours in a chamber at room temperature, 12 hours at 120°F, or 14 days if no aeration chamber is available before reusing. Most endotracheal or tracheostomy tubes should not be autoclaved.

The use of sterile appropriately sized tubes with gentle intubation and extubation and soft inflation of the cuff will aid in avoiding damage to the upper airway.

References

1. Stoelting RK, Miller RD: *Basics of Anesthesia*. New York, Churchill Livingstone, 1984.
2. Minimum Performance and Safety Requirements for Components and Systems of Continuous Flow Anesthesia Machines for Human Use. ANSI Z-79.8. New York, American National Standards Institute Inc, 1979.
3. Dorsch JA, Dorsch SE: *Understanding Anesthesia Equipment*, ed 2. Baltimore, Williams & Wilkins Co, 1984.
4. Steffey EP, Hodgson DS, Kupershock C: Monitoring oxygen concentrating devices (Letter). *J Am Vet Med Assoc* 184:626–638, 1984.
5. Lumb WV, Jones EW: *Veterinary Anesthesia*, ed 2. Philadelphia, Lea & Febiger, 1984.
6. Schreiber P: *Anesthesia Equipment*. New York, Springer-Verlag, 1972.
7. Haskins SC, Sansome AL: A timetable for exhaustion of nitrous oxide cylinders using cylinder pressure. *Vet Anesth* 6:6–8, 1979.
8. Linde HW: The physics and chemistry of general anesthetics. In Soma LR (ed): *Textbook of Veterinary Anesthesia*. Baltimore, Williams & Wilkins Co, 1971.
9. Schreiber P: *Safety Guidelines for Anesthesia Systems*. Telford, PA, North American Drager, 1984.
10. Eger EI II, Hylton RR, Irwin RH, Guadagni N: Anesthetic flowmeter sequence—a cause for hypoxia. *Anesthesiology* 24:396–397, 1963.
11. Hill DW: The design and calibration of vaporizers for volatile anesthetic agents. In Scurr C, Feldman S (eds): *Scientific Foundations of Anesthesia*. Chicago, Yearbook Medical Publishers, Inc, 1974.
12. Thurmon JC, Benson GJ: Inhalation anesthetic delivery equipment and its maintenance. *Vet Clin North Am Large Anim Pract* 3:73–95, 1981.
13. Soma LR: *Textbook of Veterinary Anesthesia*. Baltimore, Williams & Wilkins Co, 1971.
14. Chilcoat RT: Hazards of mis-filled vaporizers: summary tables (letter). *Anesthesiology* 63:726–727, 1986.
15. Hamilton WK: Nomenclature of inhalation anesthetic systems. *Anesthesiology* 25:3–5, 1964.
16. Eger, EI II: *Anesthetic Uptake and Action*. Baltimore, William & Wilkins Co, 1974.
17. Tevik A, Sharpe J, Nelson AW, Berkley WE, Lumb WV: Effect of nitrogen in a closed circle system with low oxygen flows for equine anesthesia. *J Am Vet Med Assoc* 154:166–170, 1969.
18. Klide AM, Krumm SJ: A comparison of the consumption and cost of halothane and isoflurane in dogs anesthetized with a low flow technique. *Proceedings of the Second International Congress of Veterinary Anesthesiology*, Sacramento, CA, October 7–10, 1985, p 56.
19. Klide AM, Hopskin JL, Quast LS: A comparison of high and low flow anesthesia techniques: halothane in the dog. *Proceedings of the Annual Meeting of the American College of Veterinary Anesthesiologists*, New Orleans, LA, October 12, 1984, p 8.
20. Hartsfield SM, Sawyer DC: Use of nonrebreathing systems for small animal inhalation anesthesia. *J Am Anim Hosp Assoc* 8:355–362, 1972.
21. Hartsfield SM, Sawyer DC: Cardiopulmonary effects of rebreathing and nonrebreathing systems during halothane anesthesia in the cat. *Am J Vet Res* 37:1461–1466, 1976.
22. Carmichael JA: Small animal inhalation anesthesia using the Magill system. *J Am Vet Med Assoc* 160:1492–1495, 1972.
23. Manley SV, McDonell WN: A new circuit for small animal anesthesia: the Bain coaxial circuit. *J Am Anim Hosp Assoc* 15:61–65, 1979.
24. Manley SV, McDonell WN: Clinical evaluation of the Bain breathing circuit in small animal anesthesia. *J Am Anim Hosp Assoc* 15:67–72, 1979.
25. Sawyer DC: *The Practice of Small Animal Anesthesia*. Philadelphia, WB Saunders Company, 1982.
26. Manley SV, McDonell WN: Anesthetic pollution and disease. *J Am Vet Med Assoc* 176:515–518, 1980.
27. Manley SV, McDonell WN: Recommendations for reduction of anesthetic gas pollution. *J Am Vet Med Assoc* 176:519–524, 1980.
28. Hartsfield SM, Thurmon JC: Reduced anesthetic vapor concentration in a breathing circuit related to a leak in the oxygen flush apparatus. *Vet Anesth* 5:35–38, 1978.

CHAPTER 15

Controlled Ventilation and Pulmonary Function

RICHARD V. SHAWLEY, D.V.M., M.S., D.A.C.V.A.

Artificial Ventilation

HISTORY

The first account of artificial ventilation is in the Bible; the prophet Elisha restored respiration and life to a child using a form of mouth-to-mouth resuscitation (1). Artificial ventilation was used in veterinary medicine by Vesalius in 1555 to maintain respiration in a dog with an open chest (2). However, it was not until the 1930s that artificial ventilation became an accepted and utilized technique in human anesthesia (2). This extreme delay in adapting a research technique used by Vesalius over 400 years ago illustrates the communication lag that existed in medicine before this century.

In veterinary medicine, the use of artificial ventilation during anesthesia and intensive care has become widespread only in the last 20 years. Among other reasons, the reluctance of veterinarians to adopt this technique has been due to lack of adequate anesthesia personnel and the fact that the great majority of veterinary general anesthesia cases do not require artificial ventilation to have a successful outcome.

RESPIRATORY DEAD SPACE

Before a discussion of artificial ventilation begins, it is necessary to review the anatomy and physiology of the respiratory dead space. Dead space is that volume of gas that does not contribute to the exchange of oxygen and carbon dioxide. There are three types of dead space that are important to the anesthesiologist.

Anatomical dead space is that volume of the respiratory tract extending from the external nares to the bronchioles where no gas exchange occurs. Many anesthetic agents, as well as other drugs such as atropine and isoproterenol used in anesthetic procedures, contribute to bronchodilation and increased anatomical dead space. Narcotics (3) and barbiturates (4) may reduce dead space due to bronchoconstriction.

Mechanical dead space is simply an extension of anatomical dead space. It occurs whenever masks or tracheal tubes extend beyond the nares of the animal. Increased levels of carbon dioxide occur with these devices. The awake animal will increase the tidal volume to eliminate the increase in carbon dioxide, but the anesthetized animal cannot respond as readily.

Alveolar dead space is represented by areas of the lung where no gas exchange occurs but where gas exchange normally occurs (5). Alveolar dead space and anatomical dead space together form physiological dead space.

The alveolar dead space can be ventilated, but blood flow may be reduced or eliminated (pulmonary embolism) so that gas exchange does not occur. The opposite situation may occur when ventilation is reduced (bronchial obstruction) but blood flow remains the same. Both of the situations are extreme examples of ventilation/perfusion mismatching.

Because there are regional differences within the lung that affect ventilation/perfusion (V/Q) relationships, there is some degree of V/Q mismatch in the normal animal (6). General anesthesia increases the degree of V/Q mismatching, particularly in large animals (7). The V/Q mismatch due to anesthesia has many causes, but it has been attributed to the gravitational effect, atelectasis, and loss of the sigh reflex.

If arterial blood gas values are available, the alveolar dead space ventilation can be determined. Because alveolar dead space does not participate in gas exchange, its composition is equal to that of inspired gas, being high in oxygen and low in carbon dioxide. When dead space gas mixed with expired gas from a normal portion of the lung, the exhaled gas oxygen composition (combination of the two areas) increases toward that of inspired gas. By using arterial CO_2 as a measure of alveolar gas and sampling the end expired gas for CO_2 tension, the ratio of dead space ventilation to total ventilation can be determined. The formula is:

$$\frac{\text{(Dead space volume) } V_D}{\text{(Tidal volume) } V_T} = \frac{PaCO_2 - P_ECO_2}{P_aCO_2}$$

with $PaCO_2$ being arterial CO_2 and P_ECO_2 being end expired CO_2 tension. Ratios less than 15% are considered normal. Acceptable ratios during anesthesia for small animals may be as high as 30% and for large animals as high as 50% (8).

Blood flow in the lung may result in blood bypassing alveoli and going directly to the left side of the circulation (right-to-left shunt). Causes of shunt include disease states that compress alveoli, but blood flow remains near normal. Examples are pneumothorax, diaphragmatic hernia, or packing of the lung lobes during thoracic surgery. The resulting shunt lowers the oxygen content of the arterial blood. The amount of shunt can be determined using the formula:

$$\frac{QS}{QT} = \frac{Cc - Ca}{Cc - Cv}$$

where Qs is shunt flow, Qt is total cardiac output, Cc is pulmonary capillary blood, Ca is arterial blood, and Cv is mixed venous blood.

A more clinically useful formula if blood gas data is available is:

$$\frac{QS}{QT} = \frac{(P_AO_2 - P_aO_2)0.003}{(P_AO_2 - P_aO_2)0.003 + 4}$$

P_AO_2 is determined mathematically by:

$$P_AO_2 = 713\ (\%\ \text{inspired } O_2) - (P_aCO_2 \times 1.25)$$

The 0.003 is the amount of oxygen dissolved in 100 ml of blood at 1 mm Hg pressure of oxygen tension. P_aO_2 and P_aCO_2 are the arterial oxygen tension and carbon dioxide tension, respectively, determined by a blood gas machine. The number 4 is the arterial-venous oxygen content difference of normal blood. The figure 1.25 is derived from dividing the respiratory quotient (0.8) into 1.

Percent shunt flow values of 15% or less are considered normal. However, in large animals, values of 25 to 50% are commonly seen (8).

Torr is the measurement unit for pressure. It is equivalent to millimeters of mercury. For practical purposes, 1 torr equals 1 mm Hg. Centimeters of water are also used to measure pressure; 1 torr equals approximately 1.3 cm of water pressure.

Compliance has been defined as a measure of the distensibility of the lungs and of the restriction to expansion imposed by the surrounding structures (9). Compliance is also the change in volume per unit increase in intrapulmonary pressure. Compliance of the lung and thorax can be altered by disease or during surgery by instruments or procedures that interfere with the normal expansion of the chest. Neonates and very thin patients may have less muscular development of the thoracic musculature which may increase thoracic compliance. The use of muscle relaxants may also result in an increase in compliance.

Airway resistance must be overcome for air to move through the respiratory tree. The pressure required to move air depends on several factors, but airway size is very important. Poiseuille's law states that the volume flow is proportional to the radius of the tube and inversely proportional to the length and the viscosity.

$$V = \frac{Pr^4}{8\ n\ l}$$

where V is volume flow rate, P is driving pressure, r is radius of tube, n is viscosity, and l is length of tube. Resistance is the inverse of flow, so:

$$R = \frac{8\ n\ l}{r^4}$$

Note that if the radius is halved, the resistance increases 16 times! Cross sectional area or radius of the respiratory tree can be altered by neural stimulation, chemical (CO_2), respiratory secretions, and anesthetic equipment.

Neural stimulation by sympathetic nerves may produce bronchodilation and decrease resistance. Parasympathetic stimulation (vagus) may constrict airways. This effect may be minimized with atropine.

Carbon dioxide has been shown to have a direct dilating effect and decreases resistance when applied as a enriched mixture, but high levels of arterial carbon dioxide were shown to increase constriction and resistance (10). Respiratory secretions narrow the airway as well as creating more turbulence to airflow, thereby increasing resistance. Tracheal tubes and other anesthetic equipment represent a great potential for increasing resistance. Simply stated, the larger the tracheal tube, the less the work required in breathing.

Definitions

Spontaneous ventilation refers to breathing without any assistance from a mechanical ventilator or the anesthetist squeezing the rebreathing bag. With assisted ventilation the patient initiates respiration, but the tidal volume is increased or assisted by the ventilator or the anesthetist may assist by squeezing the rebreathing bag. Controlled ventilation refers to the breathing function of the patient being done entirely by the mechanical ventilator or the anesthetist using the rebreathing bag. The ventilator or anesthetist can control the rate of respiration, the pressure applied during inspiration or expiration, and the tidal volume. Intermittent positive pressure breathing or ventilation (IPPB or IPPV) is the technique utilized in controlled ventilation or assisted ventilation to force air into the lungs during inspiration and lower it to atmospheric pressure or slightly below during expiration.

Why Use Controlled or Assisted Ventilation?

Certainly the great majority of veterinary patients do not require the use of controlled or assisted ventilation to survive a routine anesthesia procedure. However, as veterinary surgical procedures have become more sophisticated, improvements have also been made in anesthesia care and intensive care. To maintain near-normal acid base status and oxygenation during these longer procedures, the use of controlled or assisted ventilation became more frequent. Initially, these techniques were used only for thoracotomy procedures. Later, because they contributed to smooth recoveries and increased survival, their use became more widespread. Today, controlled or assisted ventilation is used for depression of the respiratory center due to drugs, increased intracranial pressure, and cerebral ischemia; cardiac or respiratory arrest; thoracic disease, including diaphragmatic hernia, pleural effusion, and pneumothorax; paralysis of the respiratory muscles due to neuromuscular blocking drugs or toxins; and inadequate respiratory exchange due to respiratory obstruction, debilitation, or alveolar-capillary membrane changes (edema), among others.

Objectives of Successful Ventilation

The objectives of successful ventilation are effective ventilation of normal and abnormal lungs and minimization of effect on the cardiovascular system. To evaluate the effectiveness of positive pressure ventilation, careful monitoring of arterial blood pressure, electrocardiogram, and capillary refill time is indicated. Arterial blood gases can quantitate the effectiveness of the lung in supplying the red blood cells with oxygen. For a better understanding of the effect of IPPV on the cardiovascular system, let us look at normal breathing first.

Normal Breathing

Understanding the changes that occur during normal breathing is essential before attempting to understand controlled ventilation. Figure 15.1, *A*, shows examples of pressure changes that occur during normal breathing and positive pressure ventilation.

During normal breathing, the pressure in the pleural cavity is always slightly negative. It is this negative pressure that keeps the lung from collapse and the alveoli open. Surfactant also plays a role in the prevention of alveolar collapse (Fig. 15.1, *A*) (11).

At the end of exhalation, the pleural pressure is approximately −5 torr when the alveolar and ambient pressures are zero (Fig. 15.1, *B*). On inspiration due to the expansion of the thorax, the pleural pressure (−12 torr) becomes even more negative, as does the alveolar pressure (−5 torr). This negative alveolar pressure creates the inward movement of air. During exhalation, the alveolar pressure becomes positive, but the pleural pressure remains negative (Fig. 15.1, *C* and *E*). With artificial ventilation, the alveolar pressure becomes becomes positive (7 torr) on inspiration and the pleural pressure becomes zero or positive depending upon the amount of pressure applied (Fig. 15.1, *D*). On expiration with artificial ventilation, the values are the same as with exhalation during normal spontaneous breathing (Fig. 15.1, *E*).

Because exhalation is due to elastic forces and requires no vigorous contraction of muscle except in extensive pulmonary disease, it is considered passive; inhalation is considered the active process. Possible causes for muscular activity required during the exhalation process include airway obstruction, disease of the chest, or narrowing of the airway due to disease.

Mechanical Ventilators

Because ventilators are somewhat complicated at first glance, there is a great deal of apprehension on the part of the inexperienced anesthetist in using them. In this text, the basic types of ventilators will be explained, but to really understand ventilators and their uses, only hands-on experience will suffice.

Ventilators are generally designed so that the inspiratory phase is active (air is forced into the lungs by pressure) and passive during expiration (elastic forces of the lung and chest wall return the airway pressure to the ambient pressure). Ventilators are driven by either a pneumatic or electrical power system. The pneumatic type uses either gas or liquid to control the on or off switching.

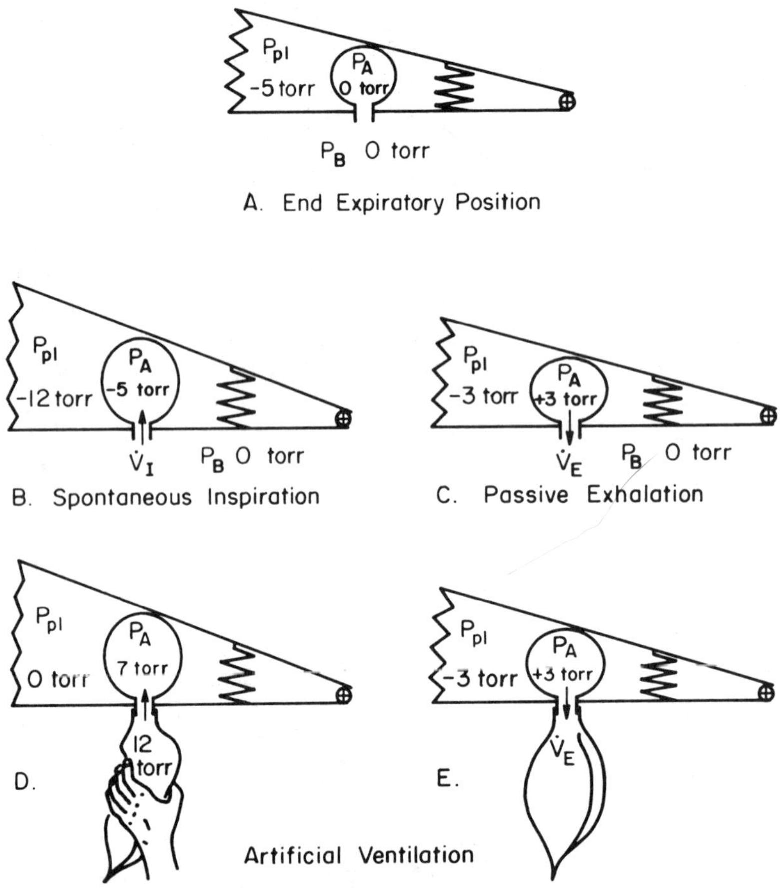

Figure 15.1. During all phases of spontaneous ventilation the intrapleural pressure remains negative. The size of the lung is proportional to the transpulmonary pressure (P_A-P_{pl}). Therefore, *B* and *D* show the same lung size, even though one is a positive and one is a negative difference. (From Soma LR: *Controlled Ventilation of the Veterinary Patient*. Washington Crossing, NJ, Pitman-Moore, 1973, with permission.)

Inspiration can be initiated by the ventilator or by the patient. The negative pressure created by the patient during an attempted inspiration may trigger the ventilator to cycle. This patient-initiated form of ventilation is referred to as assisted ventilation. If the machine or the anesthetist controls inspiration, it is referred to as controlled ventilation. Some ventilators can perform in both the assist or control mode, whereas others work only as controllers. Ventilators are also classified as either flow generators or pressure generators. If the inspiratory flow is maintained in spite of forces interfering with flow, the ventilator is classified as a flow generator. If flow is reduced by pressure forces, the ventilator is classified as a pressure generator.

Ventilators are also classified as either volume limited or pressure limited. The term "cycled" can also be used in place of the term "limited" in the previous sentence. With a volume-limited ventilator, the preset tidal volume can be delivered regardless of pressure, as shown in Figures 15.2 and 15.3. With the pressure-cycled machine, changes in resistance may alter the volume delivered as in the bird corporation ventilations.

Guidelines for Using Mechanical Ventilators

When using a ventilator, there are four basic variables that must be managed by the anesthetist. These are volume, pressure, rate, and inspiratory:expiratory time ratio.

VOLUME

The normal tidal volume for domestic animals is approximately 10 ml/kg of body weight. However, when using a ventilator, because of the compliance of the breathing hoses of the anesthetic machine and the patient's trachea and bronchi, a volume greater than the tidal volume must be used. In small animals, approximately twice the normal tidal volume or 20 ml/kg is usually recommended. In large animals, 1½ times the tidal volume or approximately 15 ml/kg is utilized. These are rules of thumb for average patients; adjustments may have to be made depending on the clinical situation. In clinical practice, the anesthetist can do an adequate job of ventilation by simply observing the

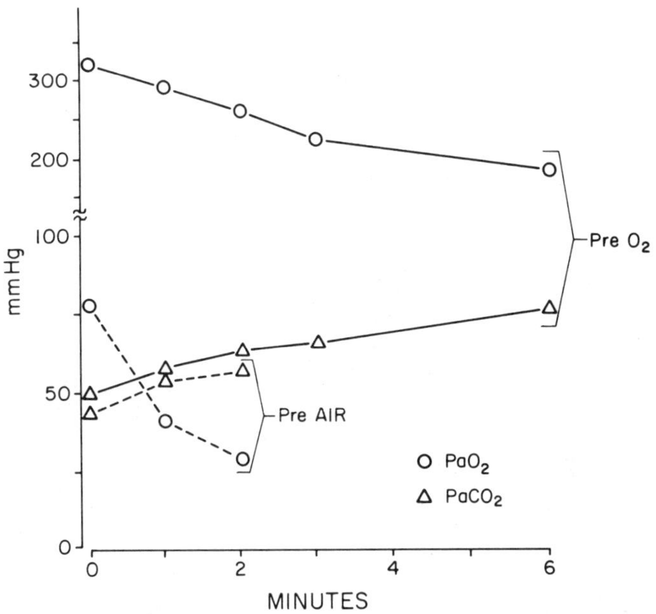

Figure 15.2. The average rate of decrease in P_aO_2 and rise in P_aCO_2 in horses (425 kg average weight) following acute endotracheal tube obstruction. The *dotted* and *solid lines* represent results of at least 15 minutes preobstruction air (F_IO_2 of .20) or O_2 (F_IO_2 of .95) breathing. (From Steffey EP: *Veterinary Clinics of North America*, Equine Respiratory Symposium. Philadelphia, WB Saunders, 1979, with permission.)

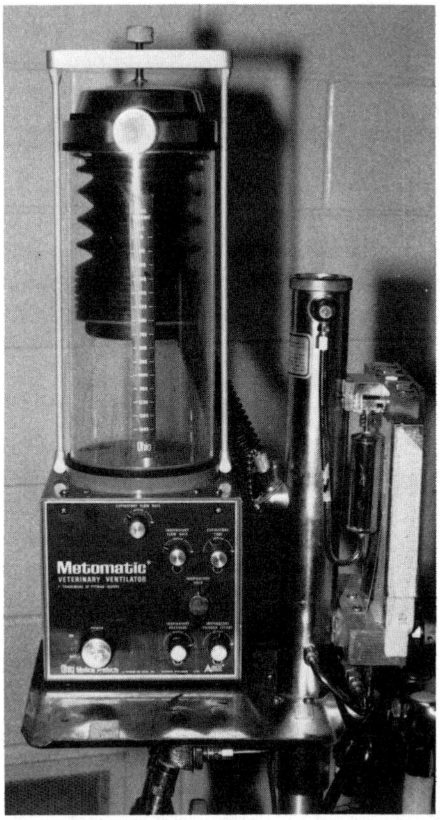

Figure 15.3. Pitman-Moore (Ohio Medical Products, Madison, WI) Metomatic Veterinary Ventilator for small animal anesthesia.

animal's chest rise. If full expansion of the lungs is occurring, the chest should rise accordingly.

PRESSURE

Many anesthetic machines are equipped with a pressure manometer within the airway circuit. Peak pressures of 15 to 30 cm H_2O are usually adequate to expand the lung (12). Airway resistance due to pulmonary disease (stiff lung) or airway secretion and gastrointestinal distention may increase the pressure necessary to expand the lung.

RATE

Because of the great variability in size within species, guidelines for breaths per minute or rate of ventilation have a wide range. Commonly used guidelines are dog, 8 to 14 breaths/min; cat, 10 to 14 breaths/min; horse, 6 to 10 breaths/min; cow, 6 to 10 breaths/min; goats and sheep, 8 to 12 breaths/min; and pig, 8 to 12 breaths/min.

INSPIRATORY:EXPIRATORY TIME RATIO

To minimize interference with venous return, the inspiratory time should be relatively short in comparison to expiratory time. Also, it is important that the peak pressure not be prolonged. To allow adequate filling time of the vena cava and right atrium, it is necessary that the inspiratory to expiratory time ratio (I:E ratio) be approximately 1:2 or 1:3 (13). For example, if an animal on a ventilator is being ventilated at a rate of 10 breaths/min, then each complete inspiratory/expiratory cycle would be 6 seconds in length. A 1:2 I:E ratio would mean an inspiratory time of 2 seconds and expiratory time of 4 seconds. A 1:3 ratio would allow 1.5 seconds for inspiration and 4.5 seconds for expiration. Expiratory time includes not only the period of actual expiration, but also the time until the next inspiration is initiated. To accurately monitor I:E time ratios, it is necessary to use a stopwatch. However, a reasonable estimate can be made with a conventional watch. Newly developed ventilators allow selection of desired I:E time ratios.

Clinical Problems with Ventilator Use

There are three main problems that occur with the clinical use of ventilators. These are the abolishment of spontaneous ventilation, re-establishment of spontaneous ventilation after a prolonged period on positive-pressure ventilation, and effects of positive pressure on the circulation.

ELIMINATION OF SPONTANEOUS VENTILATION

Spontaneous ventilation can usually be eliminated by the use of an adequate level of anesthesia and hyperventilation. This eliminates the carbon dioxide stimulus to respiration. Additional doses of barbiturates to eliminate the patient's respiratory efforts are extremely hazardous and are not recommended.

Muscle relaxants can also be used to eliminate spontaneous ventilation. Succinylcholine can be used at a dose of 0.1 to 0.2 mg/kg i.v. in the anesthetized dog or 0.2 mg/kg i.v. in the anesthetized horse. In the dog, succinylcholine can produce bradycardia, so its use may need to be preceded by atropine or glycopyrollate. Other muscle relaxants can be used. For further information, see the chapter 9.

RETURN OF SPONTANEOUS VENTILATION

Because the carbon dioxide stimulus to respiration has been lowered below normal stimulatory levels when an animal is on a ventilator, there frequently is a delay after the cessation of positive pressure ventilation and the return of spontaneous ventilation. Other causes of this delay include deep anesthesia, muscle relaxant drugs still present, muscle weakness and debility, hypothermia, and lack of painful stimuli.

After a ventilator is removed, the carbon dioxide level in the blood begins to rise during apnea at a rate of approximately of 2 to 10 torr/min (14). However, oxygen levels begin to fall rapidly, particularly if the animal is breathing air rather than 100% oxygen (Fig 15.4) (15). The usual procedure after removing the animal from the ventilator is to periodically breathe for the animal by squeezing the rebreathing bag every 15 to 20 seconds until the animal initiates respiration.

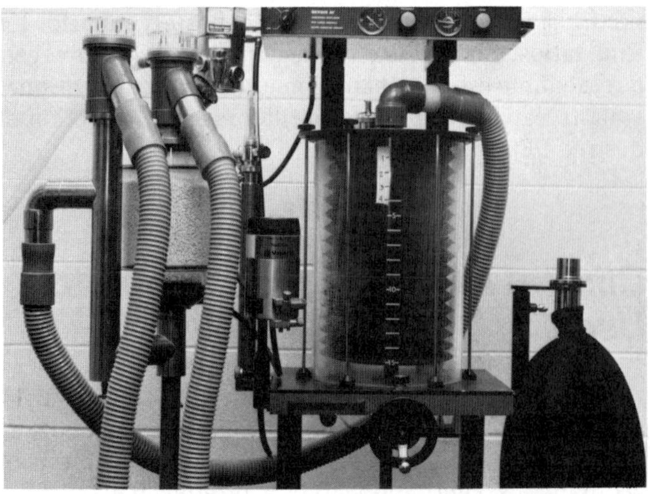

Figure 15.4. Narkovet E Large Animal Control Center. Manufactured by North American Drager, Telford, PA.

Assisted ventilation can also be used after spontaneous respiration begins.

If nondepolarizing muscle relaxants have been used, their effect on respiration may be reversed with the use of antagonists (See Chapter 9). Muscle weakness of the respiratory muscles rarely occurs except in the severely debilitated geriatric patient; however, decreased inspiratory effort and volume is a common problem. Hypothermia is a common problem in small animal patients (16). Careful attention must be paid to patients who are shivering due to hypothermia and breathing poorly because of the development of hypoxemia. Hypoxemia and hypothermia may predispose to cardiac arrhythmias (17). Supplemental oxygen and possibly positive pressure ventilation may be required.

External stimulation during recovery may help to initiate spontaneous respiration. In the horse, stimuli such as pushing on the abdomen behind the last rib with the fist or twisting the ear may elicit a respiratory stimulus. In small animals, rubbing the body, pinching the foot pad, opening the mouth, or slightly moving the tracheal tube during recovery may serve as a stimulus to initiate respiration. Excessive movement of the endotracheal tube should be avoided to reduce likelihood of laryngeal spasm or vagal stimulation and bradycardia.

CIRCULATORY CHANGES WITH IPPV

The negative pressure within the thoracic cavity that is produced on inspiration not only is responsible for moving air into the lung but also aids return of blood to the right atrium (18). This negative pressure also helps dilate the vena cava to assist in the movement of blood.

With the use of positive pressure ventilation, the intrapleural pressure becomes positive. This positive pressure is transmitted to the vena cava and the right atrium and ventricle. This increase in pressure reduces normal venous return. The lowered venous volume in the right atrium ultimately results in a decrease in cardiac output (19) and arterial blood pressure (20). During the exhalation phase, return blood flow to the right atrium increases. This change in blood pressure and cardiac output can be detected in the horse by palpating the mandibular artery and feeling the rise and fall in pulse character when the horse is receiving positive pressure ventilation. The reduction in blood pressure that occurs with positive pressure ventilation will be partially compensated for by a reflex sympathetic vasoconstriction, but it may take several minutes for compensation to occur (8).

The ability of an animal to compensate with vasoconstriction is variable. Factors such as anesthetic depth, blood volume, and drug-induced sympathetic blockade (epidurals or phenothiazine tranquilizers) may alter this ability (21, 22).

The depression in cardiac output and arterial pressure is proportional to the length of time the positive pressure is applied. Therefore, to lessen cardiovascular compromise, the amount of time either inspiratory or expiratory positive pressure is applied must be minimized; however, it must be combined with adequate time for proper ventilation of the lung.

High Frequency Ventilation

In recent years, there has been a great deal of research in the use of high frequency ventilation (23). There has been particular interest among veterinary anesthesiologists because of the problems that occur in large animals when conventional positive pressure ventilation is used. These problems include hypotension, decreased cardiac output, and variable levels of oxygenation in spite of normocapnia.

The term high frequency ventilation (HFV) refers to any form of ventilation operating at a frequency at least four times higher than the natural breathing frequency. Further classification of HFV includes the following three methods. With high frequency positive pressure ventilation, conventional mechanical ventilators are used to deliver 60 to 150 breaths/min (1 to 2.4 Hz). A frequency of 1 Hz equals 1/second. High frequency jet ventilation uses rapid delivery of small breaths through a canal in the upper airway. Rates used range from 2.5 to 5 Hz/min. High frequency oscillation (HFO) uses a pump mechanism to oscillate fresh air into and out of the lungs. Rates up to 50 Hz have been used.

The postulated advantages of HFV include the ability to achieve adequate ventilation based on arterial blood gas data without high inspiratory pressures being required. By using lower pressure, less cardiovascular compromise is produced. HFV can also be used to advantage in surgical procedures involving the trachea when the standard tracheal tubes cannot be used in the surgery site. At this writing, it appears that HFV offers little advantage over conventional ventilation, although, as one anesthesiologist has suggested (24), adequate equipment for large animals may need further development.

Positive end expiratory pressure (PEEP) to improve oxygenation in humans has been used. This has not become a common technique in veterinary medicine. When used, careful monitoring should be done because PEEP values over 5 mm Hg may produce an undesirable reduction in returning blood flow to the right side of the heart. This can be a major factor in reducing cardiac output during mechanical ventilation.

References

1. Kings II, Chapter 4, Verses 34–35. *The Living Bible.* Wheaton, Illinois, Tyndale Home Publishers, 1971, p 310–311.
2. Soma LR: *Controlled Ventilation of the Veterinary Patient.* 1:1, Washington Crossing, N.J., Pitman-Moore, 1973.
3. Soma LR (ed): *Textbook of Veterinary Anesthesia.* Baltimore, Williams & Wilkins, 1971, p 127.
4. Collins VJ: *Principles of Anesthesiology*, Philadelphia, Lea & Febiger, 1976, p 1360.
5. Severinghaus JW, Stupful M: Alveolar dead space as an index of distribution of blood flow in pulmonary capillaries. *J Appl Physiol* 10:335, 1957.
6. West JB: *Respiratory Physiology—The Essentials*, ed 2. Baltimore, Williams & Wilkins, 1971, p 43.
7. Gillespie JR, Tyler WS, Hall LW: Cardiopulmonary dysfunction in anesthetized laterally recumbent horses. *Am J Vet Res* 30:61, 1969.
8. Finlayson JK, Huria MN, Yu PN: Some circulatory effects of thoracotomy and IPPV in dogs. *Circ Res* 9:862, 1961.
9. Collins VJ: *Principles of Anesthesiology*, ed 2. Philadelphia, Lea & Febiger, 1976, p 1057.
10. Patterson RW, Sullivan SF: Inter-relation between alveolar and arterial CO_2 in the control of the mechanics of breathing in man. *NY Acad Med* 44:1265, 1968.
11. Guyton AC: Pulmonary ventilation, In *Textbook of Medical Physiology*, ed 6. Philadelphia, WB Saunders, 1981, p 477.
12. Gordon AS, Frye CW, Langston HT: *Thorac Cardiovasc Surg* 32:431, 1956.
13. Collins VJ: *Principles of Anesthesia*, ed 2. Philadelphia, Lea & Febiger, 1976, p. 409.
14. Eger EI, Severinghaus JW: The rate of rise of $PaCO_2$ in the apneic, anesthetized patient. *Anesthesiology* 22:419, 1961.
15. Steffey EP: *Veterinary Clinics of North America*, Equine Respiratory Symposium. Philadelphia, WB Saunders, 1979, p. 117.
16. Evans AT, Sawyer DC, Krahwinkel DJ: Effect of a warm water blanket on development of hypothermia during small animal surgery. *Am Vet Med Assoc* 163:147, 1973.
17. Covino BG, Charleson DA, D'Amato HE: Ventricular fibrillation in the hypothermic dog. *Am J Physiol* 178:148, 1954.
18. Beecher HK, Bennett HS, Bassett DL: Circulatory effects of increased pressure in airway. *Anesthesiology* 4:612, 1971.
19. Richards DW: Cardiac output by catheterization techniques in various clinical conditions. *Fed Proc* 4:215, 1945.
20. Pontoppidan H: Terminology. *Anesthesiology* 35:439, 1971.
21. Carr DT, Essex HE: Effect of positive pressure respiration on circulatory and respiratory systems. *Am Heart J* 31:51, 1946.
22. Price HL, King BD, Elder JD, Libien BH, Dripps RD: Circulatory effects of raised airway pressure during cyclopropane anesthesia in man. *J Clin Invest* 30:1243, 1951.
23. Froese A: High frequency ventilation: uses and abuses. *ASA Refresher Course Lecture*, Lecture 331, 1985.
24. Wilson DV, Soma LR, Klein LV: High frequency ventilation in the equine. *2nd International Congress Vet Anes Proc*, Vet Practice Pub Co. 1985, p. 188.

CHAPTER 16

Cardiovascular Medications and the Autonomic Nervous System

WILLIAM J. TRANQUILLI, D.V.M. M.S., D.A.C.V.A., AND STEPHEN A. GREENE, D.V.M., M.S.†

Introduction

The autonomic nervous system (ANS) plays an important role in maintaining homeostasis when a cardiotherapeutic agent is administered. Many cardiovascular drugs either alter the function of or elicit an indirect (reflex) response from the ANS; digitalis is an example. Cardiovascular therapy is often based upon modulation of adrenergic and/or cholinergic receptor activity located in the heart or peripheral vascular system. Cardiovascular agents will be reviewed in terms of their mechanisms of action, interaction with the ANS, and major clinical indications.

The anatomical and functional divisions of the ANS are the sympathetic and parasympathetic nervous systems. Emphasis will be placed upon neurotransmitter-receptor pharmacology and modulation of cardiovascular function by autonomic agents. The actions of the sympathetic nervous system are mediated by the release of norepinephrine and epinephrine, which interact with a variety of adrenergic receptors. The parasympathetic nervous system is mediated by the release of acetylcholine, which interacts as muscarinic and cholinergic receptors.

Based upon their clinical use, cardiovascular drugs can be divided into the three major categories of antiarrhythmic, inotropic, and vasodilator agents. Antiarrhythmic agents have been subdivided into four categories based upon their ability to alter the electrophysiology of healthy and diseased cardiac tissue. Inotropic agents enhance myocardial contractility and are important for the treatment of congestive heart failure or low cardiac output syndromes. Peripheral vasodilating agents increase venous capacitance, decrease peripheral vascular resistance, or both; they are often used in conjunction with inotropic therapy to reduce overall myocardial work and improve response to treatment. Because the diagnosis and treatment of excessive vascular resistance unrelated to heart failure is uncommon in veterinary medicine, vasodilator therapy alone is rarely implemented.

The Autonomic Nervous System

The ANS is referred to as the general visceral, involuntary, or vegetative motor system. The effector organs and tissues innervated by the ANS are associated with visceral functions over which there is little or no conscious motor control. Regulation of visceral function is essential to maintaining a stable internal environment. The ANS has been divided into the sympathetic and parasympathetic subdivisions. Both subdivisions consist of preganglionic efferent fibers originating in the central nervous system (CNS) and postganglionic efferent fibers originating from ganglia outside the CNS. Preganglionic fibers are myelinated, and postganglionic fibers are nonmyelinated. Although rarely noted, the ANS also contains sensory or general visceral afferent fibers (1).

The sympathetic system regulates activities associated with mobilizing the organism for emergency or stress situations (e.g., fight or flight responses). In contrast, the parasympathetic system regulates activities that conserve and restore body resources (e.g., gastrointestinal function of digestion and absorption of food). Anatomically, sympathetic fibers originate from the thoracolumbar spinal cord, whereas parasympathetic fibers arise from the midbrain, medulla, and sacral spinal cord and are referred to as the craniosacral system (Fig. 16.1)

NEUROANATOMY OF SYMPATHETIC DIVISION

Sympathetic neurons originate from the intermediolateral cell column of the spinal cord, exit from the cord with somatic spinal nerves, pass to the sympathetic trunk in the white rami communicantes, and pass up or down the sympathetic chain where they synapse at different segments. After branching, preganglionic fibers terminate by synapsing within paravertebral ganglia (sympathetic chain), prevertebral ganglia (celiac, mesenteric ganglia), or terminal ganglia near the bladder or rectum. Postganglionic fibers arising from the paravertebral ganglia pass via the gray rami

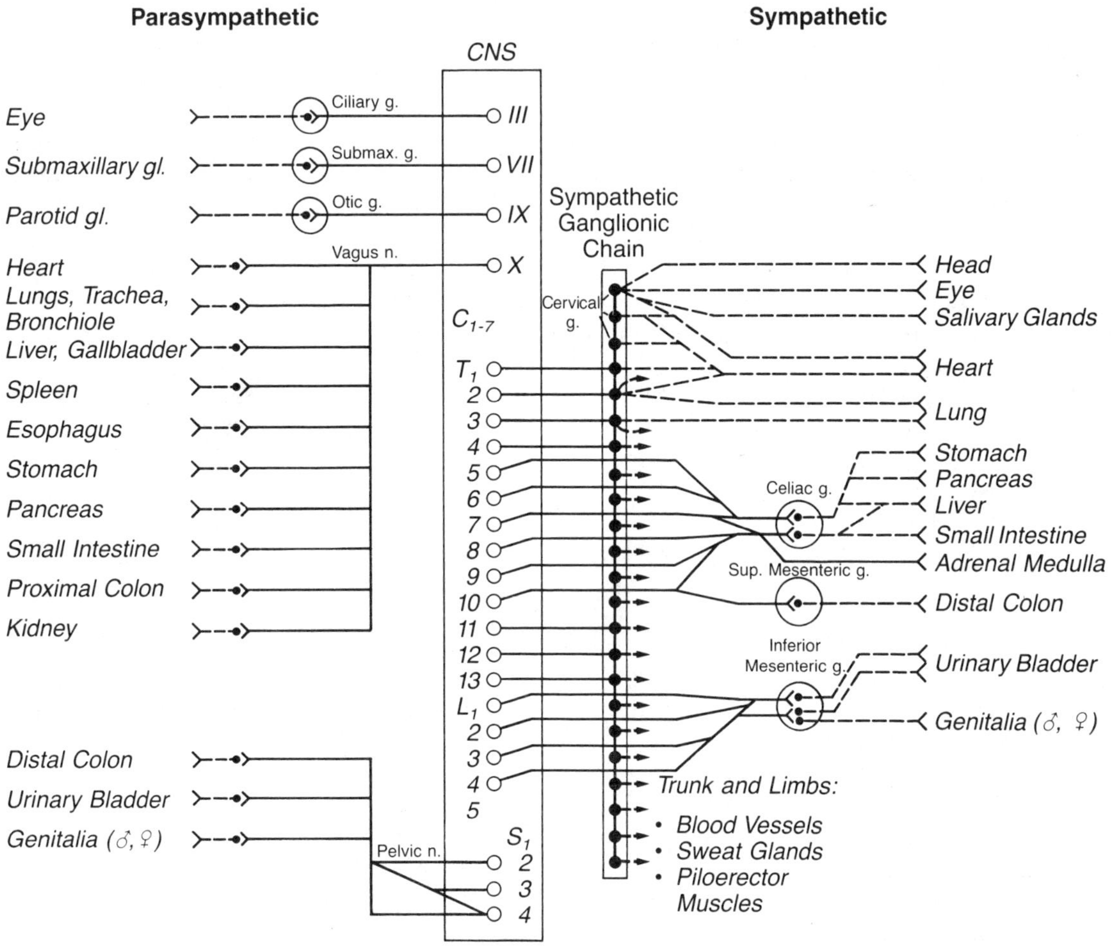

Figure 16.1. Schematic representation of the parasympathetic and sympathetic involuntary motor system to various organs and tissues of the body. Parasympathetic fibers originating from the third, seventh, ninth, and tenth cranial nerves and the sacral outflow are on the left. Sympathetic fibers from the thoracolumbar region are shown on the right. O, CNS preganglionic cell bodies; ●, ganglionic cell bodies. *Solid lines* are preganglionic fibers; and *dashed lines* are postganglionic fibers. The arrows from the sympathetic ganglionic chain depict postganglionic fibers to blood vessels, sweat glands (cholinergic), and piloerector muscles of trunk and limbs that travel with spinal nerves to the periphery. Modified from Adams (14).

communicantes and spinal nerves to sweat glands, vascular smooth muscles, and erector pili muscles of the limbs and body wall. From sympathetic fibers of the upper thorax, the cervical sympathetic chain is formed to supply sympathetic innervation to the head and neck (sudomotor, pilomotor, vasomotor, secretory, and pupilodilator innervation). The upper thoracic nerves also synapse with postganglionic fibers that supply sympathetic innervation to cardiac, esophageal, and pulmonary tissues. The splanchnic nerves consist of preganglionic fibers that terminate within prevertebral ganglia. Postganglionic sympathetic fibers from prevertebral ganglia (celiac and mesenteric) innervate the abdominal and pelvic viscera (Fig. 16.1).

The sympathetic division contains both cholinergic and adrenergic fibers. The neurotransmitter substance released by sympathetic preganglionic fibers, including fibers to the adrenal gland, is acetylcholine. Nicotinic receptors mediate postsynaptic stimulation in sympathetic ganglia. Postganglionic sympathetic fibers originating from symmpathetic ganglia release norepinephrine, which is deactivated rather slowly by catechol-o-methyl-transferase and actively taken up by nerve terminals.

The cells of the adrenal medulla are specialized postganglionic sympathetic neurons that secrete epinephrine into the blood stream when stimulated by sympathetic preganglionic cholinergic fibers. This release of epinephrine is coordinated with norepinephrine release from sympathetic postganglionic fibers to produce a coordinated sustained action. The ratio of postganglionic to preganglionic neurons is large, and each postganglionic fibers forms a diffuse network with numerous neuroeffector junctions. When the sympathetic system is activated, this arrangement produces a diffuse generalized effect.

NEUROANATOMY OF PARASYMPATHETIC DIVISION

Parasympathetic neurons originate from the tectal (midbrain), bulbar (medulla), and sacral regions of the CNS. Cranial nerves supply parasympathetic innervation to the head and thoracic and abdominal viscera. The sacral cord supplies innervation to the lower abdominal and pelvic viscera (Fig. 16.1). Tissues of the body wall and extremities are not innervated by parasympathetic fibers.

The cranial outflow of the parasympathetic nervous system is associated with four cranial nerves: the oculomotor (III), facial (VII), glossopharyngeal (IX), and vagal (X) nerves (Fig. 16.1). Preganglionic fibers within the oculomotor nerve originate from the midbrain and terminate in the ciliary ganglion where they synapse with postganglionic fibers. These parasympathetic postganglionic fibers innervate sphincter muscles (constrictor) of the eye and ciliary muscles (accomodation) of the lens. Preganglionic fibers of the facial nerve originate from the lower medulla and terminate in the pterygopalatine and submandibular, sublingual, and lacrimal glands and the secretory glands of the nasal and pharnygeal cavities. The glossopharyngeal nerve carries preganglionic fibers from the medulla to the optic ganglion where postganglionic fibers arise to innervate the parotid gland and mucous glands of the nose, mouth, and pharynx. The vagal nerve carries long preganglionic fibers that arise from the vagal nucleus in the medulla and pass via the vagosympathetic trunk to terminal ganglia near thoracic and abdominal visceral organs (Fig. 16.1). Short parasympathetic postganglionic fibers arise from these ganglia to innervate adjacent organs, such as heart, lungs, pancreas, and gastrointestinal tract. The left and right vagus nerves may supply different tissues within an organ. For example, the left vagus innervates the atrioventricular (AV) node and the right vagus innervates the sinoatrial (SA) node of the heart. Sacral parasympathetic preganglionic fibers arise from cell bodies in the sacral cord (S-2–S-4) and pass with pelvic nerves to terminal ganglia (Fig. 16.1). Parasympathetic postganglionic fibers innervate the distal colon, rectum, and urinary and genital viscera and are associated with the mechanisms of urinating and defecating.

Preganglionic parasympathetic fibers are long, synapsing with relatively few postganglionic fibers in ganglia near or in the effector organ. Transmission within parasympathetic ganglia is mediated by nicotinic and muscarinic receptors. Post ganglionic parasympathetic stimulation is mediated by muscarinic receptors on or within cells of the effector organs. Parasympathetic pre- and postganglionic fibers release acetylcholine, which is rapidly broken down by acetylcholinesterase. Thus, unlike the diffuse general effects of sympathetic stimulation, the effects of parasympathetic stimulation tend to be localized and of shorter duration.

PHYSIOLOGICAL RESPONSES TO AUTONOMIC STIMULATION

The physiological response of an organ or tissue to stimulation by the ANS is dependent upon a variety of factors. Many organs are innervated by both sympathetic and parasympathetic fibers. Within an organ, innervation may be tissue-specific. For example, the heart is innervated by sympathetic fibers to the atria and ventricles, whereas parasympathetic innervation is restricted to the atria and conducting system. Other organs or tissues are innervated by only one division of the ANS (e.g., vasculature of the body wall is only innervated by sympathetic fibers). The physiological actions induced by either system can stimulate or inhibit organ or tissue function depending upon the organ or tissue innervated. For example, during a fight or flight response, the sympathetic nervous system induces vasoconstriction of the cutaneous vasculature (α receptor mediated) while simultaneously inducing vasodilation in skeletal muscle (β_2 receptor mediated). An example of opposing actions induced by parasympathetic stimulation is the relaxation of the muscle of the pyloric sphincter coupled with simultaneous contraction of duodenal smooth muscle. Consequently, neither system exerts purely stimulatory or inhibitory actions throughout the body. However, when dual innervation to a specific tissue does exist, actions modulated by parasympathetic stimulation are most often opposed by the actions induced by sympathetic activation (1).

NEUROHUMORAL TRANSMISSION

The sequence of events that constitutes neurohumoral transmission is complex but can be simplified into conduction and transmission phases. Conduction is the passage of an impulse along an axon, whereas transmission refers to the passage of an impulse across a synaptic cleft or neuroeffector junction between cells. Local anesthetics may influence conduction along autonomic fibers, but the majority of pharmacotherapeutic agents modify autonomic function by altering transmission of impulse from nerve to tissue (2).

The arrival of an action potential at the neuronal terminal initiates a series of events that constitutes transmission of an excitatory or inhibitory impulse either presynaptically or postsynaptically at the effector cell. Neurotransmitter substance is synthesized in neuronal terminals and stored in vesicles. Depolarization of the neuronal terminal by an action potential results in calcium (Ca^{2+}) influx, which triggers the mobilization and release of neurotransmitter substance. Neurotransmitter then diffuses across the synaptic cleft and combines with specialized receptors on postjunctional membranes. In general, the response elicited by transmitter-receptor interaction will cause either depolarization or hyperpolarization of the effector cell membrane. Depolarization of the postsynaptic effector cell is referred to as the initiation of excitatory postsynaptic potential, whereas hyperpolarization of the effector cell membrane initiates an inhibitory postsynaptic potential (2). In addition, cholinergic and adrenergic presynaptic receptors have been identified and characterized as being either inhibitory (e.g., muscaranic or α_2) or facilitatory (e.g., β_2) to neurotransmitter release. The termination of transmission at cholinergic junctions results from rapid metabolism of acetylcholine; at adrenergic junctions, it results from the combination of reuptake, metabolism, and diffusion of neurotransmitter away from the synaptic cleft.

ADRENERGIC TRANSMISSION

From the amino acids phenylalanine and tyrosine, dopamine, norepinephrine, and epinephrine are synthesized. Within the cytosol of neuronal terminals, dopamine is synthesized, enters granules, and is then converted to norepinephrine. In the adrenal medulla, norepinephrine is converted to epinephrine. Epinephrine is stored in granules until released. A good portion of the norepinephrine found within neuronal terminals results from the reuptake of norepinephrine by active transport (3). Reuptake by neuronal terminals may be the major factor in terminating the effects of norepinephrine.

A variety of pharmacological interventions have been used to alter the processes involved in neurotransmitter metabolism and adrenergic transmission. These include altering presynaptic processing of neurotransmitter substance and modifying postsynaptic stimulation or inhibition of effector cells with agonists and antagonists, respectively. Adrenergic agonists are referred to as "sympathomimetic agents," whereas antagonists are termed "sympatholytic agents." Table 16.1 lists some agents and their mechanism(s) of action in altering the processes of adrenergic transmission. A diagrammatic representation of endogenous adrenergic neurohumoral transmission achieved with norepinephrine and epinephrine is shown in Figure 16.2. The major physiological effects upon cardiopulmonary function associated with each receptor type are also depicted.

CHOLINERGIC TRANSMISSION

Acetylcholine is synthesized within the cytoplasm of axonal terminals and sequestered within synaptic vesciles. The final step in the synthesis of acetylcholine is catalyzed by acetyltransferase. This enzyme acetylates choline with acetyl coenzyme A. When an action potential arrives at the axonal terminal, Ca^{2+} ions are mobilized, and acetylcholine is released. Actions induced by cholinergic transmission differ between skeletal muscle, parasympathetic postganglionic nerve terminals, and autonomic ganglia. These differences have been attributed to a variety of factors, including differences in effector cell cholinoreceptors, variation in cellular response, and distribution or location of acetylcholinesterase. Skeletal muscle cholinergic transmission is characterized by localized depolarization of a motor end plate that triggers or initiates an action potential and thus contraction. In contrast, postgan-

Table 16.1
Pharmacological Agents and Their Mechanism of Action in Altering Adrenergic Transmission

Agent	Mechanism of Action	Major Action
	Presynaptic Mechanisms	
α Methyltyrosine	Interferes with synthesis of transmitter	Depletion of NE[a]
Methyldopa	Produces α methylnorepinephrine	Forms a false neurotransmitter
Cocaine Imipramine	Inhibits active transport or reuptake of NE	Increased neurotransmitter available for receptor interaction
Reserpine	Blocks storage within granules	Causes increased degradation of NE by MAO[b] and depletion of neurotransmitter[c]
Bretylium	Prevents release of neurotransmitter	Decreases NE receptor interaction
Amphetamines	Induce a relatively rapid brief release of neurotransmitter	Increases NE release to induce a stimulatory action
	Indirect-Acting Sympathomimetics	
Ephedrine Mephentermine	Induces release of adrenergic neurotransmitter (NE) and has minor α agonistic action	Induces both α and β_1 agonistic actions via release of endogenous NE
	Postsynaptic Mechanisms	
Sympathomimetics		
Epinephrine	Stimulates all adrenergic receptors (α_1 and α_2, β_1 and β_2)	Induces universal adrenergic receptor stimulation
Methoxamine	α_1 agonist	Some of these agents (dobutamine, methoxamine, salbutamol) have restricted adrenergic action. They are used for very selective therapeutic effects and are referred to as second generation adrenergic agonists
Xylazine	α_1 and α_2 agonist (central-acting)	
Dobutamine	β_1 agonist	
Isoproterenol	β_1 and β_2 agonist	
Terbutaline or salbutamol	β_2 agonist	
Sympatholytics		
Phentolamine and phenoxybenzamine	α_1 and α_2 antagonists	Nonselective peripheral α blockade (antihypertensive) CNS stimulant
Tolazoline	(central acting)	
Prazosin	α_1 antagonist	Selective α adrenergic blockade (vasodilator)
Yohimbine	α_2 antagonist (central acting)	Selective α adrenergic blockade (CNS stimulant)
Propranolol	β_1 and β_2 antagonist	Nonselective β blocker used as an antiarrhythmic agent
Metoprolol	β_1 antagonist	Selective β adrenergic blockade (cardiac selective)

[a] NE, norepinephrine.
[b] MAO, monoamine oxidase.
[c] In the presence of MAO inhibitors, reserpine is no longer effective.

glionic parasympathetic cholinergic transmission mediated by muscarinic receptors modifies existing activity by partially depolarizing cell membranes (e.g., intestinal muscle) or by hyperpolarizing cell membranes and inhibiting activity (e.g., cardiac conduction). The inhibitory actions of acetylcholine in the heart likely result from a selective increase in potassium (K^+) permeability (4). Autonomic ganglionic transmission is primarily mediated by nicotinic receptors and appears to be a complex process combining features of cholinergic transmission found in both skeletal and smooth muscle activation. The nicotinic and muscarinic receptors found in autonomic ganglia differ from receptors found in skeletal muscle and in peripheral organs.

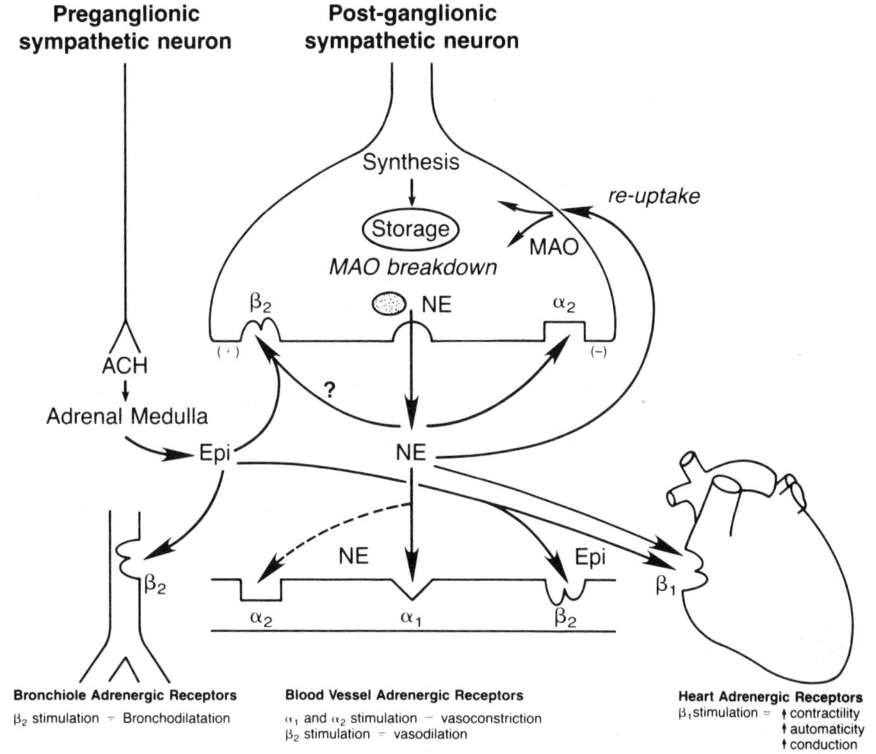

Figure 16.2. Diagrammatic representation of peripheral sympathetic neuronal terminal and a variety of effector cell receptors located in major organs and tissues. The predominant adrenoreceptor subtypes (α_1, α_2, β_1, and β_2) and associated physiological responses of the bronchiole, blood vessels, and heart are shown. In addition, adrenoreceptor stimulation by epinephrine (EPI) is depicted for these organs. Norepinephrine (NE) is released from the neuronal terminal and interacts with postsynaptic α_1 and β_2 receptors and perhaps α_2 receptors (*dashed line*) on effector cells of the vasculature and heart. NE also stimulates presynaptic α_2 receptors, which inhibits release. Presynaptic β_2 receptors are facilitatory to further NE release. Because NE does not possess a strong β_2 agonist action, EPI may play a major role in facilitating further NE release. EPI has potent β_2 actions on postsynaptic effector cells of the brionchioles and blood vessels as well, causing bronchodilation and vasodilation, respectively; α_1 and α_2 postsynaptic stimulation causes vasoconstriction; β_1 stimulation by either NE or EPI increases contractility, heart rate, and conduction velocity. NE has a weak β_2 agonistic effect when compared to EPI.

Acetylcholinesterase rapidly metabolizes acetylcholine, which is found in high concentrations in all three sites of peripheral cholinergic transmission (postganglionic parasympathetic, preganglionic autonomic, and somatic motor). The duration of cholinergic transmission is likely a result of the strategic location of acetylcholinesterase at synaptic junctions (2).

Cholinergic transmission can be altered in a variety of ways. Table 16.2 lists some agents and their mechanisms of action in modifying cholinergic transmission. Agents that enhance cholinergic actions are termed "cholinomimetic agents," whereas agents that inhibit cholinergic actions are termed "cholinolytic" or "anticholinergic agents." Cholinomimetic and anticholinergic agents can be further subdivided into nicotinic- or muscarinic-acting agents.

Sympathetic Pharmacology

Alterations in organ and tissue function resulting from adrenergic neurohumoral transmission were initially characterized by Alhquist by observing actions induced by specific catecholamines in tissues (5). He used endogenous and synthesized catecholamines to either stimulate or inhibit vascular smooth muscle contraction. The responses observed differed depending on the site, dose, and catecholamine chosen. He proposed to separate the observed effects by attributing responses to two types of receptors, α and β; α receptor activation induced vasoconstriction, whereas β receptor activation was associated with vasodilation. Isoproterenol produced the reverse pattern of activity (dilation) to norepinephrine (constriction) (Fig. 16.3). Epinephrine appeared to induce both α and β actions depending upon the dose used and specific vasculature infused. It was thus demonstrated that a catecholamine given at a specific dose could induce opposing actions in one organ or vascular bed versus another (Fig. 16.3). Lands et al. expanded Alquist's classification in 1967 by further subdividing β receptors into β_1 and β_2 subtypes (6). This division was based upon the observed selective actions achieved with various β agonists and antagonists (6). Subsequently, α adrenoceptors were

Table 16.2
Pharmacological Agents and Mechanisms of Action in Altering Cholinergic Transmission

Agent	Mechanism of Action	Effect
	Presynaptic Mechanisms	
Hemicholinium	Interferes with synthesis of transmitter	Depletion of acetylcholine
Carbachol	Displace transmitter from neuronal terminal	Cholinomimetic
Botulinus toxin	Prevents release of neurotransmitter	Anticholinergic
	Postsynaptic Mechanisms	
Muscarinic Receptor		
Methacholine	Stimulate muscarinic receptor	Cholinomimetic
Atropine	Blocks muscarinic receptor	Antimuscarinic
Nicotinic Receptor		
Nicotine	Stimulate nicotinic receptor	Cholinomimetic
Hexamethonium	Blocks nicotinic receptor	Anticholinergic
Neostigmine	Inhibits enzymatic breakdown of neurotransmitter	Cholinomimetic

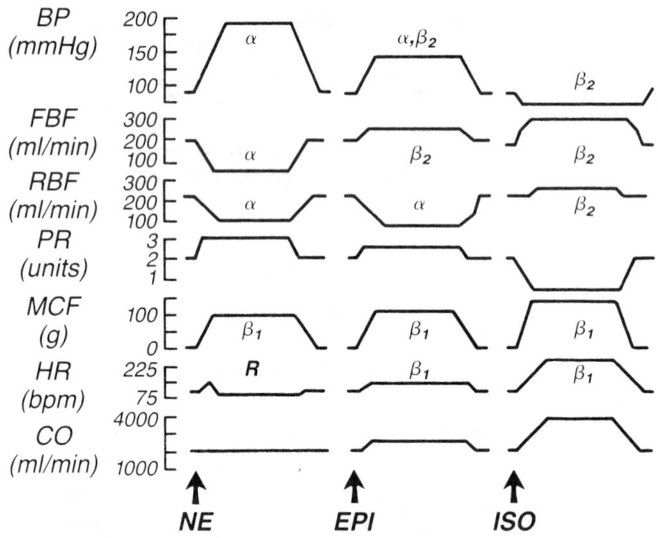

Figure 16.3. Differences in cardiovascular effects of intravenously administered norepinephrine (NE), epinephrine (EPI), and isoproterenol (ISO). Schematics represent relative effects on blood pressure (BP), femoral blood flow (FBF), renal blood flow (RBF), peripheral vascular resistance (PR), myocardial contractile force (MCF), heart rate (HR), and cardiac output (CO). Primary responses are noted as either α, β_1, or β_2 receptor-mediated; R, reflex-mediated. Differences in cardiovascular effects of these catecholamines are due to variation in α and β selectivity for each agonist. Modified from Adams (14).

also subdivided into α_1 and α_2 subtypes based upon the effects achieved with selective α agonists and antagonists.

Each adrenergic agent's effect upon a specific receptor can be attributed to the two basic properties of affinity and intrinsic activity. Affinity is defined as the neurotransmitter's ability to occupy the receptor. Intrinsic activity is the agent's ability to alter receptor configuration, thus eliciting a cellular response. Adrenergic agents with affinity and intrinsic activity for a specific receptor are termed agonists, whereas agents with little intrinsic activity but good affinity are termed antagonists or competitive blockers. This dual system of receptors (i.e., α or β) and neurotransmitter (i.e., agonist and antagonist) classification has been used to categorize and quantitate physiological responses mediated by the sympathetic nervous system and elicited by administration of endogenous or exogenous adrenergic agents (7). Many physiological responses elicited by adrenergic agents can now be explained based upon their α_1 to α_2, β_1 to β_2, or α to β receptor activity ratio (selectivity) and the adrenoreceptor population within the organ(s) or tissue(s) under scrutiny. In addition, with the introduction of central-acting α_2 agents to control blood pressure (clonidine) and induced sedative actions (xylazine), another important criterion in assessing the complete action of adrenergic agents is their central versus peripheral effects. It also appears plausible that in some tissues, adrenergic agents may actually possess a preferential presynaptic versus postsynaptic specific receptor selectivity (e.g., α_2 receptor). Thus, the actions of adrenergic agents and their resulting pharmacotherapeutic profile depend upon the predominance of a specific receptor subtype within the organ or tissue of interest and the spectrum of adrenergic stimulation exerted by a specific dose of adrenergic agonist or antagonist. Selectivity for specific receptor subtypes may be lost with increasing doses of catecholamines or synthetic agents. This dose-specific adrenergic action undoubtedly varies between and even within species, and every attempt should be made to closely monitor response of each patient to confirm whether the desired spectrum of adrenergic action is achieved.

Tissues may be characterized by specific receptor-mediated functions. The β and α adrenergic receptor subtypes found in a variety of tissues are shown in Tables 16.3 and 16.4, respectively. Dopaminergic receptor subtypes are shown in Table 16.4. Finally, it should be emphasized that modulation of neurohumoral transmission by receptor up- or down-regulation can occur. Chronic stimulation of adrenergic receptors decreases receptor numbers or affinity for agonists (down-regulation), whereas reduced levels of adrenergic receptor stimulation by chronic administration of receptor antagonists may lead to increased receptor numbers or sensitivity (up-regulation). This may result in patient refractoriness after chronic stimulation with agonists or supersensitivity to endogenous catecholamines after withdrawal of chronic blockade with antagonists (e.g., discontinuation of propranolol therapy prior to anesthesia).

Table 16.3
Some Tissues and Organs Showing the Major Alpha Adrenergic Receptor Subtype and the Effector Response to Catecholamine Stimulation

Effector Organ	Receptor Subtype	Effector Response
Eye (aqueous humor)	β_1	Increase production
Heart (SA node, atria, AV node, His Purkinje system, ventricles)	β_1	Increase contractility heart rate, conduction, and arrhythmogenic activity
Kidney	β_1	Renin release
Fat cells	β_1	Lipolysis
Posterior pituitary	β_1	Antidiuretic hormone secretion
Intestine	β_1	Decrease motility
Arterioles (coronary, skeletal, pulmonary, renal)	β_2	Dilation
Veins	β_2	Dilation
Bronchioles	β_2	Relaxation
Stomach	β_2	Decrease motility and tone
Gallbladder ducts	β_2	Relaxation
Uterus	β_2	Relaxation
Spleen capsule	β_2	Relaxation
Skeletal muscle	β_2	Contractility and glycogenolysis
Pancreas (B cells)	β_2	Increase insulin secretion
Eye (ciliary muscle of lens)	β_2	Relaxation (accomodation; far vision)
Sympathetic neuronal terminal	β_2	Increase NE release[a]
Liver	β_1 and β_2	Gluconeogenesis
Intestinal motility	β_1 and β_2	Decrease activity

[a] NE, norepinephrine.

Sympathomimetic Agents

The neuronal neurotransmitter norepinephrine, dopamine, and the vasoactive secretory product of the adrenal medulla, epinephrine, are the three endogenously produced catecholamines. Other currently used sympathomimetic agents are synthetic catecholamines, isoproterenol, dobutamine, and the noncatechol-phenylethanolamines such as phenylephrine and methoxamine (8). Beta adrenergic activity correlates with substitution on the amine portion of the side chain, whereas less substitution favors α agonism. The relative α and β activity of a variety of adrenergic agonists is shown in Table 16.5. Direct- and indirect-acting agents are listed. Indirect-acting agents produce a major portion of their agonistic action by enhancing the release of endogenous norepinephrine from sympathetic neuronal terminals to induce both α and β adrenergic effects. Consequently, actions produced by indirect-acting agents are partially dependent upon adequate stores of endogenous norepinephrine. As seen in Table 16.5, relatively few adrenergic agents are adrenoreceptor-specific (e.g., selective for only β_1 receptors).

ALPHA ADRENERGIC AGONISTS

Phenylephrine and methoxamine are relatively selective for α_1 receptors, whereas clonidine, xylazine, and detomidine induce relatively potent central α_2 agonistic actions when administered in low doses. Although α_2 activation induces vasoconstriction in vitro, the major effect induced by central-acting α_2 agonist agents in intact animals is sympatholytic because increased CNS α_2 stimulation readily depresses normal sympathetic outflow from medullary pressor centers (8).

Alpha 1 agonists can induce profound vasoconstriction and traditionally have been used as pressor agents to reverse hypotension associated with shock. However, the pathophysiology of hypovolemic shock actually results from reflexive hyperactive sympathetic stimulation. Therefore, fluid or volume replacement has become the primary therapeutic intervention in the treatment of hypovolemic shock. One remaining indication for a direct α adrenergic pressor action is reversal of severe hypotension when death is imminent. This circumstance often occurs during cardiovascular resuscitation efforts when adequate diastolic coronary perfusion is deemed essential. Any drug with strong α agonistic properties is indicated in this circum-

Table 16.4
Some Tissues and Organs Showing the Major Alpha Adrenergic Receptor Subtype and the Effector Response to Catecholamine Stimulation

Effector Organ	Receptor Subtype	Effector Response
Sympathetic neuronal terminal (presynaptic)	α_2	Inhibit NE release[a]
Platelets	α_2	Aggregation
Kidney	α_2	Inhibit renin release
Fat tissue	α_2	Antilipolysis
Pancreas (B cells)	α_2	Inhibit insulin release
CNS (medullary structures)	α_2	Inhibit cardiovascular center and sympathetic outflow
Stomach	α_2	Decrease motility
Arterioles	α_1 and α_2	Vasoconstriction
Veins	α_1	Contraction
Liver	α_1	Glycogenolysis
Uterus	α_1	Contraction (pregnant)
Male sex organs	α subtype unknown	Ejaculation
Pilomotor muscles	α subtype unknown	Contraction
Spleen	α subtype unknown	Contraction
Urinary bladder (sphincter)	α subtype unknown	Contraction
Intestine (sphincters)	α subtype unknown	Contraction
Stomach (sphincters)	α subtype unknown	Contraction
Lung (bronchial glands)	α_1	Inhibit secretion
Eye (radial muscle)	α_1	Contraction (mydriasis)
Mesenteric and renal vasculature	DA[c]1	Vasodilation
Sympathetic or parasympathetic neuronal terminals	DA 2	Inhibit NE and ACH[b] release

[a] NE, norepinephrine.
[b] ACH, acetylcholine.
[c] DA, dopaminergic receptor.

Table 16.5
Adrenergic Agonists[a]

Agent	Direct	Indirect	Adrenoreceptors				Dose
			α_1	α_2	β_1	β_2	
				Natural			
Norepinephrine	+++		+++	+++	++	±	0.05–0.3 μg/kg/min
Epinephrine	+++		++	++	+++	+++	0.05–0.2 μg/kg/min
Dopamine	+++		Dopaminergic stimulation				1–5 μg/kg/min
	++	+	+	?	++	++	5–15 μg/kg/min
	++	+	++	?	+	+	>15 μg/kg/min
				Synthetic			
Isoproterenol	+++				+++	+++	0.01–0.2 μg/kg/min
Dobutamine	+++				+++		1–5 μg/kg/min
Prenalterol	+++				+++	+	5–10 μg/kg/min
Ephedrine	+	++	++	?	++	?	0.2–1.0 mg/kg
Mephentermine	+	++	++	?	++	?	0.1–0.5 mg/kg
Metaraminol	±	++	++	?	+	?	10–100 μg/kg
Phenylephrine	+++		+++		+		1–10 μg/kg/min
Methoxamine	+++		+++				0.05–0.2 mg/kg
Clonidine			±	+++			

[a] +++, strong acting; ++, moderate acting; +, mild acting; ?, unknown. I, may or may not produce action. Modified from Lawson and Wallfisch (9).

stance, but epinephrine has been the agent of choice to induce a transient vasoconstriction and increase blood pressure (9).

In recent years, α agonists have occupied a different role in the therapeutic management and maintenance of adequate blood flow (9). This has been made possible by our increasing knowledge of the dose-dependent vascular selective actions of adrenergic agents. Recent work has documented that various adrenergic agents or even variations in doses of a single agonist can induce differential effects upon arterial and venous capacitance vessels (9). For example, norepinephrine is a potent venous and arterial constrictor, whereas methoxamine does not produce venoconstriction while inducing a potent arterial constricting action. In contrast to methoxamine, dopamine can produce significant venoconstriction at a dose that does not produce either cardiac or arterial vasoconstrictive actions. Knowledge of agent and dose differences in effects on venous and arterial vessels is important when selecting an adrenergic agonist agent. Venoconstriction produces the opposite effect of arterial constriction upon cardiac output. Venoconstriction decreases venous capacitance, increasing preload and cardiac output, while arterial constriction increases arterial resistance and afterload, most likely decreasing cardiac output. Thus, α agonists can be more appropriately selected with knowledge of their dose-dependent spectrum of venous to arterial constrictor actions. An adrenergic agonist that increases preload by inducing venoconstriction while possessing good inotropic properties appears beneficial in distributive or septic shock. For example, the use of dopamine in periods of low cardiac output improves mesenteric and renal blood flow selectively (dopaminergic receptors) while increasing cardiac output through venoconstriction and increased preload. This is feasible because low doses of dopamine have been shown to increase cardiac output via a selective increase in preload (9). Increasing doses of dopamine induce cardiac β_1 effects and eventually α_1-mediated arterial constriction (Table 16.5).

Ephedrine also induces a differential α-mediated arterial-venous constrictor action. Ephedrine is a weak, indirect-acting sympathomimetic that can be used to induce cardiotonic and venoconstrictor actions. Thus, ephedrine also increases preload and cardiac output while inducing relatively little arterial constriction. Ephedrine's actions appear preferable in pregnant patients with low cardiac outputs caused by excessive spinal block or neurogenic shock. These actions are especially important because a rise in cardiac output to increase blood pressure is essential in maintaining uterine blood flow (9). In contrast, increased arterial blood pressure achieved with a direct-acting arterial α agonist such as methoxamine drastically increases arterial resistance and afterload, reducing cardiac output. This action, while increasing blood pressure, is associated with decreased blood flow to the fetus and is contraindicated.

BETA ADRENERGIC AGONISTS

Beta adrenergic agonists have been used sparingly in veterinary medicine. Isoproterenol possesses strong nonselective β adrenergic activity. However, when used to induce specific actions such as bronchodilation or cardiac stimulation, it is associated with unwanted potent β_1-induced tachyarrythmias and inotropic cardiac actions or β_2 vasodilation and hypotension, respectively. Epinephrine induces strong β adrenergic actions but is accompanied by some α adrenergic activity in therapeutic β adrenergic doses. Epinephrine's complete spectrum of adrenergic action is desirable when treating anaphylaxis but unnecessary when treating conditions confined to specific organs or tissues (e.g., pulmonary bronchoconstriction or depressed cardiac contractility).

In recent years, the development of specific β_1 or β_2 agonists to replace nonselective agonists such as isoproterenol and epinephrine has been important in controlling the multiple actions associated with universal β receptor activation. Dobutamine is one such agent that induces relatively selective β_1 cardiac actions. Dobutamine's selective β_1 inotropic action spares the excessive β_1 chronotropic action and β_2 vasodilation seen with isoproterenol. This selective β_1 inotropic action is desirable because excessive increases in heart rate and hypotension observed after nonselective β receptor stimulation with isoproterenol often lead to increased myocardial oxygen consumption, decreased coronary perfusion, and eventual myocardial ischemia. In contrast to isoproterenol, norepinephrine's β_1 actions are accompanied by a strong α agonistic action, inducing undesirable increases in afterload. Dobutamine is thus preferable to isoproterenol or norepinephrine for the stabilization of patients suffering from acute or chronic cardiac failure because increases in heart rate (isoproterenol) or afterload (norepinephrine) are undesirable responses in these patients. Dobutamine is administered by intravenous infusion. As with all adrenergic agonists, the cardiac β_1 selectivity of dobutamine is lost with increasing doses. The lack of chronotropic action with dobutamine administration is dependent upon intact autonomic vagal reflexes to slow sinoatrial firing. Thus, adminstration of atropine before dobutamine therapy blocks vagal reflex inhibition associated with increased cardiac output and blood pressure and may result in unwanted tachycardia (10). Another selective β_1 agonist that can be used for chronic therapy is prenalterol. Its β_1 activity is similar to that of dobutamine, but prenalterol has a longer half-life and can be administered orally for the management of chronic heart failure.

Several selective β_2 agonists are now available for use in veterinary patients. Terbutaline, salbutamol, and clenbuterol induce a relatively selective β_2 agonistic action. These agents have been classified as selective bronchodilators. Although cumbersome, aerosol administration of the selective β_2 agonists is preferred when treating pulmonary conditions because fewer unwanted β_2 side effects such as hypotension are observed (8). Isoxsuprine also possesses β_2 agonist activity and has been advocated for relief of vasoconstriction or vasospasm associated with laminitis. These agents can be given orally and have long half-lives, making treatment of chronic disease more feasible but the responses are not as pronounced as when given by intravenous injection. However, prolonged therapy with β_2 agonists has resulted in attenuation of their effects (i.e., β receptor down-regulation).

High doses of β_2 agonists can result in β_1 receptor stimulation and concomitant cardiac effects. Beta adrenergic down-regulation (reduced sensitivity) associated with chronic β_2 agonist therapy has been observed. In these circumstances, the combined therapy of a β_2 agonist that increases cyclic adenosine monophosphate (cAMP) and a methylxanthine that inhibits cAMP breakdown has been advocated (11). Another therapeutic use of β_2 agonists in humans is induction of uterine smooth muscle relaxation (tocalytic therapy) to inhibit premature labor and parturition (8). This mode of β_2 agonist therapy has not been extensively implemented in veterinary medicine, and information is insufficient to advocate clinical treatment.

Table 16.6
Adrenergic Antagonists[a]

Agent	Adrenoreceptors			
	α_1	α_2	β_1	β_2
Alpha Antagonists				
Phentolamine	+	+	−	−
Phenoxybenzamine	+	+	−	−
Prazosin	+	−	−	−
Yohimbine	−	+	−	−
Tolazoline	+	+	−	−
Beta Antagonists				
Propranolol	−	−	+	+
Metoprolol	−	−	+	−
Atenolol	−	−	+	−
Practolol[b]	−	−	+	−
Oxprenolol[b]	−	−	+	+
Pindolol[b]	−	−	+	+
Mixed Antagonists				
Labetalol	+	−	+	+

[a] +, activity at clinical dosage; −, minimal or no significant activity at clinical dosage.
[b] Indicates intrinsic sympathomimetic activity.

Sympatholytic Agents

ALPHA ADRENERGIC ANTAGONISTS

Commonly used α adrenoceptor antagonists can be classified as nonselective α_1 and α_2 blockers or relatively selective antagonists for either α_1 or α_2 adrenoceptors (Table 16.6). Alpha antagonists have been used with varying success to reduce afterload, visceral ischemia during shock, hypertension, and pheochromocytoma. Two of the older nonselective α antagonists are phentolamine and phenoxybenzamine. Phentolamine and phenoxybenzamine are relatively short-acting and long-acting α blocking agents, respectively. Their actions have been associated with paradoxical sympathomimetic effects. This action has been attributed to reflex increases in sympathetic activity after the hypotensive phase of α blockade and more recently to the nonselective blockade of presynaptic α_2 receptors (Fig. 16.2) (11). Blockade of presynaptic α_2 adrenoreceptors inhibits normal negative feedback modulating effects at neuronal terminals and adrenal chromaffin cells. Presynaptic α_2 blockade thus augments neuronal release of norepinephrine to act on available unblocked adrenergic receptors (i.e., β_1 receptors). Thus, increased stimulation of β_1 receptors by norepinephrine (via the cardioaccelerator nerve) may explain the accentuated cardiac response observed after α blockade with nonselective antagonists. Phentolamine has been utilized to prevent sloughing of tissue after inadvertent norepinephrine extravasation or to test for pheochromocytoma. This agent has no notable action upon central α_2 adrenoceptor activity. Phenoxybenzamine has been used to induce long-term urinary bladder sphincter relaxation.

In contrast to the nonselective α antagonists, selective α_1 receptor antagonists such as prazosin do not possess presynaptic α_2 blocking action. Consequently, little or no cardiac sympathomimetic action is initiated by α_1 blockade achieved with prazosin. In addition, because postsynaptic α_2 adrenoceptors within the vasculature are unblocked with selective α_1 agonist agents, these receptors remain available for stimulation by catecholamines. Consequently, vasomotor tone is better maintained, and orthostatic hypotension is not prevalent after selective α_1 blockade. Prazosin may prove useful in unloading the failing heart and has been recommended as a vasodilator agent for treatment of heart failure.

During the last few years, the selective α_2 antagonist yohimbine has been used in veterinary medicine to reverse CNS depressant effects associated with the central-acting α_2 sedative actions of xylazine. A second nonselective α antagonist that has demonstrated efficacy in reversing CNS α_2-mediated sedation and sympathetic depression is tolazoline (12). Undoubtedly, with increased knowledge of α_2 adrenoceptor modulation of specific organ and tissue function, the indications and contraindications for α_2 antagonist therapy will be modified.

BETA ADRENERGIC ANTAGONISTS

Beta antagonists are used extensively in human medicine to treat a variety of conditions, including hypertension, angina, dysrythmias, cardiomyopathies, hyperthyroidism, glaucoma, and myocardial ischemia. These agents are not widely used or prescribed in veterinary medicine. Propranolol has been advocated to reduce myocardial work and oxygen consumption in obstructive cardiomyopathies or chronic heart failure of dogs and cats. However, β blocking agents may precipitate failure if compensatory sympathetic mechanisms are not present. The β antagonist actions of propranolol are nonselective and may be detrimental to some patients. In contrast, selective β_1 antagonists provide the cardiac therapeutic actions of propranolol while allowing for continued β_2 activation. Thus, selective β_1 blockade is preferred in patients with concomitant cardiac and bronchoconstrictive disease or in insulin-dependent diabetics where continued β_2-mediated bronchodilation or glucose metabolism respectively are important homeostatis functions (13).

Many new β_1 antagonists have been developed in recent years and are relatively cardioselective. Examples of β_1 antagonists are metoprolol, atenolol, and practolol (Table 16.6). In contrast to propranolol and most β_1-selective antagonists, some β antagonists have been developed that possess β_1 and β_2 blocking activity while maintaining a slight basal β adrenergic activation. This lessens the likelihood that heart failure or bronchoconstriction might be induced by cardiac β_1 or pulmonary β_2 blockade, respectively (8). The β antagonists that possess this minimal intrinsic sympathomimetic activity include practolol, oxprenolol, alprenolol, and pindolol (Table 16.6). In addition, maintenance of baseline β adrenergic stimulation may help in preventing the occurrence of β adrenergic up-regulation (increased sensitivity) after discontinuation of therapy. The β_1 antagonists have not been extensively used in veterinary medicine. However, it appears that there may be clear advantage to their use in any patient exhibiting symptoms worsened or exacerbated by nonselective β blockade, such as the use of propranolol in patients with bronchoconstrictive disease (8).

In recent years, new adrenergic antagonists have been developed that block both α and β receptors. For example, labetalol selectively blocks α_1 receptors while nonselectively blocking β receptors. Although the use of labetalol in the management of pheochromocytoma would appear advantageous in any species, the indications for mixed α and β adrenergic antagonist therapy in veterinary patients have yet to be completely defined.

Parasympathetic Pharmacology

Based upon the selectivity of certain muscarinic antagonists, such as pirenzepine, distinct subtypes of muscarinic receptors have been determined and designated as M_1 and M_2 receptors. Cholinergic agents used clinically for alteration of parasympathetic nervous system activity are usually restricted to peripheral muscarinic (M_2) receptor stimulation. Cholinergic stimulation of nicotinic receptors is observed within the motor end plate of skeltal muscle and within the ganglia of the ANS. Muscarinic receptors of M_1 sensitivity are also found in autonomic ganglia and the CNS. Thus, specific modulation of parasympathetic actions can only be achieved by stimulating or blocking muscarinic receptors (M_2) located near postganglionic parasympathetic fibers. Increased muscarinic stimulation can be achieved with anticholinesterase agents such as neostigmine and physostigmine, but the actions of increased acetylcholine levels are not confined to postganglionic parasympathetic-muscarinic receptors. Similarly, increases in acetylcholine release induced by agents such as 4-aminopyridine produce generalized central and peripheral cholinergic actions.

MUSCARINIC AGONISTS

Methylcholine, bethanechol, and carbachol are three commonly used muscarinic agonists. They have decreased susceptibility to cholinesterase hydrolysis and thus may induce a rather prolonged duration of effect (8). Methylcholine and bethanechol are muscarinic agonists, whereas carbachol possesses some nicotinic agonist action as well. Carbachol is administered topically in the eye to induce rapid constriction in the treatment of glaucoma and to stimulate gastrointestinal motility. Bethanechol can be used to stimulate gastrointestinal function and genitourinary smooth muscle contraction. A fourth muscarinic agonist, pilocarpine, has also been used as a miotic.

MUSCARINIC ANTAGONISTS

Parasympathetic antagonists may be either nicotinic-acting or muscarinic-acting. However, nicotinic receptor antagonists produce either ganglionic blocking action, such as trimethaphan, or neuromuscular blocking actions and thus do not confine their actions to specific parasympathetic functions (8). In contrast, the belladonna alkaloids, atropine and scopolamine, have specific antimuscarinic actions. Some muscarinic antagonists can cross the blood-brain barrier to induce a sedative-like action (scopolamine) as well as peripheral effects. Glycopyrrolate is a long-acting muscarinic anticholinergic agent that does not cross the blood-brain barrier and is thus considered by some clinicians to be preferable to atropine. Atropine blocks muscarinic actions whether they are excitatory (intestine) or inhibitory (heart). Atropine can induce excessive increases in heart rate that may be detrimental in some patients. This action is thought to be due to atropine blockade of muscarinic receptor-mediated cholinergic inhibition of sympathetic neuronal-release of norepinephrine (Fig. 16.4) (8).

Antiarrhythmic Agents

NORMAL RHYTHMICITY

The rhythm of the heart is initiated by a single pacemaker (SA node) and maintained by the rapid and uniform spread of an impulse through normal conduction routes. Conduction of an impulse is regulated by the uniform duration of action potential and refractory period of various cardiac conduction pathways (14). Purkinje fibers normally have a longer action potential duration (Fig. 16.5) than does normal myocardial muscle. This prevents re-entry and re-excitation of the Purkinje system by myocardial electrical activity. Disturbances in any of the factors responsible for maintaining normal rhythmicity can lead to arrhythmogenic activity (i.e., abnormal automaticity or increased spontaneous depolarization of normally subordinate pacemaker foci changes in the action potential duration or refractory period of cells responsible for normal impulse conduction, or a slowing of impulse through

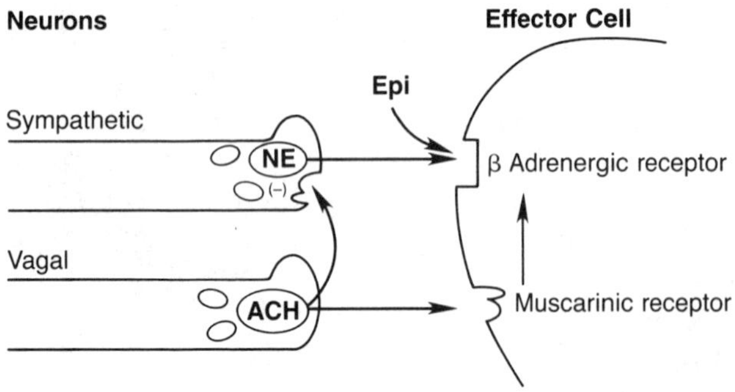

Figure 16.4. Diagrammatic representation of the interaction between sympathetic and parasympathetic nerve terminals at effector cell. Acetylcholine (ACH) release from vagal nerve terminal interacts with muscarinic receptors presynaptically on the sympathetic neuronal terminal and on the effector cell. Muscarinic stimulation is inhibitory to norepinephrine (NE) release from the sympathetic neuron. Postsynaptic muscarinic stimulation further modifies the effector cell's response to β receptor stimulation by NE and epinephrine (EPI). Modified from Watanabe and Bailey (46).

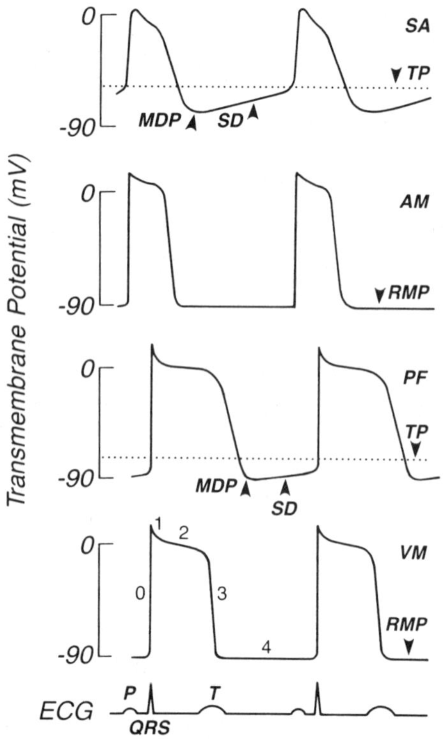

Figure 16.5. Schematic diagram demonstrating relationship between the action potentials recorded from cells of the sinoatrial node (SA), atrial muscle (AM), Purkinje fibers (PF), and ventricular muscle (VM) in relation to an ECG recording. The P wave of the ECG corresponds to depolarization of the SA and AM tissues, and the QRS complex and T wave correspond to depolarization and repolarization of VM, respectively. In the *top tracing*, it can be seen that the automatic cells of the SA node do not exhibit a Phase 4 resting membrane potential (RMP) of nearly −90 MV. Spontaneous depolarization (SD) begins immediately after attaining maximal diastolic potential for the SA tissue until threshold potential (TP) is reached, initiating another action potential. Subordinate automatic tissue is found in a variety of other tissues in the atrium, AV node, AV values, and Purkinje system. The SA node usually attains threshold potential first, propagating impulse to other pacemaker tissue before it reaches threshold. Note the duration of action potential from the PF tissue versus that of VM. Five phases of the action potential are labeled *0*, *1*, *2*, *3*, and *4* on the first action potential of VM. Modified from Adams (14).

cells or tissue). Arrhythmias are associated with imbalances in ANS activity, abnormalities in K^+ and Ca^{2+} concentrations, acidosis (hypercapnia), trauma or ischemia, infection (myocarditis), stretch (congestive heart failure), anesthetic drugs (thiamylal or halothane), and rapid change in hemodynamic function (heart rate or high blood pressure).

ARRHYTHMOGENIC MECHANISMS

Arrhythmias have traditionally been attributed to abnormal propagation (re-entry) and automaticity. The determinants of cardiac excitability responsible for abnormal propagation and automaticity reside in a complex matrix of active and passive membrane properties that have been adequately characterized for fast and slow response cardiac tissues. Table 16.7 lists some of these properties (15). The complete explanation of arrhythmogenic activity is extremely complex and will involve the unveiling of matrices of interacting variables in both normal and injured cardiac tissues. Understanding the mechanisms of action of the antiarrhythmic drugs will require knowledge of additional matrices of electrophysiological action in normal and damaged cardiac tissues. Until these complex interactions are completely characterized, re-entry and abnormal automaticity are concepts that will have to suffice as simplified explanations of arrhythmogenic activity upon which antiarrhythmic therapy can be based (15).

RE-ENTRY

Re-entry-type arrhythmias require the presence of unidirectional block in conducting pathways. This is usually due to an area of localized injury. Conduction velocity is decreased and the refractory period is prolonged in injured tissue. Normal antegrade impulses are unable to penetrate the injured area due to prolongation of the refractory state. Impulses proceed in a normal fashion along uninjured fibers and proceed in a retrograde fashion through the injured area (Fig. 16.6). Re-entry arrhythmias occur when retrograde impulses re-excite abnormal or normal tissue that is no longer refractory (Fig. 16.6).

ABNORMAL AUTOMATICITY

Impulse generation or automaticity can be divided into normal or abnormal mechanisms. Figure 16.7 is a schematic representation of the transmembrane action potential of cardiac cells with the property of spontaneous depolarization. These cells are normally found in the SA node, certain atrial or AV junctional cells, and Purkinje fibers. The potential mechanisms by which antiarrhythmic agents may suppress spontaneous depolarization are also shown in Figure 16.7. Automaticity by abnormal mechanisms may result from a decrease in membrane potential of normally depolarized cardiac fibers. Working atrial and ventricular myocardial cells do not normally possess the property of spontaneous diastolic depolarization and do not initiate spontaneous impulses. However, when the resting membrane potential is experimentally reduced to −60 mV, spontaneous diastolic depolarization may occur, resulting in repetitive impulse initiation (16). This abnormal automaticity can occur in atrial and

Table 16.7
Characteristics of Fast and Slow Response Cardiac Tissue[a]

	Fast Response Tissues	Slow Response Tissues
	Passive Membrane Properties	
Normal resting potential	−80 to −90 mV	−40 to −65 mV
Subthreshold membrane conductable	gK^+	Probably gK^+
	Active Membrane Properties	
Threshold voltage	−60 to −75 mV	−40 to −60 mV
Current responsible for Phase 0 depolarization	i Na^+	i_{si} (mixed current of Ca^{++} and Na^+)
Activation and inactivation kinetics of channel responsible for Phase 0 depolarization	Fast	Slow
Maximal rise velocity of Phase 0 (Vmax)	300 to 1000 + V/sec	1 to 50 V/sec
Peak over shoot	+20 to +40 mV	−5 to +20 mV
Overall action potential amplitude	90 to 135 mV	−30 to +70 mV
Refractoriness and reactivation	Partial reactivation during Phase 3; complete reactivation 10 to 50 msec after return to normal resting potential	Partial and complete reactivation returns after attaining resting potential (>100 msec)
Conduction velocity	0.5 to 5 m/sec	0.01 to 0.1 m/sec
Characteristics conducive to re-entry	Only with inactivation of the Na^+ system	Yes, even in normal slow response tissues
Automaticity	Yes	Yes
Automaticity depressed by physiological increased in K^+	Yes	No
Location of fast vs. slow response tissues	Working and specialized atrial; specialized intranodal conduction system (Purkinje fibers); ventricular muscle	SA and AV nodes; valves; coronary sinus; injured tissue in which Na^+-dependent tissues are converted to i_{si} (Ca^{++} and Na^+)-dependent Phase 0

[a] Modified from Arnsdorf (15).

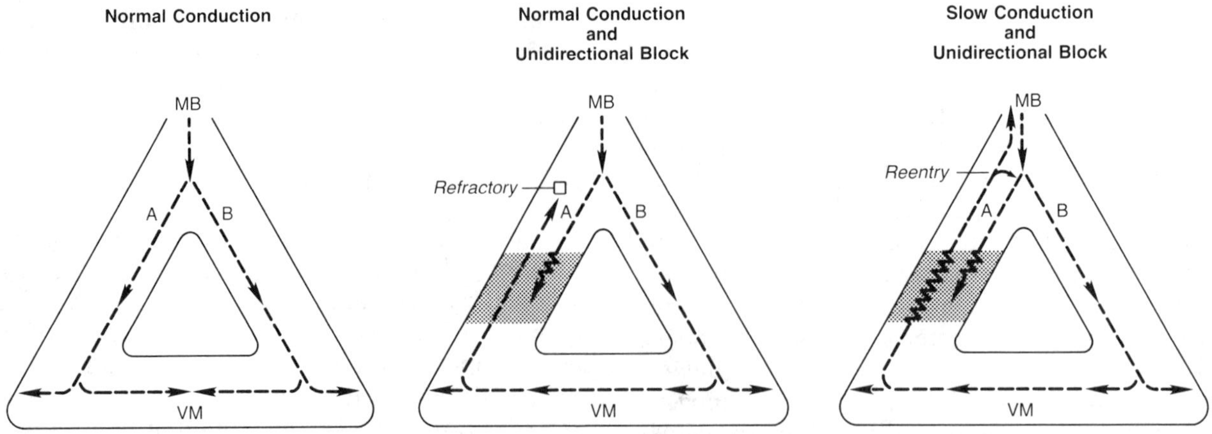

Figure 16.6. Schematic drawing of the electrophysiological mechanism responsible for re-entry arrhythmia formation. In the figure on the left, normal conduction progresses down a main bundle (MB) of the Purkinje system into Branches A and B. The impulse uniformly and rapidly excites ventricular muscle (VM) and is unable to travel retrograde into the MB because of the refractory state of the recently excited tissue. The middle figure depicts normal conduction through the Purkinje system after unidirectional block in Branch A (*shaded*). A retrograde pathway of impulse occurs, but conduction is normal and refractory tissue is encountered. In the right figure, slow conduction (*jagged line*) and unidirectional block results in a retrograde impulse through Branch A and re-entry arrhythmia formation. This occurs because refractory tissue is not encountered when the slowed impulse traverses the block area in Branch A. Modified from Adams (14).

ventricular tissue or Purkinje fibers. Abnormal automaticity is differentiated from normal diastolic depolarization and action potential upstroke by the significant involvement of slow inward current. Slow channel blocking drugs (Ca^{2+} antagonists) may induce part of their antiarrhythmic action by depressing this type of arrhythmic mechanism (17). Paradoxically, abnormal automaticity might also occur as a consequence of the toxic actions of antiarrhythmic drugs. For example, quinidine and procainamide can cause cardiac cells to depolarize, enhancing automaticity of some nonpacemaker cardiac tissue (18).

Triggered activity is caused by after-depolarizations, which are secondary depolarizations that occur either during repolarization (early after-depolarization) or after repolarization is nearly complete or just completed (delayed after-depolarization) (18). Early and delayed after-depolarizations are often referred to as "triggered impulses." Early after-depolarization usually occurs during Phase 3 of repolarization (Fig. 16.5) in cells with high maximum diastolic potential. The action potential of early after-depolarization may be caused by slow inward current and occurs prior to complete repolarization of the first action potential. Because early after-depolarization action potentials occur at a low membrane potential, they are likely caused by the same current responsible for abnormal automaticity of partially depolarized fibers. If triggered activity exceeds the rate of the sinus node, a paroxysm of tachycardia may result. Drugs that suppress abnormal automaticity (e.g., Ca^{2+} channel blockers) should theoretically prevent early after-depolarization because both arrhythmic mechanisms are a result of low membrane potential and slow inward current (Ca^{2+}) action potentials (18). Theoretically, drugs that accelerate repolarization may also prevent early after-depolarization (19). Some antiarrhythmic agents, such as procainamide, can paradoxically cause early after-depolarization by prolonging action potential duration.

Delayed after-depolarizations occur at the termination of repolarization and are induced by that action potential. If the after-depolarization is large enough to reach membrane threshold potential, a triggered impulse arises. The mechanism for delayed after-depolarization differs considerably from the mechanism thought to be responsible for abnormal automaticity and early after-depolarization. Calcium uptake into cells enhances the amplitude of delayed after-depolarizations. This occurs with increased rate of stimulation, hypercalcemia, increased catecholamines, or excessive glycoside administration. In contrast, agents that decrease Ca^{2+} uptake depress amplitude of delayed after-depolarizations. Thus, altered intracellular Ca^{2+} levels appear to be involved in the genesis of this type of arrhythmic action.

Delayed after-depolarizations and triggered activity can be caused by cardiac glycoside-induced increases in intracellular Ca^{2+} within Purkinje fibers and may be responsible for the frequently observed digitalis-induced arrhythmia (20). Antiarrhythmic agents such as the Ca^{2+} antagonists have prevented this form of triggered activity (21). Decreasing intracellular Ca^{2+} influx by accelerating repolarization or shortening the action potential duration may decrease the amplitude of delayed after-depolarization and prevent triggered activity. Similarly, depression of sodium (Na^+) influx

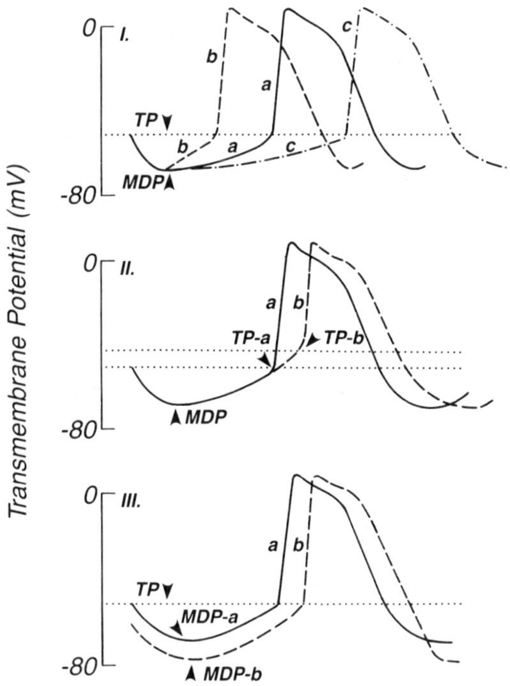

Figure 16.7. Schematic drawing of cardiac cell with property of spontaneous depolarization and automaticity. In the upper tracing, the maximal diastolic potential is near −70 mV, and the normal slope of Phase 4 spontaneous depolarization is depicted by the *solid line* (*a*). Automaticity is enhanced when the slope of depolarization goes from *a* to *b*, reducing the time required to reach threshold potential (TP). Some antiarrhythmic agents increase the time to reach threshold potential by reducing the slope of Phase 4 spontaneous depolarization (*c*), thereby depressing ectopic foci. Other antiarrhythmic agents raise the TP to a less negative value from TPa to TPb, as seen in the middle tracing, again increasing the time required to achieve TP and depressing automaticity. A third mechanism by which antiarrhythmic agents can depress automaticity is seen in the bottom tracing, where the maximal diastolic potential (MDP) is increased from −70 mV (MDP-a) to −80 mV (MDP-b) requiring more time to reach TP even though the slope of Phase 4 depolarization is unchanged. Modified from Adams (14).

with local anesthetics such as lidocaine can decrease delayed after-depolarization amplitude and abolish triggered activity (22).

CLASSIFICATION OF ANTIARRHYTHMIC AGENTS

Antiarrhythmic drugs have been presented and evaluated at the rate of one new drug about every 6 months for the last decade. Many of these new drugs were initially developed for alternative therapeutic interventions (e.g., melperone and mexiletine) and were only later discovered to possess antiarrhythmic actions. This method of discovering antiarrhythmic agents is common. In recent years, all antiarrhythmic agents have been shown to possess at least one of four basic electrophysiological actions capable of suppressing abnormal cardiac rhythm. Classification of antiarrhythmic agents has subsequently been based upon these electrophysiological antiarrhythmic properties (Table 16.8). These subdivisions not only help in classifying antiarrhythmic agents but also provide a methodology for understanding mechanisms of abnormal cardiac rhythmicity (23). New information has required that additional antiarrhythmic mechanisms or matrices be considered and has resulted in further subdivision of Class I antiarrhythmic drugs (23).

All Class I agents exert some electrophysiological action upon the fast inward Na^+ current. Class I antiarrhythmic agents have been divided into three subgroups and include quinidine, procainamide, disopyramide, and lidocaine and the new agents mexiletine, tocainide, lorcainide, encainide, and flecainide (Table 16.2). The older compounds, quinidine, procainamide, and disopyramide, became Group Ia. These agents have moderate actions on prolonging effective refractory period (ERP) and the Q-T interval and widen the QRS complex of the electrocardiogram (ECG) at high concentration. Quinidine lengthens action potential duration (APD) by delaying repolarization. In addition, both quinidine and disopyramide possess anticholinergic properties unrelated to their Class I electrophysiologic effect (23). Lidocaine, mexiletine, and tocainide (Group Ib) shorten APD in vitro and shorten monophasic action potentials and Q-T intervals in vivo (Table 16.8). They do not lengthen conduction time or QRS in sinus rhythm but prolong the ERP. The most recently introduced Class I agents are flecainide, encainide, and lorcainide (Group Ic) (Table 16.8). These agents have little effect on APD, Q-T interval, or on ERP, but they increase conduction time and widen the QRS complex (23). The basic electrophysiological antiarrhythmic mechanism of all Class I drugs can be attributed to their attachment to inactivated Na^+ channels, prolonging inactivation (23, 24). However, because the clinical indications and use of Class I antiarrhythmic agents can be quite different, many clinicians doubt that a single fundamental mode of action exists. Most antiarrhythmic agents have additional properties that distinguish their use and can explain the disparity in their clinical actions. Some of the important additional properties of Class I agents are (*a*) anticholinergic actions (e.g., quinidine and disopyramide); (*b*) variations in distribution into the CNS due to solubility and molecular size differences; (*c*) variation in metabolism and excretion rates; (*d*) shortening of action potential duration (i.e., lidocaine, mexiletine, and tocainide); and (*e*) variation in rapidity of drug attachment and release from Na^+ channels (23). The latter property is a function of each agent's solubility and dissociation constant. Many Class I agent in vitro studies have indicated a close correlation between duration of drug-

Table 16.8
Electrophysiological Classification of Antiarrhythmic Agents[a]

Class	Electrophysiologic Effects	Clinical Indications
I. Local anesthetics and membrane stabilizers		
Class Ia		
Quinidine	QRS widen with high concentration	Supraventricular and ventricular arrhythmias
Procainamide	Conduction ↓ with high concentration	
Disopyramide	ERP ↑ duration	
	APD ↑ at high concentration	
	ERP/APD ↑ ratio	
	TP ↑	
	Rate of slow and rapid depolarization ↓	
Class Ib		
Lidocaine	QRS none in sinus rhythm	Ventricular arrhythmias only
Mexiletine	Conduction none in sinus rhythm	
Tocainide	ERP ↓	
Phenytoin	APD ↓	
	ERP/APD ↑ ratio	
	Rate of rapid depolarization ↓	
Class Ic		
Lorcainide	QRS widen with low concentrations	Supraventricular and ventricular
Encainide	Conduction slowed with low concentrations	
Flecainide	ERP little change	
	APD little change	
II. Antiadrenergic beta blockers (acute effects)		
Propranolol	Rapid depolarization ↓	Re-entrant and automatic supraventricular and ventricular arrhythmias
Metroprolol	ERP ↑	
Oxyprenolol	APD ↓	
Alprenolol	ERP/APD ↑ ratio	
Atenolol		
Sotalol		
Bretylium	(Inhibits release of NE)	
III. Agents that prolong action potential		
Bretylium	Rapid depolarization no change	Atrial and ventricular arrhythmias
Amiodarone	ERP ↑ APD ↑	
Propranolol (chronic)	Prolongs repolarization	
Sotalol (acute)	ERP/APD ↑ ratio	
Melperone		
IV. Calcium channel or slow response blockers		
Verapamil	Rapid depolarization, no change	Predominately supraventricular arrhythmias
	APD ↓	
	Slow depolarization ↓	

[a] TP, threshold potential; NE, norepinephrine.

Na^+ channel interaction and the observed clinical differences in action. Thus, quantitative disparities in rapidity of attachment to and removal from Na^+ channels may account for a considerable portion of the differences observed in the clinical profiles of Classes Ia, Ib, and Ic agents (Table 16.8) (23). In general, all Class I drugs have the ability to decrease membrane responsiveness. Class I agents inhibit spontaneous depolarization (i.e., automaticity), controlling arrhythmias caused by enhanced automaticity, whereas the prolongation of the ERP can effectively abolish re-entry arrhythmias.

The Class II antiarrhythmic agents depress automaticity by inhibiting the action of catecholamines on cardiac tissues (Table 16.8). It has been demonstrated that β adrenergic stimulation increases the rate of depolarization and shortens the APD and absolute refractory period. Hyperactivity of the sympathetic nervous system is an important factor in the pathogenesis of ectopic pacemaker foci. By reducing the influence of sympathetic stimulation on the heart, β blocking drugs can be effective in controlling arrhythmias caused by excessive sympathoadrenal discharge. Beta blocking agents also possess some quinidine-like or membrane-stabilizing properties when given in high concentrations. As seen in Table 16.8, this class includes agents that prevent norepinephrine release from sympathetic nerves (e.g., bretylium), as well as those that block postsynaptic myocardial β receptors (e.g., propranolol). Thus, agents that reduce centrally mediated anxiety and indirectly decrease sympathetic activity, such as tranquilizers, and anesthetic agents, should be considered as having some Class II antiarrhythmic action.

The Class III antiarrhythmic agents exert their effect by prolongation of APD and ERP (Table 16.8).

Amiodarone is the prototypical Class III agent. Initially, it was used clinically as an antianginal agent. Recent electrophysiological results have demonstrated that amiodarone caused a prolongation of APD with only a minor sympatholytic effect (Class II action) and very minimal action as a membrane-stabilizing agent (Class I action) (25). Amiodarone has a remarkable antiarrhythmic action for control of certain pre-excitation arrhythmias, such as Wolff-Parkinson-White (WPW), and arrhythmias associated with hypertrophic cardiomyopathy that are unresponsive to Class I agents such as lidocaine (26, 27). Differences in efficacy may be associated with the preferential lengthening of APD by amiodarone in the bundle of His and ventricular muscle where abnormal pathways occur in patients with WPW. In contrast, lidocaine, which is of little value in WPW syndrome, preferentially shortens APD in distal Purkinje cells where APD is normally longest (Fig. 16.5). Thus, the lengthening of APD in specific conduction pathways may constitute an antiarrhythmic action that is selective for specific arrhythmias (23). Bretylium is also considered a Class III antiarrhythmic because it induces prolongation of APD. Beta blockers may also induce a Class III antiarrhythmic action after acute or chronic administration (Table 16.8). Recent information indicates that acute therapy with some β blockers (e.g., sotalol) can prolong APD. Similarly, chronic β blockade achieved with propranolol causes a prolonging of the APD. Propranolol-induced prolongation of APD presumably represents a secondary adaptation to long-term β blockade because prolongation of APD is observed even after termination of therapy (23).

The Class IV antiarrhythmic agents alter cardiac electrophysiology by restricting normally subordinate slower Ca^{2+} inward current (Table 16.8). These agents are often referred to as Ca^{2+} channel blockers or Ca^{2+} antagonists. In clinical practice, Ca^{2+} antagonists are most effective in controlling supraventricular arrhythmias and have shown little promise in preventing ventricular arrhythmia formation (28, 29). These agents decrease the rate of depolarization by inhibiting Ca^{2+} influx into cells, particularly at the SA and AV node. After myocardial insult, diastolic potential of myocardial cells may become partially depolarized, resulting in progressively inactivated fast Na^+ channels (23). Myocardial cells may then generate action potentials via secondary slow Ca^{2+} channels rather than through fast Na^+ channel activation. Slow channel-generated impulses are associated with slow conduction that may initiate ventricular re-entry arrhythmias (Table 16.7; Fig. 16.6). Consequently, it has been postulated that abolition of ventricular arrhythmias with Ca^{2+} antagonists is associated with the prevention of slow inward Ca^{2+} current depolarization (23). However, in a more recent study, Ca^{2+} antagonists were shown to improve conduction in Purkinje and myocardial cells. Thus, it has been alternatively hypothesized that Ca^{2+} antagonists exert their antiarrhythmic action in ventricular tissue by decreasing intracellular Ca^{2+}, which opens gap junctions between cells, decreasing resistance to conduction (23). Improved conduction would then reduce the likelihood of re-entry arrhythmia formation where unidirectional block exists (29). With faster conduction, refractory cells or tissues are more likely to be encountered abolishing re-entry arrhythmias generated through retrograde pathways (Fig. 16.6). This mechanism of action appears to be an additional viable explanation for the calcium antagonist verapamil's occasional effectiveness in treating ventricular arrhythmias (23).

CLASS I AGENTS

Quinidine is the prototype Class Ia antiarrhythmic agent. It can successfully depress atrial and ventricular ectopic premature ventricular activity. In therapeutic doses, quinidine usually spares the automaticity of the SA node. Thus, quinidine prolongs the effective refractory period (Table 16.8) of both atrial and ventricular muscle with less effect on normal pacemaker tissue. Prolongation of the ERP of atrial tissue accounts for quinidine's effectiveness in converting atrial fibrillation to sinus rhythm. A loss in cholinergic activity also causes a lengthening of the refractory period, further damping atrial tachyarrhythmias. Quinidine's indirect vagolytic effect often results in increased heart rate. Pronounced increases in ventricular rate may occur after quinidine treatment of atrial flutter or fibrillation. This is believed to be due to decreased refractoriness of the AV node as the atrial rate decreases and quinidine's vagolytic action, which allows a greater number of impulses to traverse the AV node to the ventricles (30). It has been recommended that pretreatment with digitalis for its cholinergic effect to slow AV conduction is beneficial in preventing ventricular tachycardia during quinidine therapy. This can be considered a beneficial pharmacodynamic interaction. However, an additional potentially dangerous pharmacokinetic interaction between quinidine and digitalis may also occur (14, 31). Quinidine can substantially increase the plasma concentration of digoxin by altering tissue distribution, decreasing the volume of distribution and elimination of digoxin (31). A second drug interaction observed during concomitant quinidine and verapamil therapy in man is the occurrence of profound hypotension (32). Quinidine induces a direct relaxing effect upon vascular smooth muscle, whereas verapamil inhibits Ca^{2+} influx into smooth muscle and also depresses vascular tone. It has been suggested that both quinidine and verapamil possess additional α receptor blocking properties. Thus, because the potential for inducing profound hypotension is great, the safety of simultaneously administering these two agents has recently been questioned (32).

The dose of quinidine necessary to successfully abolish atrial fibrillation may vary greatly among patients (14, 30). Intravenous quinidine administration may cause severe side effects and is not recommended. Quinidine toxicosis is manifested as gastrointestinal upset, nausea, vomiting, diarrhea, and depression. Acute toxicosis associated with intravenous administration can induce nonselective depression of electromechanical function of the heart, including first, second, or third degree AV block; SA block; slowed conduction; arrhythmia formation; hypotension; decreased contractility; decreased cardiac output; and prolongation of ECG complexes. Consequently, oral dosing is the preferred method of administration.

Quinidine is the drug of choice for frequent atrial premature depolarizations and atrial fibrillation in the horse (33). In general, quinidine is very effective for short-term treatment of both supraventricular and ventricular arrhythmias in the horse. Quinidine has also been effective in prolonging the PR interval in horses and dogs exhibiting ventricular pre-excitation syndrome and is of some diagnostic and therapeutic value for this condition (34, 35). In contrast, digitalis and verapamil are contraindicated in patients with ventricular pre-excitation because these agents may block normal AV conduction, enhancing conduction through abnormal accessory pathways (36).

Procainamide is a Class Ia antiarrhythmic agent with qualitative electrophysiological actions similar to quinidine (Table 16.8). Procainamide increases the effective refractory period, slows conduction, and can suppress both abnormal automaticity (ectopic foci) and re-entry arrhythmias. Paradoxically, procainamide's varying effects upon different specialized conducting pathways may also contribute to arrhythmogenesis. Procainamide's cardiac and vascular-depressant effects are similar to quinidine's actions. It also possesses a similar vagolytic effect. Because procainamide and quinidine increase refractoriness and slow conduction in the AV node and Purkinje system, they may potentiate first, second, or third degree heart block. These agents are contraindicated in patients with widened QRS complexes or heart block (30). Oral procainamide therapy, like quinidine, is used in the chronic management of ventricular arrhythmias. Unlike quinidine, procainamide is also used intravenously to terminate ventricular arrhythmias. Procainamide is the drug of choice for unwanted ventricular activity if lidocaine is ineffective. Larger doses of procainamide are needed to terminate supraventricular arrhythmias. Toxic signs are similar to those seen with quinidine therapy (30). A systemic lupus erythematosus syndrome has been associated with chronic procainamide therapy in humans and dogs.

Disopyramide is the third Class Ia antiarrhythmic agent of some recent interest and use (Table 16.8). It has been used in dogs, but is contraindicated in heart failure due to its myocardial depressant effect and an observed increase in peripheral vascular resistance. Disopyramide also possesses vagolytic actions and is not recommended for use in cats (37).

Lidocaine is a local anesthetic agent with Class Ib antiarrhythmic activity (Table 16.8). Lidocaine effectively abolishes both automatic and re-entry ventricular arrhythmias in all species. Because it has little effect on atrial conduction or refractoriness, lidocaine is not recommended for treatment of supraventricular arrhythmias. It is often the first agent used for treating premature ventricular arrhythmias associated with acute trauma, surgery, or anesthesia. It may be as effective as phenytoin in treating digitalis-induced arrhythmias. Lidocaine is given intravenously and has an extremely short half-life. It is not often used for chronic control of ventricular arrhythmias but has been administered as a constant intravenous infusion in dogs and cats. Toxic side effects include emesis, CNS depression, and seizures, which are more likely to be observed in the cat. Lidocaine should be used cautiously in animals with AV block or ventricular conduction disorders (37). Purkinje tissues appear to be the most sensitive to lidocaine's actions. Lidocaine is more effective when K^+ levels are normal or elevated, indicating the importance of this ion in lidocaine's mechanism of action (30).

Tocainamide and mexiletine are two new orally administered lidocaine analogues. They possess Class Ib local anesthetic (Na^+ channel blocking) effects (Table 16.8). Both drugs are well absorbed after oral administration and have long half-lives. They appear to be among the safest of the newer antiarrhythmic drugs (38). These agents have minimal inotropic and hemodynamic depressant effects (39). They may prove useful in patients whose ventricular tachyarrhythmias are uncontrolled with or who cannot tolerate currently available agents (38). Side effects appear to be minimal. Arrhythmia aggravation is unusual, but thrombocytopenia with mexiletine and pulmonary fibrosis with tocainide have been reported (38).

Diphenylhydantoin is a structural analogue of the barbiturates and is used primarily as an anticonvulsant in the treatment of epilepsy. However, its antiarrhythmic action results from a Class Ib action that is similar to lidocaine's effects (Table 16.8). It can be effective in treating a variety of ventricular arrhythmias; because of its sporadic efficacy, however, it is often overlooked. Phenytoin is not recommended for the acute treatment of ventricular arrhythmias but may be given prophylactically to patients with arrhythmias resulting from digitalis intoxication (30, 37). Phenytoin demonstrates particular effectiveness against atrial and ventricular arrhythmias resulting from digitalis toxicity. Because lidocaine is safer to administer to dogs and cats, lidocaine is often preferred for the acute control of digitalis-induced arrhythmias (36). When phenytoin is administered intravenously, heart rate may increase due to its vagolytic action. Phenytoin may also decrease sympathetic activity by its CNS-depressant effects (30).

Aprindine is an experimental Class I agent that has been used successfully in dogs. It has been effective in converting atrial and ventricular tachycardia to sinus rhythm after unsatisfactory results with standard therapy (40). Aprindine is not effective in controlling arrhythmias attributed to slow channel (Ca^{2+}) mediated activity. Toxic effects observed have included emesis, ataxia, salivation, and nystagmus. In addition, aprinidine has been combined with other Class I agents to achieve additional suppression of ventricular arrhythmias. In dogs, it has been effective in treating digitalis-induced and ischemia-related arrhythmias and increases the threshold for ventricular fibrillation.

The Class Ic agents include encainide, flecainide, and lorcainide (Table 16.8). These agents differ entirely from lidocaine in their molecular structure. They, like all Class I agents, interact with the fast inward Na^+ current (Phase 0) during depolarization. They contrast with Class Ia agents (prolonged AP) and Class Ib agents (shortened AP) because as they have little or no effect upon APD. In some patients, these agents appear effective in treating ischemia-related ventricular arrhythmias and chronic recurrent ventricular tachyarrhythmias refractory to the more conventional antiarrhythmic agents (quinidine, procainamide). However, they have been associated with some arrhythmogenic action. Encainide appears to have the greatest potential for aggravating or even initiating life-threatening ventricular arrhythmias (41). These agents have not been widely used in veterinary medicine, but they hold promise in improving the efficacy of Class I antiarrhythmic therapy.

CLASS II AGENTS

The Class II antiarrhythmic agents include propranolol and other β blocking agents (e.g., metoprolol), bretylium, and guanethidine (Table 16.8). Because stress and anxiety cause increased catecholamines and may precipitate cardiac arrhythmias, in certain circumstances, drugs that antagonize the effects of catecholamines on the heart are effective antiarrhythmic agents. Class II agents either block myocardial β receptors (propranolol) or prevent the release of norepinephrine from sympathetic nerve terminals (bretylium, and guanethidine). The controversy over whether β blockers exert their antiarrhythmic action via a local anesthetic membrane-stabilizing action (Class I) has been resolved. It is now agreed that they exert the major portion of their antiarrhythmic effect via a sympatholytic action. Propranolol can be effective in treating both atrial and ventricular arrhythmias. It depresses automaticity and conduction in abnormal ventricular myocardium. Propranolol is effective in treating high ventricular rates associated with atrial flutter or fibrillation and can abolish supraventricular arrhythmias associated with AV nodal reentry. Propranolol decreases cardiac output, myocardial work, and myocardial O_2 consumption and suppresses hypoxia-related arrhythmias. This is the rationale for its administration in hypertrophic obstructive heart disease. Because of its direct sympatholytic effect, propranolol therapy is implemented to control supraventricular and ventricular arrhythmias associated with pheochromocytoma and thyrotoxicosis (37). It can be administered orally or intravenously; intravenous administration should be carried out cautiously to prevent depression of myocardial contractility. Beta blockers also appear to be effective in treating arrhythmias associated with myocardial-sensitizing anesthetic agents such as halothane and possibly xylazine. Propranolol has been effective in controlling digitalis-induced arrhythmias when alternative therapy has been ineffective.

The toxic effects of propranolol are a result of excessive β_1 and β_2 blockade. Bradyarrhythmias and cardiac failure may occur due to direct β_1 blockade and resultant cardiac depressant effects. The β_2 blockade can be associated with bronchoconstriction and hypoglycemia and thus should be avoided in patients with airway diseases such as asthma or in diabetics receiving insulin. If cardiac failure does ensue after propranolol administration, catecholamine cardiotonic therapy will likely be ineffective. Thus, Ca^{2+}, glucagon, or digitalis therapy is preferable and should be instituted (37).

CLASS III AGENTS

Bretylium and amiodarone are prototypical Class III antiarrhythmic agents; their major effect is to increase APD and prolong repolarization (Table 16.8). Bretylium is considered the first-line agent for treatment and prophylaxis of ventricular fibrillation or for life-threatening arrhythmias that have not responded to lidocaine (42). Bretylium is not recommended for treatment of ventricular ectopy. However, bretylium has been used to successfully abolish "torsades de pointes" initiated by quinidine therapy (delayed repolarization). Bretylium has not been widely used in veterinary medicine and may be contraindicated during halothane anesthesia. Severe ventricular arrhythmias may result.

Amiodarone has been used in patients with ventricular pre-excitation (WPW) syndrome with remarkable success. It has been effective in treating both atrial (paroxysmal supraventricular tachycardia and atrial fibrillation) and ventricular (tachycardia or fibrillation) arrhythmias caused by a variety of cardiac diseases (43). However, numerous adverse effects have been reported after amiodarone therapy, including pulmonary fibrosis, hyperthyroidism, and photosensitivity. These complications have limited amiodarone's usefulness as an antiarrhythmic agent (44).

CLASS IV AGENTS

The Class IV antiarrhythmic agents, such as verapamil and diltiazem, inhibit Ca^{2+} and Na^{+} influx via slow inward channels. Arrhythmias resulting from reentry or enhanced automaticity may be initiated by the emergence of slow inward current. This current is mediated primarily by Ca^{2+} ions (Table 16.7). Of the Class IV agents, only verapamil is approved for use as an antiarrhythmic drug. Verapamil induces myocardial depressant action and flattens the plateau (Phase 2) of the action potential. It is effective in treating atrial arrhythmias and reduces ventricular response to atrial fibrillation or flutter by slowing AV conduction. Because synergistic action between verapamil and β blockers has been demonstrated, concomitant therapy with these agents should be guarded against to prevent the occurrence of complete heart block (45). Verapamil depresses contractility and may induce vasodilation. In contrast, nifedipine induces vasodilation with little cardiac depressant action. Adverse effects of Ca^{2+} channel blockade including hypotension and bradycardia can be reversed with Ca^{2+} or catecholamines.

DIGITALIS

The beneficial actions of digitalis on cardiac rate and rhythm result from its actions upon atrial tissues and atrioventricular conduction. In general, digitalis glycosides are considered the agents of choice for atrial arrhythmias (fibrillation and flutter) when congestive heart failure is present (14). By alleviating congestive failure with digitalis therapy, arrhythmias are often abolished. Generally, the therapeutic inotropic actions of digitalis occur before significant direct changes in cardiac electrophysiology are induced. The antiarrhythmic actions of digitalis are modified by a variety of factors including serum K^{+} concentration, prevailing autonomic tone, and alterations in cardiac intracellular electrolytes (30). Direct electrophysiological changes induced by digitalis are cardiac tissue-specific and dose-dependent. The only direct myocardial antiarrhythmic electrophysiological effect of digitalis in therapeutic concentrations is a slight prolonging of repolarization, making the myocardium more refractory to ectopic impulse formation.

Through indirect vagomimetic effects mediated by the ANS, therapeutic doses of digitalis hyperpolarize atrial cells, decrease the slope of atrial spontaneous depolarization, increase intra-atrial conduction, slows AV conduction, and prolongs AV node ERP (30). Thus, most atrial arrhythmias can be effectively treated, whereas increased AV refractoriness decreases ventricular rate. In contrast, in animals given atropine or high doses of digitalis that stimulate sympathetic activity, automaticity is actually enhanced in Purkinje cells and conducting pathways, leading to ectopic ventricular beats as an early sign of toxicity. Increasing digitalis doses may also decrease action potential and repolarization duration, inducing toxicity manifested as ventricular arrhythmias and atrial after-depolarizations or excitability. Patients with heart block should not be treated with digitalis because of its action upon the atrioventricular conducting system and potential for producing ectopic impulse formation (30). The cardiac tissue-specific and dose-dependent electrophysiological actions induced by digitalis do not lead to easy classification of this agent into one of the four major classes of antiarrhythmic agents (Table 16.8).

AUTONOMIC INTERACTION WITH ANTIARRHYTHMIC AGENTS

Cardiac function is partially regulated by the ANS. Sympathetic stimulation enhances cardiac function, whereas parasympathetic stimulation depresses it. Interaction between these two opposing systems is complex and occurs both within the CNS and in the periphery. Peripherally, sympathetic and parasympathetic interaction can be subdivided into prejunctional and postjunctional activity (Fig. 16.4) (46). Prejunctionally, acetylcholine can damp the release of norepinephrine from the sympathetic nerve terminal. Postsynaptically, cholinergic stimulation may further modify the effects of myocardial receptor effector-cell interaction. Thus, the ANS may modify the actions of antiarrhythmic drugs, both centrally and peripherally (pre- and postsynaptically) (Fig. 16.4). Many antiarrhythmic agents such as digitalis reflexly alter ANS function, modifying any direct electrophysiological effects. Another agent that exerts a dual action is propranolol, which exerts a sympathetic efferent nerve traffic damping effect, along with its direct β blocking action on the heart. Diphenylhydantoin possesses both a CNS and a sympathetic nervous system-depressant effect, as well as a direct myocardial membrane-stabilizing action. Lidocaine has been shown to reduce sympathetic nerve activity, as well as producing a direct Class 1b electrophysiological action. Quinidine and dysopyramide interact with peripheral autonomic muscarinic receptors at the level of the myocardium, modifying their electrophysiological actions. Consequently, to the extent that any given arrhythmia is influenced by prevailing autonomic tone, alterations in autonomic tone produced by an antiarrhythmic drug will modify the effects of the antiarrhythmic agent (46).

In contrast to known antiarrhythmic agents possessing both sympathetic nervous system-depressing effects and direct membrane-stabilizing actions, other classes of drugs, not usually thought of as having antiarrhythmic properties, may also prevent or alter arrhythmia formation through reduction of efferent sympathetic nerve activity. A variety of commonly used major and minor tranquilizers can induce this type of CNS antiarrhythmic effect. These include phenothiazine (acepromazine and promazine), butyrophenone (haloperidol, droperidol, and lenperone), and benzodiazepine tranquilizers (diazepam). Indeed, acepromazine has been indirectly advocated for the prevention of arrhythmias induced by the sensitization of myocardial tissue to catecholamines by halothane (47, 48). Agents that centrally inhibit sympathetic nerve activity, such as the antihypertensives methyldopa, clonidine, or perhaps xylazine, might also exert an antiarrhythmic effect in certain individuals with excessive myocardial sympathetic stimulation (46). Additionally, evidence has accumulated indicating that many central-acting sympathetic depressant agents, such as clonidine, may possess direct peripheral effects mediated by myocardial α receptors (49). Enhanced myocardial α receptor stimulation has been shown to increase arrhythmogenic activity, whereas blockade decreases arrhythmogenesis (50). This may help explain the seemingly paradoxical arrhythmogenic actions of the α agonist agent xylazine. Xylazine's central actions depress sympathetic efferent activity and produce a profound sedative effect while inducing a direct peripheral α_1 and α_2 agonistic action.

Inotropic Agents

HEART FAILURE

With chronic myocardial failure, the heart's ability to pump adequate quantities of blood to tissues is impaired. Reductions in stroke volume, cardiac output, and blood pressure occur, resulting in the initiation of compensatory mechanisms. The sympathetic nervous system is activated, increasing heart rate, contractility, and peripheral vasoconstriction. Activation of the renin-angiotensin-aldosterone axis results in further vasoconstriction and volume expansion via salt and water retention. Ventricular end diastolic volumes increase, causing an increase in ventricular dilatation and some improvement of cardiac output through the Frank-Starling mechanism. These responses momentarily compensate for failing myocardial function but eventually become disadvantageous and are associated with the symptoms or signs of chronic heart failure, venous congestion and edema. The result is a dilated, poorly contracting ventricle, with elevated filling pressures and reduced stroke volume being ejected against a constricted vascular bed. Increased end diastolic volumes and pressures (preload) coupled with increased systolic wall tension (afterload) increase myocardial oxygen consumption even though cardiac output is reduced.

Myocardial failure results from the inability of cardiac muscle to contract and relax normally and is associated with abnormal Ca^{2+} utilization by the myocardial cell. This abnormality can result from primary dysfunction (e.g., congestive cardiomyopathy) or can be secondary to pressure or volume overloads (e.g., mitral regurgitation). Patients may show clinical signs of heart failure associated with pressure and volume overload (e.g., mitral regurgitation or patent ductus arteriosus) or noncompliant failure (e.g., hypertrophic cardiomyopathy) even though actual myocardial failure has not yet developed (51).

The rationale for treating heart failure and, more specifically, myocardial failure is based upon restoring stroke volume and cardiac output, lowering ventricular filling pressure, and relieving symptoms of congestion. Symptomatic treatment with diuretics reduces high preload and relieves congestive symptoms but may actually result in a further reduction of cardiac output (52). When diuretic therapy is insufficient and cardiac enlargement persists, digitalis traditionally has been used to improve myocardial contractility. However, digitalis is a relatively weak inotropic agent with considerable toxic potential. Newer inotropic agents are becoming available that may be more effective while inducing fewer side effects. Vasodilator therapy is becoming more common in refractory heart failure. Arteriodilator-induced decreases in afterload can increase cardiac output and reduce myocardial oxygen consumption, whereas venodilation may decrease preload. Reduction in preload and afterload by venodilation and arterial dilation, respectively, can reduce myocardial oxygen consumption while maintaining contractility and improving cardiac output (52, 53).

Physiology of cardiac contraction and the development of tension in ventricular muscle depends on the interaction between contractile proteins (actin and myosin) located in the thin and thick filaments of the sarcomere (54–56). The energy for this contractile process is derived from ATP. The initiation of cardiac contraction depends upon Ca^{2+} delivery to contractile proteins such as troponin and tropomyosin in the thin filaments (56). For contraction to begin, Ca^{2+} must reach a critical level in the cytosol. However, extracellular Ca^{2+} influx makes only a minor contribution to the pool of activator Ca^{2+} used in contraction (56). The heart utilizes intracellular stores of Ca^{2+} located in the sarcoplasmic reticulum. The release of Ca^{2+} from the sarcoplasmic reticulum is likely triggered by extracellular influx of Ca^{2+} during the action potential down an electrochemical gradient. Extracellular Ca^{2+} enters the cell during the plateau phase of the action potential by a voltage-sensitive Ca^{2+} channel that opens in response to depolarization by fast inward Na^+ current (56). It is thought that this small amount of Ca^{2+} triggers the release of stored Ca^{2+} located in the sarcoplasmic reticulum. A second method of Ca^{2+} entry is via the Na^+/Ca^{2+} exchange system that couples outward Na flux with Ca^{2+} influx. Although this Ca^{2+} movement is not responsible for initiation of contraction, it likely determines the quantity of intracellular activator Ca^{2+} and thus indirectly regulates contractility (56). Regulation of myocardial contractility is achieved by altering mechanisms influencing Ca^{2+}-contractile protein interactions. All cardiotonic drugs interact with one or more of the steps involved in Ca^{2+}-mediated contraction and relaxation of the heart.

CARDIAC GLYCOSIDES

Cardiac glycosides remain the standard agents for long-term management of heart failure. It is generally accepted that these agents lead to an increase in activator Ca^{2+} within the cell. These agents interact with and inhibit Na^+-K^+ ATPase activity (54–56). The inhibition of Na^+ transport out of the cell results in increased Na^+/Ca^{2+} exchange and a net increase in intracellular Ca^{2+} (Fig. 16.8) (54, 55). In recent years, an alternative explanation for digitalis-induced increases in intracellular Ca^{2+} has emphasized the influence of increased intracellular Na^+ upon the inhibition of Ca^{2+} efflux via the Na^+/Ca^{2+} exchange system (55). No matter the mechanism, the resulting increase in intracellular Ca^{2+} is responsible for digitalis-induced inotropic effects in both normal and failing hearts.

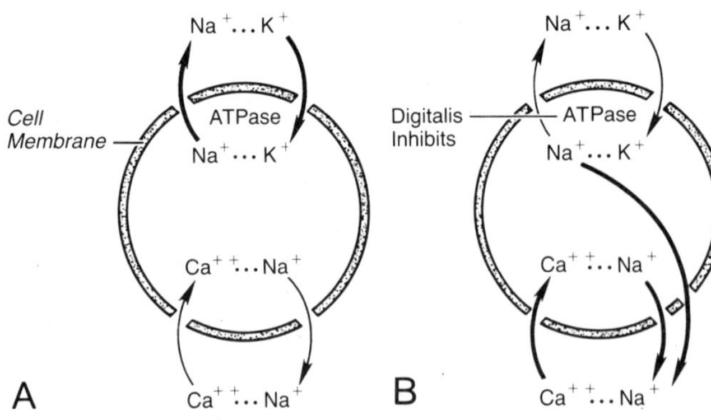

Figure 16.8. Diagrammatic representation of one proposed mechanism for positive inotropic response of cardiac glycosides. Na^+/K^+-ATPase pump activity is normally dominant in controlling efflux of Na^+ from within the cell during Phase 4 of the action potential (*A*). Inhibition of Na^+/K^+-ATPase by digitalis results in increased intracellular concentrations of sodium (*B*). This leads to an increase in Na^+-Ca^{2+} exchange (depicted by the *heavier arrows* in *B*) and an increase in intracellular calcium. Modified from Parker and Adams (53).

In addition to the direct cardiac effects of glycosides, they also affect vascular tone. Cardiac glycosides constrict isolated arterial and venous segments and vascular beds in vivo (56). Thus, the predominant action in animals with normal cardiovascular function and autonomic tone is to increase vascular resistance, which often decreases cardiac output and increases myocardial oxygen consumption (56). Cardiac failure most often induces a net increase in sympathetic activity as a compensatory mechanism for maintaining arterial pressure. By increasing intracellular Ca^{2+} levels, digitalis enhances contractility, increasing cardiac output and partially depressing the reflex-enhanced sympathetic tone. In patients with heart failure, this indirect influence of ameliorating enhanced sympathetic tone overrides the small direct vasoconstrictor actions of digitalis and reduces systemic vascular resistance (56). Thus, in congestive failure, the primary action of digitalis is to increase contractility and decrease vascular resistance. The net effect of these actions is increased cardiac output, reduced heart rate, and decreased myocardial oxygen consumption as afterload or vascular resistance is lessened (56). Digitalis has been used alone and in combination with other therapeutic methods in a variety of species for treatment of congestive failure (54, 57, 58).

BETA 1 ADRENERGIC DRUGS

The inotropic effects of the catecholamines is achieved primarily through β_1 adrenoreceptors. Epinephrine, norepinephrine, isoproterenol, dopamine, and dobutamine stimulate myocardial β_1 receptors to induce an inotropic action. The force of contraction increases very rapidly with these agents; more importantly, the duration of contraction is also decreased. This "relaxant effect" is shared by agents which increase cAMP. Rapid relaxation is important for adequate ventricular filling during periods of rapid heart rate (55).

The mechanism for β adrenergic inotropy is thought to be associated with an increase in the slow Ca^{2+} inward current during Phase 2 of the action potential. Increases in Ca^{2+} influx during depolarization may cause increased Ca^{2+} release from sarcoplasmic reticulum by acting as a greater trigger for release of "activator Ca^{2+}" (55). Beta 1 agonists also increase Ca^{2+} uptake by the sarcoplasmic reticulum, explaining the "relaxant effects" of β_1 agonists. These actions are mediated by increased adenylate cyclase and subsequently cAMP levels. Cyclic AMP activates protein kinases, changing the ability of Ca^{2+} to bind with proteins (55). A number of agents possessing β_1 adrenergic agonist activity have been used in veterinary medicine to manage acute heart failure.

Norepinephrine has β_1 agonistic effects but causes intense arteriolar vasoconstriction via its α agonistic actions (Fig. 16.3). Prolonged administration may lead to hypoperfusion and tissue acidosis. The α adrenergic vasoconstrictor effect of norepinephrine often increases blood pressure dramatically, resulting in a vagally mediated bradycardia in spite of its β_1 actions (Fig. 16.3).

In contrast to norepinephrine, epinephrine not only stimulates β_1 and α receptors but β_2 receptors as well (Fig. 16.3). The inotropic action of epinephrine is often accompanied by an increase in heart rate, because vascular resistance and blood pressure are not drastically increased, and reflex slowing of the heart does not occur (Fig. 16.3). Low doses of epinephrine induce β adrenergic effects such that vascular resistance may actually decrease and tachycardia occurs. High doses of epinephrine induce an α agonistic action and are associated with vasoconstriction and hypertension (56). Renal blood flow is decreased with high doses of epinephrine (α-mediated). Prolonged epinephrine administration has been associated with massive vasoconstriction and gangrene of the extremities. Because of these actions, epinephrine, like norepinephrine, is best utilized in acute phases of cardiac resuscitation and not for chronic inotropic therapy.

Isoproterenol is a potent β_1 and β_2 agonist that dramatically increases contractility and heart rate while decreasing vascular resistance through β_2-mediated vasodilation (Fig. 16.3). These actions lead to increases in cardiac output, but arrhythmias are common. The adequacy of coronary perfusion during periods of tachycardia and reduced blood pressure induced by isoproterenol is questionable. Isoproterenol therapy has been used to reverse the low cardiac output associated with atropine-insensitive bradycardia or to temporarily increase heart rate in patients with severe heart block (56).

Dopamine induces a rather complex and dose-dependent action upon the cardiovascular system. Low doses stimulate dopaminergic receptors in renal and mesenteric vasculature and increase renal blood flow. Higher doses induce β_1 effects and increase cardiac output and blood pressure. Dopamine may also induce release of endogenous norepinephrine, but the occurrence of dopamine-induced arrhythmias appears to be minimal. During dopamine infusion, coronary perfusion pressure is maintained as myocardial oxygen consumption increases. Dopamine may also induce coronary vasodilation via dopaminergic receptors in the coronary vasculature. High doses of dopamine, as with epinephrine, result in an α agonistic vasoconstriction response. The beneficial effects of dopamine in low and medium doses makes it an effective cardiotonic agent for acute cardiac failure when carefully administered intravenously (56).

Dobutamine has a rather selective β_1 cardiac action. It can induce a strong inotropic effect with only a minimal chronotropic action. Because tachycardia can lead to excessive increases in myocardial oxygen consumption, the ability to strengthen contraction and not induce tachycardia is beneficial. When compared with dopamine, intravenous dobutamine infusion produces improved hemodynamics with much smaller increases in heart rate. Dobutamine has been used to support the failing heart but, as with dopamine, is limited to acute therapy because it must be administered as an intravenous infusion. When administered at proper infusion rates, dobutamine's α_1 (vasoconstrictor) and β_2 (vasodilatation) agonist activities are of equal action (56).

Partial β_1 agonists (e.g., prenalteral) possess both agonist and antagonist properties. These drugs stabilize the inotropic state of the heart at a level equal to the partial agonist's β_1 activity while preventing further possible harmful sympathetic stimulation. These agents hold much promise in the treatment of ischemic heart failure (59). Such β_2 adrenergic agonists as salbutamol and terbutaline, used to induce bronchodilation in patients with bronchoconstrictive disease, also possess minimal β_1 inotropic activity. Vasodilation induced by these β_2 agonists may result in reduced afterload of the heart while increasing cardiac output. The chronotropic action of β_2 agonists is minimal when compared to the potent nonselective β agonist.

OTHER CARDIOTONICS

Other agents which have been used for their cardiotonic actions are glucagon, histamine, the methylxanthines, and the new nonglycoside noncatecholamine Class 3 phosphodiesterase inhibitors amrinone and milrinone. All of these agents influence intracellular Ca^{2+} metabolism. Glucagon increases cAMP similar to the actions of catecholamines but does so by binding to receptors other than the β_1 adrenoceptor. Glucagon directly stimulates adenylate cyclase and thus increases intracellular cAMP (55). Glucagon treatment of myocardial failure appears limited because it is relatively ineffective in patients with advanced congestive failure. It may be beneficial in acute heart failure resulting from surgery/anesthesia, cardiogenic shock, or β blockade toxicity. Histamines, like glucagon, induce an inotropic effect unrelated to β adrenoceptor stimulation. However, the usefulness of histamines as cardiotonic agents are restricted by their serious side effects (55).

Methylxanthines such as theophylline induce inotropic actions and vasodilation. The inotropic effect of theophylline is much weaker but similar in action to that induced by β agonists. The inotropic actions of methylxanthines are independent of the Na^+/K^+ pump mechanism but are influenced by Ca^{2+} channel blockers and thus are indirectly dependent on Ca^{2+} influx from extracellular spaces. Methylxanthines induce their inotropic action by inhibition of phosphodiesterase activity normally responsible for cAMP degradation. This mechanism of increasing cAMP contrasts with β agonist receptor-mediated increases in cAMP, but similarly results in increases in Ca^{2+} levels and contractility (56). Methylxanthine (e.g., theophylline) therapy has also been associated with direct catecholamine release, direct increases in Ca^{2+} entry, and inhibition of Ca^{2+} sequestration by sarcoplasmic reticulum (56). Excessive doses of phosphodiesterase inhibitors may induce arrhythmia formation.

The newest class of inotropic agents are the Class 3 phosphodiesterase inhibitors, which include amrinone and milrinone. These agents are bipyridine compounds possessing positive inotropic and arterial vasodilating properties (55–57, 59). The inotropic actions of these agents are not antagonized by β or α antagonists, reserpine, or histamine (H_1 and H_2) blockers. Milrinone is a derivative of amrinone and is 20 to 50 times as potent as the parent compound (60). Inotropic actions induced by these agents result from phosphodiesterase inhibition (increased cAMP) and may augment Ca^{2+} influx or Ca^{2+} uptake by contractile protein. Heart rate and blood pressure are not significantly affected. These agents are administered orally and have relatively long durations of action. Tachyphylaxis or acute tolerance has not been observed. However, serious side effects have been reported with amrinone therapy (hypotension, thrombocytopenia, nausea, and vomiting), which has limited its usefulness (56). Milrinone therapy has not been associated with these severe side effects. A recent study in dogs with myocardial failure has demonstrated milrinone's efficacy in improving left ventricular function (61). Milrinone therapy was not associated with clinically detectable hemodynamic abnormalities or arrhythmogenesis when given in doses of less than 1.0 mg/kg (61). Recent discussions have also centered around the potential for noncontinuous therapy with milrinone. It has been observed that short-term milrinone therapy (2 days), reverses the salt-avid state (Na^+ and water retention) accompanying congestive failure. This reversal may exist for several days after discontinuation of milrinone. If intermittent administration of milrinone proves sufficient in reversing the enhanced sympathetic action and pathophysiology associated with pump failure for several intervening days, this mode of therapy would appear advantageous.

In recent years, α_1 adrenergic receptors have been identified in myocardial tissue. Stimulation of these receptors may lead to increased contraction. However, α-mediated inotropic actions appear to differ from β adrenergic-induced contraction. In contrast to β stimulation, α adrenergic-mediated contractility develops slowly and prolongs contraction rather than shortening it. Thus, α activation does not induce a relaxant effect. Increases in heart rate are not observed. Alpha-mediated inotropic action is not associated with increases in cAMP or Na^+/K^+ ATPase activity (55). In addition, myocardial α_1 receptors may differ from α receptors in other tissues, allowing for an inotropic action unaccompanied by vasoconstriction. Alpha adrenergic-induced inotropic action may thus provide some advantage in conditions where the potential for β-mediated contractility appears minimal (e.g., hypothyroidism or hypothermia).

In summary, an ideal cardiotonic agent should improve cardiac contractility and increase oxygen supply to tissues without inducing tachycardia, arrhythmias, or increases in myocardial oxygen requirements (59). The advantages of some newer agents, such as milrinone, are that they possess a potent inotropic action coupled with vasodilating activity. Vasodilation theoretically offsets increased myocardial oxygen consumption associated with improved contractility. Vasodilation reduces oxygen utilization by reducing the excessive myocardial wall tension that results from increased afterload and venous return to the heart (59). In general, cardiotonic agents implemented in chronic heart failure should be relatively free of side effects, be consistent in their action, be orally effective, and have a reasonably long duration of action.

Vasodilator Agents

During the last 10 years, a number of new vasodilating agents have been developed. The efficacy of vasodilator therapy in the treatment of congestive failure has been promising. These agents can be classified by their mechanism(s) of action into five categories: direct-acting vasodilators (nitrates, hydralazine, and minoxidil); neurohumoral antagonists (prazosin, captopril, and enalapril); Ca^{2+} channel blockers (nifedipine and verapamil); β adrenergic agonists with vasodilator activity (salbutamol and terbutaline); and noncatecholamine-nonglycoside inotropic agents with vasodilatory actions (amrinone and milrinone; see previous section) (62). Differences in regional distribution of blood flow are observed after the administration of different vasodilating drugs. Therefore, a second method of classifying vasodilators is based upon their major site of action within the peripheral vasculature. Some vasodilators induce arterial relaxation, while others cause dilatation of the venous capacitance bed. For example, within the direct-acting group of vasodilators, hydralazine is primarily an arterial dilator, whereas the nitrates are venodilators. The acute hemodynamic effects of venodilation differs greatly from those of arterial vasodilation. Preload or cardiac filling pressure decreases with venodilation, often decreasing stroke volume and forward flow, whereas cardiac output is usually increased with arterial dilatation (63). Thus, rational vasodilator therapy is based upon understanding the mechanism of action of each vasodilating agent and differences in each agent's efficacy as a venous and/or arterial dilator.

Increased pulmonary venous pressure and low cardiac output are the two major hemodynamic changes responsible for the clinical signs of chronic myocardial heart failure (64). Dyspnea during exercise results from pulmonary congestion, whereas fatigue or exercise intolerance indicates a restriction of forward blood flow or cardiac output. Thus, the two major therapeutic objectives of vasodilator therapy are to relieve elevated pulmonary wedge pressure and to increase cardiac output. Reductions in cardiac output can result from myocardial failure (depressed contractile force) or, as seen with early mitral or aortic regurgitation, pump failure without depressed contractile function. Another mechanism that can reduce cardiac output, even though contractility is intact, is excessive resistance to left ventricular outflow. This can occur in patients with aortic stenosis or excessive peripheral vascular resistance (hypertension). Decreased cardiac output in these patients initiates further increases in vascular resistance as a means of maintaining pressure-regulated circulatory homeostasis. Elevated arterial resistance increases myocardial afterload further, adversely affecting ventricular performance.

Increased systemic vasoconstriction results from several interrelated neurohumoral changes. During heart failure, elevated circulating norepinephrine levels have been observed that increase peripheral α_1 adrenoceptor stimulation. The renin-angiotension-aldosterone system is activated as renal perfusion decreases. Angiotension II is produced; it is a potent vasoconstrictive substance. Increased aldosterone levels promote salt and water retention, contributing to elevated vascular resistance values. Increased concentrations of vasopressin have been observed in heart failure patients and may play a role in increasing vascular resistance as well. Increased tissue and vessel pressure associated with edema and vessel fluid content may also contribute to the rigidity of the circulatory system. Consequently, when cardiac output remains inadequate after diuretic-digitalis therapy, the use of vasodilators to decrease vascular resistance appears to be an appropriate method of therapy (51).

DIRECT-ACTING VASODILATOR AGENTS

Hydralazine is a direct-acting arteriolar dilator that has induced beneficial acute hemodynamic effects in dogs with congestive heart failure. It has been recommended for patients with either myocardial failure or volume-overloaded heart failure. In patients with severe myocardial failure, hydralazine can be used to decrease vascular resistance and to improve cardiac output when patients do not respond to digitalis and diuretic therapy (65). In patients with severe mitral regurgitation or left to right shunts where contractility is still normal, arteriolar vasodilators such as hydralazine and minoxidil have been advocated to improve cardiac output and reverse pulmonary congestion associated with volume overload (66).

Hydralazine therapy may be supplemented with or used as a supplement to venodilator or diuretic therapy. Hypotension can be induced by hydralazine therapy, which may lead to increased aldosterone release. If this occurs, diuretics are recommended to control water retention. Spironolactone and triamterene are effective aldosterone-inhibiting diuretics that can reverse aldosterone-induced edema and excessive K^+ loss (58).

In contrast to hydralazine, the nitrates are potent direct-acting venodilators with only a moderate arteriolar dilating action. Thus, nitrates are primarily used to reduce preload by increasing venous capacitance. They do not increase stroke volume as do the arterial dilators. Nitroglycerin and isosorbide dinitrate are the two most commonly used nitrates in man. These agents have not been used extensively in the dog or cat. The major indications for nitrate therapy are to relieve pulmonary congestion and edema in left-sided failure and tissue edema and ascites in right-sided failure.

Some patients with severe or advanced heart failure will require both arteriolar and venodilator therapy because of coexisting pulmonary congestion (dyspnea) and inadequate cardiac output (exercise intolerance). These patients may be best treated by combining venous and arteriolar dilators such as a nitrate compound and hydralazine or by using a direct-acting agent that possesses both actions. Nitroprusside has a direct smooth muscle relaxant effect on both arterial and venous vasculature. It has a short half-life, must be given intravenously, and is extremely potent. Because nitroprusside can induce severe hypotension, blood pressure should be monitored closely during infusion. In addition, when nitroprusside administration is prolonged, it can be metabolized into cyanide and thiocyanate, causing severe toxicity (58).

NEUROHUMORAL ANTAGONISTS

Prazosin and captopril are two relatively new neurohumoral antagonists possessing arterial and venous dilating properties. These agents have been used in dogs with severe signs of heart failure. These agents induce vasodilation by two very different actions. Prazosin blocks peripheral α_1 adrenoreceptors, whereas captopril inhibits angiotension-converting enzyme, thereby decreasing elevated levels of angiotensin II and aldosterone. In patients with severe myocardial failure, both prazosin and captopril have been effective in relieving congestion and/or edema while increasing stroke volume.

Subacute or delayed tolerance to prazosin therapy has been reported in humans and may occur in veterinary patients as well (67). Prazosin's specific α_1 action is beneficial in preventing reflex tachycardia in the face of reduced pressures. In general, prazosin therapy has not been associated with serious side effects (67).

Captopril inhibits the increase in plasma angiotensin II concentration that normally occurs during heart failure. Aldosterone levels are also reduced by captopril therapy, reducing salt and water retention. Thus, both the congestive signs of severe failure and cardiac output improve. Captopril may also induce changes in bradykinins and norepinephrine levels. Bradycardia may occur after captopril administration. Captopril significantly decreases renovascular resistance and increases renal blood flow (68). Unlike prazosin, tolerance has not been noted after captopril administration (67). Preliminary studies of captopril therapy in dogs with congestive cardiomyopathy have been encouraging (58). However, in some cases of mitral insufficiency, cardiac output actually decreased as preload was reduced after captopril administration. Inhibition of aldosterone release with captopril therapy may result in hyperkalemia. Consequently, electrolytes should be monitored carefully after captopril administration (58).

In summary, the selection of the most appropriate vasodilator agent for treatment of chronic congestive failure, irrespective of the etiology of left ventricular dysfunction, can be simplified by observing signs of failure after conventional therapy with digitalis and diuretics. The choice of agent is then made by noting the remaining hemodynamic deficits and symptoms and matching the potential of alleviating remaining signs with the hemodynamic response elicited by a given vasodilator. In general, when elevated pulmonary pressure or congestion is present and cardiac output is adequate, venodilators such as the nitrates are indicated. When cardiac output is decreased and systemic vascular resistance is elevated with only minimal signs of excessive pulmonary pressures, arteriolar dilators (e.g., hydralazine) are indicated. When cardiac output is low and pulmonary congestion is present, as is often the case in severe failure, mixed vasodilators such as prazosin and captopril or combinations of venodilators (nitrates) and arteriolar dilators (hydralazine) can be used to produce the most beneficial effects. As a precautionary note, vasodilator therapy should always be carefully administered, especially when signs of hypotension are present. While carefully monitoring cardiovascular signs, initial doses of any vasodilator should be low and gradually increased to optimize its effect. In addition, chronic vasodilator therapy with some agents may be associated with development of tolerance (e.g., prazosin) such that alternative vasodilators may be needed to maintain a favorable hemodynamic response (67).

The best time to institute vasodilator therapy in the treatment of chronic heart failure remains equivocal. Some reports have indicated that early treatment with vasodilators before the development of severe signs may actually prevent further myocardial deterioration. Thus, vasodilators may not only ameliorate the symptoms of severe heart failure, but by early initiation of therapy, myocardial degeneration may be slowed and longevity increased (69).

VASODILATOR THERAPY IN ACUTE FAILURE

In contrast to chronic heart failure, the use of vasodilators for acute cardiac or circulatory failure has not been well documented (70). Vasodilators have been recommended in cardiogenic shock when blood pressure was maintained and tachycardia prevented. However, constant, vigilant, sophisticated monitoring of circulatory function is required. In hypovolemia, sepsis, or neurogenic shock, acute circulatory failure is noncardiogenic in origin, but cardiac dysfunction rapidly results secondary to decreased coronary perfusion and increased myocardial oxygen demand (increased heart rate). In hypovolemic shock, vasoregulation is intact, and excessive vasoconstriction often results. Consequently, arteriodilator therapy to reduce resistance and improve tissue perfusion may be beneficial during hypovolemic shock when administered in conjunction with rapid fluid replacement. In contrast, during septic or neurogenic shock, vasodilation is often enhanced to a pathological state, making additional vasodilation inappropriate. Vasodilators that have been used in acute cardiogenic failure include phentolamine, salbutamol, nitroglycerin, and nitroprusside (70). Nitroprusside appears to be most useful in man because it induces a balanced arterial-venous dilating effect and is readily controlled. Nitroglycerin is advocated when severe pulmonary edema is the most prominent feature of acute cardiac failure and venodilation alone is indicated (70). The use of captopril in acute shock has not been adequately evaluated, but recent studies have indicated its potential usefulness in hemorrhagic shock (71).

References

1. Noback CR, Demarest RJ: *The Nervous System: Introduction and Review*, New York, McGraw-Hill, 1972, pp 140–152.
2. Mayer SE: Neurohumoral transmission and the autonomic nervous system. In Gilman AG, Goodman LS, Gilman A (eds): *The Pharmacologic Basis of Therapeutics*, ed 6. New York, Macmillan Publishing Co Inc, 1980, pp 56–90.
3. Weiner N, Taylor P: Neurohumoral transmission and the auto-

nomic nervous system. In Gilman AG, Goodman LS, Rall TW, Murall F (eds): *The Pharmacologic Basis of Therapeutics*, ed 7. New York, Macmillan Publishing Co Inc, 1985, pp 66–99.

4. Twautwein W, Kuffler SW, Edwards C: Changes in membrane characteristics of heart muscle during inhibition. *J Gen Physiol* 40:135–145, 1956.
5. Alquist RP: Study of the adrenotropic receptors. *Am J Physiol* 153:586, 1948.
6. Lands AM, Arnold A, McAuliff JP, Luduena FP, Brown RG: Differentiation of receptor systems activated by sympathomimetic animals. *Nature* 214:597–598, 1967.
7. Tranquilli WJ, Thurmon JC: Alpha adrenoreceptor pharmacology. *J Am Vet Med Assoc* 184(11):1400–1402, 1984.
8. Merin RG: Pharmacology of the autonomic nervous system. In Miller RD (ed): *Anesthesia*, ed 2. New York, Churchill Livingstone, 1986, pp 945–982.
9. Lawson NW, Wallfisch HK: Cardiovascular pharmacology—a new look at old drugs. In: *Review Course Lectures*. Las Vegas, International Anesthesia Research Society, pp 140–156, 1986.
10. Liang CS, Hood WB Jr: Dobutamine infusion in conscious dogs with and without autonomic nervous system inhibition. *J Pharmacol Exp Ther* 211:698–705, 1979.
11. Adams RH: New perspectives in cardiopulmonary therapeutics: Receptor selective adrenergic drugs. *J Am Vet Med Assoc* 185(9):966–974, 1984.
12. Tranquilli WJ, Thurmon JC, Corbin JE, Benson GJ, Davis LE: Halothane sparing effect of xylazine in dogs and subsequent reversal with tolazoline. *J Vet Pharmacol Therap* 7:23–28, 1984.
13. Nelson H: Beta adrenergic agonists. *Chest* 82 (Suppl):533–538, 1982.
14. Adams HR: Antiarrhythmic agents. In Booth NH, McDonald LE (eds): *Veterinary Pharmacology and Therapeutics*, ed 5. Ames, Iowa State University Press, 1982, pp 458–471.
15. Arnsdorf MF: Basic understanding of the electrophysiologic actions of antiarrhythmic drugs. Symposium on cardiac arrhythmias II. *Medical Clinics of North America* 68:1249–1279, 1984.
16. Surawicz B, Imanish S: Automatic activity in depolarized guinea pig ventricular myocardium: characteristics and mechanisms. *Circulation Research* 39:571–579, 1976.
17. Cranefield PF, Aronson RS, Wit AL: Effect of verapamil on the normal action potential and on a calcium-dependent slow response of canine purkinje fibers. *Circulation Res* 34:204–213, 1974.
18. Wit AL: Electrophysiological basis for antiarrhythmic drug action. Drug Mechanisms, 8th Ann Meet. NACB, Washington, DC, 1984. *Clin Physiol Biochem* 3:127–134, 1985.
19. Arnsdorf MF: The effect of antiarrhythmic drugs on triggered sustained rhythmic activity in cardiac purkinje fibers. *J Pharmac Exp Ther* 201:689–700, 1977.
20. Ferrier GR: Digitalis arrhythmias: role of oscillatory after potentials. *Prog Cardiovasc Dis* 19:459–474, 1977.
21. Henning B, Wit AL: Multiple mechanism of antiarrhythmic drug action on delayed after-depolarizations in canine coronary sinus (abstract). *Am J Cardiol* 49:912, 1982.
22. Rosen MR, Danilo P: Effects of tetrodotoxin, lidocaine, verapamil, and AHR-2666 on quabain-induced delayed after-depolarizations in canine purkinje fibers. *Circulation Res* 46:117–124, 1980.
23. Vaughan Williams EM: A classification of antiarrhythmic actions reassessed after a decade of new drugs. *J Clin Pharmacol* 24:129–147, 1984.
24. Nestico PF, Depace NL, Morganroth J: Therapy with conventional antiarrhythmic drugs for ventricular arrhythmias. Symposium on Cardic Arrhythmias II. *Med Clin North Am* 68(5):1295–1319, 1984.
25. Singh BN, Vaughan Williams EM: The effect of amiodarone, a new antianginal drug, on cardiac muscle. *Br J Pharmacol* 39:657–668, 1970.
26. Rosenbaum MB, Chiale PA, Ryba D, Elizari MW: Control of tachyarrhythmias associated with the WPW syndrome by amiodarone hydrochloride. *Am J Cardiol* 34:215–233, 1974.
27. Vaughan Williams EM, Salako L, Wittig JH: The effect on atrial and ventricular intracellular potentials and other pharmacological actions of L9146, a nonhalogenated benzo (b) thiophene-related amiodarone. *Cardiovasc Res* 11:187–197, 1977.
28. Krikler DM, Goodwin JF: *Cardiac Arrhythmias*. London, Saunders, 1975.
29. El Sherif N, Lazzara R: Reentrant ventricular arrhythmias in the late myocardial infarction period. 7. Effect of verapamil and D-600 and the role of "slow inward current." *Circulation* 60:605–615, 1979.
30. Muir WW: Applied cardiac pharmacology. *Proc Am Anim Hosp Assoc* 43:168–210, 1976.
31. Wenger TL, Strauss HC: Interaction between digitalis and antiarrhythmic drugs. *NCMJ* 1:25–28, 1985.
32. Maisel AS, Motulsky HJ, Insel PA: Hypotension after quinidine plus verapamil. Possible additive competition at α adrenergic receptors. *New Engl J Med* 312:167–170, 1985.
33. McGuirk SM, Muir WW: Diagnosis and treatment of cardiac arrhythmias. In Symposium on Cardiology. *Vet Clin N Amer: Equine Pract* 1(2):353–370, 1985.
34. Muir WW: Ventricular preexcitation in two horses. *J Am Vet Med Assoc* 183(5):573–576, 1983.
35. Hill BL, Tilley LP: Ventricular preexcitation in seven dogs and nine cats. *J Am Vet Med Assoc* 187(1):1027–1030, 1985.
36. Bonagura J. Therapy of cardiac arrhythmias. In Kirk RW (ed): *Current Veterinary Therapy VII, Small Animal Practice*. Philadelphia, WB Saunders Co, 1983, pp 360–372.
37. Kittleson M: Drugs used in the therapy of cardiac arrhythmias. In Kirk RW (ed): *Current Veterinary Therapy, VII. Small Animal Practice*. Philadelphia, WB Saunders Co, 1983, pp 297–301.
38. Roden DM: Tocainide and mexiletine, orally effective lidocaine analogues. *Arch Intern Med* 145:417–418, 1985.
39. Kutalek SP, Morganroth J, Horowitz LN: Tocainide: A new oral antiarrhythmic agent. *Ann Intern Med* 103:387–391, 1985.
40. Muir WW, Bonagura JD: Aprindine for treatment of ventricular arrhythmias in the dog. *Am J Vet Res* 43:1815–1819, 1982.
41. Hellestrand KJ: Comparison of the efficacy of newly developed antiarrhythmic drugs for the treatment of ventricular tachyarrhythmias. *Eur Heart J* 5s:87–94, 1984.
42. Anderson JL: Bretylium tosylate: Profile of the only available Class III antiarrhythmic agent. *Clin Therapeut* 7(2):205–224, 1985.
43. Heger JJ, Pstowsky EN, Zipes DP: Clinical efficacy of amiodarone in treatment of recurrent ventricular tachycardia and ventricular fibrillation. *Am Heart J* 106:887–893, 1983.
44. Mead HR, Harrison DC: Therapy with investigational antiarrhythmic drugs. Symposium on Cardiac Arrhythmias II. *Med Clin North Am* 68(5):1321–1337, 1984.
45. Muhiddin KA, Turner P: Is there an ideal antiarrhythmic drug? A review with particular reference to Class I antiarrhythmic agents. *Postgrad Med J* 61:665–678, 1985.
46. Watanabe AM, Bailey J: The role of the autonomic nervous system in medicating and modifying the action of cardiac antiarrhythmic drugs. In Garfein OB (ed): *Clinical Pharmacology of Cardiac Antiarrhythmic Agents: Classical and Current Concepts Reevaluated*. New York, New York Academy of Sciences, 432:90–102, 1984.
47. Muir WW, Werner LL, Hamlin RL: Effects of xylazine and acetylpromazine upon induced ventricular fibrillation in dogs anesthetized with thiamylal and halothane. *Am J Vet Res* 36:1299–1303, 1975.
48. Rezakhani A, Edjtehadi M, Szabuniewicz M: Prevention of thiopental and thiamylal/halothane cardiac sensitization to epinephrine in the sheep. *Can J Comp Med* 41:389–395, 1977.

49. Maze M, Smith CM: Identification of receptor mechanism mediating epinephrine-induced arrhythmias during halothane anesthesia in the dog. *Anesthesiology* 59:322–326, 1983.
50. Spiss CK, Maze M, Smith CM: Alpha adrenergic responsiveness correlates with epinephrine dose for arrhythmias during halothane anesthesia in dogs. *Anesth-Analg* 63:297–300, 1984.
51. Kittleson M: Concepts and therapeutic strategies in the management of heart failure. In: Kirk RW (ed): *Current Veterinary Therapy VII, Small Animal Practice*. Philadelphia, WB Saunders Co, 1983, pp 279–284.
52. Sharpe ND: Newer inotropic agents. *Meth Find Exptl Clin Pharmacol* 6(4):215–218, 1984.
53. Parker JL, Adams HR: Drugs and the heart muscle. *J Am Vet Med Assoc* 171:78–84, 1977.
54. Adams HR: Digitalis and other inotropic agents. In: Booth NH, McDonald LE (eds): *Veterinary Pharmacology and Therapeutics*, Ames, Iowa State University Press, 1982, pp 435–457.
55. Scholz H: Inotropic drugs and their mechanisms of action. In Katz AM (ed): *Basic Concepts in Cardiology*. JACC 4(2):389–397, 1984.
56. Smith LDR, Oldershaw PJ: Inotropic and vasopressor agents. *Br J Anaesth* 56:767–780, 1984.
57. Detweiler DK, Knight DH: Congestive heart failure in dogs: Therapeutic concepts. *J Am Vet Med Assoc* 171:106–114, 1977.
58. Kittleson M: Drugs used in the management of heart failure. In Kirk RW (ed): *Current Veterinary Therapy VIII, Small Animal Practice*. Philadelphia, WB Saunders Co, 1983, pp 285–296.
59. Carlier J, El Allaf D: Old and new inotropic drugs. *Resuscitation* (11):217–231, 1984.
60. Farah AE: Positive inotropic agents. *Ann Rev Pharmacol Toxicol* 24:275–328, 1984.
61. Kittleson MD, Pipers FS, Knauer KW, Keister DM, Knowlen GG, Miner WS: Echocardiographic and clinical effects of milrinone in dogs with myocardial failure. *Am J Vet Res* 48(8):1659–1664, 1985.
62. Packer M: Vasodilator and inotropic therapy for severe chronic heart failure: passion and skepticism. *JACL* 2(5):841–852, 1983.
63. Cohn JN: Unloading the heart in congestive heart failure. *Amer J Med* August:66–70, 1984.
64. Chatterjee K: Vasodilator agents in chronic heart failure. *Danish Med Bull* 30(1):1–9, 1983.
65. Hamlin RB, Kittleson MD: Clinical experience with hydralazine for treatment of otherwise intractable cough in dogs with apparent left-sided failure. *J Am Vet Med Assoc* 180:1327–1329, 1982.
66. Kittleson MD, Johnson LE, Oliver NB: Acute hemodynamic effects of hydralazine in dogs with chronic mitral regurgitation. *J Am Vet Med Assoc* 187(3):258–261, 1985.
67. Schwartz AB, Chatterjee K: Vasodilator therapy in chronic congestive heart failure. *Drugs* 26(2):148–173, 1983.
68. Faxon D, Halperin J, Creager M, Garras H, Schick E, Ryan T: Angiotensin converting enzyme inhibitor in severe congestive failure—acute and limb hemodynamics of captopril and observations on sustained oral treatment. *Amer Heart J* 101:548–555, 1981.
69. Braunwald E, Colucci WS: Vasodilator therapy of heart failure. Has the promissary note been paid? *New Engl J Med* 310(7):459–461, 1984.
70. Blakely C, Tinker J: Vasodilators in acute circulatory failure. *Intensive Care Med* 9:5–11, 1983.
71. Trachte GJ, Lefer AM: Beneficial action of a new angiotensin converting enzyme inhibitor (SQ 14,225) in hemorrhagic shock in cats. *Circ Res* 43(4):576–582, 1978.

CHAPTER

17

Monitoring the Anesthetized Patient

STEVE C. HASKINS, D.V.M., M.S., D.A.C.V.A.

Anesthetic drugs, the state of general anesthesia, and operative procedures impose great stress upon the homeostasis of both normal and debilitated patients. The more that is known about the mechanisms by which the disease, the anesthetics, and the surgery interact, the more appropriate the anesthetic drug selection and perioperative monitoring and the more effective the patient support.

Intraoperative monitoring is the link between preoperative evaluation and stabilization of the patient and postoperative care and support. Intraoperative monitoring can be accomplished with greater specificity and intensity because of the immobility of the patient. This is the time when anesthetic drugs are having their greatest effect on compensatory mechanisms and surgical procedures are having their greatest effect on the physiology and anatomy of the patient. It is the time when intense monitoring is most necessary. It is, however, a waste without proper attention to the pre- and postoperative needs of the patient.

The outcome of the disease-patient-operation interaction is not a predictable thing. Anesthetic complications are, of course, best treated by preventing them in the first place, but this is not always possible. The second line of defense is to recognize problems early, when they are not too severe and can be corrected easily. The importance of monitoring so as to detect unpredictable happenings cannot be overemphasized. The third line of defense is a fire engine brand of emergency medicine that is best avoided if at all possible.

The focus of the monitoring procedures should be the cardiovascular and pulmonary systems, the central nervous system, and body temperature because this is where anesthetic drugs and surgical procedures have their greatest effect. Specifically disordered visceral organ systems, including fluid, electrolyte, and acid-base abnormalities, may require monitoring procedures. Normal ranges for monitored parameters are shown in Tables 17.1 and 17.2.

Monitoring the Cardiovascular System

Each individual cardiovascular parameter has a specific significance. However, the overall significance of cardiovascular function can only be fully appreciated by correlating the measurement with the trend of previous measurements, by integrating it with other cardiovascular variables, and by considerating the recent past history of the patient. Any one parameter can be quite within its normal range in a patient whose cardiovascular system is otherwise falling apart.

HEART RATE

Heart rate can be monitored by an electrocardiograph (ECG), by electric heart rate meters (which sound an audible beep with each R wave), by an esophageal stethoscope attached to an indwelling ear piece or a heart sound amplifier (A. M. Bickford, Inc., East Aurora, New York; Praser-Harlake, Inc., Cleveland, Ohio; Summit Hill Laboratories, Avalon, New

Table 17.1
Normal Ranges for Commonly Measured Cardiovascular and Respiratory Parameters and Body Temperature in Common Domestic Species

	Dog	Cat	Rabbit	Sheep	Goat	Calf	Pig	Horse
Heart rate (min^{-1})	70–140[a,b,c,d]	110–140[c,d,e]	200–325[b,d,f,g]	70–130[b,d,h]	70–120[d,i]	90–160[b,j,k,l]	$216 \times kg^{-0.178}$[m] 60–200[b,m,n]	35–60[b,o]
Mean arterial pressure (mm Hg)	90–110[a,b,e,j]	100–150[d,p,e]	70–105[b,d,f,g]	80–110[b,d,h]	90–120[d,i]	90–160[b,j,k,l]	49 (46 × log kg)[m]	85–120[b]
Cardiac output ($ml \cdot kg^{-1} \cdot min^{-1}$)	100–200[a,b,d,o]	120[p]	200–350[b,q]	110–160[b,h]	60–230[d]	80–240[b,j,k,l]	60–150[b,n,r,j]	66–184[j]
Blood volume ($ml \cdot kg^{-1}$)	75–90[c,o,s]	47–66[c,o,s]	57–65[f,g,s,e]	55–70[c,s]	55–90[c,o,s]	60–100[c,s]	<25 kg = $9.5 \times kg^{0.922}$[m] >25 kg = $17.9 \times kg^{0.73}$[m] 50–100[c,m,n,s]	65–70[c]
Total plasma proteins (g/dl^{-1})	6.0–7.8[s,t,e]	6.0–7.5[s,t,e]	5.4–8.5[f,g]	6.0–8.0[s,t,e]	6.5–7.5[t,e]	6.7–7.5[e]	6.5–8.5[t,e]	6.0–8.0[s]
Packed cell volume (%)	40–55[s,u,e]	25–45[s,e]	35–48[f,g,s]	30–45[h,s,e]	20–38[s,e]	24–46[s,k]	32–50[m,n,s,e]	32–53[s]
Hemoglobin (g/dl^{-1})	14–17.5[s,e]	8–15[d,s]	8.5–15.5[d,g,s]	8–16[s,e]	8–14[n,s,e]	8–15[s,e,k]	10–16[n,s,e]	11–19[s]
Red cell diameter (μ)	6.7–7.2[s]	5.5–6.3[s]	6.5–7.5[d,g,s]	3.2–6.0[s]	2.5–3.9[s]	4.5–8.0[s]	4.0–8.0[s]	6–8[s]
Breathing rate (min^{-1})	10–30[c,d,e]	24–42[c,e]	30–60[d,f,g,e]	15–40[c,h,o]	15–25[c,i]	12–35[c,o,j]	10–45[c,m]	8–15[c]
Minute ventilation ($ml \cdot kg^{-1} \cdot min^{-1}$)	170–350[u,e,j]	200–350[o,e]	190–240[f,e]	100–133[o,h]		150–600[o,k]	300–400[m]	
Oxygen consumption ($ml \cdot kg^{-1} \cdot min^{-1}$)	4–11[d]	3–8[d,o]	7.8–14.2[f,o]	3.3–4.2[h,o]	3–5[d,o]	4–10[k]	2.7–4.7[b]	2–3[o]
Arterial PO_2 (mm Hg)	85–105[v,j]	100–115[v]	70–90[b]	75–100[b,h,o]	85–95[i]	80–110[o,j]	75–80[b]	85–90[b]
Hemoglobin P_{50} (mm Hg)	28–31[d,o,e]	36–38[d,o,e]	31–32[o,e]	34–37[d,o,e]	28–33[d,o,e]	31[o]	31–34[d,o,e]	25[o]
Arterial Pco_2 (mm Hg)	30–44[v,j]	28–35[v]	25–40[b,o]	30–40[b,h,o]	33–38[i]	30–50[o,j,k]	30–40[b,j]	38–40[b]
Arterial pH	7.36–7.46[b,v,j]	7.34–7.43[v]	7.36–7.44[b]	7.43–7.53[b,d,h]	7.42–7.48[i]	7.34–7.45[o,j,k]	7.38–7.50[b,j]	7.40–7.45
Bicarbonate (meq $liter^{-1}$)	20–25[v]	17–21	15–25[o]	21–28[d]	24–27[i]	20–28[o]		24–32[b]
Base deficit (meq $liter^{-1}$)	0 to −4[v]	−1 to −8[v]	0 to −8[o]	0 to +2[o]	0 to +2[i]	0 to 3[o]		0 to +4
Core temperature (°C)	37–40[d,e]	37–40[d,e]	38–40[d,f,e]	37–40[d,e]	38–40[d,i,e]	38–39[d,e]	38–40[d,r,e]	37–38[d]

[a] O'Rourke RA, Bishop VS: Cardiovascular hemodynamics in the conscious dog, *Am Heart J* 81:55–60, 1971.
[b] Gross DR: *Animal Models in Cardiovascular Research*. Boston, Martinus Nijhoff Pub., 1985.
[c] Phyllis JW: *Veterinary Physiology*. Philadelphia, W.B. Saunders Co, 1976.
[d] Spector WS: *Handbook of Biological Data*. Philadelphia, W.B. Saunders Co, 1956.
[e] Fox JR, Cohen BJ, Loew FM (eds): *Laboratory Animal Medicine*. New York, Academic Press, 1984.
[f] Harkness JE, Wagner JE: *The Biology and Medicine of Rabbits and Rodents*. Philadelphia, Lea & Febiger, 1983.
[g] Weisbroth SH: *The Biology of the Laboratory Rabbit*. New York, Academic Press, 1974.
[h] Hecker JF: *The Sheep as an Experimental Animal*. New York, Academic Press, 1983, pp 33–117.
[i] Kumar A, Thurmon JC, Nelson DR, et al: Response of goats to ketamine hydrochloride. *Vet Med Sm Anim Clin* 78:955–960, 1983.
[j] Harmison LT (ed): Research animals in medicine. National Institutes of Health, DHEW Pub No. (NIH) 72-333, Washington, DC, 1973.
[k] Kuida H, Brown AM, Lange RL, et al: Cardiovascular studies on normal calves. *Am J Physiol* 200: 247–252, 1961.
[l] Weber KT, Dennison BH, Fuqua JM, et al: Hemodynamic measurements in unanesthetized calves. *J Surg Res* 11:383–389, 1971.
[m] Mount LE, Ingram DL: *The Pig as a Laboratory Model*. New York, Academic Press, 1971, pp 65–78.
[n] Pond WG, Houpt KA: *The Biology of the Pig*. Ithaca, NY, Cornell University Press, 1978.
[o] Altman PL, Dittmer DS: *Biology Data Book*. Fed Am Soc Exp Biol: 1974.
[p] Adams BB, Baccelli G, Mancia G, et al: Cardiovascular changes during naturally elicited fighting behavior in the cat. *Am J Physiol* 216:1226–1235, 1969.
[q] Warren DJ, Ledingham JGG: Cardiac output in the conscious rabbit: an analysis of the thermodilution technique. *J Appl Physiol* 36:246–251, 1974.
[r] Stone HL, Sawyer DC: Cardiac output and related measurements in unanesthetized miniature swine. In Bustad LK, McClellan RO (eds): *Swine in Biomedical Research*. Battelle Memorial Institute, 1966, pp 411–418.
[s] Schalm OW: *Veterinary Hematology*, Philadelphia, Lea & Febiger, 1965.
[t] Swenson MJ (ed): *Duke's Physiology of Domestic Animals*, ed 10. Ithaca, NY, Cornell University Press, 1984.
[u] Andersen AC: *The Beagle as an Experimental Dog*. Ames, IA, Iowa State University Press, 1970.
[v] Haskins SC: Blood gases and acid-base balance. In Kirk RW (ed): *Curr Vet Ther VIII*. Philadelphia, WB Saunders Co, 1983.

Jersey; United States Surgical Corp., New York, New York; or Vetko, Colorado Springs, Colorado), or by a Doppler blood flow detector (Parks Electronic Lab, Beaverton, Oregon). Bradycardia, tachycardia, changes in heart rate, and irregular rhythm can be recognized. The first two methods monitor electrical activity of the heart and may be completely normal in the face of totally inadequate mechanical function. The ideal heart monitor provides a continuous, automatic, audible monitor of mechanical heart function, as do the later two above.

The importance of heart rate is in the effect that it has on cardiac output and blood pressure. A simultaneously measured cardiac output or blood pressure helps to interpret the physiological significance of an abnormal heart rate. In the absence of these measure-

Table 17.2
Normal Preoperative, Intraoperative, and Postoperative Heart Rate, Breathing Rate, and Intraoperative Systolic Blood Pressure in Normal Dogs and Cats Undergoing Elective Surgery at the University of California, Davis, Veterinary Medical Teaching Hospital[a]

Small dogs (<10 kg)	21	116 ± 20[b] (80–160)[c]	109 ± 14 (86–139)	129 ± 27 (95–180)	28 ± 10 (12–42)	24 ± 8 (12–38)	31 ± 9 (16–46)	121 ± 22 (82–161)
Large dogs (>15 but <35 kg)	66	110 ± 21 (76–160)	118 ± 19 (86–166)	136 ± 26 (80–200)	28 ± 8 (12–42)	19 ± 7 (8–43)	26 ± 9 (12–68)	135 ± 20 (93–187)
All dogs	94	111 ± 21 (76–160)	115 ± 18 (86–166)	134 ± 26 (80–200)	28 ± 8 (12–42)	20 ± 7 (8–43)	27 ± 9 (12–68)	132 ± 22 (82–187)
Cats receiving ketamine	37	166 ± 30 (90–220)	151 ± 20 (120–198)	182 ± 39 (100–260)	42 ± 14 (20–80)	25 ± 11 (10–52)	41 ± 15 (20–80)	115 ± 22 (81–159)
Cats not receiving ketamine	14	175 ± 42 (110–240)	138 ± 16 (112–159)	182 ± 22 (140–220)	38 ± 14 (20–72)	30 ± 11 (8–50)	38 ± 11 (20–60)	99 ± 21 (72–144)
All cats	51	168 ± 33 (90–240)	148 ± 20 (112–198)	182 ± 35 (100–260)	41 ± 14 (20–80)	26 ± 11 (8–52)	40 ± 14 (20–80)	108 ± 23 (72–159)

[a] No specialty breeds (such as giant breeds, sight hounds, or brachycephalics) were included. Anesthetic agents included atropine and acepromazine or meperidine for premedication, thiamylal for induction of dogs and thiamylal or ketamine for induction of cats, and halothane or methoxyflurane for maintenance. Only young healthy patients were included.
[b] Mean ± 1 SD.
[c] Range.

ments, a heart rate below 50 to 60 bpm in the dog or cat or 25 bpm in the horse or ruminant is considered to be too low and a heart rate above about 250 bpm in the dog, 300 bpm in the cat, or about 75 bpm in the horse or ruminant is considered to be too high. If possible, treatment directed at the underlying cause of the abnormal heart rate should be rendered.

Bradycardia may be caused by:

1. excessive anesthetic depth;
2. excessive vagal tone (precipitated by endotracheal intubation, traction or pressure on the eyeball or rectus muscles, visceral traction, urinary bladder distention, or periosteal stimulation);
3. terminal hypoxia;
4. narcotics, xylazine, or anticholinesterase agents;
5. hypothermia (decreased tissue metabolic requirements);
6. exogenous toxemias (digitalis);
7. endogenous toxemias (hypothyroidism, hyperkalemia, or visceral organ failure); or
8. myocardial conduction disturbances.

If the specific cause of the bradycardia cannot be determined and it is judged to have a deleterious effect on cardiac output or blood pressure and has not responded to anticholinergic therapy, it may be necessary to administer a sympathomimetic agent.

1. Dopamine (Arnar-Stone Laboratories, Inc., McGraw Park, Illinois) (40 to 200 mg in 250 to 500 D_5W or saline; administered to effect (2.5 to 20 $\mu g \cdot kg^{-1} \cdot min^{-1}$)).
2. Dobutamine (Eli Lilly & Co., Indianapolis, Indiana) (40 to 200 mg in 250 to 500 D_5W or saline; administered to effect (2.5 to 20 $\mu g \cdot kg^{-1} \cdot min^{-1}$)).
3. Mephenteramine (Wyeth Laboratories, Philadelphia, Pennsylvania) (0.1 to 0.75 mg/kg i.v.; duration 15 to 30 minutes).
4. Ephedrine (Bristol Laboratories Syracuse, New York) (0.05 to 0.5 mg/kg i.v.; duration 15 to 30 minutes).
5. Isoproterenol (Winthrop Laboratories, New York, New York) (0.4 to 1.0 mg in 250 to 500 D_5W or saline; administered to effect (5 to 10 $\mu g \cdot kg^{-1} \cdot min^{-1}$)).

Tachycardia is a response to an underlying stress, and therapy is usually directed towards alleviating the underlying abnormalitie rather than the tachycardia per se. Tachycardia may be due to a light level of anesthesia; hypovolemia; hypotension; hypoxia; hypercapnia; hyperthermia; ketamine, anticholinergic, or sympathomimetic therapy; hyperthyroidism; or pheochromocytoma.

HEART RHYTHM

Supraventricular and ventricular ectopic pacemaker activity is common during general anesthesia. There is a wide variety of arrhythmias that may manifest themselves, aside from sinus bradycardia and tachycardia and atrioventricular conduction block, which has the same causes and treatment as bradycardia. However, premature atrial (PAC) and ventricular (PVC) pacemaker activity and bundle branch blocks (BBB) are the most common (Fig. 17.1). In general, they should be considered to be a sign of an underlying disease process and should not be treated specifically. Premature ventricular contractions (PVC) may progress in severity (frequency, multifocal) and predispose to ventricular tachycardia and fibrillation and usually requires specific therapy.

The details of arrhythmia identification can be found elsewhere (2). The salient questions to answer from the rhythm strip are:

1. Is the rate too slow or too fast?
2. Is the rhythm regular?
3. Is the PQRST waveform consistently present and or approximatley normal in size and shape?

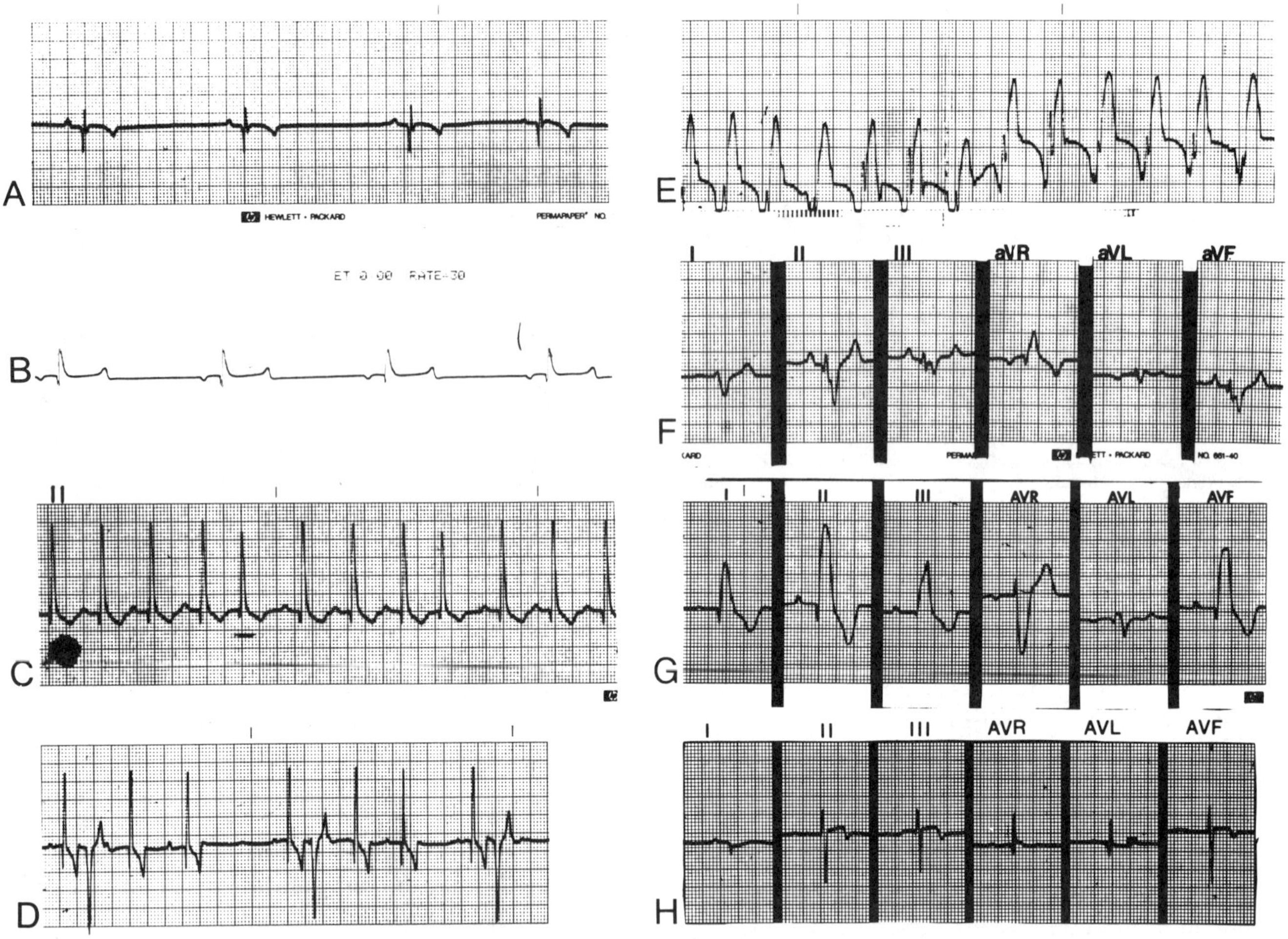

Figure 17.1. Common arrhythmias during general anesthesia. *A*, normal rate and rhythm in a dog. *B*, normal rate and rhythm in a horse. *C*, premature atrial contractions in a dog. *D*, premature ventricular contractions in a dog. *E*, ventricular tachycardia in a dog. *F*, right bundle branch block in a dog. *G*, left bundle branch block in a dog. *H*, right ventricular hypertrophy in a dog.

4. Is there synchrony between the ECG and the palpated pulse? Are all of the pulses of equal quality? Pulse deficits may be caused by:
   a. premature atrial contractions,
   b. premature ventricular contractions,
   c. variable diastolic ventricular filling, especially with high heart rates (administer 10 to 40 ml/kg of lactated Ringer's), or
   d. electromechanical dissociation (correct fluid and electrolyte abnormalities; calcium and glucocorticosteroids may be beneficial).
5. Is there a P wave prior to each QRS or is the P-R interval shortened? Absence of a P wave differentiates VPCs from right BBB and right ventricular hypertrophy (all three are associated with wide, bizarre-looking QRS complexes (Fig. 17.1)).
6. Is there a compensatory pause after the PQRST waveform in question? (Premature atrial and ventricular contractions are usually followed by a pause.)
7. Are the T waves abnormally large (normally less than 25% of the height of the R waves; be sure to measure the actual height because small R waves may make the T wave appear to be tall)?
   a. T waves may normally be a positive or a negative deflection or may be biphasic.
   b. Abnormally tall tented T waves may be due to hyperkalemia, hypoxia, or atrial dilatation (excessive venous return).
8. S-T segment depression is usually attributed to myocardial hypoxia or potassium or calcium abnormalities but commonly occurs in dogs with no other demonstrable cardiopulmonary problems.

Precise placement of the ECG leads is not necessary for monitoring purposes. The major concern is whether the PQRST waveforms appear to be approximately normal at the beginning and whether they change during the course of the surgery. In small animals, the right arm lead may be placed on the right arm or anywhere on the body rostral to the heart. The left leg lead may be placed on the left leg or anywhere on the body caudal to the heart. The left arm lead (ground) can be placed anywhere on the body not in contact with the other leads. The lead selector switch should be set to monitor Lead 2. If it is desirable to look at several specific leads during the operative period, the leads should be placed as marked.

The electrodes are placed somewhat differently in large species. The right arm lead (the negative pole) is attached low on the chest (toward the sternum); the left leg lead (the positive pole) is attached high on the chest above the spine of the scapula, and the left arm lead (ground) is attached anywhere, usually on the neck. The resultant Lead 2 ECG resembles the normal wave patterns as seen in other species.

Alligator clips provide satisfactory patient attachments if the teeth have been filed and the jaws bent or padded so as to reduce the pressure ischemia to the underlying tissue as much as possible and if they are not to be left in place for too long a period of time. Prolonged monitoring might be less traumatically achieved by the use of human electrode plates or by disposable adhesive electrodes (Silvon ECG electrode, NDM Corp.; Dayton, Ohio; or Red Dot, 3 M Corp., St. Paul, Minnesota).

Poor quality ECGs will result if the electrode-patient contact has high impedance. Usually this is minimized by using an electrolyte gel such as commercial ECG paste, Phisohex soap, ultrasound coupling gel, or alcohol (which dries fast and is not recommended). Skin resistance can be reduced by defatting the skin with acetone and de-epithelializing it by scrubbing.

Skin impedance problems can be bypassed with the use of esophageal leads. Esophageal leads may be obtained commercially (Summit Hill Laboratories) or may be homemade (Fig. 17.2). The ECG tracings obtained via esophageal leads are extremely variable, and normal guidelines with regard to waveform do not apply. Evaluate the rhythm and the waveforms to assure that they are approximately representative of a PQRST complex. If you do not like the appearance of the ECG, change the position of the esophageal lead. If the waveform changes during the course of the surgery, make sure that it is not due to a change in the position of the esophageal lead. Improper grounding of other electrical equipment (such as the electrosurgical unit) simultaneously attached to the patient may cause current to flow through the ECG electrodes and the ECG to ground, if the ECG is grounded. This causes focal points of intense energy and heat at the point of exit (the electrode), which may cause focal esophageal necrosis. Esophageal ECG monitoring should be used only with battery-operated or isolated ECG machines.

The ECG measures electrical activity in the heart and serves to identify the existing arrhythmia. It does not measure myocardial performance, cardiac output, or blood pressure and can appear quite normal in the face of miserable mechanical performance of the heart.

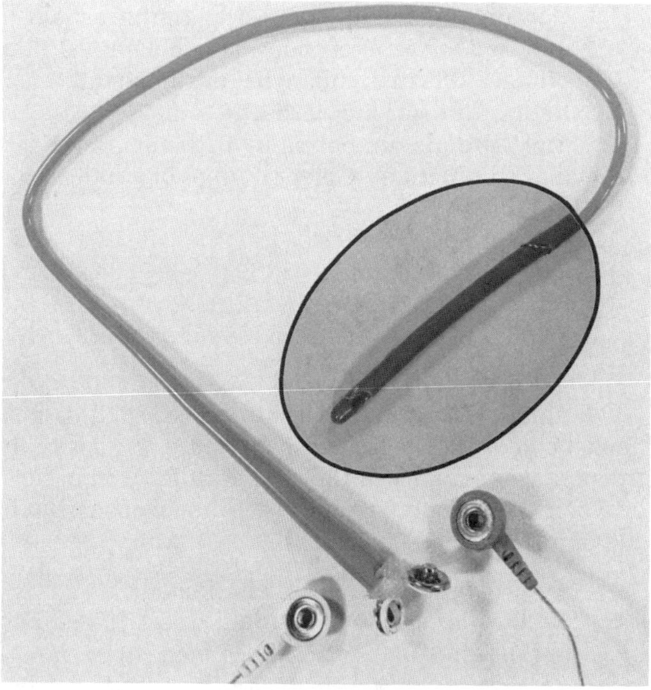

Figure 17.2. A homemade esophageal lead system for monitoring the ECG during surgery. Two stainless steel wires, isolated from one another by passing one through a plastic tube, are threaded through an appropriately sized rubber feeding tube. The distal ends exit the tube at different points and are wrapped around the tube; all wire ends must be well protected. The proximal ends are fitted with connectors to the patient cable. Silicone glue is used to seal both ends of the feeding tube. The reference electrode (third lead) can be attached anywhere on the patient's body.

The ECG is an adjunct to, but not a replacement for, other monitors of cardiovascular status.

Atrial and ventricular premature contractions may be caused by a wide variety of abnormalities, and the underlying problem should be sought and remedied whenever possible.

1. Too light (endogenous release of catecholamines) or too deep (hypercapnia or hypoxia) a level of anesthesia is commonly associated with ectopic pacemaker activity;
2. Hypoxia or hypercapnia;
3. Hypovolemia or hypotension;
4. Exogenous catecholamine therapy;
5. Digitalis toxicity, which is potentiated by hypokalemia and hypercalcemia;
6. Hypokalemia, which is potentiated by respiratory or metabolic alkalosis, glucose, or insulin therapy;
7. Hyperkalemia, which is potentiated by acidosis, hypocalcemia, or succinylcholine or may be iatrogenic;
8. Hypercalcemia, which is potentiated by respiratory or metabolic acidosis or may be iatrogenic;

9. Certain anesthetics that lower the threshold to endogenous or exogenous catecholamines (halothane, xylazine, thiamylal, or thiopental);
10. Endocarditis or myocarditis;
11. Endocardial stimulation by catheters or epicardial stimulation by pleural tubes or surgical manipulation;
12. High preload or afterload;
13. Severe hypothermia (<26°C);
14. End-stage visceral organ failure;
15. Intracranial disorders (increased pressure or hypoxia).

Premature ventricular contractions should, perhaps, be specifically treated if they are increasing in frequency or severity, if they are multifocal in nature, or when their instantaneous heart rate exceeds 180 to 200 bpm.

1. Obvious causes should be eliminated.
2. The level of anesthesia should be evaluated and appropriate vaporizer changes made. The vaporizer should not automatically be turned off because too light a level of anesthesia is often the underlying cause.
3. Maximize the inspired oxygen concentration and institute intermittent positive pressure ventilation (IPPV).
4. Check the anesthetic machine and ventilator to make sure that they are operating properly and that the oxygen supply is not depleted.
5. Begin rapid fluid administration.
6. If the PVCs persist, discontinue the administration of agents that may cause or lower the threshold to the arrhythmia.
7. If the PVCs persist, consider the administration of an antiarrhythmic agent:
   a. Lidocaine (Astra Pharmaceutical Products, Worcester, Massachusetts) (1 to 5 mg/kg i.v.)
   b. Procainamide (Squibb Pharmaceutical Co., Princeton, New Jersey) (1 to 5 mg/kg i.v.)
   c. Propranolol (Ayerst Laboratories, to New York, New York) (0.05 to 0.3 mg/kg i.v.)
   d. Verapamil (Searle Pharmaceuticals Inc., Chicago, Illinois) (0.05 to 0.15 mg/kg i.v.)

VENTRICULAR PERFORMANCE

Ventricular performance (the contractile force of the heart) can be roughly gauged by auscultation of the loudness of each heart beat. The routine use of esophageal stethoscopes and heart sound amplifiers may be useful in this regard. Diminution of the heart sounds may be due to myocardial weakness, hypovolemia, movement of the esophageal stethoscope, or weak batteries.

Mechanical performance also can be roughly estimated by the steepness or the rate of upsweep of the arterial pressure waveform or palpated pulse. The whole waveform, as well as the overall quality of the palpated pulse, is more a reflection of the stroke volume, which is the result of both end-diastolic ventricular volume and contractility. Pulse pressure and pulse quality may be minimal if the patient is hypovolemic while ventricular performance per se is quite good.

Ventricular performance can be estimated noninvasively from systolic time intervals, which are indices calculated from simultaneous recordings of central arterial blood pressure, ECG, and phonocardiogram (3–8) (Fig. 17.3). The electromechanical systole is first

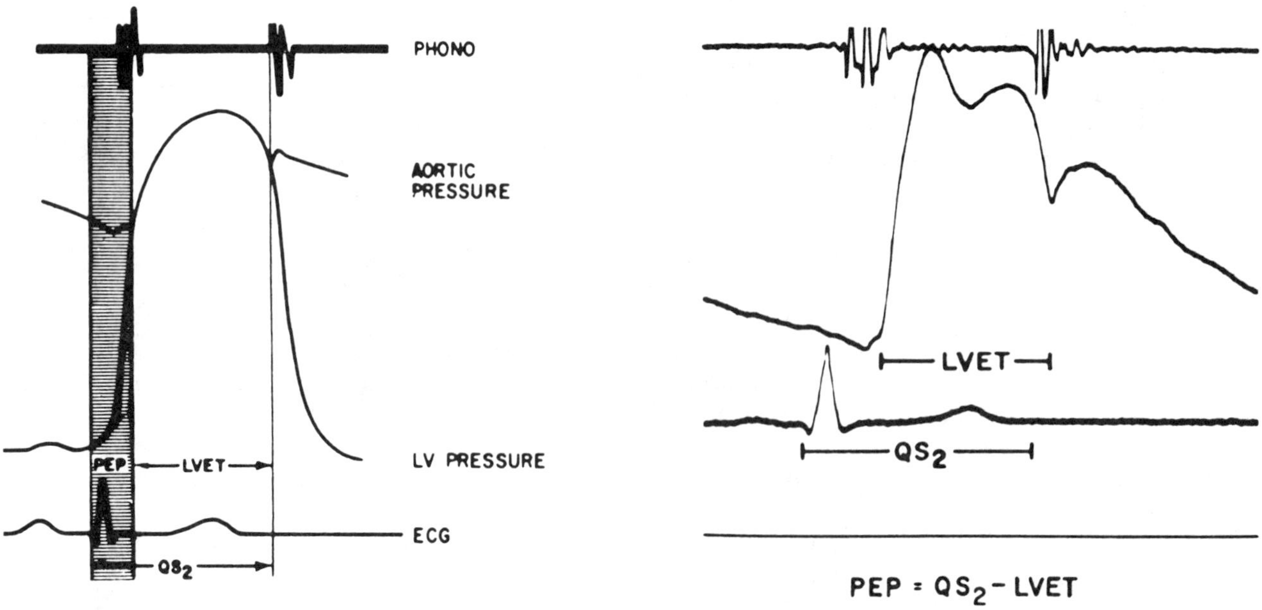

Figure 17.3. Three components of STIs. *Left*, a schematic of the left ventricular events that comprise the STI. *Right*, a recording of a phonocardiogram, external carotid pulse, and ECG at 100 mm/sec paper speed. The subintervals of the STI are indicated on both. Reprinted from Lewis RP, et al: A critical review of the systolic time intervals. *Circulation* 56:146, 1977, and by permission of the American Heart Association, Inc.

calculated as the time from the beginning of the Q wave to the first high frequency sound of aortic closure (QS_2). The left ventricular ejection time is calculated as the time from the onset of the pressure curve to the dicrotic notch (LVET). The pre-ejection period (PEP) is determined by subtracting LVET from OS_2 and provides a close approximation of isovolemic contraction time and ventricular performance. The QS_2 is prolonged with left BB and antiarrhythmic drugs and is shortened by positive inotropic drugs. The LVET is prolonged by decreased afterload and positive inotropic drugs and is shortened by decreased preload and myocardial failure. The PEP is prolonged by left BBB, negative inotropic drugs, heart failure, and decreased preload; it is shortened by positive inotropic drugs, decreased afterload, or increased period. LVET, but not PEP, varies inversely with heart rate in the human being where regression equations have been established (3). Such a relationship has been found in rabbits (6); however, it could not be established for dogs (5). PEP/LVET is a more sensitive index of left ventricular function than are any of systolic the systolic time intervals (STIs) alone and is independent of heart rate but is sensitive to preload and afterload.

Another systolic time interval, the QF interval, is the measured time from the beginning of the Q wave to the beginning of the upstroke of the peripheral pulse (8). QF includes PEP and transmission time of the pressure pulse to a peripheral site (which is proportional to the distance between the heart and the peripheral artery and is inversely related to arterial compliance or diastolic pressure). QF is considerably easier to measure than PEP, but is closely correlated with PEP.

Ventricular performance can also be determined by the maximum velocity of contraction at zero load (V max) and by the first or second derivative of the maximum rate of the ventricular pressure change during systole with respect to time (dP/dt) (9–13). The measurements require left ventricular catheterization that may not be feasible in a clinical patient.

Ventricular performance can be determined by the end-systolic pressure-volume relationship (10, 14–15) or by the end-diastolic/end-systolic relationship (16). Ventricular volume estimates may be derived from preimplanted ultrasonic crystals, a technique which does not lend itself to bedside measurements, or by transthoracic echocardiography.

Whether or not contractility is actually measured, its impact upon cardiovascular performance cannot be denied. Impaired ventricular performance is a common cuase of hypotension in critically ill patients. Contractility is adversely affected by most anesthetics, severe metabolic disturbances, hypoxia, severe pH and electrolyte disturbances, endogenous or exogenous toxicities, intrinsic myocardial disease, and excessive or insufficient end-diastolic filling volume.

Ventricular performance can be improved by the administration of one or more of the following drugs.

1. Beta-receptor agonist catecholamines
   a. Dopamine (Arnar-Stone Laboratories, Inc.) (40 to 200 mg in 250 to 500 ml D_5W or saline; administered to effect (2.5 to 20 $\mu g \cdot kg^{-1} \cdot min^{-1}$).
   b. Dobutamine (Eli Lilly & Co.) (40 to 200 mg in 250 to 500 ml D_5W or saline; adminstered to effect (2.5 to 20 $\mu g \cdot kg^{-1} \cdot min^{-1}$).
   c. Mephenteramine (Wyeth Laboratories) (0.1 to 0.75 mg/kg i.v.; duration 15 to 30 minutes).
   d. Ephedrine (Bristol Laboratories) (0.05 to 0.5 mg/kg i.v.; duration 15 to 30 minutes).
2. Calcium
   a. Calcium chloride (Bristol Laboratories) (10%) (0.1 mg/kg)
   b. Calcium guconate (Tech America Group, Inc., Elwood, Kansas; Haver, Shawnee, Kansas; or Fort Dodge, Iowa) (10%) (0.5 mg/kg)
3. Digitalis (Coopers Animal Health, Inc., Kansas City, Missouri; EVSCO Pharmaceuticals, Buena, New Jersey; Elkins-Sinn, Inc., Cherry Hill, New Jersey; or Burroughs Wellcome, Research Triangle Park, North Carolina)
4. Amrinone (Withrop-Breon Labs, New York, New York) and Milrenone are a new class of inotropic agents that have an action that is not fully understood but is distinct from digitalis preparation or catecholamines. They have some vasodilatory activity via a direct relaxant effect on smooth muscle; 0.75 to 3 mg/kg i.v. develops a peak effect in within 10 minutes with a duration of 30 to 120 minutes.

CARDIAC OUTPUT

Cardiac output is the product of stroke volume and heart rate; stroke volume is the product of end-diastolic ventricular filling volume and contractility. Whether or not cardiac output is actually measured, its importance to cardiovascular performance cannot be denied.

Cardiac output can be estimated by indicator-dilution techniques that involve the injection of an indicator of a known concentration into the right atrium and the measurement of the change in concentration of the indicator at a downstream location (pulmonary artery or aorta). Although a variety of indicators have been used, the two most common are indocyanin green dye (17, 18) and room temperature or iced saline (19–25). Of the two, the thermodilution technique more readily tends itself to clinical cardiac output measurement. Thermodilution catheters and computers are commercially available (Instrumentation Laboratory Inc., Lexington, Massachusetts; Edwards Laboratories, Santa Ana, California; Electronics for Medicine, White Plains, New York; Columbus Instruments, Columbus,

Ohio; Gould Medical Products, Oxnard, California; or Hewlett-Packard, Palo Alto, California), and the flow-directed catheters are relatively easy to introduce (26).

Pulmonary artery catheters may be inserted with the aide of fluoroscopy or blindly by observing the changes in pressure wave form as the catheter progresses from the anterior vena cava to the right ventricle to the pulmonary artery (Fig. 17.4). A commercially manufactured ballon-tipped flow-directed catheter Electro-Dianostic Instruments, Burbank, California; Vita-Stat, Chatsworth, California; Industrial & Biomedical Sensors Corp., Waltham, Massachusetts; or Medical Systems Corp., Great Neck, New York). The catheter should be flexible and have a gentle curve at the tip to facilitate passage through the right ventricle.

A wide area over the jugular vein is clipped and scrubbed with antiseptic solution. The neck should be draped and sterile gloves should be worn. The jugular vein may be surgically exposed, or a commercial or homemade introducer (a 14-gauge medical catheter slit lengthwise so that it will expand when the hermodilution catheter is passed) is percutaneously placed. The catheter is inserted into the vein and advanced toward the heart while the pressure is monitored. The transducer should be placed at the level of the right atrium for a standard zero reference level. The distance between the skin puncture site and the heart should be approximated at the start of the procedure (approximately 30 cm in a 20-kg dog). The catheter often travels down the postcava rather than entering the right ventricle. Once the catheter has been inserted 5 to 10 cm beyond the estimated distance to the heart, it should be withdrawn, rotated, and reinserted. The procedure is repeated until the tip of the catheter falls into the right ventricle. It may be helpful to partially inflate the balloon when the catheter tip is thought to be in the right atrium. The flow of blood may carry the catheter tip into the right ventricle. The catheter softens at body temperature; flushing with room temperature or iced saline will stiffen the catheter and may facilitate passage.

When the catheter enters the right ventricle, there will be a dramatic change in the measured pressure tracing. The ECG should be monitored throughout the procedure. Catheter stimulation of the endocardium may cause arrhythmias. The catheter is then slowly and gently advanced. If the catheter has a balloon, it should be inflated at this time, enabling the flow of blood to carry the catheter tip into the pulmonary artery.

When the catheter enters the pulmonary artery, there will be another abrupt change in the pressure tracing. Cardiac output is measured by the bolus injection of 3 to 10 ml of room temperature or iced saline. The area under the curve of the measured temperature change of the downstream thermistor may be computed automatically or may be hand-computed by planimetry (27) or the fore-n-aft method (28).

Cardiac output can also be estimated by computer-generated pulse contour methods (29–32). Several methods and formulas have been devised for estimating stroke volume from the pulse contour, and they are remarkably reproducible over a short period of time when compared to cardiac output determined by dye or thermal dilution. Unfortunately, the accuracy of the technique declines with time and with changing hemodynamic status (arterial wall compliance or systemic vascular resistance); without periodic recalibration, it is no more accurate than simply measuring blood pressure or pulse pressure (29, 32).

Cardiac output can also be measured experimentally by a variety of techniques including electromagnetic flowprobes (33), Doppler ultrasonic probes (34), and microsphere techniques (35).

Cardiac output may be reduced by:

1. Insufficient venous return and end-diastolic ventricular filling volume (hypovolemia, positive air-

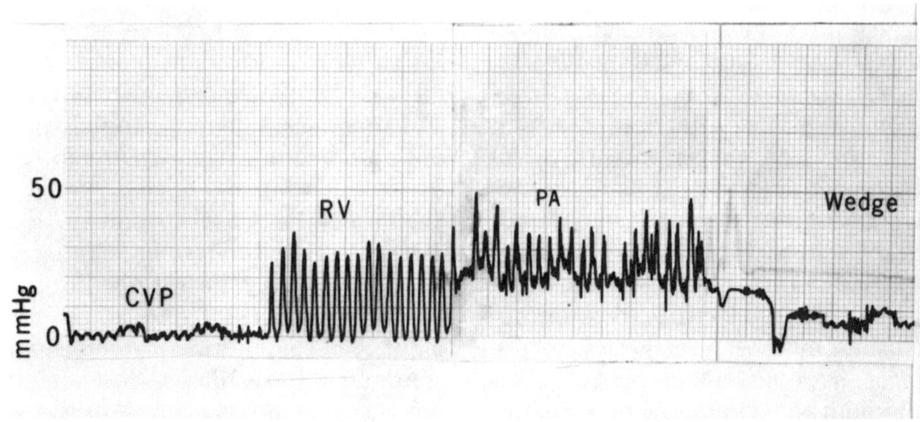

Figure 17.4. Changes in pressure wave form as the flow-directed catheter advances from the anterior vena cava (systolic/diastolic pressures average 5/0 mm Hg) to the right ventricle (20 to 40/0 mm Hg) to the pulmonary artery (20 to 40/10 to 20 mm Hg).

way and pleural pressure, or disease-induced or surgical inflow occlusion;
2. Ventricular restrictive disease (hypertrophic or restrictive cardiomyopathy, pericardial tamponade, or pericardial fibrosis);
3. Decreased contractility (as previously discussed);
4. Excessive bradycardia, tachycardia, or arrhythmias;
5. Regurgitation (retrograde flow) of part of the end-diastolic blood volume due to insufficient atrioventricular valve function; or
6. Outflow tract obstruction (stenosis).

Poor cardiac output should be improved by correcting the underlying problem when possible. When it is not possible, cardiac output may be improved by the administration of positive inotropic drugs to enhance ventricular performance.

PERIPHERAL PERFUSION

Perfusion of visceral and other peripheral organs (muscle, skin, and mucous membranes) is dependant upon a arterial-to-venous pressure gradient but is primarily regulated by vasomotor tone. Vasodilation improves peripheral perfusion but, if excessive, causes hypotension. Vasoconstriction decreases peripheral perfusion and can be easily recognized by pale mucous membrane color (when not due to anemia) and a prolonged capillary refill time (the rate at which blood flows back into a capillary bed after it has been digitally compressed). Vasoconstriction is also heralded by pale color and a lack of bleeding at the operative site, anuria, or a decrease in peripheral (skin, muscle, or toe web) temperature (36, 37). Regional blood flow can be determined experimentally by microsphere techniques (38), ultrasonic Doppler instrumentation (38), electromagnetic flow probes, radionuclide imagery (39), nuclear magnetic resonance, and position emission tomography (40).

Vasoconstriction may be induced by any stress-induced increase in sympathetic tone: hypovolemia, low cardiac output for any reason, excitement, fear, pain, or the excitement phase of recovery. Exogenous alpha-receptor agonist catecholamine therapy or smooth muscle agonists (vasopression, calcium, or oxytocin) may also cause vasoconstriction. Vasoconstriction is usually not treated specifically, therapy is directed at the underlying problem.

ARTERIAL BLOOD PRESSURE

Arterial blood pressure is the product of cardiac output, vascular capacity, and blood volume. Impairment of one of these is usually compensated for by the other two so as to maintain an adequate blood pressure, which is important for cerebral and coronary perfusion. Adequate cerebral and coronary perfusion is considered to require a mean systemic blood pressure of 50 to 60 mm Hg. If, however, the impairment is severe or if the compensatory processes are themselves exhausted or debilitated by disease, hypotension will develop.

Digital palpation of the quality of the pulse amplitude in a peripheral artery reflects stroke volume and may bear little correlation to the arterial blood pressure. The weak, thready pulse that occurs with hypovolemia is due to small stroke volume; these patients may be normotensive.

Arterial blood pressure can be measured in animals by indirect and direct techniques (41–46). Indirect, sphygmomanometry involves the application of an occlusion cuff over an artery in a cylindrical appendage. The occlusion cuff should be placed snugly around the leg. If it is applied too tightly, the pressure measurements will be erroneously low because the cuff itself will partially occlude the underlying artery. If the cuff is too loose, the pressure measurements will be erroneously high because excessive cuff pressure will be required to occlude the underlying artery. Inflation of the cuff applies pressure to the underlying tissues and will totally occlude blood flow when the pressure exceeds the systolic blood pressure. As the cuff pressure is gradually decreased, blood will begin to flow intermittently when the extraluminal pressure falls below the luminal systolic pressure.

The appearance of needle oscillations on the manometer during cuff deflation is caused by the pulse wave hitting the cuff and corresponds approximately to systolic blood pressure; however, the values are slightly higher than those derived by direct arterial measurement. Digital palpation of a pulse distal to the cuff corresponds approximately to the systolic blood pressure, although measurements are usually lower than corresponding direct arterial measurements. Auscultation of Korotkoff sounds (the first occurrence of sounds represents systolic pressure; the sudden muffling or disappearance of sounds represents diastolic pressure) in the metatarsal or coccygeal arteries of horses had been reported (46, 47). A microphone may be useful in this and smaller species (Abbott Medical Electronics Co., North Chicago, Illinois). A xylol pulse detector has been reported to be useful for the dog and horse (48).

In oscillometric instrumentation (49) (Applied Medical Research, Inc., Tampa, Florida) the lowest pressure associated with maximal oscillation of the cuff pressure corresponds approximately to mean arterial blood pressure. Plethysmographic techniques (Electro-Diagnostic Instruments; Vita-Stat; Industrial & Biomedical Sensors Corp.; Medical Systems Corp.) have been used; however, accuracy hs not been verified. Doppler instrumentation involves the application of a small piezoelectric crystal over an artery (Parks Electronics Lab; Roche Medical Electronics Division, Hoffman-La Roche, Inc., Cranbury, New Jersey). Energy is transmitted into the underlying tissue. The energy frequency reflected from moving tissues is shifted slightly from that which was transmitted, and this frequency difference is converted electronically to an audible signal. Some Doppler instruments measure blood flow and are used for the measurement of systolic blood pressure; other instruments generate signals from the movement of the arterial wall and can be used to measure both systolic and diastolic blood pressures. Doppler instrumentation has been shown to correlate closely with direct arterial measurements in a variety of animal species (46, 49–53).

All external techniques are least accurate when vessels are small, when the blood pressure is low, and when the vessels are constricted. Direct measurement of arterial blood pressure is more accurate and continuous compared to indirect methods but require the introduction of a catheter into an artery by percutaneous or cutdown procedure. For percutaneous catheterization, we have used the dorsal metatarsal artery most commonly in dogs and the facial artery in the horse (Fig. 17.5). The metatarsal artery can be used in the horse if the facial artery is not available. The subcutaneous tissues around all of the above arteries are relatively tight so that hematoma formation after

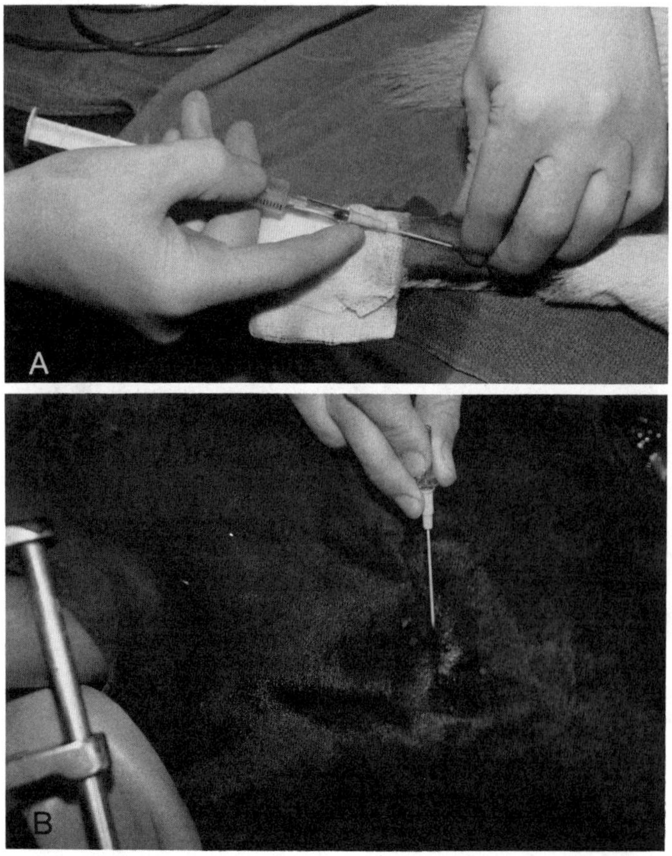

Figure 17.5. *A*, percutaneous catheterization of the dorsal metatarsal artery in a dog. *B*, percutaneous catheterization of the facial artery in a horse.

catheter removal is rarely a problem. Catheters placed in appendage arteries can easily be taped in place. Catheters on large flat surfaces must sutured in place or glued (Super Glue , Woodhill Permatex, Cleveland, Ohio) or both. We have maintianed metatarsal arterial catheters in place for several days without complications.

After a wide depilation and surgical scrub of the area over the artery, the artery to be percutaneously catheterized is palpated with one or two fingers of one hand. A relief incision is made completely through the skin with the beveled edge of a hypodermic needle without entering the artery. A thin-wall catheter outside the needle system (Angiocath, Deseret Co., Sandy, Utah) (20 gauge, 2.5 inch is positioned subcutaneously on top of the artery with the bevel up. The needle tip and the artery are simultaneously palpated with the finger(s) of the opposite hand, and the catheter is inserted into the artery, steeply at first just so that the tip of the needle penetrates the upper wall of the artery and then flat against the skin surface and parallel with the longitudinal axis of the artery so that the bevel of the needle and the end of the catheter lie entirely within the lumen of the artery without penetrating the deep wall. The presence of the needle tip within the lumen can be verified by the reflux of blood into the hub of the needle and by feel. At this point neither vessel nor needle should be moved while the catheter is gently rotated into the artery to its full length. The needle is then rapidly removed, replaced with a three-way stopcock or an infusion plug, and flushed with heparinized saline.

Femoral arteries may be catheterized percutaneously or by cutdown, carotid arteries may be cutdown in any species, and lingual arteries may be catheterized percutaneously in anesthetized dogs. For cutdown procedures, the artery is surgically isolated, and a catheter outside the needle system (Angiocath) (16 gauge, 5.5 inch) is inserted into the lumen of the artery. The needle is removed and replaced with an infusion plug, and the catheter flushed with heparinized saline. No circumferential sutures are placed around the artery. The incision is closed, and the catheter hub is sutured or glued to the skin at the puncture site.

Once the catheter is placed, it is connected to a monitoring device. The catheter must be flushed with heparinized saline hourly or continuously (Intraflo, Sorenson Research Co., Salt Lake City, Utah). The measuring device could be comprised of a long fluid administration set suspended from the ceiling and operated like a central venous pressure movement. Fluid is instilled into the tubing via a three-way stopcock to a very high level and then allowed to gravitate into the artery until the hydrostatic pressure of hte column of fluid equalizes with the mean arterial blood pressure of the patient. Never allow blood to flow into the catheter because it will clot; always make the measurement by allowing fluid to flow into the catheter. Because mean blood pressure oscillates, leaving the system open will allow blood to enter the catheter.

The measuring device could be an aneroid manometer. Water or blood must not be allowed to enter the manometer. The manometer can be attached to the catheter by a couple of lengths of extension tubing (1, 42, 45, 46). Saline is injected into the tubing via a three-way stopcock toward the manometer until the compressed air increases the registered pressure to a level above that of mean blood pressure, and then the pressurized manometer system is allowed to equilibrate with the mean blood pressure of the patient. The aneroid manometer can be further separated from the fluid column by using a collapsible diaphragm such as the cut end of a glass plunger in the glass syringe or a finger cot (Fig. 17.6). The pressure measurement is made by closing the stopcock to the patient, filling the syringe with saline to some high pressure, and then opening the system to the patient, allowing the pressurized unit to equilibrate with the mean pressure of the patient.

The arterial catheter can also be attached to a commercial transducer and recording system (Spacelabs, Hillsborough, Oregon; Datascope Corp., Paramus, New Jersey; Tektronic Inc., Beaverton, Oregon; Air-Sheilds Inc., Hatboro, Pennsylania; Carultron/KDC Medical Sales, Anaheim, California; or Electronics for Medicine); although more expensive than the homemade systems described above, these are much easier to use for continuous pressure recordings.

Normal systolic, diastolic, and mean blood pressures are approximately 100 to 160, 60 to 100, and 80 to 120 mm Hg, respectively. Systolic pressures below 80 and mean pressures below 60 are assumed to result in inadequate cerebral and coronary perfusion and warrant restitution therapy. When hypotension develops during general anesthesia, the anesthetic should be decreased as much as possible compatible with the completion of the surgical procedure. If excessive movement occurs before restoration of an acceptable blood pressure, the anesthetic should be changed to one that is less hypotensive, such as oxymorphone/diazepam or ketamine/diazepam. A bolus of crystalloid extracellular replacement solution such as lactated Ringers' (10 to 40 ml/kg) should be rapidly administered over 10 to 30 minutres. Hypotension may be due to hypovolemia, peripheral vasodilation, or reduced cardiac output.

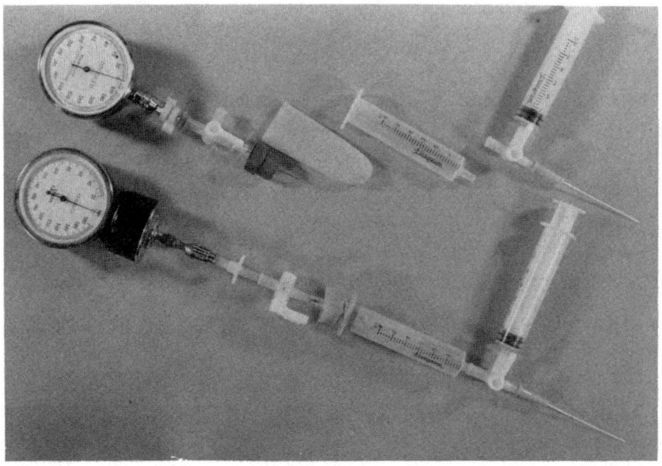

Figure 17.6. A homemade blood pressure measuring apparatus. The aneroid manometer is made to fit tightly into an appropriately sized rubber stopper. The other end of the stopper is fitted with a cut-off finger from a surgical glove, and the assembly is fitted into a 6- to 12-ml syringe barrel. The barrel is fitted with a three-way stopcock and filled with saline. The upper stopcock is opened, and saline is withdrawn until the finger cot is maximally inflated at zero pressure. The unit is then ready to attach to the arterial catheter.

Hypovolemia is the most common cause of hypotension. Pre-existing fluid deficits may be unmasked by the induction of general anesthesia. Extracellular fluid deficits may result from inadequate intake, diarrhea, vomition, diuresis, or third-space fluid accumulations. Interstitial volume deficits (which are associated with an obligatory vascular volume deficit) are heralded by decreased skin turgor and an acute loss of body weight. Vascular volume deficiencies may, in addition, be due to whole blood or plasma losses or hypoproteinemia. The signs of vascular volume deficits are the familiar signs of shock—tachycardia, weak pulse, and peripheral vasconstriction.

A multielectrolyte sodium-containing crystalloid replacement solution such as lactated Ringer's or an equivalent solution is usually the fluid of choice to start replacement therapy. These fluids are relatively economical, can be administered fairly rapidly, and are good extracellular fluid volume expanders. A suggested rate of administration during routine surgery is 10 $ml/kg^{-1}/hr^{-1}$, plus a volume two to three times that of the estimated blood loss. A volume of 20 $ml/kg^{-1}/hr^{-1}$ should be administered to animals subject to large fluid transudation from extensive thoracotomies, laparotomies, or fracture repair when active diuresis is desirable and when signs of mild hypovolemia or hypotension develop. If signs of moderate or severe hypovolemia or hypotension develop, 10 to 40 ml/kg should be rapidly administered over 10 to 30 minutes in quantities sufficient to alleviate the signs.

Anemia and hypoproteinemia constitute the primary limiting factors to the administration of crystalloid fluids. When the packed cell volume decreases below 20% and further volume therapy is needed, the infusion of red blood cells is indicated. When the total plasma proteins decrease below 3.0 to 3.5 g/dl (assuming a normal albumin/globulin (A/G) ratio) and further volume therapy is needed, the infusion of plasma or dextran 70 (Pharmacia Laboratories, Piscataway, New Jersey; Abbott Laboratories; Traverol Labs, Inc., Deerfield, Illinois; or American McGraw Labs, Santa Ana, California) is indicated.

Decreased cardiac output may be due to a variety of causes previously discussed. The underlying cause should be corrected if possible. The immediate management of heart failure may require sympathomimetic therapy in addition to correction of the underlying systemic disease. An appropriate sympathomimetic agent that causes minimal peripheral vasoconstriction should be utilized for prolonged support (dobutamine, dopamine, or mephenteramine). These agents may cause excessive hypertension and arrhythmias, and their use should be monitored closely.

Most anesthetic drugs cause peripheral vasodilation and may cause hypotension. Fluid therapy to refill the expanded vascular volume should be the primary focus of therapy. Alpha receptor agonists may be indicated initially to support blood pressure pharmacologically and provide time for blood volume restitution.

CENTRAL VENOUS PRESSURE

Central venous pressure (CVP) is the luminal pressure of the intrathoracic anterior vena cava. Peripheral venous pressure is variably higher than CVP (1) and is not a reliable indicator of CVP. Catheters should be positioned via the jugular vein into the anterior vena cava. It may be necessary to reposition the neck and forelimb several times in order to make the bend at the thoracic inlet. Contact with the endocardium of the right atrium or the right ventricle should be avoided because this may stimulate ectopic pacemaker activity. Verification of a well-placed, unobstructed catheter can be ascertained by observing small fluctuations in the fluid meniscus within the manometer synchronous with the heart beat and larger excursions synchronous with ventilation. Large fluctuations synchronous with each heart beat may indicate that the end of the catheter is positioned within the right ventricle. Measurements should be made between ventilatory excretions because changes in pleural pressure affect the luminal pressure within the anterior vena cava. A horizontal line is drawn between the estimated level of the end of the catheter (the manubrium and thoracic inlet) and the manometer to establish the "zero" reference level. This can be determined by eyeball alignment, by a string and level, or by a fluid-filled extension set (Fig. 17.7). The CVP can be roughly determined by lowering the bottle of infusion fluids to a level at which it stops dripping. The horizontal difference between the zero level and the meniscus of fluid in the deep chamber represents the CVP.

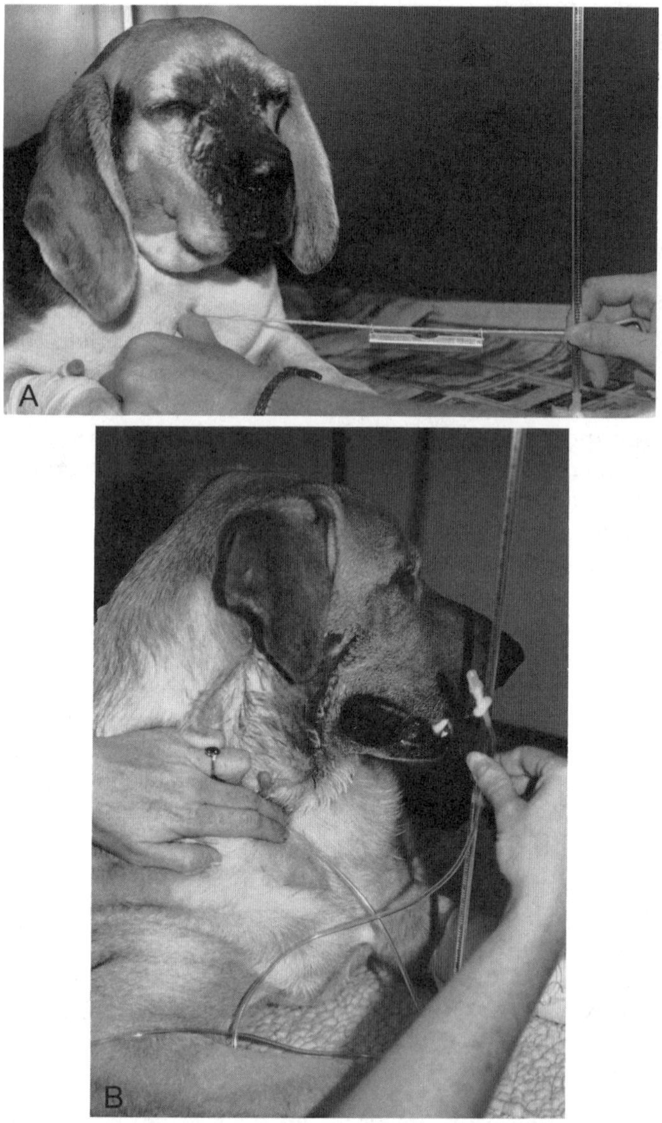

Figure 17.7. A level attached to a string (*A*) or an extension set filled with water (*B*) could be used to locate the zero level on the CVP manometer.

The normal CVP in small animals is 0 to 10 cm H_2O (awake or anesthetized); it is 5 to 15 cm H_2O in awake horses and 25 to 35 in anesthetized laterally recumbent horses (54). The CVP measurement should be correlated with previous measurements and the immediate past history of the patient. It may be zero cm H_2O in an animal that is otherwise normal and 5 cm H_2O in an animal in hypovolemic shock. Fluid therapy should be directed at improving all parameters of cardiovascular function, including an increase in the CVP from the baseline measurement. CVP is a measure of the ability of the heart to pump the quantity of fluids being returned to it and is an estimate of the relationship between the blood volume and the blood volume capacity. It should be measured whenever heart failure is suspected or when fluids are to be rapidly administered in order to better define the end-point for fluid administration. The CVP will increase if the pump begins to fail, with venoconstriction, and with hypervolemia. The CVP will decrease with vasodilation, with hypovolemia, and with obstructions to venous return peripheral to the site of measurement (upper abdominal or thoracic surgery).

PULMONARY ARTERY PRESSURE AND WEDGE PRESSURE

CVP is a measure of the filling pressure to the right side of the heart and may not accurately reflect events on the left side of the heart. Obtaining information about the performance of the left heart necessitates the passing of a silastic, a polyethylene, or a commercial ballooned-tipped flow-directed catheter into the pulmonary artery via the jugular vein, as previously described. The balloon-tipped catheter is ideal for this purpose because it can be positioned such that when the balloon is deflated pulmonary artery pressure is measured and when it is inflated wedge pressure is measured.

Once the catheter is in the pulmonary artery, it is further advanced until it wedges into a branch of the pulmonary artery. If the catheter has a balloon, it should be deflated at this time. Any difference between wedge and pulmonary diastolic pressure should be noted. If the catheter does not have a balloon, it should be withdrawn slightly (2 to 4 cm in the 20-kg dog) so as to allow free blood flow around the catheter and a clear pulmonary artery pressure tracing.

Indwelling catheters tend to migrate inward. If the pressure tracing becomes damped and the catheter is not obstructed, the catheter should be withdrawn slightly until a good pressure tracing is re-established.

If the catheter has a balloon, it can be intermittently inflated with air to obtain a wedge pressure measurement. Because vessel size and balloon position vary, a standard volume of air should not be instilled. Overexpansion of the vessel wall should be avoided because pulmonary artery rupture has been reported and is likely to be lethal (26). The balloon should be inflated to a volume that is just sufficient to obtain the wedge pressure measurement and then deflated immediately.

Ventricular arrhythmias, ventricular tachycardia, and fibrillation may occur during the introduction of the catheter. The catheter should be inserted gently and carefully, and the ECG should be monitored. Antiarrhythmic therapy may be necessary, and a defibrillator should be immediately available.

Catheter coiling in the ventricle may occur if excessive lengths of catheter are introduced. If the catheter does not enter the pulmonary artery after insertion of an adequate length, it should be withdrawn, rotated, and re-inserted. Pulmonary artery rupture and fatal hemorrhage may occur if the cuff is overinflated or remains inflated or if the catheter is left in the wedged position.

The pulmonary artery catheter may be used to measure pulmonary artery pressure, which is normally 20 to 40 mm Hg systolic, 5 to 10 mm Hg diastolic, and 10 to 20 mm Hg mean, and pulmonary capillary wedge pressure, which is 3 to 8 mm Hg.

When it is not possible to obtain an actual wedge pressure measurement and in the absence of marked tachycardia or high vascular resistance, pulmonary arterial diastolic pressure may approximate wedge pressure. It is normally slightly higher than wedge pressure (less than 5 mm Hg). Any differences between the two should be ascertained when the catheter is first inserted to determine whether or not the diastolic measurements can be reliably used to approximate wedge pressure.

Spontaneous ventilation will lower the pulmonary artery and wedge pressure values, whereas positive pressure ventilation and positive end-expiratory pressure will increase them. The pressure should be measured between breaths during the expiratory pause. If end-expiratory pressure is used, the wedge pressure should be measured occasionally without the end-expiratory pressure to determine its effect and then all subsequent measurements should be adjusted accordingly.

Falsely elevated wedge pressure measurements may occur with overinflation of the balloon; mitral insufficiency, which produces large V-waves; positive pressure ventilation; or end-expiratory pressure in excess of pulmonary venous pressure. Because effective vascular filling pressure is dependent more upon transmural than intraluminal pressure, it may be helpful to measure pleural (esophageal) pressure during the application of positive airway pressure and subtract it from the measured vascular pressure (transmural pressure). The wedge pressure is often assumed to be indicative of left ventricular diastolic filling pressure and volume. Left ventricular end-diastolic volume may be excessive even though the pressure is normal if the pericardial sac is open or if atrial contraction contributes greatly to ventricular filling during left heart failure, which produces a large A-wave. Pulmonary artery diastolic pressure may be elevated with pulmonary arterial vasoconstriction or pulmonary thromboembolism even though the wedge pressure and left atrial pressure are normal.

The pulmonary artery catheter may also be used to collect mixed venous blood samples for oxygen measurements; some catheter tips are equipped with an oximeter for the continuous measurement of hemoglobin saturation. Mixed venous oxygen is a summation measurement of all of the factors responsible for oxygen delivery to the tissues. The normal $P\bar{v}O_2$ in the dog is 50 ± 5 (55). High values indicate reduced tissue utilization (septic shock, hypothermia, cyanide intoxication, and arteriovenous shunting); below 30 values indicate reduced oxygen delivery to the tissues (hypoxemia, anemia, methemoglobinemia, and low cardiac output) or high tissue utilization (hyperthermia and sepsis).

Monitoring the Pulmonary System

Each individual pulmonary parameter has a specific clinical importance, but its contribution to the overall adequacy of pulmonary function can only be assessed by correlating the current measurement with previous trends, with other pulmonary measurements, and in consideration of the recent past history of the patient.

BREATHING RATE

Breathing rate as an isolated measurement provides little information about the adequacy of ventilation. A slow rate may be associated with adequate ventilation as long as each breath is large enough. A change in rate may signify a change in the underlying status of the patient that may, in turn, require investigation and correction.

Abnormally slow breathing rates (bradypnea) are associated with organic (cerebral edema, neoplasia, or hematoma) or metabolic (anesthetic depression, severe hypoxia, hypo- or severe hypercapnia, or visceral organ failure) dysfunction of the medullary respiratory center.

Medullary dysfunction may be manifested in breathing patterns other than bradypnea.

1. Apnea shows medullary dysfunction.
2. In diaphragmatic breathing, the diaphragmatic component precedes the thoracic component and predominates the inspiratory effort (normally the diaphragm (abdomen) and thorax expand simultaneously).
3. Cheyne-Stokes breathing is characterized by cyclic hyperventilation and hypoventilation and is attributed to greater than normal delays in the medullary response to changing carbon dioxide levels.
4. Biot's breathing is characterized by cyclic hypoventilation and apnea and is a sign of a serious medullary disturbance.
5. Apneustic breathing may be associated with brainstem disease and is commonly seen after ketamine administration.
6. Agonal gasps are characterized by periodic retraction of the hyoid apparatus and a gaping of the mouth. There may or may not be movement of a small amount of air associated with a spasmotic diaphragmatic contraction. It is always a very serious sign.

Carbon dioxide is the primary chemical stimulant of the respiratory center, and hypocapnia in an anesthetized patient results in apnea. Many patients hyperventilate just prior to induction due to excitement and apprehension. Most anesthetics are potent respiratory depressants, especially when given as large loading doses, as is required for induction of general anesthesia. Patients that are intubated and artificially ventilated to assure proper cuff inflation will be even more hypocapnic. Apnea or bradypnea may therefore occur after anesthetic induction even though the subject is lightly anesthetized. Serious hypoxemia may develop before spontaneous ventilation resumes unless the patient is attached to an enriched oxygen source. Spontaneous breathing usually resumes when the carbon dioxide levels have increased to a level sufficient to stimulate the depressed medulla. If insufficient quantities of inhalation anesthetic are taken up during this apneic period, premature awakening will occur once the induction agent has been redistributed. The patient should be artificially ventilated once every 30 seconds to assure adequate delivery of oxygen and anesthetic to the patient. If spontaneous ventilation has not commenced within 10 to 15 minutes, full support IPPV (10 to 12 breaths/minute) should be started and some other cause of the apnea should be sought. For some reason, for some patients, apnea is a normal response to the particular induction and maintenance drugs utilized, and resumption of spontaneous ventilation will have to await the end of the operation when the patient can be awakened, at which time spontaneous breathing commonly resumes.

Apnea may develop during the surgical procedure:

1. If spinal cord edema occurs secondary to cerebrospinal fluid (CSF) tap or surgical trauma;
2. When the radiopaque material is injected into the subarachnoid space;
3. If the CSF tap causes herniation;
4. If neuromuscular blocking agents are used;
5. Rarely, if aminoglycoside antibiotics are used; or
6. If the animal becomes too deeply anesthetized.

Tachypnea refers to a rapid rate of breathing without regard to volume and may be associated with hyperventilation, normoventilation, or hypoventilation depending on the nature of the disturbance. Exaggerated efforts to breath are correlated to the subjective feeling of dyspnea and are indicative of respiratory stimulation and difficulty.

Hypercapnia, hypoxemia, hypotension, and hyperthermia are important causes of tachypnea and should be identified early since the consequence of their unchecked progression is severe. Too light a level of anesthesia may be associated with tachypnea and hyperventilation. Too deep a level of anesthesia may be associated with tachypnea, exaggerated but shallow breathing efforts, and hypoventilation; positive pressure ventilation should be instituted until the anesthesia is light enough to maintain a coordinated and adequate minute ventilation.

Upper airway obstruction may cause tachypnea, exaggerated breathing efforts and hypoventilation. If the obstruction occurs before intubation, it might be due to a nasal, pharyngeal, or laryngeal filling defect or collapse. Intubation will usually provide for an open airway. If the obstruction occurs after intubation, the tube might be in the esophagus or one main stem bronchus, cuff might be overinflated or might have pushed the level of the tube against the tracheal wall, the tube might have kinked, or its lumen might be plugged. Check the proper position of the tube, deflate the cuff, withdraw it, and rotate it slightly. If these maneuvers do not alleviate the obstruction, replace the tube.

The presence or worsening of pleural filling lesions such as pneumothorax, hydrothorax, chylothorax, hemothorax, or diaphragmatic hernia may cause respiratory compromise heralded by increased breathing rates, decreased tidal volumes, decreased compliance, and abnormal ausculatory or percussion findings. The presence of pneumothorax preoperatively should red flag a potential problem because it can be rapidly progressive with PPV or exaggerated ventilatory efforts.

Excessive obesity may restrict ventilation secondary to either mediastinal fat accumulations and/or the extra weight upon the thoracic wall and the diaphragm. PPV should be instituted for the duration of the anesthesia.

Space-consuming abdominal abnormalities such as gastric or intestinal tympany, ascites, neoplastic masses, a gravid uterus, or pyometra may restrict diaphragmatic excursions and cause tachypnea and hypoventilation. Small airway collapse and atelectasis may cause tachypnea and is often relieved by administering a few deep breaths. All anesthetized patients should be artificially ventilated at 5-minute intervals to minimize the inevitable small airway and alveolar collapse that occurs during general anesthesia. More frequent sighs may be indicated if the breathing pattern is shallow of if mild to moderate parenchymal lung disease exists.

The pulmonary and thoracic effects of general anesthesia will exaggerate the respiratory compromise of parenchymal diseases such as edema, pneumonia, contusion, neoplasia, or aspiration. IPPV should be instituted to re-expand collapsed small airways and alveoli.

Narcotic drugs occasionally cause a panting breathing pattern. Anesthetic agents that stimulate the central nervous system, such as ketamine, diazepam, or narcotics, may cause tachypnea. Anesthetic agents that are pungent or stimulate airway irritant receptors may cause breath holding or tachypnea.

The normal respiratory response to general anesthesia in some patients is rapid and shallow in nature. If none of the aforementioned complications can be documented and the patient appears to be oxygenating satisfactorily, no treatment need be instituted except that the patient should be sighed once every minute to compensate for any deficiencies that may exist in minute ventilation and to prevent excessive small airway and alveolar collapse.

THE NATURE OF THE VENTILATORY EFFORT

The ventilatory effort should be smooth, easy, regular, and comprised of both thoracic and diaphragmatic excursions. Exaggerated breathing efforts, including tachypnea and hyperventilation, are indicative of respiratory stimulation that may be due to respiratory disease. Stertorous (upper airway obstruction) or wheezing (lower airway narrowing) breathing sounds, crepitation or bubbling fluid sounds, intercostal retraction during inspiration (upper airway obstruction), predominance of the diaphragmatic component during inspiration (deep anesthesia), and the abnormal rhythms previously discussed for medullary disease are all indicative of specific respiratory disorders.

AUSCULTATION

Auscultation should incorporate all areas of the lung field and the upper airway. Abnormal sounds should be localized as much as possible. An increased volume or harshness of normal vesicular sounds may indicate hyperventilation or airway narrowing. Additional harshness to lung sounds, stridor, snoring, or whistling sounds are indicative of more severe airway narrowing. Terminal expiratory/early inspiratory crepitation is indicative of an accumulation of a small amount of fluid in the small airways. Bubbling fluid sounds are indicative of a large amount of fluid. Localized areas of diminished lung sounds may be due to lobar consolidations; a more generalized dullness may be caused by a pleural filling defect.

MEMBRANE COLOR

Cyanosis may be indicative of severe hypoxemia. Cyanosis requires an absolute amount of unoxygenated hemoglobin (5 g/dl). If a patient is moderately anemic, death from hypoxia could occur without manifesting cyanosis. When cyanosis occurs during general anesthesia, first check the function of the mechanical apparatus to which the animal is attached. Is the oxygen source depleted? Is the flowmeter still registering at least 10 $ml/kg^{-1}/min^{-1}$ for circle systems or 200 $ml/kg^{-1}/min^{-1}$ for nonrebreathing systems? Are the nonrebreathing valves in the circle system operating properly? Is the endotracheal tube plugged or misplaced? The underlying problem should be corrected when it is found. If the cause is not immediately apparent, the anesthetic machine and endotracheal tube should be exchanged.

If the proper performance of the anesthetic machine, ventilator, and endotracheal tube can be verified, check the animal. Are there abnormal airway sounds? Is there evidence of a pleural space air or fluid accumulation? Is ventral small airway and alveolar collapse likely (prolonged positional stasis particularly with preexisting airway fluid accumulation)? A deep sigh breath should alleviate much of the alveolar collapse in small animals, although less so in the horse.

Cyanosis may also be due to peripheral stagnation of blood flow during shock, hypothermia, or cardiac arrest even though pulmonary function is normal. Drug-induced methemoglobinemia (acetominophen in cats (56) and benzocaine in dogs and cats (57)) causes severe cyanotic discoloration and reduced blood oxygen content even though pulmonary function and the measured PaO_2 are normal. The treatment for methemoglobinemia is acetylcysteine (140 mg/kg p.o. or i.v. every 8 hours) (58), glutathione to conjugate the toxic hydroxamic acid metabolite, and cimetadine to slow the hepatic P450 metabolism of the acetaminophen. Methemoglobin may be reduced by the administration of methylene blue (1 to 2 mg/kg) (57), but this agent causes Heinz body hemolytic anemia in cats (59).

VENTILOMETRY

Ventilation volume can be estimated by visual observation of chest or rebreathing bag excursions or by ventilometry. A shallow tidal volume that is associated with a faster ventilatory rate is acceptable as long as an adequate alveolar minute volume is the product. Tidal volume and minute ventilation can be measured with in-circuit portable ventilometers (Anesthesia Associates, Inc., San Marcos, California; Fraser-Harlake, Lancaster, New York; Boehringer Laboratories, Wynnewood, Pennsylvania; or North American Drager, Telford, Pennsylvania) (Fig. 17.8) or with a measurement grid on the side of the bellows canister. IPPV causes compression of gases within the ventilator circuit and causes expansion of the expansible circuitry. Some or all of this volume will be measured by the ventilometer (depending upon where it is located in the circuitry). The measured volume will therefore be variably larger than that actually received by the patient. If the ventilometer is located on the inhalation side of the circuitry (such as the canister grid) and if there are leaks between the ventilometer and the patient, this leaked volume will be recorded as leaving the ventilator and may incorrectly be assumed to be entering the patient. It is for this reason that ventilometers should be placed on the expiratory side of the patient whenever possible. The volume of compression, expansion, or leak can be determined by disconnecting the patient circuit at the endotracheal tube and plugging the patient port with the thumb at the same ventilator settings being used on the patient. This will account for all except leaks occurring around the endotracheal tube. The measured volume during this procedure should be recorded and subtracted from the subsequently measured volumes.

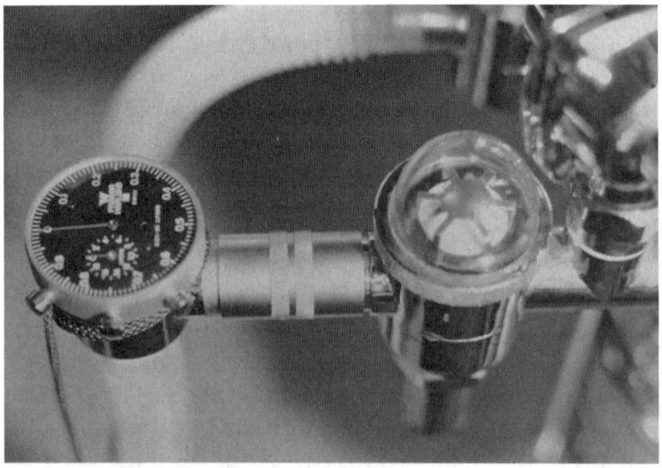

Figure 17.8. A portable ventilometer attached to the exhalation side of the anesthetic circuit.

The normal tidal volume ranges between 10 and 20 ml/kg. A smaller than normal tidal volume may be acceptable if the breathing rate is fast enough to accomplish a normal minute ventilation. The normal minute ventilation ranges between 150 and 250 $ml/kg^{-1}/min^{-1}$. A minute ventilation below 100 $ml/kg^{-1}/min^{-1}$ may not be associated with adequate ventilation, and positive pressure ventilation may need to be instituted. Values above 300 $ml/kg^{-1}/min^{-1}$ may be associated with excessive hyperventilation. Alveolar minute ventilation is of greater importance than is total minute ventilation. Alveolar minute ventilation may be as low as 35% of the total in animals with rapid and shallow breathing or added upper airway dead space and may be as high as 70% of the total if an animal is breathing slowly and deeply, particularly if it is also endotracheally intubated (60).

Ventilometry measures the amount of air moving in and out of the lungs; however, due to lung pathology, normal ventilation measurements do not preclude hypoxemia. Arterial blood gas measurements provide more precise evaluation of pulmonary function. These measurements should be correlated with the physical signs of pulmonary function, because a respiratory-compromised patient can maintain normal blood gases for a short time by exerting an extreme effort.

BLOOD GAS ANALYSIS

The analysis of carbon dioxide and oxygen in an arterial blood sample defines the adequacy of pulmonary function. Venous samples interpose a tissue bed; although not without value, they relay little information about pulmonary function. The dead space of a 3-ml glass or plastic syringe should be filled with heparin. An artery is located and percutaneously punctured using a 22- to 25-gauge needle. A consistent volume of blood (usually 3 ml) is slowly drawn into the syringe. Negative pressure should be minimized so as to avoid reductions in oxygen and red cell lysis and to reduce the introduction of air bubbles into the syringe. The needle is removed from the artery; the puncture site is digitally compressed for a minute or two to prevent any hematoma formation. All bubbles are removed from the sample. The needle is corked or the needle guard is replaced and the sample is immediately placed in ice water. The sample can be maintained and transported in ice water for several hours before in vitro metabolism significantly changes the initial pH and gas values (61).

PARTIAL PRESSURE OF CARBON DIOXIDE (PCO_2)

The arterial PCO_2 ($PaCO_2$) is a measure of the ventilatory status of the patient and is normally regulated within fairly narrow limits by the medullary respiratory centers. The normal $PaCO_2$ is 40 mm Hg (range, 35 to 45 mm Hg); a $PaCO_2 < 35$ mm Hg indicates hyperventilation and an excessive elimination of carbon dioxide; a $PaCO_2 > 45$ mm Hg indicates hypoventilation. A $PaCO_2$ in excess of 60 mm Hg is associated with a severe respiratory acidosis, may be associated with severe hypoxemia if the animal is breathing room air, and is usually considered to represent sufficient hypoventilation to institute ventilation therapy. $PaCO_2$ values below 20 mm Hg are associated with severe respiratory alkalosis and decreased cerebral blood flow, which may impair adequate cerebral oxygenation and should be avoided.

$PaCO_2$ is normally measured with a blood gas analyzer (Instrumentation Laboratory; Corning Medical, Medfield, Massachusetts; Radiometer America, West Lake, Ohio; AVL Scientific Corp., Roswell, Georgia). It may, however, be estimated by measuring the carbon dioxide concentration (% CO_2) in a sample of gas taken at the end of an exhalation (Beckman Instruments Co., Fullerton, California; Puritan-Bennett Corp., Kansas City, Missouri; Datascope Corp.; or Hewlett-Packard) (62). Although there is some variability in the correlation between end-tidal % CO_2 and $PaCO_2$ in patients with rapid breathing rates or with pulmonary disease (63), the correlation is sufficient for most clinical purposes. Venous PCO_2 ($PvCO_2$) measurements represent some combination between $PaCO_2$ and tissue metabolism and are usually 2 to 5 mm Hg greater than $PaCO_2$. $PvCO_2$ may bear no correlation to $PaCO_2$ during phases of dynamic change or anemia; however, a $PvCO_2$ in excess of 60 mm Hg in a patient with a disease that is fairly stable is indicative of hypoventilation.

Hypercapnea may be caused by hypoventilation due to medullary, cervical, or neuromuscular disease; upper or lower airway obstruction; pleural filling disorders; pulmonary parenchymal disease; and abdominal or thoracic restrictive disorders. Excessive dead space rebreathing (large face mask; nonfunctioning directional valves in the anesthetic circuit; insufficient fresh gas flows with nonrebreathing circuits; nonrebreathing circuits that are attached backwards) or exhausted soda lime within the anesthetic circuit may also cause hypercapnia.

Elevated $PaCO_2$ may be measured if the blood sample is taken shortly after the administration of sodium bicarbonate, particularly if the patient has marginal ventilation. Failure to correct the measured PCO_2 for differences in temperature between the water bath and a colder animal will result in an elevated PCO_2.

THE PARTIAL PRESSURE OF OXYGEN (PO_2)

The arterial PO_2 (PaO_2) is a measure of the oxygenating efficiency of the lungs. The PO_2 is only one of three expressions of arterial blood oxygen, the other two being percent hemoglobin saturation and oxygen content. The three are interrelated but are not synonymous (65). The PO_2 is the most commonly measured, is an ideal way to evaluate the lung's ability to oxygenate the blood, and will be used here to define hypoxemia. It must be recognized that an animal may have a normal PaO_2 and yet have a reduced oxygen content, as with anemia and methemoglobinemia. Oxygen-hemoglobin saturation analyzers are commercially and economically available (Orange Medical Products, Costa Mesa, California; Oximetrix, Inc., Mountain View, California; Radiometer America, West Lake, Ohio; Instrumentation Laboratory; or American Optical Corp., Buffalo, New York) and are easy to operate. They could be used to evaluate blood oxygenation if the cost of a blood gas analyzer is prohibitive.

The normal PaO_2 is considered to range between 90 and 100 mm Hg. Hypoxemia becomes an important respiratory stimulant at PaO_2 values below 60 mm Hg. A PaO_2 of 50 to 60 mm Hg is a commonly selected minimum value to institute respiratory therapy. It is assumed that values below 60 mm Hg represent a significant stress to the patient, and support procedures such as enriching the inspired oxygen concentration and/or ventilation therapy should be instituted to maintain the PaO_2 above 60 mm Hg.

The above guidelines assume that the $PaCO_2$ is in the range of normal; alterations in $PaCO_2$ may, however, affect the PaO_2 measurement, and therefore the PaO_2 should always be interpreted within the context of the $PaCO_2$. A change in the $PaCO_2$ will cause a similar (quantitatively slight greater ~1.1) change in PaO_2 in the opposite direction. For example, a PaO_2 of 60 mm Hg could be solely due to hypoventilation if the $PaCO_2$ is about 70 mm Hg and the animal is breathing room air, not dead-space rebreathing (an increase in the $PaCO_2$ of 30 mm Hg (70 to 40) causes a decrease in the PaO_2 of about 33 mm Hg (30×1.1)). If the measured $PaCO_2$ is between 40 and 70 mm Hg, then the hypoxemia is partly due to hypoventilation and partly to a decrease oxygenating efficiency of the lungs (venous admixture). If the $PaCO_2$ is below 40 mm Hg, then the animal is hyperventilating, and the hypoxemia is due solely to venous admixture.

Patients breathing an enriched oxygen mixture should have an elevated PaO_2 regardless of the $PaCO_2$; the PCO_2 effect can be disregarded with a high PO_2. Although the alveolar air equation provides a more accurate prediction regarding the expected PaO_2 at any given inspired oxygen concentration, a rough estimate can be obtained by multiplying the inspired oxygen concentration by 5 (66). A PaO_2 measurement below this value indicates the presence of venous admixture.

Hypoventilation is always associated with hypoxemia when the patient is breathing room air but not when breathing an enriched oxygen mixture. When hypoxemia is due to hypoventilation, improvement of the ventilatory status, not oxygen therapy, is the treatment of choice.

Hypoxemia may be due to pulmonary parenchymal complications such as pulmonary edema, pneumonia, contusion, or atelectasis. Some combination of oxygen and ventilation therapy is often required to restore acceptable blood oxygen levels. Hypoxemia may be associated with excessive dead space rebreathing and with insufficient fresh oxygen flow or excessive nitrous oxide flow. The decrease in temperature of a blood sample taken from a hyperthermic patient and measured in a normothermic blood gas analyzer will decrease the partial pressure of the measured gases (64).

Carbon dioxide elimination and oxygen uptake are functions of the same lung; however, both functions are not necessarily accomplished with the same degree of efficiency. $PaCO_2$ defines the ventilatory status of the patient and should be used to guide ventilation therapy. PaO_2 defines the oxygenating capabilities of the lung and should be used to guide the percent inhaled oxygen concentration and the level of the end-expired airway pressure when this technique is used.

Metabolic Acidosis

Metabolic acidosis occurring in the perioperative period is usually attributed to lactic acidosis secondary to inadequate tissue perfusion, usually due to vasoconstriction; however, it may also be due to hypotension, hyperthermia, or the infusion of acidotic fluids. The base or bicarbonate deficit could be calculated from measurements made with a blood gas analyzer (Instrumentation Laboratory; Corning Medical; Radiometer America; or AVL Scientific Corp.), ion-specific electrode (Gilford Instrument Laboratories, Inc., Oberlin, Ohio; or Nova Biomedical, Waltham, Massachusetts), Total CO_2 Analyzer (Harleco, Gibbstown, New Jersey), or a colorimetric titrator (Oxford Labs, Foster City, California).

The first order of therapy in known or suspected metabolic acidosis is to correct the underlying disturbance and to maximize tissue perfusion with appropriate fluid therapy. Alkalynizing therapy should be conservative and should be reserved for those patients with moderate to severe metabolic acidosis. If the base or bicarbonate deficit calculation is available, the meq of bicarbonate to administer is calculated by the formula: base or bicarbonate deficit $\times$ 0.3 $\times$ body weight (kg). If the base or bicarbonate deficit calculations are not available, the extent of the acidosis can only be estimated by a subjective interpretation of the severity of the disease process. If it is judged to be mild to severe, 1 to 5 meq/kg body weight, respectively, of sodium bicarbonate could be administered. The bicarbonate dose, regardless of how it is calculated, should be administered no faster than over 20 to 30 minutes or more slowly for less aggressive acidosis. Too rapid an infusion of bicarbonate causes excessive alkalemia, hypokalemia and decreased ionized calcium, hypotension, nausea, vomition, collapse, and possibly cardiac arrest.

Temperature Monitoring

Core body temperature is an important parameter to monitor in anesthetized patients due to the almost inevitable decrease that occurs. Hyperthermia may, however, also develop. Alterations in body temperature alter the patient's response to anesthetics and, if severe, may have primary deleterious effects. Core temperature can be measured with deep rectal or esophageal thermometers. Thermometers may be of the restrictive, nonrestrictive, or electronic (thermocouple or thermistor) types. Short restrictive thermometers may be taped with a long tag so that they may be inserted into the esophagus. Deep rectal or thoracic esophageal positions provide essentially the same measurement in the stable state. Rectal temperatures may lag behind esophageal temperature in an unstable state. Esophageal temperatures are often decreased during thoracotomy and may therefore provide misleading measurements. Estimates of core temperature may also be derived from measurements taken in the cervical esophagus, pharynx, under the tongue, or in the axilla or femoral fossa.

HYPOTHERMIA

Hypothermia during general anesthesia is the consequence of anesthetic-induced decreases in basal metabolic rate and muscular activity coupled with the increased rate of heat loss associated with depilation, the application and evaporation of antiseptic solutions, exposure to cold table surfaces, and open body cavities. The largest problem of hypothermia is nonrecognition of it. The continued administration of normothermic quantities of anesthetics to hypothermic patients will result in an anesthetic overdose. When appropriate support measures are instituted, hypothermia is safe to quite low temperature levels (67).

Temperatures above 35°C (95°F) have no deleterious effects except for postanesthetic shivering. Shivering increases oxygen consumption and decreases ventilatory capacity, which predisposes to hypoxemia in patients debilitated by anesthetic drugs or pulmonary disease.

Temperatures in the low thirties C (low nineties F) reduce anesthetic requirements due to the hypometabolic effects of the hypothermia. Recovery will probably be prolonged. Thermoregulation may be impaired, and artificial rewarming may be necessary.

Temperatures in the high twenties C (middle eighties F) cause such profound CNS depression that little or no anesthetic is required for the maintenance of anesthesia. Recovery will be prolonged, and artificial rewarming will be necessary. Cold-induced ventilatory depression may be in excess of the hypometabolism, and PPV should perhaps be instituted. Metabolic acidosis due to inadequate tissue perfusion will occur upon rewarming.

Temperatures in the middle twenties C (or high seventies F) cause cold-induced ECG changes of prolonged P-R interval and widened QRS complexes. Increased automaticity of heart predisposes the occurrence of arrhythmias such as premature ventricular contractions or fibrillation. Bradycardia in excess of the cold-induced hypometabolism results in an insufficient cardiac output. Microcirculatory sludging due to excessive blood viscosity may also occur.

Heat loss may be reduced by protecting the patient from his cool environment with blankets or towels; by minimizing the duration of the surgical procedure; and by actively warming the patient or his immediate environment. A circulating warm water blanket may be placed under and/or over the patient. The efficiency of the blanket in maintaining or restoring core temperature is determined by the body surface contact area. Thermal burns may be associated with these blankets if they are operating improperly (68).

An electric blanket may overheat the body surface contact area, causing burns and extensive skin sloughs. This is most likely to occur in patients that are hypothermic or in shock and have a vasoconstricted skin radiator system. If used, the blanket should either be well insulated with towels or placed around the patient so as to avoid direct contact with the skin. The temperature between the skin and the blanket could be measured to assure that it is less than 42°C (108°F).

Hot water bottles may be placed around the patient and under the drapes but should not contact the patient if the water temperature exceeds 42°C (108°F). The bottles should be changed when their measured temperature is below that of core temperature because at this point they will reabsorb heat from the patient.

Infrared heat lamps may be used during or after the operative period. The optimum distance between the lamp and the patient is about 75 cm; a distance of 50 cm was associated with excessive skin heating, whereas a distance 100 cm was associated with ineffective warming (69). Excessive drying of the tissues at the operative site must be prevented. Radiant-heat infant warmers are available commercially (American Hospital Supply, McGaw Park, Illinois; or Gaymar Industries Inc., Orchard Park, New York).

Warming and humidification of the inspired air may help prevent hypothermia (70) and has been used to rewarm hypothermic patients (71, 72). Open body cavities may be flushed with warm sterile saline (<42°C). Intravenous fluids may be warmed but cannot be administered in sufficient quantity to have much influence on core temperature.

In the recovery ward, the animal's environment can be warmed by infrared heat lamps, surgical lamps, electric floor heaters, forced-air hair dryers, heating blankets, or hot water blankets. Care should be taken to avoid excessive environmental temperatures and overheating of the patient. A warm water bath may be used, but care should be taken to protect the surgical incision from wound contamination.

HYPERTHERMIA

Hyperthermia occasionally occurs during general anesthesia (73–76). High metabolic activity associated with light levels of anesthesia, large or obese patients, insulation by surgical draping, and breathing a fully humidified gas mixture contribute to an increased core temperature. When recognized, it is usually easily treated by removing the offending causes and by increasing conductive heat loss. Malignant hyperthermia syndrome (MHS) is a rapid and progressive hyperthermia (77–80) that is often associated with the administration of halothane and/or succinylcholine, but virtually any anesthetic may trigger the syndrome (81). In people and swine, the disorder is related to a genetic functional defect resulting in the accumulation of calcium within the myoplasma (77, 82). Although the basic cause is unknown, the muscular defect is associated with abnormal calcium fluxes, increased muscle enzyme activity, and heat and carbon dioxide production. Muscular rigidity may or may not occur, depending upon the cytoplasmic calcium concentration. The syndrome is very rapid in onset and is associated with a high mortality rate. Muscle biopsies from suspected individuals can be tested in vitro (83; personal communication, S. Hildebrand).

The harmful effects of hyperthermia are primarily related to high metabolic activity and cellular oxygen consumption. When the body temperature rises above 42°C (108°F), the oxygen utilization exceeds the oxygen supply and cellular hypoxia occurs (84). The organs that most commonly manifest damage are the brain, kidneys, liver, and blood (85–87). Temperatures below 42°C may require monitoring but may not require specific treatment.

Severely hyperthermic patients should breathe an enriched oxygen mixture. Rapid administration of crystalloid fluids helps restore an effective circulating blood volume and cool the patient. Corticosteroid and sodium bicarbonate therapy should be considered if the hyperthermia is severe or prolonged. Brain, liver, kidney, gastrointestinal, and endocrine function should be monitored by appropriate clinical and laboratory tests for several days after severe hyperthermic episodes.

Evaporative heat loss can be enhanced by soaking the skin with water or alcohol, and conductive heat loss can be enhanced by placing ice water packs around the patient or, after surgery, by immersing the patient in cold water or ice water bath. The choice of therapy primarily depends upon the extent of the hyperthermia and the rate at which the temperature is to be decreased. Infusion of cold fluids intravascularly or into an open body cavity and ice water enemas or gastric lavage may also be used. Surface cooling techniques may have a substantial peripheral effect before much core cooling is noted. The core temperature will continue to decrease as the core and peripheral temperatures equilibrate. Because the extent of the afterdrop is unpredictable, aggressive cooling techniques such as ice water baths should cease as soon as the core temperature decreases below 40°C (104°F). Additional cooling can be applied if necessary after the core and peripheral temperatures have equilibrated.

Antipyretics such as dipyrone (Haver, Shawnee, Kansas) may directly lower hypothalmic thermostatic settings or inhibit the release of pyrogens and thereby lower body temperature. Dipyrone may cause excessive hypothermia. If malignant hyperthermia is suspected, the offending agent should be removed and aggressive attempts to lower the body temperature should be made. Dantrolene sodium (Norwich-Eaton Pharmaceuticals, Norwich, New York) reduces mortality rates in pigs, humans, and dogs (77, 88).

MONITORING URINARY OUTPUT

Urinary output is an indirect measure of major visceral organ perfusion and is particularly indicated in patients with compensated renal disease. The hormonal responses to anesthetics and the state of general anesthesia decrease renal blood flow and urinary output. If the decrease is severe enough, hypoxic cellular damage may occur and may precipitate renal failure. When renal function is known to be compromised before surgery, it is always recommended to monitor the urinary response to the stresses of general anesthesia and operation.

Urinary catheters must be placed in an aseptic manner so as to minimize the incidence of urinary tract infection. Hair around the prepuce or vulva should be clipped and the orifice and surrounding area washed with betadine scrub and solution (Purdue Frederick Co., Norwalk, Connecticut). The prepuce and vulva should then be flushed with a dilute betadine solution. In male animals, the penis is exposed and positioned by an assistant and an appropriately sized, soft catheter (Argyle, St. Louis, Missouri) is aseptically and atraumatically introduced. In female animals, the urethral orifice is more difficult to isolate. It can be palpated with a sterile gloved hand in large animals or finger in small animals. In very small animals, the urethra can sometimes be catheterized blindly by caudal retraction on the lower edge of the vulva and sliding the catheter along the floor of the vestibule. The urethra can be visualized in small animals with an otoscope or an antiseptic laryngoscope; the blade lifts the roof of the vestibule and the light enables direct visualization of the orifice (Fig. 17.9). Once the catheter is in place, it should be sutured securely to the prepuce or vulva and connected to a closed-system urine collection bag (Argyle).

The goal for intraoperative urine output is 1 to 2 $ml \cdot kg^{-1} \cdot hr^{-1}$. If urine output is inadequate, fluids (lactated Ringer's or an equivalent solution) should be administered (20 to 40 ml/kg) rapidly to induce a physiological diuresis. Once the patient is volume-loaded, if urine output is still inadequate and it has been verified that the drainage system is not obstructed, diuretic therapy should be instituted. It may consist of furosemide (Astra Pharmaceutical Products, Inc.; Elkins-Sinn Inc., Parke-Davis, Morris Plains, New Jersey; or Wyeth Laboratories) (5 mg/kg; diuresis should occur within 5 to 10 minutes; the dose may be repeated once); glucose

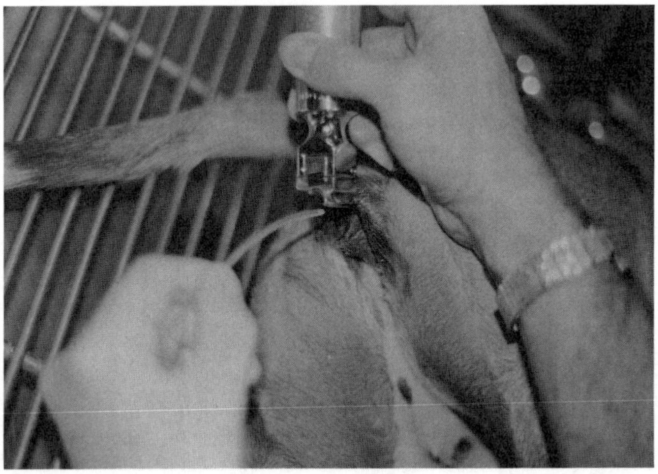

Figure 17.9. A disinfected laryngoscope blade may be used to lift the roof of the vestibule to visualize the urethral orifice.

or mannitol (Anpro Pharmaceutical, Arcadia, California; or American McGaw Labs) infusion (0.5 g/kg over 20 to 30 minutes); or dopamine (Arnar-Stone Laboratories) (1 to 5 $\mu g \cdot kg^{-1} \cdot min^{-1}$).

Monitoring the CNS

There are three aspects of central nervous system function that it would be advantageous to monitor under certain circumstances if the techniques were well established. First, the level of anesthesia (light, medium or deep) as determined by spontaneous or reflex movement, palpebral and ocular reflex activity, and mandibular muscle tone is imperative to monitor as a matter of routine to assure proper dosing of anesthetic agent so that the patient does not awaken before the end of the surgical procedure and yet awakens as soon as possible after the completion of the surgical procedure.

Secondly, electroencephalography (EEG) is a useful intraoperative monitor for the detection of excessive anesthetic depth and global ischemia (89). As cerebral hypoxia (hypoglycemia, hypothermia, hyponatremia, and anesthetic depth) worsens, the EEG loses the low voltage, high frequency activity of the activated state, leaving the high voltage, low frequency activity. The EEG then becomes intermittently isoelectric (burst suppression) and finally completely inactive. EEG monitoring is useful in any disease or surgical procedure in which cerebral blood flow may be compromised, such as intracardiac surgery, extracorporeal circulation, and deliberate hypotension.

Finally, intracranial pressure measurement would be highly informative in the management of patients with increased intracranial pressure. The technique for insertion of intraventricular catheters has not been well worked out in the clinical arena. Until such time as it is, it might be wise to make the worst case presumption: assume that intracranial pressure is elevated in all patients at risk and treat accordingly. Moderate hyperventilation, the maintenance of low normal arterial blood pressure and body temperature, restricted fluid infusion, and the prevention of venous outflow occlusion and hypoxia are the mainstays of management of such patients (90).

Monitoring the Equipment

It is, of course, imperative that the equipment used to support and monitor the patient be in good working order and be properly calibrated. Mechanical equipment has a propensity to fail when it is least expected and least desirable. The corollary, of course, is to always expect it to fail and be prepared to fix it when it does—and it never will.

Routine cleaning and preventative maintenance of anesthetic machines, vaporizers, and ventilators is paramount to their continuous proper operation (91). If a machine has just been cleaned or "fixed," be sure to evaluate it carefully before attaching it to a patient. The list of equipment-related failures is limitless (91), but a partial list of common mishaps is included below to remind us all that equipment monitoring at frequent intervals during the time that the patient is attached to it is integral to patient monitoring and to the successful outcome of the whole endeavor.

1. The oxygen supply may become depleted.
2. The flowmeter may be accidentally turned off.
3. The flowmeter tube may develop a leak (oxygen and anesthetic are not delivered to the circuit).
4. The anesthetic liquid in the vaporizer may become depleted.
5. The vaporizer may cease to function properly (usually leads to a decrease in the anesthetic output but may lead to an increase).
6. The wrong anesthetic was put into the vaporizer.
7. Connectors between the vaporizer and the circuit may loosen and leak.
8. The rubber or plastic parts of the circuit may be aged and leaky.
9. The soda lime may be exhausted (do not rely on color).
10. The nonrebreathing valves in the circle system were not replaced or are stuck in the open position.
11. The nonrebreathing circuit is attached backward.
12. The Y-piece becomes disconnected from the endotracheal tube.
13. The endotracheal tube becomes dislodged, obstructed, or kinked.

References

1. Haskins SC: Standards and techniques of equipment utilization. In Sattler FP, Knowles RP, Whittick WG (eds): *Veterinary Critical Care*. Philadelphia, Lea & Febiger, 1981.
2. Tilley LP: *Essentials of Canine and Feline Electrocardiography: Intepretation and Treatment*, ed 2. Philadelphia, Lea & Febiger, 1985.
3. Lewis RP, Ritters SE, Forester WF, et al: A critical review of the systolic time intervals. *Circulation* 56:146–158, 1977.
4. Lewis RP: The use of systolic time intervals for evaluation of left ventricular function. In Fowler NO (ed): *Noninvasive Diagnostic Methods in Cardiology*. Philadelphia, FA Davis Co, 1983, pp 335–353.
5. Pipers FS, Andrysco RM, Hamlin RL: A totally noninvasive method for obtaining systolic time intervals in the dog. *Am J Vet Res* 39:1822–1826, 1978.
6. Long JH, Diamond SS, Burningham RA, et al: Systolic time interval recordings as a measure of cardiac function in healthy rabbit: reference values. *Am J Vet Res* 43:1497–1499, 1982.
7. Spodick DH, Yoshinou LD, Bishop RL, et al: Systolic time intervals reconsidered. Reevaluation of the preejection period: absence of relation to heart rate. *Am J Cardiol* 53:1667–1670, 1984.
8. Reitan JA, Levine NA: A comparison of the PEP and QF interval as a monitoring variable. In List WF, Gravenstein JF, Spodick DH (eds): *Systolic Time Intervals*. New York, Springer-Verlag, 1980, pp 273–280.
9. Lambert CR, Wilmer WN, Pepine CJ: Indices of ventricular contractile state: comparative sensitivity and specificity. *Am Heart J* 106:136–144, 1983.
10. Goldfarb RD: Cardiac mechanical performance in circulatory shock: a critical review of methods and results. *Circ Shock* 9:633–653, 1982.
11. Stein PD, Blick EF: The physiological meaning and clinical significance of diverse indicators of ventricular performance: an integrated clinical concept. *Angiology* 24:325–331, 1973.
12. Mirskey I (ed): *Cardiac Mechanics: Physiological, Clinical and Mathematical Considerations*. New York, John Wiley and Sons, 1974.
13. Smith NT: Myocardial function and anaesthesia. In Prys-Roberts C: *The Circulation in Anaesthesia*. Oxford, Blackwell Scientific Publications, 1980.
14. Sodums MT, Badke FR, Starling MR, et al: Evaluation of left ventricular contractile performance utilizing end-systolic pressure-volume relationships in conscious dogs. *Circ Res* 54:731–739, 1984.
15. Ross J: Applications and limitations of end-systolic measures of ventricular performance. *Fed Proc* 43:2418–2422, 1984.
16. Kittleson MD, Eyster GE, Knowlen GG, et al: Myocardial function in small dogs with chronic mitral regurgitation and severe congestive heart failure. *J Am Vet Med Assoc* 184:455–459, 1984.
17. Bloomfield DA: *Dye Curves: The Theory and Practice of Indicator Dilution*. Baltimore, University Park Press, 1974.
18. Steffey EP, Howland D: Cardiovascular effects of halothane in the horse. *Am J Vet Res* 39:611–615, 1978.
19. Ganz W, Swan JHC: Measurement of blood flow by thermodilution. *Am J Cardiol* 29:241–246, 1972.
20. Isoyama T, Sato T, Tanaka J, et al: Measurements of cardiac output in small animals by aortic thermodilution. *J Surg Res* 33:170–176, 1982.
21. Allen DG, Nymeyer D: A preliminary investigation on the use of thermodilution and echocardiography as an assessment of cardiac function in the cat. *Can J Comp Med* 47:112–117, 1983.
22. Hayes BE, Will JA, Zarnstorff WC, et al: Limitations of thermodilution cardiac output measurements in the rat. *Am J Physiol* 246:H754–760, 1984.
23. Dyson DH, Allen DG, McDonell WN: Evaluation of three methods for cardiac output determination in cats. *Am J Vet Res* 46:2546–2552, 1985.
24. Warren DJ, Ledingham JGG: Cardiac output in the conscious rabbit: an analysis of the thermodilution technique. *J Appl Physiol* 36:246–251, 1974.
25. Muir WW, Skarda RT, Milne DW: Estimation of cardiac output in the horse by thermodilution techniques. *Am J Vet Res* 37:697–700, 1976.
26. Sprung CL: *The Pulmonary Artery Catheter. Methodology and Clinical Applications*. Baltimore, University Park Press, 1983.
27. Prys-Roberts C: Measurement of cardiac output and regional blood flow. In Prys-Roberts C (ed): *The Circulation in Anaesthesia*. Oxford, Blackwell Scientific Publications, 1980.
28. Bradley EC, Barr JW: Fore-n-aft triangle formula for rapid estimation of area. *Am Heart J* 78:643–648, 1969.
29. Jurado RA, Matucha D, Osborn JJ: Cardiac output estimation by pulse contour methods: validity of their use for monitoring the critically ill patient, *Surgery* 74:358–369, 1973.
30. Bourgeois MD, Gilbert BK, von Bernuth G, et al: Continuous determination of beat-to-beat stroke volume from aortic pressure pulses in the dog. *Circ Res* 39:15–24, 1976.
31. Cibulski AA, Lehan PH, Raju S, et al: Pulmonary arterial pressure method for estimating the ventricular stroke volume. *Am Heart J* 88:338–342, 1974.
32. English JB, Hodes MR, Sentker C, et al: Comparison of aortic pulse-wave contour analysis and thermodilution methods of measuring cardiac output during anesthesia in the dog. *Anesthesiology* 52:56–61, 1980.
33. McCutcheon EP. *Chronically Implanted Cardiovascular Instrumentation*. New York, Academic Press, 1973.
34. Lust RM, Lutherer LO, Cooper MW: Applicability of echocardiography in volume determinations in experimental animals. *J Appl Physiol* 56:1670–1674, 1984.
35. Arvidsson SP, Bergqvist P, Haglund V, et al: Cardiac output measurements with thermodilution and radioactive microspheres. A comparative study in cats. *Scand J Clin Lab Invest* 43:617–620, 1983.
36. Kolata RJ: The significance of changes in the web temperature in dogs in circulatory shock. *Proc Gaines Symposium* 28:21–26, 1978.
37. Joly HR, Weil MH: Temperature of the great toe as an indication of the severity of shock. *Circulation* 39:131–138, 1969.
38. Spelman FA: Regional blood flow in laboratory animals. In Herd JA, Gotto AM, et al (eds): *Cardiovascular Instrumentation*. NIH Publication No. 84-1654, 1984, pp 195–205.
39. Heymann MA, Payne BD, Hoffman JIE, et al: Blood flow measurements with radionuclide labeled particles. *Prog Cardiovasc Dis* 20:55–79, 1977.
40. Bergmann SR, Ter-Pogossian MM, Sabel BE: Positive emission tomography In Herd JA, Gotto AM, et al (eds): *Cardiovascular Instrumentation*. NIH Publication No. 84-1654, 1984, pp 239–247.
41. Anderson DE, Kearns WD: Blood pressure monitoring in laboratory animals during behavioral experiments. In Herd JA, Gotto AM, et al (eds): *Cardiovascular Instrumentation*. NIH Publication No. 84-1654, 1984, pp 5–19.
42. Hall LW, Clarke KW: *Veterinary Anaesthesia*, ed 8. London, Baillière-Tindall, 1983.
43. Geddes LA: *The Direct and Indirect Measurement of Blood Pressure*. Chicago, Year Book Medical Publishers, 1970.
44. Apple HP: Automatic noninvasive blood pressure monitors: what is available. In Gravenstein JS, Newbower RS, Ream AK, et al (eds): *Essential Noninvasive Monitoring in Anesthesia*. New York, Grune & Stratton, Inc, 1980.
45. Manley SV: Monitoring the anesthetized horse. In Steffey EP (ed): *Veterinary Clinics of North America*, vol 3, 1981, pp 111–113.
46. Riebold TW, Evans AT: Blood pressure measurements in the

anesthetized horse. Comparison of four methods. *Vet Surg* 14:332–337, 1985.
47. Smith M: Indirect measurement of blood pressure in anaesthetized horses using the sounds of Korotkow. *Nord Vet Med* 21:312–317, 1969.
48. Glen JB: Indirect blood pressure measurement in anaesthetized animals. *Vet Rec* 87:349–354, 1970.
49. Latshaw H, Fessler JF, Whistler SJ, et al: Indirect measurement of mean blood pressure in the normotensive and hypotensive horse. *Eq Vet J* 11:191–194, 1979.
50. Krart, C: An ultrasonic method for indirect blood pressure measurement in the horse. *J Eq Med Surg* 3:16–23, 1979.
51. Freundlich JJ, Detweiler DK, Hance HE: Indirect blood pressure determination by the ultrasonic Doppler technique in dogs. *Curr Ther Res* 14:73–80, 1972.
52. Reichle FA: Noninvasive blood pressure measurement in the rat by ultrasonic auscultation. *J Surg Res* 11:539–544, 1971.
53. Hochberg HM, Saltzman MB: Accuracy of an ultrasound blood pressure instrument in neonates, infants and children. *Curr Ther Res* 13:482–488, 1971.
54. Klein L, Sherman J: Effects of preanesthetic medication, anesthesia and position of recumbency on central venous pressure in horses. *J Am Vet Med Assoc* 170:216–219, 1977.
55. Haskins SC, Farver TB, Patz JD: Ketamine in dogs. *Am J Vet Res* 46:1855–1860, 1985.
56. Finco DR, Duncan JR, Schall WD, et al: Acetaminophen toxicosis in the cat. *J Am Vet Med Assoc* 166:469–472, 1975.
57. Harvey JW, Sameck JH, Burgard FJ: Benzocaine-induced methemoglobinemia in dogs. *J Am Vet Med Assoc* 175:1171–1175, 1979.
58. Kujala C, Randall JW: Iatrogenic acetaminophen poisoning. *Fel Pract* 11:12–14, 1981.
59. Smith RP, Olson MV: Drug-induced methemoglobinemia. *Semin Hematol* 10:253–268, 1973.
60. Haskins SC, Patz JD: Effects of small and large face masks and translaryngeal and tracheostomy intubation on ventilation, upper-airway dead space and arterial blood gases. *Am J Vet Res* 47:945–948, 1986.
61. Haskins SC: Sampling and storage of blood for pH and blood gas analysis. *J Am Vet Med Assoc* 170:429–433, 1977.
62. Moens Y, Verstraeten W: Capnographic monitoring in small animal anesthesia. *J Am Anim Hosp Assoc* 18:659–678, 1982.
63. Raemer DB, Francis D, Philip JH, et al: Variation in PCO_2 between arterial blood and peak expired gas during anesthesia. *Anesth Analg* 62:1065–1069, 1983.
64. Gabel RA: Algorithms for calculating and correcting blood-gas and acid-base variables. *Respir Physiol* 42:211–232, 1980.
65. Haskins SC: Blood gases and acid-base balance: clinical interpretation and therapeutic implications. In Kirk RW (ed): *Current Veterinary Therapy VIII*, Philadelphia, WB Saunders Co, 1983, pp 201–215.
66. Shapiro BA, Harrison RA, Walton JR: *Clinical Application of Blood Gases*, ed 2. Chicago, Year Book Medical Publishers, Inc, 1977, p 131.
67. Blair E: *Clinical Hypothermia*. New York, McGraw Hill Co, 1964.
68. Crino MH, Nagel EL: Thermal burns caused by warming blankets in the operating room. *Anesthesiology* 29:149–150, 1968.
69. Haskins SC: Hypothermia and its prevention during general anesthesia in cats. *Am J Vet Res* 42:856–861, 1981.
70. Haskins SC, Patz JP: Effect of inspired-air warming and humidification in the prevention of hypothermia during general anesthesia in cat. *Am J Vet Res* 41:1669–1673, 1980.
71. Hayward JS, Steinman AM: Accidental hypothermia: an experimental study of inhalation rewarming. *Aviation Space Environ Med* 46:1236–1240, 1975.
72. Shanks CA: Heat gain in the treatment of accidental hypothermia. *Med J Aust* 2:346–349, 1975.
73. DeJong RH, Heavner JE, Armory DW: Malignant hyperthermia in the cat. *Anesthesiology* 41:608–609, 1974.
74. Short CE, Paddleford RR: Malignant hyperthermia in the dog. *Anesthesiology* 39:462–463, 1973.
75. Waldron-Mease E, Klein LV, Rosenburg H, et al: Malignant hyperthermia in a halothane anesthetized horse. *J Am Vet Med Assoc* 179:896–898, 1981.
76. Manley SV, Kelly AB, Hodgson D: Malignant hyperthermia-like reactions in three anesthetized horses. *J Am Vet Med Assoc* 183:85–89, 1983.
77. Gronert GA: Malignant hyperthermia. *Anesthesiology* 53:395–423, 1980.
78. Marchildon MD: Malignant hyperthermia, current concepts. *Arch Surg* 117:349–351, 1982.
79. Gallant EM: Malignant hyperthermia: responses of skeletal muscles to general anesthetics. *Mayo Clin Proc* 58:758–763, 1983.
80. O'brien PJ, Cribb PH, White RJ: Canine malignant hyperthermia: diagnosis of susceptibility in a breeding colony. *Can Vet J* 24:172–177, 1983.
81. McGrath CJ, Rempel WE, Jessen CR, et al: Malignant hyperthermia-triggering liability of selected inhalant anesthetics in swine. *Am J Vet Res* 42:604–607, 1981.
82. Stadhouders AM, Viering WA, Verburg MP, et al: *In vivo* induced malignant hyperthermia in pigs. III. Localization of calcium in skeletal muscle mitochondria by means of electronmicroscopy and microprobe analysis. *Acta Anaesthesiol Scand* 28:14–26, 1984.
83. Rosenberg H, Reed S: *In vitro* contracture tests for susceptibility to malignant hyperthermia. *Anesth Analg* 62:415–420, 1983.
84. Pettigrew RT, Galt JM, Ludgate CM: Clinical effects of whole-body hyperthermia in advanced malignancy. *Brit Med J* 4:679–682, 1974.
85. Malamud N, Haymaker W, Custer RP: Heat stroke, a clinicopathologic study of 125 fatal cases. *Milit Surg* 99:397–449, 1946.
86. Shibolet S, Lancaster MC, Danon Y: Heat stroke: a review. *Aviat Space Environ Med* 47:280–301, 1976.
87. Krum SH, Osborne CA: Heatstroke in the dog: a polysystemic disorder. *J Am Vet Med Assoc* 170:531–535, 1977.
88. O'brien PJ, Forsyth FW: Preparation of injectable dantrolene for emergency treatment of malignant hyperthermia-like syndromes. *Can Med J* 24:200, 1983.
89. Levy WJ, Grundy BL, Smith NL: *Monitoring the Electroencephalogram and Evoked Potentials during Anesthesia*, ed 2. Boston, Butterworth, 1984, pp 227–267.
90. Shapiro HM: Neurosurgical anesthesia and intracranial hypertension. In Miller RD (ed): *Anesthesia*, ed 2. New York, Churchill Livingstone, 1986.
91. Dorsch JA, Dorsch SE: *Understanding anesthesia equipment: construction care and complications*, ed 2. Baltimore, Williams & Wilkins, 1984.

CHAPTER

18

Fluid Therapy, Electrolyte and Acid-Base Balance, and Blood Replacement

MARC R. RAFFE, D.V.M., M.S., D.A.C.V.A.

The value of supplemental fluid, electrolyte, and acid-base administration during the perianesthetic period has been widely documented in man and domestic animals. Pre-existing lesions in water, electrolyte, acid-base balance, erythrocyte mass, and coagulation profiles may have life-threatening consequences unless identified and managed in a timely and accurate manner. Recognition and management of disturbances in fluid, electrolyte, and acid-base balance during the perioperative period may be critical to the successful outcome of the surgical procedure. It is imporant to recognize that no time period can be isolated in the management of these disturbances; an integrated approach initiated during the preoperative period and carried through the postoperative phase is necessary for greatest success. Although acute resuscitation of one or more of these components may be necessary in specific cases, the rate of success diminishes if other time components are disregarded. For these reasons, a working knowledge of fluid therapy, acid-base management, and blood therapy is necessary for appropriate management of the anesthetic case.

Fluid Therapy

GENERAL PRINCIPLES

Body Water

Water is the largest component in any species. The overall percentage of body composition varies with age. Newborns have 90% body water composition at birth. This value decreases with age until it reaches 50 to 70% of total body weight at maturity. Total water composition varies with the degree of body fat content, with obese animals having a lower body water content (1).

Total body water is divided into two "functional" compartments, the extracellular and intracellular spaces. The extracellular space may be further subdivided into the intravascular and interstitial spaces. The relative contribution of each compartment to total body water balance varies with species and age. In general, the intracellular compartment contributes 30 to 40% of total body water, with the extracellular compartment contributing 20 to 30%. The intravascular compartment contributes approximately 5% of total body water, and the interstitial compartment contributes approximately 15% of total water (1–4).

Intercompartmental water balance is maintained by an equilibrium between pressure gradients. Water per se is a freely diffusible substance the distribution of which is related to tissue and vascular forces related to the Starling equation. Factors that affect hydrostatic pressure (blood pressure) or oncotic pressure (plasma protein) will disturb the normal distribution of water between tissue compartments. In general, an equilibrium is maintained between hydrostatic and oncotic pressures such that water distribution is consistently maintained between the compartments. Disturbance in hydrostatic or oncotic pressure may result in redistribution of water across cell membranes. Depletion of plasma water increases the oncotic pressure generated by plasma proteins and will result in redistribution of remaining water from the intracellular and interstitial spaces into the vascular compartment. Conversely, depletion of plasma protein may result in redistribution away from the vascular compartment toward the interstitial and intracellular space. Thus, water is redistributed on the basis of balancing the hydrostatic and oncotic forces affecting compartmental distribution. (1, 2, 4, 5).

An additional role in water distribution is controlled by electrolyte species in the extracellular and intracellular space. Sodium and chloride ions contribute to water balance by their presence in the intravascular and interstitial spaces. These ions exert osmotic pressure that contributes to water balance. Their role assumes greater importance in areas of low pressure as represented by the interstitial matrix and intracellular compartment. Sodium is considered to play a predominant role in transcellular fluid flux. In normal state, the force generated by sodium, chloride, and bicarbonate ions in the extracellular compartment is balanced by potassium, magnesium, and phosphate ions in the intracellular compartment. The net forces of water transfer relate to plasma protein and hydrostatic pressures. Lymphatic drainage plays an important role in overall water balance by removing excess fluid from the interstitial compartment (2, 5, 6).

Disturbance in water balance may be the result of an insult affecting one or more of the factors discussed above. As previously noted, alteration in plasma protein levels or hydrostatic pressure forces can result in redistribution of water from the intravascular space to the interstitial compartment. The initial flux of water into the interstitial space rapidly changes the interstitial tissue pressure and helps to prevent further pooling. Lymphatic drainage may be increased to remove excess water back to the plasma compartment and further aid in re-equilibration. A small change in local tissue pressure also inhibits redistribution; however, the contribution is small compared to other factors (5, 6).

Vascular injury may result in increased tissue permeability, which leads to transcapillary fluid flux. The difference is colloidal oncotic pressures is lost in proportion to the increase in endothelial permeability to plasma protein. Redistribution of water across cell membrane boundaries occurs in rapid fashion, with little time for compensatory mechanisms to occur. Thus, "pooling" of water in the interstitial space may result with the formation of edema (5).

Alteration in electrolyte concentration between water compartments may favor redistribution between tissue spaces. Disturbance in extracellular sodium and chloride levels has been shown to alter osmotic pressure and water retention capacity within the extracellular fluid compartment. When significant change in salt concentration is present, redistribution of water occurs. Reduction in salt concentration in the extracellular space causes redistribution of free water to the intracellular compartment. Water redistribution is in response to alteration in extracellular osmotic pressure, which results in re-establishing basal osmotic state in the extracellular space. As water is shifted between compartments, the intracellular osmotic pressure falls until it equals the extracellular pressure. At this point, a new equilibrium is established. This redistribution is accompanied by elevation in concentration of plasma protein and electrolyte values. Conversely, presence of increased salt concentration in the extracellular space will facilitate water redistribution from the intracellular to extracellular compartment (6–8).

Lymphatic injury or water redistribution in excess of lymphatic pump capacity can result in interstitial space water accumulation. Water balance will be affected by factors that inhibit this regulatory component (5, 6).

Other factors related to certain disease states may contribute to disturbance in water balance. Alteration in intravascular osmolality has been noted with hyperglycemia, hyperlipemia, azotemia, ketonemia, intoxication with ethylene glycol or salicylates, diabetes insipidus, or iatrogenic fluid administration. In these examples, an increase in plasma osmotic pressure results in redistribution of water between the intracellular and extracellular compartments. Measurement of sodium levels in these cases demonstrates a relative reduction in values resulting from fluid redistribution. Absolute values of sodium may not be reduced (7, 8).

Evaluation of water balance can be performed by a combination of clinical and laboratory methods. Under controlled conditions, measurement of fluid consumption by all routes (input) and elimination (output) can be measured or estimated by quantitative techniques. The degree of dehydration can be estimated by clinical evaluation of body weight changes, skin turgor, mucus membrane moisture, pulse quality, orbital prominence, and signs of shock (Table 18.1). Abnormalities in vascular, interstitial, and intracellular water balance will be reflected by evaluation of these parameters. Several laboratory parameters offer aid in evaluating water balance. It is important to appreciate that all techniques are sampled from the vascular compartment, with inference about interstitital and intracellular water balance gained from the results. Measurement of plasma protein and packed cell volume is frequently performed to aid in evaluation of water balance in the intravascular compartment. Disturbance in the relationship of these two parameters may indicate water loss from the vascular space (Table 18.2). Evaluation of blood urea nitrogen (BUN), glucose, and electrolyte levels can yield information regarding water balance. Calculation of serum osmolality can be useful in assessing the state of overall water balance. Several formulas are available for calculation depending on the laboratory values available (see below). Direct evaluation of water balance may be measured by plasma osmolality. Several laboratory techniques have been described to measure plasma osmolality. The most common technique is based on a freezing point depression method whereby the freezing point of plasma changes relative to solute (protein and electrolyte) concentration. This permits direct measurement of plasma osmolality for evaluation of water balance. Alteration in osmolality can reflect water balance disturbance, but it can also indicate solute loss (protein), sodium imbalance, and abnormalities in urea nitrogen or glucose concentrations. Normal values in most species are considered to be in the range of 270 to 300 mOsm/liter (1, 3, 5, 6).

Daily requirements for water are normally met through ingestion and metabolic processes. Water requirements vary with body weight, age, environmental factors, pregnancy, and pre-existing disease states that affect ingestion, transport, or regulation of water. Conditions that demand additional water metabolism as represented by fever, trauma, infection, peritonitis, ascites, edema, shock, hemorrhage, and excessive sweating must also be considered in overall water demands. Basal water requirements have been de-

Table 18.1.
Clinical Signs of Dehydration

Dehydration	Mucus Membrane Dryness	Skin Turgor	Slowed Capillary Refill Time	Sunken Eyes	Tachycardia	Poor Pulse Quality
%						
3–5	+	0	0	0	0	0
5	+	+	0	0	0	0
6–8	+	++	+	+	+	0
9–12	++	+++	++	++	++	+
12–15	+++	+++	+++	+++	+++	++

Table 18.2.
Sodium and Water Changes Associated with Some Common Clinical Conditions

Clinical Condition	Extracellular Fluid (ECF)		Intracellular Fluid		Packed Cell Volume	Total Plasma Protein	ECF Sodium Balance	ECF Water Balance
	Volume	Tonicity	Volume	Tonicity				
Predominant water loss	↓	↑	↓	↑	↑	↑	↑	↓
Surgical site evaporation								
Pulmonary evaporation								
Preoperative dessication								
Sodium and water loss	↓	N, ↓	N	N	↑↑	N, ↑	↓	↓
Gastrointestinal lesion								
Pancreatitis								
Peritonitis								
Anorexia								
Shock								
Predominant sodium loss	↓↓	↓	↑	↓	N, ↑	N, ↑	↓	↓↓
Nephritis								
Vomiting								
Diarrhea								

scribed. As an overall equation, the daily water requirement is equal to 150 × weight (kg) 0.82. Additional requirements must be considered for the disease states listed above. These requirements will be considered in fluid plan formulation (5).

Electrolytes

Electrolytes play a central role in maintenance of intercompartmental water balance as well as contributing to critical cell functions. Abnormalities in electrolyte concentrations are frequently present in various diseases; left unattended, they may result in morbidity and mortality. Laboratory evaluation of common electrolyte components is widely available and is useful in diagnosis and management of electrolyte disturbances. Rapid identification and management of electrolyte disorders will aid in overall fluid management. For these reasons, electrolyte evaluation should be performed routinely in cases that demonstrate fluid disturbance.

Sodium. Sodium is the most plentiful cation in the body, with approximately 45 meq (1 g) distributed per kilogram of body weight. Sodium acts as the osmotic skeleton of the extracellular compartment. Sodium is regulated by the kidney, and its concentration is related to the extracellular volume and controlled principally by aldosterone and other complementary factors. The presence of a large sodium concentration in the interstitial fluid compartment enables this tissue space to maintain water balance with the vascular and intracellular compartments. Osmotic concentration is tightly regulated through mechanisms that govern sodium balance. As a result of these interactions, sodium assumes a central role in overall water distribution and balance. Changes in sodium balance initially affect extracellular fluid volume. In most cases, water and sodium disturbances occur simultaneously (Tables 18.2 and 18.3). For this reason, sodium evaluation is valuable for assessing overall fluid balance. In domestic animals, plasma sodium concentration ranges from 132 to 152 meq/liter. As an overall index, a value of 142 meq/liter may be used as a guideline for normal value (1, 6–9).

Table 18.3.
Electrolyte Concentration of Fluids Lost by Common Routes

Route of Fluid Loss	Electrolyte Concentration (meq/L)			
	Na+	K+	Cl–	pH
Gastrointestinal				
Saliva	10–40	10–20	6–30	5.5–7.8
Stomach	60–120	10–20	10–30	1.5–7.5
Duodenum	90–140	2–10	70–120	5.8–7.5
Jejunum/ ilium	125–140	5–10	100–130	6.5–7.6
Colon	65–148	6–12	60–140	7.8–8.0
Bile	130–155	2–12	80–110	6.2–8.5
Pancreatic	150–155	5–10	30–50	7.8–8.8
Renal	50–120	5–10	60–130	5.0–8.0
Surgical site	140	5–7	100–120	7.4

Hyponatremia (sodium levels less than 132 meq/liter) results from water and sodium balance in the plasma space. In the absence of exogenously administered or endogenously accumulated solutes that affect sodium balance (mannitol, urea, glucose, or lipids), hyponatremia is a result of low sodium concentration or water retention in response to changes in solute concentration. The causes of hyponatremia are diverse. Lesions in the gastrointestinal or renal systems may be primary factors in development. Physiological response mediated through liberation of antidiuretic hormone (ADH) may be contributory. Factors related to ADH release in surgical cases include pain, anesthetic drugs, metabolic response to injury, hemorrhage, shock, and sepsis. Endocrine lesions related to adrenal and thyroid function may result in development of hyponatremia by impairing sodium conservation. Pre-existing edema, cardiac failure, and hepatic disease have also been reported to cause hyponatremia. Continuous routes of sodium loss represented by gastrointestinal fistula, dermal burns, and excessive sweating may also be contributory. Iatrogenic administration of parenteral fluids that are sodium-poor may also induce hyponatremia (1, 7, 9).

Clinical signs related to hyponatremia may include generalized weakness, mental depression, inappetence, and hypotension. The serum level of sodium necessary to produce clinical signs is classically considered to be less than 130 meq/liter, although clinical signs may be absent with lower values when the time course of the underlying lesion is chronic in nature. Therapy is directed at re-establishing normal sodium and water ratio in the vascular space, with re-equilibration across other compartments. This is accomplished by correction of the underlying disease process and administration of saline-containing solutions in cases that require replacement therapy. Solutions that contain sodium levels greater than plasma concentration are generally used for replacement therapy. Hypertonic saline solution (3 or 5%) is infused for deficit therapy. The amount required for replacement may be calculated based on the following formula:

$$\text{meq Na needed for replacement} = \frac{(140 - \text{Measured plasma Na})}{3} \times \text{body weight (kg)}$$

Saline also contains chloride ion that may contribute to development of metabolic acidosis. Use of saline is not recommended when pre-existing acidosis is present (1, 7).

Hypernatremia occurs when the sodium level exceeds 155 meq/liter in the plasma space. Hypernatremia is usually a result of water loss or salt gain. Water loss may be subdivided into either pure or hypotonic fluid loss. Pure water loss may result from water deprivation, water loss through sweat or the pulmonary tract, or loss of renal regulation as in diabetes insipidus. Hypotonic fluid loss may accompany gastrointestinal lesions; sweat; salivary secretions; osmotic diuresis from glucose, urea, or mannitol administration; and serosal cavity loss during surgery or peritoneal dialysis. Salt gain may be through dietary provision; response to neurohumoral substances represented by corticosteroids; epinephrine, vasopressin, and adrenocorticotropic hormone (ACTH) liberation; or inappropriate administration of saline-rich fluids. Hypernatremia is often treated by administration of free-choice water. If this is not appropriate, then parenteral administration of hypotonic solutions such as 0.45% NaCl in 2.5% dextrose, hypotonic maintaince solutions, or 5% dextrose may be indicated. Discontinuation of exogenous therapy that is contributory to salt retention is recommended (1, 8). The quantity of water deficit present may be calculated based on the following formula as determined by Feig (8):

$$\text{Water deficit} = 0.6 \times \text{Body weight (kg)} \times \frac{(1 - 140)}{\text{Plasma Na}}$$

Potassium. Potassium is the predominant intracellular cation; 98% of total body potassium is located within the cells. For this reason, potassium may be considered as the "osmotic skeleton" of the intracellular space. Evaluation of potassium can be challenging because large fluctuations in total body potassium can occur without causing corresponding changes in plasma levels. Interactions of potassium with acid-base balance, hormonal influence, renal regulation, nutritional factors, tissue injury, and various medications make evaluation and therapy complex. Unfortunately, evaluation of serum values can only indirectly reflect overall potassium balance. Thus, a working knowledge of potassium physiology is essential for proper interpretation and therapy (1, 9–12).

Potassium is essential for maintenance of several body functions. Potassium is involved in cell membrane potentials, with significant contribution to the function of skeletal and cardiac muscle, as well as nerve impulse transmission. Transcellular shifts in parenchymal organs are essential for maintenance of ion balance of the kidney and gastrointestinal systems. Potassium has an affiliation with glucose metabolism in the liver, with uptake of potassium occurring in the presence of glucose during glycogen formation. Finally, potassium is involved in transcellular ion shifts and electroneutrality related to a variety of neurohumoral modulators. Disturbance in one or more of the factors previously noted may directly or indirectly affect potassium balance and distribution between water compartments. Potassium imbalance will be clinically detected by disturbance in physiological function as reflected by alteration in neuromuscular physiology, cardiac rhythm and function, renal balance, or overall metabolic balance. Normal serum values in most species range from 2.5 to 5.5 meq/liter. The normal range is influenced by diet, gastrointestinal physiology, and renal physiology (Table 18.3). As a geneal rule, trends in potassium are opposite from sodium. Thus, elevation in potassium is usually accompanied by reduction in sodium values and vice versa (6, 9–11).

Hyperkalemia is defined as serum values in excess of 5.5 meq/liter. Hyperkalemia may result from direct or indirect effects on potassium balance. Internal redistribution of potassium may accompany acid-base disturbances, hypertonicity, insulin deficiency, hypoaldosteronism, pharmacological agents, and cell necrosis. Failures of potassium regulation include exogenous administration of potasium-rich solutions or diet, renal insufficiency, hypoaldosteronism, and renal tubular lesions. The primary danger associated with hyperkalemia is development of life-threatening cardiac arrhythmias and myocardial depression. The level of potassium required to produce these arrhythmias varies with the presence of metabolic acid-base disturbance. In most species, progressive changes in P wave configuration occur at approximately 7 meq/liter. Changes in QRS complex configuration and conduction time begin at 8 to 9 meq/liter and ultimately exhibit configurational prolongation and slurring, culminating in asystole or fibrillation at 10 to 12 meq/liter (1, 6, 10–12).

Therapy for hyperkalemia is directed at correction of the underlying lesion. Unfortunately, in many cases, the time course for correction exceeds the immediate requirements. In these cases, several approaches to management have been reported. Correction of acidosis by administration of sodium bicarbonate is useful in correction of potassium balance. The rationale for this technique is transcellular relocation of potassium to the intracellular compartment by correction of hydrogen ion excess. Administration of glucose solutions with supplemental insulin have been noted to be successful in correction. Both glucose and insulin have metabolic capacities to enhance transcellular uptake of potassium by cells. Last, administration of calcium salts at a rate of 0.25 to 0.5 meq/kg/hr has been reported to be effective in counteracting cardiac effects of potassium on a temporary basis. Correction of underlying disturbances is still critical for overall success with use of these therapies [1, 10–12).

Hypokalemia may be defined as serum potassium levels less than 3.5 meq/liter. Hypokalemia may be associated with alterations associated with acid-base balance, gastrointestinal sequestration or loss, abnormal potassium excretion from renal or gastrointestinal sites, administration of pharmacological agents, administration of potassium-poor fluids or diet, and overzealous administration of sodium-containing fluids or drugs. Tissue catabolism accompanying certain disease or injury states may result in hypokalemia if rapid elimination of liberated intracellular potassium occurs. Clinical signs referable to hypokalmia include muscle weakness and paralysis, intestinal ileus, and, infrequently, alteration in electrocardiographic complexes. Early changes have been noted in anorexia, with muscle weakness noted as early as 4 to 7 days after withdrawal of food. For this reason, early therapy of hypokalemia is recommended if serum levels are less than 2.5 meq/liter (1, 10–12).

Therapy is directed at replacing potassium salts. If oral methods are available, administration of supplemental potassium chloride is appropriate at a rate of 1 meq KCl/kg/day. If parenteral routes are necessary, then administration of supplemental potassium chloride in glucose or maintenance composition fluids is preferred. Inclusion of 20 to 40 meq/liter of potassium chloride per liter of fluid is safe if normal renal function is present. In cases of acute replacement, it is recommended that potassium administration not exceed 0.25 to 0.5 meq/kg/hr. The duration and intensity of the underlying lesion is important to consider for overall evaluation of potassium deficit. Constant re-evaluation of serum potassium levels should be performed to evaluate therapy. Correction of coexisting disturbances in acid-base balance, water balance, and drug support should also occur simultaneously to aid in correction of hypokalemia (1, 10–12).

Calcium. Calcium is an essential inorganic element that plays an important role in neuromuscular activity, cell membrane function, coagulation, lactation, and bone formation. Most calcium stores are unavailable for immediate use due to inclusion in bone matrix. Serum calcium divides into ionized and protein-bound (nonionized) fractions. Ionized calcium is physiologically important to the anesthetist because of its effects on the cardiovascular and coagulation systems. Calcium regulation is under the control of two hormones, parathormone and calcitonin. Parathormone maintains serum calcium levels by regulating resorption of calcium from bone sources. Calcitonin inhibits this process. The response of calcitonin is faster than parathormone; therefore, precise regulation of plasma calcium levels is generally associated with this hormone (6).

Hypercalcemia is considered to be serum levels greater than 11.5 mg/dl. Hypercalcemia can occur secondary to a variety of disease entities. In general, hypercalcemia can be associated with neoplasia, renal disease, and endocrine disorders represented by hypoadrenocorticism or primary hyperparathyroidism. Hypercalcemia has also been noted with severe hypothermia, osteomyelitis, and inflammatory disorders. Some of these etiologies may be encountered in the anesthetic patient. Organ systems affected by hypercalcemia include the renal, gastrointestinal, cardiovascular, and central nervous systems. Of the affected systems, the anesthetist must be concerned with cardiovascular, renal, and central nervous system problems. Alteration in electrical impulse conduction through the myocardium may result in prolonged P-R intervals and a shortened Q-T interval. The myocardium may be predisposed to development of ventricular fibrillation. Many cases exhibit hypertension associated with the inotropic actions of calcium on the myocardium. Renal function is compromised due to a reduction in glomerular filtration rate and vasoconstriction. Progressive mineralization of the renal tubular cells will contribute to presence of tubular casts and disturbance in potassium and hydrogen ion balance. Central nervous system signs may include depression and fatigue. Vomiting and inappetence may also be noted. Therapy for hypercalcemia is dependent upon the presence of clinical signs. Not all cases with elevated serum calcium levels require therapy prior to anesthesia. If significant clinical signs are present, then therapy includes fluid administration of a composition that does not contain calcium, diuretic administration to promote diuresis, and direct reduction of serum calcium levels by administration of supplemental phosphate, sodium bicarbonate, glucocorticoids, and, in severe cases, intravenous sodium EDTA (1, 6, 12–14).

Hypocalcemia is recognized when serum levels are less than 9.0 mg/dl. Hypocalcemia may be associated with a variety of conditions. Those that may affect anesthetic and surgical management include hypoalbuminemia, renal failure, soft tissue injury, calcium-free fluid administration, acidosis, and blood transfusion (citrate chelation). Body systems associated with hypocalcemia are similar to those listed for hypercalcemia. Clinical signs may include seizures, muscle tremors, gait abnormalities, hyperthermia, and electrocardiographic changes represented by tachycardia and prolonged Q-T interval. Therapy is by administration of calcium salts available as calcium chloride, calcium gluconate, or calcium borogluconate. The recommended administration is 0.25 to 1.0 meq/kg for initial administration. The dose may be higher in the dog; administration rates of 10 to 15 mg/kg/hr have been reported. Response to therapy includes improved cardiovascular function, improved musculoskeletal function, and return of normal consciousness (1, 6, 13, 14).

Magnesium. Homeostasis and metabolism of magnesium is not well understood. Magnesium plays an essential role in energy transfer related to ATP utilization. Magnesium also plays a role in neuromuscular function, thermoregulation, and protein synthesis. Distribution of magnesium between extracellular and intracellular compartments is related to acid-base balance, calcium, and aldosterone (6).

Hypermagnesemia is rare. Serum levels in excess of 3.2 mg/dl are interpreted as hypermagnesemia. In many cases, hypermagnesemia is associated with renal failure. Clinical signs associated with hypermagnesemia include neuromuscular weakness, central nervous system depression, hypotension, bradycardia, prolonged P-R intervals, and S-T segment changes. Therapy is through administration of calcium salts (1, 6, 12).

Hypomagnesmia occurs when plasma levels are less than 1 mg/dl. Hypomagnesemia may result from dietary insufficiency, diarrhea, environmental exposure, hyperparathyroidism, and diuretic administration. Clinical signs associated with hypomagnesemia include incoordination, hyperesthesia, muscle tremors and clonus, depression, and convulsions. Clinical appearance is similar to hypocalcemia. Therapy is directed at magnesium replacement through diet or parenteral means. Intravenous administration of 1 to 2 g (8 to 16 meq) of magnesium sulfate in 5% dextrose solution has been reported. Caution should be exercised in cases with compromised renal function (1, 6, 12).

Chloride. Chloride is the predominant anion of the body and also functions as an extracellular base (Table 18.3). Chloride is a relatively weak base when compared to bicarbonate, phosphate, and the plasma proteins. For this reason, solutions that have a high concentration of chloride ions are mildly acidic in composition. Chloride is controlled by mechanisms similar to those that regulate renal sodium balance. Renal regulation of electroneutrality usually causes interaction of chloride with bicarbonate ions to maintain anion equilibrium. For this reason, interaction between chloride and bicarbonate ions is important. A primary deficit in one anion species will be compensated for by an increase in the other component. In most domestic species, normal values range from 95 to 111 meq/liter. Sites of high chloride concentration include extracellular water, and renal tubules. Chloride concentration exceeds sodium levels in the upper gastrointestinal system (1, 6).

Hyperchloremia occurs when serum levels exceed 110 meq/liter. Hyperchloremia is most commonly seen with overadministration of chloride-rich fluids by oral or parenteral routes. Hyperchloremia may also be noted with renal tubular acidosis and salvage procedures requiring ureter transplantation. Reduced renal function may also precipitate hyperchloremia. Clinical signs include gastrointestinal irritation, anorexia, weight loss, lethargy, and persistent hyperventilation. Metabolic acidosis is noted due to excess bicarbonate excretion by the renal tubules. Therapy consists of removing the source of chloride ions, administration of sodium bicarbonate by oral or parenteral routes, and use of buffer-containing fluids (1, 6).

Hypochloremia is noted when plasma values are less than 94 meq/liter. Frequently, a gastrointestinal lesion is the underlying cause of hypochloremia, although metabolic lesions chracterized by elevated bicarbonate levels and hypokalemia may cause hypochloremia. Administration of diurectics with chloride loss in excess of sodium and concurrent potassium loss may also play a role. Primary renal disease may produce similar effects. Effects of hypochloremia are mediated through the effects on acid-base regulation. A metabolic alkalosis will be noted with clinical signs associated with this disturbance. In many cases, linkage with sodium ion is present with correction occurring with sodium balance. Therapy is directed at supplying chloride ion-rich fluid, such as sodium or potassium chloride. Discontinuation of such inciting therapy as diuretics is also recommended (1). A protocol for calculating chloride replacement determined by Donawich (1) is as follows:

$$\frac{\text{Body weight (kg)}}{3} \times \text{Plasma Cl}^- \text{ deficit} = \text{Meq Cl}^- \text{ required}$$

$$\frac{\text{Meq Cl}^- \text{ required}}{3} = \text{Liters of 0.9\% saline required}$$

Bicarbonate. Bicarbonate is a principal extracellular anion. Although there is more chloride, bicarbonate is the more effective buffer base because of its strength and buffering capacity. Biocarbonate is regulated by renal conservation and interconversion to carbon dioxide for pulmonary excretion. The pulmonary route is most significant on a daily basis, accounting for 70% of bicarbonate balance. Normal values and disturbances in bicarbonate balance will be covered under acid-base regulation.

Phosphorus. Phosphorus is an element essential to life. It is distributed extensively throughout the body, primarily as a constituent of bone and cellular protoplasm. The vast majority of phosphorus is stored in bone, with lesser quantities in protoplasmic spaces. About one-half of the intracellular phosphorus is in the high-energy phosphate bonds of ATP and creatinine phosphate. Normal serum values of phosphorus are age-related, with young animals having a range of 5.4 to 10 mg/dl during growth. Mature animals have a range of 2.0 to 6.0 mg/dl, with lower values expected as age increases. Plasma phosphates are filtered by the glomerulus, and about 90% are reabsorbed by the proximal tubule. If plasma phosphate levels fall below 2.5 mg/dl, virtually all phosphate will be reabsorbed. Thus, phosphorus excretion depends on dietary intake, diurnal variations in glomerular filtration rate, and tubular function. Parathormone reduces phosphate reabsorption by the proximal tubule; this increases the urinary phosphate level and decreases the serum phosphate concentration (6, 13).

Hypophosphatemia is present when serum levels fall below 2.5 mg/dl. Hypophosphatemia may be a result of dietary insufficiency; malabsorption; renal disease; diabetes mellitus; hyperparathyroidism; translocation associated with tissue trauma, acid-base disturbance, or hypoalbuminemia; or of an undefined cause. In one study in dogs and cats, 69% of all hypophosphatemia was related to surgery, hypoalbuminemia, or undefined causes. Clinical signs related to hypophosphatemia are usually mild or absent. Serious signs are not noted until serum levels fall below 1.0 mg/dl. Most clinical signs are related to reduced neuromuscular function manifested by weakness, coma, tremors, paresis, and seizures. Effects on the erythropoietic system may include hemolytic anemia, decreased oxygen-carrying capability, and inhibition of leukocyte chemotaxis and phagocytosis. Treatment includes dietary supplementation, and parenteral administration of potassium phosphate at a rate of 0.5 mg/kg/hr for 6 hours. Slow infusion is recommended to prevent hypocalcemia and hyperkalemia (1, 6, 13).

Hyperphosphatemia is usually associated with renal disease, although tissue trauma, fracture repair, and metabolic disease may also affect phosphate balance. Hyperphosphatemia is age-related; young animals will demonstrate high serum levels compared to mature animals. Therapy involves correction of the underlying disease entity (13).

Other Anions. Plasma proteins, organic acids, and sulphates are also considered as plasma anions. Plasma proteins are the third largest source of serum anions. They also contribute to acid-base balance by buffering hydrogen ion, as well as their role in maintaining water balance across plasma membranes. Organic acids are present in small quantities in normal circumstances. They may become elevated during disease states. Sulphates are a result of oxidation of sulphur-containing amino acids and are not clinically significant (6).

FLUID PLAN FORMULATION

Fluid Balance

Estimation of fluid balance in the preoperative patient is based on clinical, laboratory, and physiological parameters previously outlined. Fluid requirements can be divided into two major components, replacement and maintainence therapy. Replacement therapy is aimed at correcting pre-existing or ongoing losses from a variety of sources. The magnitude of loss is based on the parameters listed above, as well as additional information concerning anticipated continuation of fluid loss. Maintenance therapy is judged on the basis of known obligatory water metabolism and routes of loss that are common to all surgical patients (Table 18.4). Withdrawal of oral water sources during the preoperative period; insensible water loss through the skin, pulmonary, gastrointestinal, and surgical sites; and sensible water loss through urine production are common sources of water turnover. Provision of exogenous water sources is essential to prevent deficits during the perioperative period. The quantity of water required to replace or supplement these obligatory processes varies with species. Animals with relatively low body weight or young animals appear to have higher requirements on a weight basis. Additional consideration must be given to the impact of anesthetic agents on autoregulation of the peripheral circulation. Many anesthetic drugs render the animal suspectible to a fluid volume disturbance in the circulation versus vascular capacity. Supplemental fluid administration is considered to expand the circulating fluid volume to ameliorate the effects of anesthetic agents on autonomic vascular tone. Many authors support this aspect as an essential component of fluid administration during the perioperative period (1, 2, 5, 12).

A variety of protocols have been developed to fulfill the above-listed criteria. Replacement therapy should be calculated and added to maintenance requirements for the perioperative and postoperative periods. For small animal species, we use a maintenance protocol of 20 ml/kg for 1 hour, followed by 10 ml/kg for each additional hour. The basis on which we have developed this protocol is to satisfy obligatory water loss of approximately 1.5 to 3.0 ml/kg/hr plus supplemental therapy to compensate for loss from the surgical wound. Studies in man suggest that surgical trauma can be classified as mild, moderate, or severe and that incremental administration doses of 2, 4, and 8 ml/kg/hr may be administered to adjust for evaporative loss from the surgical site. The additional quantity administered during the first hour is to accommodate for the

Table 18.4.
Fluid Plan Formulation

Volume of fluid
Pre-existing losses, body weight (kg) × % dehydration = replacement volume (liter) per hour
Maintainence, 2–4 ml/kg/hr
Contemporary losses
Concentration of fluid
Osmolality
Sodium concentration
Composition of fluid
Potassium and chloride concentration
Buffer base and pH
Energy sources, such as carbohydrates, lipids
Vitamins and trace elements
Amino acids

effects of anesthetic drugs on vascular capacitance. In large animal species, we initiate fluid therapy at 10 ml/kg/hr based on data that indicates horses may safely tolerate fluid administration rates of 12 to 16 ml/kg/hr without ill effects. Supplementation is provided for preexisting losses as necessary. Rapid infusion rates should be monitored for signs of overhydration, although data indicate that the horse may safely tolerate rapid administration rates with minimum difficulty (12).

Deficit therapy should be titrated to some desirable end point, such as improvement in clinical status, skin turgor, weight gain, and remission of signs of hypovolemia and shock. Contemporary losses are estimated on the basis of the daily expected losses, which are derived from the preceding day's measured or estimated losses. Deficit therapy should be administered over a 24-hour period. Only that fraction of the daily deficit therapy that normally would be administered during the surgical period should be administered. Conveniently, the deficit volume may be delivered on a time basis (i.e., as milliliters per hour). The volume per hour is added to the maintenance requirement, resulting in the total volume of delivery. Similarly, contemporary losses may be added to the hourly infusion rate based on their anticipated volume loss (5).

Electrolyte Balance and Fluid Composition

Electrolyte balance in fluid therapy probably evokes the most controversy with respect to optimum composition and concentration. Most authors agree that several points are important: sodium is the essential extracellular electrolyte species; most fluid losses are hypotonic (sodium poor) in nature, with the exception of the gastrointestinal tract; and during the perioperative period, water balance disturbance may occur due to neuroendocrine response to anesthesia and surgery resulting in redistribution of extracellular fluid volume and electrolytes. Based on these points, electrolyte composition for replacement and maintenance fluid has been divided into two philosophies. These are replacement and maintenance therapy with isotonic electrolyte solutions and maintenance therapy with hypotonic (low sodium) fluids with isotonic fluids for replacement of isotonic losses. The dichotomy of opinion is based on personal preference, lack of objective data for the perioperative period in species other than man, and composition of available fluids (15–20).

Despite the divergence of data and personal opinion, it appears that inclusion of electrolytes in the fluid composition offers advantages over electrolyte-free fluids. The advantage is noted especially in the postoperative period, where residual effects of anesthesia and surgery are still evident. Several studies in man comparing use of lactated Ringer's solution and 5% dextrose on postoperative water and electrolyte balance demonstrate better maintenance of preoperative parameters during the perioperative period when a balanced electrolyte solution is compared to electrolyte-free solutions. This is attributed to a reduced stress response with lower levels of antidiuretic hormone and aldosterone (20–23).

If minimal blood loss is anticipated during the surgical procedure, then use of a hypotonic maintenance solution appears acceptable in mature animals. With the exception of upper gastrointestinal tract (Table 18.3), most losses encountered during anesthesia and surgery are hypotonic in composition with predominant water loss. Replacement with a hypotonic electrolyte solution replaces both water loss and sodium-poor electrolyte losses documented to occur during surgery and anesthesia. Contemporary loss through hemorrhage should be replaced with isotonic balanced electrolyte solutions such as lactated Ringer's solution. In young animals, sodium conservation mechanisms are immature. Most authors recommend isotonic balanced electrolyte solutions in these animals because the composition of loss more closely approximates an isotonic composition (12, 20, 24).

Specific electrolyte disturbances may be incorporated into the overall fluid plan (Table 18.4). Supplemental electrolytes may be added to balanced electrolyte solutions or "customized" fluids may be prepared for specific purposes. For example, documented disturbances in sodium, chloride, and potassium may be therapeutically treated by selecting appropriate fluid base (i.e., 0.9% NaCl) and supplementing the deficient electrolyte (potassium) as an aqueous salt. This fluid composition is used as the replacement therapy, with maintenance therapy provided by a balanced isotonic solution. Deficit calculations for specific electrolyte species should be performed as previously described and replaced on a schedule as noted above. Replacement therapy should be initiated prior to anesthesia and surgery, with continuation through the perioperative into the postoperative period.

Additional Therapy Considerations

Although replacement therapy cannot be entirely administered during the perioperative period, consideration for provision of essential aspects of replacement therapy should be recognized. In cases where electrolytes, energy, or acid-base disturbances are noted, incorporation of that portion of replacement therapy calculated for the perioperative period should be administered. Addition of water-soluble vitamins may also be included in the replacement fluid solution. Provision of other deficits represented by amino acids, lipid, and trace elements is reserved for the postoperative period unless the animal is already on supplementation prior to surgery. In these cases, hourly infusion rates are maintained during anesthesia.

Considering the variety of goals that fluid therapy can help achieve during the perioperative period, a priority rank must be assigned as to which goals are most critical (Table 18.4). The priority rank associated with fluid therapy may be summarized as follows: 1, replacement volume of fluid; 2, hemoglobin or packed cell volume, albumin or total protein; 3, osmolality, sodium concentration; 4, potassium concentration; 5, pH; bicarbonate concentration; 6, chloride concentration; 7, water soluble vitamins; 8, energy supplied as carbohydrates or lipids; 9, amino acids for tissue repair; and 10, trace elements. By keeping these goals focused, appropriate volume and composition of fluid may be appropriately administered (5).

Monitoring Response to Fluid Therapy

Response to fluid therapy requires time. It is unreasonable to anticipate that correction will be complete in the relatively brief intraoperative period. Many methods of monitoring will require delay until the postoperative period. Intraoperative monitoring is generally confined to essential aspects of water and electrolyte balance. Water balance may be evaluated by monitoring urine production as well as estimation of fluid loss from the surgical wound. Provision of replacement water volume usually approximates urine loss. Evaluation of packed cell volume and total solids also aids in assessing water balance. Serial determinations will provide information on trends in fluid balance when interpreted along with urine production. Pulmonary water loss may be evaluated by quantitating water condensation within anesthetic delivery circuits. In large animal species, drainage of the anesthesia machine through the moisture valve can provide information concerning water loss (4, 5, 22, 25).

Electrolyte status is evaluated by serum analysis. Generally, sodium, potassium, and chloride levels are the essential components during the intraoperative period. Values determined to be abnormal should be treated by the methods presented above. Adjustment or change in fluid composition or supplementation of specific electrolytes may be indicated to restore values to normal levels. Calculation of plasma osmolality is possible when electrolyte values for sodium, potassium, and chloride are available. Several formulae have been presented for osmolality calculation. The traditional formula for calculated osmolality is noted in the first equation. Many authors shorten the formula to the one presented in the second equation.

$$\text{mOsm/kg} = 1.86\ \text{Na} + \frac{\text{Glucose}}{18} + \frac{\text{BUN}}{2.8}$$

$$\text{mOsm/kg} = 2\ \text{Na} + \text{K}$$

Monitoring of acid-base balance will be presented in the following section.

Products Available for Fluid Therapy (Table 18.5)

Polyionic Fluids. Polyionic fluids of hypotonic or isotonic composition are probably most frequently used in maintenance fluid therapy. All fluids contain sodium and chloride; many include potassium, magnesium, phosphate, and other ion species in a variety of combinations that differ by manufacturer. Two classes of potassium-containing fluids are available, plasma equivalent and enriched variety. The goal of enriched potassium fluids is to partially aid in correction of pre-existing deficits. As noted above, the composition of the fluids is to approximate that of blood and extracellular fluid or to approximate the types of contemporary losses that may be anticipated during surgery. Many fluids have the additional feature of buffer base inclusion. Acetate, lactate, gluconate, or a combination of these salts is included to contribute to overall acid-base balance. Polyionic fluids may also include sugars as a fluid component. Fluids that contain sugars may be isotonic or hypertonic in composition.

Saline. Sodium chloride is available in a variety of concentrations. Most frequently, 0.9% NaCl or 0.45% NaCl is used for fluid therapy during the perioperative period depending upon the requirement for isotonic or hypotonic fluid composition. Replacement of large sodium losses in large animal species may require administration of hypertonic saline solution of 3 or 5% concentration. Use of the hypertonic product will permit sodium replacement in a comparably small fluid volume, thereby reducing the potential for overhydration. Hypertonic fluids may also be beneficial in vascular resuscitation of the hypovolemic patient.

Sugars. Hypotonic and isotonic sugar solutions are commercially available for fluid therapy. The overwhelming favorite is dextrose. Dextrose is available in a variety of concentrations. The most popular concentrations are isotonic or mildly hypertonic 5% and 10% concentrations. Dextrose is useful for replacement for support of blood glucose values during the perioperative period. Therapeutic uses are varied according to the underlying disease process.

Buffer Base Solutions. These will be discussed in the next section. They may come as prepared solutions that may be added to the base fluid composition.

Combination Products. A variety of products are available that incorporate one or more of the above-listed components. Generally, a consideration for overall osmolality is incorporated into the formula, and compromises are made to prevent excessive hypertonic composition. Combination fluids generally consist of a

Table 18.5.
Commercially Available Fluids for Intravenous Use

Solution	Tonicity[a]	Manu-facturer	pH	Carbo-hydrate	meq/liter					HCO₃-	HPO₄-
					Na+	K+	Ca^{+2}	Mg^{+2}	Cl−		
Plasma	282.6–303.7		7.5	5.6% dextrose	144	5	5	1.5	107	27	2
5% dextrose	I	Various	5.0	5% dextrose (50 mg/ml)							
0.9% NaCl	I	Various	5.4		154				154		
Maintainence solutions											
Ionosol MB	H	Abbott		5% dextrose	25	20	5	3	22	23 (lactate)	3
Isolyte H	H	McGaw		5% dextrose	40	13		3	40	24 (acetate)	
Normosol M	H	Abbott		Plain and 5% dextrose	40	13		3	40	16 (acetate)	
Polysal M	H	Cutter		2.5, 5, and 10% dextrose	40	16	5	3	40	24 (lactate 12) (acetate 12)	
Plasmalyte 56	H	Travenol	5.5	Plain and 5% dextrose	40	13		3	140	16 (acetate)	
Replacement solutions											
Ringer's	I	Several	5.8	Plain, 2.5, and 5% dextrose	147	4	5		156		
Lactated Ringer's	I	Several	6.5	Plain, 2.5, and 5% dextrose	130	4	3		109	28 (as lactate)	
Hartmann's	I	Several	6.8	Plain and 5% dextrose	131	4	4		111	27 (as lactate or acetate)	
Normosol R	I	Abbott	6.4–7.4	Plain and 5% dextrose	140	5		3	98	50 (acetate 27) (gluconate 23)	
Isolyte S	I	McGaw		Plain and 5% dextrose	140	5		3	98	27 (acetate) 23 (gluconate)	
Plasmalyte 148 Plasmalyte A	I	Travenol	5.5 7.4	Plain, 5% dextrose, and 10% invert sugar	140	10	5	3	103	55 (acetate 47) (lactate 8)	
Polysol	I	Cutter		Plain and 5% dextrose	140	10	5	3	103	55 (acetate 47) (lactate 8)	
Isolyte E	I	McGaw		Plain and 5% dextrose	140	10	5	3	103	55 (acetate 47) (acetate 8)	
0.45% NaCl + 25% dextrose	I	Various	4.8	2.5% dextrose	77				77		
Special purpose											
5% NaCl	Hy				855				855		
Na HCO_3 (8.4%)	Hy		7.8		1000					1000	
Dextrose (10–50%)	Hy	Various	4.2	Dextrose							
0.9% NaCl + 5% dextrose	Hy	Various	4.7	Dextrose	154				154		

[a] H, hypotonic; Hy, hypertonic; I, isotonic.

carbohydrate source combined with saline, a carbohydrate source combined with a hypotonic polyionic maintenance fluid, or a carbohydrate combined with an isotonic polyionic maintenance solution. When formulating fluids, the issue of osmolality should be kept in mind, and excessive tonicity of fluid should be avoided.

COLLOID THERAPY

Colloids are substances that are not freely permeable to vascular endothelium due to molecular size or structure. Their presence, based on the Starling equation and principles governing solute balance, aid in maintaining osmotic pressure in the intravascular compartment. Maintenance of osmotic pressure has been identified as a principal factor in preserving intercompartmental water balance. Transcompartmental water balance may be affected by modifying one or more of the following factors: capillary membrane filtration rate, capillary perfusion pressure, interstitial tissue hydrostatic pressure, plasma oncotic pressure, and tissue oncotic pressure (26, 27).

In general, disturbance in intercompartmental fluid balance noted during anesthesia and surgery is associated with capillary membrane injury or imbalance in plasma and tissue oncotic pressure. Under normal conditions, albumin plays a vital role in maintenance of intercompartmental fluid balance by acting as the major source of colloidal oncotic pressure. Reduction in albumin levels associated with disease, capillary injury, or administration of large volumes of crystalloid solutions may predispose the patient to intercompartmental shifts in water balance. Redistribution of water to extravascular tissue locations may result in edema formation. In surgical patients that exhibit a profile that places them at risk for transcompartmental water shifts, administration of colloidal solutions is beneficial to preserve compartmental water balance (5, 26, 27).

Colloids Available for Use

Colloids are both byproducts of naturally occurring substances and specifically synthesized molecules (Table 18.6). Natural colloid substances include plasma protein solutions and albumin. Synthetic preparations include dextrans and hydroxyethyl starch. Properties desirable for any colloid substance include stability for long-term storage, freedom from antigens, and relatively long half-life in vivo. Colloid metabolism should not cause hemolysis or erythrocyte agglutination. None of the commercially available or self-prepared colloids fulfill all the above-listed criteria. The limitations will be noted under individual preparations (27).

Plasma Protein. Plasma protein is a byproduct of whole blood. Plasma protein is produced by separation of erythrocytes from a stored blood unit. This may be accomplished by sedimentation and separation or by centrifugation. Plasma is an admixture of albumin, globulins, platelets, and clotting factors. The main component for colloid replacement is albumin. Plasma protein may be frozen and stored for up to 3 months at standard freezer temperature. It may be stored for up to 1 year at −70°C. If plasma proteins are frozen, then a gentle thaw in warm water is recommended prior to administration. If use is anticipated within 24 to 48 hours, then refrigeration is acceptable (27, 28).

Plasma protein has several advantages over synthetic substances. It is relatively inexpensive to produce, has a long intravascular half-life (4 to 15 days), and provides vascular compartment stabilization associated with chronic disease states. It has disadvantages related to antigenicity. Direct protein allergy, anticolloid antibodies, complement activation, and histamine release have all been noted with plasma protein administration. Transient reduction in coagulation profile has also been noted after albumin administration. Despite the potential drawbacks, plasma protein remains popular in medicine as a replacement substance due to its cost effectiveness and physiological properties. Recommended administration rates in humans are 6 to 10 ml/kg infused at a rate similar to whole blood. No formal guidelines have been established in veterinary medicine (27–29).

Dextrans. Dextrans are synthesized from microbiological activity of *Leuconostioc mesenteroides* B512 strain. Two forms of dextrans are commercially available; these are low molecular weight (mean molecular weight 40,000 or Dextram 40) and high molecular weight (mean molecular weight 60,000 to 75,000 or Dextran 70). The molecular size has a direct influence on the useful intravascular half-life, with low molecular weight having a 2-hour half-life and high molecular weight having a 6-hour half-life. Dextran 70 has an excellent vascular retention, with 30% of the infused dose still present in the intravascular space 24 hours after administration. Elimination of dextrans is predominantly by renal filtration, although gut elimination and metabolism do occur. Dextrans are refined during processing and reattached to other polysaccharides to aid in stability of preparation and to improve intravascular half-life (26).

Anaphylactoid reactions have been associated with administration of dextrans. Dextrans can act as haptens associating with IgG class immunoglobulins to trigger adverse reactions. Complement fixation may also be a component of this response. The incidence of these reactions occurring in humans appeared to be no different from other colloid substances. Administration of antihistamines prior to dextrans reduces the incidence of adverse reactions. Hemostasis may be affected through reduced platelet adhesiveness, reduction in Factor VIII activity, and increased clot lysability. This is offset by an increased peripheral blood flow after administration in hypotensive or shock states (28, 30).

Table 18.6.
Comparison of Colloidal Plasma Substitutes

Substitute	Production	Mean Molecular Weight	Intravascular Life Span	Infusion Rates	Immune Reaction	Severity
Plasma protein	Blood separation	Variable (50,000)	4–15 days	10–20 ml/kg/hr	Allergic	Mild-Severe
Dextran	*Leuconostoc mesenteroides* (B512)	40,000 or 75,000	2–6 hours 6–24 hours	Up to 20 ml/kg over 24 hours	Antidextran antibodies	Mild-Severe
Starch	Acid hydrolysis treatment of soya and corn-ethylene oxide	450,000	6 hours	Up to 100 ml/kg for shock	Complement activation	Immediate-Severe

For resuscitation purposes in cases of hypovolemia, administration rates of 40 to 50 ml/kg/hr have been suggested. Reduction in infusion rates should occur when response is noted by blood pressure evaluation. Restoration of blood pressure to 90% of baseline values is the criteria for reduction in administration rate. Some authors caution against overadministration of dextrans due to their interference with hemostasis (26, 31, 32).

Starch. Hydroxyethyl starch is prepared by hydrolysis of sorghum substrate to amylopectin. Amylopectin is then attached to glucose units to provide a satisfactory half-life within the vascular compartment. Hydroxyethyl starch is commercially available as a 6% solution under the trade name of Hetastarch. Hetastarch has been shown to be favorable in resuscitation of hypovolemia associated with trauma or disease. Hetastarch has a volume expanding effect that lasts 24 to 36 hours. It has been shown to elicit in vivo immune reactions. The reactions are characterized by complement activation upon administration. The frequency is low and is no different than other colloids (26).

Hetastarch is administered on a unit-replacement basis. In humans, administration of 1 liter of hetastarch expands plasma volume approximately 710 ml. Hetastarch is metabolized by a complex series of pathways. Hydrolysis and renal filtration, as well as phagocytosis appear to play role in excretion. Hetastarch may remain in the body as long as 17 to 48 days postadministration (26).

Indications for Use

Colloids can be used for vascular space resuscitation in the acutely injured patient or as a supplemental replacement therapy in chronic disease. The advantage of colloids for these applications is that a lower total volume may be administered to achieve intravascular resuscitation when compared to crystalloid solutions. Colloids are not a substitute for crystalloid solutions to restore water balance in the dehydrated animal, but they are useful in assisting in volume re-expansion of the vascular space associated with acute hypovolemia. Colloids are also beneficial when given in conjunction with crystalloid solutions to prevent translocation of free water from the vascular to the interstitial compartments. Colloids have been shown to improve tissue oxygen utilization, cardiac index, and left ventricular stroke work when compared to crystalloid solutions in resuscitation protocols. Preservation of myocardial function and improved oxygen delivery indicate merit for inclusion of colloids in resuscitation of acute hypovolemia (12, 26, 28).

The choice of colloid for a specific application is based on the therapeutic goals. From the previous discussion, it may be noted that different colloid preparations have variations in useful in vivo half-life. The goals for use of colloids must be considered, and the colloid selected should be based on the characteristics of the various colloid types. For long-term application or resuscitation of chronic disease, albumin remains the best choice available. Short-term vascular resuscitation may be safely accomplished with dextrans or starches. These points must be considered as therapy is initiated.

Controversies in Colloid Administration

Colloid therapy has not enjoyed a more widespread use in clinical practice for several reasons. The availability and cost of colloids have prevented their inclusion in resuscitation protocols. Albumin must be provided as a byproduct of blood collection. Other synthetic colloids are commercially available, although their cost is greater than crystalloid solutions. These factors have, in part, prevented greater use of colloids in fluid therapy.

Incompatibility reactions have been noted with colloid use. As described above, all colloid products have a small, but significant, incidence of immune-mediated reactions. The clinical significance of this may be noted by hypotension associated with administration of dextrans and starches. Fever, erythema, and cardiovascular collapse have also been reported. Complement activation and presence of anticolloid antibodies may also exacerbate the clinical signs. Clotting abnormalities have been associated with colloid administration. Dextrans appear to have a significant impact on hemostasis, as previously noted. Albumin studies in dogs have likewise demonstrated clotting profile changes for several days after administration (28).

The major controversy of colloid use centers around acute volume resuscitation in shock. A concern has been expressed that colloid leakage through injured vascular endothelium may predispose the patient to edema formation in critical tissue beds. The issue remains unresolved as to the best choice of resuscitation fluid. Most evidence supports hemodynamic integrity playing an important role in pulmonary edema formation during resuscitation. Maintenance of capillary perfusion pressure as well as intravascular colloidal pressure has been shown to be important in preventing translocation of water into the interstitium. Most studies indicate that intravascular colloid dilution related to crystalloid infusion is well tolerated during vascular resuscitation. Complications related to resuscitation appear to be associated with elevations in pulmonary capillary pressure. In addition, experimental studies have not supported an increased risk of pulmonary edema formation with colloid use after endothelial injury. Both crystalloid and colloid solutions appear to improve hemodynamics in both healthy and compromised patients. Colloids are favored if restriction of resuscitation fluid volume appears to be an issue in the compromised patient. Their administration is also indicated in cases of pre-existing or fluid-induced hypoproteinemia to stabilize colloid oncotic pressure in the intravascular space (26, 33–37).

BLOOD AND BLOOD COMPONENT THERAPY

Blood is a heterogenous substance composed of red and white cell lines, platelets, clotting factors, albumin, immunoglobulins, and water. Because of its complex composition, administration of whole blood has been described as a therapeutic procedure for a wide spectrum of disease. The reasons for the popularity of blood administration are that no synthetic substitute capable of performing the above-mentioned functions has been identified. In addition, many cases may require one or more blood components for a specific application. Despite the numerous reports regarding techniques for collection, storage, and administration of blood, the information available regarding techniques of administration and indications for specific therapy is still incomplete. Recent reports provide an excellent overview of blood products. The goal of the present discussion is to address the issue of blood use during the anesthetic period (29, 38).

Indications for Blood Therapy

Preoperative Transfusion. Preoperative transfusion is indicated in anemic patients. In general, preoperative transfusion is not considered if the patient's hematocrit is greater than 25%, corresponding to a hemoglobin level above 7 g/dl, and if the patient's cardiac, pulmonary, hepatic, and renal functions are normal. If hemoglobin levels are below this value, compensatory mechanisms may be inadequate to support cardiovascular function. Reduction in ventricular function secondary to anemia may result from inadequate myocardial oxygenation. Reduction of coronary blood flow has been shown at a hematocrit value of 20% in awake animals (39, 40).

Preoperative blood transfusion should be done at least 24 hours prior to surgery to achieve optimal results. This is particularly important if stored blood products have been administered. As a result of in vitro storage, a reduction in adenosine triphosphate occurs, with an increase in cell rigidity. In addition, a reduction in the activity of 2,3-diphosphoglycerate causes an increased affinity of hemoglobin for oxygen. Preoperative transfusion permits restoration of this activity with 50% return to baseline activity in 24 hours and complete return of activity in 48 hours. During media storage of blood, leakage of potassium into the extracellular space occurs. It has been suggested that transfusion should occur early to permit restoration of baseline electrolyte values prior to surgery (39).

In cases in which coagulation may be a problem, use of fresh blood is preferred to stored units. However, if stored units must be used, then a reduction in Factors V and VIII should be anticipated. Under these conditions, early transfusion is indicated to restore clotting factors (39).

Intraoperative Transfusion. Use of blood and blood products during the intraoperative period is usually associated with acute loss associated with the surgical procedure. In many cases, frank hemorrhage is encountered; under these circumstances, whole blood replacement is indicated to replace the volume loss. Replacement of whole blood becomes a critical issue when more than 20% of the total blood volume is lost from the vascular compartment. Losses less than this value may be safely replaced with crystalloid and colloid solutions in previously healthy patients with minimal consequence. If pre-existing disease or anemia is present, then replacement with blood or blood products may be necessary to maintain homeostasis. This is especially true in cases demonstrating pre-existing cardiovascular or pulmonary disease (39, 40, 41).

Blood losses in excess of 20% will require replacement blood products irrespective of previous health status. Animals that have pre-existing chronic anemias will be intolerant of further insult associated with blood loss during surgery. Replacement therapy should be directed at restoring the oxygen-carrying capacity lost through the surgical wound. Administration of whole blood or packed red cell preparations is the most efficient methods for replacement therapy (39–41).

Intraoperative defects in coagulation may respond to replacement therapy with plasma or platelet preparations. Administration of erythrocytes may be unnecessary and may be undesirable in these cases. Plasma infusion is also indicated in low protein states that may not be associated with reduction in red cell mass (39, 41).

Postoperative Transfusion. The indications for postoperative administration of blood and blood products are similar to those presented under intraoperative transfusion. Most losses encountered during the postoperative period are associated with continuation in hemorrhage from the surgical site. The therapy for hemorrhage may be one or more of the blood components listed above or administration of whole blood.

Components Available for Blood Product Therapy (Table 18.7)

Whole Blood. In veterinary practice, the most common blood product used for therapeutic purposes

Table 18.7.
Available Blood Products[a]

Name	Volume	Contents	Clinical uses
Whole blood	500 ml (1 unit)	Red cells, plasma leukocytes, platelets	Massive blood loss
Packed red blood cells	300 ml	Red cells, some plasma leukocytes, platelets	Anemia, blood loss
Fresh frozen plasma	200 ml	Plasma, coagulation factors	Provide clotting factors
Platelet-rich plasma	50 ml	Platelets, lymphocytes, some plasma	Bleeding due to thrombocytopenia

[a] Adapted from Steinbronn K, Huestis DW: Rational for blood therapy. In Brown, BR (ed): *Fluid and Blood Therapy in Anesthesia*. Philadelphia, FA Davis, 1983, p 154.

is whole blood. Whole blood is popular because it provides essential components required for therapy and is relatively easy to collect and handle. Although whole blood has these desirable properties, there are some drawbacks to its use that must be considered during therapy. Antigenicity, changes in coagulation, metabolic effects of in vitro storage, transfusion reactions, and changes associated with collection techniques and handling have all been reported to occur with blood transfusions. These potential risks must be addressed and minimized for successful blood transfusion to occur (29, 38).

All species have been shown to have red cell-specific antigens that may evoke an immune response after transfusion. Eight major blood group markers have been identified in the dog, with A antigen the most likely to evoke an immune reaction. Three major feline blood groups have been described in the literature. All large animal species have at least one antigen system capable of evoking immune-mediated response. A variable percentage of a species have naturally occurring isoantibodies in serum capable of evoking response. Because of the presence of potential antigens, preadministration screening is indicated to prevent hemolytic reaction. In the dog, commercial screening of potential donors for the presence of A antigen is available. Unfortunately, commercial sources for screening other species are not currently available on a widespread scale. A modified cross match procedure will detect the interaction of major hemolytic antigens. An aliquot of both donor and patient blood is separated by centrifugation. The donor red cells are admixed with recipient plasma and checked for agglutination. This is the major component of the cross match procedure, which will permit the clinician to detect the presence of major antigen groups. The procedure should be continued to check the donor plasma with recipient red cells. If no agglutination is present, then the samples should be incubated at both 4 and 37°C and rechecked in 15 to 20 minutes for the presence of agglutination. If both examinations are negative, then transfusion may be safely performed (38, 42–44).

Many problems associated with blood transfusion are a result of collection, handling, and storage techniques. Problems associated with collection techniques include inappropriate preparation of vascular puncture site, selection of container medium for collection, and method of collection. Collection sites should be aseptically prepared; removal of hair and preparation with surgical scrub solutions should occur prior to collection.

Handling of blood after collection is critical to successful blood therapy management. Blood collection receptacles of glass and plastic may affect whole blood stability. Activation of coagulation factors and platelets have been reported with both plastic bags and glass bottles. Plastic appears to have better preservation of both platelets and coagulation factors than glass. The material of the collection receptacle will affect how blood is collected. Glass bottles are evacuated for collection. Collection under vacuum may cause more injury to erythrocytes than gravity collection techniques. Pump devices permit vacuum collection for plastic bags as well. Similar caution should be observed when using this approach (29, 38).

Storage medium composition will affect viability of blood during the in vitro period (Table 18.8). Both acid-citrate dextrose (ACD) and citrate-phosphate-dextrose (CPD) media are used for long-term storage. Heparin may be used as an anticoagulant for acute transfusion. Blood stored in ACD or CPD has a progressive change in pH; 2,3 DPG activity; potassium levels; platelet viability; and coagulation factors. Microaggregates of platelets and cellular debris also increase with time. Because of these progressive changes, a definite storage time is recommended for whole blood. For ACD media, a limit of 3 weeks is recommended by most authors. For CPD media, up to 4 weeks can be anticipated. A new variant of CPD includes adenine as a component of the medium. Up to 6 weeks storage can be obtained without the development of significant cell lesions. Heparin has the disadvantage of activating platelets, resulting in clumped thrombocytes in the microcirculation. Heparin is not recommended for storage of blood in excess of 48 hours (29, 38, 45–47).

Coagulation defects may be associated with storage

Table 18.8.
Storage Media Characteristics

Name	Composition	Medium pH	70% Erythrocyte Survival Time	Milliliters Solution to Preserve 100 ml of Blood
Acid-citrate-dextrose (ACD)	1.47 g dextrose, 1.32 g citrate salt, 0.48 g citric acid	5.0	28 days	6.6
Citrate-phosphate-dextrose (CPD)	1.61 g dextrose, 1.66 g citrate salt, 0.206 g citrate acid, 0.14 g monobasic sodium phosphate	5.5	28–35 days	7.15
Citrate-phosphate-dextrose-adenine (CPD-A)	CPD components plus 0.25–0.5 mM adenine	5.5	35+ days	7.15
SMB	2.55 g dextrose, 2.63 g sodium citrate, 0.325 g citric acid, 0.222 g sodium debasic phosphate, 0.406 g trisodium phosphate	7.0	49 days	17.5
Sodium heparin	1000 I.U./ml heparin sodium	5.0	48 hours	0.5

and transfusion. Platelet viability and activity diminishes rapidly with in vitro storage. Reduction in platelet activity may be noted as early as 48 hours after storage. Coagulation Factors V and VIII are reduced with time to approximately 50% activity after 21 days of storage. Most authors do not feel that this fact by itself predisposes to coagulation defect. Disseminated intravascular coagulation (DIC) and fibrinolysis have been associated with administration of stored blood. The precise mechanism is unknown; however, multiple factors have been proposed. The inclusion of heparin as the anticoagulant may impair the precipient's coagulation system (41, 47).

Transfusion reactions may occur despite all precautions. Minor transfusion reactions are characterized by fever, chills, and urticaria. These are generally associated with leukocyte antibodies. Supportive therapy and antihistamines are usually satisfactory therapy. Hemolytic reactions are considered a major life-threatening problem. In humans, mortality rates of 40 to 60% have been reported. The principal problems associated with hemolytic reactions include DIC and renal failure. Cardiovascular collapse may be noted during anesthesia. Treatment consists of diuresis, alkalinizing the renal tubules, and cardiovascular support (47).

Plasma. Separation of red blood cells will result in plasma protein fraction. Plasma protein fraction will contain albumin, globulins, coagulation factors, and platelets if acutely prepared. Plasma collection may be performed as a separate procedure from donor animals, or plasma may be harvested from blood units that become outdated. In either case, separation of erythrocytes from plasma must be performed. This may be accomplished by gravitational sedimentation of previously collected blood units, centrifugation of whole blood in anticoagulant medium at 375 × g for 20 minutes, or by use of a constant pressure source, the plasma press. If plastic bags are used to collect blood, they may be purchased with a second accessory pouch into which plasma may be separated. Alternately, an evacuated bottle system with an aspirator-tip tubing set may be used in collecting plasma from whole blood units that have been separated (29).

If further fractionization of plasma into platelet-rich and platelet-poor fractions is desired, then a secondary centrifugation at 2000 × g for 40 minutes is required. Fresh collected blood must be used for this procedure to insure platelet viability. Platelet concentrations should be stored at 4°C to ensure early activity after transfusion (29, 38).

After collection, it is recommended that plasma be stored at −20°C. If maintenance of clotting factors is important, then freezing at −40 to −70°C is recommended. Plasma may be safely stored for up to 1 year. The storage interval of specific components should be restricted to 6 months (29).

Packed Red Blood Cells. Separation of whole blood units immediately after collection results in a concentrated red cell fraction. Hematocrits of 60 to 70% are not unusual after plasma separation has occurred. Packed red cells are indicated for cases in which significant hemorrhage has occurred without development of hypovolemic shock. Many instances in which whole blood is administered for replacement of red cell mass can be managed safely by packed red cell replacement (39, 41).

Administration of packed red cells is facilitated by reconstitution with a crystalloid solution. The selection of the crystalloid solution is based on osmolality and absence of calcium. The best crystalloid solution for reconstitution is 0.9% sodium chloride. The volume used for reconstitution is that necessary to normalize the hematocrit of the packed red cells. If the hematocrit of the stored cells is 70%, then 1:1 normal saline reconstitution should yield a hematocrit of approximately

35% (39, 41). Complications associated with administration of packed red cells are the same as those with whole blood.

Administration

Perioperative administration of blood or blood products should be performed through a vascular catheter. In small animals, a 18G × 2″ catheter should be considered the minimum for dogs and a 20G × 2″ catheter is the minimum for cats for peripheral veins. Jugular catheters are frequently used in larger dogs. In large animal species or in cases where large volume loss is anticipated, placement of a large-gauge catheter in the jugular vein is preferred. Catheter material is secondary if short-term placement is anticipated. If chronic placement is desired, use of Teflon or silastic materials is recommended. A surgical cut-down may be needed in cases of severe hemorrhagic hypovolemia for placement of catheters.

Blood products should be warmed to at least room temperature or, preferably, to 37°C prior to administration. Warming should be by a technique that does not provide excessive heat that may coagulate protein. Temperatures in excess of 56°C may initiate this process. Warm water baths or in-line heating devices serve this purpose in most cases. If massive transfusion is anticipated, whole-unit warming is preferred (29, 38, 48, 49).

The use of in-line filtration is controversial. All commercially available blood administration sets have a mesh filter of approximately 160 μ size. This filter will trap gross clots that have formed in the unit of blood. Stored blood products may form platelet-based aggregates. These microaggregates may, in theory, predispose the recipient to microembolus formation. For this reason, it has been suggested that stored products be filtered as they are administered. This point remains inconclusively proven. Little evidence of clinical sequelae to transfusion of unfiltered blood exists. Small diameter filters may inhibit rapid administration rates. If filters are to be effective, they should be in the 20 to 40 μ range. As a rule of thumb, fresh products do not require filtration; stored products should be filtered (27, 41).

Administration rates will vary with procedure (Table 18.9). Most replacement protocols will be of an acute nature during the perioperative period. Massive, acute replacement of blood during the intraoperative period will amplify complications associated with transfusion therapy. These will be discussed subsequently. As a greater percentage of the patient's blood volume is replaced, the characteristics of blood will approximate the transfusion units. Depletion of coagulation factors and platelet number may occur with acute massive replacement. Replacement therapy with red cell concentrates may result in specific deficiencies in Factors V and VIII. The quantity of blood necessary to produce these effects is variable but will exceed replacement of one blood volume in most cases (41, 47, 50).

Table 18.9.
Formula for Blood Transfusion Volume

Recipient weight = 40 kg
Recipient packed cell volume = 15%
Donor packed cell volume = 45%
Desired packed cell volume = 30%
Total blood volume of recipient, 90 ml/kg × 40 kg = 3600 ml
Existing erythrocyte mass, 3600 ml × 15% = 540 ml
Desired red cell mass, 3600 ml × 30% = 1080 ml
Required red cell mass, 1080 − 540 = 540 ml
Transfusion volume, 540 ml $\times \frac{1}{0.45}$ = 1200 ml

During administration, monitoring for signs of transfusion-associated reactions should be performed. Nausea, vomiting, facial chemosis, coughing, erythema, electrocardiographic changes, and hypotension have all been reported with blood transfusion. Administration should be reduced or stopped if these signs are noted, and the underlying cause should be determined and treated prior to further therapy (41, 47).

Complications of Transfusion

Collection, handling, and storage of blood in vitro may pose potential problems with subsequent reinfusion. Problems associated with transfusion may be subdivided into in vitro changes, coagulation defects, physiological response to administration, and compatibility reactions. Each of these problems may be minimized or treated if there is prior knowledge of their occurrence.

In Vitro Changes. Storage media do not maintain ideal conditions. Changes in ATP concentration and activity of 2,3 DPG occur. The change in 2,3 DPG activity shifts the oxyhemoglobin dissociation curve to the left, theoretically inhibiting oxygen delivery to tissues under in vivo conditions. The magnitude of this change is related to volume and storage time. Experimental studies confirm the inhibition of oxygen delivery for as long as 9 hours after transfusion. Observation of increased cardiac output and cardiac work after transfusion in humans has been noted. However, no specific evidence of tissue organ injury from hypoxia has been documented in any species (47).

Progressive changes in blood pH occur during storage. Both ACD and CPD storage media have pH values in the acid range (Table 18.8). Addition of blood to either medium changes blood pH to approximately 7.0 to 7.1. Erythrocyte metabolism further lowers pH by accumulation of lactic and pyruvic acids as end products of glycolysis. Blood pH declines to 6.6 by 21 days of storage. Part of this change is due to elevated PCO_2 levels of 150 to 220 mm Hg. This is a result of a closed container without provision for escape of CO_2 accumulation. Even when restoration of normal PCO_2 values occur, acidosis is still present. However, buffering will occur in vivo and usually does not require supplemental bicarbonate administration. Metabolism of citrate from the anticoagulant may produce alkalosis. Therefore, empirical administration of bicarbonate with transfusion is not recommended unless coexisting metabolic acidosis is documented prior to transfusion (45, 47, 51).

Coagulation Defects. Dilutional thrombocytopenia is the most frequent coagulation defect in man. At storage temperatures of 4°C, platelets are damaged sufficiently to be absorbed by the reticuloendothelial system soon after infusion. Remaining platelets have a reduced survival time. Platelet activity diminishes by 50% within 6 hours postcollection in cold blood. Platelet activity 24 to 48 hours after storage is only 5% of normal. Multiple unit transfusion accentuates this observation, with hemorrhagic diathesis occurring if platelet levels fall below 50,000/mm^3. Acutely induced thrombocytopenia appears to be less tolerated than chronically induced disease. Hemorrhagic tendencies must be monitored during multiple unit transfusions (47).

Most coagulation factors remain stable during blood storage. Factors V and VIII have been shown in humans to decrease to 15 to 50% of normal after 21 days of storage. The decrease per se has not been shown to cause clinically significant hemorrhagic diathesis; however, such deficiencies may be additive to other causes of bleeding (47).

DIC has been reported after shock and massive blood replacement. The pathogenesis of DIC differs little from other inciting causes. Release of tissue products, toxins, and thromboplastin may lead to generalized activation of the coagulation system. Hemolytic transfusion reaction may also be signaled by hemorrhagic diathesis (47).

Diagnosis of coagulation defects is limited to laboratory evaluation. Thrombocytopenia, as previously noted, is the most frequent cause. Platelet count and administration of platelet-rich plasma can reverse the course of hemorrhage. Plasma fibrinogen levels may indicate the presence of DIC. Heparin therapy and consumed clotting factors (Factor VIII) may be indicated. Factor provision should be deferred until the effectiveness of heparin therapy is determined by reevaluating platelet numbers and fibrinogen levels. If a return toward normal values is noted along with decreased bleeding intensity, response to therapy is confirmed (31, 47).

Physiologic Responses. In addition to the development of in vitro acidemia during blood storage procedures, in vivo acidosis has been suggested. Massive blood transfusion (greater than five units in man) necessitates evaluation of arterial pH and PCO_2 levels. Correction should be performed only if severe metabolic acidosis is noted (31, 47).

Citrate intoxication has been documented during blood transfusion. Intravascular binding of ionized calcium is the mechanism involved. Rapid multiple unit transfusion increases risk. Signs referable to citrate intoxication include hypotension, poor pulse quality, elevated central venous pressure, electrocardiogram abnormalities, and clotting deficiencies. These signs, if present, are transient; serum calcium levels return to normal as citrate is metabolized by the liver. Infusion rates of 1 unit of blood/10-minute time period appear to increase risk. Slower infusion rates have a low incidence of citrate intoxication. If citrate intoxication is suspected, administration of calcium salts will minimize the clinical signs (47).

Potassium levels also increase in stored blood and may be as high as 32 meq/liter in blood stored for 21 days. Elevation in serum potassium levels may be noted if administration rates exceed 120 ml/min. Extravascular diffusion and renal elimination account for potassium ion balance during transfusion (31, 47).

Infusion of cold (4°C) blood can decrease the recipient's body temperature. If core temperature decreases to less than 30°C, ventricular dysrhythmias and cardiac arrest can occur. Warming blood to body temperature prior to administration minimizes this risk. Immersion of the intravenous line in a warm water bath or attachment of a tubing length to a heating pad are two methods of adding heat. Warm baths to raise the blood temperature prior to administration is also effective (47, 48).

Transfusion Reactions. These were discussed under whole blood therapy.

Sepsis. Improper handling of blood permits bacterial contamination and growth. Administration of contaminated blood may be accompanied by endotoxin production, resulting in endotoxic shock and DIC. Blood cultures should be performed if contamination is suspected after transfusion. Discard blood that may be contaminated prior to administration (27, 52).

AUTOTRANSFUSION

Autotransfusion is the technique of collection, processing, and reinfusion of the animal's own blood in order to maintain circulatory volume. Autotransfusion may be performed by several methods. Preoperative collection and storage can be performed on an elective, short-term basis, until the animal's surgical requirements arise. Immediate preoperative collection and hemodilution with crystalloid solution is another method described. Probably the most common form of autotransfusion in veterinary medicine is intraoperative blood salvage and retransfusion to decrease the necessity of homologous blood transfusion (31).

Advantages

Autotransfusion may be performed under circumstances in which adequate quantities of stored homologous blood or typed donors are not available. Salvage of blood from body cavities or surgical sites minimizes the risk of transmitting infectious agents; prevents isoimmunization to cell, platelet, or protein antigens; minimizes graft-versus-host transfusion reactions; and provides a ready source of warm, fresh, compatible blood. Reinfusion of humoral agents may afford a greater immunological response to the introduction of infectious agents than homologous blood transfusion.

The viability of erythrocytes is better maintained with autotransfusion. Experimental studies demonstrate similar survival times between erythrocytes subjected to autotransfusion and normal erythrocytes. Levels of 2,3 DPG have also been shown to be no different in autotransfused blood. Autotransfusion in many cases circumvents the complications related to administration of hypothermic blood. Finally, reinfusion of collected blood is valuable when the blood bank is inadequate and massive hemorrhage related to surgery is anticipated. Reinfusion of collected blood may prove life-saving in those cases (53, 54).

Techniques of Autotransfusion

Under most circumstances, elective precollection for future use will not occur. Most indications for autotransfusion will be related to acute, closed cavity hemorrhage from trauma or surgery. Autotransfusion is considered when sterile, uncontaminated wound hemorrhage is present, malignant cells are absent, and minimal contact of blood with the wound surface is anticipated. Several different techniques have been described for autotransfusion. Some systems and technologies are not feasible for the average veterinary practice. The techniques described here are adaptable to many practice settings (53, 54).

Autotransfusion requires a vacuum source for blood collection. In the simplest form, a large capacity sterile syringe is acceptable. A basic approach involves a collection catheter, intravenous tubing, a multiple port stopcock (four-way), and a blood filter. The syringe acts as an aspirator and infusion pump. A second syringe containing heparin is used to provide anticoagulant for collected blood. Additional details of the procedure are described by Crowe (53).

Most other techniques require the availability of an adjustable vacuum device. Electrical, water faucet, or central vacuum pumps can be a vacuum source. Several relatively inexpensive devices can be made or purchased; 500-ml glass bottles can be adapted for this purpose and are commercially available as chest drainage bottles. After sterilization, 37.5 ml of ACD solution of 2% sodium citrate is added. Attaching this bottle in series with the vacuum source and collection of blood by suction handle or implanted drain is performed. After collection, reinfusion occurs using in-line filtration of macroaggregates. Commercially available units (Sorenson Labs, Salt Lake City, Utah) use similar principles of collection and reinfusion. Their advantage is the use of plastic containers in place of glass. Cost is higher for the commercial apparatus. Other devices, used for humans, incorporate suction devices and options for cell separation and washing. Their cost is prohibitive in veterinary medicine at the current time (53, 54).

Complications of Autotransfusion

Complications arise from the handling of blood during collection and reinfusion. In-line filtration of blood is recommended to prevent infusion of cell debris and microaggregates represented by fat, plasma lipoproteins, platelet and leukocyte clumps, and red cell-fibrin complexes. A dual filter technique using a 170 μ filter followed by a 40 μ filter has proven effective in this application. However, chemically active substances represented by serotonin, histamine, kinins, and catecholamines liberated from cell injury may interact to impair lung function in the posttransfusion period (53).

Hemoglobinemia and hemoglobinuria may result from erythrolysis and hemoglobin liberation from mechanical injury. High negative pressure, foaming, and suction line turbulence are contributory. Therapy to prevent nephrotoxicity from free hemoglobin is described elsewhere (53, 54).

Alteration in coagulation may be noted posttransfusion. The potential for coagulation activation and development of DIC has been reported from autotransfusion. Thrombocytopenia, depression of Factors V and VIII, and hypofibrinogenemia have been reported. However, the overall incidence is low (53).

Sepsis and infusion of neoplastic cells have been documented with autotransfusion. Adherence to aseptic technique and knowledge of tumor presence minimizes risk (53, 54).

COMPLICATIONS OF INTRAVENOUS THERAPY

Specific contraindications and precautions have been described as a part of individual therapies. In addition, complications common to intravenous therapy have been documented. These factors are highlighted in the subsequent discussion.

Volume Overload

Acute overhydration may be encountered in aggressive fluid therapy protocols. Small weight animals may have a greater disposition toward overhydration because the margin of error in fluid administration is less than in larger animals. Studies in normal dogs and cats suggest that administration rates of 45 ml/lb/hr (90 ml/kg/hr) may be tolerated for brief time intervals of about 1 hour without adverse reactions. Higher rates may be tolerated in healthy dogs for brief intervals if hemodynamic monitoring is used. Cats do not tolerate overhydration as well as dogs. Animals with significant cardiovascular disease, renal disease, Cushing's disease, pulmonary disease, or chronic depletion of fluid and electrolytes will be intolerant of high administration rates. The use of isotonic fluids such as 0.9% NaCl or lactated Ringer's solution may induce overhydration by retention of administered fluids within the intravascular space. Selection of fluid composition and administration rates should be made with a concern for these factors (25, 55).

Fluid administration rate must be monitored in high risk patients. Measurement of central venous pressure will provide information regarding response to fluid administration rate. Central venous pressure (CVP) measurement has limitations in cases of isolated left heart failure or biventricular failure. Placement of a catheter into the pulmonary artery and monitoring of pulmonary capillary wedge pressure are valuable in these cases. The normal mean value for CVP is 0.5 cm H_2O, with values up to 10 to 15 cm H_2O noted in high administration rate volume replacement therapy. In general, it is best not to exceed CVP values of 10 to 12 cm H_2O except in emergency replacement protocols. Pulmonary capillary wedge pressures range from 2 to 20 mm Hg, and measurements can be used to estimate the tendency to form pulmonary edema by subcategorizing low (<7 mm Hg), optimal (10 to 14 mm Hg), or elevated (>20 mm Hg) venous pressures and adjusting administration rates appropriately (56).

Clinical signs of overhydration may include cough, moist rales on pulmonary field auscultation, tissue chemosis, hypothermia, and alteration in mental status (water intoxication). Re-evaluation of fluid therapy goals, calculated administration rate, and current patient status is imperative to prevent further complications. Therapy may include discontinuation of fluids, treatment for pulmonary edema (with oxygen, bronchodilators, or diuretics), thermal support, and assessment of serum electrolyte values (56, 57).

Air Embolus

Venous air embolism is a dramatic complication of parenteral fluid administration. In people, infusion of 70 to 100 ml/sec for 2 to 3 seconds may produce sudden death from cor pulmonale. Peripheral venous infusion using a nonpressurized system is unlikely to create conditions of large volume air introduction. However, smaller quantities may be introduced and can create complications under specific conditions. Use of flexible, nonventilated containers has been reported to minimize this complication; however, administration set-catheter disconnection may allow air entrance. Central venous catheters pose a greater risk of air embolism. Aspiration of air during initial venipuncture can occur if the site of introduction is elevated relative to the level of the right atrium. Disconnection of the catheter hub-administration set interface may produce a similar complication (58, 59).

Particulate Matter

Particulate contamination occurs in commercially prepared solutions. The presence of rubber, metal fragments, fibers, mold, and plastics has been reported. The introduction of glass fragments from ampules opened to mix in the administered fluids and coring of rubber injection ports from large-bore needles have been described. Improved manufacturing techniques have diminished production-related contamination. Particles as small as 12 μ may become entrapped in the pulmonary vacular bed (58).

Few data regarding the implication of particulate matter infusion have been reported. Probably pulmonary entrapment of particles occurs in most cases. Reports have appeared regarding pulmonary hypertension and respiratory failure related to parenteral fluid administration. Particulate-mediated pulmonary edema in certain patients has been anecdotally suggested in the absence of other possible etiologies. The frequency of these findings has not been documented. This complication has been minimized by the use of in-line microfiltration (58, 59).

Chemical Contamination

Plasticizers used in the production of polyvinyl chloride containers have been reported to leach from the plastic into the solution and to accumulate in tissues. The significance of this finding and long-term implications of plasticizer toxicity have not been established (58, 60).

Admixture Incompatibility

Numerous studies of component incompatibility with added pharmacological agents, electrolytes, acidifying or alkalinizing agents, and antimicrobials have been reported. Various charts and tables have been prepared by fluid manufacturers and others detailing admixture incompatibility. As a general rule, dextrose preparations are safe to add in most instances; electrolyte-containing solutions appear to be least compatible. The reader is referred to the references cited for further information on this topic (58, 59).

CHRONIC CATHETERIZATION AND INFUSION CARE

Administration of long-term intravenous therapy requires management and care of the implanted catheter. Depending upon the composition of the fluid to be infused and the goals of therapy, either peripheral or central implantation sites may be used. Irrespective of the site selected, the materials for catheter construction are the same for all commercial catheter designs, and knowledge of their biological reaction is useful in their selection and use.

Presently, materials available for catheter construction are derivatives of plastic monomers (polyethylene or polyvinyl) or fluorinated hydrocarbon derivatives (Teflon) and silicone (Silastic). All classes of material are flexible and biologically inert during chronic tissue implantation. However, numerous reports suggest that intravascular catheterization can be associated with complications, some of which may be related to the thrombogenic potential of these materials. Experimental data suggest that intraluminal introduction of any material evokes a rapid, platelet-mediated fibrin deposition of the external surface of the catheter. This may be noted as soon as 15 minutes after catheter placement and may plateau by 40 minutes. The fibrin sheath remains for the duration of catheter implantation and dislodges upon removal. The freed thrombi may migrate in the venous blood, resulting in subclinical pulmonary emboli. Heparin bonding to the catheter surface may briefly impede this fibrin aggregation; however, little advantage is realized with long-term implantation. Of the three materials, silicone has the lowest complication rate (61, 62).

The cephalic and lateral tarsal peripheral veins may be selected as cannulation sites when isotonic solutions are used. Hypertonic solutions using a dextrose base should be given at a central venous site. Percutaneous or surgical catheter implantation of the anterior vena cava via the external jugular vein is recommended (63).

Placement techniques for long- and short-term cannulas differ. Wound care and implantation under aseptic conditions are critical to prevent complications. The proposed implantation site is prepared aseptically using three successive surgical scrubs of povidone-iodine with a water rinse after each scrub. After the final scrub, povidone-iodine solution or tincture of iodine should be applied. The site of venipuncture is barrier draped, and aseptic surgical technique is used for catheter placement. The operator wears surgical gloves and performs catheter venipuncture using standard technique. An occlusive dressing with povidone-iodine ointment is placed over the venipuncture site, and the catheter is secured by either single ligature fixation to the skin using monofilament suture material or incorporation into a bandage dressing. A protective cover made of materials with minimal absorptive properties is applied, and continuous care is given. Every 1 or 2 days (or more frequently, if gross soiling is observed), the dressing is removed, and the venipuncture site is examined for erythema, induration, or other signs of infection. Using aseptic technique and surgical gloves, the skin around the wound is cleansed, and antibiotic or antimicrobial ointment and a new occlusive dressing is applied. Changing administration sets and venipuncture sites may be considered at this time (64).

If wound care is appropriate and no clinical signs of catheter-related sepsis are noted, sequential venous rotation on a regular basis is not mandatory. Central venous placement of catheters in humans has been maintained for as long as 55 days at one site with minimal complications when good catheter care was observed. Catheters have been implanted in dogs for as long as 100 days with appropriate care. Complications associated with chronic cannulation of peripheral veins have not been reported. If intimal injury from hypertonic solutions occurs, thrombophlebitis may be noted as soon as 48 to 72 hours after catheter placement (65, 66).

Continued nursing care is critical to maintenance of aseptic cannulation. The entire administration apparatus should be considered a closed system. Infusion catheters should not be used for the administration of pharmacological agents, blood sampling, and physiological measurements such as CVP. All connections and the administration set should be continuously disinfected. Each reservoir change should include cleaning of both the administration part of the bottle or bag and the coupling terminal of the administration apparatus with povidone-iodine. Each time a junction is disconnected, both ends should be cleansed prior to reattachment. The administration set and in-line filter should be changed every 24 hours or whenever it is contaminated. Any accidental disconnection should be treated as a septic break, and the administration apparatus and solution must be replaced. Contamination of the catheter site merits either replacement or rotation of the catheter to an alternate site. Although these procedures may seem extreme, sepsis in the debilitated patient has extreme consequences (67).

Catheter-Related Complications

Sepsis. Chronic catheter implantation has been reported to be associated with numerous complications, many of which are preventable with good catheter care. Catheter-related sepsis is the more frequent complication. Inadequate preparation or maintenance of the catheter site may result in bacterial or fungal sepsis. In the dog, Gram-negative species account for the majority of contaminations in inadequately prepared venipuncture sites. Antibiotic ointments in the occlusive dressings inhibit bacterial growth but allow fungal multiplication. Occlusive dressings with antimicrobial agents (tame iodophor ointment) have been recommended to inhibit both bacterial and fungal sepsis (67–69).

Unexplained pyrexia, leukocytosis, chills, glucose intolerance, alterations in level of consciousness, and generalized deterioration of the patient's condition are all clinical signs noted with sepsis. Hematogenous dissemination from a septic anatomical site may be an additional factor. It should be determined whether sepsis is catheter-related or whether it arises from a secondary anatomical site. Catheter-related sepsis is usually noted shortly after implantation. Fibrin sheaths surround the catheter during the first 3 to 5 days after implantation. After this time, bacterial colonization of the catheter from remote sites is difficult. Introduction of cutaneous organisms during venipuncture and migration from the venipuncture site down the catheter shaft have been suggested. Removal of the administration system and solution container is mandatory. Antibiotic infusion through a contaminated catheter is not therapeutic. After removal, culture of the catheter, administration apparatus, and solution is suggested. In humans, removal of a contaminated catheter is accompanied by remission of pyrexia in 12 to 24 hours. A new catheter is aseptically implanted at an alternate site. In cases of a refractive pyrexia (greater than 24 hours) or secondary catheter sepsis from a remote anatomical site, antibiotics should be administered, if not previously initiated for other reasons. Blood cultures should also be considered in cases of refractive fever (67–69).

Thrombophlebitis. Thrombophlebitis and vascular occlusion have been associated with chronic catheterization. Chemical and mechanical factors may predispose the patient to this complication. Hypertonic solutions may induce endothelial irritation and stimulate platelet accumulation. Peripheral veins are especially susceptible, owing the disparity between the catheter diameter and the venous lumen. This disparity results in low blood flow and retarded dilution of hypertonic solutions, causing vascular irritation and thrombophlebitis. Mechanical injury to the endothelium from catheter placement may be interactive (66, 67, 70).

Several recommendations have been proposed to minimize thrombophlebitis. A study comparing four catheter materials showed a lower incidence of complications when fluoroethylenepropylene or Silastic was used as a catheter material. These materials are superior to plastic, polyvinylchloride, and tetrafluoroethylene as a catheter material. The addition of heparin (500 units) and hydrocortisone (1 mg/liter or parenteral solution) decreased thrombophlebitis in peripheral veins. In-line filtering to prevent infusion of particulate matter was reported to decrease vascular complications. Venipuncture may also create mechanical injury and tissue thromboplastin release. This injury secondarily creates platelet aggregation and promotes thrombus formation (71).

Acid-Base Balance

COMPONENTS OF ACID-BASE REGULATION

Maintenance of cellular function requires an exacting environment. Temperature, osmolarity, electrolyte concentration, nutrients, and oxygen all must be maintained within narrow limits to permit normal metabolic function. One of the most important factors in this environment is the hydrogen ion concentration (H^+), a byproduct of normal metabolism. Substances that can donate hydrogen ion are called *acids*; substances that can receive hydrogen ion are called *bases*. A constant interaction between acids and bases occurs in vivo to maintain systemic homeostasis. A substance that prevents extreme changes in free hydrogen ion concentration within a solution is called a *buffer*. Buffers allow normal cell function to continue unimpeded when cells are subjected to significant changes in hydrogen ion number (72–78).

Although pH reflects static results, it does not contribute to an understanding of dynamics and quantification of acid-base balance. This relationship is described by the Henderson-Hasselbach equation. This equation expresses a relationship of acids and conjugate base substances:

$$K = \frac{(H^+)(A^-)}{(HA)}$$

describing a relationship between dissociated and undissociated components of a chemical buffer system. K is the ionization constant of that system. Transformation of this equation can be performed to yield:

$$(H^+) = K\,\frac{(HA)}{(A^-)}$$

which in turn can be expressed in log form as:

$$-\text{Log}\,(H^+) = -\text{Log}\,K + \text{Log}\,\frac{(A^-)}{(HA)}$$

or

$$pH = pK + \log \frac{(Base)}{(Acid)}$$

This last form, the Henderson-Hasselbach equation, is the foundation for discussion of acid-base physiology.

Most domestic species have a blood pH near 7.4. If blood pH falls (hydrogen ion increase), this is acidemia. Elevation in blood pH (hydrogen ion decrease) is alkalemia. The terms "acidosis" and "alkalosis" are commonly interchanged with "acidemia" and "alkalemia" to describe biochemical alteration. Acidosis refers to a medically significant gain in acid or loss of base from the body. Alkalosis means a medically significant loss of acid or gain of base by the body. Gains and losses are not necessarily paralleled by blood pH, which only measure net effect. It is possible to have an alkalemia in an animal with a generalized intracellular acidosis.

Metabolism produces a continuous source of acidic byproducts that challenge the buffering capacity of any species. The predominant species generated is hydrogen ion; short chain organic acids also contribute to acidity. To maintain homeostasis, acid production is constantly "neutralized" by a series of buffer systems. The buffers involved in response to acid production include bicarbonate, hemoglobin, plasma protein, and phosphates.

Bicarbonate

The bicarbonate system is the predominant and most quickly responding buffering mechanism. It is, in addition, the most complex and integrated system for buffering of both volatile and fixed acid components. The bicarbonate system is the only "open" buffer system. Buffered acids may be subsequently excreted by pulmonary or renal routes. The bicarbonate system can be represented as follows:

$$CO_2 + H_2O \rightleftharpoons H_2CO_3 \rightleftharpoons H^+ + HCO_3^-$$

This equation is referred to as the hydration equation. An interrelationship between metabolic acid (H^+ ion) and carbon dioxide allows for chemical transformation of a metabolic product (fixed acid) into a volatile product (carbon dioxide). In addition, production of carbon dioxide (volatile acid) can be transformed to a fixed product for more efficient systemic transport to the organs of excretion. Owing to physical laws governing gas solubility in fluids, much less carbon dioxide carrying capacity can exist from solubility than can occur by transformation of carbon dioxide into a chemical byproduct. Thus, carbon dioxide can be transformed into bicarbonate at the cellular level for transportation to sites of elimination. When the sites of excretion are reached, reconversion to volatile acid can occur for ultimate elimination by ventilation. Virtually all produced acid is handled in this manner. Various ratios of excretion by pulmonary and metabolic routes have been reported; however, the lung is at least 1000-fold more active in acid excretion than other routes in the homeostatic situation. Free bicarbonate is re-established upon elimination of carbon dioxide.

The bicarbonate system can be represented in the generalized Henderson-Hasselbach equation. The relationship of carbon dioxide value (pCO_2) and H_2CO_3 in body fluids is such that H_2CO_3 is proportional to pCO_2 (in torr). The factor of 0.03 is the proportionally constant of carbon dioxide (H_2CO_3) that relates CO_2 and carbonic acid. Relatively little CO_2 can be carried by physical solution. Thus the equation becomes:

$$pH = 6.1 + \text{Log} \frac{(HCO_3)}{(H_2CO_3) + (CO_2)} = \frac{(HCO_3)}{0.03 \times pCO_2}$$

Assuming a normal pCO_2 value of 40 torr:

$$pH = 6.1 + \text{Log} \frac{(HCO_3)}{40 \times 0.03} = 1.2$$

Observed values of bicarbonate are approximately 24 meq/liter at pH of 7.4. Thus, a constant relationship:

$$7.4 = 6.1 + \text{Log} \frac{24}{1.2}$$

$$1.3 = \text{Log } 20$$

is established for the bicarbonate system. Stated alternatively:

$$pH_\alpha \frac{(HCO_3)}{(CO_2)}$$

This ratio is useful in interpretation of blood gas data and will be referred to later.

Hemoglobin

The bicarbonate-carbonic acid system is important in regulation of acid-base balance and is easily sampled for in vitro analysis. However, early investigations determined that separated blood plasma was not as efficient in buffering acid as whole blood and that some metabolic acids could not be volatilized. Therefore, alternate systems must exist to deal with these observations. Other systems observed in blood include phosphate, plasma protein, and hemoglobin buffers.

Hemoglobin is a complex molecule with 540 amino acid residues in its structure, 36 of which are histidine. The imidizole subunit of histidine possesses chemical properties that allow for combination of hydrogen ion on an amine group. This combination is a reversible process and has pK values in the physiological range. In addition, N-terminal valine groups have a pK of 7.8 and can serve as buffer sites. When fixed acids are buffered, approximately 60% of the buffering capacity resides in the hemoglobin buffer system, with 30% in the bicarbonate buffer system. The remaining 10% is provided by organic phosphate buffers that are intracellular. The hemoglobin buffer system is integral in buffering carbonic acid.

Addition of oxygen onto the hemoglobin molecule changes the pK of the hemoglobin buffer system. This change is a result of differences in stereochemical configuration of the hemoglobin molecule. Hemoglobin stereochemistry is related to interactions between oxygen, carbon dioxide, and hemoglobin. This stereochemical change facilitates smooth uptake and delivery of oxygen and carbon dioxide. Buffering capacity is slightly affected as the system pK is altered.

The erythrocyte has the enzyme carbonic anhydrase to facilitate bicarbonate and carbonic acid interaction. Because CO_2 is freely diffusible through cell membrane surface, diffusion into the erythrocyte initiates the mass action equation with formation of new bicarbonate ion. This ion migrates to the extracellular space in exchange for chloride ion (chloride shift), representing new bicarbonate formation.

Protein

Plasma proteins provide a broad spectrum of histidine residue buffer pairs with a range of pK ranging from 5.5 to 8.5. Their function is similar to that in the hemoglobin system. Plasma proteins are a heterogenous group of buffers that are generally conceptualized as a single entity. The contribution of this sytem to total buffering capacity is relatively small, however. Proteins can buffer acids of both respiratory and nonrespiratory origin, making them valuable in counteracting effects of carbonic acid in plasma spaces.

Phosphate

The phosphate buffer system is qualitatively similar to the bicarbonate buffer system. This system is capable of buffering both strong and weak alkali components. However, its contribution is limited by its relatively low concentration of phosphate in plasma. Its main importance is acid-base balance in renal tubules. It is also an important buffer system in intracellular fluids due to increased concentration of phosphate.

Distribution of Buffers

Buffering systems are not equally distributed in all body spaces. Extracellular fluid has the bicarbonate, protein, and phosphate systems. Intracellular fluid (including erythrocytes) has hemoglobin, phosphate, and protein buffering systems. Bicarbonate buffer does not occur in significant amounts except in cells in which carbonic anhydrase activity is present, such as erythrocytes, renal tubular cells, and choroid plexus. Interstitial fluid (lymph) has a high concentration of bicarbonate buffer. In bone, the calcium hydroxyapatite matrix can participate in buffering of hydrogen ion in acute or chronic acidosis. This occurs at the expense of solubilizing bone minerals and conversion of one insoluble salt form to another.

PULMONARY ACID-BASE BALANCE

Regulation of Ventilation

Maintenance of carbon dioxide partial pressure (pCO_2) under physiological conditions requires a feedback control mechanism to regulate carbon dioxide levels and, indirectly, acid-base balance (79–83). This regulation necessitates an integrated neurological response of both central and peripheral chemoceptor components sensitive to carbon dioxide. Extreme sensitivity to changes in carbon dioxide is apparent in the immediate response in effective ventilation to fluctuations in blood carbon dioxide levels. The control mechanism is comprised of both peripheral (carotid and aortic body) and central components; the relative contribution of each is still uncertain. Central chemoceptors located on the ventral surface of the medulla are sensitive to alteration in cerebrospinal fluid pH changes mediated by carbon dioxide tension. Elevated carbon dioxide levels diffuse across the blood-brain barrier and interact to influence hydrogen ion concentration. This mechanism is thought to be the predominant stimulus for augmented ventilation. Peripheral chemoceptor response to elevation in carbon dioxide is mediated through cranial nerve reflexes that augment ventilatory response. Thus, an integrated response is initiated when arterial carbon dioxide levels increase. This response is blunted during use of anesthetic drugs. Many preanesthetic, induction, and maintenance agents decrease the central and peripheral sensitivity to carbon dioxide levels, which will be effectively increased during the use of these agents.

Arterial Carbon Dioxide Tension

Arterial carbon dioxide tension is the direct and immediate reflection of alveolar ventilation in relation to metabolic rate. Elevated carbon dioxide tension can usually be attributed to increased metabolic rate or diminished effective ventilation. If blood carbon dioxide level is higher than normal, a decreased elimination due to hypoventilation is assumed to be the cause. Conversely, an increased elimination (hyperventilation) is assumed if the measured blood carbon dioxide is low.

In contrast to oxygen, the shape of the carbon dioxide dissociation curve is relatively linear over the physiological range. This permits a greater compensatory capacity of the lung to balance pCO_2 values between areas of high and low ventilation-perfusion disturbance. Thus, $PaCO_2$ values may be relatively normal in the presence of even moderately severe lung disease resulting from ventilation-perfusion abnormalities.

Pulmonary elimination of carbon dioxide (volatile acids) is a major component in acid-base balance. The excretion of volatile acid (CO_2) is mediated through the mass action equation:

$$CO_2 + H_2O \rightleftharpoons H_2CO_3 \rightleftharpoons H^+ + HCO_3^-$$

Carbon dioxide is carried as bicarbonate, carbaminohemoglobin, carbonic acid, and physically dissolved gas in both arterial and venous blood. An increase in one component of the above equation causes a proportional elevation in all other component concentrations. Ineffective alveolar ventilation creates retention of carbon dioxide and effectively induces retention of hydrogen ion (acidosis). Conversely, increased alveolar ventilation enhances removal of carbon dioxide and effectively reduces hydrogen ion concentration (alkalosis). Thus, the pulmonary system plays an indispensible role in moment-to-moment regulation of acid-base balance. This can be appreciated by comparing the effects of respiratory and metabolic lesions. Apnea (ventilatory failure) is accompanied by a rapid deterioration in acid-base balance; renal failure requires several hours to days to achieve similar effects. Thus, respiratory acid-base balance is integrally linked to effective alveolar ventilation. Normal values for arterial carbon dioxide in the awake animal are 36.8 ± 3.0 in the dog and 31.0 ± 2.9 in the cat.

METABOLIC ACID-BASE BALANCE

Renal Regulation of Acid-Base Balance

Acute alterations in pCO_2 are of pulmonary origin, whereas changes in bicarbonate ion concentration and, indirectly, buffer base reflect renal regulation and excretion of fixed (noncarbonic) acids. Both processes are interrelated through the Henderson-Hasselbach equation, with pulmonary regulation controlling the denominator and metabolic regulation controlling the numerator. The net result of extracellular fluid bicarbonate buffering is the formation of acid anions. The anion generated in this process ultimately undergoes renal elimination. The overall process would deplete whole body buffer base unless regeneration or conservation of bicarbonate occurs. The pathways associated with this process interact by eliminating fixed acids intact and conserving bicarbonate buffer (75, 78, 82, 84–88).

Acid Excretion. There is a continuous production of hydrogen ion as a result of normal metabolism. Hydrogen ion initially interacts with plasma buffer base, resulting in consumption of bicarbonate and other buffers. The kidneys are principally responsible for excretion of the hydrogen ion resulting from endogenous metabolism. As hydrogen ion is eliminated, conservation of bicarbonate occurs on a 1:1 basis. The kidney thus regenerates the bicarbonate used in neutralization of endogenous acid. This process occurs in a balanced manner providing the animal is normal in acid-base balance initially and is constant in dietary intake.

The quantity of hydrogen ion excreted can be measured by titrating the urine to neutral pH (7.4) and adding the amount of ammonium ion present in the urine. The amount of alkali required to titrate hydrogen ion carriers is the titratable acidity (TA) of the urine. The sum of TA and ammonium ion excreted is the total urinary acid excretion. This amount is also equivalent to the quantity of bicarbonate ion lost in this process. In people, 50 meq/day of hydrogen ion is removed by this process. This represents approximately 0.2% of total hydrogen ion loss per day. Hydrogen ion eliminated by this route, as reflected in urine pH, is approximately 400 to 800 times more acidic than plasma, thus signifying a steep concentration gradient. The quantity of hydrogen ion lost through the urine is proportional to the quantity of urinary buffers available to bind protons.

In addition to excretion of hydrogen ion, the kidney generates approximately 5000 meq of bicarbonate per day be reabsorption of filtered bicarbonate load. The kidney excretes hydrogen ion through resorption of bicarbonate, excretion of ammonium ion, and excretion of titratable acidity. In addition, potassium ion and extracellular fluid volume have significant influence on renal acid-base balance.

Bicarbonate Reabsorption. Bicarbonate undergoes a dynamic, interrelated regulation in the nephron unit. Reabsorption takes place through hydrogen ion secretion and selective recirculation of bicarbonate ion. Bicarbonate is delivered, primarily as the sodium salt, to the renal tubular lumen by glomerular filtration. Hydrogen ion present in the lumen interacts with bicarbonate ion to form water and carbon dioxide. These products are membrane permeable and diffuse into the proximal tubular epithelium and eventually venous blood. In the proximal tubular cell, bicarbonate and hydrogen ions are reformed by the corollary reaction, and differential transfer of bicarbonate ion to plasma occurs. As hydrogen ion is excreted, disturbance in electroneutrality occurs, which is rectified by resorption of sodium ion from the tubular lumen. The exact mechanism of this sodium-hydrogen exchange is not fully understood. Sodium may play a role in initiating an exchange with hydrogen ion, thus providing a driving pressure for the reaction. This reaction is rate-limited, as plasma bicarbonate values in excess of 27 to 28 meq/liter are accompanied by increased excretion of bicarbonate ion.

Bicarbonate resorption is related to a variety of regulatory factors. Extracellular volume (ECV) is a major controlling factor. Expansion of ECV inhibits sodium and, secondarily, bicarbonate resorption. Potassium is interrelated to bicarbonate levels and appears to control bicarbonate resorption intrinsically independent of ECV. Plasma pCO_2 affects bicarbonate resorption by changes in intracellular hydrogen ion concentration. Glucose levels affect bicarbonate resorption by unknown mechanisms. Elevated blood glucose levels enhance bicarbonate resorption in normal dogs. Parathyroid hormone (PTH), calcium, and phosphorous also influence bicarbonate resorption. Elevation in PTH levels depress and increased calcium levels enhance resorption by alteration in hydrogen ion secretion. Phosphorous responds in similar fashion. Aldosterone enhances acid excretion and indirectly enhances bicarbonate resorption.

Ammonium Ion. Bicarbonate conservation may also occur in distal renal tubules where intraluminal volumes are diminished and the previous interaction is exhausted. To further conserve bicarbonate, ammonia (NH_3) formed from amino acid deamination diffuses into the tubular cells and combines with hydrogen ion to form ammonium (NH_4^+). By this process, ammonia is acting as a urine buffer. Once NH_4^+ is formed, it penetrates cell membrane poorly and remains in the tubular lumen. Thus, a unidirectional flow is established.

Ammonium excretion is influenced by urine pH and metabolic acidosis. Infusion of sodium bicarbonate or acetazolamide has been shown to reduce NH_4^+ formation. Chronic metabolic acidosis favors greater deamination of glutamine furthering NH_3 production. This enhances the contribution of ammonia to acid excretion and attenuates further bicarbonate loss.

Titratable Acidity. Weak anions of mono- and di-basic phosphate interact with hydrogen ions to further preserve bicarbonate loss. The interaction of this group is commonly considered titratable acidity. In general, a majority of phosphates in the tubular lumen are of the dibasic variety that become monobasic by the acceptance of hydrogen ion. Titratable acidity can be influenced by buffer system pK, buffer quantity, and urine pH. Buffer system pK and pH interact in a manner where the system is most efficient at urine pH in the range of 6.8 to 7.4. As urine pH diminishes, a lower proportion of dibasic phosphate is present, diminishing buffering capacity of this component.

Potassium Ion. Potassium ion is also regulated by renal tubular cells and has an important role in acid-base physiology. Potassium is inversely exchanged with hydrogen ion on a one-to-one basis. Potassium is resorbed in proximal renal tubular cells in passive process and is reabsorbed in the loop of Henle as an active process. When plasma potassium concentration is elevated from hydrogen ion entry into the intracellular space, liberation of sodium and potassium in the extracellular space occurs. Acid secretion by the kidney is depressed, along with low bicarbonate retention, which results in hypokalemic alkalosis.

Extracellular Fluid Volume. The kidneys can regulate the bicarbonate concentration in plasma indirectly by altering extracellular fluid volume. This effect occurs only in extreme cases because other non-bicarbonate buffers generally attenuate bicarbonate system disturbance. Rapid volume expansion with sodium-containing fluids may create a dilutional acidosis and serve as a stimulus for bicarbonate conservation by the kidney. Conversely, and more clinically significant, loss of extracellular fluid volume may induce contraction alkalosis with elevation in bicarbonate buffer base.

Measurement of Acid-Base Balance

A variety of measurement techniques have been used to evaluate the metabolic contribution to acid-base balance. Presently, the indirect evaluation of bicarbonate concentration and base excess is the most common technique. Indirect analysis and confirmation by anion gap measurement are also useful.

Base Excess. Base excess specifies the number of milliequivalents of acid or base required to titrate 1 liter of blood to pH 7.40 at 37°C with constant pCO_2 of 40 mm Hg. The concept includes the buffering contribution of bicarbonate corrected for pCO_2 plus the buffering capacity of hemoglobin, phosphates, and other blood proteins. Base excess may be determined by actual titration or it can be derived from nomogram calculations after measurement of pH, pCO_2, and hematocrit values. Nomograms are based on titration of blood samples with different hemoglobin concentrations to standard pH values using acid or alkali. Various nomograms have been described; however, the most common in clinical practice is the Siggard-Anderson nomogram. The in vitro analysis of blood differs from in vivo dynamics of the extracellular fluid compartment. To minimize this difference, the Siggard-Anderson nomogram has been modified to include effective hemoglobin concentrations. The effective hemoglobin concentration is the contribution of hemoglobin to the buffer base capacity of the extracellular compartment. This amounts to about 20% of the actual hemoglobin concentration. Accurate measurement of in vivo base excess/deficit may be obtained by using the modified isobars representing effective hemoglobin concentration. Base excess is altered only by nonvolatile acids and measures the true nonrespiratory acid-base status.

Expression of base excess allows for assessment of

metabolic contribution to acid-base balance. The terminology can be confusing because the adjectives "negative" and "positive" are used in conjunction with the concept. A negative base excess implies a base deficit; a positive base excess signifies a base excess. Base excess is expressed in milliequivalents per liter above or below the normal buffer-base range. Thus, a normal value has been assigned. This value varies with species and is summarized in the dog as -1.5 ± 1.1 meq/liter. In the cat, values of -5.9 ± 3.9 meq/liter are suggested as normal. Once the base excess value is known, calculation of replacement base therapy (if required) can be performed.

Carbon Dioxide Content (Total CO_2). Carbon dioxide content represents the total amount of CO_2 that can be recovered from a plasma sample collected under anaerobic conditions. As a quantity factor, it is equal to bicarbonate plus carbonic acid concentrations. Because the bicarbonate to carbonic acid ratio is 20:1, the carbon dioxide content is also a relatively good index of total bicarbonate activity. Measurement of carbon dioxide content is an estimate of the metabolic component of acid-base balance. No inferences of respiratory contribution may be drawn by this measurement. Correlation with clinical signs and pathophysiology must be performed for accurate interpretation.

Several techniques may be used to perform the evaluation. A vaccine vial kit for individual tests is commercially available. Alternatively, direct titration technique is also described (Oxford titrator). Either method produces satisfactory results under appropriate conditions. The limitations of measurement are: (*a*) a constant temperature requirement for testing, (*b*) evaluation of only metabolic acid-base profile, (*c*) absence of blood pH data requires the clinician to appreciate the effects of underlying disease contributing to the acid-base disturbance, and (*d*) interference with accuracy by pulmonary disease that causes carbon dioxide retention. Despite these drawbacks, total carbon dioxide measurement is relatively inexpensive, technically uncomplicated, and relatively accurate. This examination can easily be incorporated into many veterinary practice environments.

Normal values for total carbon dioxide approximate those for bicarbonate measurement. Due to the incorporation of the carbonic acid component, mean values reported for normal are 24 meq/liter (HCO_3^-) + 1.2 meq/liter (H_2CO_3) = 25.2 meq/liter. The range of normal overlaps bicarbonate ion; therefore, bicarbonate values may be practically used in most cases.

Anion Gap. The anion gap accounts for the difference between measured cations and anions. Clinically, measured ions include sodium (Na^+), potassium (K^+), chloride (Cl^-) and bicarbonate (HCO_3^-). Unmeasured cations include calcium, magnesium, and gamma globulins. Unmeasured anions include phosphate, sulfate, lactate, pyruvate, alpha and beta globulins, and albumin. Generally, changes in unmeasured anion concentration are principle determinants of changes in anion gap.

The anion gap is derived from a concentration equation, which by secondary mathematical rearrangement results in:

$$\text{Anion gap (meq/liter)} = (Na^+ + K^+) - (Cl^- + HCO_3^-)$$

The normal value for anion gap in domestic species has been debated. Values in the range of 12 to 24 meq/liter have been reported, with one report of 10 meq/liter representing normal values. An elevation in anion gap represents metabolic acidosis, with a decline representing metabolic alkalosis. The value of anion gap measurement is to alert the clinician to alterations in metabolic acid-base profile not detectable by standard measurement techniques. An additional benefit is to assist in confirming the presence of acid-base disturbance. For example, a metabolic acidosis consumes bicarbonate ion, which creates an imbalance in the anion gap classified as a high anion gap metabolic acidosis. Examples of high anion gap acidosis include uremia, ketoacidosis, lactic acidosis, and intoxication with ethylene glycol, salicylate, methanol, and paraldehyde. Independently, acidosis unassociated with an increased anion gap is usually associated with a hyperchloremia relative to serum sodium concentration. Hyperchloremia can result from hemoconcentration, hyperchloremic metabolic acidosis, or chronic respiratory alkalosis.

The anion gap should be calculated whenever the necessary electrolyte concentrations have been measured to discriminate the existence of an acidosis independent of base excess. It may also be used to define the major source of the acidosis and serve as an index of the severity of the disease process and effectiveness of therapy.

Significance of Acid-Base Measurements

Disturbances in metabolic acid-base balance are important as an indication of the significance of the disease process and as an independent component reflecting potentially life-threatening disturbances. Mammalian species best function in a narrow range of hydrogen ion concentration (pH = 7.2 to 7.6). Values external to this range suggest important disturbances in physiology despite the interactive factors of compensatory mechanisms. Disturbances in hydrogen ion balance secondarily reflect on myocardial contractility, excitable membrane function (neuromuscular system), and blood pressure. Values of pH in the range of 7.2 to 7.6 have variable effects upon these parameters and more likely reflect ongoing pathology of specific organ systems. If pH values exceed this range, then corrective therapy is usually considered appropriate along with therapy of the underlying disease process.

Base excess calculations and related concepts have developed because an isolated abnormal pH measurement is only a sign of an acid-base disturbance. As such, this measurement does not quantitatively indicate the degree of magnitude of the actual amount of acid retention or depletion. Base excess is considered by some individuals to be a more accurate reflection of the quantity of noncarbonic or fixed acid present in blood than measurement of serum bicarbonate. However, bicarbonate evaluation still qualitatively reflects blood buffer capacity if coexisting respiratory disturbance is not present. The clinical history and circumstances of the patient at the time of base excess measurement, as well as a knowledge of the course and progression of the pH and pCO_2 abnormalities, are more important than any isolated numerical index. Use of the base excess concept confers an understanding of the patient's total clinical status.

ABNORMALITIES OF ACID-BASE BALANCE

Simple Acid-Base Disturbances

The Henderson-Hasselbach equation illustrates that pH is a result of the base/acid ratio or pH:HCO_3^-/CO_2. This may also be conceptualized as a renal function/respiratory function ratio. The standard "ratio" of the equation is:

$$pH_\alpha \frac{(HCO_3)}{(CO_2)}$$

during normal balance in most mammalian species. Disturbances can be categorized by alteration in HCO_3^- (metabolic component) or pCO_2 (respiratory component). Use of the equation aids the clinician in determining the component of primary imbalance and whether compensatory change is present. Acid-base disturbances may be categorized into four primary disturbances: primary CO_2 retention (respiratory acidosis), primary CO_2 depletion (respiratory alkalosis), primary HCO_3^- depletion (metabolic acidosis), and primary HCO_3^- retention (metabolic alkalosis). Two or more primary problems may exist in the same animal (72, 75, 79, 83, 84, 87–97).

Respiratory Acidosis. Under normal circumstances, production, transport, and elimination of CO_2 exist in balance as defined by the respiratory quotient. The rate of elimination is balanced primarily against the CO_2 production rate and is modulated by a neurogenic control mechanism. If an imbalance occurs at any step in the process, compensatory mechanisms are initiated. Compensation consists of increased alveolar ventilation in the initial period. This response, in general, is adequate; however, in circumstances related to CNS disease, thoracic lesions, pulmonary parenchymal disease, or related problems, inadequate elimination occurs. Production of CO_2 then exceeds elimination, resulting in elevated levels of carbonic acid (H^+ ion) and diminished pH values (respiratory acidosis).

In the initial period, CO_2 is generated more rapidly than bicarbonate and pH will fall immediately in all body fluids. The initiation of higher respiratory rate increases the metabolic component of ventilation (work of breathing) imposing another site of CO_2 generation. Increased ventilatory work will increase CO_2 production and may further exacerbate the underlying problem. The respiratory system cannot correct or adapt itself effectively for primary conditions involving ventilation. During the acute phase, acidosis is buffered by titration of nonbicarbonate tissue buffers. Carbonic acid protons are taken up by buffers such as hemoglobin, allowing HCO_3^- to be spared. Although HCO_3^- is produced through mass action, the quantity produced is limited, and little renal compensation exists. Clear and predictable changes have been demonstrated regarding changes in CO_2 and pH during this period. A relationship may be expressed as: HCO_3 increases 1 meq/liter for each 10 mm Hg pCO_2 elevation in acute phase. A similar relationship between pH and pCO_2 may be expressed as: anticipated pH changes will be 0.8 of pCO_2 alteration. This may be expressed as: 0.01 pH unit change will accompany each 1 mm Hg change in pCO_2 (Table 18.10).

If carbon dioxide retention persists, within 12 to 24 hours the plasma bicarbonate concentration will increase beyond the initial mass action response. This elevation is a result of renal conservation and synthesis of bicarbonate. The integration of bicarbonate resorption and synthesis stabilizes serum pH by permitting a sustained increase in serum bicarbonate concentration. This compensation normalizes overall balance; however, pH values do not return to normal. Pulmonary system adaptation balances oxygen and carbon dioxide levels to maximize alveolar ventilation in the presence of less than optimal circumstances. In the presence of metabolic compensation, the relationship of pCO_2 and bicarbonate is altered. Bicarbonate values increase 3 to 4 meq/liter for every 10 mm Hg elevation in pCO_2. This reflects the additional metabolic compensation that is present in the chronic period (Table 18.10).

Systemic effects of respiratory acidosis are noted in the cardiovascular and neuromuscular systems. The overall hemodynamic status associated with respiratory acidosis usually reflects mixed influences of hypoxemia, hypercapnia, and acidosis. Ventricular dysrhythmias have been associated with severe respiratory acidosis. During anesthesia, the interaction of acidosis and anesthetic agents renders the animal more susceptible to development of cardiac dysrhythmias

Table 18.10.
Summary of Responses to Simple Acid-Base Disorders

Primary Disturbance	Acid-Base Abnormality	Compensatory Response	Predicted Compensation Range of Values
Metabolic			
Acidosis	Loss of HCO_3^- or gain of hydrogen ion	Increase in ventilation (chemical buffering)	$PaCO_2 = (1.5 \times [HCO_3^-]) + 8$
Alkalosis	Gain of HCO_3^- or loss	Decrease in ventilation	$PaCO_2 = (0.9 \times [HCO_3^-]) + 9$
Respiratory			
Acidosis	Hypoventilation (↑ pCO_2)	Production of HCO_3^- (cell buffering)	Acute, HCO_3^- increase 1 meq/liter for 10-mm Hg increase in pCO_2 Chronic, HCO_3^- increases 3.5 meq/liter for every 10-mm Hg increase in pCO_2
Alkalosis	Hyperventilation (↓ pCO_2)	Consumption of HCO_3^- (cell buffering and renal)	Acute, HCO_3^- falls 2 meq/liter for each 10-mm Hg decrease in pCO_2 Chronic, HCO_3^- falls 5 meq/liter for each 10-mm Hg decrease in pCO_2

and hypotension. Respiratory acidosis has also been noted to increase susceptibility to digitalis intoxication.

Hypercapnia has been associated with a spectrum of neuromuscular lesions. Altered mental status, delirium, seizures, papillary edema, stupor, and coma have been observed. Tremors, myoclonus, and altered deep tendon reflexes also occur. Signs are more frequently noted in cases of chronic hypercapnia, especially if intercurrent hypoxemia is present.

Etiologies of hypercapnia reflect conditions that reduce effective alveolar ventilation (Table 18.11). In a general sense, any underlying pathology related to carbon dioxide elimination may predispose to hypercapnia and acidosis. Alteration in pulmonary perfusion, parenchymal ventilation, thoracic integrity, muscle lesions, central and peripheral nerve lesions, and improper ventilatory support have all been noted to result in respiratory acidosis. In many cases, hypoxemia may also be present as a result of hypoventilation.

Diagnosis of respiratory acidosis is made by clinical signs described above and arterial blood gas analysis. Typically, a pH value in the acidotic range is present, as well as elevation in pCO_2 levels. Alteration in bicarbonate and base excess values will vary with time course. In the acute phase, limited response will be noted, as has been suggested by experimental data. A more chronic time course will include renal compensatory mechanisms and may involve a greater change in bicarbonate values.

Respiratory Alkalosis. Respiratory alkalosis is frequently noted in animals and people. Blood gas studies from intensive care units demonstrate respiratory alkalosis in 46% of samples analyzed, the highest frequency of all acid-base disorders. Respiratory alkalosis may be a net result of multiple factors; pain and excitement are two common causes. Arterial pCO_2 (hypocapnia) falls whenever pulmonary CO_2 excretion (increased alveolar ventilation) exceeds CO_2 production. The enhanced rate of CO_2 excretion is self-limiting because the reduced pCO_2 acts to offset increased ventilation.

Hypocapnia and reduced carbonic acid levels characterize respiratory alkalosis. Nonbicarbonate cellular and extracellular buffers respond to the elevated HCO_3:CO_2 ratio by consuming HCO_3^- to attenuate pH changes. Laboratory data demonstrate hypocapnia ($pCO_2 < 35$ mm Hg), alkalemia (pH > 7.45), and low bicarbonate values (<20 meq/liter). Mild hypokalemia may also occur, reflecting renal potassium wasting. Chloride is renally retained to offset bicarbonate loss and maintain electroneutrality. Mild hypokalemia and hyperchloremia are characteristic electrolyte changes associated with respiratory alkalosis. It is unusual to note serum HCO_3^- values less than 15 meq/liter in respiratory alkalosis; lower values may reflect concurrent acidosis of metabolic origin. In severe cases, hyperventilation also results in tissue release of lactic acid and pyruvic acid, producing a base deficit that contributes to the compensatory mechanisms.

The acute phase of respiratory alkalosis is characterized by alteration in bicarbonate values that are independent of renal function. An adaptive fall in bicarbonate values occurs within minutes and is unassociated with any significant renal bicarbonate loss. Within hours, a diminution in renal acid excretion occurs, resulting in retention of endogenous acid and consumption of reserve bicarbonate. The changes associated with respiratory alkalosis mirror those noted with acute respiratory acidosis. Guidelines relating alteration in bicarbonate and pCO_2 have been established. Bicarbonate (HCO_3^-) increases 3 to 4 meq/liter for every 10-mm Hg increase in pCO_2 (Table 18.10).

Table 18.11.
Etiologies of Simple Acid-Base Disturbances

Metabolic origin	
Acidosis	Alkalosis
Normal anion gap (hyperchloremic acidosis)	Gastric loss
Gastrointestinal lesion	Emesis
Diarrhea, emesis	Renal origin
Pancreatic lesion	Mineralocorticoid excess
Ingestion of acid or potential acid	Hypercapnia compensation
Parenteral nutrition	Hypokalemia, hypochloremia
NH_4Cl, $CaCl_2$, HCl	Diuretics
Dilutional acidosis (rapid saline infusion)	Hypoparathyroidism
Carbonic anhydrase inhibitor (acetazolamide)	Bicarbonate
Renal tubular acidosis	Base infusion
Secondary to prolonged respiratory alkalosis	Volume depletion
Hypoaldosteronism	Secondary to respiratory Acidosis
Increased anion gap	Contraction Alkalosis
Generalized renal failure	
Diabetic ketoacidosis	
Lactic acidosis	
Toxicity	
Methanol	
Ethylene glycol	
Paraldehyde	
Salicylate	
Pulmonary origin	
Respiratory alkalosis	Respiratory acidosis
Cortical influences	Pulmonary-mediated
Anxiety	Perfusion
Pain	Pulmonary embolism
Fever	Cardiac arrest
Primary CNS disease	Ventilation
Hypoxemia	Pulmonary edema
Altitude	Pneumonia
Pulmonary shunts	Airway obstruction
Pulmonary V/Q imbalance	Interstitial fibrosis
Diffuse disease	Thorax, lung restriction
Hypotension	Flail chest
Pulmonary edema	Pneumothorax
Physical stimuli	Hemothorax
Decreased chest wall or diaphragm movement	Hydrothorax
Interstitial fibrosis	Abdominal distension
Inflammatory lesions	Muscular defects
Drugs or hormones	Hypokalemia
Salicylates	Myasthenia gravis
Thyroid hormone	Control-mediated
Progesterone	CNS
Catecholamines	Anesthesia
Xanthines	Analgesics, sedatives
Primary disease	Trauma, tumor
Septicemia	Spinal cord and peripheral nerves
Pregnancy	Cervical injury
Hyponatremia	Guillain-Barré syndrome
Heat exposure	Neurotoxins (i.e., tetanus)
Compensation for metabolic acidosis	Drugs (succinylcholine, pancuronum)
Mechanical ventilation	Diaphragmatic paralysis
	Failure of mechanical ventilation

Hypocapnia in excess of 6 hours results in renal adjustment to increase bicarbonate excretion and reduce loss of ammonium and titratable acid. A new steady state is reached within 1½ to 3 days. This response is directly related to pCO_2 and is independent of pre-existing metabolic state. The magnitude of change in bicarbonate values associated with chronic respiratory alkalosis is greater than the acute period. A change in bicarbonate values of up to 5 meq/liter occurs for every 10-mm Hg change in pCO_2. Respiratory alkalosis is unique in simple acid-base disturbances in its ability to return pH to normal. This occurs in people over a period of 7 to 9 days. The underlying mechanism of the complete compensation has not been determined.

Systemic effects of respiratory alkalosis mirror those associated with respiratory acidosis. Alteration in mental status, syncope, and seizures have been reported in humans. Paresthesia, muscle clonus, tetany, and exaggerated deep tendon reflexes may also be present. Tachycardia, S-T segment depression on EKG, and arrhythmias have also been demonstrated. Nausea and vomiting have been reported in extreme cases. Many of these signs disappear with persistence of low $PaCO_2$.

Etiologies of respiratory alkalosis are diverse (Table 18.11). CNS factors, hypoxemi, physical stimuli, pharmacological agents or intoxication, and specific physiological insults may all be involved. Specific factors can be appreciated from the accompanying table.

Diagnosis is made by history and physical evaluation and is confirmed by blood gas analysis. Typically, elevated pH and diminished pCO_2 and bicarbonate values are noted in the acute period. Chronic respiratory alkalosis may not affect pH values as compensation occurs. Diminished pCO_2 and bicarbonate values will persist until correction occurs.

Metabolic Acidosis. Nonrespiratory-related acidosis is frequently referred to as metabolic acidosis, although primary metabolic changes per se often have little influence on development. In acidosis of this type, plasma bicarbonate values diminish significantly with development of an acidic pH. The diminished bicarbonate level may be caused by secretory loss (diarrhea or renal disease) or by consumption of bicarbonate in response to nonvolatile acids (ketoacidosis or lactic acidosis). Buffering of nonvolatile acid will result in transformation of hydrogen ion to carbon dioxide and permit elimination by ventilation. If the fixed acid is not fully buffered by bicarbonate, then pH initially falls without respiratory response. A delay of 12 to 24 hours may exist until full ventilatory response is developed. This reflects delayed penetrance of hydrogen ion across the blood-brain barrier to stimulate central ventilatory control mechanisms. Despite the delay, cerebrospinal fluid (CSF) pH will ultimately reflect blood pH values initiating ventilatory drive. The degree of ventilatory response is proportional to the underlying metabolic component. The compensatory process will stop short of normalizing pH; this may be a reflection of the interrelated aspects of hydrogen ion and carbon dioxide on control of respiration.

With low plasma bicarbonate concentration, less bicarbonate is filtered through the glomeruli. Increased bicarbonate absorption will occur in the proximal tubule to maintain a higher blood level of HCO_3^-. The additional hydrogen ion will appear in the urine as titratable acid. The lower the plasma bicarbonate levels, the more acid the urine. The acid loss, in effect, adds buffer to the blood, and pH rises in the presence of normal renal function. Increased excretion of ammonium ion will also occur. This process will be more active as the duration of acidosis persists. In many cases, potassium ion is shifted into the extracellular space and may be lost through renal elimination.

Metabolic acidosis may be a component of a variety of medical and surgical problems (Table 18.11). The gastrointestinal tract and the kidney can excrete bicarbonate. Excessive bicarbonate loss from either source can contriute to metabolic acidosis. Diminished microcirculation from hypoperfusion allows for accumulation of metabolic acids. Factors contributing to development of metabolic acidosis may be divided into those occurring with normal renal function and those occurring with abnormal renal function.

With normal renal function, bicarbonate losses are confined to gastrointestinal losses. Copious quantities of bicarbonate are secreted on a daily basis by the pancreas and small intestine. The presence of diarrhea, emesis, or fistula drainage can lead to acid-base disturbance. The kidney attempts to secrete excess acid load to compensate for the bicarbonate loss but is not successful in all cases, especially if the loss is large and occurs rapidly. Dehydration may further contribute to the severity of acidosis. Administration of ammonium chloride, salicylates, paraldehyde, and ethylene glycol may result in metabolic acidosis. Disturbances in normal metabolism may result in production of acidic compounds in excess of renal excretory capacity. Altered substrate metabolism (diabetes) and the inability to utilize oxygen for metabolism (exercise, shock, cyanide intoxication, lactic acidosis) are factors in acid production during abnormal metabolic states.

Functional disturbance in renal hydrogen ion secretion and bicarbonate conservation produces or exacerbates metabolic acidosis. Functional disturbance may be broadly subcategorized into disturbance in renal tubular balance and reduction in parenchymal mass. Disturbances in renal tubular balance may occur in either the proximal or distal tubule, with renal tubular acidosis (RTA) the result.

Signs of metabolic acidosis reflect cardiovascular and CNS changes. Severe acidosis ($pH < 7.1$) will predispose myocardial tissue to arrythmia development. Diminished myocardial contractility (ionotropy) and alterations in vascular tone have been reported. Signs of altered mental status have been documented, but the incidence appears lower than respiratory-mediated disturbance. Ventilatory response is noted a short time after initiation of the disturbance. Serum HCO_3^- levels will decrease approximately 1 meq/liter for every 1 meq/liter increase in the anion gap (elevated anion gap acidosis); pCO_2 decreases 1.2 mm Hg for every 1 meq/liter reduction in HCO_3^- (Table 18.10).

Two groups of metabolic acidosis can be identified on the basis of the anion gap equation. A normal gap of measured cations and anions exists reflecting the presence of unmeasured species. Using this principle, two classes of acidemia, elevated anion gap and normal anion gap or hyperchloremic acidosis, have been identified (Table 18.11). Acidosis of elevated anion gap origin may reflect uremia, ketoacidosis, lactic acidosis, or intoxication with ethylene glycol and salicylates. Hyperchloremic acidosis reflects diarrhea, RTA, carbonic anhydrase agents, and rapid intravenous therapy. Elevated anion gap usually reflects direct or indirect losses of bicarbonate ion. Hyperchloremic acidosis generally reflects accumulation of hydrogen ion by incomplete elimination or bicarbonate loss with cloride retention.

Metabolic Alkalosis. Metabolic alkalosis is a common acid-base disorder characterized by primary elevation of plasma bicarbonate concentration with a reciprocal reduction in plasma chloride concentration. Development of metabolic alkalosis generally reflects increased activity of buffer base or buffer base precursors as well as loss of nonvolatile acid. Contributory factors in the development of metabolic alkalosis include administration of exogenous base substances, gastrointestinal loss or sequestration of nonvolatile acid, and increased loss of urinary hydrogen ion from multiple causes. Regardless of underlying disturbance, most compensatory mechanisms are renally mediated. Renal integrity, electrolyte values, and therapeutic course must be evaluated to prevent further metabolic disturbance.

With excess bicarbonate load, the normal kidney excretes bicarbonate in order to eliminate excess base buffer. The renal response to elevations in blood bicarbonate is rapid under these circumstances. However, certain factors can contribute to cause the kidney to maintain bicarbonate. These factors, including chloride and potassium deficiencies and hypermineralocorticoidism, cause excess resorption of bicarbonate and prevent bicarbonate loss; metabolic alkalosis is thus sustained. Three mechanisms participate in the retention of bicarbonate in the setting of high blood bicarbonate concentration. First, glomerular filtration rate (GFR) may fall reciprocally as arterial bicarbonate concentration rises; if GFR remains constant, then, secondly, enhanced proximal tubular resorption of bicarbonate or, thirdly, distal nephron conservation must occur. One or more of these factors can be activated by potassium and chloride deficiencies or hypermineralocorticoidism. The role of potassium in maintenance of alkalosis is unclear; however, the interaction of hypokalemia and hyperchloremia to sustain metabolic alkalosis is well established. Mineralocorticoids promote distal tubular acidification. Whether hyperadrenocorticoidism is a primary or secondary event, however, the net result is development of sustained alkalosis.

Clinical examples of metabolic alkalosis include overalkalinization in acidosis therapy, gastric alkalosis from emesis, overadministration of thiazide or potent loop diuretics (fuorsemide), and secondary response to chronic respiratory retention of carbon dioxide. Primary hyperadrenocorticism (aldosteronism) has also been shown to induce metabolic alkalosis (Table 18.11). Signs noted with metabolic alkalosis are uncommon; however, they may mimic those of hypocalcemia. These signs include alteration in mental status, seizures, paresthesia, and tetany. Dysrythmias may be seen. Signs attributable to coexistent electrolyte abnormalities, such as hypokalemia and hypophosphatemia, may also occur. Slight respiratory depression may occur in severe cases.

Diagnosis is made on the basis of blood gas parameters and coexisting electrolyte changes. Urine pH may be beneficial in discriminating the disorder. PCO_2 increases 0.5 to 1.0 mm Hg for every 1-meq/liter increase in HCO_3^- (Table 18.10).

Mixed Acid-Base Disturbances

The previous discussion defined the four primary alterations in acid-base disturbance and indicated the expected response. Changes in individual parameters induced by the initial disturbance provide two distinct but important conclusions. Overcompensation of the primary disorder is rare, and deviations from the guidelines may suggest coexistence of more than one primary disturbance.

Multiple disturbances are not usually encountered, but should be considered in interpretation of values. It is not possible for primary respiratory acidosis and alkalosis to exist in the same animal; however, all other combinations of acid-base disorders have been described (Table 18.12). Under rare circumstances, triple acid-base disorders have been documented. The key to recognition is an underlying comprehension of the pathophysiological effects of simple disorders. Each disorder, individually, alters acid-base and electrolyte parameters in a predictable manner.

Table 18.12.
Types of Acid-Base Disturbances

Simple
Respiratory
Acidosis (acute or chronic)
Alkalosis (acute or chronic)
Metabolic
Acidosis
Alkalosis
Mixed acid-base disorders
Mixed metabolic disorders
Metabolic acidosis + metabolic alkalosis
Anion gap acidosis + hyperchloremic acidosis
Mixed anion gap or hyperchloremic acidosis
Mixed respiratory-metabolic disorders
Respiratory acidosis + metabolic acidosis
Respiratory acidosis + metabolic alkalosis
Respiratory alkalosis + metabolic acidosis
Respiratory alkalosis + metabolic alkalosis
"Triple" disorders
Metabolic acidosis + metabolic alkalosis + respiratory acidosis
Metabolic acidosis + metabolic alkalosis + respiratory alkalosis

Compensation

The two major acid-base regulatory components, metabolic and respiratory are complimentary in their effects. Maintaince of normal acid-base equilibrium frequently results in a mixed response for compensation. Respiratory compensation is rapidly responsive to alteration in metabolic acid-base equilibrium. An adjustment in alveolar ventilation either reduces or accentuate elimination of carbon dioxide. The adjustment to alveolar ventilation is controlled by pH-sensitive receptors in the carotid bodies and respiratory centers on the ventrolateral surface of the brain. These "sensitive" areas mediate the degree of response to the metabolic abnormality. Because hydrogen ion does not rapidly transverse the blood-brain barrier, a slow equilibration of bicarbonate levels occurs between the circulation and the CSF. The CSF pH is normal at a pH level between 7.30 and 7.36. These factors result in an opposite change in CSF pH with metabolic disorders and a negative influence by the medullary centers on the attempt of the carotid bodies to compensate. An additional factor is the effect of pO_2 on the carotid body. PaO_2 values less than 70 mm Hg stimulate the carotid bodies more than pH. This partially explains the inability of the lungs to compensate effectively for metabolic alkalosis by marked hypoventilation. Although chemoceptors respond to pH, pH is determined by the $HCO_3^-:CO_2$ ratio, thus influencing ventilatory response. Transport of HCO_3^- is slow, and CSF pH requires up to 48 hours to readjust after a disturbance in $PaCO_3$. This temporal disparity blunts the maximum compensatory response initiated by the carotid body.

Metabolic compensation is mediated by the kidneys. Renal compensation requires activation and may not be fully functional for 10 to 48 hours after initial disturbance, suggesting that metabolic compensation cannot be relied upon in many cases of acute disturbance.

Respiratory compensation is seldom complete, whereas metabolic mechanisms can be restored to normal pH values. Overcompensation probably does not exist as a primary process, but may reflect additional factors. The duration of acid-base disturbance is useful in evaluating the patient's response. Metabolic compensation is deferred as long as 3 to 5 days after the initial disturbance. Respiratory compensation for nonrespiratory disorders is maximal within 8 to 12 hours.

COLLECTION OF BLOOD GAS SAMPLES

Accuracy of data provided by blood gas analysis or titration techniques depends upon adherence to appropriate collection techniques. Arterial sites are preferred. Central venous sampling will provide data with respect to acid-base status; however, no conclusions regarding respiratory function can be inferred. Peripheral capillary samples for microassay techniques may be accurate if free-flowing capillary blood is collected by appropriate methods. Use of tourniquets or flow impedance from vasoconstriction will produce inaccuracy. Warming prior to sample collection to promote local vasodialation is preferred (82, 98, 99).

Arterial site of collection include femoral and dorsal metatarsal arteries in the awake animal; the brachial, lingual, and radial arteries may be used in the anesthestized animal. Restraint-induced excitement should be minimized to prevent inaccuracies. Appropriate clipping of hair and skin preparation should be performed prior to sample collection. Indwelling catheters may be considered for multiple sampling (82, 98, 99).

Glass syringes are preferred for blood collection for gas analysis. Oxygen tension in excess of 120 mm Hg may fall in plastic syringes; however, blood pCO_2, pH, and bicarbonate are not affected. Although syringe material was reported to affect measurement, early reports of oxygen absorption by plastic syringes have been refuted. However, most authors still suggest that glass syringes are preferred for several reasons: (*a*) minimal friction between the glass barrel and plunger allows for confirmation of arterial puncture and filling pressure, (*b*) minimal plunger draw decreases the risk of air bubble introduction, and (*c*) small air bubbles are dislodged more easily from glass. Despite these theoretical advantages, most clinicians routinely use plastic syringes with acceptable results. New designs allow for collection without air bubble introduction and circumvent some of the previously stated disadvantages. Needle size varies according to personal preference, but a 25G × ⅝″ long needle is useful in all but large dogs. In large dogs, a 22G or 23G × 1″ long needle is preferred. If arterial catheterization is desired, a variety of indwelling catheters are available. Polyethylene or Teflon catheter materials are preferred; Silastic catheters are gas permeable and may affect obtained values.

Prior to collection, an anticoagulant is introduced into the syringe-needle unit. Heparin is preferred because other anticoagulants, such as (EDTA, CPD, ACD, sodium fluoride, and concentrated heparin), may induce in vitro changes in acid-base status. Sodium heparin 1000 I.U./cc (1000/ml) is introduced into the syringe and expelled until residual heparin remains only in the syringe hub (dead space). A consistent volume of blood (i.e., 2 ml) should be collected because dilution of the blood sample by heparin will induce changes in measured pH values. Consistency in technique will produce repeatable results. Newer prepackaged collection units incorporate a lypholized heparin pellet.

Sample collection should be anaerobically performed so that room air cannot influence results. Slow aspiration of the sample is preferred to minimize air entrapment. Excessive negative pressure on the syringe may cause separation of gases from the collection sample. Room air has a PO_2 of approximately 150 mm Hg and a PCO_2 of zero. Admixture with the collected sample will result in gas equilibration between the air and the blood. Significant lowering of PCO_2 and resulting alteration in pH may occur. Also, PO_2 will approach the room air value of 150 mm Hg. The greater air volume mixed in, the greater the chance of error. Therefore, collected samples with more than minor gas bubbles should be discarded. Numerous small bubbles with a foamy blood appearance indicate poor sampling technique; collection should be repeated. After the needle is withdrawn, rotation of the syringe barrel with the needle pointed up enhances dispersion of heparin and allows air to collect at the liquid surface, thereby facilitating gas expulsion. Blood is introduced to the needle tip, and a rubber or cork stopper is placed over the tip to maintain an anaerobic environment. Needle crimping is not considered satisfactory. Newer prepackaged collection units (Auto Stik or Marquest) incorporate a plunger vent to automatically expel gas bubbles during collection.

After collection, immediate analysis is preferred to provide accurate measurements. Delay in evaluation of more than 15 minutes permits continued oxygen consumption by the citric acid and cytochrome systems in leukocytes and reticulocytes as well as glycolysis in erythrocytes. Alterations in oxygen, carbon dioxide, and pH values will result. If a delay longer than 15 minutes between collection and analysis is expected, the sample should be placed in an ice bath. Failure to induce sample cooling can result in significant alteration in pO_2, pCO_2, and pH within 1 hour after collection.

INTERPRETATION

Abnormalities of Acid-Base Balance

The goal of interpretation of acid-base disorders is to establish a diagnosis on which rational treatment can be based. Prior to interpretation of laboratory values, a clinical impression should be established by reviewing presenting history and clinical evaluation and observing possible reasons for acid-base disturbance. This will prove useful in discriminating possible etiologies of acid-base disturbance. Pre-existing drug therapy, disease, and current support techniques will provide additional information. Urinalysis and plasma electrolytes will also be useful (74, 82, 83, 94, 96, 100, 101).

Blood is the most accessible medium for evaluation. Although bicarbonate/carbonic acid is not the only acid-base system present in the blood, it is extensively evaluated because: (*a*) the variables of pH, pCO_2, and bicarbonate ion are easily measured or derived; (*b*) a direct relationship exists between pCO_2 and pulmonary ventilation; (*c*) quantification of changes in metabolic acid-base balance can be expressed by bicarbonate ion change; (*d*) quantitatively the bicarbonate carbon dioxide system accounts for 50% of the body's buffering capacity; and (*e*) evaluation of oxygen dynamics in the vascular compartment can be appreciated. The most important factors in interpretation of acid-base disturbances are to determine the involvement of respiratory/metabolic components, to ascertain etiologies of the disturbance, and to devise therapeutic regimens appropriate for the underlying disturbance. From the previous discussion, recall the four primary alterations in acid-base balance. These will form the basis for data interpretation. In addition, the Henderson-Hasselbach equation is useful in determining the primary disturbance and direction or trend of response.

Analysis of obtained data should be performed in a logical, consistent manner to appropriately evaluate the animal. The interrelationship of pH, pO_2, and pCO_2 can be appreciated for evaluation of the respiratory component. Similarly, pH, HCO_3^-, and base excess values represent measured metabolic parameters. Once the primary disturbances are established, one must determine whether compension is present and evaluate the magnitude of the response (compensated, partially compensated, or uncompensated). This evaluation is the most interpretative and prone to discussion. Analytical breakdown of blood gas data follows.

The first consideration is evaluation of pH. Subsequent evaluation of the metabolic and respiratory components determines contribution to this value as described by the Henderson-Hasselbach equation. From multiple studies, a general range of pH in normal dogs and cats may be defined as 7.35 to 7.45 units. Values of pH less than pH 7.35 represent an increase in hydrogen ion concentration (acidosis); those values greater than pH 7.45 represent a decrease in hydrogen ion concentration (alkalosis).

Similar normal values have been noted for pO_2, pCO_2, and bicarbonate levels in arterial blood. Only pH, pO_2, and pCO_2 are directly measured; values of bicarbonate, base excess, and total CO_2 are derived from nomograms. The normal ranges of PO_2 in dogs and cats are 86 to 97 torr and 101 to 112 torr, respectively. Normal values of pCO_2 are 34 to 40 mm Hg in dogs and 28 to 34 mm Hg in cats. Bicarbonate levels are 20 to 24 meq/liter in dogs and 16 to 19 meq/liter in cats. Using these values for normality, one can note differences and infer underlying disorders.

Quantitation of Respiratory Disturbances

pH, pO_2, and pCO_2 values will aid in evaluation of respiratory status. Arterial pCO_2 values reflect effective minute ventilation of the lungs. Oxygen values may also reflect change if inspired oxygen concentration is not enriched. If hypoventilation occurs with retention of carbon dioxide ($PaCO_2 > 45$ mm Hg), elevation in carbonic acid concentration will emerge with development of respiratory acidosis. Conversely, augmentation of minute ventilation with elevated carbon dioxide elimination ($PaCO_2 < 35$ mm Hg) will diminish carbonic acid levels and results in respiratory alkalosis. The relationship of pH to pCO_2 is fairly predictable over a wide spectrum. Starting at a $PaCO_2$ of 40 mm Hg, for every 20-mm Hg increase in $PaCO_2$, the pH will decrease by 0.1 unit; for every 10-mm Hg decrease in $PaCO_2$, the pH will increase by 0.1 unit. Change in $PaCO_2$ is relatively slow (about 3 to 4 mm Hg per minute in apnea); the rate is limited by CO_2 production. Additional information gained from the pH and bicarbonate values indicates the chronicity of the disturbance and the primary or compensatory nature of the respiratory change.

The time course of the disturbance may be reflected in the compensation present in the metabolic component. If compensation is present, changes in metabolic parameters (HCO_3, base excess) may be noted. Bicarbonate concentration varies with ventilation because of the interrelationship noted in the mass action equation. Retention of CO_2 will elevate bicarbonate concentration; lowering CO_2 will lower bicarbonate values. The alteration in bicarbonate levels is reasonably linear and may be summarized as follows:

1. Acute changes in pCO_2 above 40 mm Hg will effect

a change in bicarbonate concentration of 1 meq/liter for each 10-mm Hg change in CO_2.
2. The change in bicarbonate concentration with an acute change in pCO_2 below 40 mm Hg is 2 meq/liter for each 10-mm Hg change in CO_2.
3. The change in bicarbonate concentration with a chronic change in pCO_2 greater than 40 mm Hg is 4 meq/liter for each 10-mm Hg change in pCO_2.
4. The change in bicarbonate with a chronic change in pCO_2 less than 40 mm Hg is 5 to 6 meq/liter for each 10-mm Hg change in pCO_2.

Change in metabolic indices in excess of these values suggests a primary metabolic component in addition to respiratory-induced changes.

Arterial oxygenation should be evaluated for presence of hypoxemia ($PaO_2 < 70$ mm Hg). This is the only direct information that can be obtained relative to ventilatory status. Hypoxemia can only be diagnosed on room air ($FIO_2 = 0.21$); however, indications may be obtained on enriched oxygen tensions. Significance of the disturbance in oxygenation may be derived by analysis of alveolar-arterial difference in oxygen values or calculation of Qs/Qt (shunt). If either of these parameters is increased, hypoventilation and/or elevation of intrapulmonary vascular shunting should be considered.

Quantitation of Metabolic Disturbance

Evaluation of metabolic disturbance relies on analysis of pH and parameters reflecting nonvolatile (metabolic) components. These components usually consist of bicarbonate and base excess values. Analysis of anion gap is also meaningful in aiding evaluation. Decreased bicarbonate levels in conjunction with lowered pH suggest metabolic acidosis. Elevated pH values with increased bicarbonate levels suggest metabolic alkalosis. Base excess values are also useful in measurement of metabolic contribution.

Analysis of pH is the cornerstone of interpretation. Interaction of pH and bicarbonate during interpretation suggests the contribution of change in metabolic parameters. A change in pH (acidosis) with simultaneous decrease in bicarbonate values suggests metabolic acidosis. A pH-HCO_3 relationship can indicate the severity of the disturbance. Conversely, elevation in pH values concurrent with an increase in bicarbonate levels may reflect metabolic alkalosis. Interactive changes in ventilation, as reflected by pCO_2 values, also indicate magnitude and duration of disturbance as well as presence or compensation. The parameter that has changed in the direction of the pH is the primary disturbance with compensation occurring through the alternate pathway.

Disturbance is one component of acid-base regulation elicits a compensatory response in the corollary parameter. If both components are altered in a similar direction, then the presence of two primary problems must be considered. pH values in the normal range may signify a totally compensated disturbance in acid-base balance. As previously noted, primary respiratory disorders seldom achieve full compensation; metabolic disorders may chronically result in full compensation. This aspect may be appreciated from the history and underlying pathophysiological processes.

THERAPY

Once an acid-base disturbance or oxygen-related disease is identified, appropriate therapy must be instituted. The progression and severity of the underlying lesion should be determined so that therapy is delivered in an appropriate manner. As a general principle, acute lesions are treated quickly and chronic lesions are treated slowly. Rapid intervention and correction of a chronic lesion may imbalance compensatory mechanisms that have occurred over a chronic time period. Likewise, conservative management of an acute lesion may not be appropriate. In certain cases, such as diabetic ketoacidosis, correction of the underlying metabolic lesion will result in restoration of acid-base balance (82, 83, 89–91, 95, 96, 102–105).

Respiratory-Related Disturbance

Primary respiratory-related disturbances are usually associated with an inadequate delivery of oxygen or retention of carbon dioxide. Compensation for primary metabolic disturbances may also be noted. Therapy is directed toward correction of the underlying lesion.

Oxygen Disturbances. If hypoxemia is confirmed by blood gas analysis, then goal-directed oxygen therapy should be utilized. The only direct effects of supplemental oxygenation are improved alveolar oxygen tensions, decreased work of breathing, and decreased myocardial work to maintain oxygenation. Clinical response to oxygen supplementation may be dramatic. Usually, concentrations less than 100% ($FIO_2 = 1.0$) will effect clinical response. A diminished respiratory rate, effort, and sense of apprehension will be noted.

Oxygen may be delivered by artificial airway (tracheostomy or endotracheal catheter), face mask, or nasal catheter. Commercially available oxygen enclosures (cages) may also improve inspired oxygen tension. Therapy may be titrated by use of air-oxygen mixer or adjustment of oxygen flow rates to entrain room air during therapy. Clinical response is indicative of adequate support as well as improvement of oxygen tension (PaO_2 greater than 60 mm Hg) on arterial blood gas analysis. Diseases related to etiologies other than true shunting will respond rapidly (15 to 20 minutes) to oxygen therapy. Failure of response suggests additional factors that should be considered. If there is no response, mechanical ventilatory support and further identification of underlying pathology should be considered. Refractory hypoxemia usually exists with cardiovascular shunts, pulmonary vascular fistulas (i.e., neoplastic metastasis), alveolar atelectasis, surfactant-related diseases, and acute pulmonary injury (respiratory distress syndrome or shock lung).

High levels of oxygen (70 to 100%) may be required acutely during cardiopulmonary resuscitation or cardiopulmonary instability. Ideally, high levels should not be administered for periods longer than 24 to 48 hours to prevent development of oxygen toxicity with pulmonary epithelial injury and fibrosis. However, high oxygen concentrations should not be withheld if they are indicated. In general, little additional benefit is achieved from oxygen concentrations greater than 50%. True shunting is not improved, hemoglobin saturation is not increased, and tissue tensions are not improved by higher concentration.

If coexistent hypercapnia is noted with diminished oxygen concentration, then ventilatory failure is present. Clinical response will not be achieved solely by oxygen administration; ventilatory support must also be provided.

Respiratory Acidosis (Ventilatory Failure). Animals that exhibit retention of carbon dioxide (hypercapnia) with or without diminished oxygenation have respiratory acidosis or ventilatory failure. These patients are unable to provide muscular work to exchange an adequate volume of air for elimination of carbon dioxide. Hypercapnia may be accompanied by a variety of clinical signs; for instance, the animal may have a rapid, labored respiratory pattern or apnea. Little response is noted with supplemental oxygen. Accompanying tachycardia, hypertension, and altered mental state may be noted.

Many insults may produce respiratory acidosis; alteration in ventilatory control mechanisms, neuromuscular disease or injury, thoracic injury, airway obstruction, pleural or parenchymal disease, anesthetic management techiques, and compensation for metabolic disturbances have all been documented. Support of ventilation must be provided until the underlying factor is reversed. Application of supplemental techniques, positive end expiratory pressure, or continuous positive airway pressure may be considered. These techniques are described elsewhere. Ventilatory support is palliative until therapy of the underlying disorder can be instituted and response is noted.

Respiratory Alkalosis. Respiratory alkalosis may be secondary to pulmonary disease. There are three primary causes of respiratory alkalosis: (*a*) chemoceptor response to hypoxemia, (*b*) ventilatory response to metabolic acidosis, and (*c*) CNS stimulation (e.g., pain, excitement, or disease-mediated response). If hypoxemia is present, then primary cardiopulmonary lesions should be considered. Alveolar disease, myocardial lesion, pulmonary edema, postoperative compromise, pregnancy, and musculoskeletal disease affecting ventilation represent possible cases in which carbon dioxide exchange is adequate, but oxygen demands are not met. In these cases, hyperventilation reflects oxygen hunger and may be corrected by oxygen therapy techniques. Respiratory alkalosis without hypoxemia is usually secondary to CNS-mediated events represented by pain and excitement. The presence of conditions affecting oxygen-carrying capacity, such as anemia or carbon monoxide poisioning, may also be reflected by respiratory alkalosis. In these cases, correction of the underlying disturbance eliminates alkalosis.

Metabolic-Related Disturbance

Metabolic Acidosis. With the exception of lactic acidosis, metabolic acidosis is rarely due to primary pulmonary disease. The main therapeutic consideration involves treating the underlying cause of the metabolic acidosis. If blood pH is 7.20 or greater, then goal-directed metabolic therapy is the only intervention necessary. However, if the pH is 7.20 or less or correction of the underlying cause cannot be attained in a reasonable time, then administration of alkalinizing salts is indicated. The bicarbonate deficit is usually derived from the formula:

$$0.3 \times \text{Body weight (kg)} \times \text{Base deficit} = \text{Net bicarbonate requirement}$$

Base deficit is derived from the base excess equation or by subtracting actual bicarbonate from desired bicarbonate values. The factor of 0.3 is a value for interstitial fluid volume. In severe acidosis, a factor of 0.6 (total body water) may be substituted for deficit calculation. If total correction is not the desired goal, then an alternative formula may be used:

$$\text{Bicarbonate dose} = (\tfrac{1}{2}\, pCO_2 - [HCO_3]) \times 0.5 \text{ body weight (kg)}$$

Alternatively, one may infuse a one-quarter to one-half portion of the total calculated deficit and remeasure parameters in 30 to 60 minutes. This time frame has been shown in humans to correlate with almost complete (98%) distribution in the interstitial space. The distribution of bicarbonate into the intracellular space is slow, requiring up to 18 hours to occur. Acid-base measurements of extracellular fluid may not reflect intracellular pH. Therefore, conservative replacement and measurement is recommended. A dynamic state occurs as therapy is administered. Therefore, the calculated requirement may be modified. Origin of acidosis, distribution of bicarbonate, and correction of the underlying disorder are all factors in therapy. Continuous bicarbonate loss, production of metabolic acids, and depletion of bicarbonate and other buffer systems in chronic, severe metabolic acidosis all have been documented to require therapy in excess of calculated values.

Potential hazards of bicarbonate infusion do exist. Hyperosmolality in a range detrimental to cerebral function has been observed due to rapid infusion of bicarbonate. An increase in CO_2 production as hydrogen ion is buffered may exacerbate pre-existing pulmonary disease and cause respiratory acidosis. Alkalinization of blood is not immediately accompanied by pH equilibrium in CSF. This paradoxic shift in CSF pH is attributed to increased pCO_2 and an absence of change in bicarbonate concentration. A decrease in minute volume due to extracellular pH change mediates retention of pCO_2 centrally with development of acidosis in CSF. Hypokalemia may result from transcellular shift in hydrogen ion in exchange for potassium. Hypocalcemia has also been noted. Hypernatremia can occur from administration of sodium salts of bicarbonate anion. Intravascular volume expansion may be noted in this case.

Metabolic Alkalosis. Metabolic alkalosis may be pure or mixed. It is compensated for by depression of ventilation with development of respiratory acidosis; however, this compensatory mechanism is limited due to activation of oxygen receptors from decreased PaO_2. Compensation may also be impaired by chronic respiratory disease, cardiac failure, and hepatic coma. Adverse effects of chronic alkalemia include: left shift of the oxyhemoglobin dissociation curve, inhibiting oxygen release; muscle irritability; blunting of hypoxic respiratory drive; and cardiac dysrythmias. Mortality increases with pH values consistently in excess of pH 7.54 and reaches 80% when pH values exceed 7.65.

Therapy of metabolic alkalosis involves correction of underlying disturbances. Administration of normal saline (0.9% NaCl) will correct volume depletion associated with alkalosis as well as replacing chloride ions. It also attenuates alkalosis associated with elevated aldosterone levels. Administration of supplemental potassium salts is beneficial. Efficacy of potassium administration without chloride ion is controversial; most studies suggest chloride ion is the therapeutic species. Saline-resistant metabolic alkalosis has also been documented and is associated with elevated mineralocorticoid production, e.g. due to Cushing's syndrome, corticosteroids, magnesium deficiency, hyperemia, and diuretic-induced potassium loss. Treatment consists of removal of the cause, correction of electrolyte balance, and blockade of mineralocorticoid activity.

Acute therapy may be provided by administration of acetazolamide or administration of dilute hydrochloric acid. These therapies are considered only if the underlying etiology cannot be corrected.

References

1. Donawick WJ: Fluid, electrolyte, and acid-base therapy in large animal surgery. In Jennings PB (ed): *Large Animal Surgery*. Philadelphia, WB Saunders, 1984, p 99.
2. Kohn CW: Preoperative management of the equine patient with an abdominal crisis. *Vet Clin N Am* 1:289–311, 1979.
3. Muir WW, Di Bartola SP: Fluid therapy. In Kirk RW (ed): *Current Veterinary Therapy VIII*. Philadelphia, WB Saunders, 1983, p 28.
4. Rose RJ: A physiological approach to fluid and electrolyte therapy in the horse. *Equine Vet J* 12:7–14, 1981.
5. Haskins SC: Fluid and electrolyte therapy. *Comp Cont Ed Pract Vet* 6:244–257, 1984.
6. Shoemaker WC: Fluids and electrolytes in the acutely ill adult. In Shoemaker WC, Thompson WL, Holbrook PR (eds): *Textbook of Critical Care*. Philadelphia, WB Saunders Co, 1984, p 614.
7. Goldberg M: Hyponatremia. *Med Clin N Am* 65:251–269, 1981.
8. Feig PU: Hypernatremia and hypertonic syndromes. *Med Clin N Am* 65:271–290, 1981.
9. Michell AR: The pathophysiological basis of fluid therapy in small animals. *Vet Rec* 104:542–548, 1979.
10. Cox M: Potassium homeostasis. *Med Clin N Am* 65:363–384, 1981.
11. Schaer M: Disorders of potassium metabolism. *Vet Clin N Am* 12:399–410, 1982.
12. Giesecke AH: Perioperative fluid therapy-crystalloids. In Miller RD (ed): *Anesthesia*. New York, Churchill Livingstone, 1981, p 865.
13. Chew DJ, Meuten DJ: Disorders of calcium and phosphorous metabolism. *Vet Clin N Am* 12:411–438, 1982.
14. Agus ZS, Goldfarb S: Clinical disorders of calcium and phosphate. *Med Clin N Am* 65:385–399, 1981.
15. Shires T, Williams J, Brown F: Acute change in extracellular fluids associated with major surgical procedures. *Ann Surg* 154:803–810, 1961.
16. Virtue RW, Levine DS, Aikawa JK: Fluid shifts during the surgical period. *Ann Surg* 163:523–528, 1966.
17. Roth E, Lax LC, Maloney JV: Ringer's lactate solution and extracellular fluid volume in the surgical patient. *Ann Surg* 169:149–164, 1969.
18. Foster PA: Intravenous fluid therapy during prolonged surgery. *S Afr Med J* 50(2):1659–1662, 1976.
19. Thoren L, Wiklund L: Fluid replacement therapy during surgical procedures. *Current Surg* 37:374–381, 1980.
20. Engquist A: Fluid and electrolyte therapy in association with uncomplicated surgical procedures. *Acta Anesthesiol Scand* 29:13–16, 1985.
21. Breviak H: Perioperative hydration with lactated Ringer's solution versus a saltfree restrictive fluid regimen. *Acta Anaesthiol Scand* 13:113–132, 1969.
22. Jenkins MT, Gieseke AH, Johnson ER: The postoperative patient and his fluid and electrolyte requirements. *Br J Anaesth* 47:143–150, 1975.
23. Immelman EJ: Routine, early postoperative fluid therapy. *S Afr Med J* 50(2):1663–1670, 1976.
24. Berry FW: Fluid and electrolyte therapy in pediatric patients. *Rev Course Lectures, IARS* 59:28–34, 1985.
25. Cornelius LM: Fluid therapy in small animal practice. *J Am Vet Med Assoc* 176:110–114, 1980.
26. Rackow EC, Falk JL: Colloid and crystalloid fluid resuscitation.

In Shoemaker WC, Thompson WL, Holbrook PR (eds): *Textbook of Critical Care*. Philadelphia, WB Saunders Co, 1984, p 733.
27. Raffe MR: Intravenous therapy and blood transfusion. In Bright RM (ed): *Surgical Emergencies*. New York, Churchill Livingstone, 1985, p 15.
28. Doenicke A, Grote B, Lorenz W: Blood and blood substitutes. *Br J Anaesth* 49:681–689, 1977.
29. Lees GE: Blood transfusion. In Slatter DH (ed): *Textbook of Small Animal Surgery*. Philadelphia, WB Saunders Co, 1985, p 74.
30. Leibold WC, Lucas CE, Ledgerwood AM, Mammen EF, Denis R, Grabow D, Staricco BA: Effect of albumin resuscitation on canine coagulation activity and content. *Ann Surg* 198:630–633, 1983.
31. Miller RD, Brzica SM: Blood, blood component, colloid, and autotransfusion therapy. In Miller RD (ed): *Anesthesia*. New York, Churchill Livingstone, 1981, p 885.
32. Gross DR, Dodd KT, Welch DW, Fife WP: Hemodynamic effects of 10% dextrose and dextran 70 on hemorrhagic shock during exposure to hyperbaric air and hyperbaric hyperoxia. *Aviat Space Environ Med* 55:1128–1129, 1984.
33. Lazrove S, Waxman K, Shippy C, Shoemaker WC: Hemodynamic, blood volume, and oxygen transport responses to albumin and hydroxyethyl starch infusions in critically ill patients. *Crit Care Med* 8:302–306, 1980.
34. Shoemaker WC: Evaluation of colloids, crystalloids, whole blood, and red cell therapy in the critically ill patient. *Clin Lab Med* 2:35–63, 1982.
35. Tranbaugh RF, Lewis FR: Crystalloid versus colloid for fluid resuscitation of hypovolemic patients. *Adv Shock Res* 9:203–216, 1983.
36. Arturson G, Thoren L: Fluid therapy in shock. *World J Surg* 7:573–580, 1983.
37. Rackow EC, Falk JL, Fein A, Siegel JS, Packman MI, Haupt MT, Kaufman BS, Putnam D: Fluid resuscitation in circulatory shock: a comparison of the cardiorespiratory effects of albumin, hetastarch, and saline solutions in patients with hypovolemic and septic shock. *Crit Care Med* 11:839–850, 1983.
38. Pichler ME, Turnwald GH: Blood transfusion in the dog and cat part I: Physiology, collection, storage, and indications for whole blood therapy. *Comp Cont Ed for the Prac Vet* 7:64–71, 1985.
39. Steinbronn K, Huestis DW: Rationale for blood component therapy. In Brown JR (ed): *Fluid and Blood Therapy in Anesthesia*. Philadelphia, FA Davis, 1983, p 151.
40. Allen JB, Allen FB: The minimum acceptable level of hemoglobin. *Int Anesth Clin* 20:1–22, 1982.
41. Stoelting RK, Miller RD: *Basics of Anesthesia*. New York, Churchill Livingstone, 1984, p 243.
42. Schalm OW: *Veterinary Hematology*, ed 2. Philadelphia, Lea & Febiger, 1975, p 631.
43. Auer L, Bell K: The AB blood group system in cats. *Animal Blood Grps Biochem Genetics* 12:287–297, 1981.
44. Auer L, Bell K, Coates S: Blood transfusion reactions in the cat. *J Am Vet Med Assoc* 180:729–730, 1982.
45. Ou D, Mahaffey E, Smith JE: Effect of storage on oxygen dissociation of canine blood. *J Am Vet Med Assoc* 167:56–58, 1975.
46. Moroff G, Dende D: Characterization of biochemical changes occurring during storage of red cells. *Transfusion* 23:484–489, 1983.
47. Miller RD: Problems posed by transfusion. In Orkin FK, Cooperman LH (eds): *Complications in Anesthesiology*. Philadelphia, JB Lippincott, 1983, p 461.
48. Copping JW, Mather GS, Winkler JM: Physiological responses to the administration of cold, room temperature, and warm balanced salt solutions in hemorrhagic shock in dogs. *Surgery* 71:206–209, 1972.
49. Van der Walt JH, Russell WJ: Effect of heating on the osmotic fragility of stored blood. *Br J Anaesth* 50:815–820, 1978.
50. Zucker HL: Massive transfusion. *Int Anes Clin* 20:157–170, 1982.
51. Smith JE, Mahaffey E, Board P: A new storage medium for canine blood. *J Am Vet Med Assoc* 172:701–703, 1978.
52. O'Rourke LG: Practical Blood Transfusions. In Kirk RW (ed): *Current Veterinary Therapy*, ed 8. Philadelphia, WB Saunders Co, 1983, p 408.
53. Crowe DT: Autotransfusion in the trauma patient. *Vet Clin N Am* 10:581–598, 1980.
54. Orr MD: Autotransfusion: Intraoperative therapy. *Int Anesthesiol Clin* 20:97–119, 1982.
55. Bjorling DE, Rawlings CA: Relationship of intravenous administration of Ringer's lactate solution to pulmonary edema in halothane-anesthesized cats. *Am J Vet Res* 44:1000–1006, 1983.
56. Bonagura JD: Fluid and electrolyte management in the cardiac patient. *Vet Clin N Am* 12:501–514, 1982.
57. Stamp GL: Metabolic response to trauma. In Zaslow IM (ed): *Veterinary Trauma and Critical Care*. Lea & Febiger, Philadelphia, 1984, p 25.
58. Lawson DH, Henry DA: Intravenous fluid therapy. *J Maine Med Assoc* 68:432–437, 1977.
59. Stephen M, Loewenthal J, Wong J: Complications of intravenous therapy. *Med J Aust* 2:557–559, 1976.
60. Rock G, Tocchi M, Ganz PR, Tackaberry ES: Incorporation of plasticizer into red cells during storage. *Transfusions* 24:493–498, 1984.
61. Peters WR, Bush WH, McIntrye RD: The development of fibrin sheath in indwelling venous catheters. *Surg Gynecol Obstet* 137:43–47, 1973.
62. Schlossman D: Thrombogenic properties of vascular catheter material in vivo. *Acta Radiol* 14:186–192, 1973.
63. Carter JM, Freedman AB: Total intravenous feeding in the dog. *Am J Vet Res* 171:71–76, 1977.
64. Deutsch S: Effects of anesthetics on the kidney. *Surg Clin North Am* 55:775–786, 1975.
65. Dudrick SJ, Wilmore DW, Vars HM: Long-term parenteral nutrition with growth in puppies and positive nitrogen balance in patients. *Surg Forum* 18:356–357, 1967.
66. Virgilio RW, Smith DE, Zarins CK: Balanced electolyte solutions: experimental and clinical studies. *Crit Care Med* 7:98–106, 1979.
67. Ryan JA, Abel RM, Abbott DM, et al: Catheter complications in total parenteral nutrition. *N Engl J Med* 290:757–761, 1974.
68. Burrows CF: Inadequate skin preparation as a cause of intravenous catheter-related infection in the dog. *J Am Vet Assoc* 180:747–749, 1982.
69. Kaminski MV, Harms DF: Prolonged uncomplicated intravascular catheterization. *Am J IV Ther* 3:19–24, 1976.
70. Wilmore DW, Dudrick SJ: Safe long-term venous catheterization. *Arch Surg* 98:256–258, 1969.
71. Turco SJ: Infusion phlebitis: pathogenesis remains unclear, but preventive measures emerge from many studies. *Crit Care Monitor* 2:6–8, 1982.
72. Brobst D: Evaluation of clinical disorders of acid-base balance. *J Am Vet Med Assoc* 166:359–364, 1975.
73. Guyton AC: *Textbook of Physiology*, ed 4. Philadelphia, WB Saunders, 1971.
74. Haskins SC: An overview of acid-base physiology. *J Am Vet Med Assoc* 170:423–428, 1977.
75. Huber GL: *Arterial Blood Gas and Acid-Base Physiology*. Kalamazoo, Upjohn Company Current Concepts, 1978.
76. Laski ME: Normal regulation of acid-base balance: renal and pulmonary response and other extrarenal buffering mechanisms. *Med Clin N A* 67:771–780, 1983.
77. Masoro EJ, Siegel PD: Acid-base regulation. In *Physiology, Pathophysiology and the Interpretation of Blood-gas Analysis*, ed 2. Philadelphia, WB Saunders Co, 1977, p 26–81.
78. Stevens JB: Teaching monograph of acid-base physiology. Col-

lege of Veterinary Medicine, University of Minnesota, St. Paul, Minnesota, 1982.
79. Comroe JH: *Physiology of Respiration*, ed 2. Chicago, Yearbook Medical Publishers, 1974.
80. Dohoo SE, McDonnell WN, Dohoo IR: A comparison of fresh gas flows during anesthesia with nitrous oxide in the dog. *J Am An Hosp Assoc* 18:900–904, 1982.
81. Haskins SC, Knapp RG: Effect of low carrier gas flows on inspired oxygen tension in anesthetized dogs. *J Am Vet Med Assoc* 180:735–738, 1982.
82. Haskins SC: Blood gases and acid-base balance: clinical interpretation and therapeutic implications. In Kirk RW (ed): *Current Veterinary Therapy VIII*. Philadelphia, WB Saunders Co, 1983, p 201.
83. Shapiro BA, Harrison RA, Walton JR: *Clinical Application of Blood Gases*, ed 3. Chicago, Yearbook Medical Publishers, 1982.
84. Arruda JAL, Kurtzman NH: Metabolic acidosis and alkalosis. *Clin Neprhology* 7:201–215, 1977.
85. Garella S, Chang BS, Kahn SI: Dilutional acidosis and contraction alkalosis. *Kidney Int* 8:279–283, 1975.
86. Holt JC: Blood pH and plasma bicarbonate determination: a practitioner's viewpoint. *J Am An Hosp Assoc* 8:448–450, 1972.
87. Polzin DJ, Stevens JB, Osborne CA: Clinical application of the anion gap in evaluation of acid-base disorders in dogs. *Comp Cont Ed Pract Vet* 4:1021–1032, 1982.
88. Sabatini S: The acidosis of chronic renal failure. *Med Clin N Am* 67:845–858, 1983.
89. Brobst D: Pathophysiologic and adaptive changes in acid-base disorders. *J Am Vet Med Assoc* 183:773–780, 1983.
90. Cogan MG, Liu F, Berger BE, et al: Metabolic alkalosis. *Med Clin N Am* 67:903–914, 1983.
91. DuBose TD: Clinical approach to patients with acid-base disorders. *Med Clin N Am* 67:799–814, 1983.
92. Kaehny WD: Respiratory acid-base disorders. *Med Clin N Am* 67:915–927, 1983.
93. Nairns RG, Emmett M: Simple and mixed acid-base disorders: a practical approach. *Medicine* 59:161–187, 1980.
94. Rosenthal MH: Acid-base equilibrium and blood-gas measurement. In Miller RD (ed): *Anesthesia*. New York, Churchill Livingstone, 1981, p 825.
95. Sabatini S, Arruda JAL, Kurtzman NA: Disorders of acid-base balance. *Med Clin N Am* 62:1223–1255, 1978.
96. Schaer M: A practical review of simple acid-base disorders. *Vet Clin N Am* 12:439–453, 1982.
97. Shoemaker WC: Fluids and electrolytes in the acutely ill adult. In Shoemaker WC, Thompson WL, Holbrook PR (eds). *Textbook of Critical Care*. Philadelphia, WB Saunders Co, 1984, p 614.
98. Haskins SC: Sampling and storage of blood for pH and blood gas analysis. *J Am Vet Med Assoc* 170:429–433, 1977.
99. Rodkey WG, Hannon JP, Dramise JG, et al: Arterialized capillary blood used to determine the acid-base and blood gas status of dogs. *Am J Vet Res* 39:459–463, 1978.
100. Adams AP, Hahn CEW: *Principles and Practice of Blood-gas Analysis*. Butter Market Ipswich, WS Cowell Ltd, 1979.
101. Bright RM, McIntosh JJ: Clinical application of arterial blood gases in companion animals. *Calif Vet* 7:20–24, 1981.
102. Hartsfield SM, Thurmon JC, Benson GJ: Sodium bicarbonate and bicarbonate precursors for treatment of metabolic acidosis. *J Am Vet Med Assoc* 179:914–916, 1981.
103. Traverso LW, Medina F, Bolin RB: The buffering capacity of crystalloid and colloid resuscitation solutions. *Resuscitation* 12:265–270, 1985.
104. Kurkendol PL, Starrs J, Gonzalez FM: The effects of acetate, lactate, succinate, and gluconate on plasma pH and electrolytes in dogs. *Trans Am Soc Artif Int Organs* 23:323–327, 1980.
105. Trudnowski RJ, Goel SB, Lam FT, Evers JL: Effect of ringer's lactate solution and sodium bicarbonate on surgical acidosis. *Surg Gynec Obstet* 125:807–814, 1967.

CHAPTER 19

Hyperthermia, Malignant Hyperthermia, and Myopathy

S.V. HILDEBRAND, D.V.M., D.A.C.V.A.

Introduction

In general, body temperature is expected to fall during anesthesia. Hypothermia can reach life-threatening levels, especially in very young or tiny patients, patients having surgery that requires an open body cavity, or patients receiving cold intravenous fluid. Such heat production mechanisms as shivering, vasoconstriction, pilorection, and muscle movement are obtunded by general anesthesia. Sweating and vasodilation, which are heat dissipation mechanisms, are caused by anesthetics. Thermoregulatory function of the hypothalamus is reduced (1). Despite this, hyperthermia can occur during anesthesia and can be due to a variety of causes, some more serious than others.

Malignant Hyperthermia

BACKGROUND AND HISTORY

In 1960, Denborough and Lovell reported a case of a young man who nearly died after general anesthesia for repair of a fractured leg (2). Before anesthesia, the man was more concerned about the anesthetic than his leg because several of his family members had died after administration of ether. The man survived his anesthetic despite a serious crisis characterized by cyanosis, hypotension, tachycardia, and hyperthermia. Subsequent surgical procedures were undergone safely using spinal anesthesia. Denborough and coworkers later described a pattern of inheritance for the hyperthermia seen in that family (3).

The hereditary nature of this intraoperative hyperthermia was reviewed (4). A number of areas were studied, but this review revealed Wisconsin had a high incidence of cases. Certain families in those areas had a high incidence of anesthetic-related hyperthermia and provided a gene pool that allowed authors to conduct systematic study. Since the early 1960's, these and many other investigators have provided understanding of the epidemiology, pathophysiology, prediction, and treatment of malignant hyperthermia (MH).

MH was discovered in a species other than humans when a muscular degeneration problem of swine was linked by a genetic relationship to unsuitable pork found at slaughter (4). Breeding patterns that produced rapid growth, feed efficiency, and superior muscling also produced animals that were likely to develop hypermetabolic states and sudden death when stressed. This became known as porcine stress syndrome (PSS). The stresses of shipping and slaughter resulted in deterioration of muscle of susceptible pigs, and the unsatisfactory carcass quality was called pale soft exudative pork (PSEP) (5, 6). The discovery that pigs so affected also developed MH reactions when anesthetized with halothane and succinylcholine meant that an animal model existed for further study of MH (7, 8).

The specific hereditary nature of MH became more complex as more was learned about the syndrome (9, 10). Early belief that MH was an autosomal dominant characteristic, with variable penetrance, has not been supported by continued investigation (3). Multiple genetic factors are involved, and there are differences in the hereditary patterns of humans and swine. Clarification of genetic factors is further complicated by the influence of environment and drugs on MH susceptibility (9). This complexity is illustrated by the wide variability of MH response, from awake episodes (11) to delayed (12–14) or partial episodes (9). Other neuromuscular disorders, including muscular dystrophy, central core disease, sudden infant death syndrome, and heat stroke, have inconsistent links to MH (15).

PATHOPHYSIOLOGY OF MH

Generalized membrane abnormality is a feature of MH. An abnormality of muscle metabolism is responsible for many of the signs of the disease (16, 17). In normal muscle, calcium is stored in the sarcoplasmic reticulum (Fig. 19.1). Muscle contraction occurs when a nerve impulse is transmitted down the sarcolemma and along the transverse tubules and transferred to the sarcoplasmic reticulum. Small amounts of calcium, called trigger calcium, are important in this process. Trigger calcium ions cause a massive release of calcium by the sarcoplasmic reticulum into the myoplasm. There calcium binds to troponin, which modifies the position of tropomyosin so that the contractile filaments, actin and myosin, can slide on each other and cause muscle shorting. "Excitation-contraction coupling" is the term used to describe the mechanism whereby the electrically excited sarcolemma is coupled to the calcium release from the sarcoplasmic reticulum (16).

In MH, there is a disturbance of intracellular calcium distribution (4, 16, 18, 19). When a predisposed

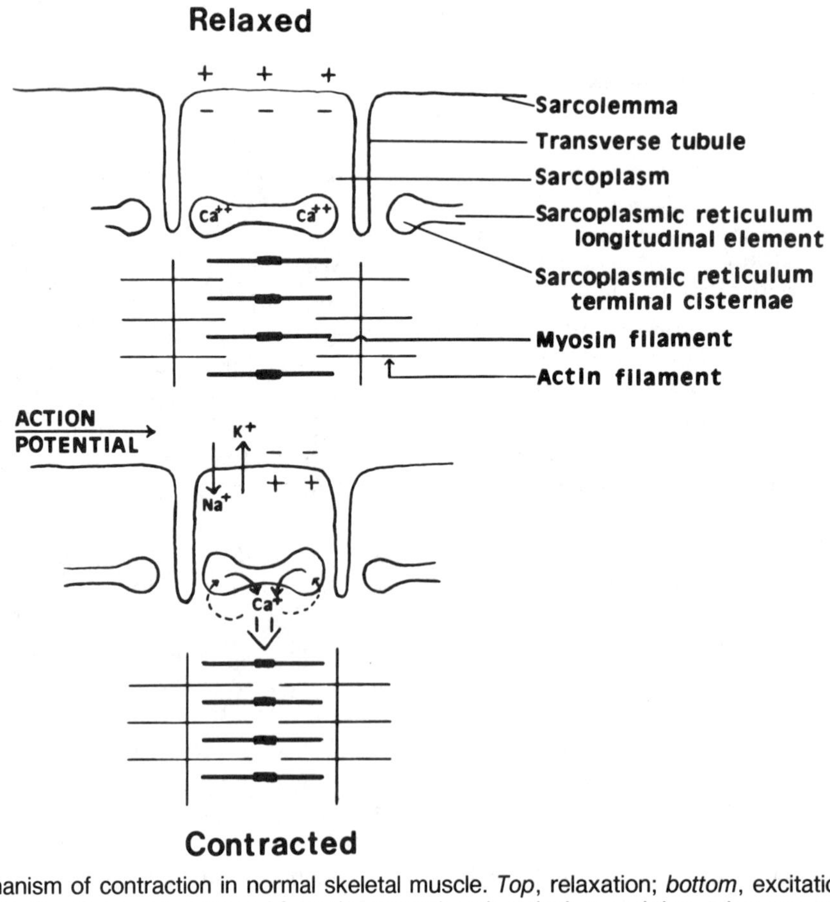

Figure 19.1. The mechanism of contraction in normal skeletal muscle. *Top*, relaxation; *bottom*, excitation-contraction coupling in response to an action potential. Calcium is released from the sarcoplasmic reticulum and then taken up again by means of a calcium pump mechanism.

individual is in a stressful situation or is exposed to initiating trigger agents, MH can occur. Initiating agents include the potent inhalation anesthetics and the depolarizing muscle relaxants. Nonanesthetic triggers include extreme emotional excitement, high environmental temperature, mild infection, and muscle injury or exercise (11, 20). The essential abnormality in the muscle cell in MH is faulty regulation of calcium by the membranes of the sarcoplasmic reticulum (17, 18, 20). In response to exposure to a trigger situation, the sarcoplasmic reticulum releases large amounts of calcium into the myoplasm (21). Pronounced and prolonged muscle contracture results. The sarcoplasmic reticulum may also be ineffective in reuptake of myoplasmic calcium (16).

The membrane defect of MH is not confined to muscle and is present in other cells of the body. Glucose induces beta cells of the pancreas to secrete higher than normal amounts of insulin in MH individuals (22). Permeability and fragility of red blood cells may be abnormal (23, 24). Platelet aggregation and ATP depletion may be abnormal (24, 25). Sympathetic nervous system responses may also be abnormal in MH-susceptible individuals, who may be hypertensive and have increased body temperature due to increased metabolism (26, 27).

CHARACTERISTICS OF MH INDIVIDUALS

Common findings in humans affected with MH include excessive muscle bulk and strength. Such individuals are not necessarily well coordinated. Spontaneous skeletal muscle cramps occur and may be very severe. Skeletal abnormalities such as joint hypermobility, kyphosis, and scoliosis may be present. Individuals tend to be short and stocky and are more anxious and apprehensive than unaffected individuals (28). Other myopathies have been noted in a few MH patients. These include familial hyperkalemic periodic paralysis, myotonia congenita, and polymyositis. Ringbinden, or ring fibers similar to those seen in myotonia dystrophia, have been seen in microscopic sections of muscle from some MH patients (28).

MH REACTION

The classic MH response occurs after exposure to a volatile anesthetic agent (4). The strongest triggers of MH are halothane and succinylcholine. The most consistent early indication of MH is tachycardia. After an intubation dose of succinylcholine, jaw rigidity or trismus may be another early warning of MH (9). Increase in end-tidal CO_2 may be useful for early detection. Other likely intraoperative signs include tachypnea, hypercapnia, metabolic acidosis, and central venous desaturation. Muscle rigidity may develop, along with cyanosis, skin mottling, fever, sweating, cardiac arrhythmia, unstable blood pressure, and hyperkalemia. Later changes include myoglobinemia, elevated serum creatine phosphokinase (CPK), elevated aspartate amino transferase (SGOT), and myoglobinurea (29).

There are many variations in the manifestation of an MH episode. Some reactions do not occur until late in the anesthetic, and some are not manifested until recovery (12). Some individuals will not be triggered until the second or third anesthesia. In addition to the rigid form of MH, Kalow, Britt, and Richter have described nonrigid MH (30). Normothermic episodes of MH have been documented (31). These variations are almost certainly due to both genetic and situational differences. In addition, species variations almost certainly play a part in the different manifestations of MH-like episodes described in equine, canine, feline, and wild animal species. MH in these species will be described elsewhere in the chapter.

DIAGNOSIS OF MH

Identification of MH-susceptible individuals has both therapeutic and economic importance. Prediction of an MH reaction allows for appropriate preventative and therapeutic measures to be taken if general anesthesia is required. Identification of affected animals allows culling of those individuals from the breeding herd, so that they will not pass on the defect, with subsequent losses due to sudden death and poor quality meat. Economic loss can be substantial (32). Identification of the MH defect in performance animals such as horses and greyhounds helps determine appropriate therapy to return those animals to high level performance and could guide breeding plans for those animals.

Unfortunately, no one test will accurately identify MH susceptibility. The following are tests that have been described. Their reliability is variable.

History

A strong suspicion of MH may be aroused if there have been a number of unexplained anesthetic or stress-related deaths in a family. A history of muscle cramping or tying-up, either after exercise or spontaneously, should also be considered suspicious. Further testing is indicated if these problems are known to have occurred (28).

Phenotype or Appearance and Physical Examination

Because heavy muscling is a common finding in MH, a heavily muscled individual may be at risk. An unusually anxious or apprehensive attitude is also a warning sign. In humans, more than one-third of MH patients have electrocardiogram (ECG) abnormalities. Most commonly observed ECG abnormalities are atrial or ventricular hypertrophy, bundle branch block, and myocardial ischemia (4, 28).

Serum Biochemistry

MH individuals may have elevated serum enzymes related to ongoing muscle damage. Resting CPK and SGOT levels may be increased. Strenuous activity causes large increases in those enzymes. However, enzyme elevation is not always present in MH individuals; normal serum biochemistry does not necessarily rule out MH (28, 33, 34).

Other serum abnormalities have been described. Solomons et al. found serum pyrophosphate to be elevated in MH patients (25).

Contracture Testing of Muscle

This invasive test unfortunately is thus far the single most reliable diagnostic test for MH. MH-suspect muscle is tested for degree of sensitivity of contracture patterns to the effects of halothane and caffeine (28, 30, 35–39). Caffeine causes release of calcium from and inhibits reuptake of calcium by the sarcoplasmic reticulum.

There is as yet considerable variation in actual technique. Dr. Beverly Britt has compiled information regarding techniques used in a number of North American laboratories (Britt, unpublished data). Differences will be noted in the following description.

Technique

Biopsy. Surgical biopsy is performed using either local or general anesthesia (Fig. 19.2, *A* and *B*). Local anesthetics of the ester group, such as procaine, are considered safe. If general anesthesia is used, any agents that trigger MH should be avoided. Choice of local or general anesthesia depends on the patient and other surgical requirements. The muscle sample is removed avoiding rough or excessive handling. A piece of muscle approximately 2 × 2 × 0.5 cm is taken by dissecting carefully along the direction of the fibers and making a clean cut at 90° to the fibers at both ends. Sloppy technique in obtaining the muscle will lead to poor test results. Unnecessary repetition of the biopsy is clearly undesirable.

The muscle used in humans is usually the vastis lateralis. Other muscles used include the rectus abdominus or any muscle near the wound edge. In horses, muscles used include omobrachialis, semimembranosus-tendinosus, and the gracilis. In pigs, the quadriceps group or the semimembranosus-tendinosus is used. Because Deuster and coworkers have shown in normal feline muscle that fiber type makeup influences contracture test results, it is important to compare results with muscle of similar fiber type makeup (40). It does not seem critical to secure the specimen in a fixed length clamp; several investigators no longer do this.

Contracture Test. The muscle is transported to the laboratory as quickly as possible. Transport medium varies with the investigator and may be room temperature normal saline, Kreb's Ringer solution, Ringer's solution, or carbogen-bubbled Kreb's. The so-

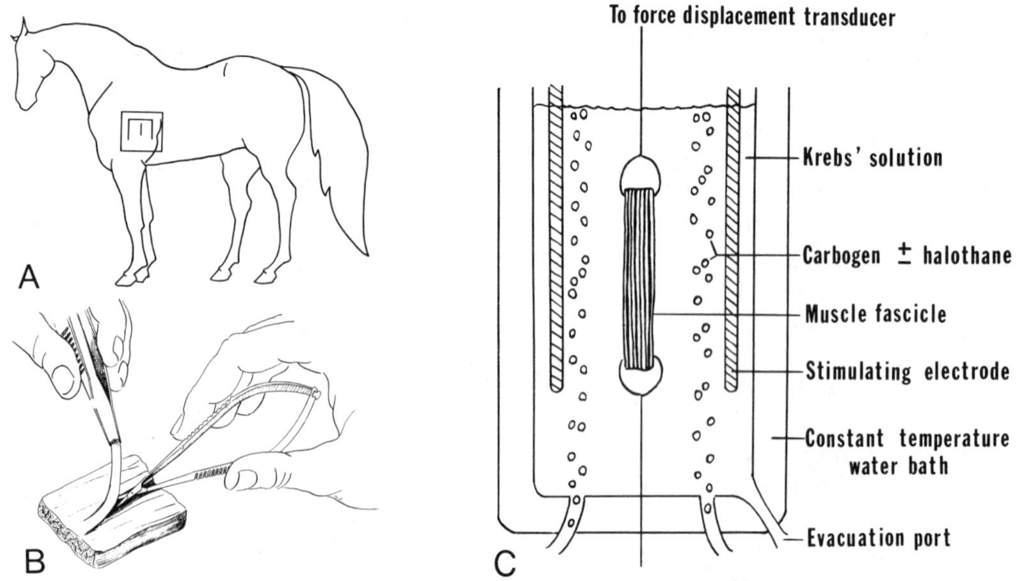

Figure 19.2. *A*, surgical site for biopsy of equine omobrachialis or triceps muscle. The area is shaved and aseptically prepared, and a local block using 2% procaine HCl is infiltrated in an inverted "U" pattern. Incision is made within the blocked area. *B*, muscle fascicles are well defined within the biopsy specimen. Dissection with small ophthalmological instruments allows dissection along the planes of each fascicles. *C*, the muscle bath is surrounded by a constant 37°C water bath. Ports into the Krebs container allow bubbling of carbogen gas, with or without halothane, and emptying of solution by gravity or suction.

lution may be previously bubbled with carbogen gas, and the sample may be transported in a beaker, a hermetically sealed jar, or a thermos.

In the laboratory, fat and fascia are trimmed from the specimen, and smaller fascicles are dissected. Size of the fascicles varies from 1 to 2 cm long to 0.2 to 0.5 cm wide. Fascicles are then placed in a carbogen bubbled Kreb's bath at 37°C (Fig. 19.2, C). Depending on facilities available, 2 to 20 facsicles are studied at once. Each fascicle or strip is secured at one end and attached to a force-displacement transducer at the other. An electrical stimulus is applied to the strip using either field or contact electrodes. Stimulus mode includes supramaximal voltage, with a duration of 2 to 20 msec and a frequency of 0.1 to 1 Hz. A stimulus booster may be required to produce sufficient current when field electrodes are used.

When a stable baseline of 0.3 to 2 g of tension is achieved (about 20 minutes), increasing concentrations of caffeine alone or in the presence of halothane are added to the bath. Caffeine concentrations increase exponentially from 0.25 to 32 mM with each exposure lasting 4 minutes. Caffeine concentrations can be increased either by adding small amounts to the Kreb's solution already in the bath or by draining the bath and refilling it with the new concentration. The strips are also exposed to halothane alone in concentrations from 1 to 4%. Some investigators use two strips only and wash out the halothane and/or caffeine before starting a new exposure. Others use new strips each time, so that any two strips will be exposed to caffeine alone or halothane alone followed by caffeine.

Interpretation. Two aspects of muscle function are noted. First, evoked tension in response to electrical stimulus increases with halothane and/or caffeine exposure. This evoked response is unrelated to contracture response, which is seen as an increase in baseline tension (Fig. 19.3, *A*). When contracture exceeds 1 g above resting tension, the caffeine concentration responsible and the absolute contracture achieved are plotted on a semilogarithmic graph to obtain the "caffeine contracture concentration" or the "caffeine-specific concentration" (CCC) (Fig. 19.4). This is the concentration of caffeine required to raise the resting tension 1 g above baseline.

The CCC for MH muscle will be significantly lower than normal muscle. CCC values less than 4.1 mM with caffeine alone or less than 1.2 mM with caffeine in the presence of halothane are considered indicative of MH vastus lateralis (Dr. Britt's laboratory, 1984). Halothane alone rarely causes a contracture of normal human muscle (28). In a study of MH-susceptible hu-

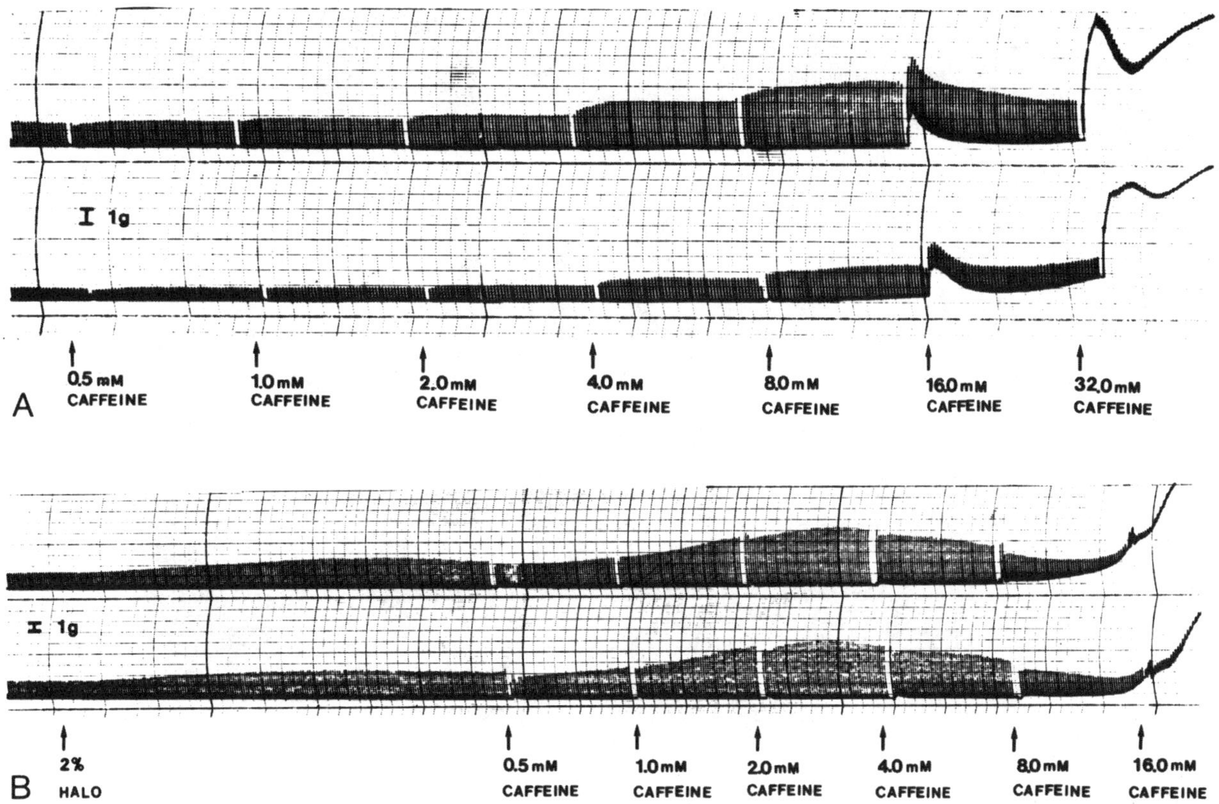

Figure 19.3. *A*, a normal contracture response of the equine omobrachialis muscle to caffeine only. The muscle is exposed to increasing concentrations of caffeine. With 8.0 mM caffeine, the baseline begins to rise. Sustained increase of greater than 1 g above baseline is achieved at 16 mM caffeine for the bottom trace, but requires 32 mM for the top trace. *B*, a normal omobrachialis response to halothane and caffeine. Halothane 2% is begun at the *arrow*. After 20 minutes of halothane exposure, caffeine is added, as in *A*. Sustained contracture is not seen until 8 mM caffeine.

man patients in Sweden and Denmark, halothane alone was the most sensitive indicator of MH-susceptible muscle (41). Response to halothane alone has been the most consistent indicator in horses studied (Hildebrand, unpublished data).

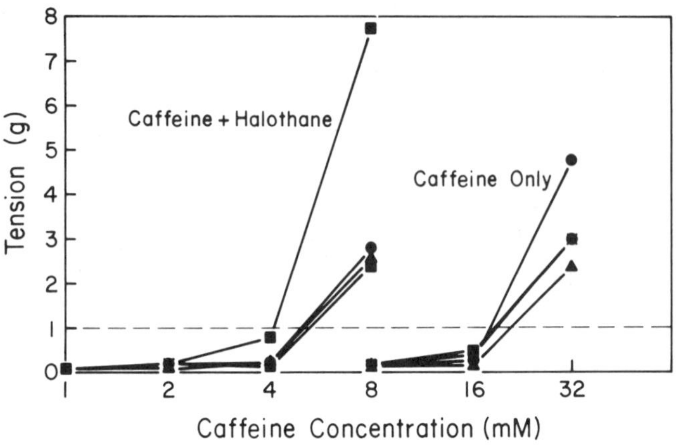

Figure 19.4. A graph plotting amount of tension (g) developed by each muscle strip with increasing concentrations of caffeine. Four fascicles are graphed. The *dotted line* at 1 g of tension crosses the plot of each strip at the CCC. For caffeine alone, an excess of 16 mM caffeine represents the CCC. The CCC for halothane plus caffeine is typically less than for caffeine alone.

Muscle fiber makeup influenced test results (40). Fiber Type 1 muscles developed contracture in the presence of halothane alone, whereas fiber Type 2 did not. Fiber Type 1 muscles were significantly more sensitive to both caffeine alone and caffeine in the presence of halothane. In the horse, contracture in the presence of halothane alone depends on the muscle group tested. For the fiber Type 2 omobrachialis of the horse, contracture in the presence of halothane is indicative of an MH-susceptible muscle (Fig. 19.5, *A*). For mixed fiber type equine muscles, contracture in the presence of halothane will occur even in normal muscle, especially at the higher (4%) halothane concentrations (Hildebrand, unpublished data). Some MH muscle will show spontaneous contracture when placed in the Kreb's bath, before exposure to either caffeine or halothane (Gronert, personal communication) (Fig. 19.5, *B*).

Microscopy. Microscopy provides a complimentary test that alone cannot be relied on for diagnosis of MH but can be useful when in vitro test results are unclear (42). Although two-thirds of MH patients have a myopathy, it is quite variable in degree and nature and seems to be associated with aging (42). The most consistent change noted in human MH muscle is the

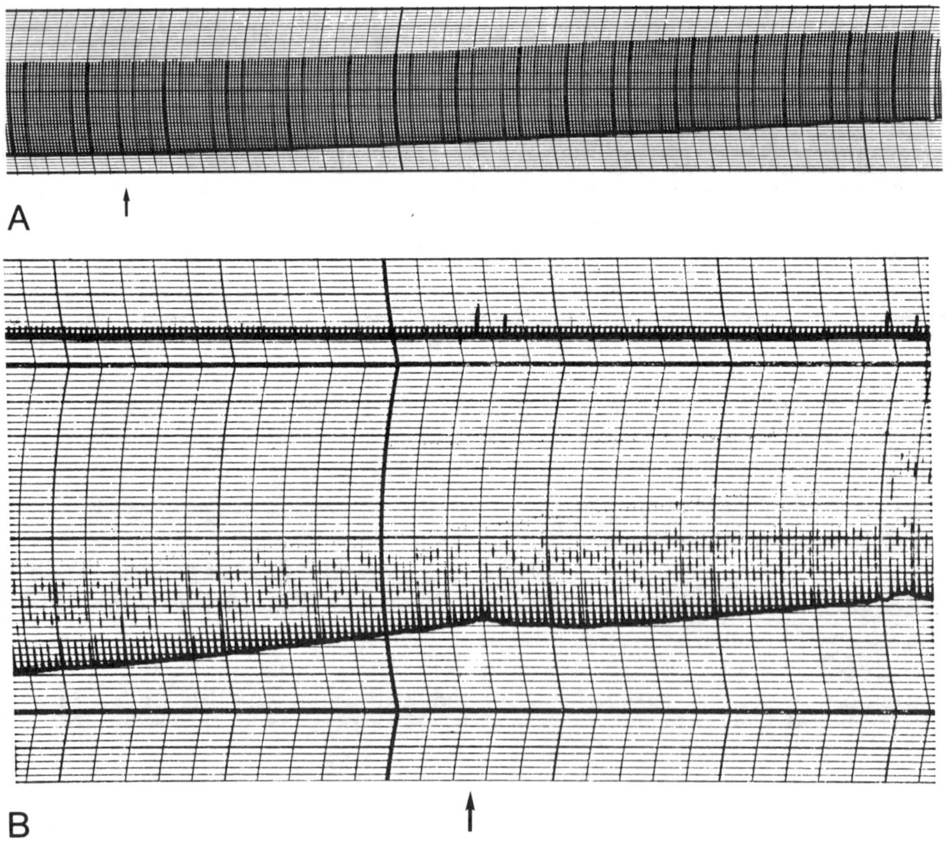

Figure 19.5. *A* and *B* are traces of contracture response from a pony which developed an MH-like reaction to halothane and succinylcholine (135). The omobrachialis muscle was biopsied on two occasions. *A* shows the left omobrachialis; *B* shows the right. In *A*, halothane 2% is given at the *arrow.* Over 20 minutes, a steady contracture results in 2 g above baseline. *B* illustrates spontaneous contracture prior to exposure to halothane or caffeine. Caffeine, 0.5 mM, is added at the *arrow.* The muscle has contracted 1.4 g above baseline before caffeine is added. For both *A* and *B*, one line represents 0.2 g tension.

presence of internal nuclei. In normal muscle, the nuclei lie at the edge of the fiber (42, 43). Single fiber atrophy; fiber necrosis and regeneration; and fibers with unstructured cores, the so-called "core-targetoid" fibers, are associated with the MH defect, but these changes can be seen in myopathies other than MH and so are considered nonspecific (42).

Histochemical Analysis. Fresh frozen sections of biopsy specimen are stained with hematoxylin and eosin, modified trichrome, periodic acid-Schiff, and oil red O or are incubated for histochemical demonstration of adenosine triphosphatase, succinic dehydrogenase, nicotinamide adenine dinucleotide-tetrazolium reductase, phosphorylase, esterase, acid phosphatase, and alkaline phosphatase (42, 44). Muscle fiber type distribution, which influences contracture test results, can be defined by these techniques. However, evidence for correlation of MH susceptibility with altered histochemical and metabolic tests is inconclusive. Adenosine triphosphate (ATP) depletion test has been described to identify MH muscle (45). Britt and coworkers found a reduced ATP depletion ratio (ATP in muscle equilibrated with carbogen plus halothane/ATP in muscle equilibrated with carbogen alone) in MH muscle (46). Allen and coworkers found that ATPase and Ca^{++} uptake were significantly reduced in MH muscle compared to control groups (47). However, Ca^{++} uptake reduction has been contradicted by more recent definitive studies (48, 49). Adenylate kinase has been studied in muscles and red blood cells from MH-susceptible humans and swine, and no abnormality in isoenzyme pattern or activity was found (50). Glucose-6-phosphate dehydrogenase deficiency has been noted in the red blood cells of MH individuals, indicating that depressed activity of a major antioxidant system may be part of MH (51, 52).

Because platelets and muscle cells have similar calcium ATP-dependent contractile apparatus, platelet bioassay has been proposed as a screening method for MH. Solomons and coworkers suggested that platelets be used as a screening test for MH (53). However, others have been unable to prove the reliability of platelet ATP depletion as a test for MH (54, 55).

Halothane-Succinylcholine Challenge. One of the best ways to accurately identify an MH-susceptible individual is to challenge that individual with halothane and succinylcholine. Obviously, this has limited application, but it is useful in research to accurately identify reactors and to verify contracture test results (18, 19). Halothane challenges also guide appropriate culling from breeding herds of swine (56). The test in swine is simple to do. Halothane is administered for 3 to 5 minutes to young pigs via face mask (56, 57). Reactions are assessed by the appearance of rigidity of the hind limbs, hyperthermia, or death with intense rigor mortis. McGrath et al. have shown that dose-response effects of halothane influence challenge results (57). False negatives were noted at halothane concentrations less than 3%, whereas increasing the halothane to 4 and 5% significantly reduced reaction times. Their conclusion was that 3% halothane was generally sufficient for MH testing. Seeler et al., in addition to halothane challenge, utilized halothane and succinylcholine together (32). Animals that did not react to 5 minutes of halothane were given 0.75 mg/kg succincylcholine i.v., and halothane and positive pressure ventilation were continued an additional 8 minutes. Reactor incidence was significantly greater with halothane-succinylcholine than with halothane alone.

Red Blood Cell Fragility. This test is done by mixing small samples (0.1 ml) of blood with saline ranging in concentration from 60 to 120 mM. A fragility curve is made by plotting the amount of hemoglobin occurring at each saline concentration. This test is much less invasive and dangerous than halothane challenge but has had variable results (22, 58, 59). A recent study by O'Brien and coworkers showed a clear increase in red blood cell (RBC) fragility in MH-susceptible Pietran swine and an intermediate increase in RBC fragility in crossbreds, compared to controls (60). Those investigators postulated a complex hereditary pattern explaining degree of response to halothane challenge, RBC fragility, and CPK activity in the crossbred versus the purebred Pietrans.

PREVENTION AND TREATMENT OF MALIGNANT HYPERTHERMIA

There is probably no "safe" anesthetic technique to prevent an MH episode, because emotional excitement and stress can initiate an episode (20, 61). Simply handling stress-susceptible pigs can precipitate a fatal crisis. The excitement of breeding, the so-called "purple porcine passion," can lead to the demise of a boar (62). MH has been described in awake (11) individuals and in patients who were administered anesthetic drugs thought to be safe (13). MH patients should be closely monitored in recovery because the episode may not occur until then (12, 13).

Certain anesthetic agents are thought least likely to trigger MH and are therefore considered appropriate for use in MH-susceptible individuals. Table 19.1 shows drugs known to trigger MH, drugs not recommended, and drugs considered safe (20, 31, 63).

All volatile anesthetic agents trigger MH, including sevoflurane, which is in the developmental stages (4, 64, 65). Of the injectable anesthetics, etomidate did not trigger MH in susceptible pigs. However, when etomidate was compared to thiopental, etomidate was thought to predispose pigs to a more rapid onset of MH when they were exposed to succinylcholine and halothane (66). The new muscle relaxants atracurium and vecuronium have been shown to be safe in MH individuals (67, 68).

Table 19.1
Anesthetic Drugs and MH

Avoid	Use	Not Recommended
Volatile anesthetic agents	Barbiturates	Ketamine
Depolarizing skeletal muscle relaxants	Narcotics	Belladonna alkaloids
Amide local anesthetics	Neuroleptanalgesia	Amide local anesthetics
	Tranquilizers	Calcium salts
	Nitrous oxide	Cardiac glycosides
	Ester locals	Catecholamines
	Nondepolarizing muscle relaxants	Quinidine

Local anesthesia techniques cannot be assumed to be safe because considerable stress may be involved and may trigger MH. Procaine and tetracaine, as ester group locals, do not affect muscle cell calcium flux. Lidocaine, mepivacaine, and bupivacaine, which are amide locals, were thought to trigger MH. However, Berkowitz and Rosenberg described a series of 103 human patients, 35 of whom were under 12 years of age, in whom femoral block with mepivacaine was used for diagnostic muscle biopsy (69). No MH episodes occurred. Wingard and Bobko went further and administered huge doses of intravenous lidocaine to MH-susceptible swine. Lidocaine toxicity was noted, but MH did not occur (70). Selection of local over general anesthetic techniques depends on such factors as the nature of the surgery, apprehension, or, in the case of domestic species, ease of handling. Heavy sedation for local or pregeneral anesthesia is appropriate.

TREATMENT OF AN MH EPISODE

Successful management of MH depends on early recognition of the crisis. If MH is suspected, the anesthetic should be stopped. All inhalation agents should be discontinued, and the patient should be ventilated with oxygen from anesthetic delivery apparatus that has not been used for volatile anesthetic agents. Sodium bicarbonate is indicated to correct metabolic acidosis and hyperkalemia. The patient should be actively cooled. This can be accomplished by placing crushed ice around the patient, administering iced intravenous fluids, and lavaging of stomach and rectum with iced saline (20, 29). Urine output should be maintained using intravenous saline or balanced electrolyte solution, osmotic diuresis with 5% dextrose in the fluids, or mannitol. Procainamide, not procaine, is indicated to control cardiac arrhythmias (29). Verapamil, a calcium channel blocker, has also been used to combat cardiac arrythmias, but recent findings have demonstrated cardiovascular collapse when verapamil and dantrolene were used in combination (71, 72). This interaction may occur with other calcium channel blockers in combination with dantrolene. After suffering an MH crisis, the patient should be closely monitored for 48 hours after an episode, because late complications or recurrence of MH is possible.

Dantrolene Sodium

Dantrolene (Dantrium, Norwich-Eaton Pharmaceuticals) is a hydantoin derivative that relaxes skeletal muscle by direct action on the muscle, but does not completely abolish contractile response even at high doses (73, 74). It is used in the treatment of neurogenic spasticity and is effective for both prevention and treatment of MH. It is the only drug that reliably accomplishes the latter. Dantrolene has little effect on cardiac muscle, but may interfere with electrical activity of Purkinje fibers (74). As noted previously, serious conduction abnormalities have been reported when dantrolene was combined with the calcium channel blocker verapamil (71, 72). Effects on intestinal smooth muscle have been reported to be negligible. A dose-dependent reduction of maximal bladder and urethral pressures indicates dantrolene may inhibit calcium movement across those membranes (74). Respiratory effects of dantrolene are negligible (73). Hepatotoxicity results from chronic therapy (74).

Dantrolene's mechanism of action is interference with excitation-contraction coupling, probably at more than one site. Dantrolene probably aborts the MH syndrome by decreasing release of calcium from the sarcoplasmic reticulum (SR), while allowing calcium uptake to continue (19, 73, 75, 76). Dantrolene may also enhance reuptake of calcium by the SR, although this has not been well defined (74). It is not clear whether dantrolene influences sarcolemmal calcium flux (19, 74).

Until recently, dantrolene was available only as an oral preparation. It is now marketed in an intravenous form in 70-ml vials that contain 20 mg of lyophilized dantrolene (74, 77). However, the commercial intravenous preparation is at present cost-prohibitive for use in large animal species. There are several "home-made" methods described for making capsule form dantrolene into a form suitable for intravenous use (78–83). We have used the method of Gronert and coworkers to prepare dantrolene powder that is readily dissolvable in sterile water, sodium hydroxide, and mannitol (82). The latter is added to correct osmolarity. Preparation of the powder is time consuming and uses a large number of filters. This is necessary in order to remove impurities in the capsule form of dantrolene. It is therefore not appropriate to assume that one can make intravenous dantrolene quickly in the event of an emergency. However, the dantrolene powder can be made by this method and stored for rapid reconstitution when needed.

Dose requirement of dantrolene varies somewhat from species to species. Oral dantrolene, given to humans at a dose of 1 to 2 mg/kg four times a day has been used for prophylaxis (84–86). Failure of that dose to prevent MH has been reported (86). An i.v. dose of 2.4 mg/kg in humans is thought to be effective in preventing and treating MH (87). Porcine dose requirement is higher. Gronert and coworkers reported that doses of 1 to 3 mg/kg only attenuated the MH response, and 5 mg/kg were needed to prevent the reaction to halothane and succinylcholine (88). Others have reported successful treatment of porcine MH with lower doses of 2 to 3.5 mg/kg (89, 90). Effective dose for other species has not been well defined. Use of dantrolene should be accompanied by other preventative and therapeutic measures cited and should not be relied on as the sole method of treatment for MH.

Other Drugs in the Treatment of MH

There is conflicting evidence regarding the ability of alpha-adrenergic antagonists such as the phenothiazines to protect against an MH episode. These drugs may increase heat loss and improve muscle perfusion by vasodilatation (4). Their ability to prevent MH may be dose-related. McGrath and coworkers found that high doses of acetylpromazine (1.65 mg/kg) prevented MH in 73% of MH swine challenged (91).

Pancuronium, initially thought to delay the MH response, may actually prevent it. Jones and coworkers used large doses of 1.5 mg/kg and prevented halothane-induced MH for 120 minutes (92).

MALIGNANT HYPERTHERMIA ASSOCIATION OF THE UNITED STATES

The Malignant Hyperthermia Association of the United States (MHAUS) is an organization formed to provide support and information to MH-susceptible patients, their families, and their physicians. A 24-hour emergency line has been established to assist physicians in treating MH episodes. MHAUS is actively involved in fund raising for continuing research on MH. One of its goals is to establish a data bank to aid research programs. For information on MHAUS, write to Box 3231, Darien, Connecticut 06820.

MH IN SWINE

MH-susceptible swine are usually found in the Poland China, Pietran, and Landrace breeds. Crossbreeds of these MH-susceptible pigs are also affected, but their genetic makeup and hence the degree of MH response can vary considerably (60). MH has also been reported in Yorkshires (Christian, Pork Quality Symposium, 1972).

Much of present knowledge of MH comes from swine. Understanding of hereditary patterns, metabolic and physiological changes, screening tests, and response to drugs is largely due to the availability of such a good animal model of the disease (93–110). The latter references are cited in addition to many others appearing earlier in the text.

MH IN DOGS

An MH-like anesthetic fatality was first reported for the canine species in 1973 when a 3-year-old pointer developed hyperthermia in response to halothane (111). Two siblings of that dog had elevated serum CPK and were therefore considered to be susceptible also. Since that time, MH-like reactions have been reported in a variety of breeds,including greyhound, border collie, Saint Bernard, and mixed breeds (112–116). One greyhound reported was the littermate of another that had died after an MH-like episode (116). Dantrolene was a part of the successful management of the Greyhound that survived. All of the dogs reported to have MH had elevated serum enzymes consistent with muscle damage. Exertional rhadomyolysis, similar to that seen in horses, has also been reported in a racing greyhound (117).

MH incidence in dogs was limited to case reports until a cross-bred Doberman pinscher suffered a fatal MH reaction at the University of Saskatchewan (118). The breeder of that dog was found, and a litter was obtained from the same dam. The dogs had many of the characteristics associated with MH in humans and swine, including hypertrophied muscles, very nervous temperaments, high resting body temperature, and mildly elevated serum muscle enzymes. Muscle biopsy samples from the dogs had positive contracture tests. Increased RBC osmotic fragility was noted (119).

Establishing a colony was difficult because a high puppy mortality resulted from attempts to interbreed the dogs. Infertility was a problem with the MH bitch. However, an MH male mated to a normal German shepherd cross female produced five puppies. Three were MH reactors, and two were nonreactors. Resting CPK levels and osmotic RBC fragility did not differentiate the MH from the non-MH offspring. Dantrolene given early and at a dose rate of 2 mg/kg was an effective treatment for the MH episodes in these dogs (120).

MH IN CATS

There is one report of MH in a cat. The episode was in response to halothane and decamethonium. Despite apparently successful attempts at cooling after the first episode, the animal died after a second attempt to recreate the episode (121).

MH IN HORSES

Equine myopathy occurs as a syndrome similar to MH. The equine syndrome includes an exercise-related myopathy or the "tying-up" syndrome, anesthetic-related myopathy, and spontaneous myopathy that can be related to stress. Although all cases of equine myopathy cannot be linked to MH, there is increasing evidence that MH is a factor in equine myopathy syndromes.

Equine Postanesthetic Myopathy

Equine postanesthetic myopathy (EPAM) continues to be a life-threatening complication of anesthesia in horses. Forelimb lameness after general anesthesia in horses was mistakenly called "radial nerve paralysis," until Trimm and Mason in 1973 showed that muscle damage was in fact the cause of the problem (122). It is now recognized that myopathy after anesthesia varies considerably. It may be a temporary condition characterized by swollen, painful muscles; inability to bear weight on the affected limb; elevated serum muscle enzymes; and myoglobinuria. Triceps, gluteals, lumbar, biceps, or semimembranosis-tendinosis muscles may be involved. Postanesthetic myopathy may also manifest as severe, fatal, generalized muscle damage. It is often not detected until the recovery phase of anesthesia, when the horse is not able to rise or the horse is unable to remain standing. The cause of postanesthetic myopathy is still not clearly understood, and the gravity of this anesthetic complication is increased by inability to predict its occurrence and lack of an experimental model to study it. At present, two possibilities seem most likely as the cause of postanesthetic myopathy.

POSITIONING, PERFUSION, AND BLOOD PRESSURE

That general anesthesia and recumbency are not innocuous and a degree of muscle damage occurs in normal horses subjected to anesthesia has been shown by several investigators who demonstrated increased SGOT, CPK, and lactic acid in horses that did not develop clinical myopathy after anesthesia (123–125). An animal as large as a horse during anesthesia is at increased risk of muscle damage caused by a possible combination of hypotension, hypoxia, acidosis, and poor perfusion to dependent muscle groups. Water beds, air mattresses, and elevation of uppermost limbs have been recommended to minimize pressure and venous occlusion (126). It has been postulated that dependent limb myopathy in the horse may be related to the compartmental crush syndrome, which refers to local muscle ischemia due to edema and increased pressure within an osteofascial compartment and is treated by faciotomy (127, 128). Lindsay et al. measured muscle pressures using a wick catheter placed in several muscle groups of anesthetized horses. The horses were subjected to lengthy deep anesthesia on a hard surface. Pressures were significantly elevated in the dependent muscles, and five out of six animals had forelimb lameness and evidence of muscle damage, which was not permanent (129). Muscle perfusion has been shown by Weaver and Staddon to decrease in anesthetized compared to awake horses, but interestingly in that study no difference was noted in perfusion of uppermost and dependent muscles (130). The horses in that study were lying on air mattresses. Efforts to create myopathies by manipulating diet and creating abnormalities such as hypoxia and hypercapnia during anesthesia, in the absence of faulty padding, have been unsuccessful in producing myopathy (125). Grandy and coworkers subjected halothane-anesthetized horses to 3 hours of mean arterial blood pressure of 85 to 95 mm Hg for one experiment, then 55 to 65 mm Hg for a second experiment 7 days later (131). The table was well padded. All the horses in the second group developed some degree of myopathy, which in three of the six was so severe as to necessitate euthanasia. Myopathy was not restricted to the dependent muscle groups.

EQUINE ANESTHETIC-RELATED MYOPATHY AND MALIGNANT HYPERTHERMIA

Increased pressure and poor perfusion do not completely explain postanesthetic myopathy that involves bilateral muscle groups in laterally recumbent horses or myopathy that is severe and generalized. MH may be responsible. In 1975, Klein reported a case of intraoperative hyperthermia and myoglobinuria in a halothane-anesthetized horse (132). Many similarities to MH were noted. There now exists clinical, laboratory, and therapeutic evidence that an MH-like muscle cell defect is a factor in equine postanesthetic myopathy.

Clinically, there are many similarities between MH and EPAM. Heavy muscling, a history of muscle cramping, an apprehensive attitude, and recent hard exercise are associated with higher risk of myopathy during anesthesia (132, 133). An increased risk of EPAM is associated with stormy induction, difficult blood pressure control, arousal and movement, widening pulse pressure, increasing end-tidal CO_2 and $PaCO_2$ despite increased ventilating volume, metabolic acidosis, and anesthesia longer than 2 hours duration (133–135). The spontaneously breathing animal may take huge tidal volumes that empty a 30-liter breathing bag, and efforts to breath may make positive pressure ventilation impossible. Such breathing efforts can occur despite use of muscle relaxants. Body temperature may or may not rise. Response to succinylcholine is similar to MH humans and swine (134–136). Prolonged muscle fasciculation, muscle rigidity, and failure to relax even with large doses may be seen. At recovery, violent behavior is accompanied by profuse sweating, pain, and hard swollen muscles. Elevated serum CPK and myoglobinuria indicate muscle damage, and postmortem findings include massive myonecrosis, the muscle being described as "par-boiled" (133, 137).

Laboratory findings also support the link between MH and EPAM. Waldron-Mease, Rosenberg, and coworkers performed contracture tests on muscle biopsies from normal and myopathy horses and found an increased sensitivity to halothane and caffeine, similar to that of MH (138–140). We have performed contracture tests on four ponies that had hyperthermia in response to halothane and succinylcholine (134) and also found an MH-like increased sensitivity. Two horses with EPAM have had similar contracture test results (Hildebrand, unpublished data).

Response to dantrolene therapy has also provided evidence for MH as a cause of EPAM (137, 141). Although controlled experimental response has not been documented, dantrolene in combination with other therapy, including analgesics, balanced electrolyte solutions, and tranquilizers, has led to recovery in horses that would, in the opinion of the clinicians, have died (unpublished data). One horse after anesthesia was unable to stand, had profuse sweating, and extreme discomfort; we treated it with 1 g of dantrolene i.v. Very shortly thereafter, she stopped sweating and within 12 hours was standing and apparently recovered. Although we have been unimpressed with the efficacy of oral dantrolene for severe EPAM, we do have one report from a practitioner who anesthetized a Thoroughbred for a carpal chip removal. Surgery, anesthesia, and recovery were uneventful until the horse returned to its stall. At that time, the horse developed severe myopathy, was unable to stand, and had a temperature of 106.8°F. Cooling with a hose, intravenous fluids, and acetylpromazine did not help, but 2 hours after 2.5 g of dantrolene orally, the horse began to stand and relax. Twelve hours later, a second 2.5-g dantrolene oral dose was given, and the horse proceeded to complete recovery.

Therapeutic dose of dantrolene for the equine is not known, but may be comparable to swine (138). Preliminary studies by Court and coworkers suggest that oral doses of 4 and 2 mg/kg i.v. may be necessary to establish effective blood levels (142).

Equine Exercise-related Myopathy

Exertional myopathy, or the "tying-up" syndrome, can vary from gait stiffness and poor performance during training to severe muscle cramping, immobility, and myoglobinuria. In MH swine, a correlation between exercise and MH is seen when exercise before anesthesia results in a more rapidly developing and more severe episode of MH (143). Heavy exercise in horses beyond the anaerobic threshold is associated with signs of muscle damage and electrolyte disturbances (144–147). These do not persist in normal horses. Consistent findings include elevated serum CPK, hypochloremia, and depletion of muscle glycogen stores. However, the "tying-up" syndrome is often associated with mild exercise that would not normally cause muscle fatigue. The cause of the "tying-up" syndrome is frequently obscure. Hypothyroidism, high grain diet, heavy exercise after a short rest (Monday morning disease), dietary deficiencies, and hormone imbalance have been implicated. Conventional therapy includes vitamin E-selenium, thiamine, estrogen compounds, and dietary manipulation. Dimethylglycine (Vetricine, Food Science Corp., Vermont) is a methyl donor that has been used as a feed supplement to lower lactate production in exercising muscles of race horses and greyhounds and so improve endurance (148, 149). In one case of equine "tying-up" syndrome, dietary supplement of sodium bicarbonate mitigated the exertional rhabdomyolysis (150).

"Tying-up" syndrome in some cases is related to MH. Failure to respond to conventional therapy and abnormal halothane-caffeine contracture tests have been reported in equine exercise-related myopathy (133). Those animals responded to 300 mg of daily oral dantrolene and were able to return to training and successful competition (151). We have also found abnormal contracture tests in horses with exertional myopathies (Hildebrand, unpublished data). Some animals that we have as yet been unable to investigate fully have histories similar to MH individuals. These are heavily muscled Quarter horses that can follow a careful training program, but tie up with the stress of showing.

Other Causes of Hyperthermia

NEUROLEPTIC MALIGNANT SYNDROME

Neuroleptic malignant syndrome (NMS) is a rare, life-threatening complication of treatment with neuroleptic drugs. NMS was first described in 1968. Agents associated with the syndrome include phenothiazines, butyrophenones, and thioxanthines. Magnitude or duration of treatment does not seem to influence the onset of NMS. Signs include hyperthermia, hypertonicity of skeletal muscles, fluctuating consciousness, and autonomic instability. NMS is differentiated from MH by using curare or pancuronium. A flaccid paralysis occurs in NMS, but rigidity persists in MH. Treatment with dantrolene, amantidine, and bromocriptine may be effective (152).

IATROGENIC BENIGN HYPERTHERMIA

During anesthesia, hyperthermia may be associated with prolonged general anesthesia, unnecessary clothing, heavy atropinization, or impermeable surgical drapes (153). These cases are differentiated from MH by lack of rigidity, normal CPK levels, and easy control of hyperthermia by exposing the body, alcohol sponging, and ice packs.

OTHER

The inflammatory response to tissue trauma can elevate body temperature for several days after surgery. Various pyrogenic bacteria can also be involved. Manipulation of infected tissues during surgery can cause febrile reactions (154). Dehydration is capable of increasing temperature by effects on the thermoregulatory centers (155). Excitement and struggling can cause elevated temperature. Postictal hyperthermia has been noted after ketamine-induced seizures (156). Pyrexia can be associated with pulmonary aspiration (154).

Capture Myopathy—Stress Hyperthermia

Hyperthermia, hyperkalemia, severe acidosis, and fatal necrosis of skeletal and cardiac muscle are part of a complex metabolic upset that occurs with the pursuit, capture, and restraint of wild animal species (157–163). The syndrome has many similarities to MH, but the mechanism of stress hyperthermia is as yet unknown. Animals often die acutely, with hyperthermia, acidemia, hyperkalemia, and pulmonary edema. Those that survive for 1 or 2 days show depression, increased heart and respiratory rates, and increased arterial CO_2 tensions. Muscle necrosis causes stiff, painful movement that progresses to paresis. Elevated CPK, SGOT, LDH, lactate, and hyperkalemia are noted. Myoglobinuria progresses to renal failure.

Supportive therapy includes intravenous fluids, oxygen, sodium bicarbonate, antibiotics, and steroids. Such treatment alone is frequently unsuccessful. A seratonin-blocking drug, ketanserin, has been partially effective in preventing the MH reaction in swine and may be effective in treating capture myopathy (164). Ketanserin 0.1 mg/kg dramatically reduced temperature and mortality in a group of stressed elk. However, on a second stress challenge that did not involve any treatment or measurements, the only animals that died were the ones that had received ketanserin for the first stress challenge 1 week earlier. Further evaluation of ketanserin in the treatment of stress hyperthermia is indicated because it was effective in prevention. Reasons for the mortality distribution on the second challenge were not clear.

Prevention of stress hyperthermia is imperative. Restricting pursuit time is critical; experienced personnel recommend that the time not exceed 1 minute. The animals must not be restrained by sacks or ropes for lengthy periods. Whenever feasible, animals should be trained ahead of time, and proper crates should be used. Stress and excitement should be avoided at all cost.

References

1. Hall GM: Body temperature and anesthesia. *Br J Anaesth* 50:29–44, 1978.
2. Denborough MA, Lovell RRH: Anesthetic deaths in a family. *Lancet* 2:45, 1960.
3. Denborough MA, Forster JFA, Lovell RRH, Maplestone PA, Villiers JD: Anesthetic deaths in a family. *Br J Anaesth* 34:395–396, 1962.
4. Gronert GA: Malignant Hyperthermia. *Anesthesiology* 53:395–423, 1980.
5. Webb AJ: The halothane test: a practical method of eliminating porcine stress syndrome. *Vet Rec* 106:410–412, 1980.
6. D'Allaire S, Deroth L: Incidence of porcine stress syndrome susceptibility at the St. Cyrille record of performance station at Quebec. *Can Vet J* 23:168, 1982.
7. Hall LW, Woolf N, Bradley JWP, et al: Unusual reaction to suxemethonium chloride. *Br Med J* 2:1305, 1966.
8. Harrison GG, Biebuych JF, Terblanche J, et al: Hyperpyrexia during anesthesia. *Br Med J* 3:594, 1968.
9. Fletcher JE, Rosenburg H: In vitro interaction between halothane and succinylcholine in human skeletal muscle: implications for malignant hyperthermia and masseter muscle rigidity. *Anesthesiology* 63:190–194, 1985.
10. Nelson TE, Flewellen EH, Gloyna DF: Spectrum of susceptibility to malignant hyperthermia—diagnostic dilemma. *Anesth Analg* 62:545–552, 1983.
11. Gronert GA, Thompson RL, Onofrio BM: Human malignant hyperthermia awake episodes and correction by dantrolene. *Anesth Analg* 59:377–378, 1980.
12. Beldavs J, Small V, Cooper DA, Britt BA: Postoperative malignant hyperthermia: a case report. *Canad Anesth Soc J* 18:202–211, 1971.
13. Grinberg R, Edelist G, Gordon A: Postoperative malignant hyperthermia episodes in patients who received "safe" anesthetics. *Canad Anaesth Soc J* 30:273–276, 1983.
14. Scheitler LE, Getzendanner L, Gussack GS, O'Neill BH, Siemen KM: Malignant hyperthermia during oral surgery. *Anesth Prog* 31:170–174, 1984.
15. Gronert GA: Controversies in malignant hyperthermia. *Anesthesiology* 59:273–274, 1983.
16. Denborough MA: Etiology and pathophysiology of malignant hyperthermia. *Int Anesth Clinics* 17:11–23, 1979.
17. Gallant EM, Godt RE, Gronert GA: Role of plasma membrane defect of skeletal muscle in malignant hyperthermia. *Muscle and Nerve* 2:491–493, 1979.
18. O'Brien PJ, Mickleson JR, Gronert GA, Louis CF: Malignant hyperthermia susceptibility hypersensitive calcium-induced calcium release mechanism of muscle. *Anesthesiology* 63:A270, 1985.
19. Allen P, Lopez JR, Jones D, Alamo L, Papp L, Sreter FS: Measurements of $[Ca^{2+}]i$ in skeletal muscle of malignant hyperthermia swine. *Anesthesiology* 63:A268, 1985.
20. Britt BA: Malignant hyperthermia. *Mod Med Can* 31:511–517, 1976.

21. Moulds RFW, Denborough MA: Biochemical basis of malignant hyperthermia. *Br Med J* 2:241–244, 1974.
22. Denborough MA, Warne GL, Moulds RFW, et al: Insulin secretion in malignant hyperpyrexia. *Br Med J* 3:493, 1974.
23. Harrison GG, Verburg C: Erythrocyte osmotic fragility in hyperthermia susceptible swine. *Br J Anesth* 45:131, 1973.
24. Zsigmond EK, Kothary SP, Penns J, et al: Normal erythrocyte fragility and abnormal platelet aggregation in MH families. In Aldrete JA, Britt BA (eds): *Malignant Hyperthermia*. New York, Grune and Stratton, 1978, pp. 213–219.
25. Solomons CC, Tan S, Aldrete JA: Platelet metabolism in MH. In Aldrete JA, Britt BA (eds): *Malignant Hyperthermia*. New York, Grune and Stratton, 1978, pp 221–225.
26. Williams CH, Stubbs DH, Payne CG, et al: Role of hypertension in fulminant hyperthermia-stress syndrome. *Br Med J* 1:628, 1976.
27. Williams CH, Shanklin MD, Hedrich HB, et al: The fulminant hyperthermia-stress syndrome: genetic aspects, hemodynamic and metabolic measurements in susceptible and normal pigs. In Aldrete JA, Britt BA (eds): *Malignant Hyperthermia*. New York, Grune and Stratton, 1978, pp 113–141.
28. Britt BA: Preanesthetic diagnoses of malignant hyperthermia. *Int Anesth Clinics* 17:63–69, 1979.
29. Ryan J: Treatment of the acute hyperthermia crisis. *Int Anesth Clinics* 17:153–168, 1979.
30. Kalow W, Britt BA, Richter A: The caffeine test of isolated human muscle in relation to malignant hyperthermia. *Canad Anaesth Soc J* 24:678–694, 1977.
31. Huckell VG, Stanloff HM, McLoughlin PR, et al: Cardiovascular manifestations of normothermic malignant hyperthermia. In Aldrete JA, Britt BA (eds): *Malignant Hyperthermia*. New York, Grune and Stratton, 1978, pp 373–377.
32. Seeler DC, McDonell WN, Basrur PK: Halothane and halothane succinylcholine induced malignant hyperthermia (porcine stress syndrome) in a population of Ontario boars. *Can J Comp Med* 47:284–290, 1983.
33. Britt BA, Endrenyi L, Peters PL, Kwong FHF, Kadijevic L: Screening of malignant hyperthermia susceptible families by creatine phosphokinase measurement and other clinical investigations. *Canad Anaesth Soc J* 23:263–283, 1976.
34. Heffron JJA, Mitchell G. Diagnostic value of serum creatine phosphokinase activity for the porcine malignant hyperthermia syndrome. *Anesth Analg* 51:536–539, 1975.
35. Nelson TE, Denborough MA: Studies on normal human skeletal muscle in relation to the pharmacopathology of malignant hyperpyrexia. *Clin Exp Pharm Physiol* 4:315–322, 1977.
36. Endrenyi L, Kalow W: Motor unit counting and the caffeine contracture test in malignant hyperthermia. *Anesthesiology* 47:490–497, 1977.
37. Moulds RFW, Denborough MA: A study of the actions of caffeine, halothane, potassium chloride and procaine on normal human skeletal muscle. *Clin Exper Pharmacol and Physiol* 1:197–209, 1974.
38. Rosenberg H, Reed S: In vitro contracture tests for susceptibility to malignant hyperthermia. *Anesth Analg* 62:415–420, 1983.
39. Ellis R, Keaney NP, Harriman DGF, et al: Screening for malignant hyperthermia. *Br Med J* 3:559–561, 1972.
40. Deuster PA, Bockman EL, Muldoon S: In vitro responses of cat skeletal muscle to halothane and caffeine. *J Appl Physiol* 58:521–527, 1985.
41. Ording H, Ranbler E, Fletcher R: Investigation of malignant hyperthermia in Denmark and Sweden. *Br J Anaesth* 56:1183–1189, 1984.
42. Harriman DGF: Preanesthetic investigation of malignant hyperthermia: microscopy. *Int Anesth Clinics* 17:97–117, 1979.
43. Huckell VF, Staneloff HM, Britt BA, Waxman MB, Morch JE: Cardiac manifestations of malignant hyperthermia susceptibility. *Circulation* 58:916–925, 1978.
44. Cardinet GH, Holliday TA: Neuromuscular diseases of domestic animals: a summary of muscle biopsies from 159 cases. *Ann NY Acad Sci* 317:290–313, 1979.
45. Gronert GA: Muscle contractures and adenosine triphosphate depletion in porcine malignant hyperthermia. *Anesth Analg* 58:367–371, 1979.
46. Britt BA, Endrenyi L, Kalow W, Peters P: The adenosine triphosphate (ATP) depletion test: comparison with the caffeine contracture test as a method of diagnosing malignant hyperthermia susceptibility. *Canad Anesth Soc J* 23:624–635, 1976.
47. Allen PD, Ryan JF, Sreter FA, Mabuchi K: Rigid vs non-rigid MH, studies of Ca^{2+} uptake and actomyosin ATPase. *Anesthesiology* 53:5251, 1980.
48. Nagarajan K, Fishbein WN, Carlin HM, Pezeshkpour G, Muldoon SM: Frozen section calcium-uptake versus halothane and caffeine contracture tests on human muscle. *Anesthesiology* 63:A307, 1985.
49. Blanck TJJ, Gruener R, Suffecool SL, Thompson M: Calcium uptake by isolated sarcoplasmic reticulum: examination of halothane inhibition, pH dependence and Ca^{2+} dependence of normal and malignant hyperthermia human muscle. *Anesth Analg* 60:492–498, 1981.
50. Marjanen LA, Denborough MA: Adenylate kinase and malignant hyperthermia. *Br J Anaesth* 54:949–952, 1982.
51. Younker D, DeVore M, Hartlage P: Malignant hyperthermia and glucose-6-phosphate dehydrogenase deficiency. *Anesthesiology* 60:601–602, 1984.
52. Schanus EG, Lovrien RE: Malignant hyperthermia (MH) in humans: deficiencies in the protective enzymes systems for oxidative damage. *Prog Clin Biol Res* 97:95–111, 1982.
53. Solomons CC, McDermott N, Mahowald M: Screening for malignant hyperthermia with a platelet bioassay. *N Engl J Med* 303:642, 1980.
54. Giger U, Kaplan RF: Halothane induced ATP depletion in platelets from patients susceptible to malignant hyperthermia and from controls. *Anesthesiology* 58:347–352, 1983.
55. Lee MB, Adragna MG, Edwards L: The use of a platelet nucleotide assay as a possible diagnostic test for malignant hyperthermia. *Anesthesiology* 63:311–315, 1985.
56. Webb AJ, Gordon CHC: Halothane sensitivity as a field test for stress susceptibility in the pig. *Anim Prod* 26:157–168, 1978.
57. McGrath CJ, Lee JC, Rempel WE: Halothane testing for malignant hyperthermia in swine: dose-response effects. *Am J Vet Res* 45:1734–17364, 1984.
58. Goden DV, Herring FG, MacLeod PJM: Malignant hyperthermia: characterization of erythrocyte membranes from individuals at risk. *J Med* 12:35–491, 1981.
59. Lampo P: Resistance osmotique des erythrocytes comme indicateur dez stress chez les porcs. *Landrace Belge et Large White Rev Agric (Brussels)* 31:843–848, 1978.
60. O'Brien PJ, Rooney MT, Reik TR, Thatte HS, Rempel WE, Addis PB, Louis CF: Porcine malignant hyperthermia susceptibility: erythrocytic osmotic fragility. *Am J Vet Res* 46:1451–1456, 1985.
61. Wingard DW, Gatz EE: Some observations on stress susceptible patients. In Aldrete JA, Britt BA (eds): *Malignant Hyperthermia*. New York, Grune and Stratton, 1978, pp 363–372.
62. Harrison GG: Porcine malignant hyperthermia. *Int Anesth Clin* 17:25–61, 1979.
63. Relton JES: Anesthesia for elective surgery in patients susceptible to malignant hyperthermia. *Int Anesth Clin* 17:141–151, 1979.
64. Shulman M, Braverman B, Ivankovitch AD, Gronert GA: Sevoflurane triggers malignant hyperthermia in swine. *Anesthesiology* 54:259–260, 1981.
65. McGrath CJ, Rempel WE, Jessen CR, Addis PB, Crimi AJ: Malignant hyperthermia-triggering liability of selected inhalant anesthetics in swine. *Am J Vet Res* 42:604–607, 1981.
66. Suresh MS, Nelson TE: Malignant hyperthermia is etomidate

safe? *Anesth Analg* 64:420–424, 1985.

67. Buzello W, Williams CH, Phool C, Watkins ML, Dozier SE: Vecuronium and porcine malignant hyperthermia. *Anesth Analg* 64:515–519, 1985.
68. Michel PA, Fronefield HP: Use of atracurium in a patient susceptible to malignant hyperthermia. *Anesthesiology* 62:213, 1985.
69. Berkowitz A, Rosenberg H: Femoral nerve block with mepivacaine for muscle biopsy in malignant hyperthermia patients. *Anesthesiology* 62:651–652, 1985.
70. Wingard DW, Bobko S: Failure of lidocaine to trigger porcine malignant hyperthermia. *Anesth Analg* 58:99–103, 1979.
71. Roewer N, Rumberger E, Bode H, Schulte Am Esch J: Electrophysiological and mechanical interactions of verapamil and dantrolene on isolated heart muscle. *Anesthesiology* 63:A274, 1985.
72. Bezer G: Dantrolene sodium intravenous-verapamil. *Anesthesia Intensive Care* 13:108, 1985.
73. Pinder RM, Brogden RN, Speight TM, Avery GS: Dantrolene sodium: a review of its pharmacological properties and therapeutic efficacy in spasticity. *Drugs* 13:3–23, 1977.
74. Britt BA: Dantrolene. *Canad Anesth Soc J* 31:61–75, 1984.
75. Morgan KG, Bryant SH: The mechanism of action of dantrolene sodium. *J Pharm Exp Therap* 201:138–147, 1977.
76. Ellis KO, Carpenter JF: Mechanism of control of skeletal muscle contraction by dantrolene sodium. *Arch Phys Med Rehabil* 55:362–369, 1974.
77. Dantrium IV. Norwich-Eaton Pharmaceutical, Medical Dept., Norwich, NY, 13815, 1985.
78. Harrison GG: Control of the malignant hyperpyrexic syndrome in MHS swine by dantrolene sodium. *Br J Anaesth* 47:62–65, 1975.
79. Fukuchi H, Kuwata N, Seki Y, Morio M: Preparation and stability of parenteral solution of 0.4 w/v % dantrolene sodium. *Hiroshima J Anesth* 15:21–24, 1979.
80. Fukuchi H, Morio M: Preparation of dantrolene sodium for intravenous use. *Hiroshima J Anesth (Suppl)* 13:119, 1977.
81. Tomonaga F, Kobayashi T, Yago K, et al: Pharmaceutical studies of dantrolene sodium. *Hiroshima J Anesth (Suppl)* 15:101–108, 1979.
82. Gronert GA, Mansfield E, Theye RA: Rapidly soluble dantrolene for intravenous use. In Aldrete JA, Britt BA (eds): *Malignant Hyperthermia.* New York, Grune and Stratton, 1978, pp 535–536.
83. O'Brien PJ, Forsyth GW: Preparation of injectable dantrolene for emergency treatment of malignant hyperthermia-like syndromes. *Canad Vet J* 24:200, 1983.
84. Free CW, Jaimon MPC: Preanesthetic administration of dantrolene sodium to a patient at risk from malignant hyperthermia. *NZ Med J* 88:493–494, 1978.
85. Pandit SK, Kothary SP, Cohen PJ: Orally administered dantrolene for prophylaxis of malignant hyperthermia. *Anesthesiology* 50:156–158, 1979.
86. Fitzgibbons DD: Malignant hyperthermia following preoperative oral administration of dantrolene. *Anesthesiology* 54:73–75, 1981.
87. Flewellen EH, Nelson TE, Jones WP, Arens JF, Wagner DL: Dantrolene dose response in awake man: implications for management of malignant hyperthermia. *Anesthesiology* 59:275–280, 1983.
88. Gronert GA, Milde JH, Theye RA: Dantrolene in porcine malignant hyperthermia. *Anesthesiology* 41:488–495, 1976.
89. Alitalo I, Schulman A: Halothane induced porcine malignant hyperthermia reversed by dantrolene. *Nord Vet Med* 35:239–242, 1983.
90. Flewellen EH, Nelson TE: Dantrolene dose response in malignant hyperthermia-susceptible (MHS) swine: method to obtain prophylaxis and therapeusis. *Anesthesiology* 52:303, 1980.
91. McGrath CJ, Rempel WE, Addis PB, Crimi AJ: Acepromazine and droperidol inhibition of halothane induced malignant hyperthermia (Porcine stress syndrome) in swine. *Am J Vet Res* 42:195–198, 1981.
92. Jones DE, Ryan JF, Taylor B, Papp L, Lopez JR, Alamo L, Sueter FA, Allen PD: Pancuronium in large doses protects susceptible swine from halothane induced malignant hyperthermia. *Anesthesiology* 63:A344, 1985.
93. Hall LW, Trimm CM, Woolf N: Further studies of porcine malignant hyperthermia. *Br Med J* 15:145–148, 1972.
94. Lucke JN, Hall GM, Lister D: Porcine malignant hyperthermia I: metabolic and physiologic changes. *Br J Anaesth* 48:297–301, 1976.
95. Hall GM, Bendall JR, Lucke JN, Lister D: Porcine malignant hyperthermia II: heat production. *Br J Anaesth* 48:305–308, 1976.
96. Lister D, Hall GM, Lucke JN: Porcine malignant hyperthermia III: adrenergic blockage. *Br J Anaesth* 48:831–838, 1975.
97. Hall GM, Lucke LN, Lister D: Porcine malignant hyperthermia IV: neuromuscular blockade. *Br J Anaesth* 48:1135–1141, 1976.
98. Hall GM, Lucke JN, Lister D: Porcine malignant hyperthermia V: fatal hyperthermia in the Pietran pig, associated with the infusion of α adrenergic agonists. *Br J Anaesth* 49:855–863, 1977.
99. Lucke JN, Denny H, Hall GM, Lovell R, Lister D: Porcine malignant hyperthermia VI: the effects of bilateral adrenulectomy and pretreatment with bretylium on the halothane induced response. *Br J Anaesth* 50:241–246, 1978.
100. Hall GM, Lucke JN, Lovell R, Lister D: Porcine malignant hyperthermia VII: hepatic metabolism. *Br J Anaesth* 52:11–17, 1980.
101. Hall GM, Lucke JN, Orchard C, Lovell R, Lister D: Porcine malignant hyperthermia VIII: leg metabolism. *Br J Anaesth* 54:941–947, 1982.
102. Gronert GA, Heffron JJA: Skeletal muscle mitochondria in porcine malignant hyperthermia: respiratory activity, calcium functions, and depression by halothane. *Anesth Analg* 58:76–81, 1979.
103. Gronert GA, Theye RA. Halothane induced porcine malignant hyperthermia: metabolic and hemodynamic changes. *Anesthesiology* 41:36–43, 1976.
104. Gallant EM, Godt RE, Gronert GA: Mechanical properties of normal and malignant hyperthermia susceptible porcine muscle: effects of halothane and other drugs. *J Pharm Exp Ther* 213:91–96, 1980.
105. Gronert GA, Theye RA, Milde JH, Tinker JH: Catecholamine stimulation of myocardial oxygen consumption in porcine malignant hyperthermia. *Anesthesiology* 49:330–337, 1978.
106. Bardsley ME, Wheatley AM, Fowler CJ, McCrodden JM, McLoughlin JV, Tipton KF: Metabolism of monoamines in malignant hyperthermia susceptible pigs. *Br J Anaesth* 54:1313–1317, 1982.
107. Gronert GA, Milde JH, Theye RA: Role of sympathetic activity in porcine malignant hyperthermia. *Anesthesiology* 47:411–415, 1977.
108. Kerr DD, Windgard DW, Gatz EE: Prevention of porcine malignant hyperthermia by epidural block. *Anesthesiology* 42:307–311, 1975.
109. Gronert GA, Milde JH, Theye RA: Porcine malignant hyperthermia induced by halothane and succinylcholine: failure of treatment with procaine or procaineamide. *Anesthesiology* 44:124–132, 1976.
110. Anderson IL, Jones EW: Porcine malignant hyperthermia: effect of dantrolene sodium on in-vitro halothane-induced contraction of susceptible muscle. *Anesthesiology* 44:57–61, 1976.
111. Short CE, Paddleford RP: Malignant hyperthermia in a dog. *Anesthesiology* 39:462–463, 1973.

112. Bagshaw RJ, Cox RH, Knight DH, Detweiler DK: Malignant hyperthermia in a greyhound. *J Am Vet Med Assoc* 172:61–62, 1978.
113. Sawyer DC: Malignant hyperthermia. *J Am Vet Med Assoc* 179:341–344, 1981.
114. Short CE: The significance of malignant hyperthermia in animal anesthesia. In Aldrete JA, Britt BA (eds): *Malignant Hyperthermia*. New York, Grune and Stratton, 1978, pp 175–182.
115. Leary SL, Anderson LC, Manning PJ: Recurrent malignant hyperthermia in a Greyhound. *J Am Vet Med Assoc* 182:521–522, 1983.
116. Kirmayer AH, Klide AM, Purvance JE; Malignant hyperthermia in a dog: case report and review of the syndrome. *J Am Vet Med Assoc* 185:978–982, 1984.
117. Bjotvedt G, Hendricks GM: Exertional rhabdomyolysis in a racing greyhound. *Vet Med/SAC* 78:1215–1220, 1983.
118. O'Brien PJ, Cribb PH, White RJ, Olfert ED, Steis JE: Canine malignant hyperthermia: diagnosis of susceptibility in a breeding colony. *Can Vet J* 24:172–177, 1983.
119. O'Brien PJ, Forsyth GW, Olexson DW, et al: Canine malignant hyperthermia susceptibility. Erythrocyte defects—osmotic fragility, glucose-6-phosphate dehydrogenase deficiency and abnormal Ca^{2+} homeostasis. *Can J Comp Med* 48:381–389, 1984.
120. Cribb PH, Olfart ED, Reynolds FB: The inheritance and prediction of malignant hyperthermia in the dog. *Proceedings 2nd International Cong of Vet Anesth* 170–171, 1985.
121. DeJong RH, Heavner JE, Amory DW: Malignant hyperpyrexia in the cat. *Anesthesiology* 41:608–609, 1974.
122. Trimm CM, Mason J: Post-anaesthetic forelimb lameness in horses. *Equine Vet Journal* 5:71–76, 1973.
123. Steffey EP, Farver T, Zinkl J, Wheat JD, Meagher DM, Brown MP: Alterations in horse blood cell count and biochemical values after halothane anesthesia. *Am J Vet Res* 41:934–939, 1980.
124. Waldron-Mease E: Postoperative muscle damage in horses. *J Eq Med Surgery* 1:106–110, 1977.
125. Johnson BD, Heath RB, Bowman B, Phillips RW, Rich LD, Voss JL: Serum chemistry changes in horses during anesthesia. *J Eq Med Surg* 2:109–123, 1978.
126. Heath RB, Redder J, Stashak T, Shaw R: Protecting and positioning the equine surgical patient. *Vet Med/Sm Anim Clinician* 67:1241–1245, 1972.
127. Mubarak S, Owen CA: Compartmental syndrome and its relation to crush syndrome: a spectrum of disease. *Clin Orthoped Rel Res* 113:81–89, 1975.
128. Rorabech CH, Bourne RB, Fowler PJ: The surgical treatment of compartment syndromes of the leg. *J Bone Joint Surg* 66:93–97, 1984.
129. Lindsay W, McDonell W, Bignell W: Equine postanesthetic forelimb lameness: intracompartmental muscle pressure changes and biochemical patterns. *Am J Vet Res* 41:1919–1924, 1980.
130. Weaver BMQ, Staddon GE: Muscle perfusion in the horse. *Eq Vet J* 16:66–68, 1984.
131. Grandy JL, Steffey EP, Hodgson D, Woliner M: The relationship between arterial hypotension during halothane anesthesia and the development of equine post anesthetic myopathy. *Am J Vet Res* (in press), 1986.
132. Klein LV: Case report: a hot horse. *Vet Anesth* 3:41–42, 1975.
133. Klein L: A review of 50 cases of post-operative myopathy in the horse-intrinsic and management factors affecting risk. *Am Assoc Eq Pract Proceedings* 24:89–94, 1978.
134. Manley SV, Kelly AB, Hodgson D: Malignant hyperthermia-like reactions in three anesthetized horses. *J Am Vet Med Assoc* 183:85–89, 1983.
135. Hildebrand SV, Howitt GA: Succinylcholine infusion associated with hyperthermia in ponies anesthetized with halothane. *Am J Vet Res* 44:2280–2284, 1983.
136. Riedesel D, Hildebrand SV: Unusual response following use of succinylcholine in a horse anesthetized with halothane. *J Am Vet Med Assoc* 187:507, 1985.
137. Friend SCE: Postanesthetic myonecrosis in horses. *Can Vet J* 22:367–371, 1981.
138. Waldron-Mease E, Rosenberg H: Postanesthetic myositis in the horse associated with in vitro malignant hyperthermia susceptibility. *Vet Sci Comm* 3:45–50, 1979.
139. Rosenberg H, Waldron-Mease E: Malignant hyperpyrexia in horses: anesthetic sensitivity proven by muscle biopsy. *Scientific Abst Am Soc of Anesthesiology* 333–334, 1977.
140. Waldron-Mease E, Klein LV, Rosenberg H, Leitch M: Malignant hyperthermia in a halothane anesthetized horse. *J Am Vet Med Assoc* 179:896, 1981.
141. Short CE, White KK: Anesthetic/surgical stress-induced myopathy (myosites) Part I: clinical occurrences. *Am Assoc Eq Pract Proceedings* 24:101–106, 1977.
142. Court MH, Engelking LR, Dodman NH, Seeler DC: The pharmacokinetics and availability of dantrolene sodium in the horse (preliminary results). *Proceedings 2nd Int Cong Vet Anesth* 103, 1985.
143. Van den Hende C, Lester D, Ooms L, Oyaert W: Malignant hyperthermia in Belgian landrace pigs rested or exercised before exposure to halothane. *Br J Anaesth* 48:832–829, 1976.
144. Snow DH, Kerr MG, Nimmo MA, Abbott EM: Alterations in blood, sweat, urine and muscle composition during prolonged exercise in the horse. *Vet Rec* 110:377–384, 1982.
145. Koterba A, Carlson GP: Acid-base and electrolyte alterations in horses with exertional rhabdonyolysis. *J Am Vet Med Assoc* 180:303–306, 1982.
146. Cardinet GH, Littrell JF, Freedland RA: Comparative investigations of serum creatinine phosphokinase and glutamicoxalocacetate transaminase activities in equine paralytic myoglobinuria. *Res Vet Sci* 8:219–226, 1967.
147. Waldron-Mease E: Hypothyroidism and myopathy in racing thoroughbreds and standardbreds. *Eq J Med Surg* 3:124–128, 1979.
148. Levine SB, Smith GL, Erb H: Effect of a nutritional supplement containing N,N-dimethylglycine (DMG) on the racing standardbred. *Eq Pract* 4:17–20, 1982.
149. Gannon JR, Kendall RV: A clinical evaluation of N,N-dimethylglycine (DMG) and disopropyl ammonium dichloroacetate (DIPA) on the performance of racing greyhounds. *Canine Pract* 9:7–13, 1982.
150. Robb EJ, Kronfield DS: Dietary sodium bicarbonate as a treatment for exertional rhabdomyolysis in a horse. *J Am Vet Med Assoc* 188:602–607, 1986.
151. Waldron-Mease E: Update on prophylaxis of tying-up using dantrolene. *Am Assoc Eq Pract Proceedings* 25:379, 1979.
152. Guzé BH, Baster LR: Neuroleptic malignant syndrome. *New Engl J Med* 313:163–165, 1985.
153. Fraser JC: Iatrogenic benign hyperthermia in children. *Anesthesiology* 48:375, 1978.
154. Crider B, Nightingale P, Hill AB: Intraoperative hyperpyrexia—keep an open mind. *Anesthesiology* 64:413, 1986.
155. Guyton AC: Body temperature, temperature regulation, and fever. In *Textbook of medical Physiology*, ed 3. Philadelphia, WB Saunders Co, 1966.
156. Lees DE, MacNamara T: Ketamine induced hyperthermia—postictal or malignant? *Anesthesiology* 47:390–391, 1977.
157. Harthoorn AM, Young E: A relationship between acid-base balance and capture myopathy in zebra (*Equus burchelli*) and an apparent therapy. *Vet Rec* 94:337–341, 1974.
158. Young E: Muscle necrosis in captive red Hartebeeste. *J So Afr Vet Med* 37:101–103, 1966.
159. Chalmers GA, Barret MW: Capture myopathy in pronghorns in

Alberta, Canada. *J Am Vet Med Assoc* 171:918–923, 1977.
160. Young E: Leg paralysis in the greater flamingo and lesser flamingo. *Intl Zoo Yearbook* 7:226–227, 1967.
161. Wobesei G, Bellamy JEC, Boysen BG, MacWilliams PS, Runge W: Myopathy and myoglobinuria in white-tailed deer. *J Am Vet Med Assoc* 169:971–974, 1976.
162. Lewis RJ, Chalmers GA, Barrett MW, Bhatragar R: Capture myopathy in elk in Alberta, Canada: a report of three cases. *J Am Vet Med Assoc* 171:927–932, 1977.
163. Haigh JC, Stewart RR, Wobeser G, MacWilliams PS: Capture myopathy in a moose. *J Am Vet Med Assoc* 171:924–926, 1977.
164. Stanley TH, Port JD, Van Der Maatin J, Kimball J: Treatment of stress hyperthermia in elk with ketanserin, a seratonin receptor blocker. *Vet Surg* 15:214–217, 1986.

CHAPTER 20

Diagnostic or Experimental Surgical Procedures

PART 1

Clinical Procedures

DEAN H. RIEDESEL, D.V.M., Ph.D., D.A.C.V.A.

Management of anesthesia during special diagnostic and surgical procedures requires an understanding of the procedure to be completed and the influence of these exercises on the animal's response to the anesthetic regime. There is an additional anesthetic risk involved in special diagnostic procedures. Due to the very nature of a procedure requiring anesthesia, for one to complete the diagnostic process implies there is incomplete diagnosis of the primary problem of the patient. Without this knowledge, less than ideal planning of anesthesia may occur. This adds to patient risk. In addition, many diagnostic procedures are completed in areas that are not convenient to monitoring equipment or emergency medications or in other circumstances that interfere with complete patient control.

Myelography

The primary anesthetic consideration for managing a patient that is to receive a myelogram is to minimize the possibility of seizures. Postmyelographic seizures are common in the canine but less frequent in the equine and feline (1–4). Metrizamide is the water-soluble contrast agent currently used. It is less neurotoxic than its predecessor, methiodal (5). However, the canine may develop seizures during the recovery period from general anesthesia after a myelogram in certain situations. The exact mechanism of the neurotoxicity is unknown but may be related to metrizamide's ability to competitively inhibit glucose transport across cell walls (6).

SEIZURE PREVENTION

Most clinical studies indicate that the canine patients with the highest risk of seizuring are heavy (>25 kg in body weight) and injected with large volumes of contrast (>7 ml of 375 mg metrizamide per ml), into the cisterna magna (1). The following may reduce the seizure incidence:

1. Prolong anesthesia.
2. Elevate the head and reduce cerebral exposure to the contrast medium.
3. Avoid using certain drugs.
4. Enhance the excretion of the contrast medium.
5. Use an anticonvulsant drug in the protocol.
6. Administer glucose.

Prolong Anesthesia

Anesthesia times of less than 30 minutes are associated with a high seizure incidence (2, 7). Thus, dogs should be kept under anesthesia for at least 30 to 60 minutes after the injection of the contrast. A delay in waking the patient probably allows more of the contrast to be absorbed from the subarachnoid space.

Reduced Cerebral Exposure

If the metrizamide can be prevented from contacting the cerebral cortex, the seizure incidence may be reduced (8). Thus, lumbar injections are less likely to cause seizures than are cisterna magna injections (1, 9). If the head can be elevated above the level of the vertebra, the contrast will tend not to enter the cranium because metrizamide has a higher specific gravity than cerebrospinal fluid. Radiographically, metrizamide can be found in the subarachnoid space for at least 60 minutes, so a patient's head should continue to be elevated after the radiographs have been taken. During recovery, the elevation of the head should be continued until the patient can roll to a sternal position and hold its head upright. Dogs that are surgical candidates immediately after the myelogram can have their heads elevated if they are to be in a sternally recumbent position. The dosage of metrizamide in a large dog should be kept to a minimum or possibly dosage should be according to body surface area rather than weight (1).

Avoid Certain Drugs

Phenothiazine-derivative tranquilizers should be avoided as a tranquilizer in dogs because they may lower seizure threshold and increase the incidence of seizures (5, 10). The short-acting opioids are a safe preanesthetic premedication (e.g., meperidine, oxymorphone, or butorphanol). Certain neuroleptanalgesic combinations (e.g., fentanyl and droperidol) can be used at a low dose for a preanesthetic medication. High doses of neuroleptanalgesics to cause unconsciousness should be avoided because they are associated with a high seizure incidence (5, 11).

It seems logical to exclude drugs that normally produce a seizure-like electroencephalogram in patients about to receive a myelogram. Drugs of this type are ketamine and enflurane (12); however, there are no studies that have evaluated these drugs in myelogram patients.

Enhance the Excretion of the Contrast Medium

Assuming that the contrast agent causes the seizures by some direct mechanism, enhanced excretion should reduce the side effects. This premise is supported by the observation that cases with abnormal retention of the contrast in the subarachnoid space of more than 24 hours were associated with seizures and other complications (1). Metrizamide is normally eliminated from the cerebrospinal fluid by absorption into the blood stream and then renal excretion. Dehydration of the patient impairs excretion of the contrast and is associated with more side effects (13). Diuresis of the patient may enhance excretion and reduce the incidence of metrizamide seizures (14).

Anticonvulsant Drugs

Several anticonvulsant drugs have been used in the anesthetic protocol. Low doses of pentobarbital have been used (0.45 to 1.35 mg/kg i.m.) as a preanesthetic medication with variable success (1). Larger dogs experienced a lower seizure incidence if they received the drug. Pentobarbital is, however, a short-acting barbiturate; when used as a premedication, it may not produce blood levels adequate to prevent seizures upon anesthetic recovery. The effect of inhalant anesthetics on the pharmacokinetics of pentobarbital is unknown but may prolong the drug's half-life, consequently retaining its anticonvulsant effects (15).

The use of phenobarbital in the protocol of canine myelogram patients may be more logical than using pentobarbital. Although most barbiturates have anticonvulsant properties, only phenobarbital can exert its maximum anticonvulsant effect at doses below those producing hypnosis (16). A retrospective clinical study in the dog showed that the preanesthetic administration of a subsedative dose (2 mg/kg) of phenobarbital i.m. reduced the seizure incidence (9).

Diazepam is another logical choice for prevention of seizures but may be of limited value because of its short half-life, slow absorption from intramuscular sites of injection, and variable neuroleptic effect (17).

Nonetheless, diazepam has been used as a pre- and postanesthetic medication resulting in a low seizure incidence (18, 19).

Glucose Administration

The mechanisms of metrizamide seizures may involve a blockade of cellular glucose metabolism. Metrizamide reduces the cellular uptake of glucose; if metrizamide could gain intracellular access, it would competitively inhibit the enzyme hexokinase (6, 20). Hexokinase is the enzyme responsible for the phosphorylation of glucose, the initial step of glucose metabolism. Glucose has been added to the metrizamide in hopes of reducing the seizure incidence but was not beneficial (21). The use of intravenous glucose in a diuresis protocol did reduce the seizure incidence, but it is not known whether the effect was from the glucose or enhanced elimination of metrizamide (14).

CANINE ANESTHETIC PROTOCOL

Preanesthetic Medication

One of the opioids is usually beneficial: meperidine (2 to 4 mg/kg i.m.), butorphanol (0.2 to 0.4 mg/kg i.m.), or oxymorphone (0.1 to 0.2 mg/kg i.m.). An anticonvulsant drug can be beneficial in the large dog (e.g., phenobarbital 2 mg/kg i.m.). Anticholinergic drugs are used only if indicated.

Induction and Maintenance

The thiobarbiturates commonly are used for a smooth and rapid induction of anesthesia. Anesthetic maintenance can be by the inhalation of methoxyflurane, halothane, or isoflurane. Nitrous oxide may be used along with one of the other more potent inhalants.

Recovery

The canine patient must be watched closely for generalized seizures as it recovers from anesthesia. The patient's head should be elevated, an intravenous catheter kept in place for possible drug administration, and an anticonvulsant drug administered. Some patients will develop isolated muscle twitches of the face, neck, or forelimbs. This muscle twitching need not be treated but should be monitored closely because it will progress in some cases to focal or generalized seizures. The seizures should be treated with incremental doses of diazepam (0.25 mg/kg i.v.) if the seizure lasts more than 60 seconds. Because of diazepam's short duration of action, seizures may reoccur in 15 minutes. These reoccurring seizures are also treated with diazepam until the patient has received 1 mg/kg total dose. Further seizures are treated with phenobarbital or pentobarbital, which are repeated until the convulsive activity subsides. In most cases, seizure will begin as the dog regains consciousness and number only one or two convulsions; the dog then recovers normally. There are, however, reports of cases with repeated seizures over a period of 12 hours postmyelography (1).

Other Complications

There are two other possible complications the anesthetist should be aware of transient apnea during the injection of the contrast medium into the subarachnoid space (1, 22) and hyperthermia (>105°F), which may develop during the first few hours of recovery (1, 23). The transient apnea may be associated with cardiac arrhythmias. Several new water soluble contrast agents (iohexol and iopamidol) are being investigated in the dog and are possibly less neurotoxic (24, 25).

FELINE ANESTHETIC PROTOCOL

Feline myelography is not performed as often as in the canine but appears to be associated with fewer complications (4, 23, 24). Phenothiazine tranquilizers should be avoided as a preanesthetic medication because they may predispose the patient to seizures. Large doses of ketamine to maintain general anesthesia should be avoided because the electroencephalographic effect of ketamine is similar to convulsive activity (12).

Preanesthetic Medication

Ketamine can be used as preinduction medication at doses of 2 to 10 mg/kg i.m. The dose is dependent on how much sedation is necessary. An anticholinergic (e.g., glycopyrolate) needs to be given with the ketamine to prevent excessive salivation.

Induction and Maintenance

Anesthesia can be induced by giving incremental doses of a thiobarbiturate or a ketamine/diazepam mixture intravenously. Mask or chamber induction with an inhalant anesthetic is also acceptable. Inhalation anesthesia with either halothane, methoxyflurane, or isoflurane is used for maintenance.

Recovery

The patient's head should be kept elevated until it is able to maintain a sternal position. An intravenous catheter should be kept in place for anticonvulsant medication should a seizure occur.

EQUINE ANESTHETIC PROTOCOL

Metrizamide myelography is also being used in the horse (3, 26, 27). Compression of the cervical spinal cord is usually suspected, and cisterna magna injections are made in the laterally recumbent anesthetized horse (28).

Preanesthetic Medication

Most of these patients are already ataxic, so it is safest to avoid using high doses of anesthetic premedications. The horse does not seem to be very prone to metrizamide seizures, so phenothiazine tranquilizers or xylazine can be used if a preanesthetic is necessary.

Induction and Maintenance

Induction of anesthesia is accomplished in a normal manner with a guaifenesin and thiobarbiturate combination. Halothane and oxygen is used for maintenance with whatever monitoring and supportive measures are needed (i.e., fluids, electrocardiogram (ECG), blood pressure, and ventilation). The horse's head should be kept in an elevated position during the injection of metrizamide.

Recovery

Recovery should take place in a quiet well-padded stall with oxygen supplementation. Postmyelogram horses may have muscle fasciculations of the muzzle, neck, pectoral, and shoulder regions as they regain consciousness. These muscle fasciculations will last for several hours and may be accompanied by jerking movements of the head and neck. Central nervous system depression is evident for about 24 hours, and many of the horses will be transiently febrile (3).

ALTERNATE INTUBATION TECHNIQUES

Occasionally, an animal has to be anesthetized for a surgical procedure of the head or neck that requires tracheal intubation through the nasal cavity or a separate surgical incision and not through the mouth. Nasal and pharyngostomy intubations are used in horses and small animals, respectively, when the surgeon needs the oral cavity devoid of extraneous apparatus (29, 30). Intubation through a tracheostomy is used for patients having certain types of laryngeal surgery (e.g., partial arytenoidectomy) and cleft palate repair (31–33).

PHARYNGOSTOMY INTUBATION

Dogs and cats can have an orally placed endotracheal tube repositioned through a pharyngostomy (Fig. 20.1) (30). The pharyngostomy incision is made after the patient is anesthetized and orally intubated in the normal manner (34). The patient is positioned in lateral recumbency, and the lateral aspect of the head and neck from the cranial edge of the ramus of the mandible to the caudal border of the larynx is clipped free of hair and surgically scrubbed. Either side can be used, although it is easier for the right-handed person to insert the tube into the patient's left pharynx. An index finger is inserted into the mouth to locate the hyoid bones. The index finger is then bent laterally and pushed outward anterior to the hyoid bones. By palpation and occlusion of the jugular vein, an area caudal to the digastricus muscle, ventral to the maxillary vein and mandibular salivary gland, dorsal to the linguofacial vein, and cranial to the epihyoid bone, lingual artery, and hypoglossal nerve is located (Fig. 20.2) (35). A skin incision is made parallel to the linguofacial vein directly over the fingertip inside the patient's mouth. A Kelly hemostat is inserted through the skin incision and pushed through the subcutaneous tissues supported by the index finger inside the patient's mouth. When the tip of the hemostat is against the pharyngeal mucosa, the index finger inside the mouth is removed and pressure is applied medially with the hemostat in order to displace part of the pharyngeal wall into the oral cavity. The hemostat is moved so that its tip is dorsal to the tongue and caudal to the tonsillar crypt. With the jaws of the hemostat spread, a scalpel is inserted into the oral cavity and the pharyngeal wall incised, allowing the tip of the hemostat to enter the oral cavity (Fig. 20.3). The jaws of the hemostat are then spread further to form a hole large enough to allow passage of the endotracheal tube. Once the hole has been enlarged, the cuff on the endotracheal tube is deflated and the adapter is removed from its end. The tube is temporarily inserted further into

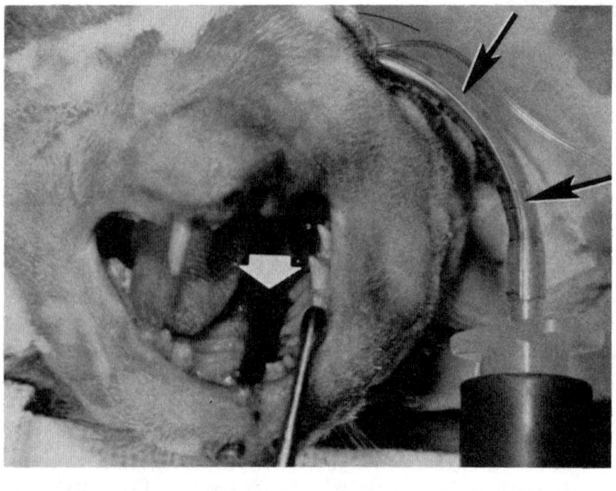

Figure 20.1. An anesthetized cat with a fractured hard palate (*white arrow*). A pharyngostomy intubation (*black arrow*) was used to facilitate surgical exposure of the hard palate.

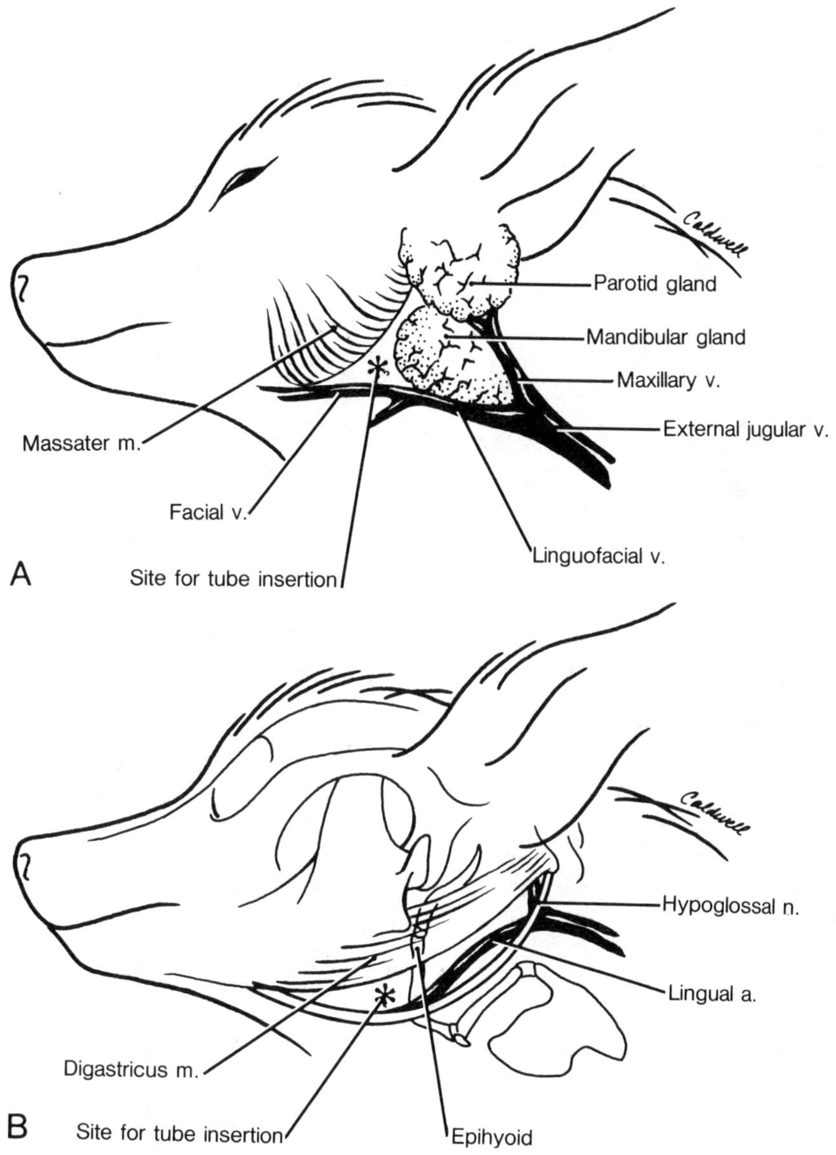

Figure 20.2. The anatomical structures adjacent to the site of a pharyngostomy intubation. *A*, superficial structures can be identified by palpation. Visualization of the venous structures is enhanced by jugular vein occlusion. *B*, the deeper structures of the pharyngeal area. The digastricus muscle and epihyoid bone can be palpated from inside the mouth. The hypoglossal nerve and lingual artery are avoided by using blunt dissection.

the trachea, and the adapter end is grasped by the hemostat and pulled through the pharyngostomy incision. Once the tube is pulled through the skin, it is repositioned in the trachea so the tip lies in the caudal cervical area. Visually inspect the tube inside the mouth for kinks and reposition the tube if necessary. The cuff can then be reinflated, if necessary, and the tube is taped or sutured in place (Fig. 20.4).

The small tube leading to the cuff of the endotracheal tube is usually left inside the mouth. If this small tube needs to come through the pharyngostomy also, it should be brought out first and then followed by the endotracheal tube. At the end of the surgical procedure, the endotracheal tube is replaced into the oral cavity and extubation is accomplished in a normal manner. The pharyngostomy is not sutured but left to heal by granulation.

TRACHEOSTOMY INTUBATION

In some surgical procedures of the larynx, the surgeon does not want an endotracheal tube interfering. In these cases, a tracheotomy is performed below the larynx and a tube is inserted (31, 36). The tracheostomy can be performed awake with local anesthesia or it can follow induction of general anesthesia and temporary orotracheal intubation.

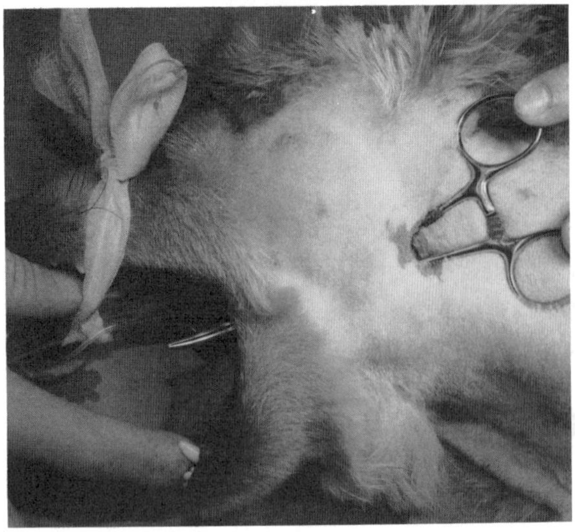

Figure 20.3. A hemostat has been inserted through a pharyngostomy incision into the oral cavity. The hemostat is used to grasp the adapter end of the endotracheal tube and to guide it through the pharyngostomy.

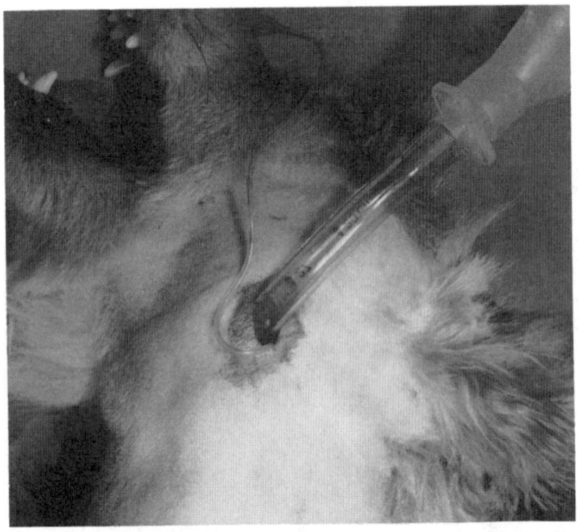

Figure 20.4. The appearance of a completed pharyngostomy intubation in a dog. The tube may be taped or sutured to the skin to prevent dislodgement.

Horse

Tracheostomy in the horse is performed at the upper one-third to middle cervical region (29). A longitudinal incision is made through the skin, and the sternocephalicus and sternothyrohyoideus muscles are separated, exposing the trachea. A transverse incision is made in the trachea between the cartilaginous rings, and the tube is inserted. The tube size is usually smaller than would be used orally. An adult horse may only allow a 20-mm inner diameter (ID) tube to be inserted.

Dog

The tracheostomy is performed in the upper one-third of the neck (37, 38). The procedure is similar to the horse with a longitudinal incision and middle separation of sternocephalicus and sternohyoideus muscles. The trachea is entered through a transverse incision between two cartilaginous rings. Be careful not to insert the tube too far and occlude one of the main bronchi. The anesthesia tube may be replaced with a specific tracheostomy tube for recovery. When the tracheostomy tube is removed, the incision is not sutured but allowed to heal by granulation.

NASAL INTUBATION

Horses of all ages can be tracheally intubated through the nose, allowing surgery or diagnostic techniques of the oral cavity without interference from the endotracheal tube (29, 39). The size of the nasal tube is usually smaller than could be used orally. A newborn foal will accept an 8- to 10-mm ID tube, while an adult horse takes only an 18- to 26-mm ID tube. The nasotracheal tube can be placed while the patient is awake with either physical or chemical restraint. Nasal intubation can be used for inhalant anesthetic induction of foals. Parenteral anesthesia can also be used prior to nasotracheal tube insertion.

A well lubricated tube is inserted into the nostril and directed along the floor of the nasal cavity with the bevel of the tube positioned dorsally. The bevel in this position will aid in sliding the tube into the nasopharynx. Once the tip of the tube is in the nasopharynx, the orotracheal axis is straightened by elevating the nose. The advancing tube will either strike the larynx and stop or enter the larynx and trachea. If intubation is unsuccessful, retract the tube 5 to 10 cm, rotate it 90°, and reinsert. Continue this procedure for several attempts before trying a smaller tube. Some foals being intubated awake, require the instillation of 3 ml of 2% lidocaine through the endotracheal tube and onto the larynx before intubation can be accomplished (39). After the tube is in place, the cuff can be inflated to form an air-tight seal, and the tube is sutured or tied in place until the patient recovers from anesthesia. Epistaxis is a potential complication if a tube size is too large.

BRONCHOSCOPY

Part of the medical workup of a small animal patient with severe or prolonged tracheal or bronchial disease may be bronchoscopy (40). General anesthesia is required before a flexible or rigid fiberoptic bronchoscope can be passed through the larynx and down the trachea (41). The benefits of bronchoscopy usually far outweigh the dangers. However, the list of possible complications should not be overlooked (40).

1. Respiratory depression of the general anesthetic. A patient with compromised pulmonary function

will be further stressed by the respiratory depression produced by general anesthesia.

2. Obstruction of the airway by the bronchoscope. The physical size of the bronchoscope is large enough in most cases to significantly increase airway resistance, resulting in hypoventilation.
3. Physical damage caused by the scope or during biopsy procedures may lead to pneumothorax or hemoptysis.

Before anesthetizing the patient, a thorough physical examination and review of the laboratory data and chest radiographs should be performed. Parenteral anesthesia is adequate in patients with mild respiratory distress. Dogs are premedicated with an opioid and/or a tranquilizer and given intermittent doses of thiobarbiturate by intravenous injection (42). Cats are premedicated with an anticholinergic (e.g., glycopyrolate 0.01 mg/kg i.m.) plus ketamine (2 to 10 mg/kg i.m.) and perhaps a tranquilizer (acetylpromazine at 0.1 mg/kg i.m.). They are then given incremental doses of a ketamine/diazepam mixture i.v. (10 mg/kg ketamine mixed with 0.5 mg/kg diazepam) for parenteral anesthesia. The larynx of the cat should be anesthetized with a local anesthetic (e.g., 2% lidocaine) before insertion of the bronchoscope to prevent laryngospasm. If possible, oxygen should be insufflated into the trachea of these patients through a side port of the bronchoscope or a separate catheter passed alongside the scope.

If the patient is in pronounced respiratory distress, it should be preoxygenated for 5 minutes by breathing into a face mask attached to an anesthetic machine with an oxygen flow rate of at least 200 ml/kg/min. No premedication is used other than an anticholinergic in cats that will receive ketamine. Anesthesia is induced by the intravenous injection of a thiobarbiturate in the dog and/or ketamine/diazepam in the cat. The patient is intubated and put onto an inhalant anesthetic. Halothane or isoflurane are preferred over methoxyflurane because the depth of anesthesia can be altered more rapidly and the recovery time is shorter. Nitrous oxide is avoided in these patients because it would significantly reduce the percentage of inspired oxygen being delivered. The bronchoscope is either passed through the endotracheal (ET) tube or the ET tube is removed and the scope is introduced directly into the trachea (43). The bronchoscope can be passed through a special adapter (Portex swivel adapter) placed on the end of the ET tube, which will provide an airtight seal and allow the continuous administration of oxygen and anesthetic. Oxygen and anesthetic can also be administered through a side port of the bronchoscope or a separate catheter passed alongside (44).

During bronchoscopy, the patient's mucous membrane color and ECG are monitored for signs of hypoxemia and arrhythmia. If respiratory failure occurs, the bronchoscope is removed and the patient is ventilated with oxygen. After the procedure, the patient is monitored during recovery for complications such as pneumothorax and hemoptysis.

LAPAROSCOPY

Laparoscopy is primarily a procedure for visually directing needle biopsy instruments into visceral organs (45). It is preferred by some over laparatomy because it is potentially a shorter procedure. There are two anesthetic considerations for laparoscopy. First, one must consider the organ system that is diseased when selecting the drug protocol. Second, the insufflation of gas (air, carbon dioxide, or nitrous oxide) into the abdomen will reduce the patient's minute ventilation. The preferred gas is nitrous oxide because air may cause vascular embolism and carbon dioxide may alter the patient's acid-base balance (46). The abdomen is inflated to a distended tympanic state. The pressure of gas inside the abdomen should not exceed 20 mm Hg; a pressure of 10 to 15 mm Hg is usually satisfactory. The pressure in the abdomen will displace the diaphragm cranially, and the respiratory minute volume will be reduced about 30% (2). A respirometer on the anesthetic machine would be a very useful monitoring device, and controlled ventilation may be necessary.

CONTROLLED DELIBERATE HYPOTENSION

Neoplasia involving the canine nasal cavity is frequently treated by surgical removal of the tumor and nasal turbinates. This type of surgery is accompanied by considerable hemorrhage that is difficult to control (47). Packing the nasal cavity with iced saline, gauze soaked in dilute epinephrine solution, and temporary occlusion of the carotid arteries have been helpful in reducing the blood loss (47, 48). Another technique to be considered is the deliberate reduction in the arterial blood pressure. This technique has been used in human surgery for a variety of procedures but is most often advocated for certain neurosurgical operations (49). There are several drugs used to lower blood pressure, including ganglionic blockers (trimethaphan), direct vasodilators (nitroprusside and nitroglycerin), and potent volatile anesthetics (halothane and isoflurane) (50). The benefits of hypotension must be weighed against the possibility of ischemia to the brain and other organs. Until more definitive studies in the dog are performed, extreme hypotension (mean arterial pressures of 40 to 50 mm Hg) should not be attempted. However, moderate reductions in the arterial pressure (mean arterial pressures of 60 to 70 mm Hg) are safe for periods of 1 to 4 hours in the dog that does not have concurrent renal or cardiac disease (50, 51).

The technique I prefer for canine nasal surgery is the administration of isoflurane with controlled ventilation. The arterial blood pressure is monitored by an arterial catheter in the dorsal metatarsal artery connected to an aneroid manometer. Approximately two times the minimal alveolar concentration (MAC) of isoflurane is required to achieve a mean arterial pressure of 60 to 70 mm Hg (52). The amount of blood loss is estimated and replaced by infusing three times that amount of lactated Ringer's. Whole blood is administered if a patient is estimated to have lost more than 25% of its blood volume or if the packed cell volume drops below 20% at any time during the surgery. Since initiating the moderate hypotensive anesthesia protocol, the estimated volume of hemorrhage in these cases has decreased. No evidence of ischemic organ damage has been seen.

Isoflurane is preferred over halothane because the former causes hypotension by reducing peripheral vascular resistance while maintaining the cardiac output (50, 52). Thus, organ ischemia should be less likely to occur with isoflurane at low blood pressures.

References

1. Adam WM, Stowater JL: Complications of metrizamide myelography in the dog: a summary of 107 clinical case histories. *J Am Vet Radiol Soc* 22:27–34, 1981.
2. Davis EM, Glickman L, Rendano VT, Short CE: Seizures in dogs following metrizamide myelography. *JAAHA* 17:642–648, 1981.
3. Nyland TG, Blythe LL, Pool RR, Helphrey MG, O'Brien TR: Metrizamide myelography in the horse: clinical radiographic, and pathologic changes. *Am J Vet Res* 41:204–211, 1980.
4. Wheeler SJ, Clayton Jones DG, Wright JA: Myelography in the cat. *J Sm Anim Pract* 26:143–152, 1985.
5. Bartels JE, Braund KG, Redding RW: An experimental evaluation of a nonionic agent amipaque (metrizamide) as a neuroradiologic medium in the dog. *J Am Vet Radiol Soc* 18:117–123, 1977.
6. Elkholm SE: Iohexol vs metrizamide in studies of glucose metabolism, a survey. *Invest Rad* 20 (Suppl):S18–S21, 1985.
7. Bartels JE, Braund KG: Experimental arachnoid fibrosis produced by metrizamide in the dog. *J Am Vet Radiol Soc* 21:78–81, 1980.
8. Le Couteur RA, Scagliotti RH, Beck KA, Holliday TA: Indirect imaging of the canine optic nerve, using metrizamide (optic thecography). *Am J Vet Res* 43:1424–1428, 1982.
9. Riedesel DH: The relationship between premedication and postmyelographic seizure activity. *California Vet* 8:23–24, 1980.
10. Maly P, Olivercrona H, Almen T, Golmen K: Interaction between chlorpromazine and intrathecally injected non-ionic contrast media in non-anaesthetized rabbits. *Neuroradiology* 26:235–240, 1984.
11. Grepe A, Widen L: Neurotoxic effect of intracranial subarachnoid application of metrizamide and meglumine iocarmate. An experimental investigation in dogs in neurolept analgesia. *Acta Radiol Suppl* 335:102–124, 1973.
12. Defalque RJ, Musunuru VS: Diseases of the nervous system. In Stoelting RK, Dierdorf SF (eds): *Anesthesia and Co-Existing Disease*. New York, Churchill Livingstone, 1983, p 305.
13. Eldevik OP, Haughton VM, Sasse EA: The effect of dehydration on the elimination of aqeous contrast media from the subarachnoid space. *Ivest Radiol* 15:155–157,1980.
14. Tamas PM, Walker MA, Paddleford RR, Tinkel SR: Prevention of postmetrizamide myelographic seizures in dogs, using 5% dextrose solution. *J Am Vet Med Assoc* 188:710–712, 1986.
15. Gray PR, Indrieri RJ, Lippert AC: The influence of anesthetic regime on post myelogram seizure incidence in the dog—a prospective study. *Proc Intl Cong Vet Anes* 2:183, 1985.
16. Harvey SC: Hypnotics and sedatives. In Gilman AG, Goodman LS, Gilman A (eds): *The Pharmacological Basis of Therapeutics*, ed 6. New York, MacMillan Publishing Co, 1980, p 339.
17. Frey HH, Loscher W: Pharmacokinetics of anti-epileptic drugs in the dog: a review. *J Vet Pharm Therap* 8:219–233, 1985.
18. Spencer CP, Chrisman CL, Mayhew IG, Kaude JV: Neurotoxicologic effects of the nonionic contrast agent iopamidol on the leptomeninges of the dog. *Am J Vet Res* 43:1958–1962, 1982.
19. Wright JA, Clayton Jones DG: Metrizamide myelography in sixty-eight dogs. *J Small Anim Pract* 22:415–435, 1981.
20. Bertoni JM, Steinman CG: Competitive inhibition of brain hexokinase by metrizamide. *Neurology* 32:320–323, 1982.
21. Northington JW, Biery DN, Glickman LT: Intrathecal dextrose to prevent seizures after metrizamide myelography in dogs. *Invest Radiol* 17:282–283, 1982.
22. Lord PF, Olsson SE: Myelography with metrizamide in the dog: a clinical study on its use for the demonstration of spinal cord lesions other than those caused by intervertebral disk protrusions. *J Am Vet Radiol Soc* 17:42–49, 1976.
23. Northington JW: Metrizamide myelography in five dogs and two cats with suspected spinal cord neoplasms. *J Am Vet Radiol Soc* 21:149–155, 1980.
24. Wheeler SJ, Davies JV: Iohexol myelography in the dog and cat: a series of one hundred cases, and a comparison with metrizamide and iopamidol. *J Sm Anim Pract* 26:247–256, 1985.
25. Cox FH, Jakovljevics: The use of iopamidol for myelography in dogs: a study of twenty-seven cases. *J Sm Anim Pract* 27:159–165, 1986.
26. Beech J: Metrizamide myelography in the horse. *J Am Vet Radiol Soc* 20:22–32, 1979.
27. Rantanen NW, Gavin PR, Barbee DD, Sande RD: Ataxia and paresis in horses Part II. Radiographic and myelographic examination of the cervical vertebral column. *Compend Contin Educ Pract Vet* 3:S161–S171,1981.
28. Stowater JD, Kneller SK, Froelich PS: Metrizamide myelography in two horses. *Vet Med Small Anim Clin* 73:177–183, 1978.
29. Steffey EP: Anesthetic management of the horse with respiratory disease. *Vet Clin North Am Large Anim Pract* 1:113–125, 1979.
30. Hartsfield SM, Gendreau CL, Smith CW, Rouse GP, Thurmon JC: Endotracheal intubation by pharyngotomy. *JAAHA* 13:71–74, 1977.
31. White NA, Blackwell RB: Partial arytenoidectomy in the horse. *Vet Surg* 9:5–12, 1980.
32. Bauman KF, Tate LP, Evans LH, Donawick WJ: Complications of cleft palate repair in large animals. *J Am Vet Med Assoc* 180:652–657, 1982.
33. Gourley IM, Paul H, Gregory C: Castellated laryngofissure and vocal fold resection for the treatment of laryngeal paralysis in the dog. *J Am Vet Med Assoc* 182:1084–1086, 1983.
34. Bohning RH, DeHoff WD, McElhinney A: Pharyngostomy for maintenance of the anorectic animal. *J Am Vet Med Assoc* 156:611–615, 1970.
35. Lantz GC: Pharyngostomy tube installation for the administration of nutritional and fluid requirements. *Compend Contin Educ Pract Vet* 3:135–142, 1981.
36. Harvey CE: Partial laryngectomy in the dog I. Healing and swallowing function in normal dogs. *Vet Surg* 12:192–196, 1983.
37. Harvey CE, Goldschmidt MH: Healing following short duration transverse incision tracheotomy in the dog. *Vet Surg* 11:77–83, 1982.
38. Harvey CE, O'Brien JA: Tracheotomy in the dog and cat: analysis of 89 episodes in 79 animals. *JAAHA* 18:563–569, 1982.
39. Webb AI: Nasal intubation in the foal. *J Am Vet Med Assoc* 185:48–51, 1984.
40. Schaer M, Ackerman N: Diagnostic approach to the patient with respiratory disease. In Ettinger SJ (ed): *Textbook of Veterinary Internal Medicine, Diseases of the Dog and Cat*, ed. 2. Philadelphia, WB Saunders Co, 1983, Vol 1, p 665.
41. McKiernan BC: Lower respiratory tract diseases. In Ettinger SJ (ed): *Textbook of Veterinary Internal Medicine, Diseases of the Dog and Cat*, ed. 2. Philadephia, WB Saunders Co, 1983, Vol 1,

p 760.
42. O'Brien JA, Roszel JF: Bronchoscopy and bronchial cytology. In Kirk RW (ed): *Current Veterinary Therapy*, ed 5. Philadelphia, WB Saunders Co, 1974, p 209.
43. Jones BD, Roudebush P: The use of fiberoptic endoscopy in the diagnosis and treatment of tracheobronchial foreign bodies. *JAAHA* 20:497–504, 1984.
44. Landa JF: Bronchoscopy: general considerations. In Sackner MA (ed): *Diagnostic Techniques in Pulmonary Disease.* New York, Marcel Dekker Inc, 1980, vol 16, p 655.
45. Wildt DE, Kinney GM, Seager SW: Laporoscopy for direct observation of internal organs of the domestic cat and dog. *Am J Vet Res* 38:1429–1432, 1977.
46. Jones BD, Hitt M, Hurst T: Hepatic biopsy. *Vet Clin North Am Small Anim Pract* 15:39–65, 1985.
47. Nelson AW, Wykes PM: Upper respiratory system. In Slatter DH (ed): *Textbook of Small Animal Surgery*. Philadelphia, WB Saunders Co, 1985, p 950.
48. Hedlund CS, Tangner CH, Elkins AD, Hobson HP: Temporary bilateral carotid artery occlusion during surgical exploration of the nasal cavity of the dog. *Vet Surg* 12:83–85, 1983.
49. Stoelting RK, Miller RD: *Basics of Anesthesia*. New York, Churchill Livingstone, 1984, p 347.
50. Newberg LA, Milde JH, Michenfelder JD: Systemic and cerebral effects of isoflurane-induce hypotension in dogs. *Anesthesiology* 60:541–546, 1984.
51. Stone EA, Rawlings CA, Finco DR, Cromwell WA: Renal function after prolonged hypotensive anesthesia and surgery in dogs with reduced renal mass. *Am J Vet Res* 42:1675–1670, 1986.
52. Steffey EP, Howland D, Jr: Potency of enflurane in dogs: comparison with halothane and isoflurane. *Am J Vet Res* 39:573–577, 1978.

PART 2

Experimental Cardiopulmonary Bypass Studies

CHARLES E. SHORT, D.V.M., M.S., D.A.C.V.A., RALPH C. HARVEY, M.S., D.V.M., AND JOSEPH N. CUNNINGHAM, JR., M.D., A.B.S., A.B.T.S.[1]

The calf is frequently used as the experimental model for studies of cardiopulmonary bypass (CPB) (1–4). The authors have used halothane as the primary anesthetic in previous studies. In the most current studies, adaptations were made to incorporate a new inhalant anesthetic, isoflurane, which shows promise for use in cardiac patients (5, 6) and in animal species (7, 8). The objectives were to determine the effectiveness of isoflurane in calves and provide additional physiological data on the combined effect of the anesthetic and other medications during cardiopulmonary bypass.

Anesthetic Management Response during CPB

Normal calves weighing between 50 and 75 kg were used in a group of studies. Each animal was pretreated with chloramphenicol 1 g/calf b.i.d. for 5 days to assure the absence of respiratory infection.

Anesthesia was induced in four animals (Group A)

[1] This study was completed at Maimonides Medical Center in Brooklyn, New York. The study was supported in part by Electro-Catheter Corporation. Isoflurane was supplied by Anaquest. An abstract of this paper was published in the proceedings of the Second International Congress of Veterinary Anesthesiologists, October 8–10, 1985, by Veterinary Practicing Publishing Co., Santa Barbara, California.

with no preanesthetic medication, using equal parts nitrous oxide and oxygen and isoflurane by mask or nasal tube. Isoflurane concentration (up to 4% setting) was increased until the animals became unconscious, and the subjects were intubated. The calves were maintained for 30- to 40-minute periods on lower concentrations of isoflurane in combination with N_2O as anesthetic levels were stabilized. At that time, N_2O was discontinued.

Anesthesia was induced in four animals (Group B) with no preanesthetic medication, using isoflurane and oxygen. Concentrations up to 4% were required. After intubation, isoflurane concentration could be reduced and still provide stable maintenance anesthesia. Sedation was induced in four animals (Group C) using xylazine, 0.06 mg/kg i.v. These calves were then intubated, and anesthesia was maintained with isoflurane.

After intubation, all experimental animals were maintained on an Ohio anesthetic unit with a precision vaporizer. Anesthesia was maintained with isoflurane given to effect (1 to 2 minimal aveolar concentration (MAC)) to produce a surgical plane of anesthesia. A minimum of 2 liters of oxygen flow per minute was provided through a semiclosed circle rebreathing system. The animals were initially breathing spontaneously, but after the establishment of surgical anesthesia, ventilation was assisted using a combination Bird 4-Bird 7 ventilator in the anesthetic circuit. The ventilator was set for 15 to 20 cm of water pressure breaths in a pressure-controlled, volume-limited method. Within 5 minutes of assisted ventilation, complete mechanical control of ventilation was possible. When it was evident by ocular rotation and no palpebral activity that surgical anesthesia was evident, pancuronium, 0.04 mg/kg i.v., was used to maintain complete relaxation.

Intravenous fluid administration was given at 10 cc/kg/hour. Fluids consisted of physiological saline or 5% dextrose in water. A urinary catheter was placed for monitoring urine production. Venous and arterial polyethylene catheters were placed in the saphenous vein and artery for drug administration and blood pressure measurements. A Baltherm Thermal Dilution Catheter (Electro-Catheter Corporation, Rahway, New Jersey) was placed via the right external jugular vein for monitoring central venous pressure and pulmonary arterial wedge pressure and for collection of mixed venous blood samples. Isoflurane anesthesia was continued via endotracheal tube until the animal was on bypass. At that time, anesthesia was maintained by connecting the delivery hose from the anesthesia unit to the cardiac bypass unit. The O_2 flow through the anesthetic unit constituted 25% of total O_2 flow. Pancuronium was given intermittently as necessary to maintain muscle relaxation. Evaluations of cardiopulmonary parameters were made during bypass to determine if sympathetic nervous system responses indicated any lack of adequate analgesia.

Before going on bypass, heparin (3 mg/kg) was administered i.v. to prevent coagulation. Activated clotting time (ACT) values were determined at 30-minute intervals with a Hemochron 400 (Trimed Corp., Huntington Beach, California), and supplemental heparin was given to maintain ACT at greater than 600 seconds.

During connection of cannulas and devices, cardiovascular responses were controlled by medications. In most instances, lidocaine (1.0 to 2.0 mg/kg i.v.) was used to control arrhythmias, atropine (0.02 mg/kg i.v.) to increase heart rate, and dopamine by dilute infusion (5 μg/kg/min) for improvement of vascular performance. Protamine sulfate (2 mg/kg i.v.) was used to reverse the effects of heparin, and furosemide (0.2 mg/kg i.v.) to control urinary output and prevent fluid overload. Nasal administration of 2% phenylephrine spray to reduce postoperative upper airway congestion was used as indicated because the calves were in a lateral recumbency for a total of approximately 5 hours.

A multichannel recorder (Honeywell, Electronics for Medicine, Pleasantville, New York) for determination of blood pressures and electrocardiogram (ECG) responses was used. Repeated samples were taken for blood gas analysis. Blood pressure was determined by direct catheterization of the saphenous artery.

Pulsatile flow cardiopulmonary bypass was used. A membrane oxygenator (Travenol LPM-50, Travenol Laboratories, Deerfield, Illinois) was used in this study. The oxygenator blood was maintained at 36 to 38°C.

The bypass circuit was primed with 1500 cc of 6% hetastarch in 0.9% sodium chloride (6). The pump rate was maintained at a mean of 85 b.p.m. in an asychronous mode. Blood flow was maintained between 3 and 6 liters/minute. Baseline and serial 30-minute measurements for activated clotting time, blood gases and pH, hematocrit, plasma hemoglobin, platelet count, and pump outputs were obtained. Protamine sulfate (2 mg/kg) was used to reverse the effects of heparin, as was potassium chloride to correct hypokalemia and furosemide to control urinary output and prevent fluid overload. Nasal administration of phenylephrine to reduce postoperative upper airway congestion was used as indicated because the calves were in a lateral recumbency for 5 hours of bypass plus time required for instrumentation, initiation of bypass, and termination of bypass.

After completion of the bypass procedure, the calves were allowed to arouse from the anesthesia by discontinuing isoflurane. When needed, residual muscle paralysis was reversed by first administering an anticholinergic (atropine 0.02 mg/kg i.v.) to prevent bradycardia and then reversing the muscle relaxant with the administration of neostigmine (0.05 to 0.1 mg/kg).

Results

Sedation with xylazine was rapid, and intubation was easily accomplished within 2 to 3 minutes after the initial injection. In contrast, mask induction with isoflurane/oxygen or isoflurane/oxygen/nitrous oxide was slower. Even though the calf does not have a keen sense of smell, some objection to isoflurane was observed during induction. There was an increase in heart rate during the induction period with mask induction. After stabilizing anesthesia at a surgical plane, the lowest concentration of isoflurane (1.8%) was observed after xylazine induction, compared to 2.1% after a nitrous oxide/isoflurane induction and 2.4% after an isoflurane/oxygen induction (Table 20.1). Within 30 minutes, the concentrations required were very similar and remained so until the animals were on bypass. The average prebypass hematocrit was 33.0%, which fell to 18.6% after hemodilution. The animals underwent 5 hours of normothermic cardiopulmonary bypass without cardiac arrest.

Table 20.1
Isoflurane Concentration (Vaporizer Settings)

	Surgical Plane Established	+30 Minutes	+60 Minutes
Isoflurane/N_2O:O_2 induction	2.1 ± 0.3[a]	2.0 ± 0.4	2.0 ± 0.4
Isoflurane/O_2 induction	2.4 ± 0.5	2.2 ± 0.6	2.2 ± 0.6
Xylazine/isoflurane induction	1.8 ± 0.5	2.0 ± 0.4	1.9 ± 0.1

Table 20.2
Myocardial Oxygen Demand Rate-Pressure Product (Systolic BP × Heart Rate)

	Surgical Plane Established	+30 Minutes	+60 Minutes
Isoflurance/N_2O:O_2 induction	10,112[a]	11,957	9,960
Isoflurane/O_2 induction	14,394	13,913	15,045
Xylazine/isoflurane induction	8,547	11,576	11,648

[a] Expressed as mean values.

As shown in Table 20.2, the myocardial oxygen demand was lowest during the early surgical plane anesthesia when xylazine was used as a preanesthetic and sedating agent and highest when isoflurane only was used for mask induction and maintenance. This is reflective of the slower heart rate and lower systolic blood pressure in animals receiving xylazine.

Blood pressure responses were stable during the first hour of anesthesia when isoflurane was used alone or in conjunction with nitrous oxide. Lower blood pressure followed xylazine induction, as shown in Table 20.3. This was corrected within 30 minutes to similar blood pressure levels in calves where xylazine was omitted before going on bypass. Slower heart rates were observed when xylazine was used, in contrast to higher heart rates with other techniques, especially after induction and maintenance with isoflurane without nitrous oxide (Table 20.4).

An analysis of the ventilation responses was made during the first hour of surgical plane anesthesia. Arterial blood pH, $PaCO_2$, and PaO_2 tensions were within anticipated normal limits with either type of mask induction and maintenance with isoflurane (Figs. 20.5 to 20.8). pH_a was initially low following the xylazine induction, even though $PaCO_2$ and PaO_2 levels were acceptable. There was compensation of pH during the anesthetic period in animals induced with xylazine.

Table 20.4
Heart Rate Changes (b.p.m.)

	Surgical Plane Established	+30 Minutes	+60 Minutes
Isoflurane/N_2O:O_2	79 ± 27[a]	91 ± 20	83 ± 13
Isoflurane/O_2	118 ± 25	105 ± 30	118 ± 17
Xylazine/isoflurane/O_2	74 ± 4	81 ± 16	81 ± 16

[a] Expressed as mean ± SD.

Table 20.3
Blood Pressure Response (mm Hg)

	Surgical Plane Established	+30 Minutes	+60 Minutes
Isoflurane induction with 1:1 N_2O:O_2, isoflurane maintenance	128 ± 31[a] 80 21	131 ± 35 74 27	120 ± 27 82 25
Isoflurane/oxygen induction and maintenance	123 ± 26 75 36	133 ± 32 93 46	128 ± 25 93 34
Xylazine induction, isoflurane/O_2 maintenance	116 ± 11 60 24	144 ± 16 70 29	144 ± 14 63 31

[a] Expressed as systolic/diastolic mean ± SD.

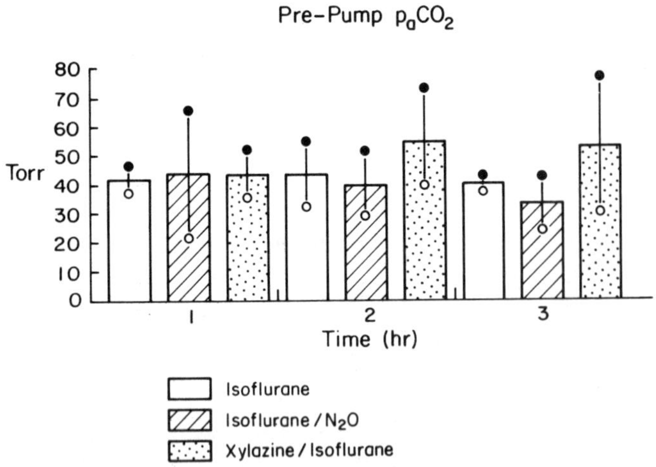

Figure 20.5. Arterial pH responses during 3 hours of anesthesia before cardiac bypass. Xylazine-sedated calves showed lower pH values than nonpremedicated groups.

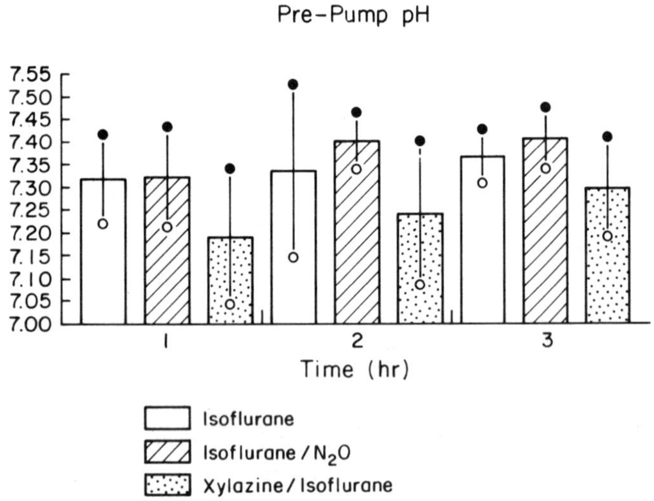

Figure 20.6. Arterial CO_2 responses during 3 hours of anesthesia before cardiac bypass. Mean values were similar during first hour with drop in the isoflurane-nitrous oxide calves by the third hour. All mean values acceptable.

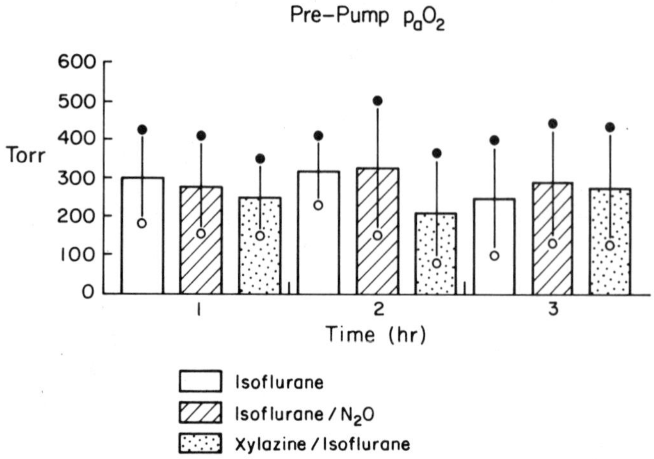

Figure 20.7. Arterial oxygen responses during 3 hours of anesthesia before cardiac bypass demonstrating acceptable oxygen levels in each procedure.

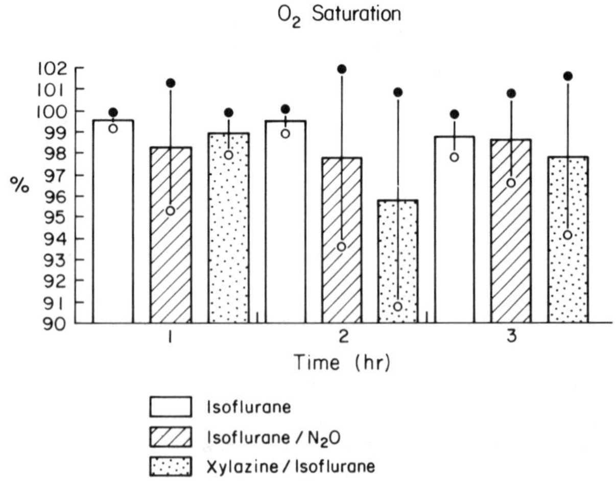

Figure 20.8. Oxygen saturation prior to cardiopulmonary bypass.

However, there was also an elevated $PaCO_2$ level during this period. Oxygen saturation values indicated the normal capability of the animals for uptake of oxygen. Less change in ventilatory responses was observed when the animals were placed on 5 hours of pulsatile flow cardiopulmonary bypass (Figs. 20.9 to 20.12).

Discussion

The induction techniques were successful in each case; however, one may conclude that induction with xylazine simplifies induction, while mask induction is more physiological. Use of supplemental oxygen to the calf before and during induction with xylazine would assist in avoiding the decrease in oxygen tension and pH levels during the early phase of induction. In contrast, it was observed that calves responded well when induced with isoflurane without preanesthetic sedation. The reduction in both heart rate and blood pressure may be attributable to xylazine, especially because it was observed to correct within 30 minutes after stabilization of anesthesia with isoflurane.

Xylazine is a non-narcotic sedative and analgetic analogue for clonidine. It is more effective in cattle than narcotics. It also has muscle relaxant properties related to central nervous system depression. As with narcotic administration in humans, xylazine administration in cattle produces analgesia and may produce significant respiratory depression.

During CPB, volatile anesthetics, such as isoflurane, may be added to the gas introduced into the bypass oxygenator by insertion of a temperature- and flow-compensated anesthetic vaporizer into the gas line (9), as used in this study. Hemodilution is common due to the fluid prime of the bypass unit but did not cause problems in maintaining anesthesia.

Membrane oxygenators have been shown to be generally superior to bubble oxygenators in limiting

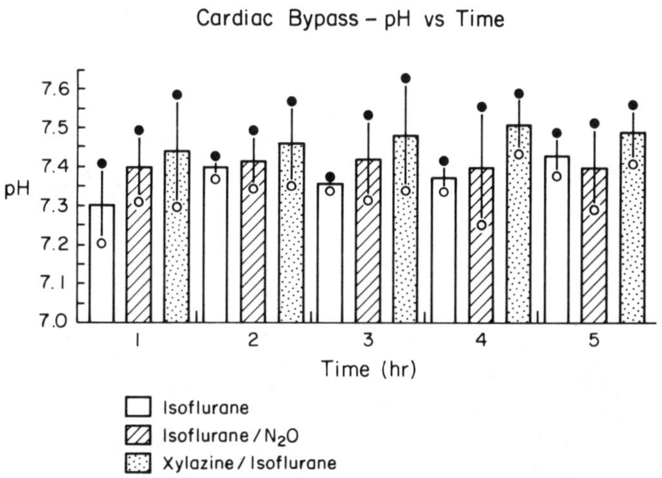

Figure 20.9. Arterial pH was maintained at a mean of 7.3 or more during cardipulmonary bypass with either prepump anesthetic technique. Standard deviation variations indicate the times adjustments were made with base (sodium bicarbonate) for adjustment.

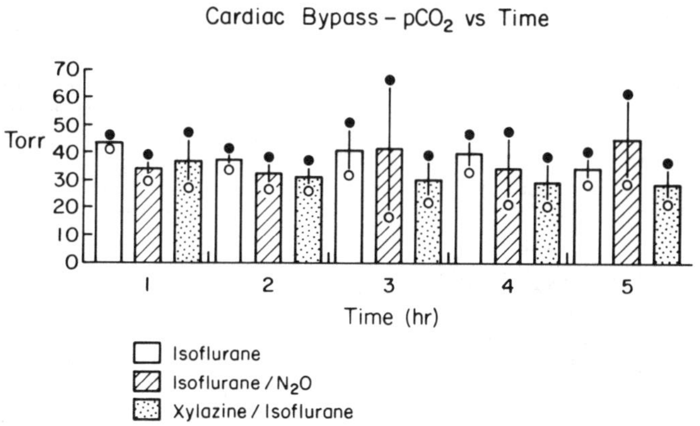

Figure 20.10. An illustration of the maintenance of oxygen levels during bypass.

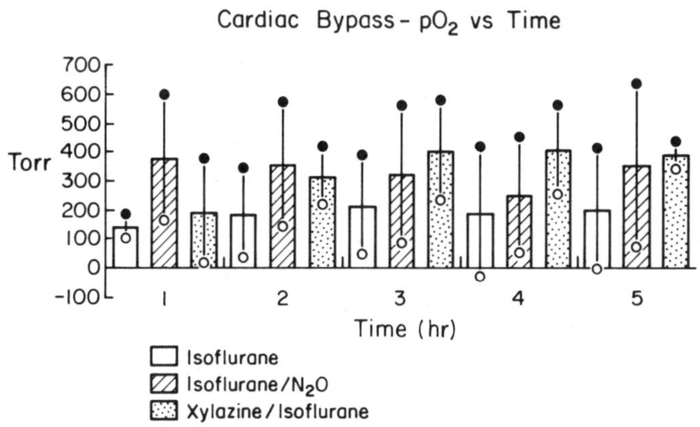

Figure 20.11. Excessive levels of $paCO_2$ were not present during cardiopulmonary bypass.

damage to erythrocytes and platelets during CPB (9). While protection of blood cells is a concern in bypass studies of such prolonged duration as 5 hours, the marked production of foam in bubble oxygenators when used with calf blood (1) led to the selection of

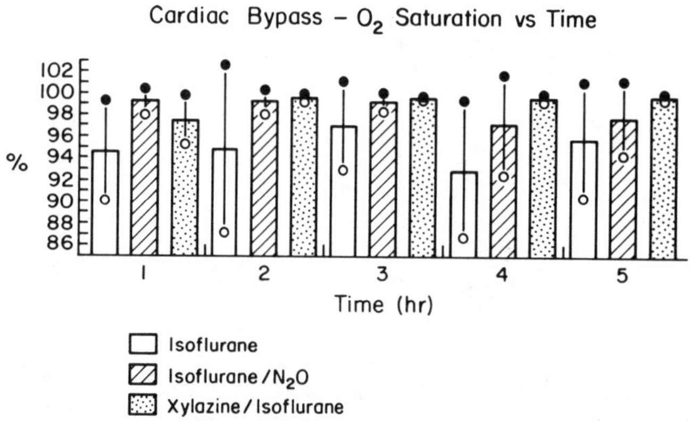

Figure 20.12. The levels of PaO_2 were influenced by the capability to obtain O_2 saturation in this group of calves. All calves were being maintained by isoflurane anesthesia. As a result, saturation levels indicate variables other than anesthetic selection.

membrane oxygenators for this study. The Travenol membrane oxygenator offers the additional advantage of requiring less priming volume than most other membrane oxygenators (9). Our circuit design avoided the need for an additional pump for the membrane oxygenator (10) by use of a gravity feed arrangement. This design eliminated a potential source of additional damage to blood cells that has been encountered with the use of membrane oxygenators in roller pump systems (10). This design helped to minimize the erythrocyte damage created by 5 hours of bypass circulation and to maintain physiologically normal conditions during anesthesia. As a result, anesthetic management was not adversely affected by the bypass technique.

Hemodilution with pump oxygenator and circuit-tube priming solutions reduced the animal's hematocrit values and plasma viscosity. Diuretic therapy (furosemide, Hoechst) was infrequently needed during pulsatile CPB. The volume of fluid used in the oxygenator, as well as supplemental fluids administered during the procedures, provided an adequate fluid load to support renal function. In each of the calves, adequate urinary output was maintained.

In these calves, undergoing experimental bypass procedures, normal systolic blood pressure of 100 to 120 mm Hg was achieved before bypass. During the bypass procedures, a flow of 3 to 6 liters of blood/minute was delivered with a mean flow of 4.5 liters/minute adjusted in coordination with the responses of the calves' circulatory systems. At these flows, systolic mean arterial pressures were maintained at more than 60 mm Hg at all times. These values in addition to the level of oxygen saturation of blood during these procedures help to assure adequate oxygenation and perfusion of the tissues. This hemodynamic status was at least partially responsible for maintenance of renal blood flow and associated renal function as evidenced by continuous production of urine throughout the procedures.

We have shown in a group of 12 calves how isoflurane can be an effective and safe anesthetic in experimental cardiopulmonary bypass studies in calves. Halothane has been successfully used in cardiopulmonary bypass studies as well (11, 12). We have attempted to provide an index to the materials and methods that may be used when anesthesia is needed for experimental procedures of this type. The principles of anesthetic responses in the cardiac patient should be considered for these special cardiac surgical procedures. In addition, refer to appropriate chapters elsewhere in this book for selection of medications to control responses or provide supplemental medications for analgesia or muscle relaxation.

The management of animals during special surgical procedures such as those requiring cardiopulmonary bypass demonstrates the complexities of veterinary anesthesia. However, the opportunity to provide anesthetic management during major experimental surgical procedures gives evidence of the advancements in anesthetic management under unusual situations.

References

1. Donawick WJ, Nara Y, Baue A: Techniques for successful cardiopulmonary bypass in the calf. *J Surg Res* 9:79–85, 1969.
2. Spratt EH, Melrose D, Bellhouse B, et al: Evaluation of a membrane oxygenator for clinical cardiopulmonary bypass. *Trans Am Soc Artif Intern Organs* 27:285–288, 1981.
3. Jarvik RK, Kessler TR, McGill LD, et al: Determinants of panuus formation in long-surviving artificial heart calves, and its prevention. *Trans Am Soc Artif Intern Organs* 27:90–96, 1981.
4. Vasku J, Cerny J, Vasku J, et al: A comparative study of a group of eight calves, surviving longer than 1 month with total artificial heart. *Artif Organs* 7:470–478, 1983.
5. Eger II EI: Isoflurane: A review. *Anesthesiology* 55:559–576, 1981.
6. Stevens WC, Cromwell TH, Halseg MJ, et al: The cardiovascular effects of a new inhalation anesthetic, Forane in human volunteers at constant arterial carbon dioxide tension. *Anesthesiology* 35:8–16, 1971.
7. Steffey EP, Howland D: Isoflurane potency in the dog and cat. *Am J Vet Res* 38:1833–1836, 1977.
8. Steffey EP, Howland D: Comparison of circulatory and respiratory effects of isoflurane and respiratory effects of isoflurane and halothane anesthesia in horses. *Am J Vet Res* 41:821–825, 1980.
9. Finlayson DC, Kaplan JA: Cardiopulmonary bypass. In Kaplan JA (ed): *Cardiac Anesthesia*. New York, Grune and Stratton, 1979, pp 393–440.
10. Boers M, van den Dungen JJAM, Karliczek GF, et al: Two membrane oxygenators and a bubbler: a clinical comparison. *Ann Thorac Surg* 35:455–462, 1983.
11. Short CE, Keats AS, Liotta P, Hall CW: Anesthesia for cardiac surgery in calves. *Am J Vet Res* 29(12):2287–2294, 1968.
12. Short CE, Harvey RC, Fisher FE, Cunningham JN Jr, Rose DM, Gelbfish J, Weiss E, Grossi E: Anesthetic and supportive management during experimental perfusion studies in calves. *Lab Anim Sci*, in press.

CHAPTER

21

Postoperative Care and Oxygen Therapy

A.I. WEBB, B.V.Sc., Ph.D., M.R.C.V.S., D.V.A., D.A.C.V.A.

Introduction

The postanesthetic period is a time when support needs to be provided for the patient as it passes the stages of anesthesia in reverse. The patient must be cared for until its reflexes have returned and the vital organ systems have been stabilized. It is a time when the animal is particularly vulnerable to the adverse effects of drugs, hypothermia, deranged pathophysiology, and pain. The postanesthetic period is one in which a significant number of complications occur; in humans, it is associated with a 20% morbidity rate (1). Despite this, it is often a time when the clinician relaxes his vigilance and is lulled into a sense of false security. To provide an adequate standard of care to animals recovering from anesthesia there are three requirements that must be met: facilities, equipment, and human resources.

Facilities

The siting of the recovery area is critical. It should be located near the operating room suite (OR) to allow the clinician to oversee the recovery. The area will then be close to essential systems such as power, oxygen, and suction. Adequate lighting is essential in the recovery area for proper observation and performance of such tasks as catheterization, venapuncture, and physical examination.

The recovery unit should be designed for maintaining a quiet environment that minimizes excessive auditory stimulation of patients which detracts from the work environment. If the area is isolated, it is important that recovery staff be able to summon help in an emergency without leaving the patient by phone or intercom system. The number and siting of electrical outputs is critical. Electrically powered equipment is heavily used in the recovery area, so these outlets should be close to the recovery cages or stalls. The outlets must be waterproofed and shockproof because recovery areas can become wet.

Large animals require special facilities for recovery from anesthesia indoors. However, recovery out of doors is suitable for short-duration anesthetics if a clean, flat surface clear of objects that could cause trauma is available. Indoor recovery facilities vary widely depending upon whether the recovery is actively assisted or not. Regardless, the recovery stall must be quiet and well padded and allow adequate observation facilities. There should also be provision for slinging horses if required.

Animals recovering from inhalant anesthetics eliminate a large portion of the anesthetic taken up by the body into the environment. This makes the recovery area a prime site of anesthetic pollution. This pollution problem can be limited by maintaining the animals on scavenged anesthetic breathing circuits as long as possible in the recovery period. It is also advisable to provide a high level of ventilation in the recovery area. This is usually achieved by high levels of air exchange by air conditioning. The recovery room temperature should be as warm as possible to limit and possibly reverse hypothermia that may develop in anesthetized patients in the operating room.

Because of the nature of cases moving through a recovery unit, there is a high risk of infection and cross-infection. Standards of cleanliness must be maintained as in the OR suite. A cleaning protocol that includes floors, cages, and all items of equipment is essential. It is desirable that the unit have its own cleaning supplies and that all items in the unit be either capable of being sterilized or disposable. Known infectious cases should not be admitted into a recovery area; they should recover in the OR suite and be taken directly to the isolation area.

Equipment

The recovery area must be properly equipped to cope with both routine situations and special emergencies. The basic equipment should include an adequate supply of oxygen, preferably with the cylinders secured outside the recovery area. There should be a variable suction unit with a full selection of suction catheters.

Respiratory support equipment includes a full range of endotracheal tubes, associated cuff inflators, laryngoscopes, face masks, Ambu-type resuscitation bags, a Mapleson D breathing circuit (T-pieces with an open bag on the expiratory limb), and a nearby mechanical ventilator. Essential cardiovascular support items of equipment include intravenous fluids, fluid administration sets and catheters, cutdown packs for placement of intravenous lines, and an electrocardiograph (ECG) monitor. ECG units that would be suitable are often battery-powered and have heavy signal filtering to minimize muscle potentials obscuring the base ECG pattern. It is desirable that ECG paper strip tracings can be obtained when necessary so that permanent records are available for review and possible use in litigation. There should also be equipment capable of cardiac defibrillation. This may be housed in either the OR or the critical care unit.

Additional equipment that should be available in the recovery area includes heating units (heat lamps, circulating hot water blankets, and builtin electrical heating; electric blankets are considered undesirable because of the potential for contact burns), a full range of needles and syringes, specimen bottles for hematology and blood chemistry, thermometers, urine collection bags, dip stick tests for blood glucose, and access to equipment and personnel to perform hematocrits and plasma protein measurements. The recovery area must also be adequately stocked with emergency drugs that are regularly rotated to avoid waste because they become out of date. A list of drugs that should be considered for the immediate postoperative area is set out in Table 21.1.

Table 21.1
Drugs Recommended for the Anesthesia Recovery Area

Central nervous system depressants	Fluids, electrolytes, and antibiotics
Acepromazine	Dextrose (both isotonic and 50%)
Fentanyl	Furosemide
Ketamine	Mannitol
Meperidine	Potassium chloride
Morphine	Sodium bicarbonate
Naloxone	Antibiotics (caution: aminoglycosides)
Oxymorphone	Intravenous fluids
Phenobarbital	Miscellaneous drugs
Thiobarbiturate	Antihistamines (chlorpheniramine)
Cardioactive drugs	Dantrolene
Atropine	Dexamethazone
Calcium (chloride or gluconate)	Doxapram
Epinephrine	Heparin
Dobutamine	Insulin
Dopamine	Methyl prednisolone
Glycopyrrolate	Neostigmine
Lidocaine	Oxytocin
Procainamide	

Personnel

Staffing of a recovery unit depends upon caseload. In a large hospital, the number of anesthesia cases may warrant a fully staffed recovery area, whereas a small practice may have only the receptionist to help the clinician care for the recovering patient. Regardless of numbers, the staffing requirements are similar; there must be sufficient personnel to provide adequate monitoring and adequate training to permit the monitoring staff to recognize and act appropriately on incipient problems. Recovery room personnel need continuous on the job training to ensure that emergency protocols are followed and decisions made in a timely manner.

Patient Care

Animals need to be carefully monitored, and thorough records should be maintained throughout the recovery period. The record can be a continuation of the anesthetic record or a separate data sheet. Such a record makes possible easy recognition of trends in the patient's vital signs and provides a legal record of the animal's condition and the treatments administered. It is imperative that, when commencing such a record or whenever staffing of the recovery area changes, the patient's identity be confirmed, the pertinent medical history be reviewed with special notice being given to past and current drug therapy, and a check of vital parameters be made. The frequency of monitoring the recovery patient is a matter of judgment; obviously the critically ill or unstable patient needs vital signs measured almost continuously, whereas the stable patient nearing the end of recovery needs less attention. The use of such continuous monitoring equipment as ECGs and indwelling thermometers allows for some automation of warning alarms when there are sudden changes in the animal. Such equipment, although expensive initially, can increase productivity of the recovery staff, result in salary savings, and enhance job satisfaction.

Vital signs that are most useful in following the progress of the postanesthetic patient include return of reflexes, chest sounds, muscular strength, mucus membrane color, pulse rate and rhythm, blood pressure, ECG, respiratory rate and depth, blood gases, and temperature. It is difficult to give normal values for these parameters during such a dynamic and changing period as anesthetic recovery; however, approximate ranges of values commonly encountered are given in Table 21.2. Attention should also be directed to the positioning of the animal, together with keeping it as clean, dry, and warm as practicable. Postoperative pain should be assessed and suitable measures taken to alleviate such discomfort. The tenets of good nursing care for recumbent patients—frequent rotation from one lateral recumbency to the other in small animals, provision of warmth, passive movement of limbs, protection of the eyes from trauma, and general cleaning and massaging of the skin—are essential components of optimal recovery from anesthesia.

Cardiopulmonary Monitoring

The importance of cardiopulmonary monitoring is illustrated by a survey of nearly 30,000 human patients recovering from anesthesia in which nearly three-quarters of all complications were related to the cardiopulmonary system (1).

Table 21.2
Expected Ranges of Physiological Parameter Values Commonly Encountered in the Postoperative Period for Cat, Dog, and Horse

	Cat	Dog	Horse
Body temperature (°C)	34–39	35–39	36–38
Capillary refill time (sec)	<2	<2	<2
Heart rate (b.p.m.)	110–150	80–130	35–55
Systemic blood pressure (mm Hg)	90–130	85–125	90–120
Respiratory rate (b.p.m.)	20–40	15–30	8–16
Blood gases (assumes breathing room air)			
P_aO_2 (mm Hg)	70–95	70–95	60–80
P_aCO_2 (mm Hg)	25–35	40–50	35–50
pH	7.3–7.4	7.3–7.4	7.3–7.4

Airway patency is of primary importance. A commonly quoted axiom is that noisy breathing is obstructed breathing. When the endotracheal tube is in place, the chance of an airway obstruction occurring is lessened, but it should not be forgotten that the endotracheal tube may become kinked or clogged with secretions or blood. An endotracheal tube is generally left in place in the trachea until the animal's protective airway reflexes have returned to normal. Brachycephalic breeds of dogs and patients who have had surgery or tissue trauma of the upper airway or pharynx should be considered at risk for airway obstruction after extubation. It is crucial to have suitable instrument packs and endotracheal tubes always in the recovery area for emergency tracheotomy.

Bilateral auscultation of the patient's chest should be performed at regular intervals to gauge adequacy and eveness of ventilation and assess heart sounds. Changes in these parameters may be more significant than isolated observations. An esophageal stethoscope may be useful in auscultation of unconscious patients.

The animal's mucus membrane color is an important guide to tissue oxygenation and perfusion. Good lighting in the recovery area is essential for subtle color changes to be appreciated. Dusky or frank cyanotic membranes are an indication of inadequate oxygenation; pale membranes may be indicative of pain, hemorrhage, shock, or any combination of these. Capillary refill time is a measure of tissue perfusion and should be brisk in all species. A gradual lengthening in the capillary refill time can be a sign of deteriorating cardiovascular function.

Attention to ensuring adequate ventilation is especially important in the recovery period because so many of the drugs associated with surgery and anesthesia have potent respiratory effects. Additionally, the inhalant anesthetics depend upon ventilation for their elimination. Arterial carbon dioxide and oxygen tensions are the best measures of ventilation and oxygenation, respectively, but may not be practicable in many practice situations. Ventilatory adequacy can be assessed indirectly by observation of breathing rate and pattern as well as the depth and strength of the ventilatory effort. Special attention should be given to those patients that receive muscle relaxants as part of their anesthetic regimen. These drugs weaken ventilatory effort and may also cause a return of muscle paralysis through interactions with other drugs concurrently administered. This is of special concern because the return to spontaneous ventilation requires only a small proportion of neuromuscular junction acetylcholine receptors to become free, and a number of drugs (e.g., neomycin, kanamycin, and aminoglycoside antibiotics) administered in the recovery period may reoccupy the receptors, causing recurarization. There are other high tech methods available for continuous monitoring of ventilation and oxygenation, such as pulse oximeters, end-tidal gas analyzers, and percutaneous and subconjuctival gas electrodes. These all give excellent quantitative data, but the clinician's and nurse's observations are adequate in most clinical situations.

In evaluating ventilatory effort, it is crucial that the effort made be matched with the production of airflow. The animal may make herculean efforts at thoracic and abdominal motion but be unable to move air because of airway obstruction or muscle weakness. In the latter, chest movements are usually paradoxical, with diaphragmatic breathing pulling the chest wall down during inspiration.

The sites for palpating arterial pulses vary with the species and the areas accessible to the recovery attendant. With training and experience, the staff monitoring recovery can gain considerable information on the animal's progress from palpation of the pulse alone. In the more critical case, some electromechanical monitoring will be required. There are many noninvasive blood pressure monitoring devices available that vary in price from less than a hundred dollars for pressure cuff and aneroid to over a thousand dollars for automated measurement of pressure and heart rate with associated definable high and low value alarms. Both gradual and sudden changes in heart rate and blood pressure are causes for concern because they are often associated with complications such as hypovolemia, shock, hypoxia, and toxemia. The ECG is an excellent method of monitoring heart rate and rhythm, but it does not reflect the pumping activity of the heart or the state of the vascular bed. Other specialized cardiovascular measurements may be indicated for particular types of cases, but that monitoring is usually a continuation of monitoring commenced before or during anesthesia.

Nervous System

The hallmark of recovery from anesthesia is the return of central nervous system function. This is demonstrated through the return of protective reflexes, response to moderate stimulation, and finally becoming ambulatory. The rate of recovery of consciousness will depend on many factors, including the anesthetic technique and drugs used and the physical condition of the patient. It is important to be able to recognize when recovery is delayed and differentiate and treat, if possible, the cause for that delay. The latter is addressed below in the section dealing with complications.

Veterinarians must provide adequate analgesia to alleviate suffering in their patients recovering from surgery. The need for postoperative analgesics will depend upon the species, the individual animal, the type of surgery, and the anesthetic technique used. Analgesics work best when administered before the onset of pain; consideration must be given to initial administration of analgesics during termination of anesthesia. Signs exhibited during anesthetic recovery that indicate pain include phonation, restlessness, hypertension, tachycardia, pallor, and, in horses, sweating. The choice of drug is wide and includes narcotic analgesics, sedative-analgesics, and nonsteroid anti-inflammatory drugs. Some suggested drug regimens are given in Table 21.3. Species variations should be noted. For example: the cat, cow, and horse can show excitement after most narcotic analgesics; other variations include the cat's inability to handle aspirin rapidly and the ruminant's sensitivity to xylazine. It is this author's view that xylazine is not suitable as a general analgesic or sedative in the cat or dog because of the prolonged cardiopulmonary depression produced.

Fluids

Account must be kept of fluids administered to or lost by patients during recovery. This includes recording any blood losses. Most animals do not have urinary catheters placed for monitoring purposes because of the inconvenience involved and the risk of introducing urinary tract infections. In those patients that do have catheters, urine output should be recorded at 30- to 60-minute intervals. During recovery, many small animals will evince signs of discomfort and even distress that subside after they urinate or defecate. If an animal has a full bladder at the end of anesthesia, recovery personnel should gently attempt to express the bladder before the patient returns to consciousness. This simple act can greatly increase patient comfort and prevent soiling of both the animal and its dressings. In the male equine, a distended bladder can cause a marked degree of colic (2).

Table 21.3
Suggested Dose Ranges for Analgesics Commonly Used to Control Postoperative Pain in Cats, Dogs, and Horses (mg/kg i.m. or s.c.)

	Cat	Dog	Horse
Butorphanol	0.05–0.1	0.05–0.1	0.05–0.1
Chloral hydrate	NR[a]	NR	10–50
Fentanyl	NR	0.005–0.01	NR
Ketamine	1–3	NR	NR
Meperidine	1–4	1–5	1–3
Morphine	NR	0.1–1.0	NR
Oxymorphone	0.01–0.02	0.05–0.2	NR
Pentazocine	1–3	1–3	1–3
Xylazine	NR	NR	0.5–1.5 (0.1–1.0 i.v.)

[a] NR, not recommended.

Fluid administration should be continued into the recovery period. This will help meet physiological fluid needs and also maintain direct access to the vascular space in the event of an emergency. The type of crystalloid fluid administered may not be critical; if a new unit of fluid has to be started during the recovery period, a one-half strength balanced electrolyte-dextrose mixture might be preferred to limit the postoperative sodium retention. When administering fluids to a patient, hydration status should be monitored to avoid possible fluid overload or, alternatively, hypovolemia. A suitable baseline rate to work from would be 5 to 10 ml/kg/hour. If blood or blood products have to be administered during recovery, they should be given through a separate intravenous line. The donor's identification should be noted on the recovery record.

Drugs and Nursing

Good nursing requires a mixture of innate compassion and common sense. One must want to protect the patient from harm while it is defenseless and weak. Similarly, recovery personnel must be able to handle and calm anxious and disorientated animals—a role that changes dramatically between both species and individual animals. The person supervising the recovery is often required to handle and comfort the patient to obviate both injury and unnecessary administration of sedatives. The animal and its immediate environs need to be kept clean of excreta and blood that could soil dressings and contaminate wounds.

Administration of drugs to animals in the perianesthetic period requires a knowledge of drug pharmacology and interactions. Drug kinetics will also be altered in this period (3). The identity, dosage, and route of all drugs should be double-checked before they are administered, and their administration should be recorded properly on the recovery sheet.

Extubation

Removal of the endotracheal tube is a critical stage in the recovery of an animal from general anesthesia. It is normally not done until the animal has recovered sufficient consciousness to have regained swallowing ability and airway protective reflexes. In equine patients, some anesthesiologists advocate leaving the oral endotracheal tube in place in the equine until it is in sternal recumbency or standing (4). The pharynx should be checked in small animals to ensure that there are no secretions or foreign materials present that could be aspirated or incite laryngeal spasm. If possible, the animal should be given one or two breaths of oxygen and the endotracheal tube cuff deflated during the last of the positive pressure breaths. This simple maneuver tends to blow out any material collected above the cuff between the tube and the upper airway. The tube should be then removed smoothly. If the tube lumen contains material suggestive of an upper airway infection, it may be advisable to sample the lumen for bacteria.

Common Postoperative Complications

The postoperative period is considered a time of restoration of physiological homeostatasis. In such a dynamic situation, it is inevitable that on occasion the process may go awry and complications ensue. The most common complications are those relating to the cardiopulmonary and nervous systems.

RESPIRATORY COMPLICATIONS

The most dramatic respiratory problem is apnea, when emergency ventilation of the patient has to be instituted. For this possible eventuality, a self reinflating resuscitator bag that incorporates oxygen enrichment should be considered an essential item in small animal and foal recovery areas. More usual sequelae of respiratory dysfunction are hypoxia and hypercarbia. These can be insidious in onset, but early detection minimizes potential irreversible effects. Early clinical signs of hypoxemia include restlessness and tachycardia, but in later stages this may develop into depression, bradycardia, and eventually coma. Hypoxemia is accompanied by cyanosis when deoxyhemoglobinemia reaches 5 g/dl. This limit to visualization of cyanosis is reached at increased levels of oxygenation in patients with higher levels of circulating hemoglobin but may be barely detected in anemic animals. Definitive diagnosis is made through arterial oxygen tensions. However, treatment should not be delayed while clinical impressions are being confirmed because oxygenation can be life-saving under such circumstances. Although increasing the F_IO_2 is a salve to the problem, the primary cause must be sought and corrected if possible. Potential causes of respiratory dysfunction during anesthetic recovery are listed in Table 21.4 below.

In Farnum's recovery room study (1), he was surprized that only 5% of the complications observed related to airway obstruction. One usually considers that upper airway obstruction is a predictable risk in the postoperative period because animals may not have regained sufficient consciousness to protect their airway. The presence of an endotracheal tube does not preclude obstruction. When an endotracheal tube

Table 21.4
Major Respiratory Problems in the Postoperative Period and Contributing Factors

Upper respiratory tract (URT) obstruction
Occluded endotracheal tube
Foreign material in pharynx and URT
URT anatomical malconformation
Laryngeal and pharyngeal swelling
External compression of pharynx and URT
Hypoventilation
Depression of central nervous system respiratory center
Residual muscle paralysis
Mechanical impairment of ventilation
Obesity
Thoracic air or fluids
Hypoxemia
Diffusion hypoxia
Mismatching of ventilation and perfusion
Hypoventilation
Increased oxygen consumption
Pneumothorax
Pulmonary edema
Airway reflexes
Laryngospasm
Bronchospasm
Sneezing
Aspiration
Chemical pneumonitis
Pneumonia

warms to body temperature, it becomes softer and more likely to become kinked or compressed. On extubation the pharynx should be inspected and suctioned clean if indicated. If pharyngeal packing has been used, the anesthetist must ensure all of it has been removed. When there is a possibility that upper airway swelling or external compression from cervical dressings or casts may result in obstruction after extubation, it may be desirable to momentarily extubate the patient before consciousness returns to assess airway patency while reintubation is still a simple process. If there are problems with the airway, a tracheotomy or replacement of the oral endotracheal tube through a pharyngotomy (small animals) (5) or nasal intubation (large animals) may be required. In brachycephalic breeds of dogs, it is best to keep the endotracheal tube in place for as long as possible. This retention of the tube, which is facilitated by minimizing stimulation of the dog, also has a role in preventing aspiration because brachycephalic dogs tend to be aerophagic and therefore are more likely to vomit.

The majority of anesthetic drugs and opioid analgesics depress the central nervous system's respiratory center. This depression is reversed as the drugs are eliminated or metabolized. The elimination of inhalant anesthetics can be enhanced by increasing the patient's ventilation. This can be done mechanically or by using a respiratory stimulant. Enhanced ventilation is most effective in inhalant agents with intermediate solubility in blood, such as enflurane, halothane, and isoflurane (6). Muscle weakness may potentiate hypoventilation. Such myasthenia could result from neuropathological causes or from incomplete reversal of muscle relaxants used as part of the anesthetic protocol. The cause of muscular weakness has to be determined and treated appropriately while ventilation is supported by assisted or controlled ventilation. Care must be taken that dressings around the thorax or abdomen do not impair ventilation. Hypoventilation during recovery from anesthesia is a common problem with obese animals. Serious impediments to ventilation are pneumothorax or hemothorax. These are indicted by marked respiratory effort with minimal achievement of air excursions. Diagnosis is made by auscultation, thoracocentesis, percussion, and radiography. Tension pneumothorax is life-threatening, and decompression is urgent. Administration of oxygen is indicated while the animal is hypoxemic.

A common cause of postoperative hypoxemia in small animals occurs immediately after cessation of the administration of nitrous oxide. This is called "diffusion hypoxia" and is caused when nitrous oxide, which is poorly soluble in blood, rapidly enters the alveoli from the blood where it was dissolved (7, 8). The rush of nitrous oxide displaces oxygen from the alveoli. Diffusion hypoxia is prevented by flushing the breathing system with oxygen and then keeping the F_IO_2 at 1.0 while assisting ventilation for 3 or 4 minutes after the nitrous oxide is turned off. In large animals, the hypoxemia associated with recovery relates to the mismatching of ventilation and perfusion that accompanies anesthesia and recumbency. During anesthesia, hypoxemia is usually avoided by keeping the animal's F_IO_2 at 1.0, but in recovery the animal is breathing air and venous admixture is so great that hypoxemia occurs. The hypoxemia can be reduced by supplemental administration of oxygen by insufflation of the upper airway. Nearly all animals seem to shiver during recovery from anesthesia; this may increase oxygen consumption so greatly that it outstrips oxygen supply and hypoxemia results. The shivering is usually related to hypothermia, especially in smaller dogs and cats, but it is most marked after inhalant anesthetics (9) and its cause is not fully understood. The solution is to correct the hypothermia if it is causing the shivering and increase the F_IO_2 using a face mask and a Mapleson D breathing system (modified T-piece). In humans, meperidine administered for postoperative analgesia has been shown to lessen shivering (10), although not improve the hypothermia. Similarly, animals with fevers or other conditions that increase metabolic oxygen consumption may develop hypoxemia that must be treated with oxygen therapy.

Aspiration can occur at any time when an animals has depressed airway protective reflexes, but the use of cuffed endotracheal tubes greatly reduces the risk. The endotracheal tube has to be removed eventually, and the airway is left unprotected. If aspiration of vomitus, regurgitated gastric contents, or foreign material in the pharynx takes place, there are two types of possible sequela; these are chemical burn if the material has a low pH and bacterial contamination. In the case of chemical pneumonitis, oxygen may be indicated during the subsequent period of pulmonary edema. The use of distending airway pressures (CPAP and PEEP) has been shown to be efficacious in humans, in animals patient compliance makes this difficult. The immediate treatment with any suspected aspiration is postural drainage and suction of the pharynx and upper airway together with pulmonary lavage if indicated. When the aspirate is particulate, the possibility of some particles lodging in an airway must be considered and bronchoscopy should be performed. Administration of antibiotics may limit the extent of bacterial infection.

CARDIOVASCULAR COMPLICATIONS

The postoperative period is often one of rapid cardiovascular dynamic changes as central nervous system depressants are being eliminated, analgesics administered, and pain sensation returning. The major cardiovascular complications encountered in the recovery area are listed in Table 21.5.

Table 21.5
Major Cardiovascular Complications of the Postoperative Period and Etiologic Factors Involved

Hypotension
Anesthetic myocardial depression
Increased vascular bed
Hypovolemia
Toxemia
Cardiac tamponade
Pain
Bradycardia
Anesthetic-related drugs
Hypothermia
Hypoxia
Excessive intrathoracic pressure
Increased intracranial pressure
Atrioventricular heart block
Tachycardia
Pain
Hypercarbia
Hypoxia
Hypovolemia
Anesthetic-related drugs
Fever
Cardiac dysrhythmias
Hypoxemia
Hypercarbia
Acidosis
Electrolyte disorders
High circulating catecholamines
Underlying cardiac pathology
Cardiac arrest

Blood pressure and heart rate are two important cardiovascular parameters used to assess patient status during the immediate postanesthetic recovery period. Changes in these parameters may reflect changes in autonomic balance and attempts by the body to regain normal function. Hypertension, which is of less concern in animals than in humans, may result from pain, hypercarbia, and drugs that increase sympathetic tone. Hypotension is caused by myocardial depression. This may be secondary to the use of anesthetic drugs and/or toxemia. Hypotension may result from insufficient blood for the vascular space due to either spinal anesthesia-induced sympathetic blockade, alpha-sympathetic blockade due to such drugs as acepromazine, hemorrhage, dehydration, or ECF sequestration of circulating blood volume.

Excessive increases in heart rate are undesirable both because of their underlying cause and the effect that tachycardia has on increasing myocardial oxygen requirements while decreasing myocardial perfusion. The principal causes of tachycardia are mediated through high sympathetic tone, either directly with increased catecholamine release or through anesthetic-related drugs such as atropine, ketamine, or epinephrine. Under the influence of anesthesia, the tachycardic response to hypoxia may be blunted so much that only late-stage bradycardia is observed. The opposite trend is seen with pain; bradycardia is the exception because pain normally produces a brisk increase in heart rate. Bradycardia is not uncommon with small dogs and cats as hypothermia develops. Bradycardia may result from improper application of controlled ventilation with prolonged or excessive positive pressure. In recovery, administration of opioid analgesics and anticholinesterases can produce bradycardia. All episodes of bradycardia should be differentiated from heart block. Parasympathoplegic drugs, such as atropine or glycopyrrolate, are excellent choices to reverse most cases of bradycardia. Care should be given in the use of atropine; first, one must administer sufficient doses to avoid central stimulation of the vagal nucleus without blocking peripheral vagal effects on the heart, which intensifies the bradycardia; second, in the equine it may be associated with gastrointestinal stasis.

Cardiac dysrhythmias are of concern because of decreased cardiac efficiency and the threat that the rhythm may progress to a more life-threatening dysrhythmia. In a study of normal dogs in the recovery room, it was found that 30% displayed cardiac arrhythmias without progressing to clinical significance (11). It is still essential that, when arrhythmias are present, the primary cause be sought and corrected if practicable. Because dysrhythmias may progress to cardiac arrest, the recovery area should be properly equipped and staffed to handle diagnosis and treatment. Cardiopulmonary resuscitation is dealt with in Chapter 22.

NERVOUS SYSTEM COMPLICATIONS

Postoperative pain in veterinary medicine appears to be of less significance than in humans. This may reflect a species difference in pain appreciation, but more likely it is a because clinicians do not recognize and appreciate the amount of pain involved in surgery for their patients. The clinician has a wide assortment of analgesics available, and the use of local nerve blocks should not be overlooked. For example, the use of intercostal nerve blocks after a thoracotomy provides major relief from an otherwise painful procedure.

Delayed Return of Consciousness

When as an animal fails to follow the expected trend of recovery, one must determine whether it is a normal recovery for this animal or a pathological delay. The possible causes for such a delay are listed in Table 21.6. In reaching a decision whether recovery is truly delayed, one must be aware of the animal's preoperative condition, the types and doses of anesthetic medication, and the duration of anesthesia. These patients, unable to display sufficient motor response to pain and stimuli, are erroneously thought to have reduced consciousness.

Hypothermia

Hypothermia during recovery is a major problem in small dogs and cats and only a minor problem in the adult large animal. The problem is caused by the depression of thermoregulation under anesthesia that causes animals to become poikilothermic (i.e., their body temperature assumes that of the environment). The situation is complicated in that operating suite temperatures are generally set to the surgeon's comfort, not patient welfare; thus the environmental temperature is usually in the 20 to 23°C range. The smaller animal develops hypothermia more rapidly and to a more profound extent. This is because it has a greater body surface area for its size, and surgical size preparations and exposure are of greater proportions. In the recovery area, one is usually better able to warm the patient, but it is a gradual process.

Complications related to hypothermia include myocardial depression (at core tempertures below 30°C ventricular arrhythmias are life-threatening); lower metabolism and drug excretion; central nervous system depression, which potentiates the effects of anesthetics and muscle relaxants; and increased bleeding tendencies. In recovery, the animal's efforts to rewarm itself by reflex shivering increases oxygen consumption; the oxygen delivery ability of the cardiopulmonary systems may be unable to meet this demand, and the result is hypoxemia.

Hypothermia is best treated by prevention. However, this is not completely possible, and so the animal must be rewarmed. The trick in rewarming is to do it as fast as possible while avoiding thermal injuries or peripheral vasodilation at the expense of perfusion of the cold core. Heat can be retained by blankets and plastic occlusive wrappings so that heat builds up. Heat can be exogenously supplied by wrapping the animal in a circulating warm water blanket (electric blankets are not safe enough to use on unconscious animals) or using overhead infrared lamps. The animal's tempertuture must be monitored during the rewarming process, which ceases as temperature approaches normal to avoid overshooting normothermia. In warm climates without air conditioning, care must be taken to avoid hyperthermia. This is a real problem in the larger species, where the effort of recovery warms the animal to the point that it can overheat. Hyperthermia is treated by wetting down the patient and placing it in a convective air current. Ice packs are ideal for cooling because they cause vasoconstriction of the mantle with reduced thermal exchange.

Table 21.6
Causes of Delayed Recovery from General Anesthesia

Central nervous system depression
Hypercarbia P_aCO_2 (above 80 mm hg is depressant to the central nervous system)
Hypothermia
Hypoglycemia (especially in neonatal or juvenile animals)
Metabolic acidosis
Uremia
Increased intracerebral pressure
Nervous cellular damage
Lack of stimuli
Shock
Drug related:
Basic overdosage (i.e., excessive for a healthy subject)
Relative overdose (i.e., dosage not appropriate to the animal's condition)
Altered kinetics (through disease or drug interactions)
Muscle weakness:
Myesthenia and general muscle weakness
Electrolyte imbalances
Poor reversal of nondepolarizing muscle relaxants
Phase II block after succinylcholine

RENAL FAILURE

Postoperatively, animals may show continued or initial manifestations of renal failure. This may reflect either exacerbation of pre-existing renal disease, current renal hypoperfusion, or intraoperative insult to the kidneys (hypoxia, toxins, myoglobinemia, or drug action such as with gentamycin). Treatment should be aimed at returning urine output toward normal. This is done first by correcting any hypovolemia, then using drugs such as mannitol, furosemide, or dopamine to stimulate urine production. While attempting to increase urine production it is important not to overload the circulation; central venous pressure should be monitored. Ideally, urine output should not fall below 1 ml/kg/hour.

BLOOD LOSS

Excessive bleeding in recovery is of concern both for the blood loss per se and also because it may indicate a coagulation defect as in hemophilia or disseminated intravascular coagulation (DIC). Appropriate blood samples should be drawn in an EDTA tube for evaluation of the hematology including platelets, citrate: bleeding times and fibrinogen, fibrin split products. If the blood loss is large and/or the patient's hemoglobin reserves are low, then blood should be drawn for cross-matching EDTA and serum. Decisions on blood replacement are based on details of past and continuing losses, hematocrit, and total plasma protein. Choices facing recovery personnel include the plasma volume expanders as well as blood and blood products.

INTEGUMENT AND MUSCULOSKELETAL COMPLICATIONS

Misadventure

During the recovery period, animal sensibility can vary between the extremes of unconsciousness to enhanced reactivity. It is not surprising therefore that accidents can occur to patients. Animals suffocating or suffering musculoskeletal trauma during recovery have been seen in even the most well-conducted facilities. Cages and stalls should be designed to have no gaps where animals can get their legs or heads caught and have no projecting edges or similar sources of trauma. Animals that are still intubated cannot be left unattended if the problem of swallowed or aspirated endotracheal tubes and esophageal probes is to be avoided. Similar care must be taken with electrical equipment so that power cords cannot be damaged and short out to burn or electrocute a patient. All recovery personnel must monitor patients closely and learn from these accidents how to develop better facilities and protocols.

Myositis or Neuropraxia

In the horse, postanesthesia muscle damage/weakness is a well-recognized complication. It has been the subject of several studies and reviews (12–15), but we are still far from knowing exactly what causes the problem and how it should be treated. After studies showing release of muscle enzymes (16), it has been assumed the problem is muscular; however, it often seems to have at least a neural dysfunction aspect as well. It is thought that the syndrome is related to inadequate muscle perfusion and the subsequent reperfusion of the affected tissue. It occurs more often in heavier horses and geldings and after long surgeries. It was first documented after the introduction of halothane, but the use of this anesthetic has permitted more invasive and longer surgeries to be performed. To reduce the incidence of the syndrome, anesthesia in the horse should be as short as possible, hypotension and hypoxia should be prevented, and adequate padding and limb positioning should be provided to avoid areas of prolonged muscle compression during anesthesia and recovery.

The myositis appears to have its onset as recovery commences (12), and it can affect upside or downside muscle as well as the muscles along the back. The affected horse is often thought initially to be having a difficult recovery and appears anxious. At this stage, fluids and some sedation seem to settle the horse that, on getting to its feet, shows lameness or stiff-gaitedness. This usually resolves over the next 24 hours. Some horses do not settle and show increasing agitation and sometimes panic. These horses need close attention to limit injury, with sedation and analgesics; phenylbutazone, meperidine, or xylazine have all been recommended. Continued attention to fluids, electrolytes, and acid-base balance is important. Some groups have used dantrolene either orally or intravenously (17). The rationale for the use of this drug is not entirely clear, and controlled studies are needed to evaluate its efficacy because it is expensive and may even prolong the crisis by increasing muscle weakness, as it does in humans. Fortunately, myositis rarely proves fatal, although the damaged muscle may cause some disfigurement or loss of performance as it fibroses.

METABOLIC DYSFUNCTION

There are numerous metabolic derangements that affect animals in the immediate postoperative period. Some of these have been alluded to already, and others are associated with the specific type of surgery or disease status of the patient. However, there are two that are common to a wide range of patients.

Acid-Base Abnormalities

It is unfortunate that most veterinary practices either do not have a blood-gas analyzer or have not made arrangements for the analyses to be carried out elsewhere. As more critical surgery and anesthesia is attempted with corresponding cost escalation, knowledge of blood gas tensions and acid-base status becomes more valuable. Acid-base status should be evaluated during recovery of all critical and unstable patients because it may be contributing to the patient's condition. If an arterial blood sample is not available, venous blood will suffice for acid-base evaluation. If metabolic acidosis is present and is severe enough to warrant treatment (best assessed using the base excess calculations), sodium bicarbonate may be slowly administered. Metabolic acidosis in the patient can be associated with an excess of lactic acid because of compromised oxygenation and perfusion. Improvement of these latter parameters often reduces the acidemia, but bicarbonate therapy is indicated in severe lactic acidosis.

Hypoglycemia

Immature animals, diabetics, and those animals with decreased carbohydrate intake or increased glucose utilization are all at risk of hypoglycemia during anesthesia and recovery. In such at-risk patients, the blood glucose levels need to be monitored with simple dip-stick techniques. Dextrose can be administered as a 5 g% in water or in combination with balanced electrolyte solutions. Hypoglycemic patients will show delayed recovery and may suffer brain damage if the hypoglycemia is profound or prolonged. Animals can be fed postoperatively when they are stable and swallowing normally unless there are specific contraindications.

Oxygen Therapy

Most small animal patients make the transition from the high F_IO_2 administered during anesthesia to breathing room air without any problem. However, any patient with systemic disease, shunting, ventilation/perfusion, $\dot{V}/\dot{Q}$, mismatching, and cardiac dysfunction should receive oxygen supplementation during recovery. In the horse, it is almost inevitable that the F_IO_2 be increased if hypoxemia is not to occur because of the extent of the $\dot{V}/\dot{Q}$ mismatching (18–20).

Prevention or correction of hypoxemia takes one or both of two steps. The first is optimization of the patient's breathing efforts by ensuring a clear and stable airway and by positioning the patient to make breathing most efficient. Routine cleaning and suctioning of the oropharynx and trachea is often necessary. This should be performed about every 4 hours in patients that cannot clear their own airway. Suction is properly performed using appropriate-sized suction catheters through which suction is applied as the catheter is withdrawn from the airway. Optimal cleaning of the airway is obtained if the catheter is rotated as it is withdrawn so the walls are cleared. Care should be taken to avoid excessively long periods of suction because this can promote lung collapse and transient but dramatic falls in arterial oxygenation (21). The second step is increasing the fractional concentration of inspired oxygen (F_IO_2) to that required to provide adequate arterial oxygenation. The simplest method of increasing F_IO_2 is insufflation using a bias flow of 100% oxygen. This replaces a portion of rebreathed dead space gases (typically 15% oxygen) with 100% oxygen. Insufflation is achieved through the endotracheal tube in initial stages of recovery and with a nasal cannula after extubation. The flows utilized for small and large animals are 2 to 3 and 10 to 15 liters/minute, respectively. Face masks are also used in small animals after extubation. In the equine, an alternative to endotracheal tube insufflation is the use of a demand valve (22) connected to the tube that delivers assisted breaths of oxygen each time the animal inspires. Small animals that require long-term oxygen supplementation should be placed in an oxygen cage or tent. The oxygen should ideally be humidified except in short-term emergency situations (23) to prevent drying of airways and reduce heat loss. A recent development that could help is the use of an artificial nose. These are small exchange humidification and filtering devices that fit on the ends of airways (24).

An arterial oxygen tension below 75 mm Hg is an objective indication of the need for an increased F_IO_2. Other signs are increased efforts to breathe, retraction of the commissures of the mouth, and cyanosis of the mucous membranes. Prolonged elevated oxygen tensions are not desired, so when PaO_2 rises above 90 to 100 mm Hg during oxygen supplementation, some reduction in F_IO_2 is indicated. Cessation of oxygen therapy is indicated when PaO_2 is sustained within normal limits, but it should be done gradually with reassurances that the patient's condition remains stable.

A cause of hypoxemia during the recovery period is hypoventilation. Hypoventilation is defined as an above-normal $PaCO_2$ (>45 mm Hg). A mild buildup of $PaCO_2$ is not necessarily harmful because the associated release of catecholamines may stimulate cardiac function beneficially. However, secondary acid-base derangements may depress such vital centers as the brain and myocardium. The only treatment for hypoventilation is to increase ventilation, either chemically or by positive pressure ventilation (PPV).

Chemical stimulation of ventilation is by doxapram hydrochloride, a respiratory stimulant that affects both peripheral chemoreceptors and medullary respiratory neurons. Doxapram can be administered as either a bolus or an infusion. Doxapram should be restricted to central nervous system depression unless it is not possible to provide PPV.

If it is considered necessary to ventilate a patient during the postanesthetic period, it is essential to monitor the progress of the patient carefully. Decisions on peak airway pressures and timing are best made by observations of the patient and evaluation of blood gas analyses. P_aCO_2 is the definitive guide to the efficacy of mechanical ventilation because it is inversely proportional to alveolar ventilation. P_aCO_2 values above 50 mm Hg indicate hypoventilation that may require some ventilatory therapy. P_aCO_2 values above 60 mm Hg that continue to deteriorate require that the patient be ventilated.

There are a number of complications that can occur during or after oxygen therapy. These range from the damage to respiratory tract mucosa from the use of cold and dry gases to the manifestations of oxygen toxicity. The risk of oxygen toxicity developing from short and medium term administration appears remote because even in humans it requires more than 24 hours of breathing 100% oxygen before the first signs of toxicity appear (25). High F_IO_2 levels may contribute to absorption atelectasis with subsequent $\dot{V}/\dot{Q}$ mismatching. Additionally, elevation of P_aO_2 may result in a decreased respiratory drive through removal of any hypoxic drive. This may result in some elevation of P_aCO_2, depending on the patient's response to carbon dioxide. There are patient and personnel risks attendant involved in the use of oxygen and compressed gases in a veterinary hospital (26), but they can be minimized by following correct handling and safety procedures.

References

1. Farnum JV: The work of the recovery room. *Brit J Hosp Med* 19:606–616, 1978.
2. McDonell WN: General anesthesia for equine gastrointestinal and obstetric procedures. *Vet Clin Nth Amer: Lrg Anim Pract* 3:163–194, 1981.
3. Elfstrom J: Drug pharmacokinetics in the postoperative period. *Clin Pharmacokin* 4:16–22, 1979.
4. Kelly AB, Steffey EP: Inhalation anesthesia: drugs and techniques. *Vet Clin Nth Amer: Lrg Anim Pract* 3:59–71, 1981.
5. Hartsfield SM, Gendreau CL, Smith CW, Rouse GP, Thurman JC: Endotracheal intubation by pharyngotomy. *J Am Anim Hosp Assoc* 13:71–75, 1977.
6. Stoelting RK, Eger EI: The effects of ventilation and anesthetic solubility on recovery from anesthesia: an in vivo and analog analysis before and after equilibrium. *Anesthesiology* 30:290–296, 1969.
7. Fink BR: Diffusion anoxia. *Anesthesiology* 16:511–519, 1955.
8. Sheffer L, Steffenson JL, Birch AA: Nitous-oxide-induced diffusion hypoxia in patients breathing spontaneously. *Anesthesiology* 37:436–439, 1972.
9. Vaughan MS, Vaughan RW, Cork RC: Postoperative hypothermia in adults: relationship of age, anesthesia, and shivering to rewarming. *Anesth Analg* 60:746–751, 1981.
10. Pauca AL, Savage RT, Simpson S, Roy RC: Effect of pethidine, fentanyl and morphine on post-operative shivering in man. *Acta Anaesth Scand* 28:138–143, 1984.
11. Buss DD, Hess RE, Webb AI, Spencer KR: Incidence of postanaesthetic arrhythmias in the dog. *J Small Anim Pract* 23:399–404, 1982.
12. Waldron-Mease E: Postoperative muscle damage in horses. *J Eq Med Surg* 1:106–110, 1977.
13. Klein L: A review of 50 cases of post-operative myopathy in the horse—intrinsic and management factors affecting risk. *Proc 24th Annual Conference Am Assoc Eq Pract, 1978* 89–99, 1978.
14. Lindsay WA, McDonell W, Bignell W: Equine postanesthetic forelimb lamness: Intracompartmental muscle pressure changes and biochemical patterns. *Am J Vet Res* 41:1919–1924, 1980.
15. White NA: Postanesthetic recumbency myopathy in horses. *Compend Contin Educ Pract Vet* 4:S44–S50, 1982.
16. Trim CM, Mason J: Post-anaesthetic forelimb lameness in horses. *Eq Vet J* 5:71–76, 1973.
17. Waldron-Mease E, Rosenberg H: Post anesthetic myositis in the horse associated with in vitro malignant hyperthermia susceptibility. *Vet Sci Commun* 3:45–50, 1979.
18. Mitchell B, Littlejohn A: The effect of anaesthesia and posture on the exchange of respiratory gases and on the heart rate. *Eq Vet J* 6:177–178, 1974.
19. De Moor A, Desmet P, Verschooten F: Influence of change of body position on arterial oxygenation and acid-base status in the horse in lateral recumbency, anaesthetized with halothane and efficiency of postanaesthetic oxygen administration. *Zbl Vet Med A* 21:525–531, 1974.
20. Steffey EP, Wheat JD, Meagher DM, Norrie RD, McKee J, Brown M, Arnold J: Body position and mode of ventilation influences arterial pH, oxygen and carbon dioxide tensions in halothane-anesthetized horses. *Am J Vet Res* 38:379–382, 1977.
21. Boutros AR: Arterial blood oxygenation during and after endotracheal suctioning in the apneic patient. *Anesthesiology* 32:115–118, 1970.
22. Waterman AE, Jones RS, Richards DLS: Use of a demand valve for postoperative administration of oxygen to horses. *Equine Vet J* 14:290–292, 1982.
23. Chalon J, Loew DAY, Malebranche J: Effects of dry anesthetic gases on tracheobronchial ciliated epithelium. *Anesthesiology* 37:338–343, 1972.
24. Weeks DB, Ramsey FM: Laboratory investigation of six artificial noses for use during endotracheal anesthesia. *Anesth Analg* 62:758–763, 1983.
25. Clark JM, Lambertson CJ: Pulmonary oxygen toxicity: A review. *Pharmac Rev* 23:37–133, 1971.
26. Webb AI, Warren RG: Hazards and precautions associated with the use of compressed gases. *J Am Vet Med Assoc* 181:1491–1495, 1982.

CHAPTER 22

Emergency Care Medicine

PETER J. PASCOE, B.V.Sc., D.V.A., D.A.V.C.A., M.R.C.V.S

Introduction

This chapter will cover three areas of emergency medicine; shock, trauma, and cardiopulmonary resuscitation. The pathophysiology of the conditions will be emphasized, and treatments that are currently recognized will be recommended. An attempt will be made to discuss recent developments and their impact on future modalities of therapy. These three topics are closely interwoven; the divisions are arbitrary. With the recent trend in the health care profession toward prevention of illness, it goes without saying that every effort should be made to prevent our patients from reaching the point where resuscitation is necessary. This requires great care and attention to detail because in many cases the cause of severe shock or cardiac arrest cannot be attributed to one incident but rather is the result of a series of minor mishaps culminating in a disaster. Nevertheless, some of our patients have serious design defects (e.g., the gastrointestinal tract of the horse, or they lack an understanding of the highway code or no trespassing signs, and or they have no comprehension of the damage that can be inflicted by leaping off tall buildings. Thus disaster cannot always be prevented, and knowledge of these subjects is a necessity for most veterinarians.

Shock

Early definitions of shock appeared to express the frustration that was encountered when dealing with this condition. It was defined as a "momentary pause in the act of death" (1) or a "rude unhinging of the machinery of life." Now the definition of shock relates to the underlying derangements, which are an "inadequate blood flow to vital organs or the inability of the body cell mass to metabolise nutrients normally" (2). This latter statement is added to account for some septic shock states in which the blood flow is normal but cellular metabolism is deranged.

ETIOLOGY

This failure of the microcirculation can be brought about by many factors. The circulation depends on three main components: a pump, fluid to pump, and tubes of the correct size and shape to deliver this fluid to the cells. The cells in turn must be able to function normally once the oxygen and nutrients have been delivered to it. Failure in any one of these components can result in a state of shock.

Hypovolemic Shock

This occurs when there is an inadequate volume of fluid being pumped around the body. It can be divided into loss of whole blood, loss of plasma, or loss of water and electrolytes. Hypovolemic shock is probably the most commonly encountered form of shock in the veterinary patient, and examples of the above divisions are often seen. Loss of whole blood externally and internally is a frequent sequela to road traffic accidents in cats and dogs. Animals with peritonitis or pleuritis may exude considerable amounts of plasma proteins into the inflamed body cavity. Neonatal animals are particularly prone to loss of water and electrolytes, and neonatal calf diarrhea will put an animal into shock if the loss is severe enough.

Clinically, an animal in hypovolemic shock may be depressed, and the eyes appear dull and lusterless. The mucous membranes are normally pale or white but may appear blue if the animal is hypoxic. The capillary refill time is slow, and the animal's extremities may feel cold. These are all signs related to poor tissue perfusion. Tachycardia is usually present, and the pulse is fast and weak. The respiratory rate is usually elevated in an effort to combat the metabolic acidosis and supply as much oxygen as possible to the blood. The body temperature may be normal or depressed depending on the length of time since the loss of volume precipitated the crisis.

Cardiogenic Shock

This occurs when the heart fails to pump enough blood to maintain an adequate supply to the tissues. The pump depends on an input and an output, so if there is severe interference with ventricular filling, cardiac shock ensues. Examples of this are cardiac tamponade and tension pneumothorax. Similarly, lesions affecting ventricular emptying, such as acute cor pulmonale, rupture of the chordae tendinae, severe toxic myocardial depression, cardiac dysrhythmias, or any severe and prolonged rise in systemic vascular resistance may induce cardiogenic shock. These lesions are uncommon in large animals and are encountered more often in small animal practice. The clinical signs associated with this are similar to those of hypovolemic shock, but there may be evidence of cardiac failure, such as distended pulsating peripheral veins, hepatomegaly, peripheral edema, pulmonary edema, cardiac dysrhythmias, or a loud heart murmur.

Vasculogenic Shock

When the vessels supplying the blood to the tissues are affected in such a way as to reduce perfusion, vasculogenic shock ensues. This can also be looked at in terms of input and output. If there is severe arteriolar constriction, then the tissues can be deprived of their blood supply. This can occur with the prolonged sympathetic stimulation associated with pheochromocytomas. In most instances, however, there is interference with the return of blood to the heart due to increases in the capacitance of the system. With some severe head injuries, one can produce vasomotor paralysis that leads to a generalized vasodilation. Endotoxic and septic shock may be classified as forms of vasculogenic shock because they produce vasodilation through the release of vasoactive substances such as histamine, bradykinin, and prostaglandins. However, sepsis and endotoxemia also impair myocardial performance and interfere with the regulation of metabolic processes so to classify sepsis of endotoxemia as vasculogenic shock is a simplistic view.

Hyperdynamic Shock

The characteristics of hyperdynamic shock are a raised cardiac output, a decreased arteriovenous oxygen difference, a decreased systemic vascular resistance, and a relatively normal blood pressure (3). The actual metabolic rate may be 1.5 to 2 times normal, so the total body oxygen consumption may be normal but there is a failure of oxygen utilization at the cellular level. This type of septic shock is seen early in the course of diseases involving localized proliferation of micro-organisms. Many animals enter a hypodynamic phase before death.

Recent comprehensive studies in humans have revealed certain physiological patterns in response to sepsis (4). The progression described by these authors is from an initial state in which there is a raised cardiac output, increased heart rate, and slightly decreased blood pressure to a subsequent stage that is characterized by a reduction in the arteriovenous oxygen difference and a slightly raised arterial blood pressure. The next stage is characterized by a normal cardiac output but a significant hypotension with a raised heart rate. A respiratory acidosis is superimposed on the existing metabolic acidosis. The final stage is one of cardiac failure in which the cardiac output decreases but the heart rate remains elevated, the arteriovenous oxygen difference increases along with the systemic vascular resistance, and the patient is still hypotensive. The use of intensive monitoring of these patients has allowed the development of characteristic circle diagrams of the physiological state. These graphic representations are easily recognizable and allow supportive therapy to be directed appropriately.

The clinical recognition of hyperdynamic shock is related to the peripheral vasodilation that causes the mucous membranes to have a brick red appearance. A pyrexia is often present due to the raised metabolic rate and the release of pyrogens from damaged leukocytes. A normal or elevated blood pressure gives an indication of hyperdynamic versus hypodynamic shock.

Hypodynamic Shock

This is the form of that which occurs late in sepsis or during endotoxin absorption and is the fourth stage mentioned in the above description. It is probably more common in veterinary medicine, especially in horses with colic or in cows with coliform mastitis. There is a vast body of literature that has used various animal models of endotoxic and septic shock (5–8); there are many differences in the responses seen. These vary with the species, the amount of toxic agent given, the route of administration, and whether the animals were anesthetized at the time, so it is hardly surprising that clinical endotoxic shock can also present in many different ways.

The main features of endotoxic shock are myocardial depression and maldistribution of blood volume. There is a tendency to increase the volume of blood in the capacitance vessels. The high peripheral resistance noted with early endotoxic shock or sublethal endotoxin administration is replaced by a paralysis of the precapillary sphincters and a low peripheral resistance in the late phases or after lethal doses of endotoxin (7). Endothelial damage is another characteristic of endotoxic shock and is manifested as infarcts in various tissues and as arterial hypoxemia in some species. The canine, which tends to clear bacteria in the liver and spleen, appears to be resistant to this acute respiratory distress syndrome (9) and does not show arterial hypoxemia as readily during endotoxic shock (10). The horse, calf, and sheep all show significant hypoxemia after endotoxin administration (11–13). An initial leukopenia and thrombocytopenia are also seen with endotoxic/septic shock (7).

PHYSIOLOGICAL RESPONSE TO SHOCK

The initial responses are homeostatic and in general are very successful at preserving life. As the injury becomes more severe, a decompensation occurs and some of the mechanisms aimed at maintaining life now become detrimental to the survival of that individual.

Baroreceptors in the arterial tree and low pressure receptors in the atrium respond to the initial effective volume depletion, and the sympathetic system is activated. This increases the resistance to flow but centralizes the distribution of the blood to the heart and brain. These two organs have almost no capacity for anerobic metabolism; they fail very rapidly when the supply of oxygen and nutrients is cut off. The release of catecholamines and stimulation of the peripheral vasculature is very rapid in onset. It occurs within seconds of the insult and continues for many hours. The release of epinephrine has a number of other effects. The first is that it produces splenic contraction. In the dog and the horse, it is quite normal for the spleen to contain 16 to 20% of the animal's red cell mass, so this reinfusion of red cells will aid in the replenishment of the lost volume (14). Epinephrine also stimulates glycogenolysis and inhibits insulin release. Thus there is often a hyperglycemia associated with shock states. This rise in blood glucose affects the osmolality of the blood and may aid the process of drawing fluids into the circulation from the interstitial fluid (15, 16). The capacitance of the venous system is reduced by catecholamine stimulation and also by a reverse stress relaxation. If a blood vessel is suddenly distended, there is an immediate increase in pressure within the lumen of the vessel, followed by a gradual decline as the cells in the vessel wall slide over each other to allow for the newly increased size. The same occurs in reverse and helps to decrease the capacitance of the venous system (17). Stimulation of the vasomotor center in response to shock radiates to other areas of the brain. The hypothalamic/pituitary axis is stimulated to release adrenocorticotrophic hormone (ACTH) and antidiuretic hormone (ADH). ACTH enhances the release of corticosteroids, which may reduce some of the effects of tissue ischemia, and ADH acts to increase renal reabsorption of water. The hypotension at the carotid baroreceptors and the reduction of circulation in the kidney also stimulate the release of renin (18), which catalyzes the formation of angiotensin I. As this passes through the lung, it is converted to angiotensin II; this substance is a very potent vasoconstrictor. It also stimulates the production of aldosterone, and the two hormones both act on the kidney to reduce salt and water excretion.

The initial responses to shock are aimed at preserving circulation to the heart and brain and restoring the effective circulating volume by stimulating the pump and filling the pipes with more fluid (drawing fluid back from the interstitium and reducing renal excretion to a minimum). These responses are not all as immediate as the initial baroreceptor responses. The renin-angiotensin vasoconstriction is activated early but may take 15 to 30 minutes to reach a peak; reverse stress relaxation may take 1 to 2 hours to achieve its maximum effect, and the fluid shifts are measurable by about 15 minutes but may take 4 to 8 hours to reach their maximum response. Renin/ADH preservation of body fluids is a relatively late event, only really being effective at 4 to 8 hours, but this system will continue to work in the face of continuing shock, whereas some of the other responses will gradually adjust to the new state so that their intensity wanes (Fig. 22.1).

The initial homeostatic mechanism in shock produces vasoconstriction in the peripheral tissues. Vasoconstriction at the arteriolar level tends to shunt blood through the tissue so that it is returned to the heart as quickly as possible. The result is that the driving pressure is lowered and less blood flows through the capillaries (Fig. 22.2). This produces two useful results: the first is that it preserves the available nutrients for the vital organs, and the second is that it reduces the capillary hydrostatic pressure, which aids in the uptake of fluid from the interstitium. The restoration of circulating volume from the extracellular fluid is thus a complicated process and requires an intact sympathetic nerve supply and release of catecholamines (19, 20). The epinephrine stimulates the hyperglycemia,

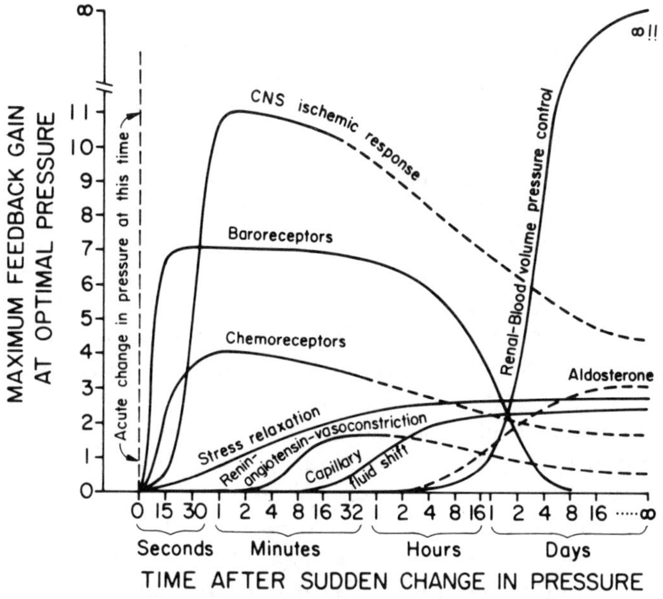

Figure 22.1. The diagram illustrates the time course of the various components of the short-term regulation of circulation. The y axis is the gain of the system and indicates the strength of each response. From AC Guyton (17).

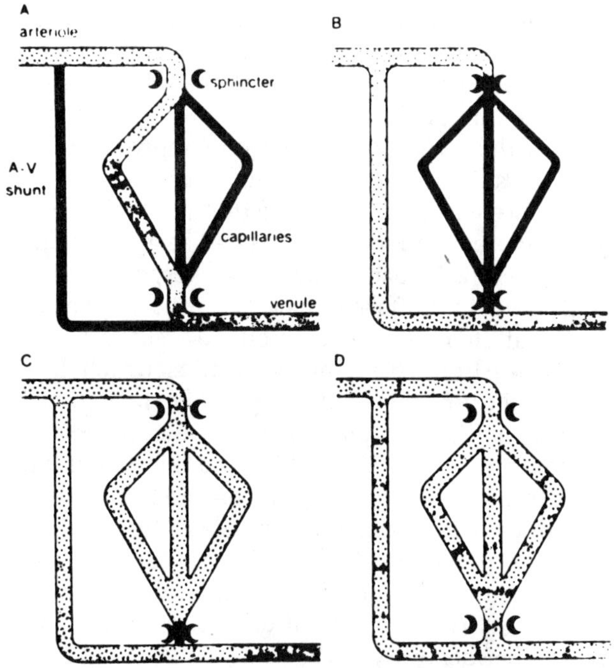

Figure 22.2. The stages of the vasoconstrictor response to hypotension. *A*, the normal state: little or no blood flows through the arteriovenous shunt and the capillaries open and close to supply the needs of the cells. *B*, the initial vasoconstricton at the arteriolar level reduces the capillary flow and the AV shunt opens up. The capillary hydrostatic pressure is reduced, aiding the uptake of fluid from the extracellular space. *C*, as metabolites accumulate, the arteriolar smooth muscle relaxes, and the capillaries all dilate for the same reasons. The sphincters at the venous end remain closed; the capillary hydrostatic pressure rises and fluids are filtered into the ECF. This is the point of decompensation. *D*, finally, the venous sphincters open when there has been further accumulation of toxic waste products. The massive increase in vascular volume caused by the dilation of all the capillaries leads to a low flow state and the acidic slow-moving blood becomes hypercoagulable. From Stoddart JC. *Trauma and the Anaesthetist*. London, Baillière Tindall, 1984.

leading to the increased osmolality, and beta$_2$ stimulation of the vasculature lowers the capillary pressure, thus encouraging a fluid shift into the blood vessels. The peripheral cells do not get an adequate supply of oxygen and nutrients, and they gradually turn over to anerobic metabolism in order to produce the necessary energy to function. It should be remembered that aerobic metabolism can produce up to 38 molecules of ATP from 1 molecule of glucose compared with only 2 molecules of ATP produced by anerobic metabolism. This progresses to the point where there is an accumulation of acid products in the area, and the pH of the tissue falls. When enough of these waste materials have accumulated, the precapillary sphincters relax. This response is part of the normal control of these sphincters in that 75% of the blood flow to a tissue is determined by its metabolic activity (21). If the use of energy outstrips the delivery, then the capillary sphincters open to allow more blood to enter that area. Many chemicals, such as lactate, histamine, adenosine, ADP, ATP, potassium, and hydrogen ions, have been implicated in this process, but none have been shown to be solely responsible for the relaxation that occurs (7). The result of this is a further reduction in blood flow to each cell because the effective volume of the capillary bed is dramatically increased by this dilation. The flow that was going through one capillary is now divided into several capillaries, thus reducing the flow for each one. The pH continues to fall, and the accumulation of waste materials results in paralysis of the arteriolar smooth muscle as well. The postcapillary sphincters seem to be more resistant to these changes and tend to remain constricted (22).

This reverses the direction of fluid movement because the capillary bed is now exposed to the full force of the arteriolar pressure. Fluid now tends to move out of the capillaries and back into the interstitium because the raised hydrostatic pressure increases outward filtration and the accumulation of waste materials increases capillary permeability. With the blood being very acid and flowing very slowly, it becomes hypercoaguable. If there are some tissue thromboplastins and/or some bacterial toxins around to trigger the coagulation cascade, the blood begins to clot in the vascular bed. This leads to the onset of disseminated intravascular coagulation (DIC), dealt with later in this chapter. Finally, the venular sphincters open, leading to further hypotension which exacerbates the poor tissue perfusion.

CELLS

The cell is the final victim in this process; it is thus pertinent to look at the progression of damage to an individual cell during shock or ischemia. Because the body is composed of cells, it is logical that as more and more are affected by shock, there is less chance of the whole animal surviving.

With the reduction in oxygen supply to the cell, there is a shift to anerobic metabolism. Because the mitochondria use over 90% of the available cellular oxygen, these organelles are affected early in the process of shock (23). In measuring the response of mitochondria during different stages of shock, it has been found that their ability to produce energy becomes depressed. Although the electron transport chain that produces most of the ATP is relatively stable, there is a reduced ability to supply the substrates necessary for incorporation in this chain (23). The increase in lactic acid within the cell reduces cytoplasmic pH, which in turn reduces enzyme activity and also alters the resting membrane potential of the cell. The catecholamines present in the circulation also alter this in the same direction, so as the potential difference drifts toward zero, the permeability of the cell membrane is altered. Sodium and calcium both enter the cell, and there is a reduction in intracellular potassium. As these ions leak into the cell, water enters passively, and the cell swells. The changes in ionic content and regulation appear to be very important to cellular function. Magnesium becomes more liable in the mitochondria, interfering with enzyme cofactor synthesis (24); high levels of calcium also depress mitochondrial function and activate phospholipase, which attacks cell membranes. For unknown reasons, cells at this stage seem to become insulin-resistant (25), and despite a good supply of glucose and insulin the cells do not utilize the substrate in a normal manner. The cell's defenses are beginning to break down, the release of arachidonic acid from the membranes provides the substrate for prostaglandin production, and these substances can produce intense local vasoconstriction, further reducing the supply of oxygen to the cells (26, 27). The production of the basic energy source, ATP, grinds to a halt, and the adenine is broken down to xanthines and then to uric acid. Once the metabolism has proceeded this far, the death of the cell is almost inevitable. Even if circulation is restored, the cell may not have enough resources left to return to normal function, because there is no mechanism for converting uric acid back to adenosine (28). Finally, the lysosomal membranes break down, releasing their toxic products into the cell. The hydrolytic enzymes released from the lysosymes are responsible for the damage to the internal and external membranes of the cell. The cell dies and releases these enzymes, which may damage cells in the surrounding area or in other areas of the body (29).

The description so far has been related to the cellular events associated with poor perfusion, which is the basic lesion in any nonseptic shock. In septic shock, however, there appears to be a primary cellular lesion caused by the bacterial toxins. The septic process increases muscle catabolism with release of amino acids into the circulation. Some of these amino acids, such as the branched chain group (valine, leucine, and isoleucine), can be used in the tricarboxylic acid (TCA) cycle in the muscle, but the others cannot and are transported to the liver. This results in an increased urea production, which is energy-consuming and gives rise to the uremia commonly seen in these patients. Alanine and glycine are use to produce pyruvate in the liver. Normally, pyruvate would be used in the TCA cycle but in the septic patient, it may either be converted to glucose and rereleased into the circulation or it may enter into a "futile" cycle in which it is converted to fructose-6 phosphate that is returned to pyruvate. This process is very wasteful of ATP, generates heat, and does not use oxygen (4).

Another major factor is the alteration in fat metabolism. Apart from the lipolysis and hypertriglyceridemia stimulated by glucagon, corticosteroids, and catecholamine, there appears to be an increase in the formation of acyl-free fatty acid-CoA complexes. These latter compounds play a significant role in altering the direction of other biochemical pathways. One of the most important of these is the inhibition of the malate-aspartate shuttle, which is involved in transporting hydrogen ions across the mitochondrial membrane. This can result in a preponderance of NADH and NADPH. The metabolism of many amino acids into energy-producing substrates is dependent on the presence of the hydrogen ion acceptors NAD and NADP, so this could account for the impairment of amino acid metabolism that occurs in late septic shock.

The result of all of these biochemical derangements is a loss of the fuels, particularly pyruvate and amino acids, used in oxidative metabolism. This accounts for the lower oxygen extraction that is characteristic of the hyperdynamic septic patient (4).

It is evident from this brief summary that the changes within the cell are very complex, but it is also clear that our increasing knowledge will enable us to treat shock with greater and greater accuracy. The concept of irreversible shock is changing, in that what was irreversible 20 years ago now stands a good chance of survival. However, when enough cells reach the point of lysosomal breakdown, the animal will die. Although we may push the frontiers forward, there will always be a stage that is irreversible (Fig 22.3).

Major Organs and Shock

Because each organ is a collection of cells, shock will affect the organ in the same way as it does the

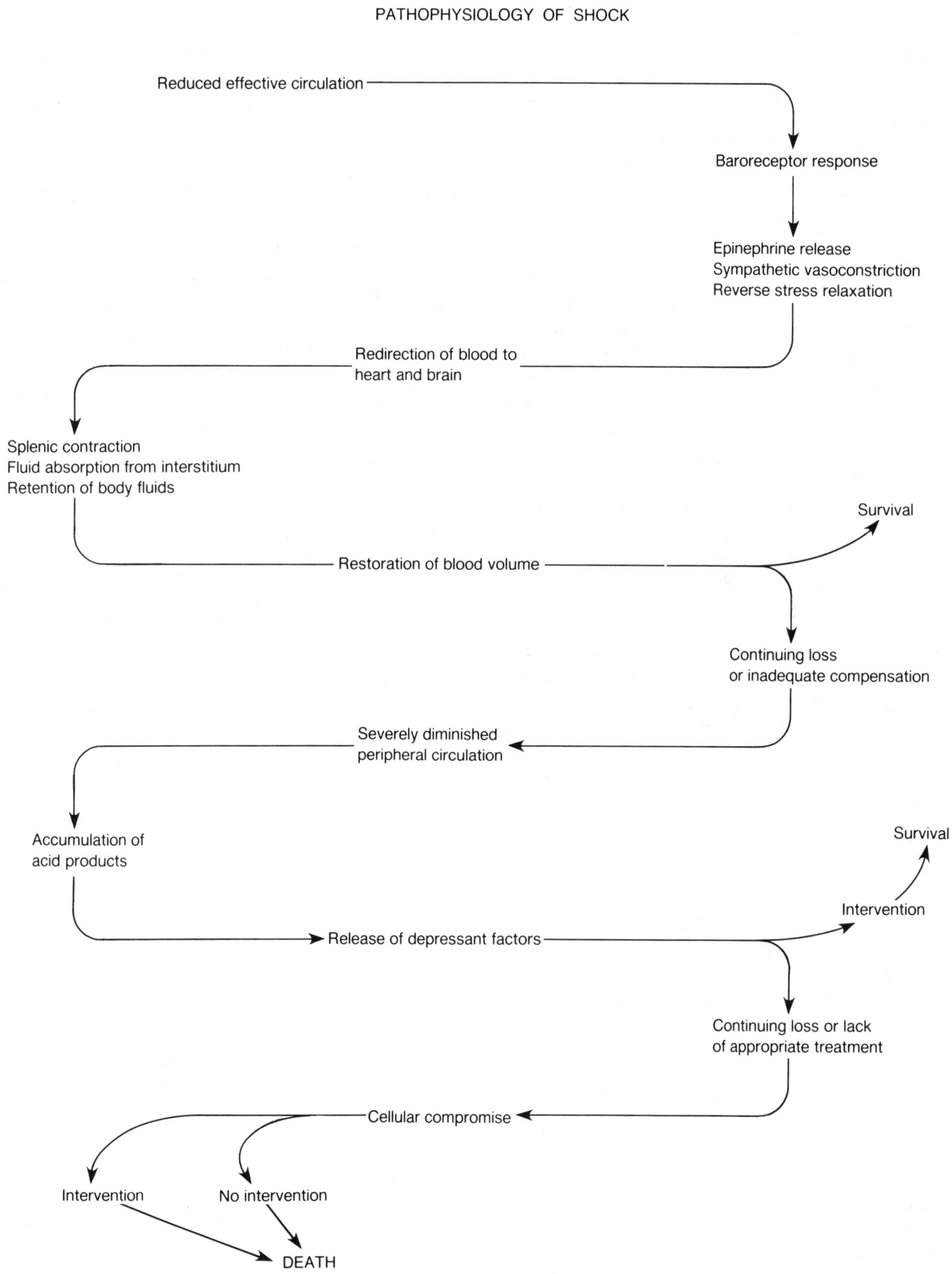

Figure 22.3. Pathophysiology of shock showing the compensatory mechanisms and the factors that lead to decompensation. Finally, an irreversible stage is reached where therapy can no longer be effective.

cells. The effect on the whole body reflects the changes occurring to each tissue.

SKIN, MUSCLE, AND BONE

These three tissues comprise a significant proportion of the body, and yet circulation is much reduced during shock. Muscle in particular has a great capacity for anerobic metabolism leading to the production of lactic acid. Because of these facts, the muscle mass makes a major contribution to total body acidosis.

VISCERA

The viscera are not well adapted for anerobic metabolism and are profoundly affected by reduced circulation. In some species the reduction in circulation is greater than in others; the dog in particular shows an intense portal vasoconstriction limiting flow to the gut (30). The intestines require an active blood supply to maintain the barrier between the mucosa and the intestinal content. The preservation of this barrier is energy-dependent, and as the energy supply is depleted, the mucosal cells are attacked by the enzymes present in the intestinal lumen. Mucosal destruction with intestinal hemorrhage is frequently seen in canine patients and does not occur if the intestinal lumen has been previously washed with saline or treated with a protease inhibitor, supporting the explanation presented above (31). The breakdown of the mucosal barrier is important not only because it is accompanied by further hemorrhage, but also because it allows bacteria and endotoxins to gain entry to the circulation. In the normal animal, small amounts of endotoxins are constantly being absorbed from the intestine. These substances are transported via the portal system to the liver, where they are removed and destroyed by the hepatocytes. The reticuloendothelial system in the liver removes most microorganisms that gain entry to the body. Because the liver is greatly dependent on the hepatic artery for its oxygen supply, the reduction occurring with sympathetic vasoconstriction significantly reduces the ability of the liver to detoxify the substances absorbed from the gut. Experimentally it has been shown that the dog in hypovolemic shock can be susceptible to $1/100{,}000$th of the dose of endotoxin that would normally kill it (32).

The reticuloendothelial system (RES) is extremely important in protecting the animal from external toxins, and any depression is highly significant. Phagocytosis by the fixed RES is reduced during shock, and this is related to the production of a reticuloendothelial depressant factor (RDF) from the splanchnic organs (33, 34) and a reduction in opsonic fibronectin (35). The latter plays a major role in modulating phagocytosis of bacterial and nonbacterial particles by leukocytes, peritoneal macrophages, blood monocytes, and Kupffer cells.

The reduction of energy supply to the pancreas appears to be the stimulus for release of another substance, myocardial depressant factor (MDF). This small peptide is a lysosomal protease present in the pancreas; as this organ suffers considerable reduction in circulation during shock, there are alterations in cell membrane permeability early in the process. When lysosomal enzymes are released from the acinar cells, they can be absorbed directly into the circulation or reach it indirectly via the lymphatic drainage. Peak levels of MDF occur between 2 and 7 hours after the onset of shock, and the half-life of MDF appears to be several hours (26). MDF has a negative inotropic effect and is a major factor in the myocardial depression occurring during shock (36). When it is given to a normal animal at levels measured during shock, MDF can induce cardiogenic shock (29). MDF also appears to intensify the vasoconstriction in splanchnic vessels, and it depresses phagocytosis by the RES; biological and chemical evidence indicates that it may be identical to RDS (37).

KIDNEYS

The effects of shock on the kidneys are related to perfusion. Initially, the glomerular filtration is preserved, but in shock autoregulation is soon lost, and a significant reduction in renal blood flow is measured (38). There is also a redistribution of blood flow within the kidney such that there is a greater reduction in flow to the inner and outer cortex compared with the outer medulla (39). This altered pattern of blood flow has the effect of washing out the medullary concentration gradient; despite the humoral changes produced by angiotensin, aldosterone, and ADH, the ability of the kidney to conserve fluids becomes very limited. In most forms of shock, this is not a problem because the severe reduction in renal blood flow restricts urine formation (prerenal failure). This reduction in renal blood flow is largely mediated by the renin/angiotensin system with limited effects produced by alpha stimulation (39).

However, in high cardiac output septic shock, or in the resuscitation phase of other forms of shock, this medullary washout can result in large volumes of urine being produced (40). In general, the kidney tolerates relative ischemia very well because oxygen consumption falls as the glomerular filtration rate falls, but acute renal failure can and does occur due to shock. It is most common after septic shock, but other high risk patients include animals that have had episodes of DIS, pre-existing renal disease, or cortical necrosis during prolonged hypotension.

CENTRAL NERVOUS SYSTEM

Because the circulation tends to be redirected toward the brain, damage to the central nervous system

(CNS) only occurs in severe hypotension. It appears that there is a general trend for the circulation to fail first in those parts of the brain that have evolved most recently (41). Thus the cerebral circulation is the first to be affected, giving rise to the depressed sensorium of the shocked patient. When circulation to the brain fails, there is a massive sympathetic release known as the CNS ischemic response that attempts to raise the blood pressure. If the circulatory failure progresses, it can lead to paralysis of the vasomotor center with ensuing vasodilation and circulatory collapse.

HEART

The heart has been implicated as one of the organs that is responsible for "irreversible" shock. Experimental evidence demonstrates clearly that prolonged hypotension can produce permanent myocardial damage (42). This may be due to reduced coronary perfusion, although the reduction in coronary flow does not parallel the reduction in cardiac output. A 70% reduction in cardiac output may only reduce coronary flow to 50% of normal (43), and there is also a reduction in the myocardial oxygen demand, but this does not match the reduction in flow (44). The distribution of flow is affected, with the subendocardial tissue suffering the most (45). As the period of shock progresses, there is a reduction in the responsiveness of the heart to sympathetic stimulation and there is a decline in myocardial norepinephrine concentrations (45). On top of all this, the heart is exposed to the toxic factors being produced elsewhere in the body, such as MDF and endotoxins, which may further compromise cardiac function.

Most of the changes noted above occur in the severely hypotensive experimental model and so can only be expected in severe clinical shock. Nevertheless, the coronary blood flow is dependent on diastolic pressure and heart rate. With the compromised coronary flow in shock, the animal may be very sensitive to stimuli that raise the heart rate (e.g., pain) or hypotensive maneuvers (e.g., rolling the animal over).

LUNGS

In uncomplicated hypovolemic shock, the only major change seen in the lungs is hyperventilation. This is stimulated by the metabolic acidosis and the existing hypoxemia. However, this form of shock is often traumatic in origin, and pulmonary damage is extremely common (46). This may take the form of pneumothorax, hemothorax, diaphragmatic hernia, or pulmonary contusion, and all of these lesions will compromise the ability of the animal to ventilate adequately.

Endotoxins damage the vascular endothelium in many parts of the body, but in the lungs this damage causes the hypoxemia that is a consistent feature of endotoxic shock (47, 48). The damage to the endothelium stimulates the attachment of leukocytes and platelets with the release of vasoactive substances (thromboxanes, prostaglandin I_2, serotonin, histamine, and platelet factor 3) causing vasoconstriction in this area. This loss of circulation to certain parts of the lung causes significant ventilation/perfusion mismatching and thus prevents the normal uptake of oxygen from the inhaled gas.

In severe shock or in shock states with complicating factors such as sepsis, emboli, DIS, trauma, or cerebral damage, a syndrome of progressive pulmonary insufficiency has been noted after initial resuscitation (49). It is characterized by a progressive pulmonary edema due to increased capillary permeability developing over the first 48 to 72 hours after initial therapy. This "shock lung" has been divided into four clinical phases. The first phase is the injury and resuscitation phase when the patient is returned to cardiovascular stability but continuous hyperventilation and borderline arterial oxygen tension. There is measurable ventilation/perfusion mismatching. Phase three is a progression of the hyperventilation with deterioration of the hypoxemia. There is radiographic evidence of diffuse interstitial pulmonary edema, and there may be auscultable crackles. Phase four is terminal hypoxia and death. Although there are many putative causes for this lesion, the basic problem is damage to the pulmonary vascular endothelium leading to an increased permeability and hence pulmonary edema (50).

BLOOD

There are many measurable changes in the blood during shock; some of these have already been mentioned. When whole blood has been lost, there may initially be no change in the hematocrit or it may rise slightly if the spleen can provide enough cells to replace the loss. However, as fluid is drawn back into the circulation from the periphery, the hematocrit falls and only tends to rise again at the point where decompensation starts. These changes, however, are not significant enough to help us in a diagnosis of prognosis for a clinical case. If the hematocrit started out in the normal range, it will probably still be within acceptable limits after a major hemorrhage. For instance, in dogs bled to 35% of their normal blood volume, the hematocrit only fell from 44% (0.44 liter/liter) to 35% (0.35 liter/liter) 60 minutes after the hemorrhage. Because a hematocrit of 35% (0.35 liter/liter) is within the normal range for the canine, one would not be able to tell from this single measurement whether this shocked dog had lost 20 or 70% of its blood volume (15).

Plasma proteins tend to rise initially and do not tend to drop as quickly as one would expect with fluid therapy. This implies that proteins are being synthesized or returned to the circulation. The source of this protein is not entirely clear.

In endotoxic/septic shock, there is usually an initial leukopenia due to increased margination and sequestration of these cells on the damaged endothelial cells. if the animal survives past 6 to 8 hours, the leukocyte numbers return to normal and may excede the normal numbers. This occurs as the bone marrow releases many granulocytes into the circulation. The leukocytes may also be suppressed in their functional capacity due to the reduction in opsonic fibronectin and the release of RDS.

Damage to the endothelium, severe acidosis, low flow state, release of thromboplastins from damaged tissue, platelet damage, catecholamines, and steroids all predispose to the initiation of the coagulation cascade. Coagulation begins in the small capillaries; because the predisposing factors are so widespread in the shocked animal, there is a great consumption of clotting factors. This process is known as disseminated intravascular coagulation (DIC). Whenever there is an initiation of coagulation, there is also an activation of fibrinolytic factors so that any clots formed are removed as rapidly as possible. Thus, depletion of clotting factors and activated clot lysis leads to an increased tendency to bleed from any tissue that has been damaged by trauma or surgery (some have been known to say that the two are synonymous). The results of DIC depend on the injury already sustained and the relative ability of the animal to produce fibrinolysin. Where there is extensive injury, there may be serious bleeding from the damaged tissue. if the clots in the microvasculature are not lysed within 20 to 30 minutes, then the cells will die. The extent of this cell death will determine whether the animal is able to survive or not (51).

Clinical Recognition of Shock

Many of the clinical signs associated with shock have already been listed and the differences between the basic types elucidated. The history of an animal presented for attention is important. In traumatized patients, the owner may be able to indicate the type of injury and its location. If they actually witnessed the accident, they will be able to give the relevant details. Because the energy from an impact is absorbed by the tissues, the higher this energy the greater the disruption of tissues. An animal injured at slow speeds in a motor vehicle event usually has less tissue damage than those injured at high speeds. Details of the health of the animal before the accident may also be given by the owner. If the dog has been treated for renal disease, then you will know that it is going to be particularly important to monitor urine output. In all animals, the duration of the crisis is very important; when combined with a physical examination, it may give a good indication of prognosis. A horse presented with a history of colic of 24 hours' duration and depression, a pronounced tachycardia, a weak pulse, and pale mucous membranes has a poor prognosis. A horse presented with the same clinical signs but with a confirmed history of colic beginning only 1 hour ago probably has a much better chance of survival.

During the time it has taken to get a quick synopsis of the patient's history, the clinician has begun to examine the animal to get an indication of the severity of nature of the condition. What is the heart rate? How does the pulse feel on an extremity versus a central vessel? What are the color and consistency of the mucous membranes? What is the capillary refill time? What is the mental status of the animal? Is there any obvious hemorrhage? What is the respiratory rate, and the breathing pattern? The blood pressure is a measurement of the vigor with which fluids are required in humans, but this technique is still not widely used in animals. In the equine colic patient, the blood pressure at the time of admission to a referral clinic has been found to have a strong correlation with prognosis (52). In the canine after hemorrhagic shock, the mean pressure can return to levels that seem quite reasonable (e.g., mean arterial pressure 80 mm Hg) even when the animal has suffered a fatal blood loss (15). Despite this example of a false-positive reading in the dog, the use of blood pressure is a useful addition to the clinical assessment of shock.

If this initial assessment indicates that the animal is in shock, then therapy can begin immediately. Given the amazing ability of the animal body to normalize after severe insults, the slightest hints should be taken as possible evidence of shock. In other words, the animal should be considered guilty until proven innocent.

Having made this initial check, the animal should now be examined in a slightly more systematic fashion to optimize rapid resuscitation. Because the supply of oxygen to the tissues is of major importance, the airway should be assessed. In trauma cases in particular, there may be severe upper airway obstruction necessitating endotracheal intubation or a tracheotomy. If there is no obvious upper airway lesion but the animal is obviously gasping for air after trauma, a rapid attempt should be made to do a thoracocentesis and remove air or fluid from the chest. Again, intubation or tracheotomy may be necessary in order to provide an oxygen-enriched inspired gas and positive pressure ventilation. If there is no problem with the airway, then the next thing is to arrest any major hemorrhage. When no major source of blood loss is immediately evident, then we must proceed to establish a large bore venous access; after taking some blood samples for future reference, therapy should be instituted.

During this initial work-up period, the animal should be handled as gently and carefully as possible. Unnecessary movement should be avoided because changes in body position can induce orthostatic hypotension that may precipitate cardiovascular collapse in an animal that is at its limit of sympathetic compensation. Sedatives and analgesics should be avoided if possible so that the response to therapy can be assessed. If these drugs are essential to enable safe handling of the patient, then drugs with a short duration of action should be chosen (e.g., diazepam, meperidine, or xylazine) and low doses given initially.

Therapy for Shock

Because the basic premise about shock is that there is a deficit in the effective circulating blood volume, the mainstay of therapy is volume replacement. There are many other things that may also be important treatments in individual cases, but without increasing the effective circulation, these therapies are doomed to failure. As with all such dogmatic statement, there is an exception that proves the rule. Anaphylaxis is an acute vasculogenic shock that can lead to death very rapidly. The animal effectively bleeds to death into its own vascular bed due to the sudden massive vasodilation. The most effective and useful therapy for this to date is epinephrine. A dose of 10 μg/kg should be given intravenously, and a further repeat dose can be given by deep intramuscular injection to sustain the response. The animal should be monitored and further doses of epinephrine administered as required. Having dealt with the exception, all other forms of shock should receive fluid volume as part of the initial therapy. The first questions that are then asked are: which fluid and how fast should it be given? In veterinary medicine, the most common fluid used initially is a balanced electrolyte solution such as lactated ringer's, Normosol (Don Mills, Ontario, or Abbott Laboratories, North Chicago, Illinois) or Plasmalyte (Travenol Laboratories, Deerfield, Illinois). These crystalloid solutions provide electrolyte concentrations that are similar to plasma and contain excess cations that will raise the blood pH. If shock is due to cardiac decompensation, then a sodium-free fluid such as 5% dextrose is indicated during the early therapy. The rate of administration has been an age-old controversy, but it has received very little scientific investigation. As with most therapies, the rate is determined by the response of the patient, but let us examine some recent data that gives a good indication as to where to start. Dogs of approximately 20 kg from which 30 to 40% of the blood volume had been removed were infused at three different rates with Normosol. The response was measured in terms of change in central venous pressure (CVP), cardiac output (CO), pulmonary arterial wedge pressure (PAWP), and mean arterial pressure (MAP). With flow rates of 15 ml/kg/min, there was an unacceptable rise in PAWP and CVP with significant elevation of cardiac output. At a flow rate of 6 ml/kg/min, there was a significant elevation of CVP and PAWP and CO, but they were acceptable. The lowest flow rate of 4 ml/kg/min gave an adequate but suboptimal response (53). In order to deliver this to the dog, the system of administration must be able to cope with the flow. The limiting factor is usually the size of the venous access. Further experimental work indicates that if we use a 1-liter bag with a maxidrip administration set (10 drops/ml), a 1¼-inch catheter is sufficient for an animal up to 6.5 kg, an 18-gauge 2-inch up to 10 kg, a 16-gauge 2-inch up to 15 kg, and a 14-gauge 2-inch up to 21 kg (54). This immediately implies that a dog over 21 kg is going to need either a larger venous access, more than one catheter, or some kind of pressure infusion set to achieve an optimal flow rate. In the horse, the author uses a maximum flow rate of 1 ml/kg/min because flow rates higher than those were shown to raise the CVP to an unacceptable level (W.N. McDonell, unpublished observation). This is usually achieved using a peristaltic pump to push the fluid through a 14-gauge 5½-inch catheter; 10-gauge and even 8-gauge catheters are now available, and rapid flow rates can be achieved with these by gravity flow alone.

The volume of fluid that is required initially should be equivalent to three times the amount of fluid lost. This statement is difficult to translate to the clinical setting because it is often impossible to know the volume deficit. With experimental hypovolemic shock in healthy animals, shock begins to occur with a volume deficit between 30 to 40% of the blood volume. Above a 40% loss, some animals will die if not treated; if more than 48% is lost, all the animals will die without treatment. Thus one must assume that for an animal to be exhibiting signs of shock, it has at least a 30% deficit in its effective circulation. The crystalloid solution that is being infused contains water and electrolytes, and these elements distribute throughout the intravascular and extravascular compartments of the extracellular fluid. Because the volume of the extravascular compartment is roughly twice that of the intravascular part, we need two more volumes of solution to be given for every unit we wish to remain in the vascular system. The final conclusion from this is that if we assume a 30% blood loss in the canine is about 30 ml/kg, the initial aim of our fluid replacement should be 90 ml/kg. With the above flow rate, this can be achieved in 15 minutes. In the cat, the blood volume is smaller, so a 30% blood loss involves about 15 to 20 ml/kg (20), which means that the initial fluid therapy should be 60 ml/kg. Recent experimental evidence suggests that this should not be given at a rate exceeding 70 ml/kg/hour. The experiments carried out have yielded conflicting results in that one study found no significant rise in extravascular lung water after an infusion of 90 ml/kg/hr of lactated ringer's when the lungs were excised soon after the infusion (eight cats) (55). In another experiment, one cat out of five died due to respiratory failure after a fluid administration rate of 70 ml/kg/hr (56). These experiments were not totally equivalent because halothane was used during the first study whereas in the second study the cats were anesthetized with ketamine. This agent tends to raise pulmonary arterial pressure. Clinically, pulmonary edema has developed in the cab with administration rates as low as 40 ml/kg. In a 500-kg horse, the volume needed would be of the order of 45 liters of fluid, but it is rare to give that much during the initial therapy.

Assessment of the effectiveness of fluid therapy is based on clinical judgement. The object of the resuscitation is to reperfuse the peripheral tissues and so any signs indicating this should be regarded as favorable, such as an increase in the strength of the pulse; decreased capillary refill time; pink, moist mucous membranes, a warming of the skin, particularly at the extremities; and reversal of cerebral depression. One of the most reliable indices of peripheral perfusion is urine production; if this returns to normal levels, then the initial resuscitation has been successful. Another measurement that is extremely useful is CVP. This provides an estimate of right heart function, because the CVP will rise if the heart is not able to pump forward the fluid being returned to it. A normal value for CVP in the dog is 0 to +5 cm H_2O; when measuring this parameter, the important factor is rate of change. It should not be allowed to rise by more than 5 cm H_2O in any 10-minute period and should not exceed a value of +15 cm H_2O. In the cat, this rate should not exceed a 2 cm H_2O rise in 30 minutes. If these values are exceeded, the rate of fluid administration should be reduced. In the canine experiment mentioned above (53), the CVP rose by about 4 cm H_2O for each 10-minute period during administration (6 ml/kg/min). In veterinary medicine, a CVP catheter is not essential for every patient admitted in shock, but it is certainly indicated in cardiogenic shock, in older animals with a history of myocardial disease, and in any patient where there is doubt as to whether therapy is proving effective.

Having completed our initial therapy, assessed the efficacy of this therapy, and placed a CVP line if necessary, a decision has to be made as to whether a balanced electrolyte solution should be continued or if other fluids are needed. Another blood sample should be drawn and a bit of time taken to get some values from this sample and the one taken before resuscitation.

CLINICAL PATHOLOGY

The minimum information that should be gleaned from these samples is the packed cell volume and the total plasma protein. The values measured initially and those measured after the end of the initial resuscitation will help determine future therapy. Other information that would be very useful includes blood/gas and acid base data, electrolytes, urea, lactate, glucose, and, in severe cases, a clotting profile.

The acid/base values give the clinician a measure of the necessity for bicarbonate therapy. During the Vietnam War, a series of blood gases was taken on soldiers being brought in wounded and in shock. The expectation was that shock produces a metabolic acidosis with a compensatory respiratory alkalosis. This pattern was only seen in 49% of the patients, and some had a distinct metabolic alkalosis (57). Without measuring blood pH, PO_2, and PCO_2, one assumes that the patient is acidotic; from the above data, such may not be the case. The measurement of electrolytes may be important in some metabolic conditions that induce shock, and those values clarify the acid/base data as well as permitting the calculation of anion gaps. The latter have been used as a prognostic indicator for shock (58).

The blood urea in the initial sample will only be above normal if shock has been severe and prolonged or if there was pre-existing renal disease. Although other explanations are possible, the existence of an elevated urea gives another indicator to the clinician that the return of urine flow is a high priority.

The lactate is one of the most underutilized measurements available to the practitioner. Lactic acid is produced during anaerobic metabolism; the higher the lactate rises, the more of an oxygen debt exists. The value of lactate has been found to be strongly correlated with prognosis. In the horse with colic, the mortality was 67% when lactate exceeded 8.3 mmol/ml (75 mg/dl); when the lactate exceeded 11.1 mmol/liter (100 mg/dl), there were no survivors (59). In a human study, the survival rate decreased from 90% with lactates less than 2.2 mmol/liter (20 mg/dl) to 10% when lactates exceeded 8.3 mmol/liter (75 mg/dl) (60). Knowing this value does not make very much difference to the therapy, but it gives the clinician help when discussing prognosis with the owner. It also gives the clinician a good idea as to the severity of the insult.

Measuring blood glucose may give an indication

as to whether glucose should be added to the fluid therapy. Initially in shock there is a hyperglycemia, but as shock progresses, the glucose precursors are depleted, and the animal becomes hypoglycemic.

Finally, in severe shock, a coagulation profile will be very helpful to determine the presence or absence of DIC. The most useful indicators of DIC are prolonged prothrombin time (PT), activated partial thromboplastin time (APTT), decreased antithrombin III activity, fibronectin and platelet numbers, and the presence of fibrin degradation products. Fibrinogen may or may not be reduced in amount.

COLLOIDS

This refers to solutions that contain elements that will remain in the vascular space for a longer period than crystalloid solutions. Many hours have been spent debating whether shock should be treated with one or the other of these fluids, and there is still no consensus on the best solution to use.

When fluids have been lost from the vascular space, then it is logical to replace only this loss and not flood the extravascular space with crystalloid solutions. Most of the circulatory abnormalities in shock relate directly to the vascular space; measurements that are made, such as blood pressure, CVP and capillary refill time, reflect the changes in the vascular space only. In an ideal world, most cases of shock should therefore be treated with colloidal solutions. In veterinary medicine, the use of colloids is somewhat restricted by cost. Whole blood is readily available for some practitioners, but if one decides to keep blood donors of any species, the cost of housing and feeding the donors makes this relatively expensive. Plasma has a similar expense because one has to harvest this from the blood. Dextrans and the other most common colloidal solutions are about ten times the cost of lactated Ringer's. Hetastarch and polygelatin solutions are also expensive. Another fact is that the domestic species appear to be able to tolerate massive blood loss better than *Homo sapiens* and it is feasible to remove 75% of the blood volume of a dog, treat it with lactated Ringer's, and have survival (15).

Nevertheless, there are indications for colloids, and they can be very helpful in certain circumstances. In the dog and cat, it is recommended that if the hematocrit is less than 25% (0.25 liter/liter) on the first sample or falls below 20% (0.2 liter/liter) during treatment, then whole blood should be given. (Refer to Chapter 19 for a discussion on blood types and anticoagulants.) If blood loss has been greater than 25% of the blood volume and is continuing, then whole blood is indicated. If the plasma protein falls below 40 g/liter then plasma or a plasma substitute should be used. Clinically, it has also been useful to give dextrans or plasma to patients when it is difficult to maintain the circulation with crystalloid. This is seen as the initial fluid is redistributed and does not remain in the vascular space. In some equine colic cases, it is difficult to maintain blood pressure despite massive fluid therapy, and the addition of dextrans or plasma can be very helpful.

SODIUM BICARBONATE

It has already been emphasized that one of the expected lesions in shock is acidosis; because an alteration in pH affects many reaction rates in the body, this can seriously impair metabolic function. As usual when this is investigated in the clinical setting, it appears that acidosis is not always present (57). When the early experimental work was done on gastric dilation/torsion in the dog, the recorded base deficits were very high (61, 62). When further clinical investigations were carried out, many of the dogs had base deficits within the normal range (63, 64). In order to treat this situation, therefore, we should know exactly what the acid-base status is. The use of blood gas measurement is becoming more widespread, and this makes rational treatment possible. Where it is not economical to invest in blood gas equipment, it may be possible to get measurements done at a local hospital, or one can use a "total CO_2" kit (Harleco CO_2 apparatus, Gibbstown, New Jersey) to give an estimate of the acid-base imbalance.

Failing this, one has to deal with the animal on an empirical basis and estimate the likely acidosis on such criteria as severity of shock, duration, and presence or absence of acute compensatory mechanisms. An example of this is the gastric dilation/torsion complex where sequestration of acid in the stomach "compensates" for the metabolic acidosis (63, 64). As a rough guideline one could assume base deficits of the following magnitude: 4 to 6 mmol/liter: mild shock; 6 to 12 mmol/liter: moderate shock; and 12 to 18 mmol/liter: severe shock.

Traditionally, these deficits have been treated with sodium bicarbonate, but it has become abundantly clear that this drug is far from innocuous and it should be used with great care. It is not entirely clear why sodium bicarbonate can kill animals, but it is certain that infusion of sodium bicarbonate can lead to fatalities. Recent studies (65, 66) indicate that the decrease in cardiac function associated with bicarbonate therapy is not a result of the hypertonicity of the solution (an 8.4% solution has an osmolality of 2000 mOsm/liter) because mannitol solutions of equal tonicity do not produce the same effect. The sodium load appears to play some part in the myocardial depression, but the combination with bicarbonate produces the most severe changes. When given by intravenous injection, there is no significant change in myocardial performance and left atrial administration induces more profound changes than right atrial administration, suggesting that the effect is produced in the coronary circulation (65). Thus the acute change in pH in the coronary circulation accompanied by the resulting changes in potassium and calcium ions results in a significant reduction in myocardial function.

Sodium bicarbonate can be used to treat a severe acidosis in shock but a mild to moderate acidosis may be treated by the lactated Ringer's or the gluconate/acetate ions present in other balanced electrolyte solutions. Lactate, acetate, and gluconate are all metabolized in the body and reduce the hydrogen ion concentration. Lactate produces about 55% of the depression caused by an equal dose of sodium bicarbonate, whereas acetate causes about the same degree of depression as bicarbonate (67). Armed with these facts, we can work out what base deficit we would treat with our initial infusion of 90 ml/kg of lactated Ringer's (LR).

$$90 \text{ ml LR contains } 0.09 \times 28 \text{ mmol lactate} = 2.52 \text{ mmol}$$

Because 1 mmol of lactate produces only 55% of the effect of bicarbonate, the effect of 2.52 mmol of lactate $= 2.52 \times 0.55 = 1.39$ mmol.

When using base deficit to calculate the amount of bicarbonate needed, we use the formula:

$$\text{Bicarbonate/kg} = \text{base deficit} \times 0.3 \text{ mmol}$$

Thus the base deficit that the above amount would treat $= 1.39 \times 0.3 = 4.6$ mmol/liter. If the precursor was acetate (27 mmol/liter), we would not have to multiply by 0.55, so base deficit treated $= (0.09 \times 27) \times 0.3 = 8.1$ mmol/liter. So an infusion of 90 ml/kg of lactated Ringers will reverse the acidosis in mild shock, and an acetate solution will reverse the acidosis in moderate shock. These solutions containing acetate also usually contain gluconate; this will potentiate this effect because it is also metabolized and reduces hydrogen ion concentration in the process.

In rare cases, once fluid therapy has begun, there may be sufficient washout of acid products from the peripheral tissues to require the use of sodium bicarbonate to reverse this acidosis. As has already been mentioned, sodium bicarbonate should be given with great care. Ideally, it should be given after an initial volume of fluids, and it should be given slowly. A rule of thumb is to give one-half the calculated dose over 15 to 30 minutes and then reassess the acid/base status or give the rest of the dose over the next 12 to 24 hours. Apart from the effect on the myocardium, rapid alkalinization of the blood can shift the oxy-hemoglobin dissociation curve to the left and may lead to cerebrospinal fluid (CSF) acidosis. This occurs as the bicarbonate combines with acid and produces carbon dioxide. The carbon dioxide can rapidly diffuse into the CSF, whereas bicarbonate diffusion takes much more time, which results in acidification of the CSF.

Sodium bicarbonate is not the only drug used for reversing acidosis. Tromethamine (THAM) is also available, and it has fewer undesirable side effects. There is no generation of CO_2 and it is a positive inotrope, but it does require renal excretion and it can produce ECG changes similar to those of hyperkalemia. Its main disadvantages are cost and the volume of solution needed for treating acidosis. (A 20-kg dog with a base deficit of 5 mmol/liter would require 110 ml of a 3.6% solution).

Definitive Treatment

The therapies considered so far are essential to get the patient on the way to recovery. After the initial fluids and reassessment, it is necessary to decide whether more fluid is indicated (and it often will be) or how one should proceed. Many other things have been proposed as being useful adjuncts to shock therapy, some of which will be discussed below. Before doing this, however, a caution should be issued. The research and clinical literature on shock is voluminous, and in the laboratory many different methods have been used to produce different types of shock. The methods used often have profound effects on the results. Were the animals awake or anesthetized? If they were anesthetized, the agent used may dramatically change the results of the experiment. In one experiment using occlusion of the superior mesenteric artery in the rat, ketamine (which is an agent recommended for use in trauma victims) produced lower survival than halothane (68). The measurements made and the time at which they are made is vitally important. If blood pressure and heart rate are the only cardiovascular parameters measured, there could be a rise in blood pressure and heart rate at the expense of cardiac output, thus giving a false impression of improved perfusion. Lastly, what is the parameter used to determine whether a particular therapy is useful? Ultimately, the bottom line is survival; the treatment must show an improved survival or decreased final morbidity if it is to be considered. A recent paper reanalyzed the results of an experiment carried out on 153 dogs in 1966 (69). This experiment was chosen because it represented one of the largest shock therapy studies carried out on a homogeneous group of dogs using a single lot of endotoxin. The analysis indicated that at the end of the first day, some treatments were more "effective" (i.e., more of the animals in the treatment group were alive than the controls). However, by the seventh day, the two groups were the same, indicating that at least this amount of time was required to determine the effect of treatment. Experimental studies can be carried out under rigid conditions, and specific questions can be answered if the correct data have been collected. Clinical studies, on the other hand, provide survival data, but there must be a rigid classification for entry into the study and great care to eliminate bias.

Corticosteroids

Given the fact that endogenous corticosteroid levels are elevated during stress and the myriad beneficial pharmacological effects of these agents, it is hardly surprising that their use has been advocated in shock therapy. That they can improve cardiac output, bind to endotoxins, and stabilize lysosomal membranes should guarantee their position in the armamentarium of shock therapy. Other benefits of corticosteroids are improved peripheral blood flow, reduced activation of the coagulation pathways, inhibition of complement activation by endotoxin, reduction of elevated ADH levels, and reduction of cerebral edema. There are many papers to support the use of corticosteroids in shock (11, 70–76), but there are also many that indicate that they have little or no overall benefit (77–82). One recent study in humans in septic shock (82) indicated that the overall mortality was not improved by corticosteroid therapy. Corticosteroids did improve short-term survival, so they may be of benefit if other therapies can be found to alter the course after initial resuscitation. Despite the masses of experimental animal data, there is no comparable clinical study in the domestic species to give evidence on the routine use of corticosteroids in shock therapy. What the experimental data does indicate is that if steroids are to have any beneficial effect, they need to be given as early as possible in the course of shock in massive doses. In hemorrhagic shock, this "therapeutic window" probably only lasts about 1 hour after the onset of shock, after which time there appears to be no beneficial effect (83). The pharmacokinetic and pharmacodynamic information suggests that prednisolone is superior to dexamethasone because of its more rapid penetration into the cells and the fact that it does not have to be metabolised first. Nevertheless, studies carried out in the clinical setting have been unable to detect a difference. In general, dexamethasone is a lot cheaper than prednisolone, and this has great relevance in veterinary practice. Doses recommended in shock therapy are: hydrocortisone sodium succinate (solu Cortef), 25 to 50 mg/kg q 4 hr; prednisolone sodium succinate (solu Delta Cortef), 30 to 60 mg/kg q 8 hr; methylprednisolone sodium succinate (solu Medrol), 15 to 60 mg/kg q 8 hr; and dexamethasone sodium phosphate (Decadron Phosphate, Hexadrol, Dexamethasone sodium Phosphate), 2 to 6 mg/kg q 8 hr.

Although no differences could be demonstrated in the above studies between dexamethasone sodium phosphate and prednisolone sodium succinate, recent experimental work has shown a clear difference for dexamethasone in propylene glycol (76). When combined with gentamicin sulfate for the treatment of *Escherichia coli* septic shock, it was clearly inferior to methylprednisolone succinate. It should also be noted that propylene glycol can produce hemolysis; although this is of little concern in the normal animal, the release of thromboplastins, associated with red cell destruction, could trigger a consumptive coagulopathy (DIC) in the shocked animal. The corticosteroid should be continued for 24 to 48 hours until the patient is stable.

Corticosteroids should be abruptly withdrawn at the end of this period without worrying about adrenal suppression. Indeed, in a recent study on endotoxic shock in the pony, dexamethasone did not even suppress cortisol while it was being administered (79). When given for this short period, it is also unlikely to interfere with wound healing.

Antibiotics

Antibiotics are an essential part of therapy when a septic focus can be identified in septic shock. If septicemia is suspected, blood should be collected for culture. When antibiotics are used in the septic patient, a broad spectrum bactericidal drug is recommended because the causative organism is unlikely to be known at this stage. Gentamicin or trimethoprim/sulfa are the drugs usually recommended with the addition of ampicillin for anaerobes if these are suspected (84, 85). Because of their bactericidal activity, these drugs may cause further endotoxin release as the causal organisms are killed. This can be fatal to the animal, and it is recommended that corticosteroids be administered at the same time to protect the animal against the effects of endotoxemia (76, 80, 81).

In the nonseptic patient, antibiotics are indicated in the animal presented in severe shock, in the patient with open wounds, and in animals that might have a reduced tolerance for infection (e.g., an animal being treated with other immunosuppressive agents). Administration of antibiotics, once started, should be continued for 3 to 5 days to ensure the best effects.

Vasoactive Drugs

Because of the hypotension associated shock, it was initially thought that alpha-adrenergic drugs could reverse this to cure shock. It is now recognized that these agents should only be used in anaphylactic shock or on a short-term basis to buy time with which to treat the underlying condition. Such short-acting compounds as norepinephrine can be given to raise the blood pressure sufficiently to sustain life while fluids are administered. Longer acting alpha-adrenergic drugs should be avoided.

Other sympathomimetic agents may be of use to support the heart and improve blood flow to the periphery. The two most common agents used in this regard are dopamine and dobutamine. The use of dopamine to improve cardiac performance and splanchnic blood flow has reached the level that in humans the dose rate forms part of the definition of shock states (86). Dopamine is the naturally occuring precursor of norepinephrine, and it acts at $beta_1$ receptors in the heart and at specific dopaminergic receptors in the kidney and mesenteric blood vessels. These latter effects have been suggested as being useful in the treatment of shock where improved renal perfusion and urinary output are desirable. Experiments in which blood pressure was held constant showed that urine production was decreased (87) in dopamine-treated animals versus controls, indicating that the improved renal production in clinical patients may be solely due to the increased blood pressure and cardiac output. Dopamine at higher doses begins to cause release of norepinephrine from presynaptic storage sites. This will cause peripheral vasoconstriction and may also predispose to cardiac dysrhythmias. If dopamine is to be used in the patient in shock to improve cardiac function and maintain perfusion, the animal needs to be monitored carefully. At the least, this should include trained personnel, an electrocardiogram (ECG), blood pressure, and urine output. One other caution should be mentioned with dopamine, and that is that severe tissue damage can occur if dopamine leaks out into traumatized tissue. There are several reports in the human literature of gangrene occurring in tissues severely vasoconstricted by the extravasation of dopamine (88). Dopamine is usually given by infusion, and doses recommended are 2 to 10 μg/kg/min.

Dobutamine is a more expensive agent and has a direct action on the $beta_1$ adrenergic receptors, but does not act at dopaminergic receptors. The commercial drug is a racemic mixture of D and L isomers, each of which have slightly different effects at the receptors. Thus its use in the shock patient is purely for its positive inotropic effect, although it is also a weak $alpha_1$ and $beta_2$ agonist. The dose recommended for dobutamine is 2 to 20 μg/kg/min, and it should be prepared in 5% dextrose because it rapidly deteriorates in solutions with a lower pH.

Many years ago, the use of alpha-adrenergic blocking agents was recommended for the treatment of hemorrhagic shock (89); this has recently been proven in the laboratory (90). The basis for this was that peripheral vasodilation would improve flow to the tissues once the initial fluid therapy was underway. This is now carried out in the medical field using alpha-adrenergic blocking agents and more specific peripheral vasodilators. Sodium nitroprusside is the most common drug used in humans, but it has not been used widely in the veterinary field. Nitroglycerine is more widely used, and the cutaneous absorption of this drug makes it simple to administer and easy to titrate. It is supplied in a petroleum-lanolin base and is formulated such that each 1-inch ribbon of cream will deliver 15 mg of nitroglycerine. A dose of 4 to 8 mg is recommended as initial therapy and can be applied every 4 hours. The person applying the cream should wear a glove to prevent absorption through their own skin.

Hydralazine is another commonly employed vasodilator that acts on the arteriolar smooth muscle but has no action on the venous system. A dose of 0.25 mg/kg can be given by slow intravenous injection every 4 to 6 hours if required. It is incompatible in solution with such drugs as furosemide, aminophylline, the sulphonamides, phenobarbital, chlorthiazide, and hydrocortisone.

The phenothiazines are commonly used in veterinary practice, but they also produce significant sedation of the animal, so nitroglycerin or hydralazine are recommended as being more appropriate therapy. Experimental evidence indicates that promethazine at a dose of 5 mg/kg improves survival in an acute hemorrhagic shock model (90). Acepromazine at a dose of 0.05 mg/kg in the dog, cat, and horse is likely to produce a similar effect. The use of alpha blocking agents in endotoxic/septic shock has not resulted in improved survival (91), but certain antihistamine agents (eg. diphenhydramine) have resulted in lower mortality (92). Since the phenothiazines are also antihistamines, it may be that this function is more important.

Recent Advances

The scientific literature is full of new approaches to the treatment of shock, which emphasizes the complexity of the syndrome. A simple problem requires a simple solution, but the changes occurring in shock are far from simple. As we can become more specific in our diagnosis of shock, so will therapy be more successful.

HYPERTONIC SALINE

Solutions containing 7.5% sodium chloride (2400 mmol/liter) have been used experimentally (66, 93, 94) and clinically (95). In an experimental study, intravenous infusion of 4 ml/kg of this hypertonic saline led to the recovery and survival for 7 days of dogs which had been hemorrhaged (40 to 50% blood loss). The control group all died. It appears that this treatment works by the passage of the hypertonic solution through the pulmonary vascular bed. Vagal blockade will remove the effect of the treatment, as will administration of the solution into the left atrium or aorta (66).

The pulmonary-vagal reflex appears to produce a redistribution of blood flow with a massive increase in mesenteric flow and a decrease in muscle blood flow. This is probably responsible for the maintained hyperosmolarity of the blood which occurs with intravenous infusions but which declines with intra-arterial injection or injection during vagal blockade. A recent article suggested that the hyperosmolar effect is important in the re-expansion of the vascular space from the extravascular fluid compartment (96). The above evidence would suggest that, while raising the osmolality by 40 to 50 mOsm/liter may be important in the initial response, the final outcome is dependent on a sustained neuronal or neurohumoral mechanism mediated through the pulmonary vascular bed and involving either afferent or efferent vagal transmission. The supporting clinical data (95) is not very rigorous, but because this therapy implies the use of very small volumes of fluids, it may be highly beneficial to large animal practices, where the volume of fluid needed for therapy is often very bulky.

NONSTEROIDAL ANTI-INFLAMMATORY DRUGS

With cell damage, there is a release of arachidonic acid; this is converted into various prostaglandins. There are several different precursors, but the main ones of clinical significance are the bisenoic (arachidonic acid) compounds. The arachidonic acid may be converted down two different pathways depending on the enzymes available. The lipoxygenase pathway converts arachidonic acid to HPETE or HETE, which are potent vasoconstrictors and may increase the adhesiveness of platelets. 5-HPETE is also the precursor in the reaction that produces the leukotrienes. These latter compounds may be involved with increasing vascular permeability. The cyclo-oxygenase pathway leads to the production of PGE_2, D_2, and F_2, as well as prostacyclin (PGI_2) and thromboxane (TxA_2). The thromboxanes are very potent vasoconstrictors and also promote platelet aggregation. The release of TxA_2 promotes the production of more TxA_2 from the platelets but it has a very short half-life of 30 seconds. Prostacyclin, on the other hand, promotes vasodilation and acts almost as a direct antagonist of the actions of TxA_2. The release of thromboxanes has been measured in various types of shock. In traumatic shock, the levels peak 4 to 5 hours after the trauma (26). In experimental models of endotoxic shock in the dog and the horse, the levels of thromboxane peak very soon after endotoxin administration (5 to 15 minutes). The levels of prostacyclin differ slightly between the horse and the dog. In the dog, there is an early peak immediately after endotoxin administration, followed by a decline and then another peak at about 2 hours. In the horse, the levels peak at about 1 hour (97, 98).

The main therapeutic approach to these effects has been to use drugs that block the cyclo-oxygenase pathway, such as aspirin, phenylbutazone, indomethacin, flunixin meglumine, and meclofenamate. As can be expected from the fact that thromboxanes peak early with an endotoxic administration, the main use for these drugs has been in septic/endotoxic shock models. So far, the protective effects have been well demonstrated in dogs, sheep, and horses. In the dog using a septic peritonitis model, flunixin meglumine at a dose of 1.1 mg/kg and gentamicin at 2.2 mg/kg (both given i.v. 15 minutes and 12 hours after the induction of sepsis) gave 100% (8/8) survival at 7 days compared with no survival in a control group and a 63% (5/8) survival in a group treated with gentamicin alone. The group treated with flunixin alone showed less clinical effect from the sepsis, but the 7-day survival is not statistically different from the group treated with antibiotics only (99). Other NSAID's such as indomethacin, flufenamic acid, phenylbutazone, aminopyrine, and ibuprofen have been shown to improve hemodynamics in septic dogs, but survival was not measured in these experiments (100, 101). In a sublethal endotoxic model in sheep, meclofenamate prevented the early pulmonary hypertension but failed to prevent the late phase of pulmonary vascular permeability. When meclofenamate (5 mg/kg plus 3 ml/kg/hr) was combined with methylprednisolone (20 to 30 mg/kg plus 10 mg/kg/hr), there was minimal pulmonary hypertension, no change in lung lymph flow, and no change in the alveolar-arterial oxygen gradient. (11).

Several studies have been carried out in ponies and horses; for this type of experiment there appears to be no difference between a pony and a horse (102). Most of the studies have used flunixin meglumine, but phenylbutazone has also been shown to be effective in reducing the effects of endotoxemia/sepsis (103). The models vary, but flunixin appears to prevent or attenuate a fall in mean blood pressure, mesenteric vasodilation, tachypnea, dyspnea, hypoxemia, damage to the cardiopulmonary vascular endothelium, colic, lactic acidosis, and diarrhea (48, 104–107). It does not prevent the leukopenia or the fall in platelets associated with endotoxemia (108). In one study that looked at survival, flunixin had improved survival, from 25% (2/8) to 75% (6/8) at the end of 7 days (106). In another study, phenylbutazone did not improve survival (103). In most of these studies, flunixin was given at a dose of 1.1 mg/kg intravenously.

The above evidence strongly supports the use of cyclo-oxygenase inhibitors in endotoxic/septic shock; because, thromboxanes are elevated in other forms of shock, it would be logical to use these drugs for general treatment of this syndrome. However, there is still no clinical evidence on the subject of survival in any of the domestic species; this information needs to be collected. On top of this, these drugs have some disadvantages. In equine colics, the very fact that flunixin prevents some of the clinical signs associated with endotoxemia means that patients with life-threatening lesions may not receive the appropriate therapy. In the canine patient, there is little information concerning the ue of NSAIDs, and the mechanism of action dictates that long-term usage is likely to be accompanied by gastric ulceration (inhibition of prostacyclin formation which is involved in controlling gastric acid secretion and blood flow) and alterations in renal function (109).

Prostacyclins have been used during traumatic shock and were able to improve short-term survival. In one study, the blood pressure did not decline as much as the control group, and there were lower levels of cathepsin D and MDF, indicating that the prostacyclin had a membrane-stabilizing effect (110). Prostacyclins have also been shown to be beneficial in endotoxic shock in several species (111). Prostaglandin E_1 has also been tried, and although it improves short term survival and has some membrane stabilizing qualities, it is not as effective as prostacylcin (112, 113).

A new generation of NSAIDs is under development, and these drugs inhibit both the lipoxygenase and cyclo-oxygenase pathways of arachidonic acid metabolism (e.g., 3-amino-1-m-(trifluoromethyl) phenyl pyrazoline). These agents will not only reduce the rise in thromboxanes but are also likely to prevent the leukopenia that still occurs with the cyclo-oxygenase inhibitors (114, 115).

NALOXONE

ACTH is stored as propiomelanocortin; when ACTH is split off from this molecule, alpha-endorphin is part of the remainder. So when ACTH is released during shock, there is also a release of B-endorphin. Proenkephalin A is found in significant amounts in the adrenal medulla, and this gives rise to leu and met enkephalin. Stimulation of the adrenal medulla will release enkephalins into the circulation. Another opiate, dynorphin, is secreted into the circulation from the posterior pituitary. The actions of these endogenous opiates is not entirely clear, but they tend to promote hypotension, sedation, hypothermia, and reduced metabolism, all of which could be considered adaptive mechanisms to promote survival (with untreated hemorrhage, hypotension may reduce further blood loss). The hypotension effects of enkephalins may be related to their ability to inhibit chronotropic and vascular contractile responses to catecholamines (116, 117). These responses may be helpful in the early stages of shock, but they become part of the decompensation that may occur later in shock. To test the hypothesis that enkephalins were involved in the hypotension associated with shock, Holaday and Faden used an endotoxic shock model in rats (118). They gave naloxone to the rats and were able to reverse the hypotension. Since then, many experiments have been carried out to confirm this effect. As with other drug therapies, the experimental evidence has been equivocal. In some of the published work, treatment with naloxone has improved survival both in endotoxic and hemorrhagic shock (119, 120). Other experiments have not been able to demonstrate either improved hemodynamics (e.g., in the horse and baboon) (119, 121) or an improvement in survival (e.g., in the pig, cat, baboon, and rat) (119, 122–124). There is little controlled clinical material that demonstrates the efficacy of naloxone. The reports so far in humans have shown no significant improvements (125, 126); indeed, there have been significant side effects (e.g., pulmonary edema and grand mal seizure). The dosages of naloxone used are also several times higher than those used for reversal of standard opiates (119, 120). Because naloxone is mainly specific for mu receptors, this suggests that one of the other receptors may be involved, and a delta receptor antagonist has been shown to reverse endotoxic shock in rats (127). Further work on kappa receptors is in progress (128). Four other factors appear to be important in using naloxone. The first is that there is a better effect if volume expansion has been carried out first (129); the second is that it is more effective if any acidosis or hypothermia has been corrected (130). The third is that the naloxone should be given after corticosteroids because there is no pressor effect in the absence of steroids (131), and the fourth is that it will reverse any analgesia present. To this end, some agonist-antagonist drugs have been used with some success (132–134).

In conclusion, because of the current cost of naloxone and the recommended dosages (2 mg/kg plus an infusion of 1.5 mg/kg/hr in the dog) (129), the clinical use of this treatment is unlikely to become common in veterinary medicine. If more specific delta or kappa antagonists are developed that can be given at economical doses, then opiate antagonist therapy may become part of the routine therapy for shock, at least in the canine. Results for other species give little room for optimism.

THYROTROPIN RELEASING HORMONE

The action of thyrotropin-releasing hormone (TRH) in supraphysiological doses is to increase respiration, body temperature, heart rate, and blood pressure. These effects are opposite to those of the enkephalins, so the use of TRH has been advocated as a physiological reversal of the opioid agonists (128). Because it does not directly antagonise the opioids, it can be used without reversing narcotic analgesia. To date, TRH has been tested in a spinal trauma model (135) and in experimental anaphylactic shock (136) with good results, and further clinical testing is in progress.

ANTIBODIES TO ENDOTOXIN CORE GLYCOLIPID

Bacterial lipopolysaccharides (endotoxins) are in general composed of three portions: the oligosaccharide side chains, the core polysaccharide, and lipid A. This latter fraction is thought to be the toxic entity, and there is little variation in the core polysaccharide-lipid A structure produced by different gram-negative bacteria. This has led to the use of a mutant *E. coli* (the J5 mutant of *E. Coli* 0111.B_4), a strain without the oligosaccharide side chains, to produce antibodies to endotoxin core glycolipid. These antibodies have been shown to give protection against gram-negative shock in a number of species. In humans, the prophylactic use of antibody before surgery with a high risk of endotoxic shock provided some protection against the effects of endotoxin (137). When used as a treatment for patients with endotoxic shock, the antibody also improved survival (138). The mechanism of action appears to involve the antibody binding to the endotoxin (139). The mechanism by which this antibody-endotoxin complex is cleared has not been elucidated. This treatment may prove to be useful in endotoxic and septic shock where the treatment can be initiated before irreversible damage occurs.

ADENOSINE TRIPHOSPHATE-MAGNESIUM CHLORIDE (ATP-$MgCl_2$)

As mentioned earlier in this review, the basic energy production of the cell is altered in shock. This is a result of the reduced supply of oxygen and glucose and the failure to remove waste products. The reduction of ATP in cells is caused by increased usage (to maintain the sodium-potassium pump) and decreased production (anaerobic metabolism). Some tissues are more resistant to these effects than others. For example, muscle cells showed no decrease in ATP levels even when the membrane potential had dropped from −91mv to −65mv (140). However, the creatine phosphate (CP) levels had fallen, implying that ATP was being maintained at the expense of CP. In the same study, the levels of ATP in the liver decreased significantly. These experiments and others with similar results were carried out in anesthetized animals (141, 142), but muscle depletion of ATP was evident in late shock in conscious animals (143). With the breakdown of the purines to uric acid, the cell cannot rebuild its energy stores even if circulation is restored.

One approach to this has been to supply ATP by an intravenous route; in combination with magnesium chloride, some success has been achieved. ATP obtained from equine muscle is made up as a fresh solution with magnesium chloride (114). The infusion of this solution at ATP dosages of 33 mmol/kg has been shown to improve survival in endotoxic shock (145), at 100 mmol/kg for hemorrhagic shock (146), and at 300 mmol/kg for the treatment of sepsis/peritonitis with the addition of glucose (147). It is not clear whether this ATP works in the cell or at the cell membrane, but recent evidence suggests that it can cross cell membrane, particularly during shock states (148, 149).

To date, the solution appears to require special preparation as a fresh solution (144), and it needs to be given very carefully to avoid tachycardia, hypotension, and a decrease in cardiac performance (144, 150, 151). Nevertheless, it is readily available and the preparation of a stable solution would greatly enhance the possibility of using this to treat clinical shock.

TRAUMA

Many of the same physiologic responses of the patient in shock will be observed in animals suffering severe trauma. Not only should one consider the local reactions and tissue damage as a result of trauma, but major trauma results in systemic responses which can influence anesthetic management or the well-being of the patient (152–155). It is not unusual to discover effects of trauma in other organ systems such as traumatic myocarditis in addition to fractures of the extremities. The responses to stress during or immediately following the injury may also carry over into the surgical period (156–163). These responses include the release of endocrines, especially adrenal responses to stress. In addition to direct hormonal effect, electrolyte disturbances may occur after trauma due to intra and extracellular fluid loss. An awareness of the extent of endocrine dysfunction following trauma will aid in the selection of anesthetic regimes. Even though more complete discussion of endocrine responses to be considered during anesthesia are detailed in other portions of this text, one should at least anticipate the alterations will effect the autonomic nervous system.

The responses to injury may result in alterations in metabolism. This change of metabolism may be part of the hypothalmic responses which in turn alters the heat production in the animal after injury (163–165). The extent of these alterations can reflect in the time delay between injury and anesthesia for corrective surgery.

As a result of the multiple systemic responses to injury, not only may one observe shock-like situations, but septic responses may occur due to the extent of trauma and alterations in responses to bacterial infection. The physiologic challenge may result in the development of septicemia (166–170). This is in part related to direct tissue damage from trauma and in part due to changes in the animal's resistance to infections as a result of alterations in the immune system (170–178).

Unfortunately, even without considerable attention to the responses to stress, injury, hemorrhagic and other forms of shock, the management of animals with severe trauma present a high anesthetic risk. The process of reducing responses to pain or the induction and maintenance of complete anesthesia for surgical correction of injuries, may result in cardiopulmonary disturbances or arrest. It is the responsibility of the veterinarian and the veterinarian's staff to maintain a current awareness of the principles and practice of the techniques and choices of medications for treatment of cardiopulmonary arrest should it occur.

Cardiopulmonary Resuscitation

An animal in cardiac arrest is dead unless we can do something about it. Thus one cannot approach this in a half-hearted manner. The knowledge of what to do must also be present because there is no time to sit down and read chapter and verse on the subject. Therapy must be rapid and accurate in order to achieve the desired goal. Cardiac arrest in humans is a much more common event than it is in animals, and over the last few years a major effort has been made to educate lay people to performing basic cardiopulmonary resuscitation (CPR). One of the efforts of basic CPR is to teach a simple but rigid protocol. The veterinarian, like the human physician, should be able to provide advanced cardiac life support, should understand the events that are occurring, and should be able to deal with each problem. To deal with this unusual event, the veterinarian must practice resuscitation and must have all the equipment set up so that it can be reached immediately. The attitude that it will never happen to me is not good enough in today's practice, because animals can be resuscitated and they can go on to lead perfectly healthy lives.

THE GOALS OF RESUSCITATION

The first aim with CPR is to restore adequate circulation. In order to do this, we need to ensure that the blood is oxygenated and that we provide external support of circulation until such time as the heart begins to beat on its own. Once the heart has started to beat spontaneously, the cardiac output must be raised so that the perfusion of the whole body is sufficient. The author has seen several cases where the initial resuscitation was not followed by vigorous support of the heart, leading to rapid demise of the animal.

The second aim after the restoration of circulation is the restoration of function, particularly with respect to the brain. Cerebral resuscitation has been the subject of intensive research over the last few years (e.g., Br J Anaesth, 57 (1), whole issue, 1985). Aggressive therapy is needed to prevent brain damage and to allow the animal to survive with normal behavior. Although these two aims are distinct, the rapid restoration of adequate circulation is the best method of preventing brain damage.

THE EVENTS LEADING TO CARDIAC ARREST

There are six main reasons for cardiac arrest:

Ischemia

This is the main cause in humans, but coronary vessel damage in animal species is relatively rare. Atherosclerotic lesions have been reported in the rabbit, chicken, pig, and hypothyroid dog (179), but ischemic arrest is a rare event in animals. Direct trauma or pressure on the heart may lead to ischemia, which could trigger fatal dysrhythmias (Fig. 22.4).

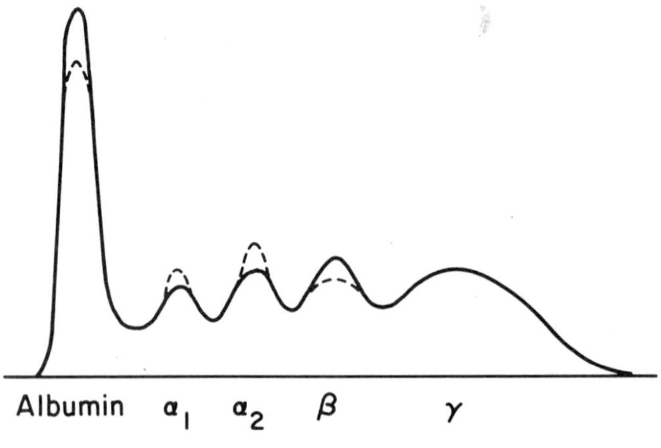

Figure 22.4. An electrophoretic strip of plasma proteins. The *dotted lines* represent the changes that occur with trauma. Gamma proteins may increase or decrease depending on the nature of the injury.

Hypoxemia

This includes any reason for either a decreased ability to take up oxygen from the lungs or a decreased supply of oxygen to the heart. The former may occur with pulmonary edema, pneumonia, airway obstruction, pulmonary hemorrhage, pulmonary embolization, or pneumothorax. A decreased supply of oxygen is caused by hypotension, and so anything which severely drops the diastolic pressure will tend to lower coronary perfusion. Examples of this include shock and severely decreased myocardial function (e.g., cardiomyopathy).

Severe Acid-Base or Electrolyte Abnormalities

Extreme acidosis or alkalosis will impair all the enzyme systems involved with energy metabolism, leading to cardiac arrest. Severe electrolyte imbalances may also produce arrest. In cats, foals, and calves, urinary obstruction and rupture of the bladder are relatively common, and the resulting hyperkalemia may put the heart into arrest. Hypokalemia may also stop the heart, and rapid changes in calcium levels can produce cardiac arrest.

Drug Toxicity

There are many drugs that are toxic to the heart. The inhalant anesthetics have a relatively narrow therapeutic index with cardiotoxicity occurring at 3.0 minimum alveolar concentration (MAC) for halothane, 3.7 MAC for methoxyflurane, 3.3 MAC for ethrane, and 5.7 MAC for isoflurane (180). The barbiturates and some local anesthetic agents are also cardiotoxic, and this is the basis for their use as euthanasia solutions. In septic shock, endotoxins may be sufficient to induce cardiac arrest.

Increased Vagal Tone

Usually the heart will "escape" from the influence of raising vagal tone, but sometimes stimulation of vasovagal reflexes such as the occulocardiac reflex may put the heart into arrest.

Electrocution

With high levels of current applied to the outside of the body (macroschock) or low levels supplied internally (microshock) via things like catheters or esophageal stethoscopes, cardiac arrest can occur. Knowledge about the cause of cardiac arrest is not essential but it may help a great deal in effective resuscitation. For example, an animal that has arrested due to excessive ocular manipulation should be easily resuscitated using basic CPR and an anticholinergic agent.

DETECTING AND PREDICTING CARDIAC ARREST

The detection of cardiac arrest should be very easy, and yet it is often not recognized early enough to be treated successfully. This failure to appreciate an impending or an actual arrest may stem from the fear of the unknown. If you don't feel comfortable dealing with a condition it will be ignored or further tests applied until there can be no doubt as to the diagnosis. Whereas this attitude may be prudent for a dermatologist, it is literally fatal for a patient in cardiac arrest. Immediate action is required and should be instituted as soon as possible. The signs associated with cardiac arrest are listed in Table 22.1.

Monitoring a patient is dealt with in another chapter of this text, but adequate knowledge of the status of the patient is the only means of predicting cardiac arrest. This may be very simple monitoring, such as the routine observation of a bitch recovering from a neutering operation to check for hemorrhage or respiratory obstruction. It may be more sophisticated monitoring with measurements being made of blood pressure, central venous pressure, urinary output, acid-base, electrolytes, blood gases, and ECG. Whatever the system used, it is ultimately dependent on the skill, training, and attention of the person who is responsible for that patient. If it appears that an animal is likely to go into cardiac arrest, then vigorous therapy is necessary. Signs that should be investigated closely include very pale or cyanotic mucous membranes (cyanosis is particularly serious if the animal is already on 100% oxygen), weak or thready pulse, irregular or agonal respiratory movements, apnea at a time when it is not expected (e.g., the brief apnea that occurs after thiopental induction is expected, but apnea 1 hour into an anesthetic is unusual), cardiac dysrhythmias that may lead to asystole or fibrillation (e.g., ventricular tachycardia, atrioventricular dissociation, or profound sinus bradycardia), and the presence of dark deoxygenated blood at the incision site.

TYPES OF CARDIAC ARREST

There are now four major dysrhythmia patterns recognized during cardiac arrest. Because these represent

Table 22.1
Signs of Cardiac Arrest

No palpable arterial pulse.
No auscultable heartbeat
Gray or cyanotic mucous membranes
Dilated pupils
No ventilatory efforts or agonal gasps
No bleeding at surgical site
Electrocardiographic diagnosis of asystole, fibrillation, or PIVR.

different electrical activities within the heart, they may require different therapies. One of the major problems with these dysrhythmias is that one needs an ECG machine to be able to diagnose them or one needs to open the thorax and look at the heart.

Ventricular Asystole

This occurs when there is a total loss of electrical activity in the ventricles. The appearance on an ECG is that of a straight line with or without P waves. If P waves are present, this is effectively an atrioventricular (AV) conduction block with no ventricular escape beats. Excessive vagal tone may cause an asystolic arrest. Because the AV node is about twice as sensitive to acetylcholine as the sinoatrial (SA) node (181), increased vagal tone initially causes an AV conduction block. As the amount of vagal efferent activity increases, this is followed by SA arrest. Electrolyte imbalances such as hyperkalemia and hypercalcemia may lead to ventricular asystole. An asystolic arrest is also seen as a terminal event after fibrillation or electromechanical dissociation (182). In humans, ventricular asystole has a poorer prognosis than other forms of arrest (183), but in veterinary practices where a defibrillator may not be available, an asystole would carry a better prognosis than fibrillation (Fig. 22.5, *A*).

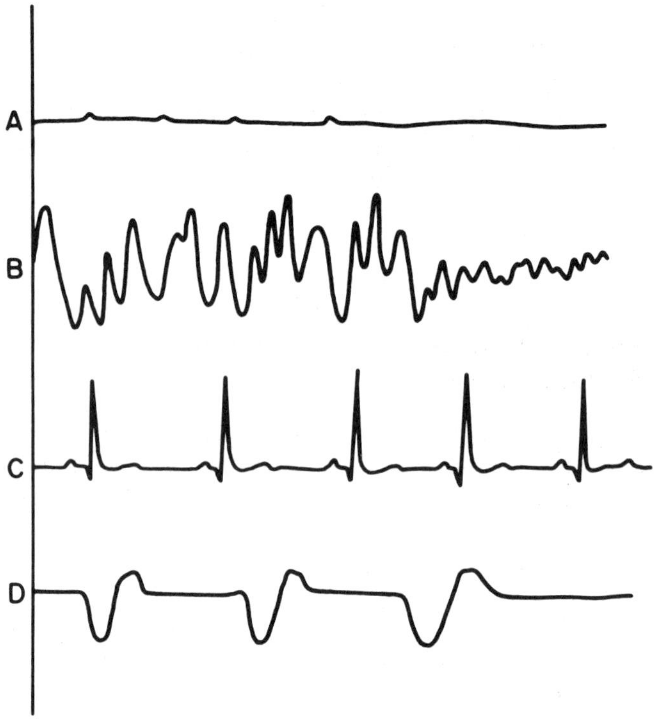

Figure 22.5. *A*, ventricular asystole. Initially there is an AV block with no ventricular escape followed by total asystole. *B*, ventricular fibrillation. Coarse fibrillation on the left gives way to a fine fibrillatory pattern to the right. *C*, electromechanical dissociation. In this instance essentially a normal ECG, but the electrical activity is not accompanied by a mechanical contraction. *D*, Pulseless idioventricular rhythm. Wide bizarre QRS complexes with a slow rate. Other idioventricular rhythms are usually faster.

Ventricular Fibrillation

Fibrillation occurs when there are totally uncoordinated sites of activation throughout the heart. Small areas of muscle contract independently of other sites. This chaotic contraction of the ventricular muscle is totally ineffective in its ability to pump blood around the body, and because there are no valves opening or closing, there are no audible sounds from the heart. Ventricular fibrillation can be diagnosed by direct visualization of the ventricle or by use of an ECG. When looking at the heart, it looks like a bag full of snakes with little bulges and dimples appearing chaotically over the surface of the ventricle. An ECG shows an irregular wavy line with no consistency in the amplitude, width, or shape of the deflections. None of the normal waves are present (Fig. 22.5, *B*). Fibrillation is arbitrarily divided into fine and coarse fibrillation, the difference between the two being the amplitude of the deflections. When looking at the heart, a fine fibrillation looks as if the heart is shivering rather than the coarse similarity to a bag of snakes. The reason for making this distinction is that it is easier to convert a coarse fibrillation back to a normal rhythm than it is to convert a fine fibrillation. Ventricular fibrillation may be seen during cardiac arrest after hypoxia, shock, direct mechanical stimulation of the heart as in trauma or surgery, and electrical shock. It may also be seen with severe electrolyte depletion such as hypocalcemia and hypokalemia and with alkalosis. Catecholamine stimulation may lead to fibrillation, particularly in conjunction with halothane, xylazine, the short-acting barbiturates, and digitalis toxicity. The mechanism for this appears to involve both alpha$_1$ and beta$_1$ receptors (184), with different effects being seen in different species. In the dog, there appears to be some involvement of both receptors, whereas in the pig the alpha$_1$ receptors are more storngly implicated. Agents that block alpha$_1$ receptors, such as the phenothiazines and butyrophenones, tend to protect the myocardium against epinephrine-induced fibrillation during halothane anesthesia. Drugs used with alpha$_1$-stimulating properties, such as norepinephrine and phenylephrine, should be used with caution during halothane administration when the patient has not had prior treatment with an alpha$_1$ blocker. Other causes of ventricular fibrillation include profound hypothermia and myocarditis.

In very small animals (<3 kg), fibrillation may revert to a normal sinus rhythm (185, 186). It would appear that a certain mass of myocardial tissue is needed to sustain fibrillation.

Electromechanical Dissociation (EMD)

This arrhythmia may be seen on an ECG as a relatively normal P, QRS, and T, but these electrical events are not associated with a musuclar contraction (Fig. 22.5, *C*). There has been an uncoupling between depolarization and contraction, probably as a result of failure in the calcium transport system. If hypoxia is the cause of an EMD, then the complexes are usually abnormal in size and configuration but in the first couple of minutes after a barbiturate overdose, the complexes may appear quite acceptable. The fact that this dysrhythmia exists means that monitoring with a device that only gives an audible signal for each QRS complex can be quite misleading. By the time there is an audible change in the rate or rhythm, the animal might have been dead for several minutes.

EMD may be mistaken for severe hypotension, particularly when heart sounds are practically inaudible. This can occur in cardiac tamponade, tension pneumothorax, myocardial rupture, severe hypovolemia, and pulmonary embolism. All of these latter conditions are usually associated with a pronounced tachycardia.

Pulseless Idioventricular Rhythm (PIVR)

The characteristic of this dysrhythmia is slow, wide, bizarre QRS complexes. The amplitude and duration of the complexes is variable, but the difference from fibrillation is the periods of quiescence in between the complexes and the fact that they usually all deflect in the same direction (187) (Fig. 22.5, *D*). PIVR is most commonly seen after prolonged hypotension as in septic or hypovolemic shock. It represents a severe disturbance of the electrolyte fluxes across the myocardial cell membranes due to changes in the energy production and distribution within the cell. Conduction is still occurring, but it is triggered from ectopic Purkinje cell electrical activity and the resulting depolarization does not result in an effective contraction. Repolarization is also slow, and so the refractory times are increased.

BASIC CARDIOPULMONARY RESUSCITATION

The fundamental aim of basic CPR is to restore the circulation. This will only work if the resuscitative efforts are instituted as soon as the arrest is recognized. Classic teaching demands that we use the A, B, C approach (A, Airway; B, Breathing; C, Circulation), but it should be recognized that these are instituted almost simultaneously.

Airway

The establishment of an airway is of the utmost importance because we must be able to supply oxgen to the lungs to reverse any hypoxemia present. Whatever the cause of the arrest, the myocardial cells are already anoxic or will become so with 2 to 3 minutes. The heart will not beat again until it is oxygenated.

In establishing an airway, the first requirement is to ensure that there is no foreign material obstructing the airway. An animal that has vomited just after extubation may have pieces of vomitus occluding the upper airway. A horse may suffer from respiratory obstruction because of nasal edema after massive fluid administration during a colic surgery. The most useful instrument for inspecting the oral cavity and larynx of small animals is a laryngoscope. The appropriate size of blade makes inspection relatively easy in small animals, but in large animals, a laryngoscope is not very useful because the herbivores cannot open their mouths very far. Once the oral cavity has been inspected, an endotracheal tube can be inserted and the animal ventilated from this tube. Even if an endotracheal tube is in place, the airway should be checked to see if it is patent. In moving animals around, the tube can get kinked or twisted such that it is not readily apparent by superficial examination. The easiest method of testing the airway is to connect the patient to a rebreathing bag on an anesthetic circuit or to a manual resuscitation bag. Once connected, it is a simple thing to give three or four breaths and feel how much pressure is required to inflate the lungs. If there is excessive resistance, this must be investigated. Ideally the gas given to the animal should be 100% oxygen; room air at 20% oxygen will be helpful, as will expired air if nothing else is available. This can be blown down the endotracheal tube in small animals, but it is not possible to ventilate a horse using this method.

When an endotracheal tube is not available, a tight-fitting mask may be used, but care should be taken to get the head and neck extended in order to maintain a patent airway. Having the head extended also reduces the risk of ventilating the stomach. As a final resort, if no equipment is available, mouth to nose ventilation can be used. The head and neck are extended, the mouth is held shut and the rescuer places his mouth over the nostrils and blows into them.

The rescuer should also consider transtracheal ventilation in situations where tracheal intubation is difficult (e.g., in an animal with a laryngeal tumor or in small species such as rats and rabbits). A tracheostomy may be performed and an endotracheal or tracheostomy tube inserted directly into the airway. If a high pressure oxygen source is available, then a catheter can be put into the trachea percutaneously and ventilation achieved with a "jet ventilation" technique. This needs a switching device on the inlet piping so that intermittent bursts or jets of oxygen can be supplied. The apparatus in Figure 22.6 consists of a dual stage regulator with a flow valve on it and some flexible

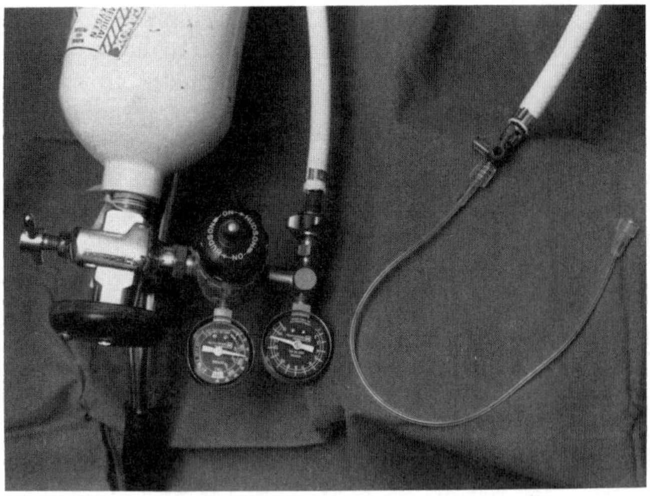

Figure 22.6. A homemade jet ventilator. The tank has a two-pressure regulator that allows the delivered flow to be adjusted. The three-way stopcock is firmly attached to the tubing so that it will not blow off when the pressure is applied. The tank is turned on, the flow turned up, and the stopcock attached to the animal's airway. When the stopcock is opened, a jet of gas is released that will entrain air and provide ventilation.

oxygen hose connected to a three-way stopcock. The flow from the tank is turned on with the stopcock closed. Pressure builds up in the flexible hose, and a jet of gas is released when the stopcock is turned on to the patient. This jet of gas entrains air from the trachea, and this augmented flow of oxygen-enriched air inflates the lungs. It is evident that the upper airway must be patent to allow gas to be inspired and expired via the larynx.

Breathing

Having established a patent airway, the next step is to start ventilating the animal. Initially four breaths should be given in quick succession; the rescuer then takes 10 seconds to check for a pulse and/or a heart beat. If the heart beat is present but the pulse is weak or absent, ventilation must be continued and support of the cardiovascular system initiated (see later). If there is no pulse or heart beat, the rescuer proceeds to C. In order to achieve adequate tidal volumes during CPR, it is better to use manual ventilating techniques rather than mechanical ventilators. In the absence of an anesthetic machine in large animals, a demand valve respirator can be used. This consists of a valve that is attached to a high pressure oxygen source (50 to 60 lbs/square inch) and which can either be triggered by the animal starting to breathe or can be tripped manually. It will deliver a flow of gas (about 50 liters/min) until a predetermined pressure is reached (20 to 25 cm H_2O). This type of equipment is essential for the practitioner who is anesthetising horses without the benefit of an anesthetic machine (188).

The rate of ventilation and the tidal volume at this stage in small animals should be about 10 to 12 breaths in a minute with a tidal volume of 20 mls/kg. When ventilating the patient, the chest excursion should be a little more than a normal breath, and the rescuer should constantly monitor the amount of chest excursion with each breath. In larger animals, the same rule applies but the tidal volume and frequency would be lower (10 to 15 mls/kg at 6 to 8 breaths per minute).

Circulation

With no return of cardiac function after ventilation, cardiac massage must be instituted. A sharp blow to the thorax (precordial thump) used to be recommended before massage was begun. The precordial thump will not defibrillate the heart, and it may convert an electromechanical dissociation to a fibrillatory pattern (189). In a practice where no defibrillator is available, this is a disaster. In cats and small dogs, cardiac massage can be achieved by compression of the ribs laterally over the heart using one hand (Fig. 22.7). In the cat, the rib cage is so compliant that the heart can usually be felt inside the thorax as compressions are instituted. If the heart is not felt as a solid object within the thorax when the chest is compressed, the rescuer should check the position of his/her hand to see if the heart can be picked up. One can also compress the chest in a ventrodorsal fashion. In the small patient, the animal is grasped by the chest with both hands. The fingers are wrapped over the dorsal spinous processes and the thumbs are applied to the sternum. In barrel-chested dogs such as the brachycephalic breeds, this ventrodorsal compression may be preferable to lateral compression. If the dog is too big for one hand, then it should be stabilized in dorsal recumbency and compression applied to the sternum with both hands.

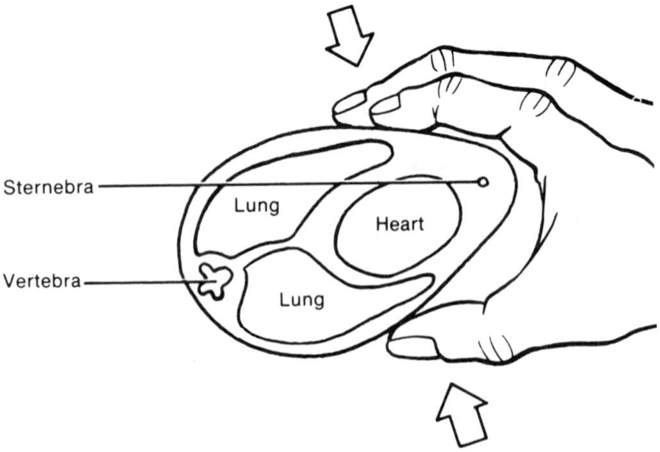

Figure 22.7. Diagram representing the chest compression in a cat or small dog. The heart is often palpable through the thoracic wall and can be compressed with external massage. From Sattler FP, Knowles RP, Whittick WG: *Veterinary Critical Care*. London, Baillière Tindall, 1981.

For other breeds, the lateral compression of the chest is the best method. The best position is probably right lateral recumbency, but this is not essential. If the table that the animal is on can be tilted slightly so that the animal's head is lower than its body, this may also help. The dog must be fixed in position so that it is not sliding around as the hand compresses the chest. This is most easily accomplished by the rescuer standing next to the back of the dog and pulling it towards his/her body with one hand. If the dog has a lot of loose skin, it is helpful to grasp a handful of this with the same hand. The other hand is used to produce a smooth uninterrupted compression and release on the chest wall using the heel of the hand. This compression should be forceful but not so vigorous that the ribs are broken. The area of compression is around the costochondral junction between the fourth and eighth ribs. If the chest is compressed further back than this, it is not as effective and there is a strong possibility of rupturing the liver. The position of the animal relative to the rescuer is also very important. The most effective compression can be achieved with a straight arm so that the whole upper part of the body is used to push down on the animal. If the table is too high for the rescuer, it may be best if the animal is moved down to the floor. A pressure of up to 35 kg may be required in the dog, and the compression phase should be from 50 to 70% of the cycle (190). The use of a longer compression phase makes a significant difference to the mean arterial pressure that can be achieved. For larger animals, one may need to use both hands (one on top of the other), as is taught for human CPR. This technique can be used in foals, ponies, and calves (191). In the horse or cow, compression is achieved by either doing knee drops on to the horse's chest or by turning around and landing on the chest with one's backside. Neither method is very successful due to the rigidity of the chest wall; although the author has resuscitated one 300-kg pony deliberately put into cardiac arrest by hypoxia with this technique and there is another report of successful resuscitation in an experimental setting (192), the chances of success in the adult equine or bovine appear to be very slim (193, 194).

It is difficult to complete compressions in small animals for prolonged periods at over 60 compressions per minute. If one considers normal heart rates, the ideal number of compressions should be about 120/min in the cat and dog under 5 kg, 100/min between 5 and 10 kg, 80/min between 10 and 30 kg, and 60/min for dogs bigger than this. In large adult animals, it is difficult to achieve rates greater than about 30 to 40/min. The breaths should be interposed between compressions, but the rescuer must not stop for the breath. If compression occurs during the ventilation, it may in fact be beneficial according to recent evidence (195). If the rescuer is working alone, then one breath should be given after every 15 compressions of the chest.

The above steps are essential if there is any hope of reversing a cardiac arrest. The equipment needed to perform basic CPR is not elaborate.

ADVANCED CARDIAC LIFE SUPPORT

Advanced cardiac life support (ACLS) implies that the rescuer has more knowledge and training than the person who is only able to provide basic CPR. It involves the ability to diagnose and treat the different dysrhythmias that may be present and to provide critical care after the initial cardiac arrest is over.

The first difference with ACLS is that immediate defibrillation is recommended, whether one has had time to diagnose this with an ECG or not. The defibrillatory current will depolarize most of the ventricular muscle, and the hope is that the sinoatrial node will take over as the pacemaker of the beat.

Defibrillation

An electrical defibrillator is a device that produces an electrical discharge with a variable energy output which is usually measured in joules or watt/seconds (1 joule (J)= 1 watt(w)/second). This electrical impulse is delivered as a damped half-sinusoidal waveform or a trapezoidal monophasic waveform (Fig. 22.8).

The discharge is released from a capacitor that is charged from the high voltage DC power supply. Older AC defibrillators are more likely to give problems with stray voltage leaks and so are not as safe as the modern DC machines. The energy output is of the order of 5 to 400 J for most defibrillators, and this shock is produced

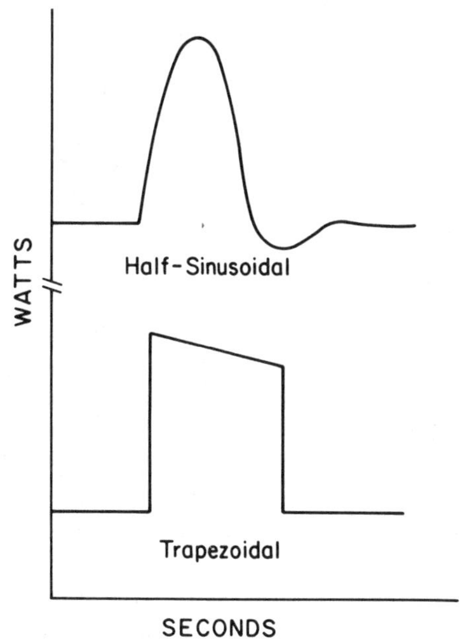

Figure 22.8. The wave forms produced by a DC defibrillator. The half-sinusoidal form is probably the most efficient at depolarizing the heart.

over a 3 to 10 ms period. It is delivered to the patient through external or internal paddles. The external paddles come in 50 to 65 cm^2 and 12 to 20 cm^2 sizes for human adult and pediatric use, respectively. The internal paddles are for use with an open chest and usually have a straight arm ending in a concave metal disc which is the contact area; again adult and pediatric sizes are available. When the external paddles are used, they are placed across the chest so as to produce a discharge through the ventricles. With the animal in dorsal recumbency, one paddle is placed at about the third or fourth interspace at the level of the costochondral junction on the right side and the other is placed close to the sternum over the fifth or sixth interspace on the left side. The discharge is produced by depressing a switch or switches which may be located on the machine or on the paddles. The safest arrangement is to have one switch on each paddle so that both have to be depressed to give a discharge (196). When using external paddles it is important to hold the paddles firmly against the body and to use a safe, effective electroconductive gel. Alcohol should not be used to improve electrical contact because of the fire risk associated with electrical discharge. The better the electrical contact with the body, the less resistance there will be to the discharge (196). Experimental work has also shown that the peak amperage may be a better measurement of the effective countershock (197). Because the current (I) is dependent on the voltage (V) and the resistance (R) ($I = V/R$), the latter obviously becomes an important determining factor in the delivered current. The electrodes should therefore be provided with a generous supply of electroconductive gel. A standard resistance used to test defibrillators is 50 ohms, but dogs probably have transthoracic resistances of the order of 40 to 100 ohms (198). Because the resistance or impedance is so important, a recent study used radiofrequency signals to measure the impedance before the first countershock is given (199). This allows the operator to choose a more appropriate electrical dose. Once the paddles have been firmly applied to the chest, the person operating the defibrillator says "All clear." This is to ensure that no one else is touching the patient or any equipment attached to the patient. If the shock is transmitted to one of the rescuers, at the least it is very unpleasant and at the worst it could cause electrocution. Before discharging the defibrillator, the operator looks all around to ensure that this instruction has been obeyed. The dose of countershock used depends on the size of the patient. There has been a long debate about this in the human literature because early work indicated that high levels of countershock were needed, particularly in individuals over 100 kg (197). Clinical evidence suggests the use of much lower currents (200–202). Based on experimental work (197, 203) in the dog, the following dosages are recommended: 2 J/kg for animals up to 7 kg; 2 to 5 J/kg for animals 7 to 40 kg; and 5 to 10 J/kg for animals over 40 kg.

This implies that a 100-kg animal should receive 500 to 1000 J, but most defibrillators have a maximum output of 400 J. In man, one recommendation is that the first countershock should be at 300 J/kg and that the maximum necessary would be 4 J/kg (202). This still means that for larger animals electrical countershocks using current equipment are not going to be as effective as they have been in patients under 100 kg. It has been suggested that sequential countershocks might achieve the same end. In one experiment, five successive 214-J countershocks given at 15-second intervals to 100-kg calves resulted in a 94% defibrillation rate (204), so it might be possible to defibrillate a horse using existing equipment by delivering sequential pulses. With shortly spaced shocks, there is a reduction in transthoracic impedance that allows a greater current density at the level of the myocardium (205). Attempts to defibrilate adult horses with single countershocks of up to 1640 W/seconds have been unsuccessful, however.

Another feature of modern defibrillators is that most have an ECG monitor as an integral part of the machine, and some have a "quick look" display. This is where an ECG signal is picked up via the paddles so that no time needs to be wasted connecting up the standard electrodes (206). Without an ECG, the first countershock is given and the rescuer proceeds with external cardiac massage. Having stated this, it is time to consider supporting the circulation with fluids and giving drugs to stimulate the heart back to life.

Fluids

The ability to administer fluids in this situation depends on the availability of a venous access or on the presence of someone who can place a needle or catheter into a vessel. The rescuer should not interrupt the massage in order to do this. The importance of having a ready venous access emphasizes the point that at least during anesthesia, a secure, large bore access should be obtained and maintained. If the vein is open, then crystalloid fluids should be administered rapidly (6 mls/kg/min) up to about 90 mls/kg initially. The amount of fluid given will depend on the state of the effective blood volume before arrest. Although acetate-containing fluids may tend to lead to a slight hypotension when given this quickly, the rapid volume replacement will counteract this effect. Virtually any isotonic crystalloid fluid can be given (saline, 5% dextrose, lactated Ringer's, plasmalyte, or normosol), but a balanced electrolyte solution is preferred. If a venous access is not present, the easiest vein to hit during external CPR in the dog is the lingual vein. The cephalic, saphenous, and jugular veins are all useful but tend to be moving in association with each compression. In order to make it easier to get a catheter into a vein, it is often more profitable to do a cut down than to waste time trying a percutaneous stab.

The only contraindications to rapid fluid therapy during cardiac arrest are when there is severe pulmonary edema or congestive heart failure. In the case of pulmonary edema, ventilation should be initiated but preferably with the addition of a positive end expired pressure (PEEP) or continuous positive airway pressure (CPAP). This will help to keep the lower airways open and may redistribute the edema fluid to the interstitial area away from the exchange surfaces (207).

Drugs

EPINEPHRINE

The use of epinephrine is definitely indicated in cases of cardiac arrest. Although the alpha-stimulating properties of this drug appear to be of major importance, in the initial part of resuscitation (208) the beta stimulation may have a role to play in improving coronary blood flow (209). The initial alpha stimulation with epinephrine will produce a generalized vasoconstriction. This rise in the systemic vascular resistance helps to direct the blood flow to those organs that are not vasoconstricted, the heart and the brain. Epinephrine will also increase venous return, and the effect of this is easy to appreciate when performing open chest massage. Before giving epinephrine, the heart often feels soft and flabby, but the administration of this drug brings the tone back to the ventricles and makes cardiac massage much more effective. The beta stimulation may have some effect on the coronary circulation, and certainly experimental results indicate an improved coronary flow (210). In the fibrillating animal, epinephrine should be used to convert fine to coarse fibrillations and to lower the defibrillation threshold.

The main disadvantage with epinephrine is that it may induce fibrillation, particularly in an animal that has been anesthetized with halothane. Pretreatment with drugs such as acepromazine or droperidol (alpha blockers) tends to reduce this risk. The mechanism behind this has been alluded to earlier in this chapter. Lidocaine has also been used as a pretreatment before epinephrine because it can raise the fibrillatory threshold (211).

The route of administration of epinephrine is also important. If a venous access is present or can be obtained easily, the epinephrine should be given by this route. If the rescuer is producing effective artifical circulation, then the drug will reach the heart. It would appear that injection into a central vein is preferable to a peripheral vein, but this is not always easy to obtain (212). If a central venous catheter is already in place, then this is the ideal route for injection. If no venous access is present, then epinephrine can be injected into the lung. In small animals, this can be achieved by passing a urinary catheter down the endotracheal tube and down into the bronchi and injecting the drug at this site. In larger animals this route is rather cumbersome, and obtaining a venous access is usually quite easy. Injecting the drug into the trachea is not as effective as injection deep into the lung in low flow states, such as cardiac resuscitation, because of the relatively poor absorption from the trachea (213). The absorption of epinephrine from the lung does not give as high a blood level as the intravenous route, so it is recommended that the dose be doubled (214). The absorption is also slower, so the blood levels are maintained for longer. This is an advantage if there is a delayed return of spontaneous circulation but may produce excessive hypertension and tachyarrhythmias if the heart starts beating promptly.

Intracardiac injections are the least favored and should be avoided if possible. With a closed chest, an intracardiac injection may tend to damage a coronary vessel, and the subsequent hemorrhage may produce a hemopericardium. In placing the needle into the heart, one has to interrupt cardiac massage, and the needle may induce ventricular fibrillation. If the injection is actually made into the myocardium, one may end up with a refractory fibrillation. On top of this, it is the least effective method of delivery. Recent research has shown that plasma levels taken from the root of the aorta were consistently lower than when the drug was given through a peripheral or central venous site (215). This is due to the absorption of the drug as it passes through the peripheral tissues and the lung. With an open chest and an open pericardium, the risk of hemopericardium is eliminated and the superficial coronary arteries can be avoided. The risk of promoting fibrillation still exists, but the amount of drug reaching the heart can be improved by occluding the base of the aorta with a finger and compressing the ventricles several times. This will increase the delivery of the drug to the myocardium and the cerebral circulation.

The dose of epinephrine required is probably quite low. An initial dose of 5 μg/kg may be all that is needed, and this can be doubled to 10 μg/kg if the first dose does not succeed. In order to give this amount, it is necessary to use solutions with concentrations of the order of 100 μg/ml (1:10,000). This can be purchased in prepackaged syringes for emergency use. By using a small dose to start with and then increasing it, the author has noticed a refractoriness to fibrillation, whereas one massive dose may convert the hypoxic myocardium to a fibrillating pattern. A dose of 10 to

20 μg/kg is recommended when the drug is injected into the lung. With small volumes, the intratracheal catheters should be flushed to ensure drug delivery into the lung and several large breaths should be given immediately afterward. The dose of epinephrine is repeated every 5 minutes.

SODIUM BICARBONATE

The acidosis that may develop during cardiac arrest is due to accumulation of carbon dioxide and the products of anerobic metabolism. This mixed metabolic and respiratory acidosis will affect the myocardium by depressing contractility (216, 217) suppressing spontaneous activity in the Purkinje fibres (218), by decreasing the threshold required to produce ventricular fibrillation (219), and by decreasing the efficacy of epinephrine. The pH of the myocardial cells will depend on three factors: the degree of hypoxia, which will determine the amount of anerobic acid production within the cells; the $PaCO_2$ because CO_2 transfers rapidly across the cell membranes; and lastly the degree of systemic acidosis. This latter is probably the least important because of the relatively slow diffusion of hydrogen ions across the cell membrane. The best methods to counteract the acidosis are adequate ventilation with 100% oxygen and effective coronary perfusion. The tendency for most people while ventilating an animal during CPR is to hyperventilate so that $PaCO_2$ values are often between 20 to 30 mmHg. Thus in the animal with no pre-existing metabolic acidosis and reasonable artificial circulation, this will prevent a severe fall in pH for the first 5 to 10 minutes of resuscitation. The dose of sodium bicarbonate should be based on blood gas and acid base analysis by using the calculations:

$$0.1 \text{ to } 0.15 \times \text{Base deficit} \times \text{Body weight (kg)} = \text{The dose of } NaHCO_3 \text{ in mmols}$$

This is one-third to one-half of the normal dose (i.e., 0.3 × base deficit × body weight) because the full dose will often cause an excessive alkalemia (220) and may produce a paradoxical CSF acidosis (221). The central compartment of the circulation is greatly reduced during resuscitation, so this dose will have a greater effect on pH than in the normal animal. If acid-base values are not available, then the administration of 0.5 to 1.0 mmol/kg of sodium bicarbonate per 10 minutes of cardiac arrest will help to prevent a metabolic acidosis. The administration of sodium bicarbonate too rapidly can produce severe hypotension (see section under treatment of shock) so it should be given intravenously and as slowly as is feasible under these dire circumstances. Sodium bicarbonate can be given by intracardiac injection but should never be given by the transpulmonary route. Because the addition of sodium bicarbonate to hydrogen ions will evolve carbon dioxide, it becomes even more important that adequate ventilation is achieved during resuscitation. Although experimental work in the dog has indicated that the defibrillation threshold is not altered by a "metabolic" acidosis (222), retrospective evidence from a clinical study has indicated that patients with a low pH (mean 7.23) are less likely to be successfully defibrillated than patients with a near normal pH (mean 7.36) (223). This evidence is rational because there are much more likely to be other toxic products (such as myocardial depressant factor) in the clinical setting than in the laboratory where the acidosis was induced with hydrochloric acid infusion.

ATROPINE/GLYCOPYRROLATE

These anticholinergics may be needed when the cause of the arrest is massive vagal stimulation. The most likely method of producing this is via the oculocardiac reflex. Traction on the muscles around the eye can result in a sinus bradycardia or even an asystolic arrest. Traction on the viscera or dissection around the vagus nerve can also do this, but the effects do not appear to be as potent as the oculocardiac reflex. (Some forms of asphyxial cardiac arrest can also produce massive vagal stimulation as a complicating factor.

Atropine and glycopyrrolate appear to give similar cardiac vagolytic activity (224), although glycopyrrolate produces better protection against neostigmine-induced bradycardia (225). This implies that it may be a better drug to use in cases with vagotonic cardiac arrest. The dose of atropine to give should be 0.02 to 0.04 mg/gk i.v. and can be repeated if the first dose does not work. Glycopyrrolate should be given at 0.005 to 0.01 mg/kg i.v. in small animals and at 0.0025 to 0.005 mg/kg i.v. in the horse. These drugs can also be given by the transpulmonary and intracardiac routes.

CALCIUM CHLORIDE/CALCIUM GLUCONATE

Since the realization that changes in cellular calcium play a major role in the damage caused by ischemia, the role of calcium salts during cardiac arrest has been a debatable issue (226). Calcium has been known as a positive inotrope for many years, and the increase in extracellular calcium produced, when this is infused intravenously, allows more calcium to enter the myocardial cells to act on the actin/myosin coupling (227, 228). Calcium is also involved in the Phase 2 repolarization of the myocardial cells, so raising extracellular calcium tends to speed this event (shorten the QT interval). These events have been seen in the nonischemic myocardium, and calcium may enhance the effects of a very weakly beating heart (e.g., electromechanical dissociation) (229). However, if arrest has been present for some time or if there has been a period of very poor perfusion before the arrest, calcium salts are contraindicated. This is because the intracellular/extracellular calcium concentrations are normally carefully regulated with a very high concentration gradient across the cell membrane (10,000:1 extracellular:intracellular). The maintenance of the gradient is ATP-dependent, and as the membranes of the cell are injured, the calcium concentration gradients throughout the cell become disorganized. A rise of ionized calcium within the mitochondria causes an uncoupled oxygen consumption such that ATP is no longer produced (230). This will obviously lead to cell death if the process is not reversed. This process appears to be part of the final common pathway for cell death (231); during a cardiac arrest it is going on in all the tissues of the body. This will be discussed further under cerebral resuscitation.

With consideration for the role of calcium in cell death the administration of this drug should be restricted to a few limited situations. Calcium should be given in hypocalcemia, hyperkalemia, and after an overdose of calcium blockers (e.g., verapamil, diltiazem, or nifedipine), and it may be of use in electromechanical dissociation (232). Calcium chloride is probably the drug of choice, but in the emergency setting the other salts (e.g., calcium gluconate) appear to be as effective. The dose of calcium chloride is 5 to 10 mg/kg (0.05 to 0.1 ml/kg of a 10% solution).

CLOSED VERSUS OPEN CHEST MASSAGE

In the 1960s and 1970s it was generally agreed that although internal massage might be slightly better, external cardiac massage was adequate for most resuscitation efforts. It is now clear that the original form of external massage is not as effective as internal massage and that even with the use of techniques such as abdominal binding and interposed ventilation, internal massage can provide better carotid and coronary flow.

Many studies have used the dog as a model for this research (233–238), but in many of these studies the methods of cardiac compression and the positioning of the animals are not those that we are likely to use directly. In several of the studies dogs were placed in dorsal recumbency and a mechanical device used to provide sternal compression. Although this may be an effective method in barrel-chested dogs such as the pug and the pekinese, it should be totally useless in a borzoi or saluki, and so we use the lateral position. Nevertheless, the overwhelming evidence from the experimental and teaching laboratory is that open chest massage can greatly improve perfusion (214, 235).

This raises the issue of exactly how external chest compression produces a blood flow. It was initially thought that when the chest was compressed, this squeezed the heart and ejected the blood into the arterial circulation. This is probably done in the small animal (less than 15 kg) (238), but it does not appear to occur in larger animals. The recent evidence (233) suggests that the blood flow is induced by the changes in pressure within the whole thorax. As the chest is compressed, the pressure builds up equally in all four chambers of the heart, thus tending to push the blood in a retrograde and anterograde fashion. However, because the veins collapse easily and there are valves in the heart and the veins (240) preventing retrograde flow, this initial flow into the vein is halted, allowing the blood to flow out into the aorta. The arteries do not tend to collapse as easily, partly because of their thicker structure and partly because of their lower capacitance. As the initial flow of blood is pushed into the arteries and veins, there is a more rapid rise of pressure on the arterial side that tends to keep these vessels open. The flow of blood through the lungs is dependent on the cascade effect from right to left sides of the heart, but emptying of the pulmonary circulation is also augmented by ventilation. This is evident in Rudikoff's study (238), where the first compression after ventilation showed augmented pressure compared with subsequent beats.

The knowledge of a thoracic pump mechanism has led to several innovations aimed at improving it. The first is the use of abdominal binding. This will raise the pressure acting on the diaphragm, thus limiting its posterior displacement during thoracic compression. This means that higher intrathoracic pressures are achieved, and there is an improvement in forward flow (238). Abdominal binding can be achieved using an elastic bandage or just a towel and some clamps in the small animal. If it is anticipated that external massage is going to be continued for several minutes, then a rubber bandage should be wrapped around the whole hind end of the body starting at the toes in order to "autotransfuse" the animal at the same time. The pneumatic military antishock trousers (MAST) are available in humans for the same purpose and have been used experimentally in the dog (241).

The second method for augmenting this effect is alternate chest and abdominal compression. Although this method has been shown to improve flow over conventional techniques, there is a greater risk of damage to visceral organs with this method.

The third method is to limit the collapse of the lungs during compression. If the lungs do not collapse or are inflated during the compression phase, then the total intrathoracic pressure change becomes greater. This can either be achieved by airway occlusion at each compression (this is not very practicable) or by ventilating at the same time as compression is applied. For this to be effective, quite high airway pressures are generated (70 to 110 cm H_2O), and this may increase the risk of barotrauma on the lung. In the author's hands, this method has been difficult to apply and has resulted in severe respiratory alkalosis. Because carbon dioxide is a significant factor in the control of cerebral circulation, this hyperventilation might lead to cerebral ischemia, and the raised venous pressure associated with high airway pressures may lower cerebral perfusion pressure. In several studies (235, 241, 242) there have been severe neurological deficits after simultaneous ventilation resuscitation despite improved carotid blood flow over the conventional interposed ventilation method.

Another reason for renewed interest in open chest massage has been the realization that it is very important to preserve the cerebral circulation as well as to get the heart started again. Cerebral preservation is mainly dependent on adequate carotid flow. Poor cerebral circulation appears to be worse than no circulation at all (243). Because of this discovery, the author recommends that, in dogs over 15 kg, if restoration of spontaneous circulation has not occurred within 2 minutes of starting external CPR, then internal massage should be performed. Other indications for internal CPR are presented in Table 22.2.

In order to perform internal cardiac massage, a thoracotomy must be performed. There is no time to clip the hair, so an incision is made along the left fifth or sixth intercostal space. Because the heart is not beating, there is minimal bleeding from the skin. The skin incision is extended from the highest point at which the rib can be felt and almost all the way down to the sternum. Once the intercostals are exposed, Mayo scissors are used when available to open the thorax. This reduces the risk of lacerating the lungs as the chest is entered; however, it is still advisable to stop the ventilation while the pleura is being cut. The incision into the chest is extended up as high as possible and down to the costrochondral junction. If it goes much lower than this, there is a very good chance of lacerating the internal thoracic artery. Use of a Finochetto self-retaining rib retractor may improve exposure if immediately available. At this point, ventilation can be resumed, and the heart can be given a few compressions by compressing it between the hand and the opposite chest wall. After two or three compressions, an incision is made into the pericardium at the apex using thumb forceps and scissors. If a scalpel is used for this purpose, then one is also likely to cut the myocardium or worse still a coronary vessel. The incision in the pericardium is extended such that the heart can be free. Opening the pericardium allows better visualization of the structures of the heart (e.g., the coronary vessels) and also allows better differentiation between fine fibrillation and other arrhythmias. In addition, it appears to allow for more effective massage (214). In order to massage the heart, it should be picked up in one hand and held so that the fingers are over the right ventricle and the thumb is over the left ventricle (in the smaller patient, one may only need a finger and thumb). The ventricular septum should be parallel to the plane of the fingers so that when the heart is squeezed both ventricles are compressed. As the hand is placed under the heart, the fingers should extend all the way up to the base, and care must be taken not to lacerate the auricle or great veins with the tips of one's fingers. In the larger animal, it is necessary to use two hands to provide the massage. The palmar surfaces of the hands should be used; the orientation of the heart is the same. The heart should feel quite turgid and should refill almost immediately. If the heart is flabby, then the patient should receive epinephrine and fluid loading if these have not already been accomplished. In order to improve cranial flow, a finger from the other hand can be pushed along the dorsal part of the inside of the thorax and occlude the descending aorta. This will help to improve both coronary and cerebral circulation.

Table 22.2
Indications for Internal Cardiac Compression

1. Animal >15 kg in which external CPR has not produced return of spontaneous circulation within 2 to 5 minutes.
2. Open chest where the heart can be massaged through the incision.
3. Open abdomen where the heart can be approached through the diaphragm.
4. Significant chest trauma (e.g., broken ribs or flail segment).
5. Suspected uncontrollable intrathoracic hemorrhage.
6. Failure to reverse mucous membranes from cyanotic/gray to pink within 2 minutes in any size animal.
7. Absence of an ECG to differentiate fibrillation from other dysrhythmias.

Open chest massage has been reported in the horse with some success (245), although neither patient survived. The technique is basically the same and is probably the only hope of achieving effective circulation in such a large animal.

The number of compressions per minute is governed by the rate of cardiac refill. The next beat can be instituted as soon as the heart refills. Ventilation should be timed to coincide with compression in order to increase pulmonary vascular resistance slightly and also to help push blood from the pulmonary veins into the left side of the heart. Because of the shapes of the ventricles, internal massage usually increases right-sided flow more than the left side so that there is a tendency to overload the pulmonary circulation. Raising the number of breaths per minute may help so ventilation frequencies of 20 to 30 per minute may be used. One should assure at least 12 breaths per minute in dogs and cats. In a dog or a cat under 10 kg, one should produce a heart rate of 100 to 120 per minute, a dog between 10 and 30 kg, 80 to 100 per minute and 30 and 100 kg a rate of 60 per minute. A minimum rate of 60 per minute should be used in small animals. In an animal the size of a horse, a heart rate of 30 per minute and respiratory rate of 12 per minute would suffice.

A mechanical ventricular assistance device has been investigated for use in CPR. This consists of a glass cup lined with a Silastic diaphragm. An alternating positive/negative pressure is applied between the Silastic and the cup in a fashion similar to a milking machine (246). This device can provide blood flows and perfusion pressures that are between 67 to 92% of the precardiac arrest values (246, 247). Another study reported results that did not achieve these levels because of technical difficulties and the experimental design, but the values were all significantly better than for either closed chest massage or open chest manual compression (248). The use of this device can thus provide very effective massage and also frees up one person in the resuscitation effort.

Once the heart has been started again, it is necessary to close the thoracic incision. Cardiac function must be effective and stable before this is attempted, and the animal should be started on a broad spectrum bactericidal antibiotic regime such as gentamycin/penicillin or trimethoprim/sulpha. The chest is packed off with a moist sterile towel, and then the hair is clipped around the wound. It may be helpful to apply a sterile water-soluble gel to the exposed tissue as this is easier to cleanse than when hair gets stuck to the fascia. The skin is then washed and prepared aseptically for surgery. Having done this, the wound can be draped as one would for a surgical approach to the thorax. The chest is lavaged with warm saline and a careful exploration is carried out for any hair that may have penetrated into the thoracic cavity. The lungs should be reexamined to ensure that no damage was done during the approach to the heart. The thorax can then be closed in a routine fashion after the placement of a chest drain. The edges of the skin and some of the fascia may need to be removed if there has been a lot of contamination, and a drain should be placed outside the thorax but under the skin to allow drainage from the subcutaneous tissues. Antibiotic therapy will need to be maintained for at least 5 days postoperatively. A relatively high incidence of infection can be observed after open chest resuscitation.

DEFINITIVE THERAPY

So far the discussion has been general in that none of the above therapies were aimed at treating a known specific cardiac dysrhythmia.

Ventricular Asystole

Drug therapy for asystole should include epinephrine, atropine, and possibly calcium chloride. In man and animals, there has been some suggestion that a fine fibrillation could be mistaken for an asystole in certain ECG leads; several leads should be checked before a decision is made not to defibrillate (249).

The use of electrical pacemakers has also been advocated in asystolic arrest. A pacemaker can either be placed transvenously or directly into the myocardium through the chest wall (250, 251). In the asystolic heart, it can be difficult to place a transvenous pacemaker into the ventricle (252), and some of the same complications may occur with the transthoracic approach as with intracardiac injections. In the study by Tintinalli and White (251), no patients survived after transthoracic pacing, and two developed cardiac tamponade before death. A failure to respond to the technique is usually indicative of severe hypoxia and acidosis.

Electromechanical Dissociation

Because there is electrical activity with a failure of mechanical contraction, the aim of therapy is to stimulate the coupling of these two events. The standard drugs epinephrine, sodium bicarbonate, and calcium chloride are used as described. In this situation, it is unlikely that the myocardium is terminally hypoxemic and so calcium chloride is indicated. The uncoupling could also be at the energy level, so corticosteroids are indicated to release ATP from the mitochondria for use at the cell membrane. Dexamethasone phosphate at 2 to 4 mg/kg or prednisolone succinate intravenously at 10 to 20 mg/kg can be used in this situation.

Pulseless Idioventricular Rhythm

This dysrhythmia occurs most frequently as a terminal event in shock (253). The usual progression of dysrhythmias in the hemorrhagic shock model is atrial arrest with a junctional bradycardia and junctional arrest followed by an idioventricular bradycardia (254). The doses for corticosteroids are given in the previous section. In one study, standard drug therapy met with 100% failure (255), but the addition of a large dose of corticosteroids to the regime has been shown to improve resuscitation to 52% (253). Further studies on the mechanisms of this treatment have shown that dexamethasone can partially reverse the uncoupling of ATP synthesis due to calcium ion influx and the presence of free HPO_4^{-2} in the mitochondria (230).

Ventricular Fibrillation

The methods and doses for external electrical defibrillation have already been discussed. It is important to differentiate fine from coarse fibrillation because the latter is much easier to convert. A fine fibrillation is usually pushed to a coarse fibrillation by epinephrine, but more than one ECG lead should be checked before deciding that the fibrillation is fine or coarse (249). The therapy for fibrillation is as for asystole with the addition of electrical countershock.

The success of defibrillation depends on a number of factors. The first is the duration of fibrillation. A second is availability of an effective defibrillator as illustrated in Figure 22.9, *A*. The longer the event, the higher the energy required for success and the poorer the prognosis (Fig. 22.9, *B*) (203). As the electrical energy is increased, there is an increased likelihood of myocardial damage (256), although there appears to be a substantial safety margin. Acidosis and hypoxia in the clinical setting also reduce the success of defibrillation (223). Certain drugs have been shown to alter the defibrillation threshold (257). Quinidine sulphate, lidocaine hydrochloride, and diphenyl hydantoin were all reported to raise the defibrillation threshold. After lidocaine administration, the dose of electrical energy required to defibrillate the heart may need to be raised by 50 to 100% (i.e., 1.5 to 2 times the initial dose). With early countershock (<2 minutes after the onset of fibrillation) epinephrine does not appear to influence success, but after this time epinephrine administration becomes increasingly important (203). If the heart has been exposed, direct defibrillation can be carried out. The electrodes are placed on either side of the ventricles, and a lower dose is required to defibrillate the heart. The recommended dose is 0.2 to 0.4 J/kg for the dog (258) and the horse. In the sheep, goat, and pig, where the heart weight is a smaller proportion of body weight, this dose should probably be reduced to 0.1 to 0.2 J/kg. When applying the internal paddles, care should be taken to ensure good contact; if the myocardium is too dry, then some sterile saline should be poured on to the heart.

Chemical cardioversion is obviously more desirable because it does not require the purchase and maintenance of expensive equipment. Although a successful technique has been described (259, 260), it is not easily applied in practice. The method described involved the intraventricular injection of potassium chloride (1 mmol/kg) and acetylcholine chloride (6.0 mg/kg) during open chest cardiac massage. This resulted in 12 of 16 animals reverting to a sinus rhythm. Potassium chloride on its own (1 mmol/kg) resulted in a 21% cardioversion (3 of 14 animals). Despite the efficacy of this regime, there are a number of problems to be solved. The first is that acetylcholine produces severe bronchoconstriction resulting in increased airway resistance and hypoxia. Crowe reported that if the root of the aorta was occluded immediately after the drugs were given, much lower doses (0.05 mmol/kg KCl and 0.3 mg/kg acetylcholine) could be used with similar efficacy. This reduced the dramatic effects on the lung and peripheral vascular bed (214). The second problem is that acetylcholine is available as a powder and has to be made up freshly, which makes it difficult to use in an emergency. Lastly, if electrical defibrillation is attempted after this, the energy required is greatly increased (259).

Other drugs such as lidocaine and bretyllium tosylate have been used without success as chemical defibrillators (261). In conclusion, potassium chloride can be used in the clinical setting for defibrillation if an electrical device is not available. This will be most effective if it is given into the heart with the chest open followed by manual compression with digital occlusion of the aorta. If the heart is successfully defibrillated, calcium chloride (5 mg/kg) should be given to counteract the effects of the potassium.

Clinical Case

The preceding pages have tried to present the information required to understand some of the patho-

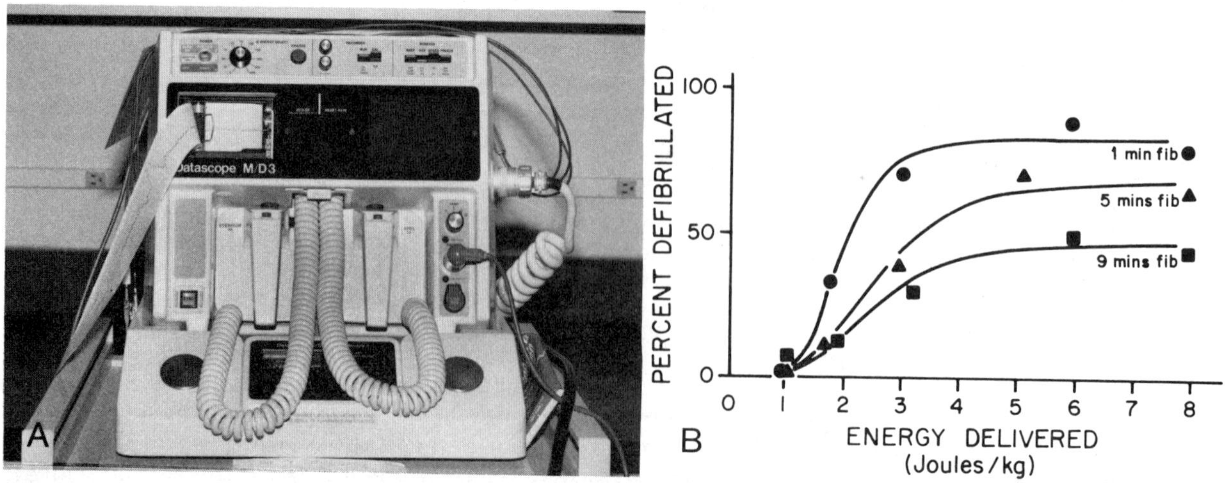

Figure 22.9. *A*, illustration of current concepts in defibrillator design with oscilliscopic capability and electrocardiographic printout. *B*, The effect of time and defibrillation dosage on dogs treated with epinephrine. The y axis indicates the percentage of successful defibrillation. Part B only from RW Yakaitis, GA Ewy, CW Otto, DL Taren, TE Moon: Influence of time and therapy on ventricular defibrillation in dogs. *Crit Care Med* 8:157–163, © Williams & Wilkins, 1980.

physiology and therapeutics of cardiac arrest and resuscitation. It is necessary at this point to try to provide an algorithm for this effort so that a clearer picture can evolve of the time constraints for resuscitation (Fig. 22.10). It is evident that such an algorithm is a simplification and the clinician needs knowledge and experience to provide the best care during this emergency. From the preceding discussion, it should be abundantly clear that provision of effective advanced cardiac life support is not a one-person job. It requires at least two and ideally three or four people to provide the ventilation, cardiac compression, and drug therapy required. In order to achieve this, a team effort needs to be developed with each member of the team understanding the things that are necessary and knowing immediately where to find the equipment. Due to the fortunate infrequency of cardiac arrest in a general practice, the staff and veterinarians need to ensure that some method is developed to enable people to practice the basic skills. The recent development of resuscitation manikins for dogs and cats (262) will make it easier to teach the basic resuscitation skills. Ideally, the equipment needed for resuscitation should be collected together and either made fully portable (a crash cart), or a table can be set aside where all the drugs and equipment are immediately available and the patient can be moved to this site.

Assuming that a team of people is available and that the equipment is present, the following approach might be used.

Rescuer 1 establishes the airway and starts ventilation. This may require any of the described methods, such as mouth to nose, mouth to endotracheal tube, oxygen demand valve to endotracheal tube, and so forth.

Rescuer 2 starts external cardiac compression and then defibrillates if a machine is immediately available and the heart is in fibrillation. If a defibrillator is not available or the arrhythmia has already been diagnosed as an EMD or PIVR, then this is not appropriate. In the dog or cat smaller than 15 kg, external massage can be continued if there is evidence of effective circulation (evenly pink mucous membranes and preferably a palpable pulse). In any animal over 15 kg, the rescuer should be prepared to do a thoracotomy after 2 to 5 minutes if external massage has not produced a restoration of spontaneous circulation.

Rescuer 3 is responsible for drug administration. If a venous access is present, then epinephrine 5 μg/kg should be given immediately and a bag of crystalloid solution attached and given at 6 mls/kg/min (1 ml/kg/min in the cat and adult large animals). If no venous access is present, a dose of 10 μg/kg of epinephrine should be given into the lung and then the rescuer should establish a large bore venous access. This person can then administer further drug therapy as required.

Rescuer 4 should attach the ECG and try to diagnose the dysrhythmia. He or she should then apply an abdominal wrap or elastic bandage to the hind end of the body. This person should also take note of the time and advise the other rescuers as to the course of events, take samples for blood gas analysis, and relieve Rescuer 2 if this individual becomes tired. When transferring cardiac massage from one person to another, care should be taken not to interrupt the rhythm. The new person should be in position and the resuscitator should give a countdown so that the rhythm and time of takeover are established.

The algorithm in Figure 22.10 gives a simple approach to CPR. It stops at the first administration and in general it is recommended that drug therapy (except for fluids, calcium, and corticosteroids) be repeated every 5 to 10 minutes of arrest.

The resuscitative effort should probably be continued for at least 25 to 30 minutes. The greater the time necessary to restore spontaneous circulation, the poorer the prognosis, but there have been a few successful cases in humans after prolonged resuscitative efforts. Because the blood flow that is achieved with CPR is not 100%, the chances of getting full neurological recovery become less and less as time goes by. Because the heart can tolerate hypoxia for longer than the brain, if the heart is not responding to any stimuli then it is likely that the brain will be severely compromised.

Postresuscitation Care and Cerebral Preservation

Once spontaneous circulation has returned, it will be necessary to provide intensive care for the patient until it wakes up. If the arrest occurred before a surgical or diagnostic procedure was started, these should be cancelled until the animal is healthy again. Return of neurological function may be immediate but is usually delayed.

The first priority is to stabilize the cardiovascular system. This may necessitate the use of antiarrhythmic drugs such as lidocaine, procainamide, or diphenylhydantoin or it may require the use of positive inotropes to raise the cardiac output and improve perfusion. The aim should be to raise the blood pressure to normal or high normal values (263). This can be achieved by putting the animal on a dopamine or dobutamine infusion. Careful monitoring is needed with these potent vasoactive drugs because they can produce severe tachyarrhythmias and hypertension if the infusion rate is too rapid. Intermittent severe hypertension may increase the neurological damage after cardiac arrest (264).

Once the heart has been stabilized and the blood

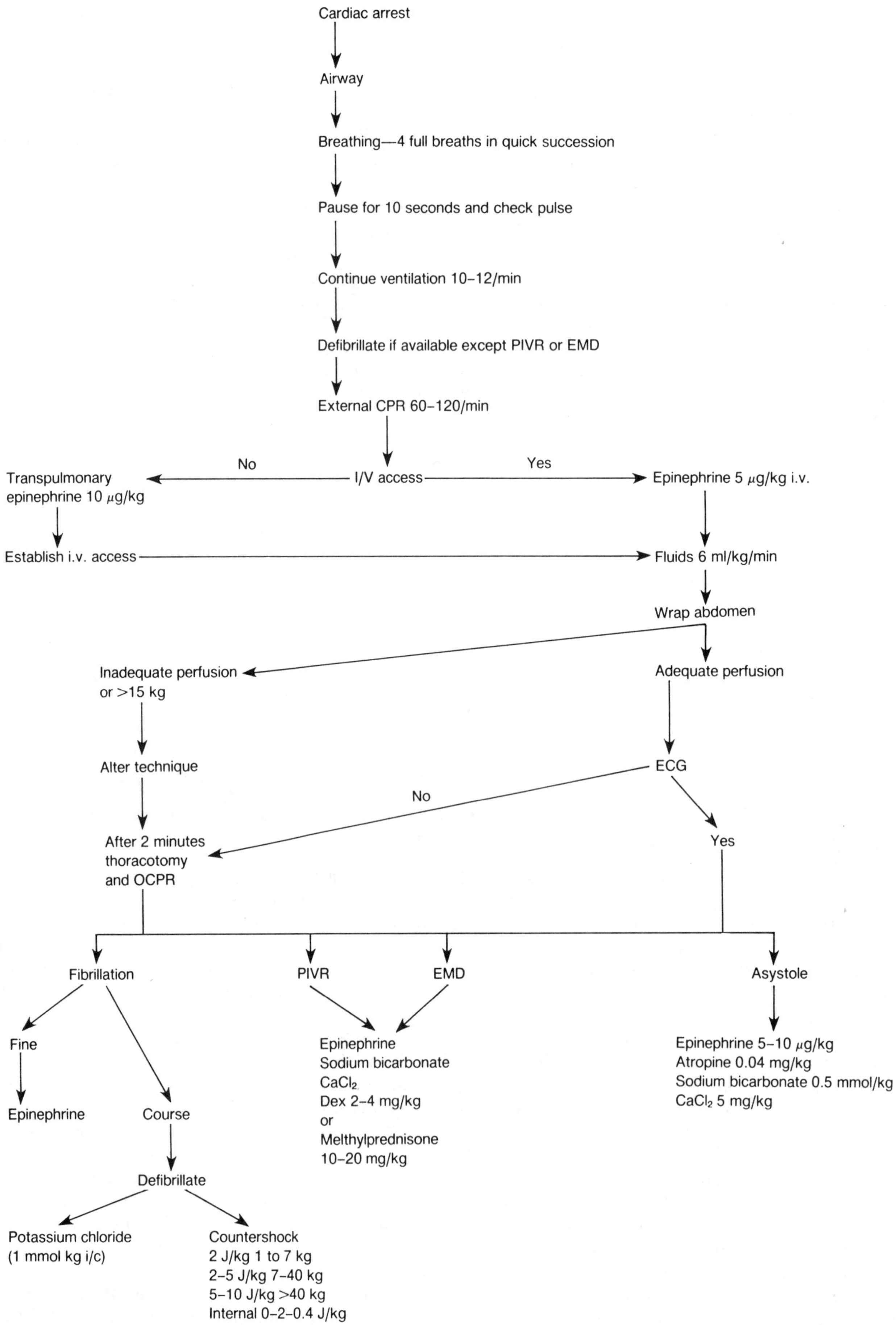

Figure 22.10. Algorithm for resuscitation. A simple but rigid protocol that can be followed for cardiac arrest. Note that a thoracotomy should be performed early in a dog over 15 kg in weight.

pressure raised to a normal level, one can concentrate on reducing neurological damage. In the past it was considered that the brain would be dead after 3 minutes of circulatory arrest. It is now established that full neurological recovery can follow periods of cardiac arrest of 12 minutes duration (265) and possibly 15 minutes of global ischemia (266). There is even some suggestion that neurones can survive up to 60 minutes of circulatory arrest (267), but it is doubtful if this recovery would be enough for normal return of function. One reason for poor recovery appears to be related to the cerebral blood flow after an ischemic episode.

During ischemia of the brain, oxygen stores are exhausted within 30 seconds and ATP stores within 5 minutes. Once the ATP levels fall, the ion pumps fail and there is an increase in cellular calcium and an efflux of potassium (268). The change in calcium concentrations is involved in the conversion of xanthine dehydrogenase to xanthine oxidase. These two enzymes both catalyze the conversion of xanthines to uric acid (the final breakdown of ATP), but the dehydrogenase uses nicotinamide-adenine dinucleotide (NAD+) whereas the oxidase can use molecular oxygen resulting in the production of superoxide radicals (269). The production of superoxide radicals is thus dependent on a source of molecular oxygen. This may explain the difference between the outcome after poor perfusion and total ischemia; with low flow states after an ischemic episode, enough oxygen is provided to produce these radicals but not enough to allow return of function. The presence of superoxide itself is not enough to cause lipid peroxidation of cell membranes because this reaction is thermodynamically unfavorable. However, low molecular weight chelates of ferrous iron (e.g., ADP-FE^{+2}) may react to produce more active oxidation species, and these will initiate lipid peroxidation thus creating damage to cellular membranes (226). This in turn allows the release of arachidonic acid with production of prostaglandins and leukotrienes. Some of these substances are potent vasoconstrictors and lead to a reduction in perfusion. This gives an explanation for the fall in cerebral blood flow that is seen after the initial reperfusion (270). Experiments have shown that between 15 to 90 minutes after reperfusion, there is a progressive increase in cerebral vascular resistance and a reduction in flow to 5 to 40% of normal. This fall in flow is not related to intravascular clotting but appears to be mediated by the prostaglandins and leukotrienes (244).

The knowledge of these mechanisms leads us to a number of possible points for therapy. The first and most important is to restore spontaneous circulation as rapdily and as effectively as possible. This will avoid the depletion of ATP and the consequences of this breakdown. This is illustrated by a recent report that shows that with a cardiac arrest time of less than 6 minutes, return of neurological function occurred in 50% of the victims if the resuscitative effort took less than 30 minutes. For arrest times longer than 6 minutes, neurological recovery was about the same if resuscitation was rapid (<5 minutes), but the prognosis deteriorated for any time longer than 5 minutes (271).

The second part of avoiding the ischemic injury is to use the most effective aid to circulation during resuscitation. Closed chest massage can be very effective, but open chest massage should be instituted early if the flow from external massage is poor.

Once spontaneous circulation has been restored, a normal or slightly high blood pressure will help to prevent hypoperfusion. The pharmacological intervention in the rest of the chain of injury then becomes important. The metabolic activity in the brain should be reduced so that there is not excessive demand on an already depleted energy reserve. This means that seizure activity must be controlled. In the late 1970s, much work was done on the use of barbiturates during the recovery period (272). These drugs, in therapeutic doses, will suppress seizures, reduce the metabolic rate of the cells, and thus reduce cerebral metabolic oxygen consumption. Thiopental even has some free radical scavenging properties (273). All of these properties may be helpful, but the available clinical (274) and laboratory evidence (275) suggests that, if seizure activity is controlled, barbiturates do not improve neurological outcome. Other agents such as diazepam, phenytoin, althesin, and etomidate may prove to be equally useful (276).

Another point of pharmacological intervention might be to prevent or reduce calcium entry into the cells. This has been achieved by the use of calcium channel blocking agents. To date, nimodipine and lidoflazine appear to be most effective and practical in this role (277, 278). Nimodipine has been shown to improve postischemic flow, whereas lidoflazine did not alter the changes during reperfusion (279). Nevertheless, lidoflazine did improve neurological outcome in these experiments (278, 280). The dose of lidoflazine for the dog is 1 mg/kg.

Superoxide radical scavenging may be another method of reducing neurological deficit, but to date no controlled studies have been done using agents such as superoxide dismutase, dimethyl sulfoxide, vitamin E, or mannitol. As with many aspects of medicine, prevention is probably the best approach; deferoxamine (an iron chelator) has been used to reduce the availability of iron in the production of the active radicals. This substance doubled the 10-day survival in rats after a 7-minute period of cardiac arrest (281) and was associated with lower levels of low molecular weight chelates of iron and malondialdehyde (a product associated with lipid peroxidation) after 15 minutes of cardiac arrest in dogs (282). The dose of deferoxamine (desferrioximine) used in the dog was 50 mg/kg.

The vasoactive prostaglandins might be reduced

by treatment with corticosteroids and/or cyclo-oxygenase inhibitors. However, other agents such as the leukotrienes may be involved, and one would need to produce an effective block of the lipoxygenase pathway as well. Some improvement in neurological function has been shown after multifocal ischemia in dogs by treating with a combination of prostacyclin, indomethacina, and heparin (282), but the role of available agents such as flunixin, phenylbutazone, and meclofenamic acid has not been assessed.

Other agents aimed at improving microcirculation are also under investigation. This includes reduction of cerebral edema with mannitol, lasix, or corticosteroids; reduction of blood viscosity by hemodilution with hetastarch (284) or dextrans and streptokinase (285); or synthetic oxygen carrying compounds (286).

Given the above information and the availability of drugs, the author's current practice is to treat the cardiac arrest victim with 2 mg/kg dexamethasone phosphate i.v. and lasix 2 mg/kg i.v. immediately after resuscitation. If there is any suggestion of seizure activity or delayed return of neurological function, the animal is given pentobarbital and put on a ventilator with the aim of reducing the $PaCO_2$ to 20 to 25 mm Hg. This helps to control cerebral blood flow and reduce cerebral edema formation. The addition of deferoxamine and lidoflazine to this regime could be helpful in reducing reperfusion injury. Hemodynamic support is provided as discussed, and the patient is monitored for signs of improvement. The return of pupillary constriction may be delayed several hours even in animals with eventual return of function (264). Beyond this, cardiovascular and renal function need to be monitored making sure that fluid loss is balanced by fluid administration. The acid/base and electrolyte status should be monitored if possible. Return of mental function may be gradual and may take 2 to 3 weeks before a full assessment can be made. However, if there is no return of midbrain reflexes within the first 12 to 18 hours, it is unlikely that full neurological recovery will occur. If an electroencephalograph (EEG) is used to assess the patient, repeated EEG silence over a 24-hour period is regarded as sufficient evidence of brain death (287), assuming that the animal is not under the influence of certain drugs or profoundly hypothermic.

When Not to Resuscitate

This has raised a lot of debate in human medicine because of the time, effort, and money spent in resuscitation and long-term care if full neurological function does not return. In general, it is not worth attempting resuscitation on an animal that has been in arrest for more than 5 minutes unless it is profoundly hypothermic or has been given drugs that might protect the brain. Animals with severe disease that cannot be cured should not be resuscitated unless this has been discussed with the owner. Lastly, the wishes of the owner should be respected in any case where a request has been made that resuscitation should not be attempted.

References

1. Warren JC: Surgical pathology and therapeutics. In Warren JC: *Shock*. Philadelphia, WB Saunders Company, 1895, p 279.
2. MacLean LD: Shock: Causes and management of circulatory collapse. In Sabiston DC (ed); *Davis-Christopher Textbook of Surgery: The Biological Basis of Modern Surgical Practice*, ed 12. Philadelphia, WB Saunders, 1981, p 58.
3. Kolata RJ: The clinical management of circulatory shock based on pathophysiological patterns. *Compend Contin Educ Pract Vet* 2:314–322, 1980.
4. Siegel JH, Cerra FB, Border JR, Coleman B, MacMenamy RH: Human response to sepsis: A physiologic manifestation of disordered metabolic control. In Cowley RA, Trump BF (eds): *Pathophysiology of Shock, Anoxia and Ischemia*. Baltimore, Williams and Wilkins, 1982, p 235.
5. Burrows GE: Endotoxemia in the horse. *Equine Vet J* 13:89–94, 1981.
6. Hardie EM, Rawlings CA: Septic shock, Part I, Pathophysiology. *Compend Contin Educ Pract Vet* 5:369–377, 1983.
7. Moore JN: Endotoxemia: Part II, Biological reactions to endotoxin. *Compend Contin Educ Pract Vet* 3:S392–S397, 1981.
8. Wichterman KA, Baue AE, Chaudry IH: Sepsis and septic shock—A review of laboratory models and a proposal. *J Surg Res* 29:189–201, 1980.
9. Crocker SH, Duane OE, Obenauf RN, Wismar BL, Lowery BD: Bacteremia: Host specific lung clearance and pulmonary failure. *J Trauma* 21:215–220, 1981.
10. Evans SF, Hinds CJ, Varley JG: A new canine model of endotoxin shock. *Br J Pharmac* 83:433–442, 1984.
11. Begley CJ, Ogletree ML, Meyrick BO, Brigham KL: Modification of pulmonary response to endotoxemia in awake sheep by steroidal and non-steroidal anti-inflammatory agents. *Am Rev Respir Dis* 130:1140–1146, 1984.
12. Moore JN, Gardner HE, Shapland JE, Hatfield DG: Lactic acidosis and arterial hypoxemia during sublethal endotoxemia in conscious ponies. *Am J Vet Res* 41:1696–1698, 1980.
13. Olson NC, Brown TT: Effects of endotoxemia on lung water and hemodynamics in conscious calves. *Am J Vet Res* 46:711–718, 1985.
14. Nelson AW, Swan H: The effects of the canine spleen on red cells and blood volume determination using ^{51}RBC. *Surgery* 71:215–244, 1972.
15. Brasmer TH: *The Acutely Traumatized Small Animal Patient*. Philadelphia, WB Saunders Company, 1984.
16. Jarhult J, Lundvall J, Mellander S, Tibblin S: Osmolar control of plasma volume during hemorrhagic hypotension. *Acta Physiol Scand* 85:142–144, 1972.
17. Guyton AC: *Textbook of Medical Physiology*, ed 7. Philadelphia, WB Saunders, 1986, p 216.
18. Jarecki M, Thoren PN, Donald DE: Release of renin by the carotid baroreflex in anesthetized dogs: Role of cardiopulmonary vagal afferents and renal arterial pressure. *Circ Res* 42:614–619, 1978.
19. Hillman J, Lundvall J: Hormonal and neurogenic adrenergic control of the fluid transfer from skeletal muscle to blood during hemorrhage. *Acta Physiol Scand* 112:271–280, 1981.
20. Hillman J, Gustafsson D, Lundvall J: ^{2}-adrenergic control of plasma volume in hemorrhage. *Acta Physiol Scand* 116:175–180, 1982.

21. Duling B: Oxygen, metabolism and microcirculatory regulation. In Kaley G, Altura BM, (eds): *Microcirculation*. Baltimore, University Park Press, vol 2, 1977, p 401.
22. Mellander S, Lewis DH: Effect of hemorrhagic shock on the reactivity of resistance and capacitance vessels and on capillary filtration transfer in cat skeletal muscle. *Circ Res* 13:105–118, 1963.
23. Chaudry IH: Cellular alterations in shock and ischemia and their correction. *Physiologist* 28:109–118, 1985.
24. Baue AE, Chaudry IH, Wurth MA, Sayeed MM: Cellular alterations with shock and ischemia. *Angiology* 25:31–41, 1974.
25. Chaudry IH, Sayeed MM, Baue AE: Insulin resistance in experimental shock. *Arch Surg* 109:412–415, 1974.
26. Lefer AM: Vascular mediators in ischemia and shock. In Cowley RA, Trump BF (eds): *Pathophysiology of Shock, Anoxia and Ischemia*. Baltimore, Williams & Wilkins, 1982, p 169.
27. Lefer AM: Leukotriorenes as mediators of ischemia and shock. *Biochem Pharmac* 35:123–127, 1986.
28. Jones CE, Crowell JW, Smith EE: Significance of increased blood uric acid following extensive hemorrhage. *Am J Physiol* 214:1374–1377, 1968.
29. Glenn TM, Lefer AM: Significance of splanchnic proteases in the production of a toxic factor in hemorrhagic shock. *Circ Res* 29:338–349, 1971.
30. Bounous G, Hampson LG, Gurd FN: Cellular nucleotides in hemorrhagic shock: Relationship of intestinal metabolic changes to hemorrhagic enteritis and the barrier function of intestinal mucosa. *Ann Surg* 160:650–658, 1964.
31. Bounous G, Menard D, De Medicis E: Role of pancreatic proteases in the pathogenesis of ischemic enteropathy. *Gastroenterology* 73:102–108, 1977.
32. Fine J: The intestinal circulation in shock. *Gastroenterology* 52:454–458, 1967.
33. Blattberg G, Levy MN: A humoral reticuloendothelial depressing substance in shock. *Am J Physiol* 203:409–411, 1962.
34. Loegering DJ: Presence of a reticuloendothelial depressing substance in portal vein blood following intestinal ischemia and thermal injury. *Adv Shock Res* 5:67–77, 1981.
35. Saba TM, Jaffe E: Plasma fibronectin (opsonic glycoprotein): its synthesis by vascular endothelial cells and role in cardiopulmonary integrity after trauma as related to reticuloendothelial function. *Am J Med* 68:577–594, 1980.
36. Okada K, Kosugi I, Tanokura Y, Tajimi K, Ohmura A, Innami H, Tsukamoto T, Inaba T: MDF—Its participation in the pathophysiology of shock. In Lefer AM, Schumer W (eds): *Molecular and Cellular Aspects of Shock and Trauma*. New York, Allan R Liss, Inc., 1983, p 125.
37. Lefer AM, Blattberg B: Comparison of the effects of two factors present in plasma of shocked animals. *J Reticuloendothel Soc* 5:54–60, 1968.
38. Passmore JC, Leffler CW, Neiberger RE: A critical analysis of renal blood flow distribution during hemorrhage in dogs. *Circ Shock* 5:327–338, 1978.
39. Hook CE, Passmore JC, Levin JI, Neiberger RE: Angiotension II and alpha adrenergic control of the intrarenal circulation in hemorrhage. *Circ Shock* 9:81–94, 1982.
40. Rosenberg IK, Gupta SL, Lucas CE, Khan AA, Rosenberg BF: Renal insufficiency after trauma and sepsis. *Arch Surg* 103:175–183, 1971.
41. Chien S, Simchon S: The sympathetic and central nervous systems in shock. In Altura BM, Lefer AM, Schumer MD (eds): *Handbook of Shock and Trauma*. New York, Raven Press, 1983, p 152.
42. Henson EC, Lockard VG, Crowell JW, Arhelger RB, Brunson JG: Recovery from a usually lethal period of hypotension. *Arch Pathol* 95:73–76, 1973.
43. Kolata RJ, Burrows CF, Soma LR: Shock—Pathophysiology and management. In Kirk RW (ed): *Current Veterinary Therapy VII. Small Animal Practice*. Philadelphia, WB Saunders, 1980, p 32.
44. Lee JC, Downing SE: Myocardial oxygen availability and cardiac failure in hemorrhagic shock. *Am J Physiol* 226:9–15, 1974.
45. Downing SE: The heart in shock. In Altura BM, Lefer AM, Schumer W (eds): *Handbook of Shock and Trauma*. New York, Raven Press, 1983, p 5.
46. Spackman CJA, Caywood DD, Feeney DA, Johnston GR: Thoracic wall and pulmonary trauma in dogs sustaining fractures as a result of motor vehicle accidents. *J Am Vet Med Assoc* 185:975–977, 1984.
47. Schaub RG, Moore JN, Garner HE, Shapland JE: Pulmonary vascular damage in the pony induced by endotoxin: effect of lidocaine. *Am Assoc Equine Pract Newslett* 2:87–96, 1982.
48. Ture JJ, Templeton CB, Bottoms GD, Fessler JF: Flunixin meglumine alteration of endotoxin-induced damage to the cardiopulmonary vascular endothelium of the pony. *Am J Vet Res* 46:591–596, 1985.
49. Lium B, Saugstad OD, Aasen AO, Guldvog I, Nordstoga K, Amundsen E: Experimental post-traumatic lung insufficiency in dogs; gross and light microscopic lesions. *Acta Vet Scand* 23:118–127, 1982.
50. Chamberlin WH, Rice CL, Moss GS: Pulmonary dysfunction in shock. In Altura BM, Lefer AM, Schumer W (eds): *Handbook of Shock and Trauma*. New York, Raven Press, 1983, p 105.
51. Hardaway RM: Pathology and pathophysiology of disseminated intravascular coagulation. In Cowley RA, Trump BF (eds): *Pathophysiology of Shock, Anoxia and Ischemia*. Baltimore, Williams & Wilkins, 1982, p 186.
52. Parry BW, Anderson GA, Gay CC: Prognosis in equine colic: a comparative study of variables used to assess individual cases. *Eq Vet J* 15:211–215, 1983.
53. Dula DJ, Lutz P, Vogel MF, Weaver BN: Rapid Flow Rates for resuscitation of hypovolemic shock. *Ann Emerg Med* 14:303–306, 1985.
54. Aeder MI, Crowe JP, Rhodes RS, Shuck JM, Wolf WM: Technical limitations in the rapid infusion of intravenous fluids. *Ann Emerg Med* 14:307–310, 1985.
55. Bjorling DE, Rawlings CA: Relationship of intravenous administration of ringer's lactate solution to pulmonary edema in halothane anesthetised cats. *Am J Vet Res* 44:1000–1006, 1983.
56. Boothe HW, Clark DR, Merton DA: Cardiovascular effects of rapid infusion of crystalloid in the hypovolemic cat. *J Small Anim Pract* 26:477–489, 1985.
57. Cloutier CT, Lowery BD, Carey LC: Acid-base disturbances in hemorrhagic shock in 66 severely wounded patients prior to treatment. *Arch Surg* 98:551–557, 1969.
58. Bristol DG: The anion gap as a prognostic indicator in horses with abdominal pain. *J Am Vet Med Assoc* 181:63–65, 1982.
59. Moore JN, Owen R.apR, Lumsden JH: Clinical evaluation of blood lactate levels in equine colic. *Eq Vet J* 8:49–54, 1976.
60. Weil MH, Afifi AA: Experimental and clinical studies on lactate and pyruvate as indicators of the severity of acute circulatory failure (shock). *Circulation* 41:989–1001, 1970.
61. Merkley DF, Howard DR, Eyster GE, Krahwinkel DJ, Sawyer DC, Krehbiel JD: Experimentally induced acute gastric dilation in the dog: Cardiopulmonary effects. *J Am Anim Hosp Assoc* 12:143–148, 1976.
62. Wingfield WE, Cornelius LM, DeYoung DW: Pathophysiology of the gastric dilation torsion complex in the dog. *J Small Anim Pract* 15:735–739, 1974.
63. Muir WW: Acid-base and electrolyte disturbances in dogs with gastric dilation-volvulus. *J Am Vet Med Assoc* 181:229–231, 1982.
64. Wingfield WE, Twedt DC, Moore RW, Leib MS, Mollie W: Acid-base and electrolyte values in dogs with acute gastric dilation volvulus. *J Am Vet Med Assoc* 180:1070–1072, 1982.
65. Dumont L, Stanley P, Chartrand C: The cardiovascular effects of hypertonic sodium bicarbonate in conscious dogs—under-

lying mechanisms of action. *Can J Physiol Pharmacol* 62:314–318, 1983.
66. Lopes OU, Pontieri V, Rocha e Silva M, Velasco IT: Hyperosmotic NaCl and severe hemorrhagic shock: role of the innervated lung. *Am J Physiol* 241:H883–H890, 1981.
67. Hartsfield SM, Thurmon JC, Benson GJ: Sodium bicarbonate and bicarbonate precursors for treatment of metabolic acidosis. *J Am Vet Med Assoc* 179:914–916, 1981.
68. Bavister PH, Longnecker DE: Influence of anesthetic agents on the survival of rats following acute ischaemia of the bowel. *Br J Anaesth* 51:921–925, 1979.
69. Beller BK, Archer LJ, Lane MM, Murray CK, Parker DE, Hinshaw LB: Preventing versus delaying death in shock therapy studies: Evaluating survival. *Circ Shock* 11:351–358, 1983.
70. Altura BM: Glucocorticoid-induced protection in circulatory shock: Role of reticuloendothelial system function. *Proc Soc Exp Biol Med* 150:202–206, 1975.
71. Frauenfelder HC, Fessler JF, Moore AB, Bottoms GD, Boon GD: Effects of dexamethasone on endotoxin shock in the anesthetised pony—hematologic, blood gas and coagulation changes. *Am J Vet Res* 43:405–411, 1982.
72. Schrauwen EM, Houvenaghel AM: Endotoxin shock in the pig—beneficial effects of pretreatment with prednisolone sodium succinate. *Am J Vet Res* 45:1650–1653, 1984.
73. Schumer W: Steroids in the treatment of clinical septic shock. *Ann Surg* 184:333–341, 1976.
74. Schumer W: Controversy in shock research Pro: The role of steroids in septic shock. *Circ Shock* 8:667–671, 1981.
75. Smith JAR, Norman JN: Use of glucocorticoids in refractory shock. *Surg Gynecol Obstet* 149:369–373, 1979.
76. White GL, White GS, Kosanke SD, Archer LT, Hinshaw LB: Therapeutic effects of prednisolone sodium succinate vs dexamethasone in dogs subjected to E. coli septic shock. *J Am Anim Hosp Assoc* 18:639–648, 1982.
77. Blaisdell FW: Controversy in shock research Con: The role of steroids in septic shock. *Circ Shock* 8:673–682, 1981.
78. Dillon R, Hankes GH, Nachreiner RF, Redding RW: Experimental hemorrhage in dogs: effects of prednisolone sodium succinate. *J Am Anim Hosp Assoc* 14:673–682, 1978.
79. Ewert KM, Fessler JF, Templeton CB, Bottoms GD, Latshaw HS, Johnson MA: Endotoxin-induced hematologic and blood chemical changes in ponies: effects of flunixin meglumine, dexamethasone and prednisolone. *Am J Vet Res* 46:24–30, 1985.
80. Hinshaw LB, Coalson JJ, Benjamin BA, Archer LT, Beller BK, Kling OR, Hasser EM, Phillips RW: Escherichia coli shock in the baboon and the response to adrenocorticosteroid treatment. *Surg Gynecol Obstet* 147:545–557, 1978.
81. Hinshaw LB, Beller BK, Archer LT, Flournoy DJ, White GL, Phillips RW: Recovery from lethal escherichia coli shock in dogs. *Surg Gynecol Obstet* 149:545–553, 1979.
82. Sprung CL, Caralis PV, Marcial EH, Pierce M, Gelbard MA, Long WM, Duncan RC, Tendler MD, Karpf M: The effects of high dose corticosteroids in patients with septic shock—A prospective, controlled study. *N Engl J Med* 311:1137–1143, 1984.
83. Shatney CH: The use of corticosteroids in the therapy of hemorrhagic shock. In Cowley RA, Trump BF (eds): *Pathophysiology of Shock, Anosmia and Ischemia*. Baltimore, Williams & Wilkins, 1982, p 465.
84. Hardie EM, Rawling CA: Septic shock. Part II—Prevention, recognition and treatment. *Compend Cont Ed Pract Vet* 5:483–493, 1983.
85. McAnulty JF: Septic shock in the dog: a review. *J Am Hosp Assoc* 19:827–836, 1982.
86. Goldberg LI: Dopamine—Clinical uses of an endogenous catecholamine. *New Engl J Med* 291:707–710, 1974.
87. Neiberger RE, Levin JI, Passmore JC: Renal effects of dopamine during prolonged hemorrhagic hypotension in the dog. *Circ Shock* 7:129–138, 1980.
88. Winkle MJ, Trunkey DD: Dopamine gangrene, association with D.I.C. *Am J Surg* 142:588–591, 1981.
89. Brasmer TH: Shock—Basic pathophysiology and treatment. *Vet Clin North Am* 2:219–233, 1972.
90. Goetsch DD, Wilson RC, Huber TL: Effects of promethazine on hemorrhagic shock in the dog. *Am J Vet Res* 43(12):2193–2195, 1982.
91. Masucci FD, Hinshaw LB: Evaluation of protection with phenoxybenzamine against lethal endotoxin shock. *Proc Soc Exp Biol Med* 116:1057–1060, 1964.
92. Hess ML, Krause SM, Kornwatana P: Myocardial failure and excitation-contraction uncoupling in canine endotoxin shock: role of histamine and the saroplasmic reticulum. *Circ Shock* 7:277–287, 1980.
93. Prough DS, Johnson JC, Poole GV Jr, Stullken EH, Johnston WE, Royster R: Effects on intracranial pressure of resuscitation from hemorrhagic shock with hypertonic saline versus lactated Ringer's solution. *Crit Care Med* 13:407–411, 1985.
94. Velasco IT, Pontieri V, Rocha E, Silva M Jr., Lopes OU: Hyperosmotic NaCl and severe hemorrhagic shock. *Am J Physiol* 239:H664–H673, 1980.
95. DeFelipe J Jr, Timoner J, Velasco IT, Lopes OU, Rocha E Silva M Jr.: Treatment of refractory hypovolemic shock by 7.5% sodium chloride injections. *Lancet* 3:1002–1004, 1980.
96. Fettman MJ: Hypertonic crystalloid solutions for treating hemorrhagic shock. *Compend Contin Ed Pract Vet* 7:915–923, 1985.
97. Bottoms GD, Johnson MA, Roesel OF: Endotoxin-induced hemodynamic changes in dogs: Role of thromboxane and prostaglandin I_2. *Am J Vet Res* 44:1497–1500, 1983.
98. Bottoms GD, Templeton CB, Fessler JF, Johnson MA, Roesel OF, Ewert KM, Adams SB: Thromboxane, prostaglandin I_2 (epporostenol), and the hemodynamic changes in equine endotoxic shock. *Am J Vet Res* 43:999–1002, 1982.
99. Hardie EM, Rawlings CA, Collins LG: Canine *Escherichia coli* peritonitis: long-term survival with fluid, gentamicin sulfate, and flunixin meglumine treatment. *J Am Anim Hosp Assoc* 21:691–699, 1985.
100. Culp JR, Erdos EG, Hinshaw LB, Holmes DD: Effects of anti-inflammatory drugs in shock caused by injection of living *E. coli* cells (35548). *Proc Soc Exp Biol Med* 137:219–223, 1971.
101. Fink MP, MacVittie TJ, Casey LC: Inhibition of prostaglandin synthesis restores normal hemodynamics in canine hyperdynamic sepsis. *Ann Surg* 200:619–626, 1984.
102. Moore JN: Comparison of the responses of ponies and horses to a sublethal dose of endotoxin. *Am Assoc Equine Pract Newslett* 2:73–76, 1982.
103. Burrows GE: Therapeutic effect of phenylbutazone on experimental acute *Escherichia coli* endotoxemia in ponies. *Am J Vet Res* 42:94–99, 1981.
104. Bottoms GD, Fessler JF, Roesel OF, Moore AB, Frauenfelder HC: Endotoxin-induced hemodynamic changes in ponies: effects of flunixin meglumine. *Am J Vet Res* 42:1514–1518, 1981.
105. Moore JN, Garner HE, Shapland JE, Hatfield DG: Prevention of endotoxin-induced arterial hypoxemia and lactic acidosis with flunixin meglumine in the conscious pony. *Equine Vet J* 13:95–98, 1981.
106. Templeton CB, Bottoms GD, Fessler JF, Turek JJ, Boon GD: Effects of repeated endotoxin injections on prostanoids, hemodynamics, endothelial cells, and survival in ponies. *Circ Shock* 16:253–264, 1985.
107. Moore JN: The effects of flunixin meglumine prior to or following endotoxin administration in ponies. *Am Assoc Equine Pract Newslett* 2:77–82, 1982.
108. Fessler JF, Bottoms GD, Roesel OF, Moore AB, Frauenfelder HC, Boon GD: Endotoxin-induced change in hemograms, plasma enzymes and blood chemical values in anesthetized ponies: effects of flunixin meglumine. *Am J Vet Res* 43:140–144, 1982.

109. Fink MP, MacVittie TJ, Casey LC: Effects of nonsteroidal anti-inflammatory drugs on renal function in septic dogs. *J Surg Res* 36:516–525, 1984.
110. Lefer AM, Sollott SL, Galvin MJ: Beneficial actions of prostacyclin in traumatic shock. *Prostaglandins* 17:761–767, 1979.
111. Trim CM, Moore JN, Hardee MM, Hardee GE, Graham DAM: Cardiopulmonary effects of prostacyclin infusion in anesthetized horses. *Am J Vet Res* 46:928–931, 1985.
112. Araki H, Lefer AM: Protective action of 6-keto-prostaglandin E_1 in traumatic shock. *Prostaglandins Med* 2:277–284, 1979.
113. Machiedo GW, Brown CS, Lavigne JE, Rush BF Jr: Beneficial effect of prostaglandin E_1 in experimental hemorrhagic shock. *Surg Gynecol Obstet* 143:433–436, 1976.
114. Higgins AJ, Lees P: The acute inflammatory process, arachidonic acid metabolism and the mode of action of anti-inflammatory drugs. *Equine Vet J* 16:163–175, 1984.
115. Jolly SR, Lucchesi BR: Effect of BW755C in an occlusion-reperfusion model of ischemic myocardial injury. *Am Heart J* 106:8–13, 1983.
116. Eiden LE, Ruth JA: Enkephalins modulate the responsiveness of rat atria in vitro to norepinephrine. *Peptides* 3:475–478, 1982.
117. Ruth JA, Doerr AL, Eiden LE: Leuenkephalin inhibits norepinephrine-induced contraction of rat aorta. *Eur J Pharm* 105:189–191, 1984.
118. Holaday JW, Faden AI: Naloxone reversal of endotoxic hypotension suggests role of endorphins in shock. *Nature* 275:450–451, 1978.
119. Hinshaw L, Beller B, Chang A, Flournoy DJ, Lahti RA, Passey RB, Archer LT: Evaluation of naloxone for therapy of *E. coli* shock: species differences. *Arch Surg* 119:1410–1418, 1985.
120. Vargish J, Reynolds GD, Gurll NJ, Lechner RB, Faden AI, Holaday JW: Naloxone reversal of hemorrhagic shock in dogs. *Circ Shock* 7:31–38, 1980.
121. Moore AB, Roesel OF, Fessler JF, Bottoms GD: Effects of naloxone on endotoxin-induced changes in ponies. *Am J Vet Res* 44:103–109, 1983.
122. Faden AI, Holaday JW: Naloxone treatment of endotoxin shock: stereospecificity of physiologic and pharmacologic effects in the rat. *J Pharmacol Exp Ther* 212:441–447, 1980.
123. Fettman M, Hand M, Chandrassena L, Cleek J, Mason R, Phillips R: Effects of naloxone therapy on lethality, hemodynamic and metabolic parameters in awake endotoxemic yucatan minipigs. *Circ Shock* 9:185, 1982.
124. Koyama S, Santiesteban HL, Ammons WS, Manning JW: The effects of naloxone on the peripheral sympathetics in cat endotoxin shock. *Circ Shock* 10:7–13, 1983.
125. DeMaria A, Hefferman JJ, Grindlinger GA, Craven DE, McIntosh TK, McCabe WR: Naloxone versus placebo in treatment of septic shock. *Lancet* 1:1363–1365, 1985.
126. Rock P, Silverman H, Plump D, Kecala Z, Smith P, Michael JR, Summer W: Efficacy and safety of naloxone in septic shock. *Crit Care Med* 13:28–33, 1985.
127. Holaday JW: Cardiovascular effects of endogenous opiate systems. *Ann Rev Pharmacol Toxicol* 23:541–594, 1983.
128. Bernton EW: Naloxone and TRH in the treatment of shock and trauma: what future roles? *Ann Emerg Med* 14:729–735, 1985.
129. Evans SF, Hinds CJ, Varley JG: Effects of intravascular volume expansion on the cardiovascular response to naloxone in a canine model of severe endotoxin shock. *Br J Pharmac* 83:443–448, 1984.
130. Gurll NJ, Reynolds DG, Vargish T, Ganes E: Body temperature and acid base balance determine cardiovascular responses to naloxone in primate hemorrhagic shock. *Fed Proc* 41:1135–1138, 1982.
131. Parton ML, Gurll NJ, Reynolds DG, Vargish T: Adrenalectomy abolishes and cortisol restores naloxones beneficial effects on cardiovascular function and survival in canine hemorrhagic shock. *Circ Shock* 10:317–327, 1983.
132. Chance E, Paciorek PM, Todd MH, Waterfall JF: Comparison of the cardiovascular effects of meptazinol and naloxone following hemorrhagic shock in rats and cats. *Br J Pharmacol* 85:43–53, 1985.
133. Gurll NJ, Reynolds DG, Vargish T, Lechner R: Naltrexone improves survival rate and cardiovascular function in canine hemorrhagic shock. *J Pharmacol Exp Ther* 220:625–628, 1982.
134. Paciorek PM, Todd MH, Wyllie MG: Restoration of mean arterial pressure in endotoxic shock by meptazinol. *Biochem Pharmacol* 32:877–881, 1983.
135. Faden AI, Jacobs TP, Holaday JW: Thyrotropic releasing hormone improves neurologic recovery after spinal trauma in cats. *N Engl J Med* 305:1063–1067, 1981.
136. Faden AI, Feuerstein G, Hayes E, Lux WE: Leukotrienes and anaphylactic shock: a therapeutic role for thyrotropin-releasing hormone. *Circ Shock* 10:246–250, 1983.
137. Baumgartner JD, McCutchan JA, Melle GV, Vogt M, Leuthy R, Glauser MP, Ziegler EJ, Klauber MR, Muehler E, Chiolero R, Geroulanos S: Prevention of gram-negative shock and death in surgical patients by antibody to endotoxin core glycolipid. *Lancet* 2:59–62, 1985.
138. Ziegler EJ, McCutchan JA, Fierer J, Glauser MP, Sadoff JC, Douglas H, Braude AI: Treatment of gram negative bacteremia and shock with human antiserum to a mutant *Escherichia coli*. *N Engl J Med* 307:1225–1230, 1982.
139. Dunn DL, Mach PA, Condie RM, Cerra FB: Anticore endotoxin $F(ab')_2$ equine immunoglobulin fragments protect against lethal effects of gram-negative bacterial sepsis. *Surgery* 96:440–446, 1984.
140. Peitzman AB, Corbett WA, Illner HM, Shires GT: Correlation of transmembrane potential with high energy phosphate levels in hemorrhagic shock in primates. *Surg Forum* 31:5–8, 1980.
141. Gallagher JF, Shires GT: Correlation of transmembrane potential difference with high energy phosphate levels in hemorrhagic shock. *Surg Forum* 28:19–21, 1977.
142. Lefer AM, Daw JC, Burne RM: Cardiac and skeletal muscle metabolic energy stores in hemorrhagic shock. *Am J Physiol* 216:483–486, 1969.
143. Chaudry IH, Sayeed MM, Baue AE: Effect of hemorrhagic shock on tissue adenine nucleotides in conscious rats. *Can J Physiol Pharmacol* 52:131–137, 1974.
144. Chaudry IH, Calmens MG, Baue AE: Alterations in cell function with ischemia and shock and their correction. *Arch Surg* 116:1309–1317, 1981.
145. Filkins JP, Buchanan BJ: Protection against endotoxin shock and impaired glucose homeostasis with ATP. *Circ Shock* 4:253–258, 1977.
146. Chaudry IH, Sayeed MM, Baue AE: Effect of adenosine triphosphate-magnesium chloride administration in shock. *Surgery* 75:220–227, 1974.
147. Chaudry IH, Hirasawa H, Baue AE: Effects of adenosine-triphosphate-glucose administration following sepsis. *J Surg Res* 29:348–356, 1980.
148. Garvin PJ, Jellinek M, Morgan R: Renal cortical levels of adenosine triphosphate—Restoration after prolonged ischemia by in site perfusion of ATP-$MgCl_2$. *Arch Surg* 116:221–224, 1981.
149. Machiedo GW, Ghuman S, Rush BF: The effect of ATP-$MgCl_2$ infusion on hepatic cell permeability and metabolism following hemorrhagic shock. *J Clin Invest* 67:1118–1125, 1981.
150. Horton JW, Landreneau RJ, Coln D: Cardiovascular effects of ATP-$MgCl_2$ in hemorrhagic shock. *Surg Forum* 34:15–17, 1983.
151. Newberg LA, Milde JH, Michenfelder JD: Cerebral and systemic effects of hypotension induced by adenosine or ATP in dogs. *Anesthesiology* 62:429–436, 1985.
152. Breznock EM: The systemic response of the traumatized patient—An overview. *Vet Clinics of North Amer: Small An Pract* 10:523–532, 1980.
153. Gordon NH, Scott DB, Robb IWP: Modification of plasma corti-

costeroid concentrations during and after surgery by epidural blockade. *Br Med J* 1:581–583, 1973.
154. Kono K, Philbin DM, Cossins CH: Renal function and stress response during halothane or fentanyl anesthesia. *Anesth Analg* 60:552–556, 1981.
155. Rosin E: The systemic response to injury. In Bojrab MJ (ed): *Pathophysiology in Small Animal Surgery*. Philadelphia, Lea & Febiger, 1981, p 3.
156. Haas M, Glock SM: Radioimmunoassayable plasma vasopressin associated with surgery. *Arch Surg* 113:597–600, 1978.
157. Fieldman NR, Forsling ML, Le Quesne LP: The effect of vasopressin on solute and water excretion during and after surgical operations. *Ann Surg* 201:383–390, 1985.
158. Cochrane JPS: The aldosterone response to surgery and the relationship of this response to postoperative sodium retention. *Br J Surg* 65:744–747, 1978.
159. Le Quesne LP, Cochrane JPS, Fieldman NR: Fluid and electrolyte disturbances after trauma: the role of adrenocortical and pituitary hormones. *Brit Med Bull* 41:212–217, 1985.
160. Barton RN: Neuroendocrine mobilization of body fuels after injury. *Brit Med Bull* 41:218–225, 1985.
161. Ryan NT, George BC, Harlow CL, Hiebert JM, Egdahl RH: Endocrine activation and altered muscle metabolism after hemorrhagic shock. *Am J Physiol* 233:E439–E444, 1977.
162. Eigler N, Sacca L, Sherwin RS: Synergistic interactions of physiological increments of glucagon, epinephrine and cortisol in the dog. A model for stress induced hyperglycemia. *J Clin Invest* 63:114–123, 1979.
163. Cuthbertson DP: Observations on the disturbance of metabolism produced by injury to the limbs. *Q J Med* 1:233–246, 1932.
164. Stoner HB: Effects of injury on the responses to thermal stimulation of the hypothalamus. *J Appl Physiol* 33:665–671, 1972.
165. Little RA: Heat production after injury. *Brit Med Bull* 41:226–231, 1985.
166. Moyer ED, Border JR, Cerra FB, Reed R, Yu L, Chernier R, Caruana J, McMenamy RH: Multiple systems organ failure—III: Contrasts in plasma amino acid profiles in septic trauma patients who subsequently survive and do not survive: effects of intravenous amino acids. *J Trauma* 21:263–274, 1981.
167. Wiles CE III, Cerra FB: The exogenous substrate support of the trauma patient. In Worth MH Jr (ed): *Principles and Practice of Trauma Care*. Baltimore, Williams & Wilkins 1982, p 312.
168. Fleck A, Colley CM, Myers MA: Liver export proteins and trauma. *Brit Med Bull* 41:265–273, 1985.
169. Polk HC: Consensus summary on infection. *J Trauma* 19:894–896, 1979.
170. Constantian MB, Menzoian JO, Nimberg RB, Schmid K, Mannick JA: Association of a circulating immunosuppressive polypeptide with operative and accidental trauma. *Ann Surg* 185:73–79, 1977.
171. Heideman M, Kaijser B, Gelin L: Complement activation and hematologic, hemodynamic and respiratory reactions early after soft tissue injury. *J Trauma* 18:696–700, 1978.
172. Bjornson AB, Altermeier WA, Bjornson HS: Complement, opsonins, and the immune response to bacterial infection in burned patients. *Ann Surg* 191:323–329, 1980.
173. McPhaden AR, Whaley K: The complement system in sepsis and trauma. *Brit Med Bull* 41:281–286, 1985.
174. Miller SE, Miller CL, Trunkey DD: The immune consequences of trauma. *Surg Clin North Am* 62:167–181, 1982.
175. Ninnemann JL: Immunosuppression following thermal injury through B cell activation of suppressor T cells. *J Trauma* 20:206–213, 1980.
176. Baker CC, Miller CL, Trunkey DD, Lim RC: Identity of mononuclear cells which compromise the resistance of trauma patients. *J Surg Res* 26:478–487, 1979.
177. Winchurch RA, Munster AM: Post-traumatic activation of suppressor cells. *J Recticuloendothel Soc* 27:83–88, 1980.
178. Salo M: Effect of anesthesia and surgery on the number of mitogen-induced transformation of T and B-lymphocytes. *Ann Clin Res* 10:1–13, 1978.
179. Robinson WF, Maxie MG: The Cardiovascular system. In Jubb KVF, Kennedy PC, Palmer N (eds): *Pathology of the Domestic Animals*, ed 13. New York, Academic Press, 1985, vol 3, p 2.
180. Wolfson B, Hetrick WD, Lake CL, Siker ES: Anesthetic indices—Further data. *Anesthesiology* 48:187–190, 1978.
181. Musgrave GE, Branch CE, Beckett SD: Relative sensitivity of the canine sinus node and atrioventricular node to acetylcholine. *Can J Physiol Pharmacol* 59:1050–1062, 1981.
182. Tilley LP: *Essentials of Canine and Feline Electrocardiography—Interpretation and Treatment*, ed 2. Philadelphia, Lea and Febiger, 1985, p 222.
183. McIntyre KM, Lewis AJ, Winslow EBJ, Parker MR, Kaye W: Sudden cardiac death. In McIntyre KM, Lewis AJ (eds): *Textbook of Advanced Cardiac Life Support*. New York, American Heart Association, 1981.
184. Tranquilli WJ, Thurmon JC, Benson GJ: Alterations in ADE following adrenergic receptor blockade in halothane-xylazine anesthetised dogs. *Veterinary Midwest Anesthesia Conference* 1:5, 1985.
185. Clark DR: Recognition and treatment of cardiac emergencies. *J Am Vet Med Assoc* 171:98–106, 1977.
186. Ederstrom HE: Ventricular fibrillation susceptibility as related to heart size and maturity. *Fed Proc* 35:221, 1976.
187. White BC: Pulseless idioventricular rhythm during CPR—An indication for massive intravenous bolus glucocorticoids. *JACEP* 5:449–454, 1976.
188. Riebold TW, Evans AT, Robinson NE: Evaluation of the demand value for resuscitation of horses. *J Am Vet Med Ass* 176:623–626, 1980.
189. Yakaitis RW, Redding JS: Precordial thumping during cardiac resuscitation. *Crit Care Med* 1:22–26, 1973.
190. Birch LH: Mechanical external cardiac compression and ventilation during cardiopulmonary resuscitation. In Safar P, Elan J (eds): *Advances in Cardiopulmonary Resuscitation*. New York, Springer-Verlag, 1977, p 94.
191. Frauenfelder HC, Fessler JF, Latshaw HS, Moore AB, Bottoms GD: External cardiovascular resuscitation of the anesthetized pony. *J Am Vet Med Assoc* 179:673–676, 1981.
192. Goldstein MA, Schwark WS, Short CE, White KK: Cardiopulmonary resuscitation in the horse. *Cornell Vet* 71:225–268, 1981.
193. Muir WW: Equine cardiopulmonary resuscitation—Part I. *Comp Cont Ed Pract Vet* 5:S228–S234, 1983.
194. Muir WW: Equine cardiopulmonary resuscitation—Part II. *Comp Cont Ed Pract Vet* 5:S287–S295, 1983.
195. Chandra N, Rudikoff M, Weisfeldt ML: Simultaneous chest compression and ventilation at high airway pressure during cardiopulmonary resuscitation. *Lancet* 1:175–178, 1980.
196. Creed JD, Packard JM, Lambrew CT, Lewis AJ: Defibrillation and synchronized cardioversion. In McIntyre KM, Lewis AJ (eds): *Textbook of Advanced Cardiac Life Support*. New York, American Heart Association, 1981, p 89.
197. Geddes LA, Tacker WA, Rosborough JP, Moore AG, Cabler PS: Electrical dose for ventricular defibrillation of large and small animals using precordial electrodes. *J Clin Invest* 53:310–319, 1974.
198. Thomas ED, Ewy GA, Dahl CF, Ewy MD: Effectiveness of direct current defibrillation: role of paddle electrode size. *Am Heart J* 93:463–467, 1977.
199. Kerber RE, Kouba C, Martins J, Kelly K, Low R, Hoyt R, Ferguson D, Bailey L, Bennett P, Charbonnier F: Advance prediction of transthoracic impedance in human defibrillation and cardioversion—Importance of impedance in determining the success of low-energy shocks. *Circulation* 70:303–308, 1984.
200. Adgey AAJ, Patton JN, Campbell NPS, Webb SW: Ventricular defibrillation: appropriate energy levels. *Circulation* 60:219–

223, 1979.
201. Campbell NPS, Webb SW, Adgey AAJ, Pantridge JF: Transthoracic ventricular defibrillation in adults. *Br Med J* 2:1379–1381, 1977.
202. Tacker WA Jr, Ewy GA: Emergency defibrillation dose: recommendations and rationale. *Circulation* 60:223–225, 1979.
203. Yakaitis RW, Ewy GA, Otto CW, Taren DL, Moon TE: Influence of time and therapy on ventricular defibrillation in dogs. *Crit Care Med* 8:157–163, 1980.
204. Gold JH, Schuder JC, Stoeckle H, McDaniel WC, Moellinger DW, Roberts SA: Transthoracic defibrillation in 100-kg calves with sequentially applied pulses. *Am J Physiol* 243:H982–H989, 1982.
205. Geddes LA, Tacker WA, Cabler P, Chapman R, Riviera R, Kidder H: The decrease in transthoracic impedance during successive ventricular defibrillation trials. *Med Instrum* 9:179–180, 1975.
206. O'Dowd WJ: Defibrillator design and development—A review. *J Med Eng Tech* 7:5–15, 1983.
207. Pare PD, Warrine B, Baile EM, Hogg JC: Redistribution of pulmonary extravascular water with positive end-expiratory pressure in canine pulmonary edema. *Am Rev Respir Dis* 127:590–593, 1983.
208. Yakaitis RW, Otto CW, Blitt CD: Relative importance of and adrenergic receptors during resuscitation. *Crit Care Med* 7:293–296, 1979.
209. Holmes HR, Babbs CF, Voorhees WD, Tacker W, De Garavilla: Influence of adrenergic drugs upon vital organ perfusion during CPR. *Crit Care Med* 8:137–140, 1980.
210. Koehler RC, Michael JR, Guerci AD, Chandra N, Schleien CL, Dean JM, Rogers MC, Weisfeldt ML, Traystman RJ: Beneficial effect of epinephrine infusion on cerebral and myocardial blood flows during CPR. *Ann Emerg Med* 14:744–749, 1985.
211. Adams HR: Cardiovascular emergencies—Drugs and resuscitative principles. *Vet Clin North Am: Small Anim Pract* 11:77–102, 1981.
212. Kuhn GL, White BC, Swetnam RE, Mumey JF, Rydesky MF, Tintinalli JE, Krome RL, Hoehner PJ: Peripheral vs central circulation times during CPR—A pilot study. *Ann Emerg Med* 10:417–419, 1981.
213. Ralston SH, Voorhees WD, Babbs CF: Intrapulmonary epinephrine during prolonged cardiopulmonary resuscitation—Improved regional blood flow and resuscitation in dogs. *Ann Emerg Med* 13:79–86, 1984.
214. Crowe DT Jr: Cardiopulmonary resuscitation and advanced cardiac life support. In Zaslow IM (ed): *Veterinary Trauma and Critical Care*. Philadelphia, Lea and Febiger, 1984, p 507.
215. Barsan WG, Levy RC, Weir H: Lidocaine levels during CPR—Differences after peripheral venous, central venous and intracardiac injections. *Am Emerg Med* 10:73–78, 1981.
216. Cancy RL, Cingolani HE, Taylor RR: Influence of sodium bicarbonate on myocardial performance. *Am J Physiol* 212:917–923, 1967.
217. Carson, Allan SA, Chorley GE, Hamilton FN, Lee DC, Morris LE: Variation in cardiac output with acid-base changes in the anesthetized dog. *J Appl Physiol* 20:948–953, 1965.
218. Hecht HH, Hulter OF: Action of pH on cardiac purkinje fibres. *Fed Proc* 23:157, 1964.
219. Gerst PH, Fleming WH, Malm JR: A quantitative evaluation of the effects of acidosis and alkalosis upon the ventricular fibrillation threshold. Surgery 59:1050–1060, 1966.
220. Haskins SC: Cardiopulmonary resuscitation. *Comp Cont Ed Pract Vet* 4:170–182, 1982.
221. Berenyi KJ, Wolk M, Killip T: Cerebrospinal fluid acidosis complicating therapy of experimental cardiopulmonary arrest. *Circulation* 52:319–324, 1975.
222. Kerber RE, Pandian NG, Hoyt R, Jensen SR, Koyanagi S, Grayzel J, Kieso R: Effect of ischemia, hypertrophy, hypoxia, acidosis, and alkalosis on canine defibrillation. *Am J Physiol* 244:H825–H831, 1983.
223. Kerber RE, Sarnat W: Factors influencing the success of ventricular defibrillation in man. *Circulation* 60:226–230, 1979.
224. Abboud T, Raya J, Sadri S, Grobler N, Stine L, Miller F: Fetal and maternal cardiovascular effects of atropine and glycopyrrolate. *Anesth Analg* 62:426–30, 1983.
225. Mirakhur RK, Dundee JW, Jones CJ, Coppel DL, Clarke RS: Reversal of neuromuscular blockade: Dose definition studies with atropine and glycopyrrolate given before or in a mixture with neostigmine. *Anesth Analg* 60:557–562, 1981.
226. White BC, Krause GS, Aust SD, Eyster GE: Postischemic tissue injury by iron-mediated free radical lipid peroxidation. *Ann Emerg Med* 14:804–809, 1985.
227. Denlinger JK, Kaplan JA, Lecky JH, Wollman H: Cardiovascular responses to calcium administered intravenously to man during halothane anesthesia. *Anesthesiology* 42:390–397, 1975.
228. Scheidegger MD, Drop LJ: Calcium ion concentration and beta adrenergic activity. Studies in the anesthetised, intact dog. *J Thoracic Cardiovasc Surg* 80:441–446, 1980.
229. White RD: Cardiovascular pharmacology, Part I. In McIntyre KM, Lewis AJ (eds): *Textbook of Advanced Cardiac Life Support*. American Heart Association, 1981, p 99.
230. White BC, Hoehner PJ, Wilson RF: Mitochondrial O_2 use and ATP synthesis—Kinetic effects of Ca^{++} and HPO_4^{-2} modulated by glucocorticoids. *Ann Emerg Med* 9:396–403, 1980.
231. Schanne FAX, Kane AB, Young EE, Farber JL: Calcium dependence of toxic cell death—A final common pathway. *Science* 206:700–702, 1979.
232. Hughes WG, Ruedy JR: Should calcium be used in cardiac arrest? *Am J Med* 81:285–296, 1986.
233. Babbs CF: New versus old theories of blood flow during CPR. *Crit Care Med* 8:191–196, 1980.
234. Babbs CF, Voorhess WD, Fitzgerald KR, Holmes HR, Geddes LA: Influence of interposed ventilation pressure upon artificial cardiac output during cardiopulmonary resuscitation in dogs. *Crit Care Med* 8:127–130, 1980.
235. Bircher N, Safar P: Cerebral preservation during cardiopulmonary resuscitation. *Crit Care Med* 13:185–189, 1985.
236. Luce JM, Rizk NA, Niskanen RA: Regional blood flow during cardiopulmonary resuscitation in dogs. *Crit Care Med* 12:874–878, 1984.
237. Niemann JT, Rosborough JP, Niskanen RA, Alferness C, Criley JM: Mechanical "cough" cardiopulmonary resuscitation during cardiac arrest in dogs. *Am J Cardiol* 55:199–204, 1985.
238. Rudikoff MT, Maughan WL, Effron M, Freund P, Weisfeldt ML: Mechanisms of blood flow during cardiopulmonary resuscitation. *Circulation* 61:345–352, 1980.
239. Wilder RJ, Weir D, Rush BF Jr, Ravitch MM: Method of coordinating ventilation and closed-chest cardiac massage in the dog. Surgery 53:186–194, 1963.
240. Fisher J, Vaghaiwalla F, Tsitlik J, Levin H, Brinker J, Weisfeldt M, Yin F: Determinants and clinical significance of jugular venous valve competence. *Circulation* 65:188–196, 1982.
241. Bircher N, Safar P, Stewart R: A comparison of standard, MAST-augmented and open-chest CPR in dogs. A preliminary investigation. *Crit Care Med* 8:147–152, 1980.
242. Arai T, Dote K, Tsukahara I, Nitta K, Nagaro T: Cerebral flow during coventional, new and open chest cardiopulmonary resuscitation in dogs. *Resuscitation* 12:147–154, 1984.
243. Bircher N, Safar P: A comparison of standard and "new" closed chest CPR in dogs. *Crit Care Med* 9:384, 1981.
244. White BC, Wiegenstein JG, Winegar CD: Brain ischemic anoxia. *JAMA* 251:1586–1590, 1984.
245. De Moor A, Verschooten F, Desmet P, Muylle E, Steenhaut M: Intrathoracic cardiac resuscitation in the horse. *Eq Vet J* 4:31–33, 1972.
246. Anstadt GL, Schiff P, Baue AE: Prolonged circulatory support

by direct mechanical ventricular assistance. *Trans Am Soc Artif Intern Organs* 12:72–79, 1966.
247. Bartlelt RL, Stewart NJ, Raymond J, Anstadt GL, Martin SD: Comparative study of three methods of resuscitation—Closed-chest, open-chest manual, and direct mechanical ventricular assistance. *Ann Emerg Med* 13:773–777, 1984.
248. McCabe JB, Ventriglia WJ, Anstadt GL, Nolan DJ: Direct mechanical ventricular assistance during ventricular fibrillation. *Ann Emerg Med* 12:739–744, 1983.
249. Ewy GA, Dahl CF, Zimmerman M: Ventricular fibrillation masquerading as ventricular standstill. *Crit Care Med* 9:841–844, 1981.
250. Kaye W: Invasive therapeutic techniques. In McIntyre KM, Lewis AJ (eds): *Textbook of Advanced Cardiac Life Support.* New York, American Heart Association, 1981, p 199.
251. Tintinalli JE, White BC: Transthoracic pacing during CPR. *Ann Emerg Med* 10:113–116, 1981.
252. Hazard PB, Benton C, Milnor PJ: Transvenous cardiac pacing in cardiopulmonary resuscitation. *Crit Care Med* 9:666–668, 1981.
253. White BC, Petinga TJ, Hoehner PJ; Wilson RF: Incidence, etiology, and outcome of pulseless idioventricular rhythm treated with dexamethasone during advanced CPR. *JACEP* 8:188–193, 1979.
254. White BC, Hoehner PJ, Petinga TJ, Moeser JC, Wilson RF: His electrocardiographic characterization of terminal arrhythmias of hemorrhagic shock in dogs. *JACEP* 8:298–303, 1979.
255. Iseri LT, Siner EJ, Humphrey SB, Mann S: Prehospital cardiac arrest after arrival of the paramedic unit. *JACEP* 6:530–535, 1977.
256. Van Vleet JF, Tacker WA, Cechner PE, Bright RM, Green JA, Raffee MR, Geddes LA, Ferrans VJ: Effect of shock strength on survival and acute cardiac damage induced by open-thorax defibrillation of dogs. *Am J Vet Res* 39:981–987, 1978.
257. Babbs CF, Yim GKW, Whistler SJ, Tacker WA, Geddes LA: Elevation of ventricular defibrillation threshold in dogs by antiarrhythmic drugs. *Am Heart J* 98:345–350, 1979.
258. Geddes LA, Tacker WA Jr, Rosborough J, Moore AG, Cabler P, Bailey M, McCrady JD, Witzel D: The electrical dose for ventricular defibrillation with electrodes applied directly to the heart. *J Thor Cardiovasc Surg* 68:593–602, 1974.
259. Breznock EM, Kagan KG, Attix ES: Chemical cardioversion of electrically induced ventricular fibrillation in dogs. *Am J Vet Res* 39:971–975, 1978.
260. Breznock EM, Kagan KG, Attix ES: Effects of ionic salts or acetylcholine, or both, on electrically induced ventricular fibrillation in dogs. *Am J Vet Res* 39:977–980, 1978.
261. Breznock EM, Kagan K, Hibser NK: Effects of bretyllium tosylate in the in vivo fibrillating canine ventricle. *Am J Vet Res* 38:89–94, 1977.
262. Short CE: Alternates to live animals in teaching of CPR and arrhythmia detection. *Proc Intl Cong Vet Anes* 2:185, 1985.
263. Safar P, Stezoski SW, Nemoto EM: Amelioration of brain damage after 12 min cardiac arrest in dogs. *Arch Neurol* 33:91–95, 1976.
264. Bleyaert AL, Sands PA, Safar P, Nemoto EM, Stezoski SW, Moossy J, Rao GR: Augmentation of postischemic brain damage by severe intermittent hypertension. *Crit Care Med* 8:41–47, 1980.
265. Gilroy BA, Rockoff MA, Dunlop BJ, Shapiro NM: Cardiopulmonary resuscitation in the non-human primate. *J Am Vet Med Assoc* 177:867–874, 1980.
266. Nemoto EM, Bleyaert AL, Stezoski SW, Moossy J, Rao GR, Safar P: Global brain ischaemia: a reproducible monkey model. *Stroke* 8:558–564, 1977.
267. Hossman KA, Sato K: Recovery of neuronal function after prolonged cerebral ischemia. *Science* 168:375–376, 1970.
268. Harris RJ, Symon K, Branston NM, Bayhan M: Changes in extracellular calcium activity in cerebral ischemia. *J Cereb Blood Flow Metab* 1:203–209, 1981.
269. McCord JM: Oxygen derived free radicals in postischemic injury. *N Engl J Med* 312:159–163, 1985.
270. Ames A III, Wright RL, Kowada M, Thurston JM, Majno G: Cerebral ischemia—II. The no reflow phenomenon. *Am J Pathol* 52:437–453, 1968.
271. Mullie A, Hedstrand U, Breivik H, Skulberg A, Tammisto T, Jastremski M, Lind B, Bozza-Murrubini M, Potter D, Canton A, Kaminski B: Effects of brain ischemia times on neurological recovery after cardiac arrest. *Crit Care Med* 13:361, 1985.
272. Shapiro HM: Barbiturates in brain ischemia. *Br J Anaesth* 57:82–95, 1985.
273. Smith DS, Rehncrona S, Siesjo BK: Inhibitory effects of different barbiturates on lipid peroxidation in brain tissue in vitro: Comparison with the effects of promethazine and chlorpromazine. *Anesthesiology* 53:186–194, 1980.
274. Abramson NS, Safar P, Detre KM, Kelsey S, Monroe J, Reinmuth O, Snyder JV, Mullie A, Hedstrand U, Tamist T, Lund I, Breivik H, Lind B, Jastremski M: Thiopental loading in cardiopulmonary resuscitation (CPR) survivors—A randomized collaborative clinical study. *Anesthesiology* 51:A101, 1983.
275. Todd MM, Chadwick HS, Shapiro HM, Dunlop BJ, Marshall LF, Dueck R: The neurologic effects of thiopental therapy following experimental cardiac arrest in cats. *Anesthesiology* 57:76–86, 1982.
276. Gisvold SE, Steen PA: Drug therapy in brain ischemia. *Br J Anaesth* 57:96–109, 1985.
277. Bircher NG: Ischemic brain protection. *Ann Emerg Med* 14:784–788, 1985.
278. Vaagenes P, Cantadore R, Safar P, Alexander H: Effect of lidoflazine on neurologic outcome after cardiac arrest in dogs. *Anesthesiology* 59:A100, 1983.
279. Dean JM, Hoehner PJ, Traystman RJ, Rogers M: Effect of lidoflazine on total and regional cerebral blood flow after global ischemia. *Stroke* 15:531–535, 1984.
280. Winegar CP, Henderson D, White BC: Early amelioration of neurologic deficit by lidoflazine after fifteen minutes of cardiopulmonary arrest in dogs. *Ann Emerg Med* 12:471–477, 1983.
281. Babbs CF: Role of iron ions in the genesis of reperfusion injury following successful cardiopulmonary resuscitation: preliminary data and a biochemical hypothesis. *Ann Emerg Med* 14:777–783, 1985.
282. Nayini NR, White BC, Aust SD, Huang RR, Evans AT, Indrieri RJ, Bialek H, Jacobs WA, Komara J: Reduction of iron delocalisation and malondialdehyde production in the brain following cardiac arrest. *Proc Intl Cong Vet Anes* 2:91, 1985.
283. Hallenbeck JM, Leitch DR, Dutka AJ, Greenbaum LJ, McKee AE: Prostaglandin I-2, indomethacin, and heparin promote postischemic neuronal recovery in dogs. *Ann Neurol* 12:145–156, 1982.
284. Ruiz E, Brunette D, Robinson E: Cerebral resuscitation of dogs after cardiac arrest. *Veterinary Midwest Anesthesia Conference* 3, 1985.
285. Lin SR, O'Connor MJ, Fischer HW, Harnish P, King A: The effect of combined dextran and streptokinase on cerebral function and blood flow after cardiac arrest—an experimental study in the dog. *Invest Radiol* 13:490–498, 1978.
286. Takagi T, Nagai H, Mabe H, Urmemura S, Yoshida T: Effect of fluozol-DA on experimental cerebral ischemia. *J Cereb Blood Flow Metab* 3:S353, 1983.
287. McIntyre KM: Medicolegal aspects of cardiopulmonary resuscitation (CPR) and emergency cardiac care (ECC). In McIntyre KM, Lewis AJ (eds): *Textbook of Advanced Cardiac Life Support.* New York, American Heart Association, 1981, p 275.

CHAPTER

23

Allergic Reactions and Immune Responses during Anesthesia

CHARLES E. SHORT, D.V.M., M.S., D.A.C.V.A.

Fortunately, allergic reactions do not occur often in animal patients; when they do occur, however, these responses may be very difficult to manage. Onset is frequently rapid, and early diagnosis and therapy is essential to avoid irreversible complications. In a recent report, 4% of all human hospital admissions were due to adverse responses to therapeutic doses of medications; 48% of the patients in this study were considered to have experienced an allergic reaction, with a mortality rate of 0.005%. The incidence of allergic reactions during anesthesia seems to be on the rise, probably due to the use of greater numbers of drugs during the intraoperative period as well as cross sensitivity between drugs (1).

The term "immediate hypersensitivity" denotes an immunological sensitivity to antigens that manifests itself by tissue reactions occurring within minutes after the antigen combines with its appropriate antibody. Such a reaction may occur in any member of a species (anaphylaxis) or only in certain predisposed or hyperreactive members (atopy).

In 1890, von Behring discovered the prophylactic use of antiserum against diphtheria toxin. In the search for other prophylactic antisera, Portier and Richet noted an immediate shock-like reaction in a dog sensitive to sea anemone toxin; this harmful reaction they called "antiphylaxis" (or anaphylaxis) (2).

Anaphylaxis

"Anaphylaxis" is a manifestation of immediate hypersensitivity resulting from the *in vivo* interaction of cellular sites with antigen and specific antibody. "Generalized anaphylaxis" is a shock-like state occurring within minutes after an appropriate antigen-antibody reaction. Upon the first exposure of an animal to an antigen, a cytotropic antibody can form that sensitizes mast cells and basophils in tissues and blood, respectively. After a second exposure to the antigen, the sensitized animal reacts to histamine and other mediators released by mast cells as a result of the antigen-antibody reaction. Histamine causes a marked vasodilatation and leakage of intravascular fluids, resulting in shock. There are smooth muscle spasms, especially in certain smooth muscle-containing organs such as guinea pig bronchi and canine liver. These are the principal specific shock organs in these two species. The extreme bronchoconstriction in the guinea pig results in respiratory obstruction, asphyxia, and death. The extreme vasodilatation and resulting leakage of fluids in the dog or in humans causes profound shock and death. Epinephrine may be a life-saving treatment in anaphylaxis (2).

"Local anaphylaxis" may occur in specific target organs, such as the gastrointestinal tract, nasal mucosa, or skin. Free histamine and serotonin exert their pharmacological effects on adjacent smooth muscles and vascular endothelial cells. Similar mechanisms probably exist for the release of other mediators, such as SRS-A, ECF-A, and bradykinin. Cromolyn sodium apparently can stabilize mast cell membranes or granules and can prevent the release of mediators.

Anaphylaxis is a reaction found in almost all vertebrate animal species (hamster excepted); it results from sensitization of tissue-fixed mast cells by cytotropic antibodies after exposure to antigen. Subsequent exposure to antigen results in complexing of an antigen molecule with two antibody molecules in mild to moderate antigen excess. Complexed antibody molecules are physically distorted and initiate an enzyme cascade ending in the release of pharmacological mediators that exert their effects upon adjacent target tissue.

Allergy and Atopy

Von Pirquet proposed the term "allergic" in 1906 to denote an immune deviation from the original state or a "changed reactivity" of an individual. An allergic individual was one who deviated from the expected immunological response. Von Pirquet included all forms of altered immunological responsiveness, encompassing reactions to toxins, bacteria, and other infectious agents; patients with pollen hay fever; and urticaria-producing foods. Coca in 1923 coined the word "atopy" to denote an abnormal state of hypersensitivity, as distinguished from hypersensitivity responses in normal individuals, i.e., contact dermatitis, serum sickness, anaphylaxis, and infection with tubercle bacilli (2).

Until recently, atopy was thought to be restricted to humans, but such conditions have now been described in dogs, rats, and even a baby walrus. In genetically susceptible individuals, atopy may affect one or more primary shock organ systems. In humans, atopy involving the respiratory system (the nasal mucosa, bronchioles, and aural mucosa) can cause hay fever, asthma, and serous otitis. With the skin as the shock organ, urticaria, angioneurotic edema, and atopic dermatitis (eczema) occur. Sensitized intestinal and urinary systems react with antigen to cause vomiting, abdominal pain, diarrhea, urinary frequency, and pain on urination. Vascular involvement, especially of the central nervous system, may result in headaches, personality changes, and other nervous system manifestations.

An allergic reaction may follow the administration of drug in any patient, but chronic broncheal problems or other drug or food allergies and sensitivities indicate a greater probability of allergic reaction to drugs administered intravenously during anesthesia. This increased susceptibility is primarily a reflection of a genetic predisposition of patients to form increased amounts of immunoglobulin E (IgE) antibodies. In normal patients, IgE antibodies are present in trace amounts in the plasma, but the concentration is elevated in some patients (1).

There are four mechanisms for allergic reaction. They are anaphylaxis (Type I hypersensitivity or immune-mediated hypersensitivity); classic pathway activation of the complement system; alternate pathway activation of the complement system; and anaphylactoid reactions, which are due to a direct histamine release (1). To have an anaphylaxis reaction requires a previous exposure to the drug or a chemically similar substance and the production of the IgE antibodies. The first exposure stimulates production of antibodies that attach to receptor sites on the cell membrane of both mass cells in tissue and basophils circulating in the plasma. These cells that are bound to antibodies are considered to be sensitized and are capable of stimulating an anaphylactic reaction (1).

Immune Mechanism

Various immune mechanisms involved in the production of tissue damage were classified in 1963 by Gell and Coombs into four basic types (3):

- Type I: Anaphylactic (immediate response)
- Type II: Cytotoxic
- Type III: Arthus type and antigen-antibody complexes
- Type IV: Delayed hypersensitivity (48 to 72 hours)

The magnitude of change in cell membrane and influx of calcium leading to the release of granules from the cells is influenced by the dose of drug injected, the affinity of the drug for cell-bound IgE antibodies, the number of cell-bound IgE antibodies, and the intracellular concentration of cyclic nucleotides. This release of granules from mast cells or release of chemical mediators from basophils produce pharmacological effects. These pharmacological effects are responsible for clinical manifestations of allergic reactions (1).

Histamine is the most important chemical mediator released and the only substance proven to be essential for anaphylaxis to occur. Stimulation of H_1 receptors is responsible for smooth muscle effects, whereas cardiac effects reflect stimulation of H_2 receptors (1). The histamine effect of these chemical mediators released by degranulation of mast cells and basophils includes an increased capillary permeability and bronchoconstriction. The release of prostaglandins can produce bronchoconstriction (prostaglandins D_2 or F_2) or bronchodilation from prostaglandins E_1 and E_2. The release of the platelet-activating factor can cause platelet aggregation and degranulation. Heparin release can cause anticoagulation and inhibition of complement system activation and slow-reacting substance of anaphylaxis and cause bronchoconstriction. It is evident that these reactions greatly influence the animals' ability to breath and can result in rapid deterioration of the patient.

An allergic reaction due to classic pathway activation of the complement system does not require previous sensitization, but can occur with the first exposure to the drug. An adverse response due to alternate pathway activation of the complement system can occur with the first or subsequent exposure to a drug.

An anaphylactoid reaction is due to direct effect of a drug on mast cells and basophils that stimulates the release of histamine. The drugs *d*-tubocurarine, succinylcholine, or the thiobarbiturates can displace basic histamine molecules from cells (1).

The manifestations of an allergic reaction include hypotension, sinus tachycardia, hyperparastylosis, bronchial spasms, arterial hypoxemia, ventricular cardiac dysrhythmias, and sometimes hyperexcitability (1).

Anaphylactic reactions to narcotics are exceedingly rare. A reaction to meperidine was reported in man in 1982 (4). This patient had facial urticaria, coughing, wheezing, and cyanosis. Profuse frothy secretions were produced in the airway. It was necessary to suction the trachea, administer epinephrine intravenously, and do cardiopulmonary resuscitation (CPR). Hypotension had developed, and there were tonic clonic seizures. The patient became acidotic, with a pH of 7.25, $PaCO_2$ of 50 mm Hg and PaO_2 of 80 mm Hg. Pulmonary edema and sinus tachycardia developed rapidly. This reaction is somewhat similar to two cases of reaction to intravenous meperidine in horses observed by the author. The horses developed sinus tachycardia, profuse sweating, vasodilatation, and hypotension.

Narcotics can produce an anaphylactoid reaction; it is normally caused by histamine release. In most instances of narcotic reaction, there may not be an ultimate diagnosis because histamine or IgE levels are not frequently determined. Antigen-specific IgE antibody can be measured by the radioallergosorbent test (RAST). Because anaphylaxis is an acute, potentially fatal reaction, prompt recognition and treatment is necessary to avoid a disastrous outcome; as a result, the specific antibody testing or histamine release is not usually evaluated (2). There have been reports of histamine release during induction of anesthesia with sufentanil or fentanyl (5) as other examples of narcotic-produced anaphylactoid reactions.

Reactions to ultrashort-acting barbiturates are also rare but have been reported. Several cases of anaphylactic-type shock in man due to thiopental have been reported (6). Some have been confirmed by basophil degranulation tests. In these cases, salivation, cyanosis, constriction of pupils, hypotension, and sinus tachycardia may occur. A similar response has been observed in three dogs after induction with sodium thiamylal. The dogs developed a thick frothy discharge from the upper airway within seconds. They were cyanotic with chest rales, labored breathing, and sinus tachycardia. Immediate intubation and supplemental oxygen along with suction produced satisfactory recoveries in each case.

Acute anaphylactoid reactions to anesthetic drugs is now sufficiently common to be considered a potential complication after the use of muscle relaxants, atropine, neostigmine, lidocaine, narcotics, and ultrashort-acting barbiturates (7). Intradermal testing, especially for the proposed utilization of muscle relaxants in human subjects, is now done in some hospitals. Presently, this does not appear to be considered necessary in animal subjects unless a previous anaphylactoid anesthetic reaction has occurred. These anaphylactoid reactions, although rare, can cause major problems (8).

In a study of 24 patients surviving life-threatening clinical anaphylaxis due to anesthesia, confirmation was made by determination of reaginic antibodies using the Prausnitz-Kustner test. This test can be done in humans and monkeys. Tests can be made for muscle relaxants and ultrashort-acting barbiturates (9). This is not a test that has been reported for use in veterinary medicine.

Antihistamines, steroids, and bronchodilators alone do not prevent reactions of an anaphylactic type to anesthetics. It is difficult to get sufficient correlation of the abnormalities of immunoglobulins and a history of allergies to anesthesic reactions (10). In a study of these reactions in Australia, the clinical features included cardiovascular collapse, bronchospasms, gastrointestinal symptoms, prolonged unconsciousness, pulmonary edema, convulsions, and occasionally death.

The use of contrast media can be incriminating in anaphylactic reactions during anesthesia (10). Intradermal testing has not been used in animals, but has been effective in predetermining potential reactions in human subjects, especially for muscle relaxants (11). Intradermal testing is safe and provides useful information, but false-negatives can probably occur. It is suggested that all induction agents should be diluted 1:100, muscle relaxants should be diluted 1:1000 (except *d*-tubocurarine, 1:10,000), and narcotics (other than fentanyl should be diluted 1:100,000. A wheal of 10 mm or more in diameter is acceptable as positive if it occurs within 10 minutes after the skin test (11). The combination of testing and history has been shown to be effective in preventing acute anaphylactic reactions (12).

General anesthesia and surgery affect cell-mediated cytotoxicity during surgical removal of primary malignant melanomas in patients. The cytotoxic ability was reduced in all patients 1 day after the operation and was not restored until approximately 6 days later (13). The distress of labor at the end of pregnancy causes an increase in maternal secretion of immunoreactive beta-lipotropin/beta-endorphin which is not related to the degree of pain. Epidural anesthesia has no effect on the plasma levels of these substances (14).

It has been shown that when halothane is used as the primary inhalant agent there is an effect on histamine released during bronchospasm in basenji-greyhound cross-bred dogs. Halothane, but not thiopental, significantly attenuates an increase in pulmonary resistance provoked by antigen challenge in these dogs. Plasma histamine levels, however, increased with either thiopenthal or halothane in this group of dogs, thus indicating the protective effect of halothane on the airways was not due to an inhibition of the release of histamine from mast cells (15). Isoflurane is also effective in attenuating increases in pulmonary resistance provoked by ascaris antigen aerosols in basenji-greyhound dog models for asthma. This supports evidence that isoflurane may be a useful alternative to halothane in patients with pulmonary edema, bronchospasm, or limited cardiac reserve (16). In the basenji-greyhound used as a bronchial asthma model, there is altered beta-adrenergic function in both airways and peripheral mononuclear leukocytes (17). Halothane was less effective than fentanyl in maintaining control or reduced levels of beta-endorphin immunoreactivity during the stress response of coronary artery bypass grafting, including cardiopulmonary bypass (18). High doses of morphine produced peripheral vasodilitation and frequently significant hypotension. These effects are thought to be due in part to the release of histamine. The greatest decrease in the systemic vascular resistance occurred in those patients with the highest level of plasma histamine. Patients receiving fentanyl have little change in plasma histamine and no decrease in arterial blood pressure or systemic vascular resistance (19). Clinically, it has been observed that morphine produced an anaphylactoid-type reaction in an aged, overweight poodle admitted for cataract surgery. The dog was hypotensive and developed pulmonary edema and bronchial spasms. Treatment with corticosteroids, oxygen through an established airway, and other supportive measures including reversal of the morphine by antagonist did not reverse the anaphylactic reaction. The dog died in congestive heart failure along with continued hypoxemia in spite of efforts to ventilate the animal. Histamine release by thiopentone may occur in animals or man (20, 21).

The inhibition of basophil histamine release has been attempted with anti-inflammatory steroids. The glucocorticosteroids inhibit the IgE-dependent release of histamine from basophils. Dexamethasone has the greatest potency, followed by betamethasone, prednisolone, and hydrocortisone. Dexamethasone inhibits IgE-induced histamine release without altering its rate. The mechanism by which steroids inhibit basophil IgE-dependent activation may be through a specific glucocorticoid receptor (22).

The three possible factors predisposing to althesin hypersensitivity are the total dose, the method of administration, and the presence of pregnancy (23). Hypersensitivity can occur even in the course of slow infusion of althesin (24).

The sustained vasodilitation in muscle produced by intravenous adrenalin may not be a local effect of adrenalin or its central reflex. It may be due to raised plasma histamine levels; intra-arterial *d*-tubocurarine infusions of 1 to 10 mg/minute into the brachial artery sometimes produced slight rises in plasma histamine. Similar responses can be seen after intravenous infusions of adrenalin at 10 to 20 mcg/minute, but no change in plasma histamine concentration was observed (25).

Penicillin appears to be one of the major causes of drug hypersensitivity in humans. Although not seen frequently in animals, this has been observed in cats, birds, and horses. During anesthesia in birds, concurrent use of penicillin should be avoided; it should be used with discretion in cats (26).

Systemic reactions are not unusual during radiological examinations requiring intravascular contrast media. The rate and manner of intravenous administration of dye for these studies can produce reactions; rapid bolus injections more frequently result in reactions than slow infusions. The procedures during which these reactions may occur include urographic, cerebral, and coronary angiography. These reactions frequently have cardiovascular and respiratory symptoms. The high iodine content of contrast media can cause several physiological effects. Contrast media are also hypertonic relative to plasma. Hemodynamic alterations may result from the administration of hyperosmotic solutions. These do not have to be related to systemic effects of contrast media producing histamine release; they may consist of an initial brief hypertensive response followed by mild hypotension. Initially, central venous, right ventricular, and pulmonary artery pressures increase, as does cardiac output. Hyperosmotic solutions may decrease systemic vascular resistance, and hemoglobin/hematocrit levels may fall. The high osmolarity may cause shrinkage and clumping of erythrocytes resembling an agglutination-thrombosis effect. There can be diuresis and potentiation of anesthesia (27). There is frequently an eventual vascular collapse marked by decreased cardiac filling pressures, compensatory ventricular tachycardia, hypotension, and other cardiac dysrhythmias. Oral, lingual, or pulmonary edema may develop, as may airway obstruction and bronchospasms. It is difficult to maintain oxygenation. There can be disruption of the blood-brain barrier, histamine release, and anxiety (27).

This phenomenon has been observed in the dog after diatrizoate meglumine and diatrizoate sodium renal graffin administered intravenously for contrast media studies of the kidney. The dog developed central nervous symptoms including seizures and eventually died in a complicated, nonreversible state including failing cardiovascular function and deterioration of the intestinal tract. Careful monitoring is needed while administering anesthetics if contrast media is to be injected intravenously. Treatment of contrast media reactions consists of adrenergic antagonist (epinephrine), aminophylline, anticholinergics such as atropine or glycopyrrolate as indicated, antihistamines, steroids, and intravenous fluids. Airway management and administration of oxygen is crucial, and the utilization of various life-support systems and monitoring are necessary.

After open-heart surgery, balanced anesthesia versus high dose fentanyl anesthesia produced only minor differences in lymphocyte proliferative responses. There was depressed immune function after open heart surgery, but not in association with anesthesia alone. The decreases were not mediated by hydrocortisone-sensitivty suppressor cells (28).

The RAST test for immediate type IgE-mediated thiopenthal hypersensitivity can result in false-positive results in patients with high serum IgE levels (29). Surgical stress can lead to depression of delayed hypersensitivity and impairment of immunofunction. These responses are not modified by epidural analgetic regimes that provide adequate pain relief (30). The partition of some parameters are cell-mediated.

The depression induced by the stress of parturition on some parameters of cell-mediated immunity of mothers and newborns can be at least partially prevented by using epidural anesthesia. There are reports of a significant increase in the T-cell count in mothers without epidural analgesia, but not in newborns (31).

Relationship between Allergies and Anesthetic Reactions

There is an ever-increasing incidence of allergies in the human population. It is reasonable that similar responses may be observed in members of various species of animals. Allergic reactions that cause asthma in man or asthma-like responses in animals are important preanesthetic considerations (32). Patients with asthma-like activity may have an immunological hypersensitivity, especially if IgE levels are above 200 IU/ml (33). A history of allergy with or without elevated IgE levels increases the difficulty of selection of anesthetic medications for either initial or repeat anesthesia (34). There is evidence for the role of IgE and anaphalactoid reactions in 70% of patients with muscle relaxant reactions. There is a related basophil histamine release to suggest that the histamine release is allergen induced (35).

From a biological viewpoint, human IgE antibodies and reaginic antibodies in experimental animals have similarities. Reaginic antibodies have been produced in the rat by immunization of antigen plus *Bordatella pertussis* vaccine. This antibody has also been found to be capable of sensitizing homologous skin in the rabbit, dog, mouse, monkey, guinea pig, and cattle. The physicochemical properties of homocytotrophic antibodies are similar to those of human IgE. It was also found that the antigenic structure of the immunoglobulin class to which the antibodies belong was different for IgG, IgA, and IgM in each species. This indicates the complexities of the use of the IgE antibody even if radio immunoassays are available as a means of determining if animals are likely to have anaphylactic reactions to anesthetics, muscle relaxants, narcotics, or other substances (36).

The influence of general anesthesia in operative surgery on immune responsiveness has been studied in blood obtained from women undergoing laproscopic sterilization and abdominal hysterectomies. There is no evidence that anesthesia or surgery impaired the immune response of the patients (37). Even so, there is concern. Etomidate has been recommended by some for its use in high-risk patients who may have allergies or who have exhibited severe anaphylactoid responses with previous anesthetics (38).

Not all immune responses in surgical patients are caused by anesthetics. The advent of transplantation of body tissues has been accelerated because of the development of immunosuppression therapy. This not only reduces immune response, but also is of concern relative to possible infection and the response to anesthetics (39).

Treatment of Life-Threatening Allergic Reactions

The use of the IgE inhibition test, leukocyte histamine release test, or RAST does not appear to be practical in animal anesthesia in the near future. Consequently, potential for allergic reactions when barbiturates, narcotics, ketamine, or diazepam are administered should be considered. This may also occur when the iodine preparations for intravenous contrast media radiographic procedures are used. Likewise, allergic reactions may occur during nontyped blood transfusion or from the administration of protomine to reverse the effects of heparin. Protomine is derived from salmon sperm and can produce anaphylactic reactions. Anaphylactic reactions can occur during administration of dextran, hetastarch, and other artificial plasma substitutes.

The treatment of life-threatening allergic reactions includes supplemental inspired oxygen, intravenous epinephrine, and intravenous infusion of crystalloid or colloid solutions. The administration of intravenous aminophilline may be indicated if bronchospasms are severe or sustained. Medications necessary to maintain tissue perfusion include steroids and anticholinergics. The beta-adenergic-stimulating effect of epinephrine relaxes bronchial smooth muscle and can be of benefit in bronchial spasm. Specific corticosteroids do not block interactions of drugs with IgE antibodies or prevent the release of chemical mediators from mass cells and basophils. Nevertheless, they do not have an adverse affect. The pure beta-adrenergic-stimulating effect of isoproterenol is frequently beneficial during allergic reactions, but the drug must be administered cautiously in the presence of hypovolemia or cardiac irritability, which commonly is associated with these reactions. The pretreatment of high risk patients with H_1 and H_2 receptor antagonists (antihistamines) may reduce the likelihood of the development of severe allergic reactions. When allergic reactions do develop, progressive and prompt treatment must be initiated (1).

Associated Immune Responses

The massive liver cell necrosis that developed in 16 patients after halothane anesthesia has been investigated by serological techniques. In some patients, a specific halothane-related antibody has been determined, indicating that these patients are sensitized to halothane-altered liver cell membrane components (40). The newborn is particularly susceptible to the immunosuppressant effects of anesthesia in surgery (41). The lymphocyte depressant effects of general anesthesia are found to be significantly less when regional epidural anesthesia is used in contrast to general anesthesia in sheep. The lymphocyte response is related to dose and length of anesthesia (42). This was further documented as T-lymphocyte depression during and after surgery under general anesthesia (43). The depressive effect of surgery under general anesthesia or monocyte cytolysis and lymphocyte proliferation is partly transferable by serum factors (44). These may be considered Type II or III immune responses.

Anesthetics and Infections

All anesthetic agents at sufficient levels to control pain probably produce reduction in the traffic of small and blast lymphocytes (45). These factors may contribute to the affect of anesthetics on viral replication. Halothane at 2% reduced the number of infectious measles virus particles produced in cultured cells (46). It was further determined that total inhibition of replication of viruses may occur at 1.6 and 2% halothane. The viruses inhibited included vesicular stomatitis virus and herpes simplex virus Type I. The virus may be reduced by at least two orders of magnitude for vasicular stomatitis and four orders of magnitude for herpes simplex virus with 2.2% halothane. The Newcastle disease virus and measles virus are most susceptible to exposure to halothane (47). This can have implications for the potential of reduced virus ability in anesthetic circuits where halothane is in use. Viruses altered during the course of their replication by anesthetic agents such as halothane may produce variants. Most of these will probably be harmless, but it has been shown that a variant of measles virus can cause a latent central nervous system disease in children called subacute sclerosing panencephalitis (48). Reports of similar problems occurring in animal species were not found (48). It appears there is increased interpulmonary shunting during anesthesia after acute viral respiratory infection in sheep; impaired air arterial oxygenation is probably due to an increased shunting (49). The effects of halothane on the measle virus are probably due to its effect on RNA synthesis (50). Anesthetics may inhibit the ability of viral proteins to interact with each other or with target molecules. Patients harboring virus infections at the time of anesthesia may have the course of their infection altered by anesthetic treatment (50). This encourages preoperative evaluation to determine animals that may have been exposed to viral infections prior to anesthesia and may explain the development of disease in the postoperative period in some cases.

Phencyclidine (PCP) and some of its derivatives are psychotromimetic and have been used for anesthesia in animals. Phencyclidine can block potassium ion channels in brain tissue, and there is a specific binding to lymphocytes. It has been shown that phencyclidine depresses hemoral and cellular immune responses when immunocytes were treated with PCP. This may contribute to postoperative infection (51).

In addition to the potential of anesthesia to alter immune responses and protective mechanisms alter viral infection responses by systems, administrative technique may contribute to infection. Careful attention must be given to anesthetic equipment (especially endotracheal tubes and other rubber goods), anesthetic machines, syringes, needles, catheters, and other devices to assure that the cross contamination with infectious agents does not occur. This is especially true when anesthesia must be administered to animals with infectious processes before the same equipment is used on other subjects. The incidence of infections associated with the administration of anesthetics is usually not reported in the scientific literature. Spinal epidural abscess, an uncommon infection of the central nervous system, was reported in 1983 after a local anesthetic injection (52). Appropriate hygiene and sterilization of equipment is indicated, and proper care of intravenous administrations sets to avoid contamination is warranted to avoid postanesthetic infections and complications. Postanesthetic infections may well be due to alterations in immune mechanisms rather than the induction of infectious material with anesthetic equipment.

References

1. Stoelting RK: Allergic reactions during anesthesia. *Anesth Analg* 62:341–356, 1983.
2. Frick OL: Immediate hypersensitivity. In Fudenberg HH, Stites DP, Caldwell JL, Wells JV (eds): *Basic and Clinical Immunology*, ed 2. Los Altos, Calif, Longe Medical Publisher, 1978, pp 246–266.
3. Wells JV: Immune mechanisms in tissue damage. In Fudenberg HH, Stites DP, Caldwell JL, Wells JV (eds): *Basic and Clinical Immunology*, ed 2. Los Altos, Calif, Longe Medical Publisher, 1978, pp 267–282.
4. Levy JH, Rockoff MA: Anaphylaxis to meperidine. *Anesth Analg* 61(3):301–303, 1982.
5. Rosow CE, Philbin DM, Keegan CK, Moss J: Hemodynamics and histamine release during induction with sufentanil or fentanyl. *Anesthesiology* 60(5):489–491, 1984.
6. Fox GS, Wikinson RD, Rabow FI: Thiopental anaphylaxis: A case and a method of diagnosis. *Anesthesiology* 35(6):655–657, 1971.
7. Fisher MMcD: The diagnosis of acute anaphylactoid reactions to anaesthetic drugs. *Anaesth Inten Care* 9(3):235–241, 1981.
8. Laxenaire MC, Monerit-Vautrin DA, Watkins J: Diagnosis of the causes of anaphylactoid anaesthetic reactions. *Anaesthesia* 38:147–148, 1983.
9. Fisher MMcD: Reaginic antibodies to drugs used in anesthesia. *Anesthesiology* 52(4):318–320, 1980.
10. Fsiher MMcD, More DG: The epidemiology and clinical features of anaphylactic reactions in anaesthesia. *Anaesth Intens Care* 9(3):226–234, 1981.
11. Sage D: Intradermal drug testing following anaphylactoid reactions during anaesthesia. *Anaesth Intens Care* 9(4):381–386, 1981.
12. Fisher MMcD: Intradermal testing in the diagnosis of actue anaphylaxis during anaesthesia—Results of five years experience. *Anaesth Intens Care* 7(1):58–61, 1979.
13. Moller-Larsen F, Moller-Larsen A, Haahr S: The influence of general anesthesia and surgery on cell-mediated cytotoxicity and interferon production. *J Clin Lab Immunol* 12(2):69–75, 1983.
14. Jouppila R, Jouppila P, Karlquist K, Kaukoranta P, Leppaluoto J, Vuolteenaho O: Maternal and umbilical venous plasma immunorective beta-endorphin levels during labor with and without epidural analgesia. *Am J Obstet Gynecol* 147(7):799–802, 1983.
15. Hermens JM, Edelstein G, Hanifin JM, Woodward WR, Hirshman CA: Inhalational anesthesia and histamine release during bronchospasm. *Anesthesiology* 61(1):69–72, 1984.
16. Hirshman CA, Edelstein G, Wayne R: Attenuation of allergic bronchoconstriction by halothane and isoflurane. *Anesthesiology* 55(3):386, 1981.
17. Hirshman CA, Downes H, Peters J, Chan SC, Hanifin J, Leon D, Margolin L: Basenji-greyhound dogs show altered beta adrenergic responses. *Anesthesiology* 55(3):385, 1981.
18. Cork RC, Hammeroff SR, Weiss JL: Effects of halothane and fentanyl anesthesia on plasma beta-endorphin immunoreactivity during cardiac surgery. *Anesth Analg* 64(7):677–680, 1985.
19. Rosow CE, Moss J, Philbin DM, Savarese JJ: Histamine release during morphine and fentanyl anesthesia. *Anesthesiology* 56(2):93–96, 1982.
20. Hirshman CA, Peters J, Cartwright-Lee I: Leukocyte histamine release to thiopental. *Anesthesiology* 56(1):64–67, 1982.
21. Lorenz W, Doenicke A, Meyer R, Reimann HJ, Kusche J, Barth H, Geesing H, Hutzel M, Weissenbacher B: Histamine release in man by propanidid and thiopentone: pharmacological effects and clinical consequences. *Brit J Anaesth* 44:355–368, 1972.
22. Schleimer RP, MacGlashan DW, Gillespie E, Lichtenstein LM: Inhalation of basophil histamine release by anti-inflmmatory steroids. *J Immunology* 129(4):1632–1636, 1982.
23. Simpson PJ, Radford SG, Lockyer JA, Sear JW: Some predisposing factors to hypersensitivity reactions following first exposure to althesin. *Anaesthesia* 40(5):420–423, 1985.
24. Benoit Y, Chadenson O, Duchoux B, Veysseyre CM, Bringuier JP, Veysseyre C, Descotes J: Hypersensitivity reactions to althesin infusion: measurement of complement involvement. *Anaesthesia* 38(11):1079–1081, 1983.
25. Mongar JL, Whelan RF: Histamine release by adrenaline and d-tubocurarine in the human subject. *J Physiol* 120:146–154, 1953.
26. Shelley WB: Indirect basophil degranulation test for allergy to penicillin and other drugs. *JAMA* 184(3):171–178, 1963.
27. Goldberg M: Systemic reactions to intravascular contrast media. *Anesthesiology* 60(1):46–56, 1984.
28. Eskola J, Salo M, Viljanen MK, Ruuskanen O: Impaired B lymphocyte function during open-heart surgeery. Effects of anaesthesia and surgery. *Br J Anaesth* 56(4):333–338, 1984.
29. Duech R, O'Connor RD: Thiopental: False-positive RAST in patients with elevated serum IgE. *Anesthesiology* 61(3):337–338, 1984.
30. Hjortso NC, Andersen T, Frosig F, Neumann P, Rogon E, Kehlet H: Failure of epidural analgesia to modify postoperative depression of delayed hypersensitivity. *Acta Anaesthesiol Scand* 28(2):128–131, 1984.
31. Ryhanen P, Jouppila R, Lanning M, Jouppila P, Hollmën A, Kouvalainen K: Effects of segmental epidural analgesia on changes in peripheral blood leucocyte counts, lymphocyte subpopulations, and in vitro transformation in healthy parturients and their newborns. *Gynecol Obstet Invest* 17(4):202–207, 1984.
32. Dundee JW, Fee JPH, McDonald JR, Clarke RSJ: Frequency of atopy and allergy in an anaesthetic patient population. *Br J Anaesth* 50:593–598, 1978.
33. Watkins, J, Clarke RSJ, Fee JPH: The relationship between reported atopy or allergy and immunoglobins: a preliminary study. *Anaesthesia* 36:582–585, 1981.
34. Fisher MMcD, Roffe DJ: Allergy, atopy and IgE. *Anaesthesia* 39:213–217, 1984.
35. Fisher, MMcD, Baldo BA: Role of IgE in anaphylactoid reactions during anaesthesia. *Ann Fr Anesth Reanim* 4(2):133–136, 1985.
36. Ishizaka T, Ishizaka K: Biology of immunoglobulin E. *Prog Allergy* 19:60–121, 1975.
37. Robertson AJ, Gibbs JH, Potts RC, Brown RA, Milne MK, Lawson JI, Beck JS: Effect of anaesthesia and surgery on the pre-S-phase cell cycle kinetics of mitogen-stimulated lymphocytes of previ-

ously healthy people. *Br J Anaesth* 44(4):338–347, 1983.
38. Watkins J: Etomidate: An "immunologically safe" anaesthetic agent. *Anaesthesia* 38:34–28, 1983.
39. Grizzle AL: Immunology, kidney transplantation and anesthesia. *AANAJ* 51(2):154–158, 1983.
40. Neuberger J, Gimson AE, Davis M, Williams R: Specific serological markers in the diagnosis of fulminant hepatic failure associated with halothane anesthesia. *Br J Anaesth* 55(1):15–19, 1983.
41. Puri P, Brazil J, Reen DJ: Immunosuppressive effects of anesthesia and surgery in the newborn: 1 short term effects. *J Pediatr Surg* 19(6):823–828, 1984.
42. Moore TC: Anesthesia associated depression in lymphocyte traffic: Less with regional anesthesia than with general anesthesia in sheep. *Am J Surg* 148(1):71–76, 1984.
43. Hole A, Bakke O: T-lymphocytes and the subpopulations of T-helper and T-suppressor cells measured by monoclonal antibodies (T11, T4, and T8) in relation to surgery under epidural and general anaesthesia. *Acta Anaesthesiol Scand* 28(3):296–300, 1984.
44. Hole A: Pre- and postoperative monocyte and lymphocyte functions: Effects of sera from patients operated under general or epidural anaesthesia. *Acta Anaesthesiol Scand* 28(3):287–291, 1984.
45. Moore TC: Anesthesia-associated depression in lymphocyte traffic and its modulation. *Am J Surg* 147(6):807–812, 1984.
46. Bedows E, Knight PR: Pressure reversal of halothane's antiviral effect. *Anesthesiology* 59(2):107–112, 1983.
47. Bedows E, Davidson BA, Knight PR: Effects of halothane on the replication of animal viruses. *Antimicrob Agents Chemother* 25(6):719–724, 1984.
48. Bedows E, Holland TC, Knight PR: Mechanism of halothane-induced inhibition of herpes simplex virus synthesis. *Anesthesiology* 57(3):358, 1982.
49. Dueck R, Prutow RJ, Richman D: Increased intrapulmonary shunt with anesthesia following acute viral respiratory infection in sheep. *Anesthesiology* 59(3):511, 1983.
50. Bedows E, Knight PR: Effect of halothane on measles virus RNA synthesis. *Anesthesiology* 59(3):385, 1983.
51. Khansari N, Whitten HD, Fudenbeg HH: Phencyclidine-induced immunodepression. *Science* 225(4657):76–78, 1984.
52. Rustin MH, Flynn MD, Coomes EN: Acute sacral epidural abscess following local anaesthetic injection. *Postgrad Med J* 59(692):399–400, 1983.

CHAPTER 24

Anesthetic Waste Gases and Your Health

ROBERT R. PADDLEFORD, D.V.M., D.A.C.V.A.

Introduction

The identification of an occupational disease often occurs after specific disease entities are identified among individuals in similar environments or similar occupations. This was the case with operating room personnel exposed to trace anesthetic waste gases.

The modern inhalant anesthetic agents came into widespread use in the late 1950s and early 1960s with the introduction of methoxyflurane and halothane. In 1967, a survey showed an unusually high incidence of headache, fatigue, irritability, nausea, and pruritus in a survey of 303 Russian anesthesiologists (1). It was also noted that 18 of 31 pregnancies among female anesthesiologists ended in spontaneous abortion. Numerous reports published after this article expressed concern over exposure to waste anesthetic gases. In 1974, a study was published in which over 49,000 operating room personnel in the United States were surveyed regarding occupational disease (2). It concluded that chronic exposure to trace anesthetic gases could be a causative factor for several disease processes, although the study did not establish a cause-and-effect relationship. Subsequent reports linked exposure to trace anesthetic gases as a possible causative factor in spontaneous abortions, congenital abnormalities, cancer, hepatic disease, renal disease, and neurological disease (3–6).

The issue of exposure to waste anesthetic gases is important to anyone using inhalant anesthetic techniques in the operating room. Although a cause-and-effect relationship has not been clearly demonstrated between the increases in certain diseases and exposure to waste anesthetic gases, there is considerable evidence to suggest that exposure to these waste gases can be a health hazard.

The toxicity of waste anesthetic gases seems to be related to metabolic degradation rather than to the parent agent. Evidence for the metabolism of a number of inhalant anesthetic agents was published in 1965 (7). Studies have indicated that metabolites of halothane can be recovered from the urine of patients for up to 20 days (8) and metabolites of methoxyflurane can be recovered for up to 10 days after anesthesia (9).

Studies of physician anesthesiologists have demonstrated traces of methoxyflurane in their expired air for as long as 29 hours, halothane for as long as 64 hours, and nitrous oxide for as long as 7 hours after the clinical administration of anesthesia to patients (10). One study showed increased fluoride ion concentration in a physician anesthesiologist following 6½ hours of occupational exposure to methoxyflurane (11).

This chapter will review what is known about the relationship between waste anesthetic gas exposure and certain disease processes and what can be done to limit or reduce this exposure.

Cellular Mechanisms of Anesthetic Toxicity

Any long-term organ toxicity caused by inhalation anesthetics is most likely related to the products of the inhalant anesthetic's biotransformation. Anesthetic biotransformation may produce cellular damage due to the accumulation of metabolites in excess of the threshold for organ toxicity, the production of reactive intermediates that form irreversible (covalent) bonds with tissue macromolecules, and/or the formation of metabolites that act as haptens that ultimately produce hypersensitivity or immune responses. Of the inhalant anesthetics, isoflurane is the most stable and least biodegradable, followed by enflurane, halothane, and methoxyflurane, which is the least stable and most biodegradable (Table 24.1).

A number of potentially toxic anesthetic metabolites have been examined, including inorganic fluoride, oxalic acid, and inorganic bromide. Inorganic fluoride is a major end product of methoxyflurane metabolism. Inorganic fluoride is responsible for the polyuric renal insufficiency syndrome that may occur after the administration of methoxyflurane anesthesia (12). This toxicity is dose-related, enhanced by enzyme induction, and attenuated by enzyme inhibition; it can be produced experimentally by the injection of inorganic fluoride in the absence of methoxyflurane anesthesia (12). Oxalic acid may also contribute to the nephrotoxicity associated with methoxyflurane, but it is not the major cause of this syndrome.

Inorganic bromide is a metabolite of halothane metabolism. The half-life of inorganic bromide in serum is approximately 11 days. Clinical signs of bromism in human patients occur when serum bromide levels reach 6 to 10 mEq/l and include headaches, sleepiness, weakness, and decreased sexual activity. Serum levels of 3 mEq/l have been reported in human patients after prolonged halothane anesthesia (13).

Under circumstances not completely understood, the halogenated anesthetics may be converted into free radicals. A free radical occurs when there is an unpaired electron in the outer molecular orbit of a compound. A free radical is highly reactive and can covalently bind to tissue macromolecules and thus alter their function. It has been demonstrated that halothane can covalently bind to liver microsomes and to tissue macromolecules (14). Unsaturated fatty acids and nucleic acids are most susceptible to covalent binding. Free radical intermediates may initiate preoxidation decomposition of the fatty acid complexes of the membranes of the hepatic endoplasmic reticulum and mitochondria. Exposure of the radical to oxygen results in cleavage of the radical. This results in severe structural and functional impairment of the adjacent fatty acid complexes and finally destruction of the cell membrane (12).

Table 24.1
Percentage of Inhaled Anesthetics Recovered as Metabolites in Humans

Agent	Structure	% Recovered as Metabolites
Isoflurane	CHF_2-O-CHCl-CF_3	0.3
Enflurane	CHF_2-O-CF_2-CHFCl	2.4
Halothane	CF_3-CHClBr	15–20
Methoxyflurane	CH_3-O-CF_3-$CHCl_2$	50

Although the inhalant anesthetic agents are nonreactive molecules and probably do not act as antigens, their metabolites could be highly reactive and could thus form stable bonds with protein which could serve as hapten-carrier complexes. Experimental data has shown that halothane metabolites can act as haptens in the rabbit (15), although the clinical significance of this has not been shown.

Rehder et al. (16) and Stier et al. (17) demonstrated that metabolites of halothane could be recovered from the urine of patients for up to 20 days after anesthesia. Metabolites of methoxyflurane have been recovered from patients up to 10 days after anesthesia (18), and nitrous oxide has been exhaled by patients for as long as 56 hours after its administration (10). Of particular interest to medical personnel exposed to waste gases is the retention of inhalant anesthetic agents in anesthesiologists after routine occupational exposure demonstrated by Corbett and Ball (19). They showed that traces of anesthetic gases could be found in the expired air of anesthesiologists for as long as 64 hours with halothane, 29 hours with methoxyflurane, and 7 hours with nitrous oxide after the administration of clinical anesthesia. This demonstrated that anesthesiologists could in fact retain inhalant anesthetics in their bodies after routine exposure to waste anesthetic gases and thus chronic exposure to metabolites might occur.

Reproductive Problems and Anesthetic Gas Exposure

The evidence that chronic exposure to waste anesthetic gases may adversely effect reproduction includes both human epidemiological studies and animal experiments. A significant and consistent finding of several epidemiological studies has been a higher than expected incidence of spontaneous abortions and congenital anomalies among operating room personnel.

The first report linking waste anesthetic gas exposure and possible reproductive problems appeared in 1967 (1). A survey of 303 Russian anesthesiologists noted that 18 of 31 pregnancies among female anesthesiologists ended in spontaneous abortion; 2 of the pregnancies ended in premature delivery, and 1 in congenital malformation. In 1970, a second report demonstrated a high rate of spontaneous abortion among anesthetists in Denmark (20). This report revealed that approximately 20% of all pregnancies ended in spontaneous abortion, compared with a rate of approximately 10% among the same group prior to working in the operating room. In 1971, Cohen et al. (21) reported a 38% abortion rate among physician anesthesiologists and a 30% abortion rate among operating room nurses. This compared to a 10% abortion rate for control groups of other female physicians and general duty nurses. Also, miscarriages occurred earlier in gestation in both physician anesthesiologists and operating room nurses compared with the control groups. This report suggested a fetal lethality that was possibly due to waste anesthetic gas exposure of the mother, although no specific anesthetic agent was incriminated, nor was a cause-and-effect relationship established.

In 1972, a report was published in which 563 married women anesthetists and 828 married women nonanesthetist physicians were studied (22). This study found the frequency of spontaneous abortion to be 18.2% when the anesthetists were working and 13.7% when they did not work. This compared to a spontaneous abortion rate in the control group of 14.7%. Also, 12% of the anesthetists suffered from involuntary infertility, compared to 6% of the control group.

In 1973, a survey of 621 female nurse-anesthetists was conducted in Michigan (23). This report indicated a high incidence of birth defects among children of nurse-anesthetists. The overall incidence of congenital anomalies was higher when the mother practiced during pregnancy (16%) than when the mother did not practice (6%).

In 1974, a national study of occupational disease among operating room personnel was conducted (2). Questionnaires were mailed to 49,585 exposed operating personnel in four professional societies (the American Society of Anesthesiologists, the American Association of Nurse Anesthetists, the Association of Operating Room Nurses, and the Association of Operating Room Technicians) and to 23,911 unexposed individuals in two professional societies (the American Academy of Pediatrics and the American Nursing Association). These latter two groups served as controls. This study provided statistically significant evidence that the risk of spontaneous abortion was increased for women exposed to the operating room environment during the first trimester of pregnancy as well as during the preceding year. The increased risk was observed in female physician anesthesiologists, nurse anesthetists, operating room nurses, and technicians. The risk was estimated to be 1.3 to 2 times that of unexposed personnel. There was also evidence that supported an increased risk of congenital abnormalities among the live-born babies of the female respondents. The exposed female physician anesthetists showed a two-fold increase in congenital abnormalities when compared to the female pediatricians in the control group. There was also an increase of 25% in the incidence of congenital abnormalities for the wives of exposed male physician anesthesiologists.

Cohen et al. (24) published a report in 1980 based on a survey of 30,650 dentists and 30,547 dental assistants. This study looked at individuals heavily exposed to nitrous oxide waste gases; heavy exposure was defined as more than 9 hours of exposure per week. For wives of male dentists heavily exposed to waste anesthetic gases during the year prior to conception, there was a 1.5-fold increase in spontaneous abortions when compared to the control group. There was a 1.7- to 2.3-fold increase in spontaneous abortions among female dental assistants when they had heavy exposure prior to conception when compared to the control group. Heavy exposure of male dentists to nitrous oxide was not associated with a measurable increase in congenital abnormalities in their children. This finding differed from Cohn's study, in which there was an increase in congenital anomalies in babies sired by male anesthesiologists (3). However, the male physician anesthesiologists in Cohn's study were exposed to both nitrous oxide and halogenated anesthetic agents; this fact might account for the difference. Analysis of the overall incidence of congenital abnormalities in children of female dental assistants showed a 1.5-fold increase when the mothers were heavily exposed to nitrous oxide. When the rates for congenital abnormalities were examined by organ systems, there was a 2-fold increase in the rate of musculoskeletal anomalies among children born to exposed dental assistants as opposed to children born to nonexposed dental assistants.

Numerous experimental animal studies have demonstrated possible adverse effects on reproduction when animals are exposed to concentrations of waste anesthetic gases as found in operating rooms. In one study, rats subjected to continuous exposure to 20% nitrous oxide for up to 35 days demonstrated injury to spermatogenic cells manifested by a reduction in mature spermatozoa and the appearance of multinucleated forms (25). Other studies have shown (*a*) abnormalities in spermatogonial cells, reduced ovulation and implantation, and retardation of fetal development in rats exposed to the same anesthetic waste gas concentrations found in unscavenged operating rooms (26); (*b*) lethal effects of nitrous oxide on rat embryos (14); and (*c*) renal and hepatic damage, degenerative cerebrocortical lesions, and learning deficits in neonatal rats whose mothers were exposed to the same concentrations of trace anesthetic gases that are found in operating rooms during gestation (27).

As early as 1955, it was postulated that inhalation anesthetic agents might interfere with the cell division process when it was observed that patients with tetanus sedated with nitrous oxide developed severe leukopenia (5). A subsequent study confirmed that nearly all inhalation anesthetics can exert a concentration-dependent inhibition of cell division with all phases of the division process affected (28). However, the mechanism is not understood, and cell division is apparently not affected at concentrations of waste anesthetic gases found in unscavenged operating rooms.

It has been argued that one cannot accurately compare nonhuman animal studies with the events actually occurring in humans and that retrospective surveys of exposed personnel suffer from potential errors of responder bias, perception, and recall as well as the use of improper control groups. However, a recent article by Buring et al. (29) statistically analyzed the major retrospective studies appearing in the literature and determined that there is a statistically significant increase of 1.3 in relative risk of spontaneous abortion among both female physicians and female nurses exposed to waste anesthetic gases. For congenital abnormalities, the relative increased risk of 1.4 was of borderline statistical significance and only for exposed physicians. The mounting evidence seems to support the fact that exposure to waste anesthetic gases does indeed increase the risk of reproductive problems in exposed personnel.

Mutagenicity and Exposure to Anesthetic Gases

A mutation is a heritable change in genetic information that may be caused by a variety of factors, including chemical agents. Mutagen testing is primarily used to determine whether a chemical has the potential to produce genetic alterations in humans. However, mutagen tests have also been used to predict potential carcinogens.

Several tests are used, including the Ames Salmonella Assay (30). This bacterial assay system utilizes strains of *Salmonella typhimurium* that are dependent on exogenous histidine for growth because of a mutation in the gene that codes for histidine synthesis. A subsequent mutation that allows the bacteria to synthesize histidine is called a "reversion" and is detected when the bacteria can grow in a culture medium lacking histidine. With this assay, 85% of known carcinogens have been mutagenic with an incidence of noncarcinogic false-positives of less than 10% (30). Utilizing this system, halothane, methoxyflurane, enflurane, and isoflurane were demonstrated not to be mutagenic (31, 32). However, one study did show that the metabolites of halothane were mutagenic (26), although other studies have supported the original findings that halothane is not mutagenic (33, 34).

In a recent article, the mutagenic effects of halothane, fluroxene, enflurane, isoflurane, and nitrous oxide were tested using the sex-linked recessive lethal assay in the fruit fly, *Drosophila melanogaster* (35). Enflurane, isoflurane, and nitrous oxide were not mutagenic at the concentrations tested. Fluroxene and halothane were found to cause a dose-dependent and statistically significant increase in the rate of sex-linked recessive lethals, although halothane was only weakly mutagenic. However, the concentrations of halothane that the files were exposed to were in excess of the levels found in most unscavanged operating rooms. The overwhelming evidence supports the fact that inhalant anesthetic agents are most likely not mutagenic, at least at levels found in nonscavanged operating rooms.

Carcinogenicity and Exposure to Anesthetic Gases

Evidence that relates exposure to waste anesthetic gases and increased incidence of cancer can be divided into epidemiological studies and experimental studies. In 1968, Bruce et al. (36) published a study of the causes of death among anesthesiologists over a 20-year period. This study was based on 441 deaths among members of the American Society of Anesthesiologists from 1947 to 1966 and revealed a higher than normal incidence of death from reticuloendothelial and lymphoid cancer. In 1974, Corbett et al (37) published the results of a survey of 621 female nurse anesthetists in Michigan that demonstrated the incidence of malignancy among the nurse anesthetists was three times the expected rate. However, Bruce et al. were unable to confirm a high malignancy rate in a later survey, and the findings of Corbett et al. were challenged on the basis of small numbers and the years selected for comparison (38). A nationwide epidemiological survey conducted by the American Society of Anesthesiologists suggested a higher incidence of cancer among female anesthesia personnel (2). The increased occurrence of cancer ranged from 1.3 to 2 for female physician anesthesiologists, nurse-anesthetists, operating room nurses, and technicians when compared to unexposed control groups consisting of pediatricians and nonoperating room nurses. Separate analysis by type and location of tumor indicated there was no statistically significant difference between types of cancer, with the exception of leukemia and lymphoma. There was no difference found between exposed and unexposed males. The results of this study were criticized because of the methods of data collection and for statistical inadequacies (39).

A survey of dentists and dental assistants demonstrated no significant increase in the rate of cancer in male dentists exposed to high levels of nitrous oxide

(3). However, the data for the female dental assistants exposed to high levels of nitrous oxide waste gas did suggest an increased risk of cancer, although it was not a statistically significant increase.

The conclusions of the statistical analysss of Buring et al. concerning risk rates for individuals exposed to anesthetic waste gases was that there was no significant increased risk among men; however, among women, the increase risk rate was 1.4. This was due entirely to an increased risk of cervical cancer and did not take into account any other predictive variables (29).

Experimental evidence utilizing animal models and cell cultures have not demonstrated halothane, methoxyflurane, enflurane, isoflurane, or nitrous oxide to be carcinogenic (33, 38, 40). At present, it appears that experimental data and critical analysis of epidemiological studies supports the fact that exposure to the commonly used inhalant anesthetics does not increase the risk of cancer.

Hepatic Dysfunction and Exposure to Anesthetic Gases

In the late 1950s, halothane was introduced into clinical human anesthesia; over the next 10 years, it became the most popular inhalant anesthetic used in human anesthesia. Within a year after its introduction into clinical practice, isolated case reports of unexplained jaundice after halothane administration began to appear in the literature, and the term "halothane hepatitis" became popular. A retrospective epidemiological study was conducted in the middle 1960s to compile data on halothane hepatitis to determine if such an entity existed and how significant it was. The National Halothane Study examined 856,000 patients who had halothane anesthesia (41). The study revealed seven episodes of unexplained massive hepatic necrosis in patients after halothane anesthesia. No casual relationship between halothane and fatal postoperative hepatitis was determined; however, this published data only fueled the controversy.

Hepatotoxicity is most likely related to the metabolites of the inhalant anesthetics produced during biodegradation. It was not until the middle 1960s that it was recognized that halothane and methoxyflurane were in fact biotransformed by the liver (42). For halothane, this metabolism can occur via an oxidative hepatic microsomal enzyme pathway (major pathway) that produces relatively harmless metabolites or it can occur via a reductive pathway (nonoxygen dependent and minor pathway) that produces potentially harmful metabolites. Therefore, the toxicity of the inhalant anesthetics, especially halothane, seems to be related to their metabolic degradation rather than to the parent compound itself.

There are three mechanisms by which reactive metabolite intermediates can cause liver damage (43). In the first, lipoperoxidation consists of hydrogen abstraction followed by oxygen incorporation into long chain polyeonic unsaturated fatty acids of intracellular membranes and organelles by action of electronegativity of free radicals. The peroxylipids break down into aldehydes and carboxylic acid derivatives; cellular necrosis can result. Secondly, there can be antioxidant depletion. Certain antioxidants in the cell, such as glutathione and alpha-tocopherol, inhibit free radical reactions, and depletion of these antioxidants can intensify free radical reactions. Finally, covalent binding can cause liver damage. Reactive intermediate metabolites can attach to proteins, lipoproteins, and lipids covalently; this changes the tertiary structure of the proteins and lipids, altering their function and resulting in necrosis. Of the three mechanisms covalent binding appears to be the most likely cause for liver damage produced by halogenated hydrocarbons such as halothane or methoxyflurane (44).

Certain factors seem to increase the risk of halothane hepatitis when human patients are anesthetized. Repeated administration of halothane has now been confirmed to be a risk factor for halothane hepatitis in humans (45, 46). Human studies have shown that obese females metabolize halothane to produce larger amounts of fluoride ion (47). In experimental rat models, mild hypoxemia along with halothane exposure has resulted in increased hepatic damage (48). Genetics may be a factor in that certain individuals seem to metabolize halothane via the reductive metabolic pathway normally as opposed to the normal oxidative metabolic pathway (49). Finally, optimal metabolism of halothane occurs with low-dose chronic exposure (50, 51). Low-dose chronic exposure is the type of exposure occurring to operating room personnel.

The above evidence supports the fact that halothane has a potential to produce hepatoxicity; however, this rarely happens. The rarity of halothane hepatitis in surgical patients is probably due to multifactorial etiology, with genetic predisposition playing a major role. Strong evidence indicates reductive metabolism of halothane is the basis of liver injury in patients anesthetized with halothane.

In 1969, Klatskin and Kimberg (52) published an article that described a case of recurring hepatitis in an anesthetist who was exposed to halothane. Although there was controversy over this report, subsequent studies have supported the fact that exposure to waste anesthetic gases does indeed increase the risk of liver disease. The retrospective study of the Ad Hoc Committee of the American Society of Anesthesiologists (2) showed that hepatic disease was more frequent in exposed female groups when compared to unexposed controls, even after excluding serum hepatitis. The rate of increase was 1.3- to 2.2-fold. There was also a statistically significant increase in hepatic disease in exposed male physician anesthesiologists compared with male pediatritions. The retrospective study of Cohen et al (3) also demonstrated a 1.6- to 1.7-fold increase in liver disease in dental assistants and male dentists exposed to waste anesthetic gas in the dental operating room. The review article by Buring et al. (29) states that the relative increase in risk of liver disease is 1.6 in men and 1.5 in women exposed to waste anesthetic gases.

In addition, there are at least two unreported cases of toxic hepatitis that have occurred in veterinarians exposed to waste gas concentrations of halothane (C. E. Short, personal communication). In each situation, the practitioner had been exposed over a number of years to halothane in the operating room. Neither practice used scavenging devices. In each case, a diagnosis of toxic hepatitis was made by a physician. Scavenging methods were incorporated in each practice, and the use of isoflurane replaced halothane. In each case, the veterinarian returned to active participation in his practice. The effectiveness of the control methods incorporated to reduce exposure in the second case has not been determined.

The mounting evidence supports the fact that halothane and possibly other halogenated inhalant anesthetics are potential hepatotoxins. In addition, chronic exposure to waste gases do in fact increase the risk of liver disease in operating room personnel.

Renal Dysfunction and Exposure to Anesthetic Gases

The first report of possible nephrotoxicity due to inhalant anesthetic agents was published by Crandell et al. (53) in 1966. They reported polyuric, vasopressin-resistant renal failure in 13 of 41 clinical patients who had received methoxyflurane anesthesia. Subsequently, Mazze and Cousins confirmed these findings (54, 55). Their reports indicated increased concentrations of inorganic fluoride and oxalic acid in serum and urine in all patients anesthetized with methoxyflurane. Inorganic fluoride can produce proximal renal tubular necrosis, and this was thought to be responsible for the nephrotoxicity. Enflurane and isoflurane can also be metabolized to fluoride ion but to a much lesser extent (56, 57). At the present time, direct nephrotoxicity in patients exposed to halothane, enflurane, or isoflurane has not been reported.

Until the early 1970s, inhalant anesthetic nephrotoxicity was associated only with clinic patients receiving methoxyflurane anesthesia. The report of the Ad Hoc Committee of the American Society of Anesthesiologists (2) was the first to demonstrate a possible link between chronic exposure to waste anesthetic gases and renal disease. This report did show a 1.2- to 1.4-fold increase in the incidence of renal disease (excluding cystitis and pyelonephritis) in exposed female groups compared to the control groups. There was no increased incidence of renal disease in exposed male physician anesthesiologists. The retrospective study of Cohen et al. (3) showed a 1.2- to 1.7-fold increase in renal disease in female dental assistants and a 1.2-fold increase in male dentists exposed to waste anesthetic gases. The review article of Buring et al. (29) confirmed a statistically significant increase in renal disease only in exposed females.

Again, published reports and corresponding statistical analysis support the fact that exposure to waste anesthetic gases increases the risk of renal dysfunction, at least in females.

Central Nervous System Dysfunction and Exposure to Anesthetic Gases

Several published reports have described an increased incidence of headaches, nausea, fatigue, and irritability in anesthetists and anesthesiologists exposed to waste anesthetic gases (1–3). Additionally, Bruce et al (58) demonstrated that 4 hours of exposure to waste anesthetic gas concentrations in volunteers decreased their psychomotor skills. They found impairment in an individual's ability to recognize a problem, make a decision on the problem, and act on that decision when exposed to trace anesthetic gas concentrations. Other studies have refuted Bruce's findings (59–61).

One of the metabolites of halothane biodegradation is bromine. Bromine has a half-life of 12 to 25 days and is slowly eliminated from the body. Bromine is known to cause mood changes, headache, ataxia, drowsiness, lethargy, psychosis, and depression when serum bromine levels of 6 to 10 mEq/l are reached (62, 63). In one experimental study (64), rats exposed to trace anesthetic concentrations of halothane for 4 to 6 weeks showed degenerative changes in cortical neurons and persistent learning deficits.

Chronic exposure to nitrous oxide has been associated with myeloneuropathies (65, 66). This may be related to an interaction of nitrous oxide and vitamin B_{12} (67). Cohen et al. (3) found a highly significant and medically important increase in the incidence of general neurological disease in male dentists (1.2- to 1.9-fold increase) and female dental assistants (1.7- to 2.8-fold increase) exposed to high levels of nitrous oxide. There was also a significant increase in tingling sensations, numbness, and muscle weakness in male dentists (1.8- to 3.8-fold increase) and female dental assistants (2.1- to 4.4-fold increase).

Again, the data support the conclusion that exposure to waste anesthetic gases may not only have short-term neurological effects (i.e., headache, nausea, depression, irritability, lethargy, and ataxia), but also long-term effects (i.e., myoneuropathies, muscle weakness, neuron destruction, and learning disabilities).

Hemopoietic Immune System Dysfunction and Exposure to Anesthetic Gases

Many studies have been conducted to determine the effects of the inhalant anesthetic agents on the hemopoietic and immune systems. Nitrous oxide is known to suppress bone marrow function (68). In patients exposed to 50% nitrous oxide for longer than 6 hours, deoxyuridine was suppressed and a megaloblastic hemopoiesis occurred. If the period of nitrous oxide exposure was less than 6 hours, the changes did not occur.

Eastwood et al. (69) demonstrated bone marrow depression in human leukemia patients from chronic exposure to nitrous oxide. Parbrook (70) was able to demonstrate bone marrow depression in normal subjects when exposed to nitrous oxide. Other studies have been unable to demonstrate hemopoietic changes in experimental animals after long term exposure to low concentrations of nitrous oxide (71).

However, in one unpublished case (C. E. Short, personal communication), a veterinarian experienced signs of fatigue and malaise. He had been using methoxyflurane for a number of years in his surgical practice. Upon examination by his physician, it was determined that his hemopoietic system was abnormal. Because there was no indication of infection, it was speculated that he was suffering from exposure to some toxin. Exposure to methoxyflurane was considered. After switching from methoxyflurane to isoflurane and scavenging waste gases, he was able to return to his practice, and the signs of fatigue and malaise have disappeared. However, no cause-and-effect relationship was ever proven in this case.

Numerous studies have examined the effects of anesthetics on the immune system (72–74). It does not appear that exposure to concentrations of waste anesthetic gases found in the operating room pose an occupational hazard (38, 72).

Magnitude of Operating Room Contamination by Waste Anesthetic Gases

In 1969, Linde and Bruce (75) documented the first occupational exposure of operating room personnel to waste anesthetic gases. They described peak levels of 27 ppm of halothane and 428 ppm of nitrous oxide in nonscavenged operating rooms. In 1970, Askrog and Peterson (76) reported average concentrations of 85 ppm of halothane and 7000 ppm of nitrous oxide in the breathing zone of the anesthesiologist when a nonrebreathing delivery system was used. Corbet and Ball (11) found 2 to 10 ppm of methoxyflurane in the area of the anesthesiologist and 1 to 2 ppm in the area of the surgeons in nonscavenged operating rooms. They then demonstrated that the methoxyflurane concentrations could be significantly reduced by placing a gas trap over the pop-off valve and venting the exhausted gases to the wall suction. Whitcher et al. (77) were able to reduce halothane contamination of the operating room by 10-fold with the use of appropriate scavenging equipment.

Several published reports have described the amount of waste gas exposure to veterinary personnel. Wingfield et al. (78) surveyed 210 practices, of which 80.8% were using inhalant anesthetics. They found waste anesthetic gas exposure was less in veterinary practices than in human hospitals. Exposure to the halogenated anesthetics ranged from 1 to 10.4 ppm for veterinarians and 1.3 to 20.9 ppm for animal health technicians. Waste anesthetic concentrations were affected by the size of patient, the type of breathing system used, and the use of scavenging systems. Ward and Byland (79) monitored halothane concentrations in 14 operating rooms and 3 treatment rooms in veterinary hospitals. All but 1 room was in a private practice. The air was monitored during regularly scheduled surgical or dental procedures under routine working conditions. The mean maximal steady halothane value for all rooms was 4.7 ppm, with a range of 1.1 to 18 ppm. Ten rooms exceeded the recommended 2 ppm maximum concentrations. Rooms with scavenging devices averaged 1.4 ppm, whereas nonscavenged rooms averaged 5.2 ppm. Milligan and Sablan (80) monitored waste gas contamination in a small animal recovery room. They found that the duration of excessive waste anesthetic gas concentrations (concentrations in excess of National Institute for Occupational Safety and Health (NIOSH) recommendations) averaged 59 minutes when halothane had been administered to dogs for 2 hours at 1.0%, 106 minutes when halothane had been administered for 2 hours at 1.5%, 30 minutes when methoxyflurane had been administered for 2 hours at 0.5%, and 30 minutes when nitrous oxide had been administered for 2 hours.

Methods to Reduce Operating Room Contamination

The NIOSH has recommended that the environmental concentration of halogenated anesthetic agents (halothane, methoxyflurane, enflurane, and isoflurane) should not exceed 2 ppm when used alone or 0.5 ppm when used with nitrous oxide; the nitrous oxide concentration should not exceed 25 ppm (81). Effective reduction of waste anesthetic gases involves effective scavenging, equipment leak prevention maintenance, and possibe alteration of anesthetic techniques.

SCAVENGING

The single most important factor in reducing operating room pollution is scavenging the waste anesthetic gases from the breathing circuit. There are three major components to a gas scavenging system: the gas-capturing system, the interface, and the disposal system (82). The gas-capturing system captures waste gases from the breathing circuit or mechanical ventilator. This system is incorporated into the "pop-off" valve (Fig. 24.1). Gas-capturing devices have also been designed for obsolete anesthetic machines still in use in veterinary practice (83). Gas-capturing systems are also available for nonrebreathing circuits (Fig. 24.2). The interface joins the gas-capturing mechanism of the breathing circuit with the disposal system (Fig. 24.3). This interface balances the positive pressure present at the site of overflow with the negative pressure existing at the disposal system. It is designed to relieve positive pressure if the scavenging system occludes and to prevent vacuum or negative pressures from reaching the patient's breathing circuit when a blower

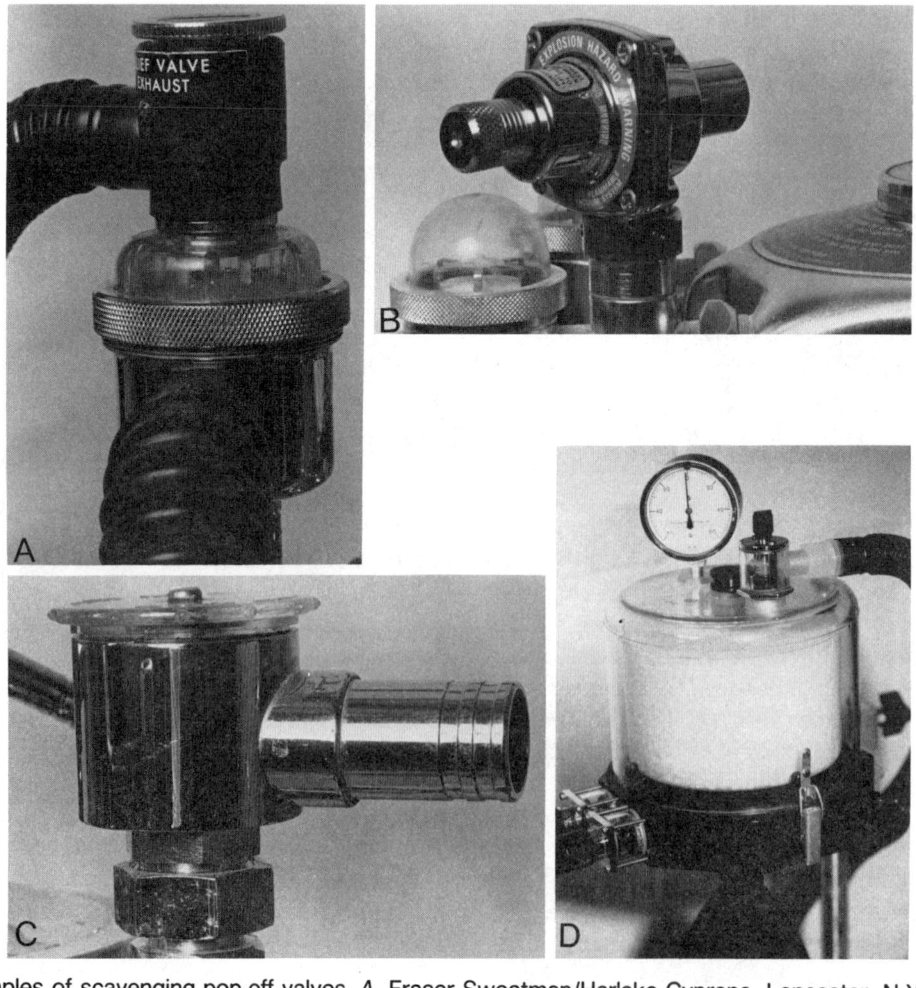

Figure 24.1. Examples of scavenging pop-off valves. *A*, Fraser Sweatman/Harlake Cyprane, Lancaster, N.Y. *B*, Omeda (formerly Ohio Medical), Madison, WI. *C*, North American Drager, Telford, PA. *D*, A.M. Bickford, Inc., Wales Center, N.Y.

or central suction is used for waste gas elimination. A resevoir bag should be provided at the interface to collect waste anesthetic gases until the vacuum system can eliminate them.

The disposal system ultimately removes the waste anesthetic gases from the operating room. Several options are available. They include exhausting the waste gases into the nonrecirculating portion of the air condition system, a central vacuum system, a dedicated suction system, a passive through-wall system, and the use of charcoal absorbers. In operating rooms with nonrecirculating ventilation systems, the scavenged waste gases can be conducted to the exhaust (return air) grills (Fig. 24.4). Flow through the grill into the ventilation system effectively removes the waste gases (82). Scavenging to an air conditioning system that recirculates the air is not recommended unless it can be exhausted before it enters the general circulation; otherwise, the recirculated air will contaminate all rooms within the ventilation system. A central vacuum system combined with surgical suction may be used to eliminate the exhausted gases. However, a better alter-

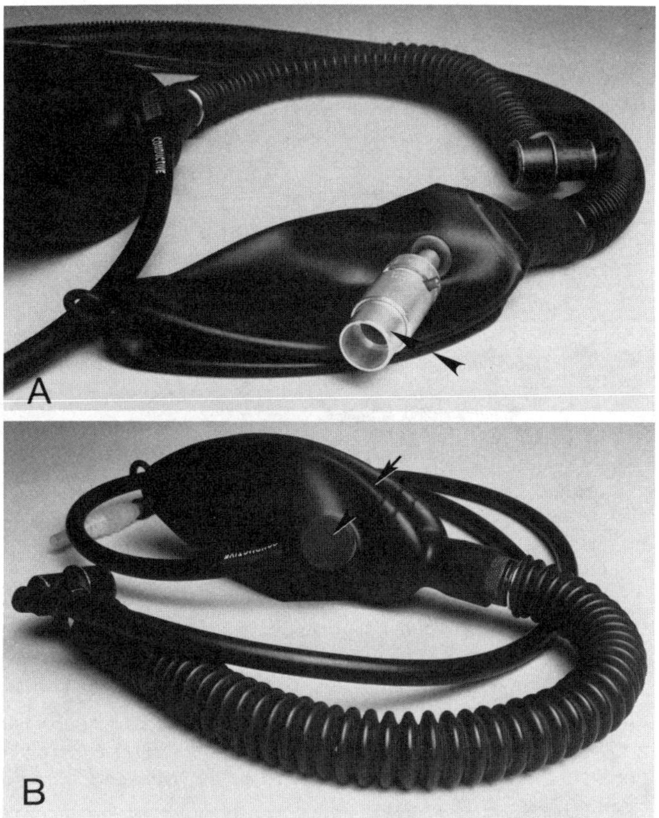

Figure 24.2. Examples of scavenging devices available for nonrebreathing delivery systems. The scavenging devices are attached to the outlet port of the nonrebreathing system and exhausted into the positive/negative interface. *A*, Dupaco, San Marcos, CA. *B*, A.M. Bickford, Inc., Wales Center, N.Y.

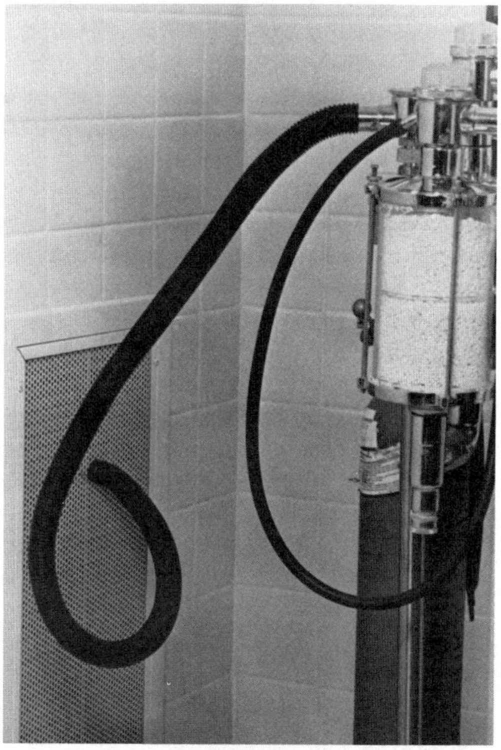

Figure 24.4. Scavenging system attached to exhaust grill of nonrecirculating air conditioning system.

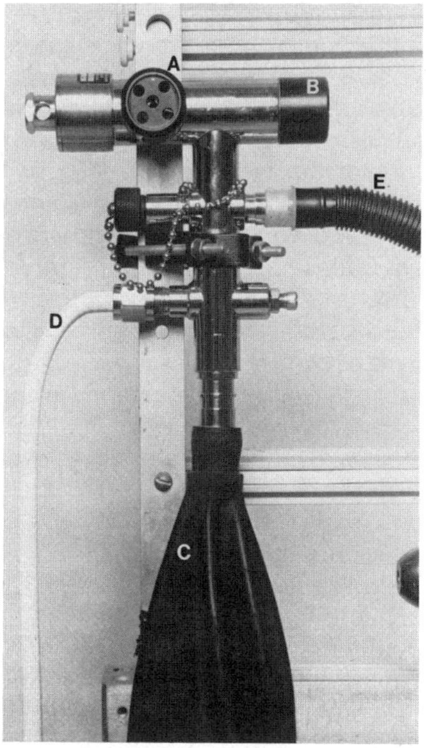

Figure 24.3. Example of a positive/negative interface for a gas scavenging system. *A*, Positive pressure relief valve designed to relieve excess pressure if scavenging system occludes. *B*, Negative pressure relief valve designed to prevent vaccum pressures from reaching breathing circuit when central suction or blower is used. *C*, Resevoir bag for collecting waste anesthetic gases until the vaccum system can remove them. *D*, Line to central vaccum system. *E*, Hose from scavenging pop off valve.

native is to utilize a dedicated or independent vacuum system to eliminate the waste gases (Fig. 24.5). The system should be readily accessible to the anesthetic machine and have a high volume flow (30 to 40 L/min) (82), although a high vacuum is not necessary. Passive systems exhausting waste gases through a wall fitting or window to the outside are also acceptable. The exhaust hose from the pop-off valve to the wall should be no more than 10 to 12 feet in length to prevent any problems with resistance to gas flow. All these systems should also have a positive pressure relief valve in case occlusion should occur.

Finally, activated charcoal absorbers can remove halogenated anesthetic gases from the waste gases (Fig. 24.6). However, these devices are ineffective in removing nitrous oxide (84), are expensive, and must be changed frequently. One method that does *not* work is to simply scavenge the waste gases to the floor. Although anesthetic gases are heavier than air, air currents in the operating room essentially mix the anesthetic gases throughout the room (82, 85).

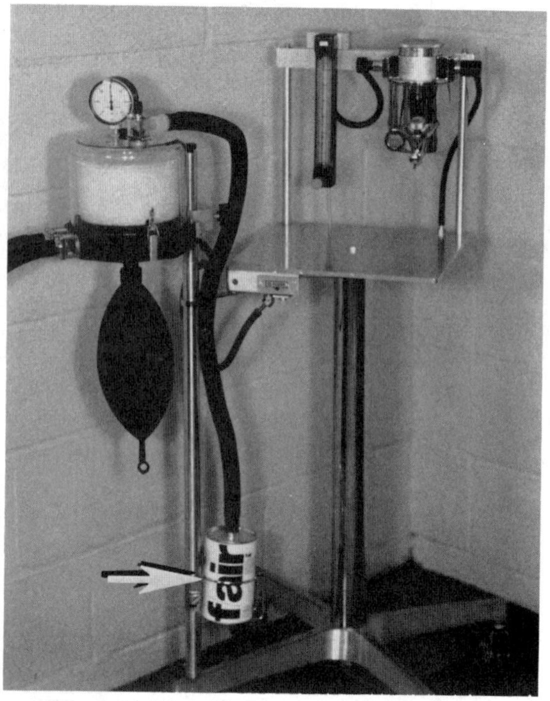

Figure 24.6. An example of a charcoal absorber attached to an anesthetic machine (*arrow*). The charcoal absorbs the halogenated anesthetics but not nitrous oxide (courtesy of A.M. Bickford, Inc., Wales Center, N.Y.).

EQUIPMENT LEAK PREVENTION MAINTENANCE

Although scavenging of waste anesthetic gases will reduce operating room pollution dramatically (11, 77–79), an ongoing maintenance program for equipment leak prevention is essential in reducing pollution. Anesthetic machines should ideally be serviced at 6-month intervals by a manufacturer's representative with continuous in-house maintenance by veterinary personnel. One report stated that significant leaks remained in 20% of the low-pressure systems and 25% of the high-pressure systems after routine manufacturer servicing (82). It is unrealistic to think that periodic maintenance by a manufacturer will keep equipment in a leak-free state.

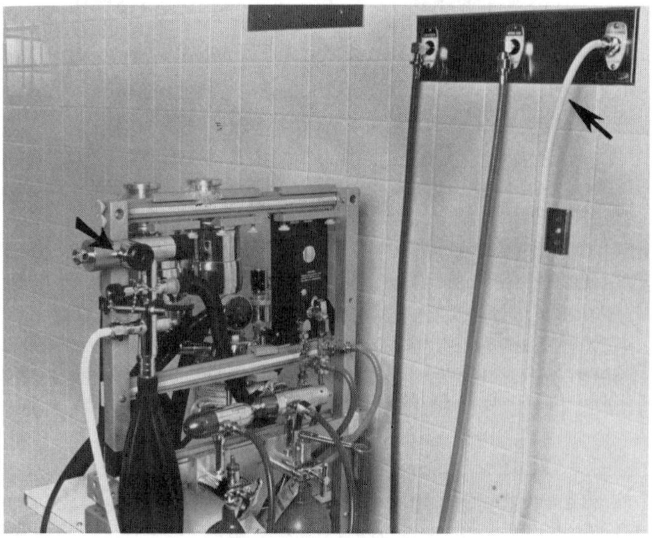

Figure 24.5. Scavenging system attached to a dedicated or independent vaccum system (*arrow*). A high volume flow is needed (30 to 40 L/min), although a high vacuum is unnecessary.

In examining for leaks, one must look at both the high-pressure and low-pressure portions of the equipment. The high-pressure portion of an anesthetic machine extends from the nitrous oxide tanks or central nitrous oxide supply to the anesthetic flowmeters. The low-pressure portion extends from the anesthetic machine flowmeters to the patient.

Leakage in the high-pressure system usually develops slowly and will continue until corrected. The most likely points of leakage include "quick connects" on the central inflow lines (crimp joints, screw joint seals and spring seals, and "O" rings), the nitrous oxide tank yolk connector, and the nitrous oxide regulator (Fig. 24.7). A 10% dilute detergent solution can be placed on joints to check for leaks. Bubbles will form at the leak sites. The high-pressure system should be checked for leaks on a regular basis. To check for leaks at the nitrous oxide cylinder yolk, turn on the cylinder, note the tank pressure reading, and turn the cylinder valve off. Recheck the gauge in 1 hour. If the pressure has bled off, there is a leak in the system. If internal tubing or reducing valves are leaking, the manufacturer will most likely need to service the machine. Lecky (82) found the average nitrous oxide background level in 20 operating rooms where anesthetics were administered was 19 ppm. This was without any an-

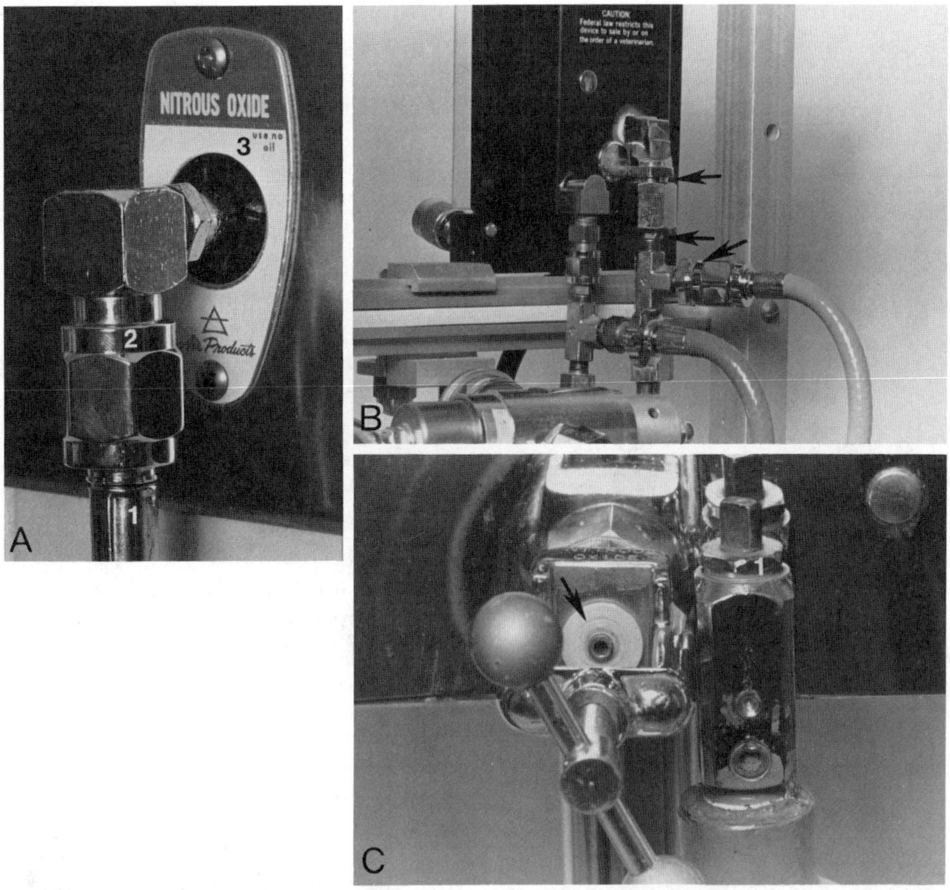

Figure 24.7. Possible sites for high pressure nitrous oxide leaks. *A*, "Quick connect" central inflow line. Leaks can occur at crimp joints (*1*), screw joint seals (*2*), or spring seals (*3*). *B*, Attachment of central inflow lines to anesthetic machine (arrows). *C*, Nitrous oxide hanger yolk. This usually occurs due to defective, omitted, or duplicated washers (*arrow*). Leaks may also occur at the cylinder valve (*1*).

esthetics being administered. Some rooms had as much as 66 ppm of nitrous oxide. After steps were taken to eliminate the high pressure leaks, the background nitrous oxide levels were reduced to an average of 0.2 ppm.

Leakage from the low pressure system extending from the flowmeters to the patient can be enough to virtually negate scavenging (82). In fact, nitrous oxide concentrations have reached 200 to 300 ppm in operating rooms from low pressure leaks alone (82). The low pressure system should be tested for leaks twice a week and/or whenever the soda lime is changed and/or prior to attaching a patient to the breathing circuit. Leaks in the low pressure system can occur at the connection between the flowmeters and vaporizers, at the unidirectional valves, at the soda lime cannister, around the endotracheal tube, from holes in the rebreathing bag and delivery hoses, and from the pop-off valve (Fig. 24.8). To test for low pressure leaks, place a stopper in the patient end of the Y piece and in the breathing bag attachment. Close the pop-off valve. The oxygen flowmeter is opened and the oxygen flow necessary to maintain circuit pressure at 40 cm H_2O for 30 seconds is determined. An oxygen flow of 200 ml/minute or less to sustain a circuit pressure gauge reading of 40 cm H_2O for 30 seconds is an acceptable rate (82, 85).

ALTERING ANESTHETIC TECHNIQUES

Many of the problems of operating room contamination can be reduced or eliminated by altering anesthetic techniques. Always make sure the waste anesthetic disposal system is attached and functional. Do not turn on the vaporizer or nitrous oxide until the patient is attached to the delivery system. Select the proper size of endotracheal tube for the patient, and make sure the cuff is adequately inflated. Once the patient is attached to the breathing circuit, disconnect the circuit as infrequently as possible. Empty the rebreathing bag into the scavenging system, not the room. Scavenge all nonrebreathing systems (Fig. 24.2). Only use chamber or mask induction when necessary, and make sure the mask fits tightly. Avoid spilling anesthetic when vaporizers are filled. It is advisable to fill vaporizers at the end of the day just before the staff

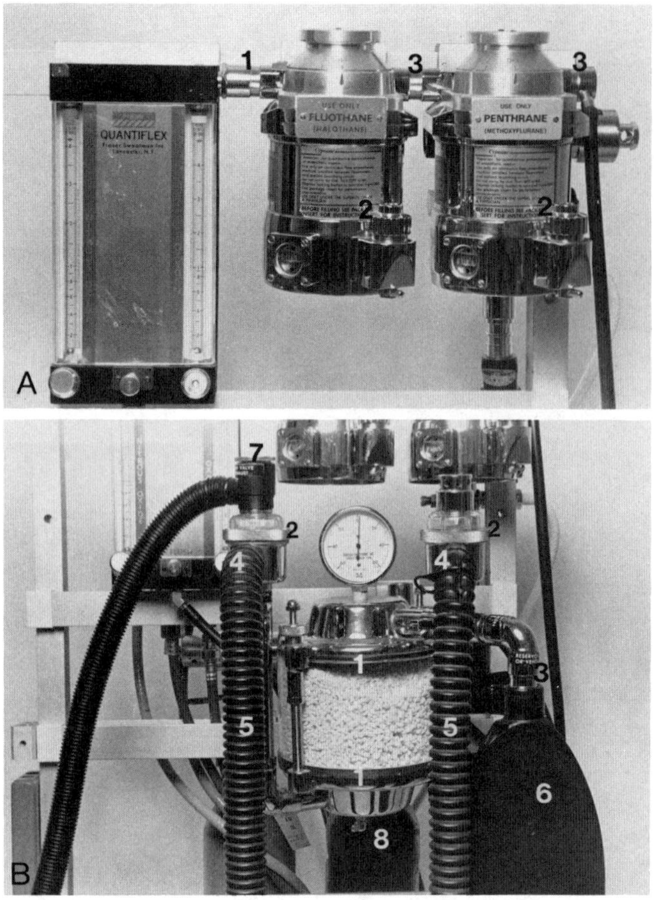

Figure 24.8. Possible sites for low pressure anesthetic leaks. *A*, Leaks may occur between the flowmeters and vaporizer (*1*), at the fill port of the vaporizer (*2*), or at the outlet port of the vaporizer (*3*). *B*, Leaks may occur in the circle delivery system. Leaks at the soda lime canister (*1*) are common and may be due to worn seals, soda lime particles on seals, or an incompletely closed canister. Leaks may occur at the dome valves (*2*) due to cross-threaded or loosely closed domes, worn seals, or cracked domes. Leaks may occur at the connection of the rebreathing bag (*3*) or the connection of the breathing hoses and the circle (*4*). Old, cracked tubing (*5*) or rebreathing bags (*6*) may leak. A leak may develop due to a faulty pop-off valve (*7*). An open drain port (*8*) will produce a substantial leak.

leaves. Recap the bottle of anesthetic after usage even if empty. At the end of the surgical procedure, keep the patient on 100% oxygen for as long as possible. Not only is this good patient care, but it allows expired anesthetic to be collected by the scavenging system. When possible, personnel should stay at least 3 feet from the anesthetic machine exhaust, the head of the recovering animal, and anesthetic spills. By observing these simple, basic precautions, operating room contamination can be greatly reduced, although it is impossible to completely eliminate it.

MONITORING WASTE ANESTHETIC GASES

Waste anesthetic gas concentrations are measured on a volume per volume basis and expressed as parts per million (ppm). The gas concentrations are determined by infrared analysis; samples can be sent to a laboratory or analyzed in-house using portable equipment (Fig. 24.9) (86). The portable equipment is expensive and may not be cost-effective for an individual veterinary practice. Companies that specialize in waste gas monitoring will monitor the operating rooms of private practices. Several samplings should be done throughout the day and at different times during the anesthetic procedure and an average contamination determined. It might be economically feasible for several practices to purchase and share an infrared analyzer. A minimal survey period of every 3 months has been recommended.

There are also nitrous oxide analyzers available that can be worn by personnel exposed to nitrous oxide (Fig. 24.10). These are dosimeters that are worn by an individual and monitor exposure to nitrous oxide; they are then analyzed for total exposure. These systems only monitor nitrous oxide exposure, not exposure to halogenated anesthetics.

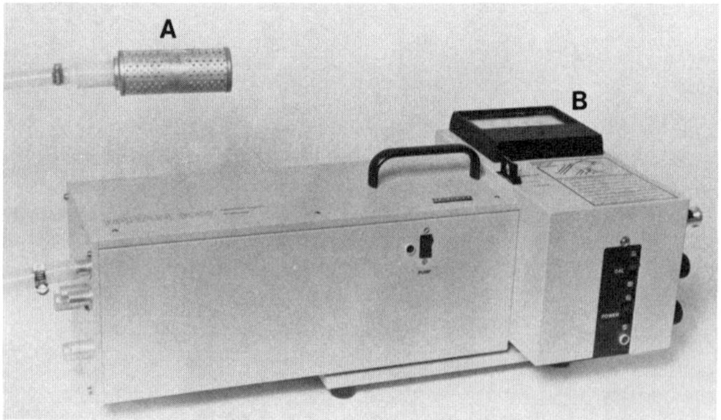

Figure 24.9. An example of a portable infrared gas analysis system. Room air is taken in at (*A*) and the parts per million (ppm) of gas is read on the scale (*B*). A separate filter and scale must be inserted into the unit for each gas monitored (Foxoboro Co., South Norwalk, CT.).

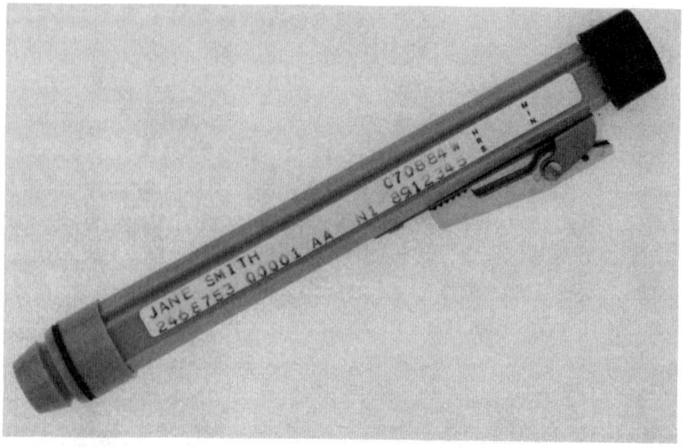

Figure 24.10. Example of a nitrous oxide dosimeter. This is worn by the individual and analyzed for nitrous oxide exposure (Courtesy of R.S. Landauer, Jr., and Co., Glenwood, IL.).

Conclusion

Published data seem to support the fact that there are potential health hazards from exposure to anesthetic waste gases. Reproductive, hepatic, renal, and central nervous system dysfunctions have all been described, as well as increased cancer rates in women. All personnel exposed to waste anesthetic gases should be made aware of the potential risks. Exposure to waste anesthetic gases can be kept to a minimum by using scavenging devices, performing preventative maintenance on equipment, and altering or improving anesthetic techniques.

References

1. Vaisman AI: Working conditions in surgery and their effect on the health of anesthesiologists. *Eksp Khir Anesteziol* 3:44–49, 1967.
2. Ad Hoc Committee of the American Society of Anesthesiologists: Occupational disease among O.R. personnel: A national study. *Anesthesiology* 41:321–340, 1974.
3. Cohen EN, Brown BW, Wu ML, et al: Occupational disease in dentistry and chronic exposure to trace anesthetic gases. *J Am Dent Assoc* 101(1):21–31, 1980.
4. Layzer RB, Fishman RA, Schafer JA: Neuropathy following abuse of nitrous oxide. *Neurology* 28:504–506, 1978.
5. Cullen BF: Cellular effects, teratogenicity and toxicity of anesthetics. Proceedings of the ASA Refresher Courses in Anesthesiology. 111:1–4, 1979.
6. Baden JM, Brown RB Jr, Cahalan MK, Dykes MHM: Hepatotoxicity and carcinogenicity. Proceedings of the ASA Refresher Courses in Anesthesiology 231:1–15, 1980.
7. Van Dyke RA, Chenoweth MB: Metabolism of volatile anesthetics. *Anesthesiology* 26:348–357, 1965.
8. Stier A, Alter H, Hessler O, et al: Urinary excretion of bromide in halothane anesthesia. *Anesth Analg* 43:723–728, 1964.
9. Holaday DA, Rudofsky S, Treuhaft PS: The metabolic degradation of methoxyflurane in man. *Anesthesiology* 33:579–593, 1970.
10. Corbett TH: Anesthetics as a cause of abortion. *Fertil Steril* 23:866–869, 1972.
11. Corbett TH, Ball GL: Chronic exposure to methoxyflurane: A possible occupational hazard to anesthesiologists. *Anesthesiology* 34:532–537, 1971.
12. Bades JM, Mazze RI: Anesthetic toxicity: A problem for everyone. Proceedings of the ASA Refresher Courses in Anesthesiology. 121:108, 1978.
13. Mazze RI, Calverley RK, Smith NT: Inorganic fluoride nephrotoxicity: Prolonged enflurane and halothane anesthesia in volunteers. *Anesthesiology* 46:265–271, 1977.
14. Howard LC, Brown DR, Blake DA: Subcellular binding of halothane-1-14C in mouse liver and brain. *J Pharm Sci* 62:1021–23, 1973.
15. Rosenburg P, Wahlstrom T: Trifluoroacetic acid and some possible intermediate metabolites of halothane as haptens. *Anesthesiology* 38:224–27, 1973.
16. Rehder K, Forbes J, Alter H, et al: Halothane biotransformation in man: A quantitative study. *Anesthesiology* 28:711, 1967.
17. Stier A, Alter H, Hessler O, et al: Urinary excretion of bromide in halothane anesthesia. *Anesth Analg* 43:723–728, 1968.
18. Holaday DA, Rudofsky S, Treuhaft PS: The metabolic degradation of methoxyflurane in man. *Anesthesiology* 33:579–593, 1970.
19. Corbett JH, Ball GL: Chronic exposure to methoxyflurane: A possible occupational hazard for anesthesiologists. *Anesthesiology* 34:532–537, 1971.
20. Askrog V, Harvald B: Teratogen effect of inhalations-anestetika. *Saertyk Nord Med* 3:490–500, 1970.
21. Cohen EN, Belville JW, Brown BW: Anesthesia, pregnancy, and miscarriage: A study of operating room nurses and anesthetists. *Anesthesiology* 35:345–347, 1971.
22. Knill-Jones RP, Moir DB, Rodrigues LV, et al: Anaesthetic practice and pregnancy—a controlled survey of women anesthetists in the United Kingdom. *Lancet* 2:1326, 1972.
23. Corbett TH, Cornell RG, Enders JL, Lieding K: Birth defects among children of nurse anesthetists. *Anesthesiology* 41:341–344, 1974.
24. Cohen EN, Brown BW, Wu MC, Whitcher CE, et al: Occupational disease in dentistry and chronic exposure to trace anesthetic gases. *J Am Dent Assoc* 101(1):21–31, 1980.
25. Kripke BJ, Kelman AD, Shah NK, et al: Testicular reaction to prolonged exposure to nitrous oxide. *Anesthesiology* 44:104–113, 1976.
26. Randall-Baker L, Milliken RA, Garro A: Halothane mutagenicity. *Anesth Analg* 58:64, 1979.
27. Chang LW, Katz J: Pathological effects of chronic halothane inhalation—an overview. *Anesthesiology* 45:640–653, 1976.
28. Sturrock JE, Nunn JF: Mitosis in mammalian cells during exposure to anesthetics. *Anesthesiology* 43:21, 1975.
29. Buring JE, Hennekens CH, Mayvent SC, Rosner B: Health experiences of operating room personnel. *Anesthesiology* 62:325–330, 1985.
30. Amec BN: The detection of chemical mutagens with enteric bacteria. In Hollaender A (ed): *Chemical Mutagens: Principles and Methods of Their Detection*. New York, Plenum Press, 1971, pp 267–282.
31. Baden JM, Brinkenhoff M, Wharton RS, et al: Mutagenicity of volatile anesthetics: halothane. *Anesthesiology* 45:311–318, 1976.
32. Baden JM, Kelly M, Wharton RS, et al: Mutagenicity of halogenated ether anesthetics. *Anesthesiology* 46:346–350, 1977.
33. Waskell L: A study of mutagenicity of anesthetics and their metabolites. *Mutat Res* 57:141–153, 1978.
34. Basler A, Rohrborn G: Lack of mutagenic effects of halothane in mammals *in vivo*. *Anesthesiology* 55:143–147, 1981.
35. Kundomal YR, Baden JM: Mutagenicity of inhaled anesthetics in *Drosophila melanogaster*. Anesthesiology 62:305–309, 1985.
36. Bruce DL, Eide KA, Linde HW, et al: Causes of death among anesthesiologists: a twenty year survey. *Anesthesiology* 29:565–569, 1968.
37. Corbett TH, Cornell RG, Lieding K, et al: Incidence of cancer among Michigan nurse anesthetists. *Anesthesiology* 41:341–344, 1974.
38. Ferstandig LL: Trace concentrations of anesthetic gases: a critical review of their disease potential. *Anesth Analg* 57:328–345, 1978.
39. Walts LF, Forsythe AB, Moore JG: Critique. Occupational diseases among operating room personnel. *Anesthesiology* 42:608–611, 1975.
40. Sturrock J: Lack of mutagenic effect of halothane or chloroform on cultured cells using azaquanine test system. *Br J Anaesth* 49:207–209, 1977.
41. Bunker JP, Forest WH Jr, Mostell F, et al (eds): *The National Halothane Study*. Bethesda, MD, National Institute of General Medical Services, 1965.
42. Van Dyke RA, Chenoweth MB: Metabolism of volatile anesthetics. *Anesthesiology* 26:348–357, 1965.
43. Brown BR, Jr: Anesthetic hepatotoxicity. Proceedings of the ASA Refresher Courses in Anesthesiology. 138A:1–4, 1981.
44. Widger LA, Gandolfi AJ, Van Dyke RA: Hypoxia and halothane metabolism *in vivo*. Release of inorganic fluoride and halothane metabolites binding to cellular constituents. *Anesthesiology* 44:187, 1976.
45. Fee JPH, Black GW, Dundee JW, et al: A prospective study on liver enzymes and other changes following repeat administration of halothane and enflurane. *Brit J Anaesth* 51:1133–1141, 1979.
46. Inman WHW, Mushin WW: Jaundice after repeated exposure to

halothane: An analysis of reports to the Committee on Safety of Medicine. *Brit Med J* 1:5–10, 1974.
47. Bently JB, Vaughan RW, Gandolfi AJ, Cork RC: Halothane biotransformation in obese and non-obese patients. *Anesthesiology* 57:94–97, 1982.
48. Brown BR, Sipes IG: Biotransformation and hepatotoxicity of halothane. *Biochem Pharmacol* 26:2091–2094, 1977.
49. Cousins MJ, Gourlay GK, Hall P, Adams JF: Genetics and halothane hepatitis. *Brit Med J* 213:1334–1335, 1981.
50. Stoyka WW, Havashi G: The effects of repeated ^{14}C halothane exposure in mice. *Can Anaesth Soc J* 24:243–251, 1977.
51. Sawyer DC, Eger EI, Bahlman SH, et al: Concentration dependence of hepatic halothane metabolism. *Anesthesiology* 34:230–235, 1971.
52. Klatskin G, Kimberg DV: Recurrent hepatitis attributable to halothane sensitization in an anesthetist. *New Engl J Med* 280:515–522, 1969.
53. Crandell WB, Pappas SG, MacDonald A: Nephrotoxicity associated with methoxyflurane anesthesia. *Anesthesiology* 27:591–607, 1966.
54. Cousins MJ, Mazze RI: Methoxyflurane nephrotoxicity: a study of dose response in man. *JAMA* 225:1611–1616, 1973.
55. Mazze RI, Cousins MJ, Kosek JC: Dose-related methoxyflurane nephrotoxicity in rats: A biochemical and pathological correlation. *Anesthesiology* 36:571–587, 1972.
56. Cousins MJ, Greenstein LR, Hitt BA, Mazze RI: Metabolism and renal effects of enflurane in man. *Anesthesiology* 44:44–53, 1976.
57. Mazze RI, cousins MJ, Barr GA: Renal effects and metabolism of isoflurane in man. *Anesthesiology* 40:536–542, 1974.
58. Bruce DC, Bach MJ, Jack A: Trace anesthetic effects on perceptual, cognitive and motor skills. *Anesthesiology* 40:453–458, 1974.
59. Cook TL, Smith M, Starkweather JA, et al: Behavioral effects of trace and subanesthetic halothane and nitrous oxide in man. *Anesthesiology* 49:434–440, 1971.
60. Garfield JM, Garfield FG, Sampson J: Effects of nitrous oxide on decision-strategy and sustained attention. *Psychopharmacologic* 42:5–10, 1975.
61. Smith G, Shirly AW: Failure to demonstrate effects of low concentrations of nitrous oxide and halothane on psychomotor performance. *Br J Anaesth* 49:65–70, 1977.
62. Johnson NE, Kennell EM, Behar MG, et al: Serum bromide concentrations after halothane anesthesia in man. *Anesthesiology* 46:498–601, 1977.
63. Tinker JA, Gandolfi AJ, Van Dyke RA: Elevation of plasma bromide levels in patients following halothane anesthesia. *Anesthesiology* 44:194–196, 1976.
64. Chang LW, Katz J: Pathological effects of chronic halothane inhalation: an overview. *Anesthesiology* 45:640–653, 1976.
65. Layzer RB, Fishman RA, Schafer JA: Neuropathy following abuse of nitrous oxide. *Neurology* 28:504–506, 1978.
66. Layzer RB: Myeloneuropathy after prolonged exposure to nitrous oxide. *Lancet* 2:1277–1280, 1978.
67. Nunn JF, Chanarin I: Editorial: Nitrous oxide and vitamin B_{12}. *Br J Anaesth* 50:1089–1090, 1978.
68. O'Sullivan H, Jennings F, Ward K, et al: Human bone marrow biochemical function and megaloblastic hematopoiesis after nitrous oxide anesthesia. *Anesthesiology* 55:645–9, 1981.
69. Eastwood DW, Green CD, Lambdon MA, et al: Effect of nitrous oxide on the white cell count in leukemia. *N Engl J Med* 268–297, 1963.
70. Parbrook GE: Leucopenic effect of prolonged nitrous oxide treatment. *Br J Anaesth* 39:117–127, 1969.
71. Cleaton-Jones P, Austin JC, Banks D, et al: Effect of intermittent exposure to low concentrations of nitrous oxide on hematopoiesis in rats. *Br J Anaesth* 49:223–226, 1977.
72. Duncan PC, Cullen BF: Anesthesia and immunology. *Anesthesiology* 45:522–538, 1976.
73. Duncan PG, Cullen BF, Calverly R, et al: Failure of enflurane and halothane to inhibit lymphocyte transformation in volunteers. *Anesthesiology* 45:661–665, 1976.
74. Nunn FJ: Editorial: Anesthesia and infection. *Br J Anaesth* 49:283–284, 1977.
75. Linde HW, Bruce DC: Occupational exposure of anesthesiologists to halothane, nitrous oxide and radiation. *Anesthesiology* 30:363–368, 1969.
76. Askrog V, Peterson R: Ferurening of operationsstuer med luft formige anaestetika og recontgenbestraaling. *Saertryk Nord Med* 83:501–504, 1970.
77. Whitcher CE, Cohen EN, Trudell JR: Chronic exposure to anesthetic gases in the operating room. *Anesthesiology* 35:348–353, 1971.
78. Wingfield WE, Ruby DC, Buchan RM, Gunther BJ: Waste anesthetic gas exposures to veterinarians and animal technicians. *J Am Vet Med Assoc* 178:399–402, 1981.
79. Ward GS, Byland RR: Concentration of halothane in veterinary operating and treatment rooms. *J Am Vet Med Assoc* 180:174–177, 1982.
80. Milligan JE, Sablan JE: Waste anesthetic gas concentrations in a veterinary recovery room. *J Am Vet Med Assoc* 181:1540–1541, 1982.
81. *Criteria for a Recommended Standard Occupational Exposure to Waste Anesthetic Gases and Vapors.* HEW Publication No. (N105H) 77-140. U. S. Department of Health, Education and Welfare, Public Health Service, Centers for Disease Control, National Institute for Occupational Safety and Health, Washington, D.C., 1978.
82. Lecky JH: The mechanical aspects of anesthetic pollution control. *Anesth Analg* 56:769–774, 1977.
83. Gallagher LV, Klavano PA: Scavenging waste anesthetic gases from obsolescent anesthetic machines. *J Am Vet Med Assoc* 179:1393–96, 1981.
84. Kim BM, Shivaji S: Adsorption characteristics of volatile anesthetics on activated carbons and performance of carbon cannisters. *Anesthesiology* 46:159–166, 1977.
85. Manley SV, McDonnell WN: Recommendations for reduction of anesthetic gas pollution. *AVMA* 176:519–524, 1980.
86. Whitcher C, Piziali RL: Monitoring occupational exposure to inhalation anesthetics. *Anesth Analg* 56:778–785, 1977.

CHAPTER

25

Veterinary Malpractice

CHARLES X. CONNICK, ESQ.

Introduction

Veterinarians, like other professionals, are becoming more and more involved in malpractice claims and litigation. These claims can result in large money verdicts and settlements, sizable legal fees, and disruption of the practitioner's personal and professional life. Veterinarians and administrators of veterinary hospitals and clinics should have an understanding of the legal process that resolves malpractice claims. This chapter will discuss the adverse effects of veterinary malpractice litigation, the basic legal concepts and theories of a malpractice case, the procedures followed in these cases, and the actions veterinarians and veterinary hospitals can take to protect their financial assets and to minimize the likelihood of malpractice actions.

This discussion will focus specifically on those claims that arise from the use of or the failure to use general, regional, or local anesthesia. Anesthesia-related claims are common; they illustrate the fundamental principles common to all veterinary malpractice cases. Further, many of the most serious cases brought against the veterinarian involve anesthesia.

Prevalence of Malpractice Claims

As of May 1981, the American Veterinary Medical Association (AJMA) Professional Liability Insurance Trust reports that 1 in 10 veterinarians were involved in claims of malpractice (1). In the period from 1976 to 1984, the total number of claims related to horses, cattle, and dogs was 5074. Of this number, 3397 were related to drug usage; of these, 364 involved anesthesia and 1486 involved surgery. The specific breakdown of drug-related claims can be seen in Table 25.1 (2). Statistics for the 7-year period from 1968 to 1974 indicate that 17.4% of the 812 claims that involved canine practice were drug-related and 57.4% of those claims were related to general anesthesia (3).

When the tremendous number of procedures that are performed in any one year is considered, the total number of claims is extremely small. Further, it must be kept in mind that all claims do not result in lawsuits. There are no published statistics on the number of lawsuits that result from these claims.

Effects of Malpractice Cases on Veterinarians

When a malpractice case is commenced, a number of events occurs. First, the veterinarian is brought into the legal system, where he or she has little or no experience. Second, the lawsuit puts the professional competence of the practitioner in question. The facts that give rise to the allegations of malpractice may form a basis for review of medical competence by the state qualification and competence board. Third, the

Table 25.1
Claims Related to Drug Usage

	Horse	Cattle	Dog	Total
Anesthesia	98 (11.0%)	24 (3.2%)	232 (11.9%)	354
Surgery	356 (39.9%)	316 (41.9%)	814 (41.7%)	1486
Medical	438 (41.1%)	414 (54.9%)	905 (46.4%)	1757
Total	892	754	1951	3597

veterinarian's personal assets, such as house, car, and savings, are put into jeopardy because the person suing (the plaintiff) is seeking to collect money damages.

INVOLVEMENT IN THE LEGAL SYSTEM

Lawsuits generally begin with an unexpected visit from a process server who hands the veterinarian papers stating that the veterinarian is negligent and owes the plaintiff a large sum of money. In addition to being an emotional shock, receipt of these papers (the Summons and Complaint) starts the lawsuit and puts in motion rules of legal procedure that can seem burdensome, a waste of time, and unreasonable. When served with papers, the veterinarian should immediately seek counsel from an attorney and refer the legal papers to the practitioner's insurance carrier. One should not expect the case to be easily or quickly resolved; cases frequently take years to conclude. Defense of a malpractice suit will result in legal fees, demands on the veterinarian's time and attention, and a verdict or settlement. If the verdict or settlement is against the veterinarian, there will be an obligation to pay money to the plaintiff. If the veterinarian wins the case, legal fees and defense cost must still be paid.

MALPRACTICE IS A CLAIM OF SUBSTANDARD PRACTICE

A malpractice suit is a negligence action against a professional. It asserts that the veterinarian was either unknowledgeable, unskilled, or careless in carrying out professional duties. It is a claim that the care and treatment rendered was substandard. The veterinarian loses a malpractice case when proven to have rendered services that fall below the care that the veterinary community accepts as standard and approved. The allegations can be such that the veterinarian's actions might become subject to close scrutiny by the state licensing board, by his or her employer, and by hospitals with which he is associated. Should the matter be brought before the state board that reviews quality and competence, the practitioner's license might be placed in jeopardy (4–7).

FINANCIAL EXPOSURE

In addition to incurring legal fees and defending his or her competence, the defendant faces a potential money judgement. The sum of money that can be awarded by a jury can be large. In New York, for example, the owners of a well-bred and successful racehorse sought $25,000,000 in damages against the hospital where the animal was euthanized after a recovery room accident. The issue in the case involved a claim that the horse's death was due to negligent anesthesia management of the horse. In another case, a veterinarian faced a claim for millions of dollars in damages when a bystander suffered brain damage after being knocked down by a horse receiving treatment. The claim in that case was that the failure to use anesthesia while performing a minor surgical procedure constituted negligence, with the result that a 47-year-old man was left totally disabled, in constant pain, and unable to work to support his wife and family. In each of these cases, the veterinarian and the veterinary hospital faced considerable financial risk directly related to their decisions on anesthesia management.

Most suits do not result in jury verdicts or settlements for hundreds of thousands of dollars. Indeed, it is encouraging to note that trials involving veterinarians frequently end with a favorable result for the defendant. A review of the jury verdict reporters from New York, Illinois, and California for the past 5 years discloses that most trials result in verdicts for the defendant veterinarians (8–10). These injury verdict reporters do not record most settlements; until recently, they have not published all verdicts. Although these jury verdict reporters are helpful in providing a general picture of the frequency of trials involving veterinarians and the results of those trials, they do not give a complete picture. The weaker cases tend to be settled before the case reaches trial; these cases are not reported. Further, the fact that most trials are successfully defended does not compensate the veterinarian for inconvenience and expense.

Legal Theory of Malpractice Litigation

Society, through the law, imposes duties, responsibilities, and standards on persons who engage in veterinary medicine. The law begins its regulation of veterinary medicine by first determining who can practice. Before an individual may practice, he or she must be qualified and licensed. The law continues its regulation of the professional activities of practitioners, in part, by allowing civil lawsuits against professionals whose practice does not meet the standards the law requires. Veterinary malpractice litigation is a lawsuit that determines whether in a particular case a veterinarian performed the duties that the law imposed on him when he practiced his profession.

REQUIREMENTS OF THE LAW

The law requires a veterinarian who uses anesthesia to possess certain knowledge and capabilities. This knowledge and skill must be used in a reasonable way, acting in accordance with the accepted and approved methods of anesthesia used in the community in which the practice is located. Where a veterinarian's care and treatment departs from standard and approved practice, an act of malpractice has been committed. To put it in layman's terms, malpractice is bad, substandard, or careless practice. This malpractice can be due to lack of knowledge, lack of skill, the careless application of knowledge or skill, or the failure of the anesthesiologist to render the best judgment after careful examination and consideration of alternate methods (11, 12).

APPROVED AND ACCEPTED PRACTICE IN THE COMMUNITY

A veterinarian using anesthesia is required to use anesthetics and make decisions with regard to anesthesia in accordance with good, accepted, and approved methods and techniques in general use in the community in which he or she practices. Certainly, the most prevalent method in use is likely to be in accordance with good practice (11, 12). However, the fact that a veterinarian is using a method, agent, or technique of a respected minority, even a very small minority, does not mean that the veterinarian is not following accepted practice (13, 14). Approved and accepted practice can and usually does include a variety of methods, techniques, and anesthetic agents. One has only to read texts on animal surgery and anesthesia to ascertain that there frequently are several acceptable ways to handle the same situation. The veterinarian should not be concerned that his methods are used only by a minority of practitioners as long as the community in which he practices regards them as a respected minority. The practitioner should be aware that a technique or agent that was once acceptable may have become unacceptable because of new information about the technique or agent or because of the development of other techniques or agents that significantly reduce risks or complications.

As far as a lawsuit is concerned, good and accepted practice is what the expert witnesses say it is. As a general rule, a party cannot prove a case against a veterinarian unless a fellow veterinarian takes the witness stand and swears under oath that there is an approved practice and that the defendant veterinarian departed from that approved practice (11, 15–17).

Experts can disagree on what the good, accepted, and approved methods and techniques are. Indeed, in Case 4 below, one of the major issues decided by the jury was identifying accepted practice for postanesthesia recovery of a horse. Because it had no experience with veterinary anesthesia, the jury based its decision solely on selection of which expert it believed as to what constituted good and accepted practice in that community.

In many cases, there is no dispute that good practice requires the veterinarian to follow a certain procedure; the issue for the jury to determine is whether the veterinarian followed good practice in that particular case. For example, there is no question that good practice requires monitoring an animal's vital signs while the animal is under anesthesia. Many cases involve nothing more than a determination of whether the veterinarian followed good practice by monitoring the vital signs.

A lawyer can evaluate the viability of a good case based on whether the plaintiff has a persuasive expert and strong literature support for his or her position. A lawyer can prepare a good defense if there are good witnesses available to support the client's anesthesia management.

The application of the concept of good and accepted practice in the context of a lawsuit can best be explained by examples of claims made against veterinarians.

Case 1

A busy local veterinarian received a phone call from a patron at a stable several miles away. One of the riding horses had a laceration of the skin under the right foreleg. The veterinarian, who was extremely busy handling office appointments, elected to send his experienced, licensed veterinary technician to suture the wound. The technician arrived and observed a quiet animal with a deep 3-inch laceration; the laceration was of a type she had frequently handled successfully in the past. The technician elected to suture the wound at the stable. Numerous bystanders were present. A twitch was used as a form of restraint; no chemical restraint was employed. No local or general anesthetic was considered or used.

The stable owner volunteered to hold the twitch, but this fellow was not as experienced as he claimed. While the wound was being sutured, the horse reacted violently, rearing back and striking the stable owner, who fell and struck his head on the concrete floor, fracturing his skull. He suffered brain damage that left him without hearing in his left ear and with partial loss of vision, loss of smell, and impotence, among other things.

The stable owner sued the veterinarian and technician, claiming that it was a departure from accepted practice not to transport the horse to a hospital for care under general or local anesthesia. He further claimed that the veterinarian departed from accepted practice by sending an unqualified person to perform the service. The plaintiff argued that good practice required the veterinarian to render his treatment under general anesthesia and away from bystanders.

Case 2

A dog underwent an orthopedic evaluation under general anesthesia. Before the dog fully recovered from the anesthesia, he was placed in a recovery cage and left unattended. He was later found dead from apparent suffocation. A malpractice claim was made based on the veterinarian's failure to follow the accepted practice of observing the dog until the animal was fully recovered from anesthesia (18).

Case 3

A veterinarian elected to perform a minor procedure on a dog without anesthesia. He asked the dog's owner to hold the animal. During the procedure, the animal bit the owner, leaving him with severe scars. The owner sued, claiming that good and accepted practice required the use of general anesthesia as restraint.

Case 4

While recovering from general anesthesia, a thoroughbred race horse attempted to stand from sternal recumbency. The horse's efforts were unsuccessful. Her rear legs splayed, and she suffered bilateral fractures of her femurs. The horse was euthanized. The plaintiffs claimed that it was a departure from good and accepted practice not to have a person pulling the horse up from a sternal to a standing position. Further, the plaintiff argued that when the horse attempted to stand, she looked groggy, and that under these circumstances good practice required the administration of xylazine in the recovery stall before the horse made attempts to stand.

Case 5

A dog owner asked a local veterinarian to groom her large and aggressive guard dog. The person that had groomed the owner's other dogs refused to handle this aggressive animal for safety reasons. The veterinarian placed the dog under general anesthesia and groomed him. The dog was sent home later that day with his owner. Three days later, the dog was brought back to the veterinarian's office in obvious distress. The animal died that day after intensive efforts by the veterinarian to save him; subsequent pathology reports confirmed that bronchial pneumonia was the cause of death. Months later, the owner sued the veterinarian, claiming that the dog had an upper respiratory infection when the general anesthesia was given and that good practice required that anesthesia not be given in such circumstances.

Of these five cases, Case 4 was tried and resulted in a defendant's verdict. Case 5 was discontinued during the course of the trial because the plaintiff was not able to secure an expert opinion, Cases 1 and 3 did not teach the trial stage, and Case 2 is taken from an article on a potential situation that may face a practitioner. These cases are reported to illustrate the type of allegations that are asserted against veterinarians, not to illustrate good or bad practice. In a lawsuit, what a jury decides is good practice may not be what the majority of the community believes good practice to be; it may be only what plaintiff's expert witness says it is. In those cases where plaintiffs offer the jury testimony from an expert who is clearly misrepresenting what is good and accepted practice, it is defense counsel's task to demonstrate these inaccurate portrayals and to present a clear picture of proper practice.

Theories on which plaintiff's attorneys will claim departures from good practice are as numerous as an attorney's mind is imaginative. Every step of anesthesia management is subject to review. Other frequently advanced theories concern failure to diagnose underlying pathology; failure to make all appropriate diagnostic tests; failure to properly interpret diagnostic tests; failure to use general anesthesia; failure to use regional or local anesthesia; improper use of anesthesia; failure to refer to a specialist; improper monitoring of a patient intraoperatively; failure to take proper corrective actions when faced with respiratory, metabolic, or cardiopulmonary complications intraoperatively; improper choice of preanesthetic agents or anesthetic agents; improper dosages; or failure to administer the agents in a timely fashion. This partial list illustrates only that each decision made by a clinician may be put into issue.

UNIVERSITY PRACTICE VERSUS PRIVATE PRACTICE

Attorneys handling veterinary malpractice cases have noted that farm, small private practice, race track, and university practice can vary greatly with respect to several aspects of veterinary care. Anesthesia is one area where practice can differ greatly. The reasons for this seem obvious. University hospitals have tremendous resources of personnel and equipment that are not available to the farm, private or track veterinarian. Frequently, economic limitations may dictate the service a practitioner may offer a dog owner or the owner of a $25,000 racehorse. These standards are not relevant to the university hospital's rendering of services. These factors can and do affect the kind of treatment rendered to an animal. The degree of difference is reflected in something as basic as record keeping. Compare the scant records kept in many nonuniversity situations to the complete charts kept at university hospitals. University hospitals are more likely to have the newest and most advanced monitoring and backup equipment. They also have the resource of personnel with a more diverse expertise. The differences in services between the university and nonuniversity situation can be dramatic.

The fact that the local practitioner does not have the resources of the larger hospitals does not mean that the local practitioner should stop using anesthesia or that if he does use anesthesia, his level of care is automatically below the accepted standard (i.e., the university hospital's standard). The local practitioner, however, must take into account the type of treatment that can be provided by these larger facilities, and failure to advise an owner of these facilities in appropriate cases may form the basis for liability. Referral of a sick dog of undistinguished pedigree to a university hospital hundreds of miles away may not be reasonable, but if the animal being treated is a show dog, then a failure to refer may create the basis of liability against the veterinarian.

An example of a situation in which nonuniversity and university practice may differ is when the local veterinarian acts as both surgeon and anesthesiologist in the performance of equine surgery. It would be unusual to find a veterinarian at a university hospital assuming this dual role, and it is certainly beyond dispute that closer monitoring of the animal can be achieved by an anesthesiologist whose attention is not diverted by the surgery itself. It has been suggested that the veterinarian who assumes this dual role is departing from accepted practice (19). It has been implied by some that to act as both surgeon and anesthesiologist prevents the veterinarian from proper monitoring. Therefore, in a situation where a horse suffered respiratory collapse and death during a castration procedure, the veterinarian was negligent in that he did not properly monitor the horse. The animal was given acepromazine as a sedative and glycerol guaicolate as a general anesthesia. Because the procedure took longer than expected, additional intravenous anesthetic was given and the respiratory collapse followed. Pathology reports were consistent with shock resulting from anesthetic death.

The defense of this veterinarian rests with the retention of an expert who believes and will testify that accepted practice in his community includes a veterinarian assuming both roles. The fact that a larger and better equipped institution would have followed different procedures does not mean that other procedures are substandard.

LEVEL OF KNOWLEDGE

A veterinarian must have a reasonable degree of knowledge for the type of practice engaged in, including accepted methods of clinical practice for the species and health problems treated. Implicit in this principle is continuing education and review of the literature in a practitioner's specialty. Knowledge of advances in medicine and changes in treatment is essential. If a clinician is a specialist, he is held to the standard of a specialist (11). For the anesthesiologist, this involves not only knowledge of the physiological and pharmacological aspects of anesthesia, but also knowledge of the use of anesthetic equipment. The practitioner must be aware of advances in the use of new anesthetic agents and equipment.

Lack of knowledge as a basis for a malpractice is illustrated by the testimony of the expert for the plaintiffs in the above-mentioned recovery room accident to the thoroughbred racehorse (Case 4). The owners who were suing the veterinary hospital for negligent anesthesia management placed on the stand a purported expert. He claimed that it was a departure from accepted practice not to have veterinarians and helpers in a 12 by 12 foot recovery stall during the entire period of recovery, including when the horse moved from a sternal position to a standing one. He explained that the anesthesiologist and helper would physically restrain the animal if it had not blown off enough anesthesia and that they would assist the animal when it attempted to stand. The experts put on the stand by the defense advised the jury that it is accepted practice not to have people present in the recovery stall at all times; one of the reasons for this is the safety of those assisting the horse. Under cross examination, the plaintiff's expert acknowledged that his experience was based on his education 15 years earlier and a small private practice; he admitted that he had not taken continuing education courses. This purported expert witness was not believed by the jury; he would face serious problems defending an action brought by an assistant who suffered personal injury when crushed by a horse in a recovery stall during a recovery he managed because he would have difficulty demonstrating to the jury that he had a reasonable degree of knowledge about the current accepted methods of anesthesia management.

ABILITY

In addition to knowing what to do, a practitioner must have a reasonable degree of skill and the ability to carry out approved methods of practice. A case in point is the example cited above in which a technician was sent to surgically repair a laceration to a horse (Case 1). This trained technician was quite skilled in the administration of local anesthesia (lidocaine and carbocaine) and the intramuscular use of tranquilizer-sedatives (xylazine) to do minor surgical procedures such as suturing. She did not have the skill or experience to give intravenous injections or general anesthesia. This lack of knowledge and skill and inability to consider alternative methods of anesthesia made the defense difficult. She knew of the procedures and methods, but she did not have the skill nor license to carry them out. Arguably, the person rendering the service did not have the requisite skill and competence to perform the services that she was engaged in.

Lack of the knowledge and skill possessed by the reasonably competent practitioner is a concern not only of the individual practitioner but also of the employer or the university hospital that asks the practitioner to perform the service. Employers and hospitals are responsible for the acts of their employees, servants, and agents (11, 12, 14, 20, 21). A veterinarian who designates another veterinarian in his employ to manage anesthesia is responsible for that employee's negligence. The legal responsibility can arise not only from the employer-employee relationship, but also from the fact that the resident or intern, for instance, did not have the requisite knowledge and skill to manage the anesthesia (14).

It is not enough that a veterinarians be knowledgeable and skillful; they must also use their best judgement and reasonable care in the exercise of their knowledge and ability. One must act as a reasonable and prudent practitioner in choosing a method of treatment and in consideration of all alternatives and options. Lack of knowledge and skill also can form the basis for liability when practitioners attempt to use new machines or drugs with which they are not fully familiar. A practitioner might be quite aware of the appropriate dosage of a drug and the manner of giving the drug, but through simple carelessness give the wrong drug or the wrong dosage; this constitutes negligence.

The law requires that the practitioner's best judgment and exercise of reasonable care be based on a careful examination. This includes taking a complete history, doing a thorough physical examination, completing laboratory tests, and monitoring appropriately. All indicated equipment and laboratory tests that are available should be used to make a complete and accurate assessment of the patient. Certainly, if an animal succumbs to cardiac, metabolic, or respiratory complications intraoperatively or postoperatively, the clinician should be in a position to describe to a jury the animal's heart rate and rhythm, blood pressure, and other vital signs customarily monitored. The clinician must be able to show that his judgement was based on a careful examination. Frequently, a case focuses on the question of whether a careful examination was done. A decision to use halothane, for example, may be very good judgement as long as there is no history of myocardial insufficiency or liver disorder (17). Failure to take reasonable steps to elicit a relevant history raises significant question as to whether treatment was based on a careful examination.

Liability for the Acts of Others

The law imposes liability on individual veterinarians and hospitals for the substandard practice of their employees, agents, and servants (11, 20, 21); this includes other veterinarians, nurses, or persons who maintain its machines. The imposition of liability encourages the profession to carefully screen those who perform acts for them. If a practitioner hires a newly licensed veterinarian and asks the new employee to induce anesthesia, and the animal dies because of the newly licensed veterinarian's lack of ability or skill, not only is the negligent veterinarian answerable for damages, but the employer is also liable. This point is illustrated in the example given earlier of the veterinarian who sent a technician to do a procedure (Case 1); that veterinarian is answerable for damages if his technician is found to be negligent.

EQUIPMENT

Advances in animal surgery in large part have been due to advances in anesthesia management, which in turn have been achieved by the development of monitoring and ventilation equipment. The careful examination, which in the past was done by eye, ear, and palpation, is today supplemented by monitoring machines and laboratory tests. Decisions about when to treat hypotension or metabolic imbalances are made based on what machines tell the veterinarian. If these machines malfunction and fail to ventilate or indicate an incorrect course of treatment, the anesthesiologist is faced with a problem. Was the failure of the machine caused by improper use of the equipment or by failure to maintain it? Should the failure have been detected based on clinical signs?

It may be that the maintenance department of the hospital or the product manufacturer is to blame in whole or in part when there is a breakdown of equipment. The veterinarian, however, must be in a position to take appropriate action in case of equipment failure. If a backup unit is unavailable, the veterinarian must be prepared to follow an alternate course of action.

In the studies by the AVMA Trust cited above, claims related to inhalation anesthesia such as halothane (Fluothane) and methoxyflurane (Metofane) were associated with poor maintenance and improper adjustment of the equipment and not to improper selection of the anesthetic agent (3).

Potential lawsuits that involve equipment include claims made by persons who are using the equipment or near the equipment. In the recent case of *Helminski v. Ayerst* (22), the parents of a developmentally retarded child brought a suit against the manufacturer of the general anesthetic, Fluothane. It was claimed that the child's in utero exposure to this anesthesia caused injury to his developing nervous system. The child was exposed while his mother worked full time as a nurse anesthetist administering the anesthesia. Although no claims have yet been asserted against veterinarians for this type of injury, increased studies in the area, as well as increased attention, may change this (23). The *Helminski* case resulted in a verdict for the defendant.

Equipment of a different type was involved in a 1985 trial in California. The issue for the jury to decide in that case was whether a recovery room accident to a valuable racehorse was caused by a defect in the floor of the recovery room or by the horse stumbling following a stormy recovery (24).

What Malpractice is Not

Unless a veterinarian promises a cure, the law does not guarantee a good result. The veterinarian is not automatically responsible for a bad result (11). A veterinarian is not responsible just because there are complications or known and accepted risks occur. The fact that a horse succumbs to hypotension during surgery does not imply liability. Postoperative myopathy or anesthetic accidents do not imply negligent anesthesia management. Anaphylactic reaction to a drug does not create liability. Every practitioner knows of anesthesia-related complications that occur despite good practice. To prove the case against the veterinarian, the plaintiff must prove that the bad result was the result of substandard practice.

A veterinarian is not held responsible for an error in judgement, provided the best judgement possible was made after a careful examination. A veterinarian who renders a careful examination and weighs alternate methods is not held responsible just because a retrospective look at the case makes it clear that the untaken alternative would have led to a better result. The question that the jury is presented with is whether the veterinarian acting with the information available after careful examination used his best judgement. Therefore, the anesthesiologist who elects to follow one course as opposed to another has not committed malpractice as long as he renders a careful examination and considers his alternatives (11, 17). The successful defense of an anesthesia case is frequently made possible by demonstrating to the jury that there was careful examination and by supporting the testimony with a clear and complete anesthesia record that is further corroborated by the results of the laboratory tests.

How Damages are Computed

Veterinary malpractice suits generally involve two types of claimed loss. The loss involves either personal injury to a bystander or assistant or property damage to an animal.

In a case involving personal injury to an assistant or bystander, the damages are awarded to the injured person for past, present, and future pain and suffering and for the financial loss from medical expenses and lost income (25). When the injured party is married, the spouse has an action for loss of services and consortium. In the example in Case 1 of the 47-year-old who suffered fractures of the skull, brain damage, impotence, loss of smell, and so forth, his damages for pain and suffering, medical expenses, and lost earnings were obviously significant.

In cases involving damage to property, such as cases involving injury or death to horses, cats, or dogs, the measure of damages is different. As a general rule, there is no recovery by an owner or an animal for pain and suffering to the animal or for the owner's loss of companionship. There are cases in which lower courts have allowed recovery for emotional distress and loss of companionship (26, 27). The measure of damage is the difference between the fair market value of the animal prior to the act of negligence and the fair market value of the animal after the negligence. The value of a mixed breed dog is small. The value of a thoroughbred racehorse is considerable (26–42).

The measure of damages takes into account the condition of the animal at the time of the negligence. A very sick animal with a poor prognosis for recovery has far less value than the same animal healthy. Therefore, if a horse undergoes general anesthesia for repair of an orthopedic condition and dies due to negligent anesthetic management, the damages paid by the veterinarian would reflect the fact that had the horse not died, racing and possibly breeding value would have been diminished by the underlying orthopedic problem.

Like the issue of damages, the value question is resolved by a jury based on the testimony of expert witnesses. In one case involving an unraced thoroughbred racehorse, plaintiff's expert testified that if the malpractice had not occurred, the horse would have recovered and been valued at $1,000,000. This expert based his evaluation on the horses's pedigree and training times. The defense expert looked at the same pedigree and training times and valued the horse at $7,500 without the underlying condition and at no value with the condition. The jury found against the veterinarian, but set his damages at a little over $8,000, which coincided with defendant's expert opinion of the animal's value plus the cost of the medical care and surgical procedure. In cases where there have been prior sales or the animal has been entered in a claiming race, the prior sale or offer of sale establishes the maximum value of the animal.

Anatomy of a Malpractice Litigation

The actual legal process and procedure in prosecution and defense of a veterinary malpractice suit varies from state to state and can vary within a particular state. For discussion purposes, the actual litigation can be broken down into three stages: pleadings, discovery, and trial. The time between the start of the lawsuit by service of the Summons and Complaint until the day of trial can be several years.

PLEADINGS

As set forth above, a party commences a lawsuit against a veterinarian by serving him or her with formal legal papers called a Summons and Complaint. The Summons gives the court jurisdiction over the veterinarian. The Complaint states in very general terms the basis for the lawsuit. The Complaint states that the plaintiff is seeking a sum of money; this frequently is large and rarely is related to the actual damages suffered.

Upon receipt of the Summons and Complaint, the defendant veterinarian must interpose a legal paper in answer to the plaintiff's Complaint. The defendant's Answer must be served within a prescribed time period. If it is not, the defendant can lose the case, jeopardize his defense, or at the very least create added cost and aggravation to himself, the defending attorney, and the insurance carrier.

Upon receiving a Summons and Complaint, a veterinarian should immediately seek the advice of counsel and give notice to the liability insurance carrier. Failure to take prompt action in this regard may jeopardize the defense and cause a carrier to deny to the veterinarian the benefits available under the professional liability policy. If the veterinarian was employed at the time of the alleged negligence, notification should be made to the employer and the employer's insurance carrier, because the defendant may be the beneficiary of the employer's insurance policy or statutory indemnification (43).

In some jurisdictions, along with the Answer a defendant veterinarian is entitled to ask for further particulars or amplification from the plaintiff concerning his claim. In New York, for example, a defendant is entitled to demand a Bill of Particulars, which requires the party suing to provide more details about the case to limit and frame the issues and prevent surprise.

DISCOVERY

The pleadings are intended to frame the issues of the lawsuit by showing what theory the plaintiff is going to proceed with against the veterinarian and informing the plaintiff of the veterinarian's defense. Once this is done, the lawsuit enters its discovery phase. The discovery phase is best thought of as a period of time before trial when each side is able to collect facts about the case from the other side to prepare a case or a defense for trial.

It is not necessary to go over all the discovery devices available to an attorney during this fact-finding part of the litigation. For the veterinarian, the particular discovery procedure that most involves him or her is the deposition. The deposition or examination before trial (EBT) is a procedure in which each side's lawyer is permitted to question the other side under oath about the facts relevant to the litigation. The EBT, in the opinion of many lawyers, is the most important part of the lawsuit and is frequently the most neglected by counsel. The veterinarian who is being sued should insist on meeting with his or her attorney well in advance of the EBT so the case can be adequately prepared.

The importance of the deposition can best be understood by knowing how it can be used. The court will instruct the jury that the EBT testimony is the same as testimony given at trial. It is evidence. In an anesthesia case, a veterinarian who testifies at an EBT without complete and careful review of the anesthesia record, the lab results, or the hospital charts is asking for trouble. Any error or misstatement caused by lack of preparation for the EBT becomes a piece of evidence that forms a basis of liability and is difficult to correct.

TRIAL

Once discovery is completed, the case is placed on a trial calendar, then the wait can be short or long. Within the New York metropolitan area, the wait on the trial calendar in one county is 6 to 8 weeks; in another, it is 1½ years.

The trial itself is inconvenient and time consuming. The courts generally cannot and do not accommodate the schedules of all the litigants; the trial may come at a time that does not fit into a veterinarian's schedule. Adjournments can be achieved, but the litigants must realize that a trial frequently requires the participation of several parties and that it is impossible to accommodate everyone.

Conceptually, a trial is nothing more than giving one's side of a claim to a jury, who are lay people from the community. This jury almost never includes people with training or experience in veterinary medicine. Indeed, in a malpractice case involving a horse in an urban area, the six members of the jury, the judge, and both lawyers may never even have ridden a horse. Juries tend to think of animal anesthesia in terms of human medicine. They do not expect the anesthetic to be the cause of injury or death.

BURDEN OF PROOF

At the trial, the plaintiff has the burden of proof. A party suing a veterinarian must place on a witness stand another veterinarian who will testify that the one being sued has departed from accepted and approved veterinary practice in the community. He must further prove that this negligence resulted in damage. With rare exceptions, if the plaintiff does not produce this expert testimony, the case will be dismissed before the defendant puts a witness on the stand. In fact, minor cases are frequently discontinued before or during trial because the plaintiff has no expert or does not with to pay for one.

In cases where a healthy animal is delivered to the veterinarian and the animal dies while in the veterinarian's possession, some cases have held that the plaintiff merely has to show that there was delivery and the burden then falls on the veterinarian to come forward with an explanation as to why the death was not a result of negligence (27). In such a case, for the plaintiff to prevail he would then have to come forward with expert testimony.

BATTLE OF EXPERTS

Once the plaintiff's expert witness testifies, the defendant will present his case and place on the stand an expert representing the defense; this expert will often disagree with what the plaintiff's expert said was accepted practice. In this situation, the jury will have to decide which expert to believe. The case will boil down to nothing more than a battle of experts, and the defendant's financial security may rest solely on which person made a better impression on the jury.

QUESTION OF FACT

Often the experts for each side do not disagree on accepted practice. The trial will turn on what the jury believes the facts in the case to be. Both experts may agree that good practice involves taking a history. The dispute in the case may be the simple question of whether the owner or the owner's agent told the veterinarian a particular fact. In one case, an owner claimed that prior to general anesthesia she had observed her dog to have a running nose and a cough. The veterinarian agreed that had the animal exhibited these signs of upper respiratory infection, he would have postponed the elective procedure. The veterinarian denied the animal had these symptoms. The issue in this case became not what accepted practice was, but whether the jury would accept the veterinarian's recollection as being true.

What the jury believes is determined by a number of factors. A defendant who is a good witness, who has clear and complete records, and who projects dedication to his profession will positively influence the jury's decision.

Avoiding Malpractice Suits

All malpractice suits cannot be avoided. Malpractice suits are started for a variety of reasons. Some of the primary reasons are the following.

1. They have merit and are justified. That is, there was substandard practice.
2. There is an extremely bad result, and plaintiff and plaintiff's counsel begin and prosecute a case hoping to discover a departure from accepted practice.
3. Lack of communication existed as to the condition of the animal, the treatment, and the reasons for treatment. The animal owner may also perceive the treatment of the animal and the owner to be uncaring, discourteous, or experimental.
4. Other veterinarians, usually subsequent treating veterinarians, comment adversely on the prior treatment without knowing all the facts and circumstances that faced the first veterinarian.
5. There was incomplete or sloppy record keeping.
6. To avoid paying a bill, when a veterinarian starts a lawsuit to collect for services rendered, a counterclaim that the veterinarian committed malpractice is made. This counterclaim is brought to excuse nonpayment as well as to collect damages.

CASES THAT CANNOT BE AVOIDED

Cases based on merit cannot be avoided. Veterinarians, like all people, have bad days and make mistakes. These cases can usually be settled promptly. Unfortunately, all nonmeritorious cases cannot be avoided, because avoidance is not under the veterinarian's control. There are known and accepted risks and complications related to the use of anesthesia. These occur despite the best practice. When the bad result involves the loss of large sums of money, some owners, injured people, and their lawyers view this as an opportunity to enhance their financial position. They sue without considering the merit of the case.

COMMUNICATION

Although all cases are not avoidable, there are ways to minimize the number of lawsuits. Good communication is probably the best way to avoid litigation, particularly unjustified litigation. Good communication means that the veterinarian must maintain a good relationship with clients both before and after an unwanted result. In one New York case, a Standardbred trotter undergoing a neurectomy died of complications related to the general anesthesia. In addition to claiming negligence with regard to the anesthesia management, the plaintiff said that he consented to the procedure with the understanding that local and not general anesthesia would be used (44). Certainly, an owner whose horse dies of anesthesia-related complications is less likely to sue if he is fully aware of the nature and risks of the anesthesia.

Anesthesiologists and veterinarians must communicate to their clients the risks and complications of surgical procedures as part of their job. It is interesting to note that at least one veterinarian seems to define surgical failure to include the clinician's failure to communicate with the client (45). Failure is not synonymous with malpractice, but the message is clear: communicate with your client. An owner who understands the prognosis, the benefits and risks of alternative methods of treatments, and the limits of what the veterinarian can do is less likely to have unjustified expectations and should not be surprised by a bad result.

Effective communication can be quite difficult and is sometimes impossible. Communicating with clients may be an easy task in a general small-animal practice in the suburbs where the owner brings the animal to the veterinarian's office and has one-on-one contact with the veterinarian. In this situation, the owner has chosen the doctor from among others and a good relationship between the two is likely. The owner frequently does not want to sue.

Communication becomes more difficult within the setting of a large university hospital, where the hospital's contact is with the referring veterinarian, the owner's representative, or the representative of the mortality insurance carrier who has taken over the medical care of the animal pursuant to the provisions of the insurance policy. As a practical matter, the treating doctors do not have any contact with the owner. Indeed, the owner may not be pleased with the decision to send the animal to the larger facility. The regular veterinarian may resent the insurance carrier's decision to refer the animal. With whom does the hospital's veterinarian communicate and from whom does he get consent?

The general answer to this question, from the point of view of a lawsuit, is that the hospital veterinarian must speak with the persons "accepted and approved practice" obligates him to speak with. It would also be prudent to have owners or their agents sign appropriate consent forms upon admission. In practice, the hospital doctor must rely on the referring veterinarian or the owner's agent to effectively communicate with the owner.

ADVERSE COMMENTS BY SUBSEQUENT TREATING DOCTORS

Professional colleagues seem to feel free to second-guess and criticize each other to owners. This generally occurs when the subsequent treating physician is in possession of an incomplete set of facts as given to him by the owner. These comments frequently are the seeds from which malpractice suits grow and are usually unrelated to successful treatment of a case. The critizing physician frequently regrets his or her comments when it is later discovered that they were not warranted and brought about litigation. Defense attorneys often learn during the course of discovery that the first criticism of their client has come from a subsequently treating physician. It is suggested that before veterinarians criticize each other, they should have a complete factual picture.

RECORD KEEPING

A clear and detailed record containing a complete history, findings on physical examination, results of laboratory tests, differential diagnosis, and plan of treatment prevents lawsuits and assists the defense of lawsuits. In an anesthesia case, a sparse, incomplete, or sloppy record makes it difficult to ascertain just what happened and why. A fair-minded owner, reviewing an anesthesia record with a retained expert, will have difficulty determining whether there is a basis for suit if the record is incomplete or illegible. The very incompleteness suggests carelessness to many, and a party may be forced to commence suit just to ascertain what happened. Some attorneys do not start lawsuits unless they have had an expert review the records and advise them that there is a departure from acceptable care. This is certainly not always the case; when it is true, however, a clear and complete record may prevent the lawsuit. Prosecution of a veterinary malpractice suit is expensive, and a prudent attorney will not start an action unless there is a reasonable basis for believing that there is a case.

A sloppy or incomplete record hampers the defense of a case in several ways. In addition to giving a bad impression, an unclear record cannot refresh a client's memory. When a clinician performs hundreds of procedures a year, it is difficult to recall the details of each case. Frequently, the anesthesiologist will not remember a significant detail. A poor record does not assist his recall; a clear record will.

An incorrect record poses serious problems for the defense of a case because this record will become evidence in the case and will have to be explained. As bad as an incorrect record may be, under no circumstances should a record be corrected, amended, or altered after a claim has been made against a veterinarian. Such a change is perceived by a jury as an improper alteration; in cases in which there is a "doctored" record, a defense is extremely difficult if not impossible even where there is no negligence (46). Prior to a lawsuit, if a correction is to be made, it is suggested that it be made as an addendum, and the corrected material not be deleted. A clear and complete record presents a wonderful first impression to a jury and is a valuable tool to the veterinarian to refresh his recollection as to his actions.

Minimizing the Effects of Malpractice Suits

The adverse effects of malpractice litigation can be minimized by education, insurance, and cooperation with your attorney. The veterinarian who understands what constitutes malpractice is able to protect himself with as little disruption to his life as possible.

INSURANCE

The single most important protection available to a veterinarian is professional liability insurance. This insurance is available through the AVMA-sponsored program. Insurance policies not only pay the amount of verdict against the veterinarian or the settlement made on his behalf up to the limits of his coverage, but also cover the cost of defending these suits. The cost of an effective defense is expensive. Expenses include not only the attorney's time, but also literature research, expert consultations, court expenses, and appeals. A meritless case taken to verdict may be lost without adequate representation; even if won, litigation costs can be great. Insurance carriers have experience in handling these types of cases and access to attorneys who specialize in defending professionals.

Insurance coverage should be greater than the value of the most expensive animal you deal with. Those practitioners and institutions treating racehorses syndicated at values in the multimillion dollar range should have coverage that will protect them in the event of loss.

Insurance contracts require prompt notification of the carrier of claims and cooperation from the insured. As a general rule, a veterinarian should provide notice to a carrier of any claim or any potential claim. Your professional liability carrier's interest is served by protecting your interests. Prompt notification to them protects your rights under the policy and allows the carrier the opportunity to take steps to protect your interest.

OTHER SOURCES OF INDEMNIFICATION

In addition to insurance coverage purchased by a veterinarian, the veterinarian may also be a named insured under a policy of insurance purchased by his employer or the hospital where he is employed. The veterinarian should make inquiry before accepting employment as to malpractice insurance with regard to defending and indemnifying employees who are sued. Contracts of employment may make specific provision for this insurance, and some jurisdictions provide by legislation for the employee's defense and indemnification (43).

DEFENSE COUNSEL

Whether a veterinarian has insurance or not, consultation and cooperation with an attorney who specializes in civil litigation is a necessity. The veterinarian should see the attorney as soon as it is believed there is a pending lawsuit; this may arise from a request by an owner's attorney for a patient's records. Legal counsel should be secured particularly when there has been personal injury to a bystander or injury to a valuable animal. The attorney will be in a position to advise concerning the release of records, notification of the insurance carrier, and any other steps that might be appropriate. As a practical matter, defense counsel is generally assigned by the insurance carrier. Despite the fact that the carrier assigns and pays counsel, the attorney is the veterinarian's attorney, not the insurance company's lawyer. The veterinarian's interests are paramount.

Conclusion

Malpractice lawsuits are a fact of life for all professionals. Litigation is society's way of resolving an injured party's claim against the veterinarian. The veterinarian is held liable for damages for a bad result only when this resulted from substandard practice. The veterinarian will not lose the case simply because a complication occurred or a retrospective analysis indicates that there was a better alternative. If the veterinarian follows the approved methods and procedures in the community in which the practice is located, this will serve to avoid most claims; for those claims that are brought, this will provide a viable defense.

The cost to the veterinarian of malpractice litigation is more than the potential exposure to a verdict of money damages. Legal fees, expert's fees, and other costs of defense are substantial. In addition, the veterinarian must take time and effort away from professional endeavors.

Fortunately, the adverse effects of malpractice litigation can be reduced by professional liability insurance. The risk of a claim being made can be minimized by good and effective communication and accurate record keeping.

References

1. Stauffer VD: Welcome to the world of malpractice. *J Am Vet Med Assoc* 178(10):1056, 1981.
2. Dinsmore JR: Drug related malpractice claims. Unpublished.
3. Dinsmore JR: Malpractice claims in small animal practice. *J Am Vet Med Assoc* 168(10):944–946, 1976.
4. *Amado v. Commonwealth State Board of Veterinary Medical Examiners* (1984, PA Commonwealth) 484 A2d 871.
5. *Brown v. Georgia State Board of Veterinary Medicine*, 134 Ga. App. 574, 215 SE2d 332.
6. *Lies v. Ohio Veterinary Medical Board*, 2 Ohio App. 3d 204, 2 Ohio BR 223, 441 NE2d 584.
7. *Eastep v. Veterinary Medical Examining Board*, 22 Or. App. 457, 539 P2d 1144.
8. *The New York Jury Verdict Reporter.*
9. *Cook County Jury Verdict Reporter: Illinois Jury Verdict Reporter.*
10. *Jury Verdicts Weekly (California).*
11. Lanzer LD, Boehm LJ, Bracken FB, Bryant BK, Leff JJ, Winter GR, Hughes HJ, Farrell RT, Thornton PW: *New York Pattern Jury Instructions and Cumulative Supplement Issued November 1984*, ed 2. Rochester, Lawyers Cooperative Publishing Co, 1968, vol 1, pp 390–403.
12. *Veterinarian's Liability for Malpractice*, Annotation, 38 ALR2d 503.
13. *Schreirher v. Cestari*, 40 A.D.2d 1025, 338 N.Y.S.2d 972.
14. *Henry v. Bronx Lebanon Medical Center*, 55 A.D.2d 476, 385 N.Y.S.2d.
15. Ytreberg D: Veterinarians. In *American Jurisprudence*, ed 2. 1985 Cumulative Supplement, vol 78, pp 1–8; Cumulative Supplement, pp 15–16.
16. *Southall v. Gabel*, 33 Ohio Misc. 194, 293 N.E. 2nd 891.
17. *Koehler v. Schwartz*, 48 N.Y.2d 807, 424 N.Y.S.2d 119, 399 N.E.2d 1140.
18. AVMA Professional Liability Trust: Could It Happen in Your Practice? *JAVMA* 169:1058, 1976.
19. AVMA Professional Liability Trust: Could It Happen in Your Practice? *JAVMA* 170:694, 1977.
20. Prosser: *Law of Torts*, ed 4, chapter 12.
21. Lanzer LD, Boehm DA, Bracken LJ, Bryant FB, Kassal B, Leff JJ, Winter GR, Hughes HJ, Farrell RT, Thornton PW: *New York Pattern Jury Instructions and Cumulative Supplement Issued November 1984*. Rochester, The Lawyers Cooperative Publishing Co, 1968, ed 2, 2 volumes. vol 1, pp. 548–566.
22. *Helminiski vs. Ayerst*, 766 F.2d 208 (6th Cir. 1985).
23. Steffy EP: Equine inhalation anesthesia. In Jennings PB (ed): *The Practice of Large Animal Surgery*. Philadelphia, WB Saunders Co, p 183. 1984.
24. *Jennings v. Baker*, *Jury Verdicts Weekly*, vol 29, no. 20, p 34.
25. Lanzer LD, Boehm DA, Bracken LJ, Bryant FB, Kassal B, Leff JJ, Winter GR, Hughes HJ, Farrell RT, Thornton PW: *New York Pattern Jury Instructions and Cumulative Supplement Issued November 1984*. Rochester, The Lawyers Cooperative Publishing Co, 1986, ed 2, 2 volumes. vol 1, pp 627–648.
26. *Knowles Animal Hospital v. Wills*, 360 So.2d 37.
27. *McDermott v. Sall*, New York Law Journal, December 9, 1985.
28. *Snyder v. Bio-Lab Inc*, 94 Misc.2d 816, 405 N.Y.S.2d 752.
29. *Melton v. South Shore U-Drive*, 32 A.D.2d 950, 303 N.Y.S.2d 752.
30. *LeBlanc v. Underwriter's at Lloyd's of London*, 402 So.2d L92, 22 ALR 4th 1040.
31. Annotation: *Livestock-Loss or Injury-Damages*, 79 ALR2d 677–750.
32. *Borousseau v. Rosenthal*, 110 Misc.2d 1054, 443, N.Y.S.2d 285.
33. *Young v. Delta Airlines*, 78 A.D.2d 616, 432 N.Y.S.2d 390.
34. *Corso v. Crawford Dog and Cat Hospital, Inc.*, 97 Misc.2d 530 415 N.Y.S.2d 182.
35. *DiMichele v. Filacchione*, 60 Misc.2d 619, 303 N.Y.S.2d 562.
36. *Miron v. Yonkers Raceway, Inc.*, 400 F.2d 112.
37. *Stettner v. Graubard*, 368 N.Y.S.2d 724.
38. *White Devon Farm v. Stahl*, 389 N.Y.S.2d 724.
39. Warren OL, Markinson GC: *Cumulative Supplement. Negligence in the New York Courts*. New York, Matthew Bender, 1984.
40. *Elements and Measure of Damages For Breach of Warranty in Sale of Horse*, 91 ALR3d 417.
41. *Measure, Elements and Amount of Damages for Killing or Injuring Cat*, 8 ALR4th 1287.
42. *Measure, Elements of Damages for Killing or Injuring Dog*, 1 ALR3d 997.
43. N.Y. Public Officers Law, p. 17.
44. *Massimo v. Woodhead*, New York Jury Verdict Reporter, 5/81-101.
45. Haynes PF: Surgical failures in upper respiratory surgery. In Milne FJ (ed): *Proceedings of the Twenty-Fourth Annual Convention of the American Association of Equine Practitioners*. St. Louis, American Association of Equine Practitioners, 1979, pp 223–249.
46. Rumore JJ, Fahri KA, Titkemeyer C: Medical Records and the Law. *J Am Vet Med Assoc* 178(3):202–205, 1981.

Index

Page numbers in *italics* denote figures; those followed by "t" denote tables.